McKusick's

Heritable Disorders of Connective Tissue

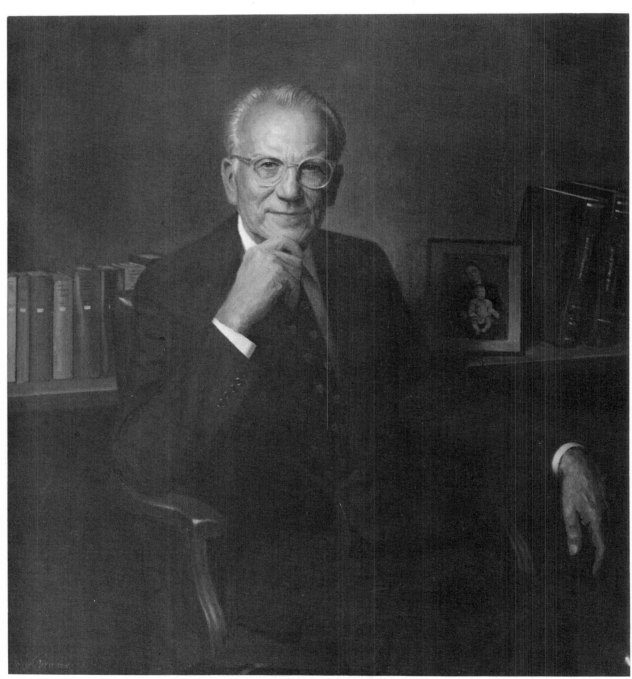

Victor A. McKusick

McKusick's

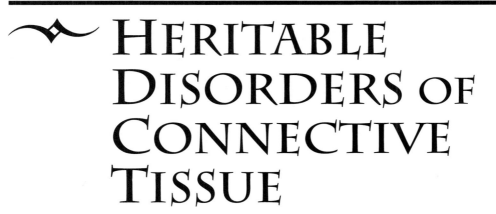

HERITABLE DISORDERS OF CONNECTIVE TISSUE

FIFTH EDITION

Edited by

Peter Beighton, M.D., Ph.D.
Professor of Human Genetics
University of Cape Town Medical School
Cape Town, South Africa

with 14 contributors

with 1072 illustrations

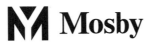 **Mosby**

St. Louis Baltimore Boston Chicago London Philadelphia Sydney Toronto

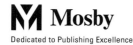

Mosby

Dedicated to Publishing Excellence

Editor: Stephanie Manning
Developmental Editor: Barbara S. Menczer
Project Manager: Patricia Tannian
Production Editor: Mary McAuley
Designer: Jeanne Wolfgeher

Printed in the United States of America

Mosby–Year Book, Inc.
11830 Westline Industrial Drive
St. Louis, Missouri 63146

Library of Congress Cataloging in Publication Data

McKusick's heritable disorders of connective tissue / edited by Peter Beighton; with 14 contributors.—5th ed.
 p.   cm.
 Rev. ed. of: Heritable disorders of connective tissue / Victor A. McKusick. 4th ed. 1972.
 Includes bibliographical references and index.
 ISBN 0-8016-6358-X
 1. Connective tissues—Diseases—Genetic aspects. I. Beighton, Peter. II. McKusick, Victor A. (Victor Almon), 1921-   Heritable disorders of connective tissue. III. Title: Heritable disorders of connective tissue.
 [DNLM: 1. Connective Tissue—physiology. 2. Connective Tissue Diseases—diagnosis. 3. Connective Tissue Diseases—genetics. 4. Connective Tissue Diseases—therapy. WD 375 M4784]
 RC924.M39 1992
 616.7'7042—dc20
 DNLM/DLC
 for Library of Congress   92-49167
                                                                    CIP

93 94 95 96 97 CL/MY 9 8 7 6 5 4 3 2 1

~~✦~~ *Contributors*

Peter Beighton, M.D., Ph.D., F.R.C.P., D.C.H.
Professor of Human Genetics,
University of Cape Town Medical School,
Cape Town, South Africa

Peter Berman, M.B., Ch.B., M.Med. (Path)
Senior Lecturer,
Department of Chemical Pathology,
University of Cape Town Medical School,
Cape Town, South Africa

Peter Byers, M.D.
Professor,
Department of Pathology and Medicine,
University of Washington School of Medicine,
Seattle, Washington

Maurice Godfrey, Ph.D.
Assistant Professor of Pediatrics,
Meyer Rehabilitation Institute,
Hattie B. Munroe Center for Human Genetics,
University of Nebraska Medical Center,
Omaha, Nebraska

Judith G. Hall, M.D.
Professor and Head,
University of British Columbia,
Department of Pediatrics,
B.C. Children's Hospital,
Vancouver, British Columbia, Canada

Ralph S. Lachman, M.D.
Professor of Radiology and Pediatrics,
Harbor—University of California at Los Angeles
    Medical Center,
Los Angeles, California

Irene H. Maumenee, M.D.
Ort Professor of Ophthalmology;
Professor of Pediatrics;
Director,
The Johns Hopkins Center for Hereditary Eye
    Diseases,
Johns Hopkins University School of Medicine,
Baltimore, Maryland

Victor A. McKusick, M.D.
University Professor of Medical Genetics,
Johns Hopkins University School of Medicine,
Baltimore, Maryland

F. Michael Pope, M.D., F.R.C.P.
Head, Medical Research Council Dermatology
    Research Group;
Consultant Physician,
Clinical Research Centre,
Northwick Park Hospital,
Harrow, Middlesex, England

Reed E. Pyeritz, M.D., Ph.D.
Professor of Medicine and Pediatrics;
Clinical Director,
The Center for Medical Genetics,
Johns Hopkins University School of Medicine,
Baltimore, Maryland

David L. Rimoin, M.D., Ph.D.
Professor of Pediatrics,
University of California at Los Angeles;
Steven Spiedlberg Chairman of Pediatrics,
Cedars-Sinai Medical Center,
Los Angeles, California

Štefan Sršen, M.D., Dr. Sc.
Professor,
Institute of Clinical Genetics;
Medical Faculty,
University of Komensky,
Martin, Czechoslovakia

Petros Tsipouras, M.D.
Professor,
Department of Pediatrics,
University of Connecticut Health Center,
Farmington, Connecticut

Denis Viljoen, M.D.
Senior Lecturer,
Department of Human Genetics,
University of Cape Town Medical School,
Cape Town, South Africa

Chester B. Whitley, M.D., Ph.D.
Assistant Professor,
Division of Genetics and Metabolism,
Department of Pediatrics and Institute of Human
    Genetics,
University of Minnesota,
Minneapolis, Minnesota

Dr. Victor A. McKusick dedicated each of the four previous editions to *Archibald E. Garrod*, the forefather of human biochemical genetics, and

to all who believe as he did, that the clinical investigation of hereditary disorders can shed light on normal developmental and biochemical mechanisms.

We who have joined in the preparation of this fifth edition repeat the dedication, with the observation that in his life's work and writings, Dr. McKusick has demonstrated that he himself has been guided by Garrod's vision.

Foreword

The publication of the fifth edition of McKusick's *Heritable Disorders of Connective Tissue* has been awaited with much anticipation by many physicians, medical geneticists, and other biomedical scientists. The fourth edition appeared over 20 years ago, and many advances have been made since 1972. Unlike the earlier editions, which were written by Victor McKusick alone, this volume is a multiauthored work, each chapter written by a recognized expert. Several of these chapter authors previously have worked with McKusick.

This book rapidly became *the* classic work for genetic connective tissue disorders in the 1960s and 1970s. The latest edition promises again to become the principal reference for this field. The first edition, published in 1956, was an important landmark in medical genetics. It was one of the first attempts to meld a large body of clinical information with genetic data for a group of diseases that were classified together. The power of the mendelian paradigm in the understanding of disease was made explicit and served as a stimulus for future biochemical and molecular studies. With this working concept the first edition heralded McKusick's future impact on the field of medical genetics, leading to his being recognized internationally as the most outstanding clinical geneticist of his generation. Over the years specific mutations of connective tissue genes that cause diseases such as the mucopolysaccharidoses, osteogenesis imperfecta, and the Marfan syndrome have been elucidated. This knowledge has then been applied for understanding and increasingly for diagnosis of these disorders. Despite these advances, we do not yet have insight in the various modifying genetic and developmental factors that make for differences in clinical expression in most of these disorders. More work must be done to allow more accurate clinical predictions regarding the severity and extent of organ involvement in these disorders.

Victor McKusick should be proud to see the culmination of his many efforts in this area in this book. The volume appropriately concludes with his ideas about the future. Many physicians, scientists, and students are grateful to the editor and chapter authors for publication of this volume. They and the patients who suffer from these conditions are looking forward to a not-too-distant time when future scientific advances will necessitate another edition of this classic of medical literature.

Arno G. Motulsky, M.D., D. Sc.
University of Washington
Seattle, Washington
Summer 1992

✦ *Preface to the Fourth Edition*

Heritable disorders of connective tissue are generalized defects involving primarily one element of connective tissue—collagen, elastin, or mucopolysaccharide—and transmissible in a simple mendelian manner.

Probably the first disorder to be interpreted as a generalized disorder of connective tissue was osteogenesis imperfecta. In 1920 Bauer[2] and in 1952 Follis[5] discussed this disorder in essentially the terms just stated. In 1931 Weve,[8] in calling the Marfan syndrome "dystrophia mesodermalis congenita, typus Marfanis," also recognized the nature of the condition. In 1955 I[7] introduced the designation *heritable disorders of connective tissue* for the class of disorders that included, in addition to those mentioned, the Ehlers-Danlos syndrome, pseudoxanthoma elasticum, and gargoylism, which Brante[4] had characterized in 1952 as a disorder of mucopolysaccharide metabolism. "Heritable disorders of connective tissue," like Garrod's[6] "inborn errors of metabolism," has gained wide currency. The term "heritable," although essentially synonymous with "genetic" and "inherited," may have the advantage that in the case at hand the disorder, although capable of hereditary transmission in the same or other patients, is not in that instance inherited, having arisen instead by new mutation.

It has been 17 years since some of the material in this monograph was first published as a series of articles in the *Journal of Chronic Diseases*. The continued interest in the heritable disorders of connective tissue and their continued importance to clinical medicine and the biology of connective tissue are notable. In the interval, understanding of these diseases from both the clinical and the biologic points of view has increased appreciably. The collagen molecule has become more familiar in its physicochemical details, although it has far to go to match that paragon of protein molecules—hemoglobin. Characterization of the nature and metabolism of mucopolysaccharides has also advanced.

In connection with the Marfan syndrome, surgi-

cal treatment of the aortic complications is entirely a development of the last 17 years. An exciting discovery is that an inborn error of metabolism (homocystinuria) is responsible for a clinical picture which, because of ectopia lentis and vascular disease, simulates the Marfan syndrome. The vascular complications of the Ehlers-Danlos syndrome have become better appreciated. The existence of a recessive form of osteogenesis imperfecta now seems certain. Evidence for involvement primarily of the elastic fiber in pseudoxanthoma elasticum has forced revision of the view held 17 years ago. Furthermore, the recessive inheritance and histopathologic features, as well as the experience with homocystinuria, suggest that an inborn error of metabolism should be sought. The example of homocystinuria also suggests that alkaptonuria deserves classification as a heritable disorder of connective tissue. Increased understanding of cutis laxa and of the Weill-Marchesani syndrome justify separate chapters in the present edition.

Nosology has advanced furthest in relation to the mucopolysaccharidoses. Whereas in 1955 the nature of gargoylism as a mucopolysaccharidosis was recognized on histochemical grounds and two genetic forms—the autosomal recessive and the X-linked—were distinguished, characterization of the mucopolysacchariduria and identification of several other distinct varieties are developments of the 1960s.

It is especially the generalist—the *general practitioner* and the *internist* and the *pediatrician* without particular subspecialization—to whom the problems related to the several syndromes discussed here are of importance and to whom this book is addressed. He is in the best position to size up the total situation in the individual patient and relate it to the family background, with which he is most likely to have firsthand familiarity. He can best evaluate what may be excessive loose-jointedness and "ganglingness" or mild pectus excavatum, pigeon breast, kyphoscoliosis, and flatfeet. In the light of the general manifestations and the family background he can best appraise the significance of internal medical manifestations, which may be integral parts of a generalized syndrome.

Asboe-Hansen[1] has made the following cogent comment: "Connective tissue connects the numer-

---

This preface to the fourth edition, in which Dr. McKusick set out his views and philosophy concerning the heritable connective tissue disorders, is retained for its historical value and to preserve continuity.

ous branches of medical science. Without connective tissue, medicine would come to pieces, even non-viable pieces, just like the cells of the human body."

The ubiquity of connective tissue is responsible for its unifying influence on medicine, referred to in the statement quoted from Asboe-Hansen. Furthermore, its ubiquity is responsible for the fact that concern with the problems of generalized and hereditary disorders of connective tissue extends also to many divisions of medical science and practice.

The *ophthalmologist* sees grave changes in the eyes in pseudoxanthoma elasticum, in the Marfan and Weill-Marchesani syndromes, and in homocystinuria and sees less serious, yet significant, alterations in osteogenesis imperfecta, the Ehlers-Danlos syndrome, and the mucopolysaccharidoses.

The *otologist* sees the patients with certain of the mucopolysaccharidoses, those with osteogenesis imperfecta, and rarely those with the Marfan syndrome.

The *orthopedist* is concerned with cases of osteogenesis imperfecta, the Ehlers-Danlos syndrome, mucopolysaccharidoses (e.g., Morquio syndrome), and sometimes the Marfan syndrome. Patients with fibrodysplasia ossificans progressiva are frequently seen by him.

The *general surgeon* repairs the hernias of the patient with the Marfan syndrome, the Ehlers-Danlos syndrome, osteogenesis imperfecta, or the Hurler syndrome.

The *hematologist* is consulted for the bruisability in the Ehlers-Danlos syndrome, for the tendency to multiple hemorrhages in patients with pseudoxanthoma elasticum, and for the multiple venous and arterial thromboses in homocystinuria.

The *gastroenterologist* is likely to encounter a case of pseudoxanthoma elasticum if he treats a sizable group of patients with gastrointestinal hemorrhage.

Increasingly the *cardiologist* is finding the Marfan syndrome of greater importance among the "causes" of aortic regurgitation and of dissecting aneurysm of the aorta than he had previously realized. In the Hurler syndrome and other mucopolysaccharidoses the cardiac involvement may bring the patient to medical attention and is frequently the cause of death at an early age. Among cases of *peripheral vascular disease*, pseudoxanthoma elasticum or homocystinuria occasionally figures as the etiologic factor.

Aside from the cardiovascular manifestations, the *chest physician* will be interested in the occurrence of cystic disease of the lung in the Marfan syndrome and of rupture of the lung with pneumothorax or mediastinal emphysema in the Marfan syndrome and in the Ehlers-Danlos syndrome.

The *dermatologist* treats patients with pseudoxanthoma elasticum and the Ehlers-Danlos syndrome.

The *plastic surgeon* is called in to provide cosmetic relief for the unsightly changes in the skin of the neck in pseudoxanthoma elasticum and of the face in cutis laxa.

The *dentist* sees abnormalities, especially in osteogenesis imperfecta and the mucopolysaccharidoses.

The *rheumatologist*, interested in connective tissues in general, is likely to see in these heritable disorders of connective tissue, derangements in purer culture and more easily analyzed form than in the acquired disorders of connective tissue such as the arthritides. Specifically, the rheumatologist may be consulted for the repeated hydrarthroses that may accompany the loose-jointedness of the Ehlers-Danlos syndrome, for the stiff joints of the mucopolysaccharidoses, and for the arthritis of alkaptonuria.

The *endocrinologist* is frequently consulted by the parents of a child with the Marfan syndrome or the Hurler syndrome and by the patient with osteogenesis imperfecta or fibrodysplasia ossificans progressiva, the incorrect supposition being that an endocrinopathy is present.

By reason of their hereditary nature, all these conditions are of interest to the *medical geneticist*.

The *pathologist*, of course, must be familiar with them, and the *radiologist* will find in every one of these syndromes diagnostic features that can be revealed by his rays.

For the *medical student* (in either the narrow sense or in the broad sense under which everyone in medicine should qualify) the disorders discussed in this book and other syndromes are important ingredients of the curriculum. They force the student to muster all his knowledge of anatomy, biochemistry, physiology, developmental biology, and genetics to account for the phenomena he observes.

Obviously, one objective of this book and of the

clinical investigations on which it is based is a synthesis of the scattered information about several conditions which have in common the facts that they are (1) generalized disorders of connective tissue and (2) heritable, even if not inherited in the individual instance. To my knowledge, only Bauer and Bode[3] have previously attempted such a synthesis.

A second objective has been to see what justification could be found for a favorite, although (witness the following quotation from Harvey as well as the dedication) far from original, notion of mine: that clinical investigation of pathologic states is as legitimate a method as any other for studying biology. Specifically, the hereditary syndromes are tools for study of the normal situation—in this case for the elucidation of connective tissue. When the clinician compares his methods as biologic tools with the electron microscope, analytical chemistry, tissue culture, and others, he tends to get an inferiority complex. I will leave it to the reader to judge whether the clinical researches, which are reported here but which are in only small part my own, demonstrate that the clinician can take his place with the so-called "pure scientists" in the group now trying to fit together the varishaped pieces of the intricate jigsaw puzzle that is connective tissue.

Nature is nowhere accustomed more openly to display her secret mysteries than in cases where she shows traces of her workings apart from the beaten path; nor is there any better way to advance the proper practice of medicine than to give our minds to the discovery of the usual law of Nature by careful investigation of cases of rarer forms of disease. For it has been found, in almost all things, that what they contain of useful or applicable nature is hardly perceived unless we are deprived of them, or they become deranged in some way.*

Victor A. McKusick

REFERENCES

1. Asboe-Hansen G, editor: *Connective tissue in health and disease*, Copenhagen, 1954, Ejnar Munksgaards Forlag.
2. Bauer KH: Über Osteogenesis imperfecta, *Dtsch Z Chir* 154:166, 1920.
3. Bauer KH, Bode W: Erbpathologie der Stützgewebe beim Menschen. In *Handbuch der Erbpathologie*, vol 3, Berlin, 1940, Julius Springer.
4. Brante G: Gargoylism—a mucopolysaccharidosis, *Scand J Clin Lab Invest* 4:43, 1952.
5. Follis RH Jr: Osteogenesis imperfecta congenita: a connective tissue diathesis, *J Pediatr* 41:713, 1952.
6. Garrod A: The lessons of rare maladies, *Lancet* 1:1055, 1928.
7. McKusick VA: The cardiovascular aspects of Marfan's syndrome: a heritable disorder of connective tissue, *Circulation* 11:321, 1955.
8. Weve HJM: Über Arachnodaktylie (Dystrophia mesodermalis congenita, Typus Marfan), *Arch Augenheilk* 104:1, 1931.

*From a letter written by William Harvey in 1657, six weeks before his death. Quoted by Garrod, Sir Archibald: The lessons of rare maladies, *Lancet* 1:1055, 1928. Also see translation of *The Circulation of the Blood* and other writings of Harvey by K. J. Franklin, Everyman's Library, New York, 1963.

Acknowledgments to the Fourth Edition

The original investigations referred to in this book were supported in part by a grant from the Daland Fund of the American Philosophical Society held at Philadelphia for Promoting Useful Knowledge and in part by grants-in-aid from the National Institutes of Health, Public Health Service.

The late Dr. Joseph Earle Moore encouraged these studies, by wise suggestions improved their published form, and in general made this book possible.

To the late Dr. Richard H. Follis, Jr., I owe the largest debt of conceptual nature; his concept of osteogenesis imperfecta as a generalized unitary defect of connective tissue probably catalyzed my own thinking along these lines.

It would be impossible to name all the individuals who have assisted in accumulating the data presented. Nor can I list all the persons whose thoughts have influenced mine during the course of analyzing these disorders.

To my fellow members of the Galton-Garrod Society, founded at The Johns Hopkins University in the early 1950s by several of us who share an interest in human genetics, I am indebted for the pleasure and profit of many stimulating exchanges of ideas. Among others, Dr. Barton Childs, Dr. Bentley Glass, and Dr. Abraham Lillienfeld have been especially helpful to me.

The course in biophysical and biochemical cytology conducted by Professor F. O. Schmitt, Dr. Jerome Gross, and colleagues at the Massachusetts Institute of Technology, June, 1955, was of great assistance in the preparation of the brief survey of the biology of normal connective tissue. In recent years Dr. Karl A. Piez and Dr. George R. Martin, as well as others of the National Institutes of Health, have continued my education in this area.

The editors and publishers of *American Journal of Human Genetics, Bulletin of The Johns Hopkins Hospital, Circulation, Bulletin of the New York Academy of Medicine, Medicine,* and *Annals of Internal Medicine* kindly permitted reuse of illustrative material.

The annual conferences on The Clinical Delineation of Birth Defects held here at Johns Hopkins beginning in 1968 have provided valuable information that has been used in this fourth edition. I am grateful to many participants and to the National Foundation–March of Dimes, which provided financial support and published the proceedings, for permission to reuse illustrative and other material here.

In recent years several of my research fellows have contributed importantly to the study of several of the heritable disorders of connective tissue. Deserving particular mention are Drs. Roswell Eldridge, Richard M. Goodman, W. Bryan Hanley, Irene E. Hussels, R. Neil Schimke, Charles I. Scott, and David Wise. Dr. A. E. Maumenee and several members of his staff at the Wilmer Ophthalmological Institute, past and present, particularly Drs. Harold E. Cross, James P. Gills, Jr., Morton F. Goldberg, Howard A. Naquin,† David Paton, Gunter K. von Noorden, and George Weinstein, have contributed in many ways to the study of these disorders of connective tissue, almost all of which seem to have ocular manifestations. I owe a particular debt to Dr. John P. Dorst, Professor of Radiology here at Johns Hopkins, for a long, stimulating, and productive collaboration in the study of skeletal disorders and for specific assistance in the analysis of radiologic aspects of the entities discussed here.

Conversations with Dr. Karl Meyer, formerly of Columbia University, have been stimulating and informative. Dr. David Kaplan, Downstate Medical Center, Brooklyn, and Dr. Elizabeth F. Neufeld, National Institutes of Health, Bethesda, contributed significantly to the biochemical study of the mucopolysaccharidoses, and Dr. B. Shannon Danes, New York Hospital, New York, to their cytologic study. Numerous colleagues at other institutions deserve acknowledgments for their assistance to me: Drs. Robert J. Gorlin (Minneapolis), Leonard O. Langer (Minneapolis), John S. O'Brien

†Died September 21, 1972.

(La Jolla, California), William B. Reed (Burbank, California), Jürgen W. Spranger (Kiel, Germany), and many others.

The late Dr. Ernst Oppenheimer, in preparing the German translation of the first edition, made several worthwhile suggestions that were incorporated in subsequent editions.

I am indebted to Professor Charles E. Dent, London, for directing my attention specifically to the simulation of the Marfan syndrome by homocystinuria. Dr. Robert A. Milch gave valuable assistance in the original preparation of the chapter on alkaptonuria and has been a constant source of stimulation and insight.

To the many others who directly or indirectly contributed to this book I extend my grateful appreciation. Essential to the successful pursuit of a study such as this, which is partly retrospective and which concerns disorders of relatively infrequent occurrence, are the careful recording of information by many individuals over a long period of time and its careful preservation in the archives of our hospitals and other institutions. I am deeply grateful for the contributions of many members of the staff of The Johns Hopkins Hospital over a period of many years.

Victor A. McKusick

Preface to the Fifth Edition

Before the publication in 1956 of the first edition of *Heritable Disorders of Connective Tissue*, no comprehensive account of this fascinating group of conditions was available. This book awakened the interest of the medical world, and successive editions have focused the attention of researchers on this field. The steady growth in size of each volume has reflected the exponential increase in knowledge concerning these disorders, and the fourth edition, published in 1972, represented a summation of all then-existing information. This book was widely regarded as the standard text on this subject.

In the two decades that have passed since the publication of the fourth edition, the manifestations and complications of the heritable connective tissue disorders have been thoroughly documented and considerable heterogeneity has been recognized. Equally, sophisticated biochemical and molecular investigations have led to dramatic advances in the understanding of the basic defect and pathogenesis of many of these conditions.

The purpose of this new edition is to provide an up-to-date review of the clinical, genetic, and biomolecular aspects of these disorders. The wealth of historical detail that was contained in previous editions has been preserved, as have many of the case reports, as these lend a special flavor to the book. The best of the numerous existing illustrations have also been retained, and these have been supplemented by much new material. Bibliographies have been expanded to encompass publications that have appeared since 1972; in some instances several hundred references are provided, and where space has permitted, the bibliographies pertaining to specific disorders are complete. The format and chapter titles are virtually unchanged, but the contents have been updated throughout the text. In particular, the opening chapters, which are concerned with basic genetics and the biology of connective tissue, have been rewritten to provide an overview of the current status of these complex subjects.

This monograph represents the definitive work in this field, and it should find a place on the shelves of every medical library and academic genetics department. Access to this book will be crucial for all medical geneticists and genetic counselors. In addition, the contents are relevant for a wide range of medical specialists, who are likely to encounter patients with the heritable connective tissue disorders; these include pediatricians, dermatologists, orthopedic surgeons, rheumatologists, and obstetricians. The text will have equal relevance for biochemists and molecular biologists who are involved in the laboratory aspects of these conditions.

This new edition has been compiled by a team of expert chapter authors, each of whom is an authority in his or her own field. In recognition of Dr. Victor McKusick's immense contribution to medical genetics and to perpetuate his name and his association with this major work, the title has been altered to *McKusick's Heritable Disorders of Connective Tissue*.

Peter Beighton

Acknowledgments to the Fifth Edition

I offer my thanks to Dr. V.A. McKusick for his encouragement and guidance, and for the example of excellence that he has set for all those who have been privileged to work with him.

Many friends, colleagues, and associates have assisted in the preparation of this book, and I am especially grateful to:

My wife, Greta, for proofreading, manuscript preparation, and library research

Gillian Shapley, for her dedicated and enthusiastic secretarial assistance

Dr. Denis Viljoen and Dr. Ingrid Winship for their personal contributions and for proofreading my own chapters

Professor Michael Connor for his guidance in the preparation of Chapter 12

Dr. Maurice Godfrey for gallantly undertaking the preparation of Chapter 3 after the untimely death of Professor David Hollister. Dr. Godfrey offers his personal thanks to Drs. Carlos Almeida, Peter Byers, Francesco Ramirez, Timothy Galbraith, Bruce McManus, James R. Neff, Mary J. Roman, Michael E. Yablonski, and to Lori Myers and Virginia Burns for their assistance

Stephanie Manning, Barbara Menczer, and Mary McAuley of Mosby–Year Book for their kindly interest and for their benign tolerance of delayed deadlines

The chapter authors for their expert contributions (There were many problems with deadlines, but all is now forgiven.)

My own work in the field of inherited disorders of connective tissue, on which my contributions to this book were based, has received long-term support from the Medical Research Council of South Africa, the Mauerberger Foundation, the Harry Crossley Foundation, and the University of Cape Town Staff Research Fund.

Contents

15   Future Prospects, 691

• *Victor A. McKusick*

Appendices

The Clinical Behavior of Hereditary Syndromes, with a Precis of Medical Genetics

Judith G. Hall

Many of the inherited disorders of humans have importance far out of proportion to their frequency because of the light they have shed on normal physiologic mechanisms, as well as on pathophysiology. The recent rapid developments in molecular genetics have moved the understanding of the heritable disorders of connective tissue to a molecular level. The isolation and mapping of genes involved in the structure and function of connective tissue and the determination of the mechanisms involved in the control of these genes have permitted increased understanding of the pathogenesis of connective tissue disorders. Despite these advances, however, many traditional genetic concepts remain important for the understanding of these and other genetic disorders.

The history of genetics as a scientific discipline is barely more than a hundred years old. In 1865 the Austrian monk Gregor Mendel defined some of the principles of genetics for the first time. Previously inheritance had been thought to be a merging of the characteristics of each parent. Mendel suggested that there were discrete units of heredity, that there was segregation of those units to offspring in a predictable manner, and that the units were responsible for independent assortment of physical traits. Those units of heredity are now termed *genes*, and many of them have been defined on a molecular basis. *Segregation* implies that two members (*alleles*) of a single pair of genes are present and will separate and that only one will be passed on to each offspring via the gamete. *Independent assortment* means that members of different gene pairs will go to gametes independently of one another.

In the early 1900s these concepts were rediscovered and applied to human disease. Inborn errors of metabolism began to be understood, and it was realized that they were the result of defects in the genetic information that coded for the components of a particular metabolic pathway. Until the ability to examine individual chromosomes was developed in the late 1950s, genetic concepts were supported on a clinical and biochemical basis.

When it became possible to visualize and determine the correct number of human chromosomes, various chromosomal abnormalities were identified. Their role in causing congenital anomalies, mental retardation, infertility, and reproductive failure was recognized for the first time. A great deal of work since then has helped to define the relative frequencies of various chromosomal aberrations among early conceptions, spontaneous abortions, stillbirths, live births, and individuals with various disorders. Lyon's formalization of the concept of inactivation of one X chromosome in each cell of females[16] helped to explain a variety of clinical observations and led to an understanding of dosage compensation and the role of the sex chromosomes in sexual differentiation. Barr had discovered that the inactivated X chromosome could be visualized in some types of cells as a condensed, deeply staining body on the nuclear membrane at interphase,[2] which became known as the *Barr body*. Before the advent of technical advances that allowed each chromosome to be visualized directly, the Barr body was of value in estimating the number of X chromosomes present in the cells of an individual.

Since the early 1970s the powerful new technologies of molecular biology have been applied to the field of human genetics with dazzling results. Enormous progress has been made in the isolation and cloning of specific genes and in the mapping of genes to precise locations on particular chromosomes. Sequencing the deoxyribonucleic acid (DNA) of the entire human genome is now a funded research goal. The implications for the study of connective tissue disorders are that the structure of the genes for various components, as well as their control mechanisms, is likely to be defined in the foreseeable future. The challenge, of course, is to understand the pathophysiologic features and the abnormal processes that underlie these diseases. These interactions are extremely complex and will require a more holistic approach than simply sequencing genomic DNA. The processes within cells and tissues and the interactions among many genes must be further understood. Nevertheless, the identification and localization of all human genes is an attainable goal.

TERMINOLOGY

Most of the disorders discussed in this book are evident on clinical examination as symptom complexes, or syndromes. Literally meaning a "running together," the term *syndrome* is applied to any consistent combination of two or more clinical manifestations. As used to describe connective tissue disorders, the term has no etiologic connotations; in other words, a syndrome need not be genetically determined or represent the effect of a single abnormal gene. *Syndrome* and *disease* are distinguishable terms, the latter referring to a specific etiopathogenetic entity and the former to a combination of manifestations that may have diverse causes. For example, it might be argued that because the abnormality of the enzyme hypoxanthine-guanine-phosphoribosyltransferase (HGPRT or HPRT) in the Lesch-Nyhan syndrome has been

identified,[23] this condition should be termed the Lesch-Nyhan *disease*. It is clear, however, that at a molecular level there are many different DNA defects that lead to the failure of production of normal amounts of the enzyme.[24] In this book *syndrome* is used in a specific sense, that is, to signify a distinct etiopathologic entity, the diverse manifestations of which result from a single primary cause (e.g., lack of a functional enzyme, although the reasons for that deficiency may be quite diverse).

The use of the term *syndrome* in this manner need not and should not obscure the issue of genetic heterogeneity. Cases that might legitimately be called the Hurler syndrome by satisfying the original criteria described by Hurler[14] are now known to be examples of distinct clinical entities and have been given completely different names, for example, Hunter syndrome[13] and Maroteaux-Lamy syndrome.[19] With further enzymatic and molecular definition each of these has been divided into different subtypes on the basis of involvement of different enzymes. In the same way, some patients who showed features of the Marfan syndrome were recognized as having a specific inborn error of metabolism that could be distinguished by the presence of homocystine in the urine.[8] The designation *homocystinuria* is now used for this disorder. Now that the fibrillin gene has been found to be abnormal in the Marfan syndrome,[20] further subcategorization of this condition may be possible in terms of the domains of the gene that are involved.

The term *heritable* (rather than *inherited* or *hereditary*) was selected for the title of this book to convey the sense that in a given individual the gene or disease, or both, although transmissible to offspring, may not have been inherited but rather may have arisen by new mutation. The terms *inherited, genetic, hereditary,* and *familial* are essentially synonymous with *heritable* but have particular shades of meaning. Down syndrome is a genetic disorder, since it results from an abnormality in the genetic material. It is also heritable but is usually not inherited from a parent. *Familial* is a general term that can refer to the aggregation of particular traits in families for other than genetic reasons.

Congenital and *hereditary* are not synonymous. Congenital simply means "present at birth"; it has no etiologic connotation. A disorder may be congenital and not hereditary (e.g., rubella syndrome, in which intrauterine infection with rubella leads to cataracts and deafness); conversely, it may be hereditary and not congenital (e.g., pseudoxanthoma elasticum, a genetic disorder that manifests only later in life).

Abiotrophy is a term suggested in the early years of the twentieth century by Gowers[9] for neurologic disorders in which a particular tissue or cell class is capable of function for only a limited time because of an innate weakness. Friedreich ataxia and Huntington disease are examples. The abiotrophies are not congenital, although they are hereditary. The changes in the aorta in the Marfan syndrome; in the skin, eye, and blood vessels in pseudoxanthoma elasticum; and in the joints in alkaptonuria are abiotrophic. Abiotrophy, as a term, means no more than the late onset of degenerative changes.

Pleiotropic (loosely meaning "many effects") is a term applied to those single genes that are responsible for multiple manifestations in different tissues and different areas of the body. Although the gene may have many phenotypic effects, the primary action of the gene is unitary because of faulty action of a single gene, that is, a specific protein is not functioning normally in many different tissues or body regions. *Polyphenic* is a useful term that is synonymous with *pleiotropic*.

It is desirable to avoid eponyms and preferable to use designations that indicate as precisely as possible the fundamental nature of the disease entity under consideration. In our present state of knowledge, however, there are good reasons to employ eponyms for many syndromes. First, eponyms neither prejudice the search for the fundamental defect nor conceal our ignorance of its nature. For example, in the Hurler syndrome the name *lipochondrodystrophy* was previously used, with the erroneous assumption that the basic defect was one of cellular fat metabolism. Second, since eponyms do not use features of a complex syndrome as designations, they avoid conveying the impression that the presence of a specific feature is a sine qua non for the diagnosis. Nevertheless, eponyms are merely tags; they often have no justification from the standpoint of historical priorities, since frequently either someone else had described the condition earlier or the person whose name is used eponymously did not describe the full syndrome or even the specific syndrome

for which his or her name is used. As the molecular basis of specific disorders becomes clear, there will surely be a move toward more precise terminology. Nevertheless, some eponyms such as the Marfan syndrome are hallowed by time and wide general use. It is likely that these will be retained and perhaps qualified by designations that reflect the underlying biomolecular defect and heterogeneity.

MOLECULAR BASIS OF GENETIC DISEASE
Gene Structure and Control

Biologically inherited characteristics, both normal and pathologic, are determined by genes carried on the chromosomes. Each gene codes for a specific protein, either an enzyme or a structural protein. Proteins frequently are modified after they have been synthesized and combine with other proteins to make complex structures. Furthermore, the genetic code itself may be modified via alternative splicing during the transcription of the DNA into messenger ribonucleic acid (mRNA), as described in the following paragraphs.

Deoxyribonucleic acid. The chromosomes lie within the nucleus of the cell and are composed of DNA and many auxiliary proteins. DNA in turn consists of four types of *nucleotides* (adenine, thymidine, cytosine, and guanine, abbreviated A, T, C, and G). Each of the nucleotides differs from the others in its *base* component. A DNA molecule can be any length (and can contain any number of genes); chromosomal DNA contains two strands of nucleotides, joined by bonds like ladder rungs, in a *double helix* configuration (Fig. 1-1). Because of the three-dimensional constraints of the double helix configuration, each nucleotide in a DNA molecule can bond, or *pair*, only with its *complementary* nucleotide partner on the other strand (i.e., A with T and C with G). This process is called *complementary base pairing*, since it is the base component of each nucleotide that forms the bond. The structure of the double helix allows the genetic information to be copied precisely and passed on from cell to cell and generation to generation: when the DNA is *replicated*, the two strands are "unzipped" and the enzyme *DNA polymerase* adds a new strand of complementary nucleotides to each original strand, producing two new, complete, and identical DNA molecules. This process

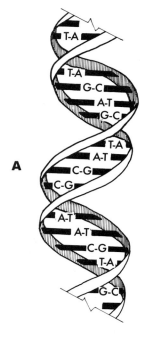

A

Fig. 1-1. A, The structure of the DNA double helix showing base pairing. G pairs only with C and A pairs only with T, via hydrogen bonding. The constraints of the helix structure determine that these complementary bases pair only with each other. Thus, given the sequence of bases on one strand, the order of the bases on the other strand is predetermined, which allows the genetic code to be maintained intact from one cell division to the next. **B,** Partial chemical structure of the base portion of the five nucleic acids (including uracil, found only in RNA). The bases are shown as they pair with their complementary base. Uracil replaces thymadine (T) in RNA, which is generally single stranded and thus does not base pair.

Purines   **Pyrimidines**

Adenine   Thymine

B

Guanine   Cytosine

Uracil (in RNA only)

is known as *semiconservative replication,* since each new molecule contains one strand from the original molecule and one newly synthesized strand. DNA sequences that are identical are said to be *homologous.*

Each individual gene is comprised of a long, highly specific *sequence* of nucleotides. Thus the four nucleotides act as the "alphabet" from which the genetic code is "written": every three nucleotides along the length of a gene constitutes a *codon;* each codon in turn codes for a specific amino acid when the genetic code, using the molecular machinery of the cell, is *translated* into protein.

Ribonucleic acid. One strand of the DNA of the gene is *transcribed* into RNA by an enzyme known as *RNA polymerase.* The portion of the DNA where the RNA polymerase first attaches is called the *promoter* region of the gene. Unique "start-and-stop" sequences in each gene limit the transcription of each of these *mRNA* molecules to the boundaries of the specific gene; thus the *transcript,* or molecule of mRNA, contains the complete code of the gene—and only that gene—in a form that is far more portable and discrete than is the DNA of the chromosome.

There are several types of RNA: *transfer RNA* (tRNA) carries specific amino acids to the protein synthesis machinery of *ribosomes* in the cytoplasm; *ribosomal RNA* (rRNA) is a structural component of the ribosomes; and the *mRNA* varies the nucleotide sequence of the gene to the ribosomes.

The question of which strand of a double helix acts as the template for the formation of the complementary mRNA is crucial, since the code of one strand differs from the code of the other strand and only one can yield a correct protein sequence. For a particular gene the strand that is actually transcribed is that which contains the specific promoter sequence. This strand is termed the *sense strand* or *coding strand;* the other, the *antisense strand,* is not used in transcription.

Not all genes in a cell are transcribed at all times. Intricate mechanisms regulate the production of numerous enzymes and transcription factors, which in turn determine which genes are "turned on." Some genes may be transcribed only during a brief period in the life cycle of an organism, such as during embryogenesis. Other genes, known as *housekeeping genes,* are consistently transcribed at low levels to maintain the viability of the cell. Certain cell-specific genes are transcribed only in a few cell types to facilitate highly specialized functions.

Introns, exons, and ribonucleic acid processing. Although the RNA polymerase "reads" the nucleotide sequence of the gene in order, it does not produce a functional mRNA transcript as a first step. Most vertebrate genes are interrupted by several *introns,* or intervening sequences of DNA, which generally do not contain any coding information for the protein to be synthesized. The coding regions of the gene are called *exons,* or expressed sequences of DNA. The initial RNA transcript must be cut to remove intron sequences, and the exon sequences must then be *spliced* before the RNA molecule leaves the cell nucleus. The splicing mechanism must be absolutely precise to conserve the codon *reading frame* for translation into protein (see the section on protein synthesis). How this high degree of precision is accomplished is not yet well understood, but it is presumed that particular sequences contained at the beginning and end of introns (called *splice junctions*) act as signals.

Splicing is one aspect of mRNA *processing* that takes place before translation. In addition to the loss of introns, a string of 50 to 200 adenine nucleotides is added to the end of the RNA transcript; this *poly(A) tail* appears to aid in transporting the RNA molecule from the nucleus into the cytoplasm. At the other end of the RNA a *cap* consisting of a modified G nucleotide is added; its function appears to be to attach the finished mRNA to the ribosome. An RNA transcript may be *alternatively* spliced, giving rise to different proteins from a single gene.

Protein synthesis. Each molecule of mRNA is translated into protein at the *ribosomes* in the cytoplasm. The ribosome "reads" along the length of the mRNA molecule and strings together amino acids into a complete, specific protein molecule according to the code of the mRNA sequence (Fig. 1-2). Transfer RNA carries the amino acids to the ribosome, each tRNA molecule coding for one specific amino acid.

Regulation of gene expression. Another advantage of the intermediate role of mRNA is that, rather than synthesizing protein directly from the chromosome, mRNA provides a second level of

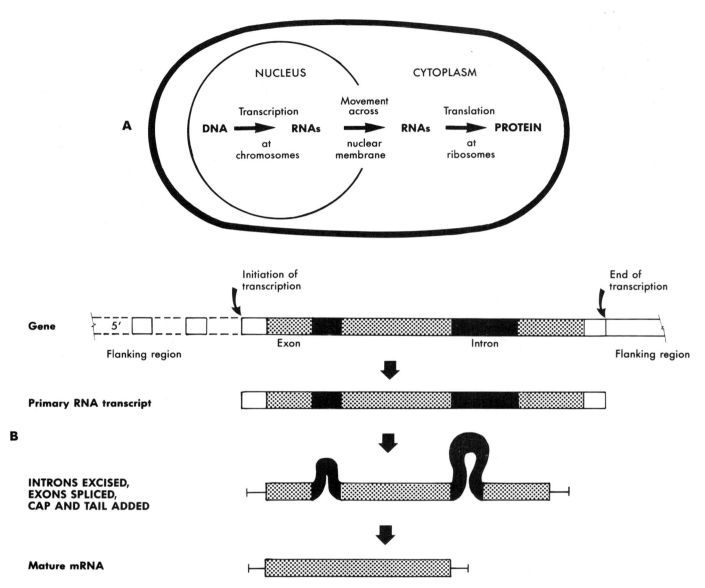

Fig. 1-2. A, The chain of events leading from DNA code to protein. Messenger RNA is transcribed from the DNA in the nucleus, where noncoding intervening sequences (introns) are cut out and the mature mRNA is spliced back together. It is then transported to the cytoplasm, where the ribosomes "read" the code and insert the proper amino acid carried by tRNA. **B,** Transcription and processing of a gene. In the nucleus, the entire sequence of the gene is transcribed into a primary RNA transcript; introns are then excised, and the exons are spliced into a mature mRNA. **C,** Translation of mRNA into a polypeptide at the ribosomes. In eukaryotic cells many ribosomes move along an mRNA molecule at once. These compounds are sometimes referred to as "polysomes." **D,** Diagram of the entire process of synthesis of a polypeptide chain, detailing the codon triplets that code for each amino acid. After synthesis of the polypeptide, it may be modified by the addition of carbohydrate moieties, assembly into complexes, and the like to form the mature protein molecule.

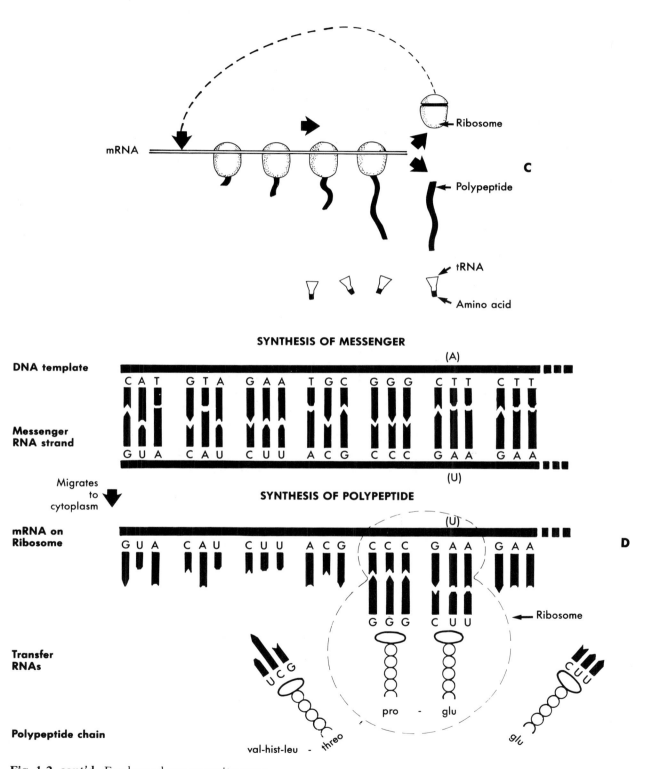

Fig. 1-2, cont'd. For legend see opposite page.

exquisitely precise control for gene expression. The first level is at the gene itself: various DNA binding factors made by different cell types (e.g., *transcription factors* and *repressor proteins*) can increase, decrease, or block the transcription of the gene by the RNA polymerase. This process is called *transacting*, or *epigenetic*, regulation, meaning that it originates at a distance from the gene. Certain DNA sequences "upstream" or "downstream" of the gene can affect transcription, presumably by altering the three-dimensional folding of the DNA and making it more accessible to the RNA polymerase. This process is *cisacting* regulation, meaning that DNA sequences adjacent to the gene are responsible. Although every gene needed by an organism is carried in every cell, entire genes can be inactivated so that they are never expressed in a particular cell or cell type. The random inactivation of one of the X chromosomes in females is an example, although it is becoming clear that only portions of that X chromosome are inactivated.[5] The mechanism(s) by which this inactivation occurs is not yet fully understood; methylation of the DNA appears to maintain the inactivated state but probably occurs secondarily.

The second level of control for gene expression is determined by the half-life of the mRNA molecule: those molecules that remain intact in the cytoplasm for a longer period will be translated into a greater number of protein molecules. Thus, additional noncoding sequences in the mRNA can effectively increase or decrease the ultimate expression of the gene by affecting mRNA half-life. This process is called *posttranscriptional* regulation.

Mutation. A mutation is a change in the DNA sequence of the gene and can be one of several types: *deletion* (actual loss of one or more nucleotides from the sequence); *missense* (a change in a nucleotide that alters the code such that a different amino acid is inserted at that position in the protein); *nonsense* (a change in a nucleotide that alters the code such that it does not code for any amino acid); or *frameshift* (in which the sequence of nucleotides is altered in a way that causes the code to fall out of the proper reading frame for the three-nucleotide codons. In other words, where the order *123-456-789-* might code for three specific amino acids, a shift to *-234-567-890-* would completely disrupt the code for that section of the gene.) Mutations can be caused by errors in replication; although the DNA polymerase has a sensi-

tive *proofreading* mechanism to detect and repair errors in copying, errors still occur at a frequency of approximately 10^{-6} per gene per cell. Mutations can also be caused by exposure to various chemicals (known as *mutagens*) or radiation. These mutations are often in the form of *strand breaks*, in which the bonds between two nucleotides on the same strand are disrupted, or *thymidine dimers*, in which two adjacent T nucleotides on a single strand become covalently linked in such a way that neither the DNA polymerase nor the RNA polymerase can recognize these bases.

If a mutation occurs in the *coding* region of a gene, the protein product is altered and this alteration may cause defective function. If the mutation occurs in the *regulatory* region of a gene, it may affect the quantity of the protein that is made or block its synthesis entirely.

Molecular Genetic Techniques

The advent of powerful laboratory techniques in molecular genetics within the last 20 years has allowed access to and manipulation of the genes themselves. It is beyond the scope of this chapter to offer a comprehensive description of contemporary molecular biology, but a brief overview should convey a sense of the capabilities of the technology.

Gene cloning. The term *recombinant DNA* refers to the ability to join genes from different species and have them be functionally expressed (i.e., transcribed into mRNA, which in turn is translated into protein). All cells—from bacterial to human—carry the enzymes and factors required to read the DNA code and synthesize protein; thus, as long as the species-specific regulatory sequences also are contained in the recombinant DNA molecule, any cell can express genes from any other cell.

An essential phenomenon in molecular genetics, *hybridization*, is based on the complementary sequences of DNA that pair in the double helix configuration (i.e., A pairs only with T, and C pairs only with G). This process occurs spontaneously at room temperature. Thus a fragment of DNA with a particular sequence can base pair, or *hybridize*, with any other DNA molecules that have a complementary sequence. This situation allows a fragment with a known sequence, for example, a particular gene, to be used as a molecular *probe* to search for that gene in any sample of DNA. This process is critical when attempting to clone a gene.

The *site-specific restriction endonucleases* ("restriction enzymes") are a set of biochemical tools that have made possible the construction of recombinant DNA molecules. Derived from bacteria, restriction enzymes cut, or *digest*, DNA at specific sequences that are from four to eight base pairs long. Thus the chromosomal, or *genomic*, DNA can be cut into smaller fragments at predictable sites, which allows the *construction* of *recombinant plasmids*. A plasmid is a small, extrachromosomal circle of bacterial DNA, which often carries genes that determine antibiotic resistance. The bacterial portion of the recombinant plasmid is called a *vector*. Viral DNA molecules from bacteriophages can also be used as vectors.

When foreign genes are inserted, or *ligated* into the vector, it can then be employed for a number of different purposes. If the vector is used to carry those genes back into bacteria, hundreds of thousands of copies of the foreign DNA can be obtained when the bacteria replicate the recombinant plasmid along with their own DNA. This process is a form of *amplification*. The bacteria can be plated onto agar and their DNA hybridized with a probe for a specific gene; this approach is useful in cloning, as will be discussed later. The vector can be used to express a gene in any type of cell, for instance, in bacteria, to produce large quantities of the protein, or into cells of the species from which the gene was obtained, to study its regulation. Such a construct is called an *expression* vector.

DNA can be *sequenced* to determine the exact order of the bases along the length of a single strand. This procedure is usually undertaken by setting up four reaction tubes, one for each of the nucleotides C, G, A, and T. The DNA is then added to the tubes with polymerase, a reaction mixture, and a radioactive label. Each nucleotide-specific reaction mixture then generates multiple copies of the DNA that are terminated at various positions containing that nucleotide, and all the copies are radioactively labelled. In this way a size "ladder" of all the variously sized fragments that can be obtained from ending at that nucleotide is generated. For example, if a sequence were ATGCCACT-GATAG, the *A* reaction tube would contain fragments that were 1, 6, 10, and 12 nucleotides in length. The products of each tube can then be run in parallel lanes on an acrylamide gel (which separates all the fragments according to size), and the

gel can be exposed to radiographic film to generate an *autoradiograph* (Fig. 1-3). The sequence can then be "read" by comparing the positions of all the fragments in each lane, that is, a 50-base long fragment in the A lane and a 51-base long fragment in the G lane would indicate a sequence of AG at this point.

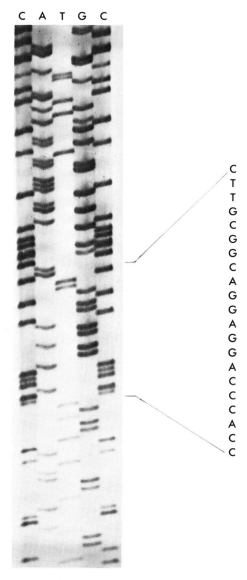

Fig. 1-3. Autoradiograph of a DNA sequencing gel produced by the method of Sanger using chain-terminating inhibitors. The DNA is sequenced to determine the exact order of the bases along the length of a single strand. (Courtesy Patrick Tippoo, Cape Town, South Africa.)

If a probe for a particular gene is available, the gene can be *cloned* in a number of ways. One approach is to digest all the genomic DNA from the desired organism or tissue with restriction enzymes and insert the resulting fragments into viral DNA vectors. The result is called a *genomic library* and contains each of the genes in individual vector molecules, much like individual books are contained in a conventional library. This genomic library can then be used to infect bacteria, and the bacteria can be plated onto agar plates, colonies allowed to grow up, and the plate pressed onto a filter that binds DNA. The bacterial DNA, which will be in the same position on the filter as on the plate, can then be hybridized with the probe for the specific gene. Only those bacterial colonies that carry the desired gene hybridize with the probe; those colonies can then be identified on the plate and grown in large quantities to amplify the gene.

A simple variation on the previously described technique involves the use of a *complementary DNA (cDNA) library.* In the construction of this type of DNA library the mRNA from a tissue or cell culture is purified, and the enzyme *reverse transcriptase* is used to generate cDNA molecules from the strands of RNA. Using mRNA for a library has the advantage that only sequences actually *expressed* in the cell are copied, not all the noncoding intron and nonspecific sequences that are contained in the genomic DNA. This approach reduces the number of bacterial colonies that must be screened with the probe and increases the probability of obtaining a complete gene in one colony. In addition, mRNA has already been spliced properly. The disadvantage is that important regulatory sequences contained only in the genomic DNA may be lost.

A number of techniques can be used to identify the DNA coding sequence for a particular protein. One such method is *polysome precipitation,* in which antibodies directed against a specific protein are used to bind that protein while it is being synthesized at the ribosomes. The mRNA from which it is being translated thus can be isolated, and from this mRNA a specific cDNA can be synthesized and used as a probe to clone the gene. Alternatively, if the DNA sequence can be deduced from the amino acid sequence of the protein, a probe can be chemically synthesized *de novo.*

Southern blots and restriction fragment length polymorphisms. Mutation may be analyzed using

Southern blots. In this method the DNA from a particular individual or cell population is digested with various restriction enzymes, run on a gel to separate the restriction fragments by size, immobilized by transfer to a nylon membrane, and hybridized with a probe for the gene in question. The same procedure is undertaken for the DNA from other individuals who do not carry a mutation in that gene. When the two sets—from the carrier of the mutation and the normal individuals—are compared, it is often apparent that they have generated DNA fragments of different lengths. This discrepancy occurs because the DNA sequence at a restriction site has been altered by the mutation; thus the restriction enzyme does not cut at that point. (Alternatively the mutation may generate a *new* restriction site; when the restriction enzyme cuts at this new site, a fragment of shorter length results.) This digestion, electrophoresis, and hybridization of a DNA probe to DNA on a membrane is known as a *Southern blot.* (The technique was developed by Southern[26] in 1975; variants of the technique have been humorously named *Northern* blots for probing RNA with a DNA probe and *Western* blots for binding antibodies to a protein gel.[18])

Southern blots can be used to detect naturally occurring variation among the nucleotides of normal individuals. For example, the genomes of two unrelated people differ from each other in roughly one of every several hundred bases, yet there may be no corresponding phenotypic differences, especially if the variable sites lie in the spacer regions between genes, in introns, or in bases where a mutation would not alter the function of the protein. Nonetheless, these genomic differences affect restriction enzyme digestion if they occur at a restriction site. In these circumstances, if the genomic DNA from two individuals is digested and run side by side on a gel, the differences in sequence are reflected in different fragment sizes, that is, in *restriction fragment length polymorphism* (RFLP) (Fig. 1-4).

Particular RFLPs are inherited with certain genetic disorders. In other words, the disease locus in most individuals affected with the condition in question cosegregates with a particular fragment when specific restriction enzymes and probes are used. In these circumstances the RFLP is said to be *linked* to that disorder; observations of this type are extremely useful in mapping the gene responsible for the condition (see the section, Linkage and Mapping). It should be emphasized that RFLP

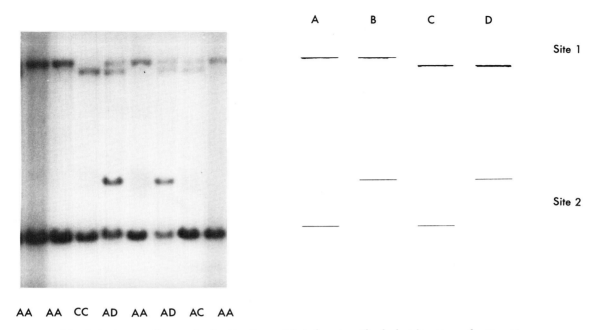

AA AA CC AD AA AD AC AA

Fig. 1-4. Autoradiograph of a Southern blot showing the hybridization of a Huntington disease–linked probe to *Hind* III-digested genomic DNA. Two "2" allele RFLP systems are indicated, *Site 1* and *Site 2. Haplotypes* A, B, C, and D have been determined from the alleles seen for each *Hind* III RFLP *(Sites 1 and 2).* (Courtesy Dr. Jacquie Greenberg, Cape Town, South Africa.)

analysis involves visualizing the DNA with any number of random probes; thus, to link that gene with an RFLP,[17] it is not necessary that the specific gene be isolated or that a probe for the specific gene be available.

Polymerase chain reactions. Most DNA techniques require at least a microgram (one millionth of a gram) of DNA, an amount not always obtainable. A recent advance allows millionfold amplification of a specific DNA fragment when only a few molecules of that fragment are present or from as little as a nanogram (1/1000 of a microgram) of mixed starting material. In the *polymerase chain reaction* a pair of synthetic *oligonucleotide* (from the Greek *oligo-*, that is, *small*) probes are used. These probes hybridize to the two DNA strands (sense and antisense) at opposite ends of the particular region to be amplified. Each probe acts as a *primer* to initiate DNA replication by a special DNA polymerase obtained from a thermophilic ("heat-loving") bacterium, which is active only at about 70° C. (The polymerase copies only the DNA with the primers attached; thus any other sequences present are not replicated.) In subsequent cycles of replication,

both old and new strands provide sites for the binding of primers, and so on. Changes in the temperature of the reaction mixture control the phases of successive cycles: a temperature of 95° C serves to *denature* the complementary strands of DNA so that they may be replicated, 40° C to attach the primers, and 70° C to extend the two strands with the polymerase.

Linkage and Mapping

Genes that lie close together on the same chromosome tend to be inherited together; they are said to be *linked* and to demonstrate *linkage. Syntenic* genes are any that are situated on the same chromosome. If they lie beyond a certain distance from one another, they fail to demonstrate linkage because of the phenomenon of *crossing over*, in which *homologous* segments of a chromosome pair are exchanged via recombination during meiosis. Thus a chromosome pair with the alleles *AB/ab* for genes *a* and *b* may become *Ab/aB*. Since meiosis results in the segregation and inheritance of only a single member of each chromosome pair by the zygote, the probability that alleles *A* and *B* will be inherited together increases as the distance between them on the chromosome decreases, that is, as the probability that a crossover will occur between them decreases.

Genes on the same chromosome are said to be *coupled;* when they lie on opposite chromosomes of a homologous pair, they are said to be in *repulsion.* The arrangement of a particular pair of genes is called the *linkage phase.* If genes are inherited together more than 50% of the time, generally they are linked. Detailed and carefully made pedigree studies are required to determine how closely they are linked. Many anonymous *markers,* or segments of DNA, are used for linkage studies, in addition to specific genes. The usefulness of a particular genetic marker can be expressed by its *polymorphism information content* (PIC). When a particular disorder is studied, complex mathematical computer programs can be used to determine linkage to genes on a particular chromosome, as well as to exclude that chromosome as a possible locus for the causative gene.

Studies of linkage have led to the mapping of the actual locus for many genes, that is, to a specific band or subband of a specific chromosome. Mapping makes use of family studies, somatic cell studies, chromosome analysis, and molecular technology. The use of recombinant DNA technology has increased the proportion of the human genome that has been mapped. Many connective tissue genes have been mapped to specific chromosomes, and many have been isolated and cloned.

Gene families. An interesting avenue of research in molecular genetics has involved the search for related genes and proteins, using DNA sequence and protein structure information to identify homologies. It has become clear that in the course of evolution some portions of the human genome were duplicated, with subsequent divergent changes resulting in the development of large families of similar proteins. The collagen genes are one such family.

Animal models. Many of the advances made in the study of the human genome have been derived from the extrapolation of animal data to human studies. Remarkable homologies are present when comparing, for example, the human and the mouse genomes. Thus it is possible, in mouse models, to produce mutations in specific genes of interest in human disease, using a technique known as *insertional mutagenesis.* In addition, it is now possible to introduce human genes into mouse embryos. If the foreign gene is introduced at a sufficiently early stage of embryogenesis, many of the tissues of this *transgenic* mouse carry and express the gene. If the gene is present in the germline of the mouse, some of its offspring express the gene in all their tissues. Thus it is possible to study the regulation of the gene and the effects of its expression *in vivo.*

CYTOGENETICS AND CHROMOSOMAL DISORDERS

Each species has a characteristic chromosomal constitution or *karyotype* with respect to number and structure. The chromosomal structure is visible at the time of cell division, when the nuclear *chromatin* material condenses to form rod-shaped organelles.

Normally the human possesses 46 chromosomes in each somatic cell; these comprise 23 *homologous* pairs. The members of a homologous pair are matched with respect to the genetic information that each carries, although they may contain different alleles of the same genes. In normal circumstances one member of a chromosome pair is inherited from the mother and one from the father, and one of each pair will be transmitted to each offspring through the gametes. Twenty-two of the pairs, the *autosomes,* are similar in males and females. One pair, the sex chromosomes, is different; females normally have two X chromosomes, and males normally have an X and a Y chromosome. The Y chromosome is always inherited from the father and passed on to the son. The Y chromosome plays a primary role in determining the male phenotype: unless the Y chromosome is present, a female phenotype results. Since females have two X chromosomes, they would produce twice the male dose of gene product for every X-linked gene unless there were a mechanism of *dosage compensation.* Random inactivation of large portions of either the maternally or paternally derived X chromosome early in embryonic development *(lyonization)* achieves equivalent X-linked gene dosage in males and females.

Cell Division

There are two types of cell division. *Mitosis* occurs in the somatic cells as the body grows and replaces cells. This process involves the precise duplication of each chromosome so that the daughter cells will be identical to the original cell in terms of genetic information. The second type of cell division, *meiosis*, is the specialized process by which germ cells or *gametes* are produced. During meiosis the *diploid* number of 46 chromosomes is reduced to the *haploid* number, in which only one copy of each chromosome pair is present. Various stages of cell division can be distinguished; this distinction is useful in determining the point at which errors in cell division occur.

Errors can occur in both mitosis and meiosis, resulting in daughter cells that contain abnormal numbers of chromosomes. Often these *aneuploid* cells cannot survive. In other instances *mosaicism* occurs, in which both *euploid* (carrying a normal number of chromosomes) and aneuploid cells are present. When an error in cell division occurs during mitosis, it may lead to *somatic mosaicism*, that is, two different cell lines in one organism. Occasionally the patchy distribution of pigment or tissue dysplasia makes it possible to suspect somatic mosaicism at the clinical level. Various tissues tolerate aneuploidy differently. Thus some types of mosaicism are encountered only in one tissue or another (e.g., fibroblasts or leukocytes). When such an error in cell division occurs during meiosis, it leads to *germline mosaicism*, and in these circumstances there is an increased risk that offspring will carry the chromosomal abnormality.

Techniques for Visualizing Chromosomes

Chromosomes can be visualized in a variety of tissues, but by virtue of accessibility and convenience cytogenetic studies are usually undertaken on white cells of the circulating blood. If chromosomal mosaicism is suspected, cytogenetic investigations should also be undertaken in other tissues such as cultured fibroblasts.

Part of the chromosome analysis involves blocking cell division so that the chromosomes can be visualized; for this reason the cells must be cultured and stimulated to divide. A *mitogen* is usually added to the cell culture to obtain sufficient numbers of mitotic cells. When the cells are dividing rapidly, further division is blocked by the ad-

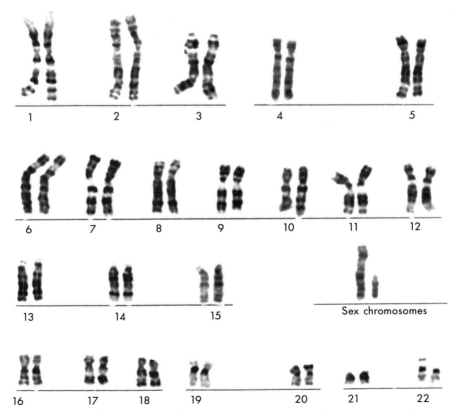

Fig. 1-5. Standard karyotype with chromosomes arranged by pairs according to size and shape.

dition of colchicine, a substance that interferes with spindle function. A hypotonic solution is then added to make the cells swell and to separate the chromosomes. At this point the chromosomes can be photographed under the microscope and arranged in pairs in order of descending size. This arrangement of chromosomes is called the *karyotype* of the cell (Fig. 1-5). Abnormalities in chromosome number and structure thus can be determined for each cell, and when enough cells have been examined, a conclusion can be drawn regarding the cytogenetic status of the patient.

A number of staining methods can be used to visualize different portions of the chromosome. Staining with quinicrine mustard and related compounds *(Q-banding)* necessitates examination with a fluorescent microscope. The Q-bands are used as the reference for the classification of banding. *G-banding* requires treatment of the chromosomes with trypsin, which denatures the chromosome protein, followed by Giemsa staining. The chromosomes show light and dark staining patterns with this method; the dark bands correspond to the bright fluorescent bands produced by Q-banding. *R-band* staining produces reverse staining, so the dark bands become the light bands. In R-banding the chromosome preparation receives a heat pretreatment followed by Giemsa staining. *C-banding* is a method used specifically to stain centromeric regions and some other areas of heterochromatin or dark staining. A method for staining the *nuclear organizing regions (NOR)* is NOR staining; a metallic silver stain is used. This method is especially applicable to the areas that contain the 28S and 18S ribosomal genes.

In the 1960s buccal smears for Barr body studies (inactivated X chromosomes) were used to determine the number of X chromosomes present in a cell. As cytogenetic techniques improved, it became clear that these investigations could be misleading and this method now is rarely used. Cytogenetic studies using bone marrow preparations can yield reliable results in a few hours in an emergency situation. As more highly sensitive molecular techniques are developed, buccal smears may again replace lymphocytes for *in situ* investigation, since the former approach does not necessitate the "invasive" procedure of drawing blood.

High-resolution banding is a technique in which the chromosomes are "stained" before they have completely condensed. The cultured cells are blocked in an early phase of the cell cycle and

then released at a later time, so most of the cells are in the prophase or prometaphase stage of cell division. With this method the chromosomes can be fixed in an extended, rather than tightly compact, configuration and many more bands can be demonstrated.

A number of *fragile sites* on chromosomes can be visualized by using folic acid– or thymine-deficient medium when culturing the cells or by adding inhibitors or thymine synthetase. Increased numbers of chromosome breaks also are seen in certain disorders.

Special culturing and staining techniques can demonstrate recombinations and rearrangements during cell division. Thus *sister chromatids* (the new copy and the old copy of a specific chromosome) may cross over and exchange segments of the chromosome arm. This crossing over between sister chromatids can be demonstrated by bromodeoxyuridine staining. An increased number of sister chromatid exchanges is seen in some genetic disorders and after exposure to particular environmental agents.

In addition to traditional cytogenetic techniques, *in situ DNA hybridization* techniques now allow visualization of specific genes and DNA sequences known as markers. DNA probes for specific genes or DNA fragments can be tagged with fluorescent or radioactive molecules that, when hybridized with the DNA of the chromosome on a slide, pinpoint the location of that gene. This technique is known as *fluorescent in situ hybridization (FISH)*. Chromosomal deletions involving several genes are known as *contiguous deletions*, which sometimes are large enough to be visualized with the cytogenetic techniques previously described. This kind of deletion also allows the identification of specific genes that have been deleted, as in the case of the dystrophin gene in Duchenne muscular dystrophy. The spatial relationship between particular genes on various chromosomes is becoming more clear as a result of the combination of mapping through linkage and direct visualization using *in situ* hybridization.

Gametogenesis

In the process of normal mitosis (the mechanism by which somatic cells divide) the nucleus undergoes a complicated series of events leading to the duplication of the chromosomal material, after which the cell cytoplasm separates into two parts. This normally leads to production of identical daughter cells with the diploid number of chromosomes. However, meiosis is a special type of cell division in which the germ cells or gametes are formed with the haploid number of chromosomes. In human females this process is largely complete at birth. In males it begins with sexual maturity and continues through the rest of life. In meiosis each daughter cell has half (haploid) the normal number of chromosomes, with one representative from each chromosome pair. Two successive cell divisions are needed to yield this result. In meiosis I the *reduction* division and the chromosome pair are duplicated, but when the duplicated pairs *disjoin*, the centromeres remain together, with the result that one complete chromosome *pair*, rather than a single copy of each of the original chromosomes, goes to each of the daughter cells. Meiosis II follows without DNA replication, and the centromeres separate from each other and divide, resulting in gamete cells with half the normal number of chromosomes (one from each original pair). During meiosis, exchange of chromatid arms can occur. The points where the chromatids cross over each other and exchange material are known as *chiasmata*. This process can be seen in preparations of germline cells, and these chiasmata are evident at least once on each chromosome arm. The end result of meiosis is a reduction in the number of chromosomes to half the somatic cell number; in this way the normal number of chromosomes can be reconstituted during fertilization.

In the male the production of sperm takes about 64 days. *Spermatogonia* with 46 chromosomes reside in the seminiferous tubules of the testes. From the time of sexual maturity *primary spermatocytes* in the testes are undergoing meiosis I to form *secondary spermatocytes*, which also have 46 chromosomes. These secondary spermatocytes then undergo cell division (meiosis II) without duplication to form *spermatids*, which contain the haploid number of 23 chromosomes. The spermatids develop without further cell division to form mature sperm. It is thought that the greater the number of cell divisions, the greater the chance of error (mutation) in a sperm. Thus older men whose spermatogonia have had more cell divisions appear to be at increased risk for errors in DNA replication, that is, new gene mutations.

In females, at about the third month of prenatal development the germ cells begin to develop into *primary oocytes*. Various germ cells enter meiosis at various points in development. However, the primary oocytes are suspended in first meiotic division until sexual maturity is reached. Each individual follicle then matures, and meiosis I is completed by the time of ovulation. During this division one of the sets of duplicated chromosomes receives most of the cytoplasm, and the other becomes the *first polar body*. The ova remain in this configuration for many years. The second meiotic division begins when the ovum passes down the oviduct but is not completed until after fertilization. Again, one of the sets of chromosomes receives all the cytoplasm and the other set remains as the *second polar body*.

Chromosomal Disorders

The union of the egg and sperm at fertilization reestablishes the normal diploid number of chromosomes. Abnormal numbers of chromosomes or rearrangements of chromosomes or of segments of chromosomes can produce major abnormalities in the affected individual. Most of these cytogenetic anomalies are thought to arise during the process of meiosis. However, it is also clear that they can arise during mitosis, either of the primary germ cells as they migrate to populate the gonad, or in somatic cells of the body during growth and development. The presence of abnormal numbers of chromosomes is known as *aneuploidy* (i.e., "not euploid"). Certain chromosomal rearrangements are not compatible with viability or are selected against by the growth of more vigorous normal cells during development. However, a wide variety of rearrangements (translocations, inversions, and the like) and extra or missing chromosome segments are tolerated.

In humans a large number of chromosomal abnormalities have been defined, and the clinical characteristics and natural history of these conditions have been well characterized. It is clear that if genes related to specific connective tissue genes are deficient or in excess, clinical defects in connective tissue may result. For example, patients with the XXXY and XXXXY Klinefelter syndromes frequently have radioulnar synostosis. Persons with 45,X Turner syndrome have large medial condyles of the femur and a complementary defect in the medial aspect of the proximal tibia. Furthermore, coarctation of the aorta, which occurs in about 10% of persons with Turner syndrome, also might be considered a connective tissue malformation. The pelvis in patients with trisomy 21 (Down syndrome) is sufficiently characteristic to aid in the diagnosis. A specific syndrome of multiple exostosis, cone epiphysis, hair and nose anomalies, and mental retardation is seen with a deletion of the long arm of chromosome 8 (8q). As is discussed in the section, Uniparental Disomy, the absence of a chromosome from one of the parents can result in growth disorders. However, affected persons tend to have multiple system involvement and multiple congenital anomalies rather than simple connective tissue disorders.

The cause(s) of chromosomal abnormalities is not well understood, although there appear to be predisposing genetic and environmental factors. The incidence of chromosomal anomalies in newborns is 0.5%, and advanced maternal age increases the risk of having a child with a chromosomal abnormality.[28]

Examination of spontaneous abortion specimens reveals that as many as 50% carry a chromosomal abnormality.[28] It is thought that a failure of chromosomes to separate during meiosis (nondisjunction) and falling behind (anaphase lag) during meiosis are major contributors to this problem.[28] Failure to cross over or form chiasmata also seems to play an important role. Because the oocytes wait suspended in the first meiotic division for longer periods with advancing maternal age, it has been thought that aneuploidy might be due entirely to problems with maternal spindle function.[26] However, it is now known that paternal nondisjunction contributes between 5% and 10% of aneuploidy cases, as demonstrated by new DNA techniques.[29] It has recently been postulated that the chromosomal aneuploidy associated with maternal aging is a result not of an increased frequency of ova with damaged chromosomes but of a failure to spontaneously abort an aneuploid embryo or fetus.[7] In addition, there may well be gene mutations that predispose to nondisjunction, since in consanguinous matings and in some families there appears to be a higher incidence of children with chromosomal abnormalities than would be expected.

Autoimmune disease may play some role in predisposing to nondisjunction, since high titers of thyroid antibody have been observed in the mothers of children with Down syndrome and in the children themselves.[28] Radiation can lead to nondisjunction in lower animals, and this factor may also be a cause of nondisjunction in humans.[29] Viruses and teratogenic agents may also lead to nondisjunction or increased crossover and structural rearrangements in animal models; this situation can be rarely demonstrated in humans. Finally, chromosomal abnormalities in the parent (e.g., a translocation) can lead to chromosomal abnormalities in the offspring.

Cytogenetic investigations are indicated in a child with multiple congenital anomalies or anomalies involving more than one organ system, since a major cause of this type of clinical picture is the presence of a chromosomal abnormality. Most children with an abnormal karyotype are short in stature and mentally retarded. Exceptions are some sex chromosome abnormalities, in which a missing or extra X or Y chromosome may produce a normal clinical appearance. With the advent of prenatal diagnosis, many parents now choose to have prenatal chromosome studies of amniocytes or chorion cells. However, those investigations are not usually of sufficient quality to rule out small deletions or chromosomal rearrangements.

Individuals with streaky pigment or regions of dysplastic, hypoplastic, or hyperplastic tissue, or both, may have somatic mosaicism for a chromosomal abnormality (i.e., some of their cells carry the abnormality, whereas others do not). In children with chromosomal abnormalities of this type it is often appropriate to undertake examination of fibroblast culture karyotypes (since cytogenetic investigations on leukocytes may yield normal findings). A region of contiguous deletions also may produce this phenotype, as in trichorhinophalangeal syndrome type II, which is caused by deletion of a short region of the long arm of chromosome 8.

GENE DISORDERS

The term *single gene inheritance* refers to the concepts that were developed by Mendel; therefore this type of inheritance is also called *mendelian inheritance*. Various genes may have multiple forms in which the DNA sequence differs, any two of which may be *carried* by an individual (since an individual normally possesses two copies of each chromosome in every cell). *Alleles* are alternative forms of a gene at a particular *locus*, or location on the chromosome. Occasionally, different mutations in the same gene (i.e., different mutant alleles) can produce phenotypes that are entirely different diseases at the clinical level. Some forms of osteogenesis imperfecta and the Ehlers-Danlos syndrome (EDS) are good examples of this situation; different mutations in the same gene can result in these quite different clinical disorders.

Two levels on which the genetic makeup of an individual may be considered are the *genotype,* or particular alleles of a given gene carried by an individual, and the *phenotype,* that is, the physical, biochemical, or physiologic characteristics determined by a gene. Before the development of DNA technology most single genes were recognized by their phenotypic effects, which in turn were regarded as inherited *traits* or disorders.

Simple mendelian traits are inherited via *autosomal transmission* (i.e., the genes for these traits are carried on one of the 22 pairs of *autosomes,* or nonsex chromosomes) or via *X-linked transmission* (i.e., genes carried on the X chromosome). With autosomal traits, in normal circumstances one copy of the gene is contributed by the mother and one by the father. X-linked traits always are derived from the mother in males (since they have received a Y chromosome from their fathers) and from either parent in females (since they have received an X chromosome from each).

Autosomal Dominant Traits

Dominant disorders are those in which a clinically recognizable abnormality is produced when only one abnormal copy (allele) of the gene is present, that is, in the *heterozygous* state. The Marfan syndrome and most types of osteogenesis imperfecta are examples of autosomal dominant traits. An autosomal dominant trait usually is characterized by an obvious phenotypic abnormality in individuals who carry the abnormal allele. This abnormality may be present at birth (congenital) or may develop over time.

An autosomal dominant trait characteristically appears in every generation and shows *vertical transmission* in a pedigree (Fig. 1-6, *A*). On average the autosomal dominant gene (i.e., the abnormal allele that determines the trait) is transmitted to 50% of the offspring of an affected individual. Conversely, unaffected individuals do not transmit the abnormal gene and their offspring are not at risk for development of the condition in question. Affected individuals have an affected parent, except in the event of a *new mutation* of the gene. New mutations may be the cause of some of the more severe genetic disorders, especially since the reproductive fitness or even the

survival of these individuals is greatly reduced and they are therefore unlikely to pass the mutation to their offspring.

New mutations occur on a regular but unpredictable basis. These are most frequently observed as dominant mutations, since the dominant nature of the gene allows phenotypic expression, although recessive mutations occur with equal frequency. It is estimated that the mutation frequency for most genes is in the range of 1 in 30,000 to 1 in 100,000 liveborn individuals. However, there are some human disorders that have far higher mutation frequencies, such as Duchenne muscular dystrophy or neurofibromatosis I (1 in 6000). This difference in mutation frequency may be influenced by the size of the gene, its nucleotide sequence, its exact position on a chromosome (e.g., at a "hot spot"), or by other as yet undefined factors.

With autosomal dominant traits the sex ratio of affected individuals is usually equal. However, there are conditions in which sex limitation or sex modification occur. For instance, testicular feminization is expressed only in males. Equally, hemochromatosis is far more likely to be expressed in males because females have reduced stores of iron as a result of regular blood loss at menstruation.

Autosomal Recessive Traits

Recessive disorders are those that usually are clinically expressed only when two abnormal copies of the gene are present *(homozygosity).* In other words, with autosomal recessive disorders individuals in whom both copies of the gene are abnormal (i.e., *homozygotes*) usually manifest the trait or disease. Conversely, autosomal recessive traits do not usually cause clinical symptoms or disease in the heterozygote (i.e., the individual with one normal allele and one abnormal allele). Examples of autosomal recessive disorders include homocystinuria and diastrophic dysplasia.

A recessive disorder is expressed clinically when no normal copy of the gene is present *(hemizygosity).* For instance, hemizygosity occurs normally in males with respect to the X chromosome; this situation leads to disease (i.e., an *X-linked disorder*) when the single normal copy of a gene carried on the X chromosome is lost or damaged. Hemizygosity also can occur for autosomal genes if one member of a chromosomal pair is lost. This process is known to be the mechanism causing

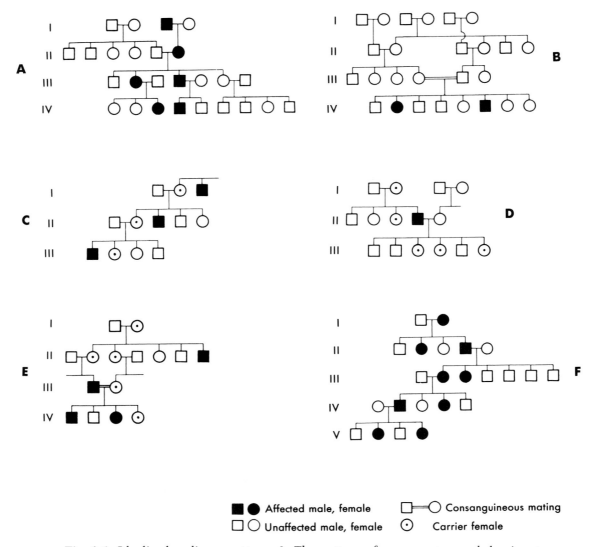

Fig. 1-6. Idealized pedigree pattern. **A,** The pattern of a rare autosomal dominant disorder. **B,** The pattern of a rare autosomal recessive disorder. **C, D,** and **E,** The pattern of a X-linked recessive disorder. **D,** All daughters of an affected male are carriers, and all sons are normal. **E,** The offspring of the mating of an affected male with a carrier female are represented. The affected son is not an exception to the rule of "no male-to-male transmission," since the gene came from the carrier mother. **F,** The pattern of an X-linked dominant trait. Although the families with affected mother suggest autosomal dominant inheritance, all daughters of affected males are affected and all sons of affected males are normal.

some cancers: an oncogene may become activated in a cell where there is one normal copy and one mutated copy of a *suppressor gene;* when the normal copy of a suppressor gene is lost, suppressor function is lost.

When an autosomal recessive condition is present in a family, there is usually a *horizontal* distribution of cases, that is, among sibs (Fig. 1-6, *B*). The abnormal copy of the gene (the abnormal allele) also may be carried by heterozygous relatives, offspring, and parents because the trait or disease normally appears only in the *offspring* of two carriers of the defect. In autosomal recessive disorders the parents of an affected individual may be related, or *consanguineous,* since this would make them more likely to have inherited the same abnormal allele. Usually both males and females are among the affected individuals in the pedigree of an autosomal recessive disorder. In a specific family with an autosomal recessive disorder, the severity of symptoms and age of onset are often similar in all affected children.

The term *recessive* generally refers to the full-blown disease or syndrome, but in some conditions manifestations in the heterozygote may also occur. For example, ataxia-telangiectasia is considered a recessive disorder, yet the heterozygous carriers of the gene for this disease are predisposed to cancer. Sickle cell anemia is another example in which carriers may show some aspects of the disease: the sickle cell *trait,* with sickling of the red cells, is observed in carriers, but severe anemia occurs only when both copies of the gene are defective.

Among the autosomal recessive disorders in which the pathogenic mechanism is known, many represent defects in an enzyme, which makes sense because a normal copy of a gene can usually produce sufficient quantities of an enzyme for normal function. Thus in many disorders for which the specific enzyme has been identified, the heterozygous carriers often have only 50% of the normal level of the enzyme. Frequently, homozygotes for autosomal recessive disorders do not reproduce because the homozygous state of the deleterious gene reduces their biologic fitness. For this reason some autosomal recessive traits must have conferred a selective advantage on the heterozygous individual during the course of evolution; otherwise the condition would not be as prevalent in the general population as it is. A relatively high frequency of a mutation in a population may be maintained by this kind of selective advantage or because of a *founder effect,* when a progenitor has had many children. Occasionally parents may carry different alleles of a particular gene; in this event the offspring could inherit two differently abnormal copies of the gene. In these circumstances the affected individual is said to be a *compound heterozygote.* This situation might result in a disorder characterized by a combination of the manifestations of two somewhat different diseases, for example, some of mucopolysaccharidoses. Alternatively the two defective alleles may compensate for each other, resulting in a normal phenotype. This mechanism is known as *complementation.*

X-Linked Traits

X-linked traits, as mentioned previously, are those in which the genes producing the abnormal phenotypes are located on the X chromosome. Because males do not pass their X chromosome on to their sons (i.e., the sons are male because they have inherited their father's Y chromosome), there will be no male-to-male transmission of an X-linked trait in a pedigree. Females, with two X chromosomes, may manifest an abnormal phenotype for an X-linked trait, depending on whether the trait is dominant or recessive. In addition, the manner in which normal X inactivation (lyonization) occurs may affect expression. Thus, if by chance the normal allele is on an X chromosome that is inactivated in a considerable proportion of the cells, a carrier female may express some phenotypic features of a recessive disorder. For instance, female carriers of the gene for Duchenne muscular dystrophy may have some enlargement of the muscles of the calves of their legs.

X-linked genes are passed from men to their daughters (i.e., they are female because they inherited their father's X chromosome), so daughters are *obligate heterozygotes* for any mutant alleles carried on the father's X chromosome. These genes in turn will be transmitted, on average, to half of the daughter's sons (since a son receives only one of his mother's two X chromosomes). Normally an X-linked trait is not transmitted from an affected father to his male children. Thus affected males in a kindred are either brothers or related to another affected male through carrier females. Unaffected males do not transmit

X-linked conditions, since the males do not carry the gene for these conditions (Fig. 1-6, *D*).

X-linked recessive disorders include Menkes syndrome, Hunter syndrome (MPS II), and EDS type V. Carrier females ordinarily do not show clinical manifestations in these conditions, and the phenotypic features are primarily seen in males.

X-linked dominant conditions are traits that are phenotypically expressed in the female carrier as well as in the male. Examples of X-linked dominant conditions include hypophosphataemic or vitamin D–resistant rickets and Alport disease. Females transmit the trait to both sexes with equal frequency, and the affected males transmit the trait to all their daughters but none of their sons. In families with X-linked dominant traits there are approximately twice as many affected females as males, since females receive twice the number of X chromosomes as do males. Affected females are usually more variably and on average more mildly affected than affected males.

A group of X-linked dominant conditions appears to be lethal in males. These conditions include focal dermal hypoplasia, Melnick-Needles syndrome, one form of the Conradi-Hünermann syndrome, and incontinentia pigmenti. The stigmata of these disorders are patchy in females, with involvement of bone, skin, and eyes. It is thought that the cells in which the abnormal gene has been inactivated via lyonization survive, whereas the cells that express only the abnormal gene die, resulting in a "patchy" phenotype. Therefore males carrying only the abnormal gene could not survive. Males who do manifest this type of disorder are presumed to be viable only because the mutation arose spontaneously during their own embryonic development, such that they are probably *mosaic* in their somatic tissues. Females affected with these conditions often have an increased rate of spontaneous abortion; this situation is thought to reflect the miscarriage of affected males.

Multifactorial Disorders

Some traits appear to have a familial predisposition but do not conform to simple mendelian inheritance. These tend to be single system disorders such as club foot and dislocated hips. It is thought that they result from the interaction of many different genetic and environmental factors; thus they are termed *multifactorial*. The recurrence risk for this type of disorder is empirically determined. The empiric risk is often in the range of 3% to 5% that first-degree relatives will have another affected child, and the risk is perhaps half that for second-degree relatives. The recurrence risk increases as the number of affected relatives increases. The sex frequency may be equal; however, some disorders of this type are more common in males, whereas others predominate in females.

A number of traits demonstrate a continuous spectrum of variability in the "normal" range, such as height, weight, and intelligence. It is postulated that these traits are determined by the combined action of a number of genes; thus they may be referred to as *polygenic* traits. However, it is obvious that a characteristic such as height is influenced by environmental factors (such as nutrition) as well as genetic ones.

Examples (drawn from conditions discussed in this book) of disorders transmitted by the various modes of mendelian inheritance are listed in the box on p. 21.

NONTRADITIONAL INHERITANCE

In addition to the mechanisms observed by Mendel, there are other ways in which genes can be passed on from parent to child. This category of inheritance includes transmission of cytoplasmic, that is, mitochondrial genes, germline mosaicism, imprinting, and uniparental disomy.

Cytoplasmic (Mitochondrial) Inheritance

The nucleus is not the only cellular organelle to carry genetic information. Cytoplasmic components are present in the ova but not in the sperm. Thus the elements of the cytoplasm, such as the mitochondria (and possibly the mitotic spindles, endoplasmic reticulum, and the like), are initially derived from the mother via cytoplasmic inheritance. The mitochondria contain a separate genome, which comprises over 16,000 base pairs. The chromosome carrying the mitochondrial genome is circular; parts of both strands of *mitochondrial DNA* (mtDNA) are transcribed and translated, in contrast to the single coding strand of the nuclear chromosomes. Each mitochondrion contains many copies of these circular genomes; thus each cell (with its many mitochondria) usually contains thousands of copies of the mitochondrial genome but only two copies of each nuclear chromosome. The mitochondrial genome is transcribed as a single mRNA that is cleaved into var-

---

Disorders Transmitted by Mendelian Inheritance

Autosomal dominant

Marfan syndrome
Ehlers-Danlos syndrome (types I, II, and III)
Cutis laxa (benign form)
Osteogenesis imperfecta (most forms)
Fibrodysplasia ossificans progressiva
Osteopoikilosis
Achondroplasia
Hypochondroplasia
Osteopetrosis (benign type)
Cleidocranial dysplasia
Multiple cartilagenous exostoses

Autosomal recessive

Homocystinuria
Ehlers-Danlos syndrome (type VI)
Cutis laxa (severe form)
Alkaptonuria
Pseudoxanthoma elasticum (most forms)
Mucopolysaccharidoses (except MPS II)
Diastrophic dysplasia
Metatropic dysplasia
Ellis-van Creveld syndrome
Asphyxiating thoracic dysplasia

Achondrogenesis
Cartilage-hair hypoplasia
Osteopetrosis, malignant type
Pycnodysostosis
Weill-Marchesani syndrome

X-linked recessive

Ehlers-Danlos syndrome (type V)
Mucopolysaccharidosis II (Hunter syndrome)
Spondyloepiphyseal dysplasia, tarda type
Menkes syndrome

X-linked dominant

Hereditary hypophosphatemia (vitamin D—resistant rickets)

Data compiled from McKusick VA: *Mendelian inheritance in man: catalogs of autosomal dominant, autosomal recessive and X-linked phenotypes*, ed 9, Baltimore, 1990, Johns Hopkins University Press.

ious genetic units. The products of the mitochondrial genes participate in a number of functions, the most important being the energy-generating synthesis of adenosine triphosphate via oxidative phosphorylation. Of the 69 separate polypeptides known to be required for oxidative phosphorylation, 13 are coded for by the mtDNA.

Because inheritance of mtDNA follows a strict maternal line of transmission, a clue to this cytoplasmic mode of inheritance is that a trait is passed only through females but all (or almost all) offspring are affected (as opposed to X-linked recessive traits, in which only half the sons are affected, or X-linked dominant traits, in which only 50% of offspring, male and female, would be expected to be affected).

A small number of clinical entities have been demonstrated to be caused by mutation in the mitochondrial genome, including Leber optic atrophy, myoclonic epilepsy with ragged red fibers, and infantile bilateral striated muscle necrosis. The mothers of affected persons are often *hetero-plasmic*, meaning that they carry some normal and some abnormal mitochondria and thus may appear to be unaffected. It seems likely that other categories of developmental anomaly may turn out to be mitochondrially determined, particularly in light of the importance of the mitochondrial genes in supplying the energy needs of the cell.[22]

Mosaicism

Somatic mosaicism refers to the presence in an individual of both normal cells and cells carrying a mutation at a particular locus or a chromosomal abnormality, caused by a mutation or nondisjunction in a somatic precursor cell early in embryogenesis. This type of mutation is not inherited from either parent and will not be passed on to the affected individual's children. Somatic mosaicism may explain certain disorders such as Albright polyostotic fibrous dysplasia, in which some cells have an abnormal genotype and others are normal, resulting in a "patchy" distribution.

Happle[12] has suggested that this sort of condition would be lethal if present in all tissues; therefore transmission between successive generations is not observed. By the use of new molecular techniques it may be possible to identify the difference between affected and unaffected tissues in this type of disorder.

In contrast to somatic mosaicism, *germline* or *gonadal* mosaicism implies that an individual carries both normal germline cells and others that carry a mutation. This mutation may be passed on to the offspring. The importance of this concept is that parents can have more than one child with the same "new" dominant mutation but be perfectly normal themselves. This situation has been demonstrated in a significant proportion of sporadic individuals with osteogenesis imperfecta whose condition is due to new mutations of the type I collagen gene. Germline mosaicism has important implications for recurrence risks in genetic counseling.

Imprinting

Imprinting is the mechanism by which certain genes produce various phenotypic effects depending on whether they have been inherited from the mother or father. A compelling body of evidence from mouse and human studies now suggests that imprinting plays a causal role in a number of human disorders. These include familial cancers, chromosome deletions, and single gene disorders, such as familial glomus tumors and Wiedemann-Beckwith syndrome.[11] Thus it is important when analyzing large pedigrees to determine whether a

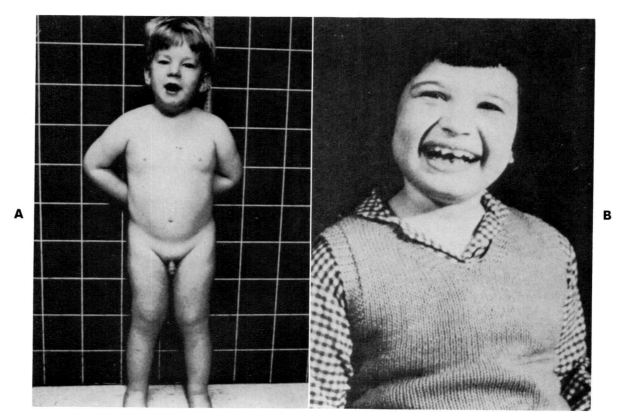

Fig. 1-7. A, The Prader-Willi syndrome (mental retardation, obesity, and characteristic facies). **B,** Angelman syndrome (mental retardation and characteristic gait). These phenotypically different syndromes are both apparently due to a deletion in the same region of chromosome 15. Each condition is associated with a deletion in the chromosome received from a different parent, which supports the theory of genomic imprinting. (From Hall JG: *Dev Suppl* 141-148, 1990.)

gene is expressed in the same way when inherited from the mother as when it has been transmitted through her sons.

Recently it has been recognized that Prader-Willi syndrome (Fig. 1-7, *A*) frequently is associated with the deletion of chromosome 15. It is always the *paternal* chromosome that has been deleted when this syndrome is present. By contrast, Angelman syndrome (Fig. 1-7, *B*) may result from a deletion of the same region of chromosome 15, yet it is the *maternal* copy that has been deleted. Therefore it appears that expression of the paternal and maternal chromosome 15 at this locus or region may be differentially regulated.[11]

Uniparental Disomy

Uniparental disomy involves the inheritance of both members of a chromosome pair from one parent. This phenomenon may result in the expression of a recessive allele, even though only one parent carries that allele.

Observations of uniparental disomy have lent further support to the theory of imprinting discussed previously: mice with uniparental disomy may show tissue hyperplasia or growth retardation, suggesting again that chromosomes inherited from each parent may have complementary but different roles to play in development.[10] Humans with uniparental disomy of chromosome 7 suffer intrauterine and postnatal growth retardation, which suggests that other forms of intrauterine growth retardation may also be influenced by imprinting.[10]

POPULATION DYNAMICS: MUTATIONS, GENETIC EQUILIBRIUM, AND SPORADIC CASES

All single gene disorders have arisen via genetic mutation at some time in recent or more distantly past generations. In this way a proportion of individuals with autosomal dominant and X-linked recessive disorders owe their abnormality to a mutation that occurred in the germ cells of one or other parent. The more severe the particular dominant or X-linked trait and the more drastically it interferes with reproduction of the affected persons as a group, the higher the proportion of cases that represents new mutations. This conclusion follows directly from an assumption of *genetic equilibrium*. If no new mutation occurred and the affected individuals reproduced less often than the average for the general population, the disorder

would disappear. If, on the other hand, new mutations continued to arise, even at low frequency, and the reproductive fitness of affected persons were not reduced, the condition would occur quite frequently. Genetic equilibrium can be compared to a bucket of water from which water (the genes) may be lost through a hole at the bottom (negative selection) but into which other genes are added from a tap at the top (new mutation). At equilibrium the loss and gain of genes balance each other.

Considerations relating to equilibrium and the proportion of cases that are sporadic and nonfamilial, having arisen by new mutation, are illustrated by X-linked recessive conditions such as Duchenne muscular dystrophy, the Hunter type of mucopolysaccharidosis (MPS) and Menkes syndrome, in which few if any affected males reproduce. It is estimated that about one-third of these individuals owe their disease to mutation affecting the X chromosome that the mother transmitted to the affected son. In the other two thirds the mutation occurred in a generation earlier than the mother's; in these circumstances other males in the family may be affected. Mutation rates (which relate to the gametes) are calculated on the basis of this principle of equilibrium. The values usually found are of the order of 1 in 100,000 gametes per generation, or, as it is more often stated, 1×10^{-6} per gamete per generation.

If a sporadic case of a heritable disorder occurs (i.e., an isolated instance, in which parents and all other relatives of the individual are normal), the following are possibilities:

1. As discussed previously, the disorder in the affected individual may be the result of new mutation. This situation is possible when the condition is autosomal dominant or X-linked recessive. The possibility of fresh dominant mutation is strengthened if paternal age is elevated. For example, the average age of fathers of individuals with sporadic, presumably new mutation in cases of Marfan syndrome, fibrodysplasia ossificans progressiva, and achondroplasia is five to seven years greater than the average age of fathers generally.

2. The affected individual may have a recessive gene in the homozygous state; if the parents are consanguineous, this possibility is strengthened. Since human families are usually small, a majority of families have only one

child affected by a recessive disorder. In the early stages of recognition of a "new" recessive disorder, genetic causation and specifically recessive inheritance may be missed because all cases are "sporadic."

3. Although no certain example in humans can be cited, it is theoretically possible that a disorder might require the existence of two collaborating but independently inherited dominant genes. Neither gene alone would produce abnormality. In such a situation the "sporadic" patient would have derived one dominant gene from each parent.

4. It is possible that the trait is in fact dominant but the parent who is heterozygous has the disorder in such subtle form that it escapes detection. This situation might result from variable expression to the extent of apparent nonpenetrance.

5. The sporadic case could be the result of germline mosaicism in either parent. In other words, during the parent's own embryogenesis more than one of the germ cells carry the mutation, which would then be passed on to the offspring derived from those germ cells.

6. Theoretically, somatic mutation can account for sporadic cases, especially when the anomaly is localized. In these circumstances the genetic change would necessarily occur in the zygote or in the embryo at an early stage of development.

7. The sporadic case could be the result of uniparental disomy. Uniparental disomy involves the inheritance of both members of a chromosome pair from one parent. Uniparental isodisomy may result in the phenotypic expression of a recessive allele because the offspring may carry two of the recessive allele copies transmitted from the one parent. In addition, an apparently abnormal phenotype could be due to the phenomenon of genomic imprinting, by which chromosomal regions inherited from the mother produce a different phenotype than does the same region inherited from the father.

8. Sporadic severely affected individuals could result from chromosomal aberration.

9. The sporadic case may represent a *phenocopy*. This term signifies the situation in which an environmental factor produces the same clinical disorder (i.e., the same phenotype) that also occurs as a genetic derangement. For example, the manifestations of

ochronosis, which are similar to those of alkaptonuria, can be produced by prolonged use of carbolic acid dressings on chronic cutaneous ulcers. Another example is the epiphyseal stippling produced by warfarin embryopathy, which closely resembles that of Conradi-Hünermann syndrome.

GENETIC MECHANISMS, CONCEPTS, AND GENOTYPE-PHENOTYPE CORRELATIONS
Penetrance and Expressivity

Autosomal dominant traits are not always expressed to the same degree in all affected individuals. In the real world of complex genetic and environmental interactions some members of a family may be severely affected, others only mildly so. Indeed, there may even be transmittors of a dominant allele who appear phenotypically normal. To describe this phenomenon, the concepts of *penetrance* and *expressivity* have been developed.

Penetrance refers to the ability to detect the presence of the faulty gene in an individual who is a member of an affected pedigree and who carries the abnormal allele. If a gene has been characterized at the level of the DNA, penetrance can be accurately determined, but when the defect can be observed only at a clinical or biochemical level, its detection can be far more difficult. Penetrance is an "all or none" phenomenon; that is, the presence of the abnormal copy of the gene either can or cannot be detected. Thus a trait or disease may have 60% penetrance; this means that 60% of the time a carrier of the dominant abnormal allele shows some phenotypic expression or observable abnormality. The unaffected carrier is described as nonpenetrant.

Expressivity refers to severity, that is, degree of expression of the abnormal gene in the phenotype. It is assumed that some features of the defect are present; i.e. that penetrance has occurred. The variety of ways in which the gene may be expressed, in terms of severity, time of onset, and affected tissues or organs, is described as *variability of expression*. Variability of expression is a characteristic of particular conditions; some disorders show great variability, whereas others show little from individual to individual.

Pleiotropism

Pleiotropism refers to the concept that a single abnormal gene may produce multiple and apparently unrelated clinical manifestations. Theoretically it is to be expected that when the pathogenic mechanisms are understood, it will be possible to trace the seemingly unrelated effects to a common "cause." Before a defect in the fibrillin gene was identified as the cause of the Marfan syndrome, the mechanism responsible for the *pleiotropic* effects in the cardiac, skeletal, and ocular systems was not known.

Epistasis

Epistasis is the influence on a gene by an allele at another locus. Clear-cut examples of epistasis are provided by the interrelationships of some of the common blood group antigens. Equally, in the heritable connective tissue disorders, interfamilial variation in the phenotypic manifestations of the same gene can be explained by this process. For instance, this mechanism might play a role in the variable clinical severity in members of the same family with conditions such as the autosomal dominant forms of EDS, osteogenesis imperfecta (OI), and Marfan syndrome.

Domains

It is possible that two different mutations in the same gene can produce different phenotypes. This phenomenon occurs when the mutations lie in different *domains* of the protein product and thus affect different functions of the same protein. For example, OI types I and II and EDS type VII are caused by mutations in the gene for the alpha 1 chain of type I collagen (COL1AI), which might not be predicted from the very different phenotypes in these disorders, especially between the two forms of OI and EDS VII. The explanation is that EDS VII is caused by a mutation in the N-pro-peptide domain, whereas the two forms of OI are due to mutations in the helical domain of the collagen protein.

Phenotypic Diversity Caused by Allelic Series

Whereas genes at different loci can give rise to similar or identical phenotypes, as in some forms of OI types I and II, different alleles at the same genetic locus can produce a change in the same enzyme or other protein product, resulting in quite a different clinical picture. A striking example is provided by two mucopolysaccharidoses: Hurler syndrome (MPS I H) and Scheie syndrome (MPS I S). These were initially considered separate disorders because of their great difference in phenotype and were called MPS I and V. They are now known to have deficiency of the same en-

zyme, alpha-L-iduronidase, and they presumably are produced by homozygosity for different alleles at the iduronidase locus.

In humans and even more in other species there is extensive precedence for this type of *allelic series* with wide phenotypic range. The various alleles at the beta hemoglobin locus can, for example, lead to phenotypes as disparate as persistent anemia with painful crises (sickle cell anemia), drug-induced anemia (Hb Zurich), or polycythemia (Hb Chesapeake). Equally, the various alleles at the alpha 1 chain of type I collagen can result in OI type I or type II.

Further phenotypic diversity arises from allelic series because of the occurrence of *genetic compounds*, in which the individual carries two different mutant alleles. (*Double heterozygote* is a term reserved for the condition of heterozygosity at two different loci.) Hemoglobins S and C are determined by allelic genes. The genetic compound, SC disease, is phenotypically distinct from both SS disease and CC disease. To return to the MPS example, if the Hurler syndrome (comparable to SS disease) is allelic with the Scheie syndrome (comparable to CC disease), among the patients with mucopolysaccharidoses some are likely to have Hurler-Scheie compounds. They are likely to have a phenotype intermediate between those of the Hurler and Scheie syndromes and have a deficiency of the same enzyme, alpha-L-iduronidase. It is possible, of course, that persons observed to have such a phenotype are homozygous for yet another allele at the iduronidase locus.

An allelic series is suspected at the MPS II locus because mild and severe forms of MPS II seem clearly distinguishable but have deficiency of the same enzyme. However, since the MPS II locus is X linked, no male can have a genetic compound.

Heterozygosity and Carrier Detection

The detection of heterozygous carriers of recessive traits, either autosomal or X-linked, has practical importance in genetic counseling. It also has scientific importance in the establishment of mode of inheritance; for example, discovery of a partial defect such as an intermediate level of enzyme activity in both parents of an affected person or in the mother only is strong support for autosomal recessive or X-linked recessive inheritance, respectively. Furthermore, the findings in heterozygotes for X-linked traits have special genetic interest in connection with the Lyon principle of X inactivation.

Methods for detecting heterozygotes consist mainly of (1) demonstration of an intermediate deficiency of a gene product, such as an enzyme; (2) demonstration of less than normal functioning when a particular metabolic step is placed under stress by a "loading test," or tolerance test; or (3) identifying the presence of an abnormal gene with DNA technology. In a number of recessively inherited inborn errors of metabolism in which the specific defective enzyme has been identified, partial deficiency of that enzyme has been demonstrated in parents. Homocystinuria is a case in point. In phenylketonuria, loading tests in which orally administered phenylalanine is used demonstrate increases in blood levels that persist longer than usual. DNA analysis requires that a particular gene has been isolated and cloned, so a molecular probe for the gene is available. However, as molecular genetic technology progresses, this analysis is possible with an ever-increasing number of genes.

Females heterozygous for X-linked recessive traits are likely to show directly or indirectly a reduced level of the particular gene product. Reduced red blood cell glucose-6-phosphate dehydrogenase (G6PD) activity in primaquine sensitivity or favism and reduced antihemophilic factor (factor VIII) in hemophilia A are examples. In addition, considerations of the Lyon principle dictate that if the phenotype is observable at the cellular level, heterozygotes for X-linked traits have a mosaic of cells with the same defect as in cells of the affected hemizygous male, together with cells that are perfectly "normal."

Mosaicism in heterozygotes has been demonstrated for several X-linked recessive traits in humans. For example, the female who is heterozygous for X-linked ocular albinism shows a mosaic pigmentary pattern of the fundus oculi. The female heterozygous for G6PD deficiency has two classes of erythrocytes: deficient and normal. In the X-linked disorder of mucopolysaccharide metabolism, the Hunter syndrome, two classes of connective tissue cells can be demonstrated in the heterozygous female.

Complex Genetic Predisposition

As mentioned in the section, Multifactorial Disorders, many defects have a tendency to run in families, but unlike those conditions that are the subject of this book, the pattern of familial occurrence does not suggest simple mendelian inheritance. Indeed, whenever a survey of the role of genetic factors in the diseases of a given system is undertaken, it is found that the entities tend to fall into the following categories (exclusive of chromosomal aberrations, whose effects are usually not limited to one system): (1) the relatively uncommon, simply inherited disorders and (2) the common conditions in which genetic factors seem to play some role but environmental factors are also involved, often in a complex manner. Rheumatoid arthritis, rheumatic fever, systemic lupus erythematosus, and scleroderma (systemic sclerosis) are generally considered "connective tissue diseases," although it can be argued that they are diseases *in* but not *of* connective tissue. In each of these some evidence for familial aggregation is available, but discussion of the genetics of these common disorders is beyond the scope of this book.

The questions that the geneticist considers are different in the two categories of disease. In the rare, simply inherited disorders, issues include gene frequency, mode of inheritance, nature of the basic defect, mechanism of the phenotypic features, mutation rate, selection factors, and so forth. In the more common conditions of multifactorial causation, in which genetic factors—themselves multiple (polygenic)—may play a role, the questions are likely to be: "How important is the genotype in determining the occurrence of the disease in question?" and "If important, by what mechanism does the genetic constitution contribute to the development of the disease?" The methods for answering these two questions, especially the first, include studies of familial aggregation, comparison of *concordance* rates of monozygotic and like-sex dizygotic twins (see the section, Twin Studies), comparison of different ethnic groups, study of the genetics of separate components in pathogenesis, search for RFLP disease association, and the genetic study of homologous disorders in experimental animals.

Association. An association is a statistical observation made when certain signs, abnormalities, or markers occur together more frequently than would be expected by chance alone. In dysmorphology the term is used to describe combinations of congenital anomalies, such as the *v*ertebral defects, imperforate *a*nus, *t*racheoesophageal fistula, and *r*adial and *r*enal dysplasia *(VATER)* association; it is also used for marker-disease associations such as the human lymphocyte antigen (HLA) specification B27 and ankylosing spondylitis.

In addition to association, some conditions are

actually linked to the HLA locus. Congenital adrenal hyperplasia with 21 hydroxylase deficiency and hemachromatosis are two examples. Not only are these disorders linked (in that the gene lies in physical proximity to the HLA locus), but also they have haplotype associations (such that a particular HLA haplotype is more likely to be present in an affected individual than in others).

Because the HLA locus is so highly polymorphic, it can be used as a marker to predict the inheritance of other abnormal genes. In addition, because each person's HLA pattern is so highly individual, it can be used to discern paternity and nonpaternity with a high degree of reliability.

Twin studies. Twin studies have been exceptionally helpful in the study of genetic influences in diseases. In these investigations identical or monozygotic twins are compared with fraternal or dizygotic twins, since they have shared the same intrauterine environment and often share the same postnatal environment. In the case of monozygotic twins the assumption is that the differences are explained on the basis of environmental influences. Twin studies are used to identify the genetic influences in particular diseases. For instance, in diabetes mellitus there is a marked difference between juvenile onset and maturity onset diabetes. High *concordance* exists among monozygotic twins for maturity onset diabetes, whereas the concordance for juvenile onset diabetes is far lower. On the other hand, there is a marked association of juvenile onset diabetes with HLA type, suggesting that infection may be a trigger. Twin studies do not rule out the possibility of a new somatic mutation, or the loss of imprinting, occurring in one twin during embryogenesis; statistical correlations can be drawn, however, if enough sets of twins are studied for a particular disorder.

HETEROGENEITY OF GENETIC DISEASE

It has happened so often in medical genetics as to be considered the rule that when subjected to careful examination, a condition that appears at first to be homogeneous is found in fact to comprise two or more separate and distinct entities. There are many examples, including mucopolysaccharidoses, OI, and EDS.

Heterogeneity of genetic disease is a corollary of the axiom that the phenotype is not a necessary indication of the genotype. Several different genotypes can lead to the same phenotype, which is to

be expected, since many steps, each separately gene-controlled, go into the determination of most phenotypes, and mutation at several different steps can lead to the same end effect. The situation has been compared to the stalling of a car, which can have many causes, although the end result, or phenotype, is identical.[27] *Genetic mimic* or *genocopy* are terms given to a genetic condition that is phenotypically similar or identical to another but has a different genetic basis. As stated earlier, phenocopy is the designation given to a phenotype that is similar or identical to a genetically determined one but is determined by exogenous factors.

Separate entities are discerned (1) by subtle phenotypic differences, (2) by genetic differences, (3) by biochemical differences, and (4) by physiologic differences. Each of these approaches is described in the following paragraphs.

Phenotypically the presence or absence of corneal dystrophy was noted to be a feature distinguishing two forms of the condition formerly known as gargoylism (i.e., the autosomal recessive type documented by Hurler and the X-linked recessive form described by Hunter). Equally, downward versus upward displacement of the ocular lenses and the presence of mental retardation can distinguish homocystinuria from Marfan syndrome.

The genetic means of distinguishing separate heritable entities include demonstration of different modes of inheritance or different linkage relationships and the study of offspring produced by the marriage of two persons with a recessively inherited disorder. Spastic paraplegia, retinitis pigmentosa, and Charcot-Marie-Tooth peroneal muscular atrophy are three disorders that are inherited as autosomal dominant in some families, as autosomal recessive in others, and as X-linked recessive in yet others. Usually in conditions with these three forms of inheritance the autosomal recessive form is most severe, the dominant form least severe, and the X-linked recessive form intermediate in severity.

At least two distinct forms of elliptocytosis (ovalocytosis), both inherited as dominant traits, have been distinguished on the basis of serologic linkage relationships, although no definite phenotypic differences are discernible. Linkage studies[21] indicate that one form is determined by a gene at a locus on the same pair of chromosomes as the locus occupied by the Rh blood group genes, whereas a second form of elliptocytosis is determined by a gene at some position far removed from the Rh locus.

In many instances congenital deafness (deaf-mutism) can be shown to be inherited as a simple autosomal recessive trait. Assortative (i.e., nonrandom) mating is often practiced by persons with deaf-mutism; persons with deafness marry other persons with deafness far more often than would occur randomly. All children of two persons with deafness, each from a family with a recessive pattern of inheritance, have deafness if the two parents are homozygous at the same locus. Families fulfilling this expectation have been observed. However, in other families the two parents, both affected by phenotypically identical and recessively inherited deafness, all children have normal hearing; the explanation is that the parents with deafness are homozygous at different loci and have genetically distinct forms of deafness.

Biochemical means of differentiating phenotypically similar genetic entities are illustrated by certain of the mucopolysaccharidoses, since differences in the pattern of urinary excretion of mucopolysaccharides can be used to distinguish entities. Biochemical or enzymatic studies may provide definitive differences, as in the recognition of the phenotypically indistinguishable forms of the Sanfilippo syndrome (MPS III) on the basis of deficiency of different enzymes involved in the degradation of the mucopolysaccharide heparin sulfate.

The physiologic method for differentiation of phenotypically similar genetic diseases is demonstrated by hemophilia. Before about 1950 all sex-linked hemophilia was assumed to be one and the same disease, although the possibility of multiple allelism had been suggested to explain the occurrence of clinically mild and clinically severe forms. It was then discovered that the blood from some persons with hemophilia would correct the clotting defect in others. The correctability was mutual. The explanation is that the location of the defect in the chain of clotting reactions is different and bloods from two persons with hemophilia complement each other, each providing an essential clotting factor missing in the other. Hemophilia A (classic hemophilia) and hemophilia B (Christmas disease) were distinguished in this way. Although both are determined by genes on the X chromosome, the genes are known to be on different parts of the chromosome; linkage studies indicate that the hemophilia A gene is fairly close

to the locus of color blindness, the G6PD locus, and the Xg group locus, whereas the Christmas disease gene is not linked to these loci. Thus evidence from genetic linkage corroborates the evidence from physiologic studies.

PATHOGENETIC MECHANISMS
Inborn Errors of Metabolism

The pathogenesis of alkaptonuria was adequately recognized, characterized, and analyzed only after it was established that the condition resulted from an *inborn error of metabolism*. Homocystinuria is another clear example of a heritable disorder of connective tissue caused by an inborn error of metabolism. Both of these conditions are autosomal recessive traits; as stated earlier, this mode of inheritance is always suggestive of the possibility of an inborn error of metabolism, that is, an enzyme defect.

As schematized in Fig. 1-8, there are at least three mechanisms by which multiple mutations resulting in various genetic enzyme blocks can produce the same phenotypic features of an inborn error of metabolism. (1) Excess substance may accumulate proximal to the block; the connective tissue manifestations of alkaptonuria have this basis. (2) Lack of the product of the chain of enzymatic reactions may lead to the phenotypic features. Albinism, several forms of congenital ad-

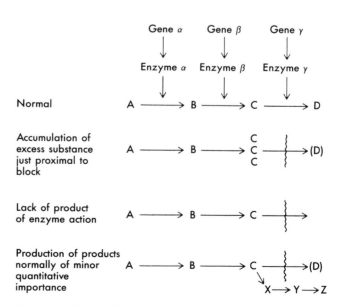

Fig. 1-8. Chains of metabolic reactions and the effects of enzyme blocks.

renal hyperplasia, and genetic defects in thyroid hormonogenesis leading to familial goiter are examples. (3) The production, through an alternative pathway, of products that normally are of minor quantitative importance may be responsible for some or all of the phenotypic features. Phenylketonuria is a case in point; some of the urinary excretory products are produced through an alternate metabolic pathway.

Yet another mechanism by which a genetic enzyme block can have pathologic consequences is a special case of the second mechanism listed in the preceding paragraph. In this situation the failure of synthesis of a product may remove a feedback control mechanism. In orotic aciduria, for example, large amounts of orotic acid are produced and result in hematuria caused by irritation of the urinary tract by orotic acid crystals. The relatively massive urinary excretion of orotic acid is due not only to the accumulation proximal to the enzyme block but also to loss of the feedback control of the first step in the pyrimidine pathway, which is exercised normally by the end products of the pathway.[25]

Defects in Membrane Transport Systems

Several hereditary syndromes have been shown to be the result of a gene-determined defect in a membrane transport system. Cystinuria, not to be confused with homocystinuria, is an example. The defect concerns transport of cystine and related amino acids (lysine, ornithine, and arginine) across the renal tubule cells; the plasma level of cystine and of the other three amino acids is normal or low. By contrast, the aminoaciduria of inborn errors of metabolism such as homocystinuria is of the overflow type; the plasma level of the amino acid that accumulates proximal to a block in intermediary metabolism is elevated or, if there is no renal threshold for the substance, unaltered.

End-Organ Unresponsiveness

A number of disorders such as the testicular feminization syndrome and nephrogenic diabetes insipidus are the result of mutations that result in loss of capacity of the end-organ to respond to a hormone (testosterone and vasopressin, respectively, in these examples). There appear to be several forms of dwarfism ("sexual ateleiosis") in which the defect is not deficiency of growth hormone but rather end-organ unresponsiveness. In one, the Laron dwarf, unresponsiveness to growth

hormone has been ascribed to a defect in the growth hormone receptor.[4] In pseudohypoparathyroidism, adenosine 3':5'-cyclic phosphate, which mediates the effects of parathormone on the kidney and on bone, is not synthesized.[3]

Disorders of Processing

Many proteins undergo extensive changes via *processing* after they are initially synthesized at the ribosome. Errors in this processing, such as a failure to cleave the procollagen molecules into collagen or to hydroxylate selected lysyl residues in the collagen chain, can result in an abnormal phenotype.

GENETICS IN CLINICAL PRACTICE

Medical genetics contributes to *diagnosis* through analysis of the family history and awareness of the implications of the phenomenon of pleiotropism. Some of the pleiotropic effects of a single gene may be important external clues to the presence of a serious internal disorder; for example, the ectopia lentis of the Marfan syndrome can be a useful clue in the differential diagnosis of aortic regurgitation. In the same way, the presence of angioid streaks in the fundus oculi, which serves as a diagnostic indicator of pseudoxanthoma elasticum, can be a valuable aid in the differential diagnosis of gastrointestinal bleeding.

Prognosis ("What is going to happen?") in the medical genetics context concerns mainly the unborn child of parents who have had a previously affected child, or the child of a parent who is affected or who has an affected relative. The art and science of gauging the risk and providing meaningful information and advice are embraced in *genetic counseling*. This process is later discussed in greater detail.

Recognition of the carrier state is particularly useful in the case of X-linked recessive disorders. Whereas the normal but heterozygous sister of a patient with homocystinuria will have affected offspring only if she marries another carrier (an unlikely possibility if she does not marry a relative), the normal heterozygous sister of a patient with the Hunter syndrome or Duchenne muscular dystrophy has a 50% risk that any son will be affected, regardless of the genotype of her husband.

Genetic Counseling

Many connective tissue disorders have a genetic basis, and members of an affected family often seek guidance concerning recurrence risks. Consultation and interaction with a kindred when a family member has severe genetic disease is not an easy matter. Families are often distraught, the information may be technical, and it is always difficult to convey bad news. But it is the responsibility of health professionals to provide the family with as much information as possible so that they may make reproductive and long-range planning decisions that are appropriate to their personal situation.

Genetic counseling is actually a process of information exchange whereby the geneticist can learn enough about the family to provide relevant information. In the process of counseling, a number of areas are discussed, although the exact order and depth of the discussion may vary depending on the disease in question and the family's situation at that time. Furthermore, the process of providing information is usually ongoing, since new developments arise and new diagnostic techniques are developed. The time at which information is provided often depends on the urgency of the situation (e.g., prenatal diagnosis of a severe disorder), the necessity to make decisions in nongenetic areas (e.g., regarding aggressiveness of treatment), or the need to collect additional information (e.g., pedigree data).

Frequently the family is as much concerned about what to expect in the future (i.e., the medical prognosis) as they are about the risks of recurrence of the disorder in the offspring of members of the kindred. The natural history of the disorder must be discussed, with elaboration on the potential range of severity. Possible future complications and their preventions should be reviewed as well. The recurrence risks for the patient, the parents, and other family members warrant attention. It often turns out that family members are worrying needlessly, and genetic counseling may alleviate a burden of concern that has been carried for many years. Sometimes steps can be taken to prevent complications or to screen for their early development. The family needs to be aware of any possibilities in this regard.

Prenatal Diagnosis and Carrier Detection

Genetic counseling has found a strong ally in the methods for prenatal diagnosis based on amniocentesis (possible at about the fourteenth week of a pregnancy), chorionic villus sampling (possible as early as the ninth week of a pregnancy), and

ultrasonography (throughout the pregnancy). In a rapidly increasing list of disorders it is now possible to recognize the affected fetus by study of the amniotic fluid itself or, more often and more reliably, by biochemical or chromosomal study of cultured amniotic or chorionic cells. Among the heritable disorders of connective tissue, homocystinuria, OI, and the mucopolysaccharidoses lend themselves particularly well to prenatal diagnosis. These methods are generally applied in high-risk families, that is, those in which the parents are known to have a significant risk of affected children, either because of family history of a specific disorder or because of advanced maternal or paternal age in the case of chromosomal conditions. By means of prenatal diagnosis and selective abortion it is possible to help such parents have unaffected children. In lethal conditions autopsy, together with biochemical and DNA analysis, may be an essential prerequisite to facilitate prenatal diagnosis in subsequent pregnancies.

A family with a genetic condition needs to know whether prenatal diagnosis and carrier detection are available. They may choose not to take advantage of these approaches at the time of consultation, but they should be informed of the options for themselves and for other family members. Frequently, potential carriers of a faulty gene wish to know the status of research or treatment, since this information may influence their decision to carry a pregnancy to term or even to risk becoming pregnant. The possibility of carrier detection should be raised, whether or not it is presently available, since with the rapid progress in molecular genetics it may become available within the foreseeable future.

Every counseling situation is unique. Each family has a unique set of personal values, cultural experience, and emotional circumstances that surround their need for information. Each disease carries a unique set of complications, diagnostic possibilities, and natural history. In addition, the health professional dealing with a genetic problem cannot always be neutral; each brings subjective values to the counseling session.

In genetic counseling it is essential to determine what the family's questions actually are, since the health provider may think they need to know one thing, when they really wish to know something quite different. It is appropriate to start any discussion by asking the family to list the questions they wish to raise. They should be reassured that no matter how irrelevant the question may seem, if it is important to them, it needs to be answered.

A number of organizations such as the National Marfan Foundation, the Little People of America, and the Osteogenesis Imperfecta Association produce excellent information booklets for affected individuals and their families. It is often helpful to put families in touch with these organizations, since talking to another person with the condition frequently has a stronger impact than talking with a physician. In addition, these organizations are able to offer a variety of practical suggestions that can be helpful to a family coping with the everyday challenges of living with a particular disorder.

Therapy

Although admittedly the "short suit" of medical genetics, treatment is rapidly becoming effective in the broad group of hereditary disorders. Modalities of therapy now include restriction of particular dietary constituents (e.g., a low-methionine diet in the treatment of homcystinuria), administration of cofactor in pharmacologic dosage (e.g., high doses of vitamin B_6, again in the treatment of homocystinuria), surgical replacement of the defective organ or tissue (e.g., the aorta in the treatment of Marfan syndrome), attenuation of physiologic stress on the genetically defective tissue (e.g., use of beta-adrenergic blockade in the treatment of Marfan syndrome). Bone marrow transplantations make it possible to introduce normal copies of genes when circulating levels of gene product could correct a metabolic defect, as with the mucopolysaccharidoses. Enzyme replacement and liver transplantation have entered the realm of reality in the treatment of Gaucher disease. Gene therapy experiments have successfully delivered cloned normal genes to tissues when their expression can correct an endogenous genetic defect. For example, a normal copy of the cystic fibrosis gene has been inserted into lung cells *in vivo* by use of adenovirus vectors.[1] As techniques for delivering corrective genes are further developed and improved, more and more disorders should become amenable to this type of therapy.[15]

SUMMARY

During the 20 years since the fourth edition of this book was published, molecular genetics has undergone explosive development. Current knowledge has progressed from a basic understanding of what a gene is and how it functions to an ability to identify, isolate, and clone the gene for almost any disorder, given enough time and resources. Many of the extremely intricate and complex mechanisms by which gene expression is regulated have been unraveled—for instance, how oncogenes are activated during development and in many cancers and how they are kept quiescent in normal adult cells; how certain cells are able to express high levels of tissue-specific genes for proteins not found in other tissues; and how the overproduction or underproduction of certain gene products can lead to specific disorders. Recombinant DNA technology has been harnessed to produce large quantities of therapeutic proteins in bacteria using human genes (for instance, insulin and human growth factor); plants and livestock have been "genetically engineered" for greater yields of food and energy products; and genes have been inserted into human cells for the purpose of direct gene therapy. It is only a matter of time before the entire human genome is mapped; this will allow all these endeavours to proceed even more quickly and efficiently and will render many genetic diseases more accessible to elucidation and treatment.

Despite these dramatic advances, most of the genetic principles established in an earlier era are still valid and are essential for the understanding and management of genetic disease.

Among the important concepts presented and discussed in this chapter are the following:

1. *Congenital* is not synonymous with *genetic*. Broadly speaking, genetic disorders fall into the following categories: single gene disorders, chromosomal aberrations, and multifactorial disorders.
2. Genes are situated on the chromosomes, which are comprised of DNA; a gene is transcribed to mRNA; the mRNA is then translated into a specific protein. At each of these steps there are many levels of control and modulation of expression. One gene codes for one protein.
3. Single gene disorders are either recessive (i.e., a normal copy of the gene prevents expression of the disease phenotype) or dominant (i.e., one abnormal copy of the gene results in the disease phenotype).
4. Gene mapping via the use of family pedigrees and restriction fragment length polymorphisms is still highly useful in localizing

and isolating the gene for a specific disorder. Genetic disorders, in particular, severe ones that interfere with reproduction, may be the result of new, as opposed to inherited, mutations.

5. A single gene can have multiple and apparently unrelated effects on different tissues; this process is termed *pleiotropism*.

6. Phenotypic diversity within a single heritable disorder can be caused by (1) environmental factors, (2) allelic series (an individual who has two alleles of a single gene with two different mutations), (3) genetic compounds (two different allelic mutations in the same gene), or (4) mutations in different domain-coding regions of the same gene.

7. Similar phenotypes can be caused by the action of any one of several genes. This situation is termed *heterogeneity* of disease.

8. Nontraditional genetic mechanisms include cytoplasmic (mitochondrial) inheritance, mosaicism, imprinting, and uniparental disomy. These mechanisms may prove to be increasingly important causal factors in disorders in which transmission does not follow classical mendelian patterns of inheritance.

REFERENCES

1. Anonymous: Cystic fibrosis: toward the ultimate therapy, slowly (editorial comment), *Lancet* 336:1224-1225, 1990.
2. Barr ML, Bertram EG: A morphological distinction between neurones of the male and female, and the behaviour of the nucleolar satellite during accelerated nucleoprotein synthesis, *Nature* 163:676-677, 1949.
3. Chase LR, Melson GL, Aurbach GD: Pseudohypoparathyroidism: defective excretion of 3'05'AMP in response to parathyroid hormone, *J Clin Invest* 48:1832-1844, 1969.
4. Daughady WH et al: Defective sulfation factor generation: a possible etiological link in dwarfism, *Trans Assoc Am Physicians* 82:129-140, 1969.
5. Davies K: The essence of inactivity, *Nature* 349:15-16, 1991.
6. Eichenlaub-Ritter U, Winking H: Nondisjunction, disturbances in spindle structure, and characteristics of chromosome alignment in maturing oocytes of mice heterozygous for Robertsonian translocations, *Cytogenet Cell Genet* 54:47-54, 1990.
7. Ezzell C: New clues to origins of Down's syndrome, *Science News* 139:292-294, 1991.
8. Gibson JB, Carson NAJ, Neill DW: Pathologic findings in homocystinuria, *J Clin Pathol* 17:427-437, 1964.
9. Gowers WR: Abiotrophy, *Lancet* 1:1003-1007, 1902.
10. Hall JG: How imprinting is relevant to human disease. In Monk M, Suranie A, editors: *Genomic imprinting*, Cambridge, 1990, The Company of Biologists, pp 141-148.
11. Hall JG: Genomic imprinting: review and relevance to human disease, *Am J Hum Genet* 46:857-873, 1990.
12. Happle R: Lethal genes surviving by mosaicism: a possible explanation for sporadic birth defects involving the skin, *J Am Acad Dermatol* 16:899-906, 1987.
13. Hunter C: A rare disease in two brothers: elevation of the scapula, limitation of movements of joints and other abnormalities, *Proc Roy Soc Med* 10:104-106, 1917.
14. Hurler G: Ueber einen Type multipler Abartungen, virwiegend am Skelettsystem, *Z Kinderheilk* 24:220-234, 1919.
15. Kelley WN: Gene therapy in humans: a new era begins (editorial), *Ann Intern Med* 114:697-698, 1991.
16. Lyon M: Chromosomal and subchromosomal inactivation, *Ann Rev Genet* 2:31-52, 1968.
17. Mange AP, Mange EJ: *Genetics: human aspects*, Sunderland, Mass, 1990, Sinauer Associates, pp 286-289.
18. Maniatis T, Fritsch EF, Sambrook J: *Molecular cloning: a laboratory manual*, New York, 1988, Cold Spring Harbour Laboratory Press.
19. Maroteaux P et al: Une nouvelle dysostose avec élimination urinaire de chondroitine-sulfate B, *Presse Méd* 71:1849-1852, 1963.
20. McKusick VA: The defect in Marfan syndrome, *Nature* 353:279-281, 1991.
21. Morton NE: The detection and estimation of linkage between the genes for elliptocytosis and the Rh blood type, *Am J Hum Genet* 8:80-96, 1956.
22. Nora JJ, Faser FC: *Medical genetics: principles and practice*, Philadelphia, 1989, Lea & Febiger, pp 70-71.
23. Seegmiller JE, Rosenbloom FM, Kelley WN: Enzymatic defect associated with a sex-linked human neurological disorder and excessive purine synthesis, *Science* 155:1682-1684, 1967.
24. Silverman LJ, Kelley LJ, Palella TD: Genetic analysis of human HGPRT deficiency, *Enzyme* 38:36-44, 1987.
25. Smith LH Jr, Huguley CM Jr, Bain JA: Hereditary orotic aciduria. In Stanbury JB, Wyngaarden JB, Fredricksen DS, editors: *The metabolic basis of inherited disease*, ed 2, New York, 1966, McGraw-Hill.
26. Southern EM: Detection of specific sequences among DNA fragments separated by gel electrophoresis, *J Mol Biol* 98:503-517, 1974.
27. Stern C: *Principles of human genetics*, San Francisco, 1949, WH Freeman.
28. Thompson JS, Thompson MW: *Genetics in medicine*, Philadelphia, 1991, WB Saunders, pp 118, 203, 216-217.
29. Vogel F, Motulsky AG: *Human genetics*, Berlin, 1986, Springer-Verlag, pp 344, 404.

CHAPTER 2

The Biology of Normal Connective Tissue

Peter H. Byers

Since the fourth edition of this book was published, 20 years ago, the advances in isolating proteins of the extracellular matrix, characterizing the sequences defining their interactions in the extracellular matrix, characterizing the genes and determining their chromosomal position, and elucidating the mechanisms of gene expression have provided a complex picture of how tissues differ and the molecular basis of these differences. In this chapter the molecular components are identified and their interactions, which are an important aspect of how the proteins produce the properties of tissues, are discussed.

Four major classes of proteins within the extracellular matrix are collagens, elastin, proteoglycans, and glycoproteins. Strictly speaking, collagens and proteoglycans are also glycoproteins, although of a highly specialized nature; since their properties are quite distinct, referring to them as separate classes is worthwhile.

COLLAGENS

The multigene collagen family has more than 25 members dispersed to more than 12 chromosomes. The proteins encoded by these genes share the following features: they form trimers that contain a triple-helical domain characterized by the repeating amino acid motif *glycine (Gly)-X-Y$_n$;* they have hydroxyproline and hydroxylysine that arise from posttranslation modification of prolyl and lysyl residues, respectively; and they reside in the extracellular matrix. (See Bornstein and Sage,[17] Bornstein and Traub,[18] and Mayne and Burge-

son[97] for detailed reviews of collagen protein structure and Vuorio and deCrombrugghe[152] for detailed review of collagen genes and gene structure.) Other proteins, including acetylcholinesterase,[98] the C1q component of the complement cascade,[125] a pulmonary surfactant protein,[13] the mannose binding protein,[36] and the macrophage surface scavenger protein,[77] contain short stretches of triple helix, probably as a structural motif. With the rise of recombinant DNA technology the genes that encode most of the human collagens that have been identified at the protein level have been isolated and partially characterized. Increasingly, new genes are identified before the proteins have been isolated and before analysis of tissue distribution, protein structure, or protein function.

As a family the collagens are the most abundant protein in the body. Most of the collagen in the body is type I collagen; collagen is the major protein in bone, skin, tendon, ligament, sclera, cornea, blood vessels, and many hollow organs. Most collagens have a tissue-limited distribution. For example, collagen types II, IX, X, and XI, are found in hyaline cartilage and the vitreous of the eye,[43,100,135,149] type IV collagen is limited to basement membranes,[54,76] and type VII collagen forms anchoring fibrils at certain epithelial-mesenchymal junctions.[21] Most collagens are synthesized only by certain differentiated cell types, but a single cell type may synthesize several collagens. Chondrocytes, for example, synthesize collagen types II, IX, X, and XI but not collagen type I or III. The mechanisms by which cell type–specific control is exerted have received considerable study, but understanding of how this control is achieved remains limited.

Collagens provide tensile strength, facilitate transparency, provide form during embryonic and fetal development, cooperate with other proteins to build tissues and organs, separate cell layers, and provide filtration barriers between spaces. Type I collagen, for example, polymerizes into fibrils that provide tensile strength in bone, skin, and tendon and are mineralized in bone to increase tissue weight-bearing properties. In addition, type I collagen fibrils are organized in the cornea to induce transparency but also contribute to the opacity of the adjacent sclera. Type IV collagens are the principal structural protein of basement membranes, where they form the interface between mesenchyma and epithelia and act as filtration barriers in multiple tissues, including the kidney. Collagen types II, IX, X, and XI form a matrix in cartilage, which, along with proteoglycans and other glycoproteins, provides a highly hydrated cushioning tissue in regions of weight-bearing stress. As in cartilage, some of the functions attributed to collagen are the direct result of protein structure; often, however, it is the interactions of collagens with other components of the extracellular matrix that determine the features of a tissue and its mechanical properties.

Gene and Protein Structure

On the basis of structure the following classes of collagen genes are apparent:

1. Fibrillar collagens (COL1A1, COL1A2, COL2A1, COL3A1, COL5A1, COL5A2, COL5A3, COL11A1, and COL11A2)
2. Basement membrane collagens (COL4A1, COL4A2, COL4A3, COL4A4, and COL4A5)
3. Fibril-associated collagens with interrupted triple helices (FACIT) (COL9A1, COL9A2, COL9A3, and COL12A1)
4. Network collagens (COL8A1, COL8A2, and COL10A1)
5. Collagens of microfibrils (COL6A1, COL6A2, and COL6A3)
6. Long-chain collagen of anchoring fibrils with an interrupted triple helix (COL7A1)

Fibrillar collagen genes (types I, II, III, V, and XI). Each fibrillar collagen gene encodes an unbroken triple-helical domain that contains slightly

more than 1000 amino acids characterized by the repeating triplet motif of Gly-X-Y, for which they employ a set of 42 exons that contain 45, 54, 99, 108, or 162 base pairs.* Junction exons at each end of the triple-helical domains encode sequences that contain proteolytic cleavage sites. The remainder of each gene is devoted to the sequence of the propeptides, the control elements (largely at the 5' ends), and transcribed but untranslated sequence (largely at the 3' ends). Each gene consists of 51 or 52 exons arrayed over a distance of 20 to 40 kb. The exons in the triple-helical domain begin with a complete glycine codon, but those in non–triple-helical regions may begin with interrupted codons. Differences in gene size reflect the differences in intron length. The similar gene structure and homologies in amino acid sequence provide strong evidence for the divergence of collagen types in the evolutionary setting of gene structure. The genes are distributed to several different chromosomes as follows:

COL1A1 on 17[69,143]
COL1A2 on 7[69,141]
COL2A1 on 12[142]
COL3A1 on 2[40,70]
COL2A1 on 9[58]
COL5A2 on 2 (in the same domain as COL3A1)[40]

Two human type XI collagen genes have been isolated and assigned to chromosomes 1 (COL11A1) and 6 (COL11A2).[60,66,79,89]

Type I procollagen, a heterotrimer that contains two pro alpha 1(I) chains (encoded by COL1A1) and one pro alpha 2(I) chain (encoded by COL1A2), forms a model for the fibrillar collagens. Type I procollagen contains seven distinct domains, each of which has one or more functions. Each pro alpha chain is synthesized with a signal sequence of approximately 20 residues that facilitates passage across the rough endoplasmic reticulum membrane and is cleaved during transit.[112] The pro alpha 1(I) chain contains a cysteine-rich globular extension of 86 residues whose function is unknown; a similar sequence is missing from the pro alpha 2(I) chain. Both chains contain a 36-residue domain (of repeating Gly-X-Y triplets) that forms a triple helix in the intact procollagen molecule. This short triple helix has a relatively high denaturation temperature and may stabilize the amino-terminal end of the molecule. A short,

---

*References 7, 22-24, 34, 104, and 134.

non–triple-helical domain contains the site of proteolytic cleavage of the amino-terminal propeptide extension and lysyl residues that become involved in intermolecular cross-link formation. The major triple-helical domain of both chains is 1014 residues in length and is characterized by glycine in every third position (Gly-X-Y$_{338}$); hydroxyproline occupies the Y position in about a third of the triplets and is often preceded by proline. Some lysyl residues in the Y position are also hydroxylated, but the extent of this modification is highly collagen-type–dependent. A 28-residue telopeptide at the carboxyl-terminal end of the triple helix contains both a lysyl residue in pro alpha 1(I), which is absent from pro alpha 2(I) and involved in interchain cross-link formation, and the sequence at which the carboxy-terminal procollagen peptidase cleaves. The final 220 residues of the pro alpha chains form globular structures that contain intrachain and interchain disulfide bonds. The domain of the globular structures facilitates chain assembly, determines the chain specificity of the type I procollagen molecule, and provides intracellular solubility.

Basement membrane collagen genes (type IV). The genes that encode the basement membrane non-fibrillar collagens are similar in size to those that encode fibrillar collagens but differ somewhat in organization.[86,133] The exons that encode the largely triple-helical domains vary widely in size, do not always begin with a glycine codon or end with a codon for a Y-position amino acid, frequently split codons, and encode interruptions of the triple helix. The interruptions of triple-helical sequence, when compared with the sequence in the fibrillar collagen genes, could be explained by small deletions, single nucleotide substitutions, and mutations at former splice junctions. Five genes that encode basement membranes have been isolated and appear to encode similar messenger ribonucleic acids (mRNAs), have similar gene structures, and have a remarkable organization. Two genes, COL4A1 and COL4A2, are located in a head-to-head array on the distal long arm of chromosome 13 and share promoter sequences during transcription from opposite DNA strands. Two other genes, COL4A3 and COL4A4, are closely linked, whereas the fifth member of the group is located on the X chromosome.[20,32,140] Given the structural relationship between basement membrane genes and the fibrillar collagen genes, it seems likely that they share an ancestral gene and that both diverged before duplication of the two arms.

Fibril-associated collagens with interrupted triple helices (types IX, XII, and XIV). Distinct from both the fibrillar and the basement membrane genes are those genes which code for collagenous proteins that appear to become associated with fibrillar genes. Of these proteins the first to be recognized was type IX collagen, now known to comprise three genes, each of which encodes chains that contain three triple-helical domains with interruptions. Each chain consists of about 900 amino acids divided into seven distinct domains: three domains that contain triple-helical Gly-X-Y repeat motifs (COL1, COL2, and COL3 domains that contain 115, 339, and 137 amino acids, respectively) and four non-collagenous domains (NC1, NC2, NC3, and NC4 domains that contain approximately 20, 30, 12, and 243 amino acids, respectively). The NC1 domain is the most carboxyl-terminal region of each chain, the NC2 domain separates COL1 and COL2, and the NC3 domain separates COL2 and COL3. The COL3 domain contains one imperfection and the COL1 domain contains two. Type IX collagen genes are expressed in concert with those of type II collagen, and the proteins are found together in cartilage and the vitreous humor of the eye. The alpha 2(IX) chain contains an attachment site for a glycosaminoglycan side chain that may facilitate interactions between collagens and proteoglycans in cartilage matrix.[150]

Two additional members of the FACIT gene family are COL12A1 and COL14A1. The type XII collagen gene draws attention to the complexity of some of the collagen-related genes in that the collagenous domains are quite small in relation to the content of other domains shared by matrix proteins. This introduces the complexity of relationships that exist between collagens and other matrix proteins.[37,56,57,158] Type XII collagen is a homotrimer of alpha 1(XII) chains and is ubiquitously distributed, paralleling the distribution of the fibrillar collagens. This ubiquitous distribution has suggested that type XII collagen may act in a manner similar to that of type IX collagens in interacting with type II collagen in cartilage in which covalent cross-links that contain sequences from both types of collagen confirm their proximity. The difference between the mass of the amino-terminal end of type XII collagen and that of type IX must raise some question about the precise correspondence of the two classes of molecules.

Filament-producing collagen (type VI). The genes for human collagens type VI[25] have been isolated and their chromosomal location determined.[53,153] The COL6A1 and COL6A2 genes reside on the long arm of chromosome 21, whereas the COL6A3 gene is located on chromosome 6. These genes encode three polypeptide chains that together have a triple helix of 335 or 336 amino acids; two imperfections are embedded within noncollagenous sequences. The COL6A1 and COL6A2 proteins encode an NC2 (amino-terminal) peptide of about 235 residues and an NC1 (carboxyl-terminal) peptide of about 430 residues. The COL3A1 gene encodes a protein with a homologous collagenous domain but with a large (1800 amino acids) NC2 (amino-terminal) domain and a NC1 domain that is twice the size of the peptides in the other two type VI collagens. The NC1 domain of the alpha 3(VI) chain contains more than six repeats of a von Willebrand-factor domain, whereas the carboxyl-terminal non-collagenous domain contains repeats of other types. Type VI collagen is assembled as a trimer of all three chains, although there are some suggestions that other forms may exist. The monomers form partial-overlap head-to-tail structures that interact with other similar structures to produce tetramers, which are the base units for forming beaded microfilaments in the matrix. These in turn form microfibrillar arrays in extracellular matrix of virtually all tissues and in cultured cells in vitro. The microfibrillar network formed by type VI collagen is probably distinct from the network that contains fibrillin.[78] The function of these microfibrillar structures is unknown.

Network-forming collagens (types VIII and X). Types VIII and X collagens have similar gene structures and appear to encode proteins that form meshworks similar, perhaps, to the meshwork produced by type IV collagens in basement membranes. The structure of these genes is, however, markedly at variance with those of the type COL4 family of genes. Type VIII collagen originally was isolated from endothelial cells but more

recently has been recognized to be an abundant component of Descemet's membrane that separates corneal epithelium and corneal stroma. Two genes of type VIII collagen have been partially characterized and localized to chromosome 3 (COL8A1) and chromosome 1 (COL8A2). Type X collagen is a component of hypertrophic cartilage; although a role for endochondral bone formation has been postulated, its function remains uncertain.[87,144] Only a single gene that encodes type X collagen chains has yet been isolated.[2,145] The three previously mentioned genes have a remarkably compact structure and encode chains that are quite similar. The two COL8 genes encode chains that have a core triple-helical domain of 454 (COL8A1) and 457 (COL8A2) residues bounded by an NC1 domain (carboxyl-terminal) of 173 and 167 residues and a slightly smaller NC2 (amino-terminal) domain. The gene contains three exons: the triple-helical and NC1 domains are encoded by a single exon, and the NC2 domain is divided between the remaining two exons. The structure of the COL10A1 gene is similar, differing only in the size of the respective domains.[107] The type X collagen protein appears to exist as a homotrimer, and it is likely that the type VIII protein is a heterotrimer of the two gene products, of which the precise proportions are uncertain.

Anchoring fibril collagen (type VII). Type VII collagen is confined to anchoring fibrils at the dermal-epidermal junction and at other basement membranes that separate epithelial and mesenchymal structures. It has been partially characterized and shown to be large, with a single-chain, precursor-sized, collagen-like domain of approximately 170 kd. Partial gene sequencing has indicated that type VII collagen is a composite protein with both triple-helical and multiple domains similar to those of other matrix proteins. The gene locus is on the long arm of chromosome 3.[113,131]

Structure and Function of the Collagen Triple Helix

The triple-helical structure of collagens has a primary sequence in which each of the alpha chains has a repeating $Gly-X-Y_n$ molecular formula: X and Y can be most amino acids other than glycine but often are proline (Pro) and hydroxyproline (Hyp), respectively (Fig. 2-1). The length of the uninterrupted repeating tripeptide

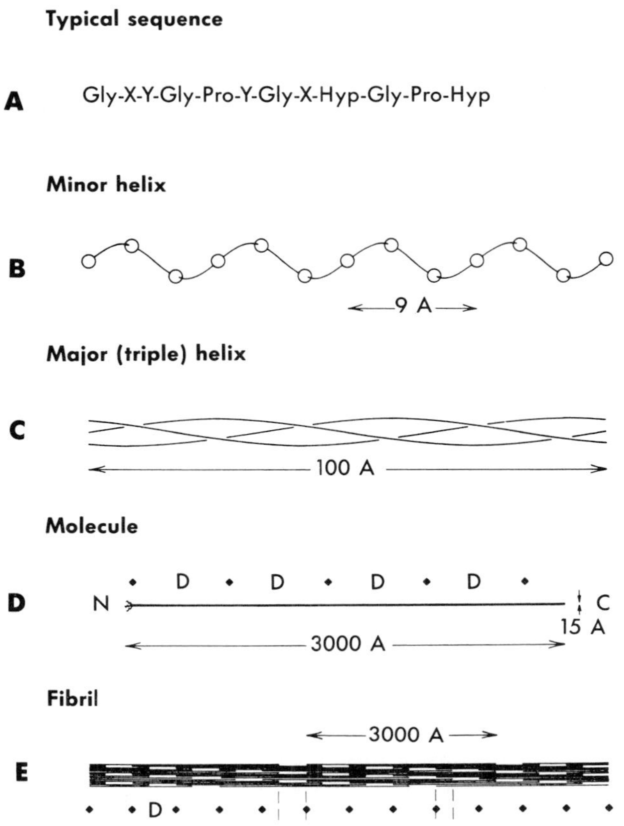

Typical sequence

A   Gly-X-Y-Gly-Pro-Y-Gly-X-Hyp-Gly-Pro-Hyp

Minor helix

B

←9 A→

Major (triple) helix

C

←————— 100 A —————→

Molecule

D   N → • D • D • D • D •   C
←——— 3000 A ———→   15 A

Fibril

←—— 3000 A —→

E
• • D • • | • • • |• • • •

Fig. 2-1. Structure of collagen. **A,** Glycine *(Gly)* occurs in every third position throughout most of the polypeptide chains. Proline *(Pro)* and hydroxyproline *(Hyp)* are abundant. *X* and *Y* represent any amino acid. **B,** Each polypeptide chain has a polyproline helical conformation. **C,** The three polypeptide chains of each collagen molecule are further coiled about one another. **D,** The NH$_2$ ends of the three chains are together at one end of the molecule. The distribution of amino acids is unique throughout the length of the molecule, but there is a pseudorepeat, *D,* with a periodicity of about 680 angstroms. **E,** Collagen fibrils are formed by association of molecules in such a way that regions of length, *D,* are in register. Length, *D,* corresponds to the repeats seen in electron micrographs. Each molecule extends 4.4 D, and a space, or "hole," of 0.6 D is left between molecules in line. *A,* Angstrom; *C,* carboxyl terminal; *D,* domain; *N,* amino terminal. (Courtesy Karl A. Piez, Bethesda, Md.)

unit varies among collagens. In the fibril-forming collagens the length ranges from 338 to 341 triplets; in the other molecules the length is substantially shorter. Glycine, which has no side chain, is required in every third position to allow a helical structure to occur. The side chains on any substi-

tuting residue disrupt the triple helix and, at least for fibrillar collagens, this disruption has highly deleterious consequences (see Chapters 6, 8, and 14). A triple helix has a relatively high thermal stability and is resistant to digestion by the majority of proteases in the extracellular matrix.[61,156] The stability of the triple helix is provided by interchain hydrogen bonds between the amide group of glycine and the oxygen of the carbonyl group of an X-position residue on an adjacent chain.[122] Additional hydrogen bonds that involve the hydroxyl group of hydroxyproline and the carbonyl backbone of the chain further stabilize the molecule. Thus in the absence of hydroxylation the triple helix of type I collagen denatures at about 27° C,[11,128] but with complete hydroxylation the denaturation temperature is about 42° C. It is likely that other factors, especially charge-to-charge interactions, contribute to the stability of the triple helix; although these factors have been recognized for some time, their importance is often overlooked. Once denatured, the exquisite sensitivity of the chains to most proteases ensures normal turnover. Triple-helical structure is required for transport of fibrillar collagens beyond the rough endoplasmic reticulum.[63,74]

Biosynthesis of Collagen

The biosynthesis of collagens is complex because of the need for coordinated transcription of genes that encode chains constituting a single protein and because of the multiple steps involved in posttranslational modifications.[46]

The mechanisms for the control of collagen gene expression probably differ for each set of genes that contribute to the distinct collagen types. The genes of type I collagen (COL1A1 and COL1A2), for example, are located on different chromosomes but in cells that synthesize both chains to assemble the type I procollagen molecules, the mRNA steady-state levels reflect the relative proportions of the two chains synthesized, although gene copy number is the same. Thus in most cells the pro alpha 1(I) mRNA and the pro alpha 2(I) mRNA are present in approximately a 2:1 ratio, although in certain cells virtually no pro alpha 2(I) mRNA is present.[33] Despite intense efforts, there is little understanding of the mechanisms by which the expression of the two genes is coordinated. In contrast, some of the other genes, notably the COL4A1 and COL4A2 genes that encode two of the basement membrane nonfibrillar collagens, share a bi-directional promotor and the relative synthesis of the two depends on binding of regulatory factors to the different strands of deoxyribonucleic acid (DNA).

Tissue-specific control of expression of type I collagen genes resides in a domain encompassing a 3.5-kb region upstream of the transcription start site, as well as in the first intron of the COL1A1 and COL1A2 genes.[19,65,91,93,130] Both upstream regions and regions in the first intron may provide negative control.[16,136] The expression of fibrillar collagen genes can be altered by a variety of growth factors[121,127] and by ascorbic acid.[103] In the COL2A1 gene, alternative splicing of a second exon provides different products during development. Similarly, alternative splicing and different transcription start sites help determine the protein product and the tissue expression of the COL6A3 and the COL9A1 genes. Translational efficiency of fibrillar collagen genes may be determined in part by stem-to-loop structures in the 5'-untranslated region of the mRNA derived from those genes.[137,157]

A feedback control of synthesis of type I procollagen has been postulated to result from peptides derived from the amino-terminal extension of the pro alpha 1(I) chains of type I procollagen[67,111] and from sequences derived from the carboxyl-terminal propeptide.[4] Although gene expression and translational effects provide the first level of control of collagen synthesis, the heteropolymeric nature of some collagens provides an additional level of control. In molecules like type I procollagen, stable molecules contain two or more pro alpha 1(I) chains. Thus, regardless of the amount of pro alpha 2(I) synthesized, the amount of type I procollagen secreted reflects the amount of pro alpha 1(I) available for trimer formation. A final editorial checkpoint in collagen production occurs in the rough endoplasmic reticulum and, perhaps, in the Golgi apparatus, where structure is assessed and more than 10% of the basal production of collagen is shunted to a pathway of intracellular degradation.[12,14] Thus the control of collagen production can be regulated at many levels: some function in an "on-off" fashion and others provide a continuous range of variation.

Collagen precursor mRNAs are transcribed in the nucleus, spliced to remove intervening sequences,[3] capped, polyadenylated, and trans-ported to the cytoplasm. The mRNAs are translated on ribosomes that become membrane bound. The signal sequences that direct the binding of the ribosomes to membranes and then the vectorial insertion of the chains through the rough endoplasmic reticulum membrane are cleaved during elongation of the pro alpha chains. Initiated during translation and lagging about 300 residues behind amino acid incorporation into chains, prolyl and lysyl residues amino-terminal to glycyl residues in the major and minor triple-helical sequences are hydroxylated by the enzymes prolyl 4-hydroxylase and lysyl hydroxylase, respectively.[81,120] The enzymes recognize only chains that are not in a stable triple-helical conformation.[82] Prolyl 4-hydroxylase, a tetramer of two alpha subunits and two beta subunits,[10,108] is an endoplasmic reticular–resident protein by virtue of sequence at the carboxyl-terminal end of the beta subunit, which is the same protein as protein disulfide isomerase.[30,118] Lysyl hydroxylase is a homodimer, the monomer of which has a molecular weight of 85,000.[148] Although the extent of posttranslational modification of prolyl and lysyl residues in various collagen types differs substantially, no available evidence argues convincingly for the activity of type-specific modifying enzymes.

The collagen hydroxylases require Fe^{2+}, 2-oxoglutarate, molecular oxygen (O_2), and ascorbate. The 2-oxoglutarate is decarboxylated and oxidized to succinate[123]; the other member of the oxygen molecule is incorporated into the prolyl or the lysyl residue, depending on the enzyme involved. The ascorbate can be replaced by other reducing agents[115] and may keep the Fe^{2+} atom reduced.

The hydroxylation of proline in the 4 position is essential to provide thermal stability to the triple helix. Hydroxylation of lysyl residues provides substrates for glycosylation; the hydroxylysyl residues form more stable covalent cross-links than do lysyl residues and are important determinants of tissue tensile strength.[42]

Once synthesis of each chain of fibrillar collagen is completed, the globular domains of the pro alpha chains fold and are stabilized by intrachain disulfide bonds,[35] interchain association occurs through domains created by the correct folding of the carboxyl-terminal propeptide sequences,[83] and the trimer is stabilized by the formation of interchain disulfide bonds. The determinants of interaction of molecules other than fibrillar and basement membrane collagens are not known. In fibrillar collagens and type IV collagens, triple-helical formation begins at the carboxyl-terminal end of the molecule and propagates toward the amino-terminal end.[6] Peptidyl proly cis-trans isomerase facilitates correct folding.[5]

The glycosylation of hydroxylysyl residues in collagen requires two enzymes, hydroxylysyl galactosyltransferase and galactosylhydroxylysyl glucosyltransferase.[80] The former transfers uridine diphosphate galactose to the oxygen on the 5' carbon of hydroxylysine in peptide linkage; Mn^{2+} is probably a cofactor for the enzyme. The latter transfers uridine diphosphate glucose, also in the presence of the metal cofactor. The distribution of monosaccharide and disaccharide is influenced by collagen type, probably by the amino acid sequence in the region of the hydroxylysyl residue. The reaction is carried out only on a non–triple-helical substrate. The functions of the carbohydrate on collagens are unknown. Carbohydrate modification may influence fibril formation, may affect collagen-cell interaction and collagen interactions with other macromolecules, and may protect modified hydroxylysyl residues from oxidation to cross-link precursors. The modification of asparagine residues by heterosaccharide occurs in several collagens, parallel to modification of other glycoproteins[1,26,59] in which carbohydrate units are synthesized on a dolichol lipid intermediate in the membrane of the rough endoplasmic reticulum and transferred intact to the pro alpha chains.[38,68,84]

Some collagens, including types V and III, undergo sulfation of some tyrosine residues in the amino-terminal propeptide extension[47,48] and phosphorylation of certain serine residues of the extension of pro alpha 1(I) in bone.[51] The function of these modifications is not known.

Procollagen molecules are translocated to the Golgi apparatus and then packaged in secretory vesicles, which fuse with the cell membrane and release their contents into the extracellular environment.

In the extracellular space some procollagens undergo proteolytic conversion by removal of one or both terminal extensions. These reactions are best understood for the fibrillar collagens, particularly for type I collagen. In those molecules the precursor-specific peptides are removed by two enzymes, procollagen N-proteinase and procollagen C-proteinase.[88,102,146,147] A preferred order for cleavage of the terminii does not appear to exist, and intermediates that contain either end intact can be found in tissues and in cultured cells.

Once cleaved, fibrillar collagen molecules rapidly aggregate into ordered structures that contain more than a single type of collagen. Indeed, the reaction of different collagens appears to be important for the regulation of fibril diameter. In cartilage, interaction of types IX and II collagens in the same fibrils provides mechanisms for integrating the complex network of extracellular matrix molecules through the proteoglycan side chain. Similar interactions involving types XII and I collagens and other macromolecules in soft tissues may also facilitate tissue organization. In fibril-forming molecules, interaction of molecules reflects the distribution of charged and hydrophobic groups at the surface of the cell membrane.[117] Collagen molecules aggregate in an ordered parallel configuration and overlap with adjacent molecules staggered by slightly less than a quarter of the length of a molecule (Fig. 2-1). Fibril formation is a nonenzymatic process, but stabilization of the fibril network depends on the formation of lysyl- and hydroxylysyl-derived cross-links. In other tissues such as basement membrane and, perhaps, in tissues containing meshworks of types VIII and X collagens the nature of the interactions of the molecules is more complex and does not depend on the triple-helical domains.

Collagen molecules in fibrillar array are substrates for the enzyme lysyl oxidase that deaminates by oxidation certain lysyl and hydroxylysyl residues in collagen and elastin.[75,139] Lysyl oxidase activity results in formation of a reactive aldehyde that condenses with lysyl or hydroxylysyl residues in adjacent molecules to form divalent cross-links.[42] Divalent cross-links are the first product but rapidly become transformed to more complex cross-links that contain histidine or additional lysyl and hydroxylysyl residues to form three-membered cross-link amino acids. Lysyl oxidase requires pyridoxyl and copper as cofactors, the latter, probably, for stability.[62,155] Cross-linking is vital for tissue tensile strength.

Collagen Degradation

Fibrillar collagens are stable molecules that have residence times of months or years in adult tissues.[101] Connective tissues are constantly being remodeled in response to mechanical stress, growth, and injury. The turnover of these macro-molecules is regulated in part by collagenases that recognize sequences in the triple helix and cleave intact molecules that are in fibrillar array.[49,61,64] Some collagenases specifically degrade most fibrillar molecules, and others are known to digest type IV collagens in basement membrane.[92] In part these proteases facilitate further degradation because, after a single cleavage, the products have

melting temperatures several degrees below that of the intact molecule[28] and become substrates for other, less specific proteases.

PROTEOGLYCAN STRUCTURE, BIOSYNTHESIS, AND FUNCTION

Proteoglycans are macromolecules that have a core protein to which is bound covalently one or more (often many) glycosaminoglycan chains; pro-teoglycans frequently contain asparagine-linked oligosaccharide and O-linked glycosides. The com-

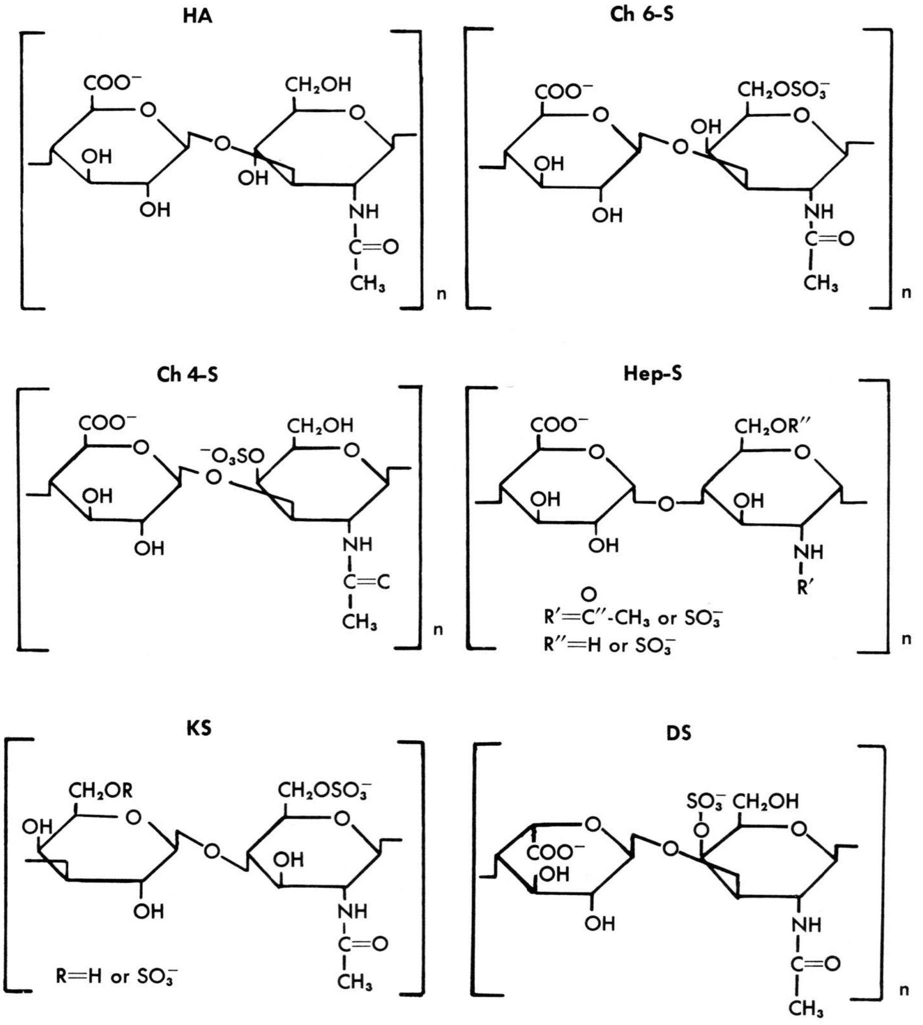

Fig. 2-2. Structure of the repeating subunits of six mucopolysaccharides. *HA*, Hy-aluronic acid; *Ch 6-S*, chondroitin-6-sulfate (formerly, chondroitin sulfate C); *Ch 4-S*, chrondroitin-4-sulfate (formerly, chondroitin sulfate A); *Hep-S*, heparan sulfate (for-merly, heparitin sulfate); *KS*, keratan sulfate (formerly, keratosulfate); *DS*, derma-tan sulfate (formerly, chrondroitin sulfate B). (From Meyer K: *Am J Med* 47:664, 1969.)

plex glycosaminoglycan chains are characterized by a repeating disaccharide unit in which one moiety is a hexosamine and the other is a uronic acid[154] (Fig. 2-2). Substantial differences in the size of the core proteins, in the tissue expression of these genes, and in the sequence of the proteins outside the glycosaminoglycan attachment domains reflect and determine the function of proteoglycans. Indeed, their functions appear complex. In cartilage, for example, aggrecan, hyaluronic acid, and link protein together provide a large proportion of the structural elements to the tissue. Other proteoglycans such as decorin are elements of soft connective tissues, are bound to collagen fibrils, and may play a role in limitation of fibril growth. As was pointed out previously, the alpha 2(IX) chain of type IX collagen contains a single glycosaminoglycan, so the distinction among proteins of different major classes can be blurred. As with collagens, the functions of individual proteoglycans probably differ substantially, reflecting their tissue distribution and structure.

The proteoglycans can be classified according to the following criteria: (1) size of the core protein (which is large and resembles aggrecan of cartilage, the fibroblast large-core protein, and the basement membrane heparan sulfate large-core protein, or small, similar to decorin, biglycan, and others), (2) whether they are cell associated by virtue of transmembrane domains (eg., syndecan or fibroblast membrane heparan sulfate proteoglycan) or free in the matrix, (3) the genetic relationship of the genes, and (4) the nature of the attached glycosaminoglycan chains.

Structure of Protein Cores

The initial studies performed on proteoglycans concentrated on the sugar structure of the glycosaminoglycans. Almost 3 decades ago, it began to become clear that these entities are synthesized on protein cores, and the interest shifted to understanding the nature of those proteins and to the characterization of protein structure, gene isolation, and determination of how expression of those genes was regulated. Furthermore, although many of the early studies concentrated on analysis of cartilage proteoglycans and their structure, more recent investigations have made it clear that all tissues contain proteoglycan molecules and that tissue structure depends in a large part on the integrity of these complex glycoproteins. Finally, although it appeared initially that each class of glycosaminoglycan polymer may reside on individual core proteins, it is now evident that some proteins are modified by the addition of more than a single type of glycosaminoglycan chain.

Large proteoglycan cores: aggrecan and versican. Cartilage provides one model of how proteoglycans function in tissues. In cartilage, aggrecan, the major core protein from cartilage that contains dozens of chondroitin-sulfate side chains and a fewer number of keratan sulfate side chains, interacts with link protein and with hyaluronic acid to produce enormous hydrated polymers that provide the tissue with mass and resistance to compression. The core protein contains just more than 2000 amino acids in which several discrete functional and structural domains can be discerned. The amino-terminal end of the protein contains a globular domain that binds both link protein, with which it shares sequence homology, and hyaluronic acid (a polymer of the repeating dimer glucuronic acid and N-acetyl glucosamine). A second globular domain is similar to the link-protein–binding domain but binds neither link protein nor hyaluronic acid. The third globular domain, in the carboxyl-terminal region, has lectin-inlike function and binds galactose and fucose. Because the ends of the molecule are a considerable distance apart (in molecular terms), binding domains at the two ends could provide the means for anchoring the large molecules or for providing the molecular means for cell-matrix or matrix-matrix interactions. The three globular domains contain oligosaccharide attachment sites. The keratin sulfate addition domain, a region of 113 amino acids that is rich in proline-serine and proline-threonine dipeptides, separates the first two globular domains from the chondroitin sulfate attachment domain. In humans the chondroitin sulfate attachment domain has three types of repeats. The first has a base motif of approximately 40 amino acids in which there are four serine-glycine dipeptides; of these, there are approximately 10 complete or partial repeats, the second has a 100–amino-acid motif in which there are 14 serine-glycine dipeptides within six complete or partial repeats, and the third has a repeating 19–amino-acid sequence that is reiterated 19 times.

Gene structure reflects the protein sequence: the globular domains are sequestered into a small number of exons, the keratin sulfate binding domain is contained largely in a single exon, and the chondroitin sulfate domain is encoded by a single large exon. The domains of the globular regions homologous to link protein share similar exon structures.

A second large proteoglycan core with substantial homology to decorin has been designated *versican*.[159] Like aggrecan, versican binds hyaluronate but is synthesized by fibroblasts and possibly other non-cartilage cells. It probably is important for matrix integrity in those tissues, perhaps to stabilize tissues subject to pressures.

A third large proteoglycan core protein is heparan sulfate proteoglycan, originally isolated from a mouse basement membrane tumor[114] and more recently characterized from human tissues.

Small proteoglycans of the extracellular matrix: decorin and biglycan. Two proteoglycans, biglycan and decorin (previously known as proteoglycan (PG) and PG II, respectively), which have small core proteins of approximately 40 kd mass, are found ubiquitously distributed in connective tissues. Decorin derives its name from its association with ("decoration of") collagen fibrils in skin and other connective tissues. Biglycan refers to the presence of 2 glycosaminoglycan side chains. The gene that encodes decorin is located on chromosome 12, and that for biglycan is on the X chromosome.[52]

Decorin is synthesized as a precursor from which the signal sequence is cleaved during transport across the membrane of the rough endoplasmic reticulum. During elongation, N-linked oligosaccharide is added[55] and a single dermatan sulfate chain is added at the serine in position 4 of the mature protein. The function of this proteoglycan is uncertain. The core protein interacts with type I collagen and affects fibrillogenesis,[138,151] whereas the chondroitin sulfate chain may interfere with cell binding to fibronectin, thus altering cell-matrix interactions. Biglycan shares motifs with decorin, including the 80% of the core sequence that contains a reiterated 24–amino-acid sequence rich in hydrophobic amino acids, and could facilitate interactions with other, similar proteins or with cell surfaces.[50]

Membrane-anchored proteoglycans. During the last few years it has been recognized that a family of proteins exists in which individual members have a characteristic transmembrane domain, an intracellular domain, and an extracellular domain that can be modified by the addition of one or more glycosaminoglycan chains. The functions of these molecules are thought to reside in their ability to mediate cell-matrix interactions.

Biosynthesis

The biosynthesis of proteoglycans is marked by the unusual features of glycosylation of the core protein that distinguish this set of macromolecules. The addition of asparagine (Asn)-linked oligosaccharide units occurs in the rough endoplasmic reticulum at Asn-X-threonine (Thr) and serine (Ser) sequences in parallel to the modification of other glycoproteins.

The chondroitin sulfate, dermatan sulfate, heparin, and heparin sulfate glycosaminoglycans are synthesized on the protein cores in the Golgi apparatus with the same initial structure. Xylosyltransferase adds xylose to serines contained within appropriate recognition motifs in a reaction using the uridine diphosphate sugar that occurs either in the cis-Golgi or in the rough endoplasmic reticulum. In general, not all the available sites are modified. Separate transferases add two galactosyl residues, a glucuronic acid, and N-acetyl galactosamine to form the core to which further additions occur. At this point two additional transferases, which add the hexosamine and the uronic acid moiety of the glycosaminoglycan, elongate the chain. The mechanisms by which chain length is determined are unknown. After chain elongation, epimerization converts some D-glucouronic acids to L-iduronic acid and sulfation of some iduronic acids leads to the different glycosaminoglycans.

Proteoglycan degradation occurs both within the matrix and in the lysosome. From the point of view of known connective tissue disorders, defects in the lysosomal degradation pathway are most significant. Hydrolysis of peptide bonds occurs in lysosomes, leaving the extended glycosaminoglycan chains. The catabolism of these macromolecules requires the sequential activity of a series of exoglycosidases and sulfatases. Because of the repeating nature of the glycosaminoglycan chains and the sequential activity of the enzymes in the degradative pathway, the loss of a single enzyme may lead to accumulation of large amounts of extended glycosaminoglycan chains that cannot be degraded further. The results of such defects are the mucopolysaccharidoses (see Chapter 11).

ELASTIC FIBER STRUCTURE, FUNCTION, AND BIOSYNTHESIS

Elastic fibers are complex structures that are present in many compliant connective tissues. Elastic fibers probably contain many proteins, a few of which have been identified and include elastin, the microfibrillar protein fibrillin, lysyl oxidase, and other proteins that are probably related to the microfibrillar system. On morphologic study the two major components of elastic fibers are an amorphous element (composed largely of the protein elastin) and a microfibrillar array (that contains fibrillin and other proteins). Elastic fibers are present in virtually all connective tissues and are particularly prominent in elastic arteries, skin, and elastic cartilage. In skin the microfibrillar elements of elastic fibers often insert into the basement membrane zone without accompanying amorphous elastin. The zonular fibers of the lens consist almost entirely of microfibrils, which in part explains the relationship between lens subluxation and abnormalities of other connective tissues seen in persons with the Marfan syndrome.

Elastic fibers first appear as arrays of microfibrils in the developing fetus during the second trimester. Elastin is then deposited on the scaffold provided by microfibrils, and the elastic fiber "matures" as the fetus develops and continues to acquire elastin during childhood. The mature elastic fiber has a long half-life in tissues and turns over largely in response to local injury.

The human elastin gene is located at the long arm of chromosome 7, band 11.2, according to recent reassignment.[41,46] The human gene is about 45 kb in size, contains 36 exons, and encodes a set of mRNA species of about 3.5 kb.[8,44] These species are generated by alternative splicing of some exons and by the presence of at least two polyadenylation sites. The coding sequence of the mRNA directs the synthesis of a protein that contains 760 amino acids.[72,73]

The cloning of the complementary DNAs (cDNAs) and their sequence determination provided the first complete sequence of the elastin protein. Because the protein is highly cross-linked in its mature form, because it resists proteolytic and chemical degradation, and because it has a highly repetitive sequence, the sequence had not been elucidated by means of traditional protein sequence determination. The protein itself is organized in alternating hydrophobic and hydrophilic regions that correspond to exon demarcations. The hydrophilic regions are characterized by a high density of lysyl residues that, in the mature protein, are engaged in polyfunctional cross-links. These alternate with regions rich in hydrophobic residues. The early attempts to characterize the elastin protein sequence depended on the isolation of the protein from copper-deficient animals in which elastin was not effectively cross-linked. Copper is a cofactor for lysyl oxidase, the enzyme that catalyzes the oxidative deamination of lysyl groups to provide the substrate for non-enzymatic condensation of modified lysyl groups in polyfunctional cross-links.

Elastin is synthesized by most connective tissue cells, including fibroblasts and smooth muscle cells, although in relatively low quantity. The precursor contains two cysteine residues near the carboxyl-terminal end of the chain, which had not been recognized in the extracted protein and are thought to have a role in binding to the cysteine-rich proteins of the microfibrillar scaffold of elastic fibers. Elastin is not a glycoprotein and contains no arginine (Arg)-Gly-Asp sequences that are common features of matrix proteins involved in cell-matrix interactions. After secretion, virtually all of the 40 lysyl residues in the molecule are modified enzymatically and become enmeshed in intrachain and interchain covalent cross-links. These create a protein meshwork that is resistant to boiling and to alkali denaturation and provides a highly compliant network. The location of the intrachain and interchain cross-links has not been determined and, given the nature of the sequence and its repetitive character, this localization may be difficult to achieve.

The best-characterized protein of the microfibrillar array is fibrillin, the protein that appears to harbor most of the mutations that result in the Marfan syndrome (see Chapter 3). Fibrillin is a 360-kd glycoprotein encoded by a gene on chromosome 15. There appear to be at least two, perhaps more, members of the fibrillin class of proteins, the functions of which are uncertain. Linkage of a second fibrillin gene on chromosome 5 to contractural arachnodactyly has been demonstrated, compatible with an important functional role for the protein product. Little, however, is known about that protein.

Fibrillin (the product of the gene on chromosome 15) is synthesized as a precursor, glycosylated within the cell, and secreted to the matrix, where there appears to be proteolytic removal of a peptide with a mass of approximately 30 kd. The large protein is aggregated in the matrix into microfibrillar structures, which are stabilized by extensive intermolecular disulfide bonds.

The fibrillin gene has been partially characterized, and more than 70% of the cDNA has been sequenced.[90,95] The cDNA sequence encodes a protein with more than 30 repeats of an epidermal growth factor (EGF) precursor-like repeat (about 40 amino acids containing cysteines in a characteristic position). These repeats occur reiteratively: 7 to 13 units are separated by a unit of about 80 amino acids that contains eight cysteine residues and is similar to sequences in a small group of proteins, including the transforming growth factor type beta binding protein (TGFβ). The complete gene probably occupies more than 100 kb and contains more than 60 exons. The role of the EGF-like repeats as more than structural elements is unclear. The protein in the matrix is a fibril structure, and alterations in the protein may have dramatic effects on tissue integrity with few apparent effects on the ultrastructural appearance of the microfibrillar network.

The physical relationship among fibrillin, elastin, and other elastic fiber proteins is not known but is currently the subject of intense scientific scrutiny.

MATRIX GLYCOPROTEIN STRUCTURE, BIOSYNTHESIS, AND FUNCTION

Basement membranes and pericellular matrix contain distinctive glycoproteins that, along with collagens, provide the integrative meshwork of connective tissues. Characteristically these proteins have multiple domains that offer binding sites for other matrix macromolecules and for cell surface proteins, thus serving to bind cells and matrix proteins.

Fibronectin

Fibronectin is the prototype adhesive glycoprotein.[71] Encoded by a gene located on chromosome 2, fibronectin is composed of two chains, which are the product of the same gene but generally differ in alternative splicing. The protein is synthesized ubiquitously and is involved in many processes, including cell adhesion and spreading to synthetic substrates, determination of cell morphologic appearance, cell migration during development and wound healing, phagocytosis, and he-

mostasis. (See Hynes and Yamada[71] for a detailed review.) Each chain has a molecular mass of approximately 250 kd. The protein is remarkable in consisting of a series of three types of repeating motifs arrayed along the chain. There are 12 type I repeats of approximately 45 amino acids, of which four are cysteine residues that permit stabilization of specific intrachain disulfide bonds. Five type I repeats are found at the amino-terminal end of the chain, where they compose heparin- and fibrin-binding domains; three occur at the carboxyl-terminal end of the molecule in another fibrin-binding domain, and the remainder are interspersed with a series of type II repeats (approximately 60 residues that contain four cysteine residues) to form a collagen-binding domain. The remainder of the protein, approximately 1700 of about 2400 amino acid residues of fibronectin, consists of a series of repeats of yet a third sequence, the type III repeat. These repeat units contain a DNA-binding motif and cell-binding and heparin-binding motifs. The type III repeats provide the domains for the majority of alternative splicing that accounts for the production of as many as 20 distinct proteins from the single gene. The central cell-binding domain of fibronectin contains the amino acid sequence Arg-Gly-Asp-Ser (*RGDS* in the single-letter amino acid code), which has come to be recognized as a ubiquitous cell-recognition motif.[116] The gene that encodes fibronectin mirrors the motif structure; indeed, some of the motifs are seen in a variety of other matrix proteins.The gene is more than 50 kb in length and contains more than 50 exons. The organization of the exons and the break sites of codons in many of the type III repeat domains permits alternative splicing to occur without change of the reading frame.

Other matrix glycoproteins, including thrombospondin and tenascin (see Bornstein and Sage[17] for a discussion of their functions), share motifs with fibronectin and may function in regulation of cell adhesion and loss of adhesion to synthetic substrates and, perhaps, to other proteins.

Basement Membrane Glycoproteins

In addition to the several species of type IV collagen molecules, basement membranes contain several major glycoproteins, including laminin (composed of three proteins, the A, B1, and B2 chains) and entactin, or nidogen, that are capable of mediating cell adherence and migration and may play important roles in defining the structure of the basal lamina.

Laminin consists of three chains, the A chain, with a size of approximately 400 kd, and the B1 (210 kd) and B2 (200 kd) chains, which combine to form a cruciate structure. This protein can bind multiple other macromolecules, including cell surface proteins, heparin, collagen, and nidogen, and thus may be one of the integrative molecules of basement membranes. The human genes for the three chains have been mapped to the short arm of chromosome 18, band 11.3 (18p11.3) (A chain, Nagayoshi et al.[106]); the long arm of chromosome 7, band 22 (7q22) (B1 chain, Pikkarainen et al.[119]); and the long arm of chromosome 1, band 31 (1q31) (B2 chain, Mattei et al.[96]). Nidogen, another protein of the basement membrane zone, interacts with laminin and binds to it in a stoichiometric fashion. A glycoprotein with a mass of approximately 150 kd, nidogen is encoded by a gene on the long arm of chromosome 1, band 43 (1q43).[110]

CONCLUSION

Building tissues is a complex process that requires the coordinated expression of hundreds of genes with precise timing and spatial representation. Extracellular matrix develops as a result of synthesis of proteins that interact with molecules of the same type and with a vast array of different molecules. Although much is known about many individual genes and proteins that contribute to the extracellular matrix, the manner in which their expression is coordinated and their interactions are controlled is little understood. The relatedness of many of the proteins in the matrix is often surprising; several motifs that are important for structure and interactions (e.g., repeated triple helices of collagens, the fibronectin repeat domains, EGF-like domains that provide elements of structure, and von Willibrand repeats that may be important for binding) are reiterated in different contexts in many matrix proteins.[15,41] The appearance of these sequences in so many proteins argues persuasively for their importance and suggests that similar motifs in different proteins may have similar functions and that these motifs may be important in the overall integration of the matrix.

Although the manner in which matrix is organized during development is poorly understood, it is likely to be a key consideration in understanding some of the more complex connective tissue disorders in which abnormalities of limb development may not be the consequence of mutations in matrix proteins but, rather, may depend on some aspect of the timing or spatial location of expression of a set of genes. (Ectrodactyly and other similar disorders are good examples.) It is likely that the interest in developmental genes and the process of development that has recently been turned toward understanding mammalian development will ultimately provide significant insights into how mutations alter extracellular matrix and the role of the matrix in forming organisms.

In many instances the functions of collagens, glycoproteins, elastin, and proteoglycans will be best demonstrated by means of analysis of naturally occurring and, increasingly, induced mutations in genes that encode components of the extracellular matrix. This course has been pursued to considerable advantage during recent years, and the identification of collagens and other matrix genes has amply demonstrated their functional importance. (See Chapters 3, 6, 8, and 14 for many examples). It is fitting to return at this point to the last paragraph of this chapter as it appeared in the fourth edition of this book, in which, as follows, the relationship between mutation and functional analysis was posed with such perspicacity by McKusick:

In the Marfan syndrome: What does the suspensory ligament of the ocular lens have in common with the media of the aorta? What controls longitudinal growth of bone? *In pseudoxanthoma elasticum:* What is the nature of Bruch's membrane of the eye and what does it have in common with elastic fibers? *In the Ehlers-Danlos syndrome:* What is responsible for the tensile strength of the skin and for its elasticity? What is the organization of collagen bundles in ligaments, tendons, and joint capsules, and what is the relationship between this organization and the stretchability of these structures? What determines the elastic properties of the collagen and elastin molecules, and of fibers of these proteins? *In osteogenesis imperfecta:* What is the normal organization of apatite on collagen, which accounts for the important structural properties of bone, and in this disease what change in collagen has occurred to disrupt the normal collagen-apatite relationship? In disorders such as osteogenesis imperfecta and the Ehlers-Danlos syndrome, is there any abnormality of amino acid sequences of collagen comparable to the abnormalities demonstrated by Ingram in the aberrant hemoglobins?

Although some of these questions have been used to help identify candidate genes for a variety of disorders, some of the questions, 20 years later, remain unanswered and the candidate genes for many disorders have yet to be determined.

REFERENCES

1. Anttinen H et al: Evidence for the transfer of mannose to the extension peptides of procollagen within the cisternae of the rough endoplasmic reticulum, *FEBS Lett* 87:222, 1978.
2. Apte S, Mattei MG, Olsen BR: Cloning of human α1(X) collagen DNA and localization of the COL10A1 gene to the q21-q22 region of human chromosome 6, *FEBS Lett* 282:393-396, 1991.
3. Avvedimento VE et al: Correlation between splicing sites within an intron and their sequence complementarity with U1 RNA, *Cell* 21:689, 1980.
4. Aycock RS et al: Posttranscriptional inhibition of collagen and fibronectin synthesis by a synthetic homolog of a portion of the carboxyl-terminal propeptide of human type I collagen, *J Biol Chem* 261:14355, 1986.
5. Bächinger HP: The influence of peptidyl-prolyl cis-trans isomerase on the in vitro folding of type III collagen, *J Biol Chem* 262:17144, 1987.
6. Bächinger HP et al: The role of *cis-trans* isomerization of peptide bonds in the coil−triple helix conversion of collagen, *Eur J Biochem* 90:605, 1978.
7. Barsh GS, Roush CL, Gelinas RE: DNA and chromatin structure of the human α1(I) collagen gene, *J Biol Chem* 259:14906, 1984.
8. Bashir MM et al: Characterization of the complete human elastin gene: delineation of unusual features in the 5'-flanking region, *J Biol Chem* 264:8887-8891, 1989.
9. Bennett VC, Adams SL: Characterization of the translational control mechanism preventing synthesis of α2(I) collagen in chicken vertebral chondroblasts, *J Biol Chem* 262:14806, 1987.
10. Berg RA, Kedersah NL, Guzman NA: Purification and partial characterization of the two nonidentical subunits of prolyl hydroxylase, *J Biol Chem* 254:311, 1979.
11. Berg RA, Prockop DJ: The thermal transition of a nonhydroxylated collagen: evidence for a role for hydroxyproline in stabilizing the triple helix of collagen, *Biochem Biophys Res Commun* 52:115, 1973.
12. Berg RA et al: Lysosomal function in the degradation of defective collagen in cultured lung fibroblasts, *Biochemistry* 23:2134, 1984.
13. Bhattacharyya SN et al: Isolation and characterization of two hydroxyproline-containing glycoproteins from normal animal lung lavage and lamellar bodies, *J Clin Invest* 55:914, 1975.
14. Bienkowski RS, Curran SF, Berg RA: Kinetics of intracellular degradation of newly synthesized collagen, *Biochemistry* 25:2455, 1986.
15. Bork P: Shuffled domains in extracellular proteins, *FEBS Lett* 286:47-54, 1991.
16. Bornstein P, McKay J: The first intron of the α1(I) collagen gene contains several transcriptional regulatory elements, *J Biol Chem* 263:1603-1606, 1988.
17. Bornstein P, Sage H: Structurally distinct collagen types, *Annu Rev Biochem* 49:957, 1980.
18. Bornstein P, Traub W: Collagen. In Neurath HG, Bill RL, editors: *The proteins,* ed 3, New York, 1979, Academic Press, p 411.
19. Bornstein P et al: Regulatory elements in the first intron contribute to transcriptional control of the human α1(I) collagen gene, *Proc Natl Acad Sci USA* 84:8869-8873, 1987.
20. Boyd CD: The genes coding for human pro α1(IV) collagen and pro α2(IV) collagen are both located at the end of the long arm of chromosome 13, *Am J Hum Genet* 42:309, 1988.
21. Burgeson RE: Type VII collagen. In R Mayne, RE Burgeson, editors: *Structure and function of collagen types,* Orlando, Fla, 1987, Academic Press, p 145.
22. Cheah KSE et al: Identification and characterization of the human type II collagen gene (COL2A1), *Proc Natl Acad Sci USA* 82:2555, 1985.
23. Chu M-L et al: Human pro α1(I) collagen gene structure reveals evolutionary conservation of a pattern of introns and exons, *Nature* 310:337, 1984.
24. Chu M-L et al: Isolation of cDNA and genomic clones encoding human pro α1(III) collagen, *J Biol Chem* 260:4357, 1985.
25. Chu M-L et al: Characterization of three constituent chains of collagen type VI by peptides sequences and cDNA clones, *Eur J Biochem* 168:309, 1987.
26. Clark CC: The distribution and initial characterization of oligosaccharide units on the COOH-terminal propeptide extensions of the pro α1 and pro α2 chains of type I procollagen, *J Biol Chem* 254:10798, 1979.
27. Clark CC: Asparagine-linked glycosides, *Methods Enzymol* 82A:346, 1982.
28. Constantinou CD et al: The A and B fragments of normal type I procollagen have a similar thermal stability to proteinase digestion but are selectively destabilized by structural mutations, *Eur J Biochem* 163:247, 1987.
29. Cotta-Pereira G, Guerra G, Bittencourt-Sampaio S: Oxytalin, elaunin and elastic fibers in the human skin, *J Invest Dermatol* 66:143-148, 1976.
30. Creighton TE, Hillson DA, Freedman RB: Catalysis by protein−disulphide isomerase of the unfolding and refolding of proteins with disulphide bonds, *J Mol Biol* 142:43, 1980.
31. Cronlund AL, Kagan HM: Comparison of lysyl oxidase from bovine lung and aorta, *Connect Tissue Res*:15:173, 1986.
32. Cutting GR et al: Macrorestriction mapping of COL4A1 and COL4A2 collagen genes on human chromosome 13q34, *Genomics* 3:256-263, 1988.
33. de Wet WJ, Chu M-L, Prockop DJ: The mRNAs for the pro α1(I) and pro α2(I) chains of type I procollagen are translated at the same rate in normal human fibroblasts and in fibroblasts from two variants of osteogenesis imperfecta with altered steady state ratios of the two mRNAs, *J Biol Chem* 258:14385, 1983.
34. de Wet W et al: Organization of the human pro α2(I) collagen gene, *J Biol Chem* 262:16032, 1987.
35. Doege KJ, Fessler JH: Folding of carboxyl domain and assembly of procollagen I, *J Biol Chem* 261:8924, 1986.

36. Drickamer K, McCreary V: Exon structure of a mannose-binding protein gene reflects its evolutionary relationship to the asiologlycoprotein receptor and nonfibrillar collagens, *J Biol Chem* 262:2582-2589, 1987.

37. Dublet B et al: The structure of avian type XII collagen: alpha 1(XII) chains contain a 190-kd non–triple-helical amino-terminal domain and form homotrimeric molecules, *J Biol Chem* 264:13150-13156, 1989.

38. Duksin D, Bornstein P: Impaired conversion of procollagen to collagen by fibroblasts and bone treated with tunicamycin, an inhibitor of protein glycosylation, *J Biol Chem* 252:955, 1977.

39. Emanuel BS et al: Chromosomal localization of the human elastin gene, *Am J Hum Genet* 37:873-882, 1985.

40. Emanuel BS et al: Human α1(III) and α2(V) procollagen genes are located on the long arm of chromosome 2, *Proc Natl Acad Sci USA* 82:3385, 1985.

41. Engel J: Domains in proteins and proteoglycans of the extracellular matrix with functions in assembly and cellular activities, *Int J Biol Macromol* 13:147-151, 1991.

42. Eyre DR, Paz MA, Gallop PM: Cross-linking in collagen and elastin, *Ann Rev Biochem* 53:717, 1984.

43. Eyre D, Wu J-J: Type XI or 1α2α3α collagen. In R Mayne, RE Burgeson, editors: *Structure and function of collagen types*, Orlando, Fla, 1987, Academic Press, p 261.

44. Fazio MJ et al: Cloning of full-length elastin cDNAs from a human skin fibroblasts recombinant cDNA library: further elucidation of alternative splicing utilizing exon-specific oligonucleotides, *J Invest Dermatol* 91:454-464, 1988.

45. Fazio MJ et al: Human elastin gene: new evidence for localization to the long arm of chromosome 7, *Am J Hum Genet* 48:696-703, 1991.

46. Fessler JH, Fessler LI: Biosynthesis of procollagen, *Ann Rev Biochem* 47:129, 1978.

47. Fessler LI et al: Intracellular transport and tyrosine sulfation of procollagens V, *Eur J Biochem* 158:511, 1986.

48. Fessler LI et al: Tyrosine sulfation in precursors of collagen V, *J Biol Chem* 261:5034, 1986.

49. Fields GB, Van Wart HE, Birkedal-Hansen H: Sequence specificity of human skin fibroblast collagenase: evidence for the role of collagen structure in determining the collagenase cleavage site, *J Biol Chem* 262:6221, 1987.

50. Fisher LW, Termine JD, Young MF: Deduced protein sequence of bone small proteoglycan I (biglycan) shows homology with proteoglycan II (decorin) and several nonconnective tissue proteins in a variety of species, *J Biol Chem* 264:4571-4576, 1989.

51. Fisher LW et al: The Mr24,000 phosphoprotein from developing bone is the NH2-terminal propeptide of the α1 chain of type I collagen, *J Biol Chem* 262:13457, 1987.

52. Fisher LW et al: Human biglycan gene: putative promoter, intron-exon junctions, and chromosomal localization, *J Biol Chem* 266:14371-14377, 1991.

53. Francomano CA et al: The COL6A1 and COL6A2 genes exist as a gene cluster and detect highly informative DNA polymorphisms in the telomeric region of human chromosome 21q, *Hum Genet* 87:162-166, 1991.

54. Glanville R: Type IV collagen. In R Mayne, RE Burgeson, editors: *Structure and function of collagen types*, Orlando, Fla, 1987, Academic Press, p 43.

55. Glossl J, Beck M, Kresse H: Biosynthesis of proteodermatan sulfate in cultured human fibroblasts, *J Biol Chem* 259:14144-14150, 1984.

56. Gordon MK, Gerecke DR, Olsen BR: Type XII collagen: distinct extracellular matrix component discovered by cDNA cloning, *Proc Natl Acad Sci USA* 84:6040-6044, 1987.

57. Gordon MK et al: Type XII collagen: a large multidomain molecule with partial homology to type IX collagen, *J Biol Chem* 264:19772-19778, 1989.

58. Greenspan DS et al: Human collagen gene COL5A1 maps to the q34.2 to q34.3 region of chromosome 9, near the locus for Nail Patella syndrome, *Genomics* 12:836-837, 1992.

59. Guzman NA, Graves PN, Prockop DJ: Addition of mannose to both the amino- and carboxy-terminal propeptides of type II procollagen occurs without formation of a triple helix, *Biochem Biophys Res Commun* 84:691, 1978.

60. Hanson IM et al: The human α2(XI) collagen gene (COL11A2) maps to the centromeric border of the major histocompatibility complex on chromosome 6, *Genomics* 5:925-931, 1989.

61. Harper E: Collagenases, *Ann Rev Biochem* 49:1063, 1980.

62. Harris ED: Copper-induced activation of aortic lysyl oxidase in vivo, *Proc Natl Acad Sci USA* 73:371, 1973.

63. Harwood R, Grant ME, Jackson DS: The route of secretion of procollagen: the influence of α,α'-bipyridyl, colchicine and antimycin A on the secretory process in embryonic-chick tendon and cartilage cells, *Biochem J* 156:81, 1976.

64. Hasty KA et al: The collagen substrate specificity of human neutrophil collagenase, *J Biol Chem* 262:10048, 1987.

65. Hatamochi A, Paterson B, deCrombrugghe B: Differential binding of a CCAAT DNA binding factor to the promoters of the mouse α2(I) and α1(III) collagen genes, *J Biol Chem* 261:11310, 1986.

66. Henry I et al: Mapping of a human fibrillar collagen, pro α1(XI), 1988.

67. Horlein D et al: Regulation of protein synthesis: translational control by procollagen-derived fragments, *Proc Natl Acad Sci USA* 78:6163, 1981.

68. Housley TJ et al: Effects of tunicamycin on the biosynthesis of procollagen by human fibroblasts, *J Biol Chem* 255:121, 1980.

69. Huerre C et al: Human type I procollagen genes are located on different chromosomes, *Proc Natl Acad Sci USA* 79:6627, 1982.

70. Huerre-Jeanpiere C et al: The pro α2(V) collagen (COL5A2) maps to 2q14→2q32, syntenic to the pro α1(III) collagen locus (COL3A1), *Hum Genet* 73:64, 1986.

71. Hynes RO, Yamada KM: Fibronectins: multifunctional modular glycoproteins, *J Cell Biol* 95:369-377, 1982.

72. Indik Z et al: Alternative splicing of human elastin messenger-RNA indicated by sequence analysis of cloned genomic and complementary DNA, *Proc Natl Acad Sci USA* 84:5680-5684, 1987.

73. Indik Z et al: Structure of the elastin gene and alternative splicing of elastin mRNA. In L Sandell, C Boyd, editors: *Genes for extracellular matrix proteins*, New York, 1990, Academic Press, pp 221-250.

74. Jimenez SA et al: Intracellular collagen and protocollagen from embryonic tendon cells, *J Biol Chem* 248:720, 1973.

75. Kagan HM: Lysyl oxidase. In Mecham RP, editor: *Biology of extracellular matrix*, vol 1, Orlando, Fla, 1985, Academic Press, p 321.

76. Kefalides NA, Alper R, Clark CC: Biochemistry and metabolism of basement membranes, *Int Rev Cytol* 61:167, 1979.

77. Kidama T et al: Type I macrophage scavenger receptor contains α-helical and collagen-like coiled coils, *Nature* 343:531-535, 1990.

78. Kielty CM et al: Isolation and ultrastructural analysis of microfibrillar structures from foetal bovine elastic tissues: relative abundance and supramolecular architecture of type VI collagen assemblies and fibrillin, *J Cell Science* 99:797-807, 1991.

79. Kimura T et al: The human α2(XI) collagen (COL11A2) chain: molecular cloning of cDNA and genomic DNA reveals characteristics of a fibrillar collagen with differences in genomic organization, *J Biol Chem* 264:13910-13916, 1989.

80. Kivirikko KI, Myllylä R: Collagen glycosyltransferases, *Int Rev Connect Tissue Res* 8:23, 1979.

81. Kivirikko KI, Myllylä R: Posttranslational enzymes in the biosynthesis of collagen: intracellular enzymes, *Methods Enzymol* 82(A):245, 1982.

82. Kivirikko KI, Myllylä R: Biosynthesis of the collagens. In Piez KA, Reddi AH, editors: *Extracellular matrix biochemistry*, New York, 1984, Elsevier, p 83.

83. Koivu J: Identification of disulfide bonds in carboxy-terminal propeptides of human type I procollagen, *FEBS Lett* 212:229, 1987.

84. Kornfeld R, Kornfeld S: Assembly of asparagine-linked oligosaccharides, *Ann Rev Biochem* 54:631, 1985.

85. Kuhn K: The classical collagens. In R Mayne, RE Burgeson, editors: *Structure and function of collagen types*, Orlando, Fla, 1987, Academic Press, p 1.

86. Kurkinen M et al: Characterization of 64–, 123– and 182–base-pair exons in the mouse α2(IV) collagen gene, *Nature* 317:177, 1985.

87. Kwan APL et al: Comparative studies of type X collagen expression in normal and rachitic chicken epiphyseal cartilage, *J Cell Biol* 109:1849-1856, 1989.

88. Lapiere CM, Lenaers A, Kohn LD: Procollagen peptidase: an enzyme excising the coordination peptides of procollagen, *Proc Natl Acad Sci USA* 68:3054, 1971.

89. Law ML et al: The gene for the α2 chain of the human fibrillar collagen type XI (COL11A2) assigned to the short arm of chromosome 6, *Ann Hum Genet* 54:23-29, 1990.

90. Lee B et al: Linkage of Marfan syndrome and a phenotypically related disorder to two different fibrillin genes, *Nature* 352:330-334, 1991.

91. Liau G et al: Restriction enzyme digestions identify discrete domains in the chromatin around the promoter of the mouse α2(I) collagen gene, *J Biol Chem* 261:11362, 1986.

92. Liotta LA et al: Preferential digestion of basement membrane collagen by an enzyme derived from a metastatic murine tumor, *Proc Natl Acad Sci USA* 76:2268, 1979.

93. Liska DJ, Slack JL, Bornstein P: A highly conserved intronic sequence is involved in transcriptional regulation of the α1(I) collagen gene, *Cell Regulation* 1:487-498, 1990.

94. Lozano G et al: A distinct class of vertebrate collagen genes encodes chicken type IX collagen polypeptides, *Proc Natl Acad Sci USA* 82:4050, 1985.

95. Maslen CL et al: Partial sequence of a candidate gene for the Marfan syndrome, *Nature* 352:334-337, 1991.

96. Mattei M-G et al: cDNA cloning, expression and mapping of human laminin B2 gene to chromosome 1q31, *Hum Genet* 79:235-241, 1988.

97. Mayne R, Burgeson RE, editors: *Structure and function of collagen types*, Orlando, Fla, 1987, Academic Press.

98. Mays C, Rosenberry TL: Characterization of pepsin-resistant collagen-like tail subunit fragments of 18S and 14S acetylcholinesterase from electrophorus electricus, *Biochemistry* 20:2810, 1981.

99. Miller EJ: The structure of fibril-forming collagen, *Ann NY Acad Sci* 460:1, 1985.

100. Miller EJ, Matukas VJ: Chick cartilage collagen: a new type of α1 chain not present in bone or skin of the species, *Proc Natl Acad Sci USA* 64:1264, 1969.

101. Molnar JA et al: Synthesis and degradation rates of collagens in vivo in whole skin or rats: studied with 1802 labeling, *Biochem J* 240:431, 1986.

102. Morris NP, Fessler LI, Fessler JH: Procollagen peptide release by procollagen peptidases and bacterial collagenase, *J Biol Chem* 254:11024, 1979.

103. Murad S et al: Regulation of collagen synthesis by ascorbic acid, *Proc Natl Acad Sci USA* 78:2879, 1981.

104. Myers JC et al: Partial covalent structure of the human α2 type V collagen chain, *J Biol Chem* 260:5533, 1985.

105. Myllylä R, Kuutti-Savolainen E-R, Kivirikko KI: The role of ascorbate in the prolyl hydroxylase reaction, *Biochem Biophys Res Commun* 83:441, 1978.

106. Nagayoshi T et al: Human laminin A chain (LAMA) gene: chromosomal mapping to locus 18p11.3, *Genomics* 5:932-935, 1989.

107. Ninomaya Y et al: The developmentally regulated type X collagen gene contains a long open reading frame without introns, *J Biol Chem* 261:5041, 1986.

108. Olsen BR et al: Collagen synthesis: localization of prolyl hydroylase in tendon cells detected with ferritin-labeled antibodies, *Science* 182:825, 1973.

109. Olsen BR et al: Short-chain collagen genes and their expression in cartilage, *Ann NY Acad Sci* 460:141, 1985.

110. Olsen DR et al: Human nidogen: cDNA cloning, cellular expression, and mapping of the gene to chromosome 1q43, *Am J Hum Genet* 44:876-885, 1989.

111. Paglia LM et al: Inhibition of procollagen cell-free synthesis by amino-terminal extension peptides, *Biochemistry* 18:5030, 1979.

112. Palmiter RD et al: NH2-terminal sequence of the chick pro α1(I) chain synthesized in the reticulocyte lysate system, *J Biol Chem* 254:1433, 1979.

113. Parente MG et al: Human type VII collagen: cDNA cloning and chromosomal mapping of the gene, *Proc Natl Acad Sci USA* 88:6931-6935, 1991.

114. Paulsson M et al: Structure of low-density heparan sulfate proteoglycan isolated from mouse tumor basement membrane, *Mol Biol* 197:297-313, 1987.

115. Peterkofsky B, Kalwinsky D, Assad R: Substance in L-929 cell extracts which replaces the ascorbate requirement for prolyl hydroxylase in a tritium release assay for reducing cofactor: correlation of its concentration with the extent

of ascorbate-independent proline hydroxylation and the level of prolyl hydroxylase activity in these cells, *Arch Biochem Biophys* 199:362, 1980.

116. Pierschbacher MD, Ruoslahti E: Cell attachment activity of fibronectin can be duplicated by small synthetic fragments of the molecule, *Nature* 309:30-33, 1984.

117. Piez KA, Trus BL: Sequence regularities and packing of collagen molecules, *J Mol Biol* 122:419, 1978.

118. Pihlajaniemi T et al: Molecular cloning of the β subunit of human prolyl 4-hydroxylase: this subunit and protein disulphide isomerase are products of the same gene, *EMBO J* 6:643, 1987.

119. Pikkarainen T et al: Human laminin B1 chain: a multidomain protein with gene (LAMB1) locus in the q22 region of chromosome 7, *J Biol Chem* 262:10454, 1987.

120. Puistola U et al: Studies on the lysyl hydroxylase reaction. II. Inhibition kinetics and the reaction mechanism, *Biochim Biophys Acta* 611:51, 1980.

121. Raghow R et al: Transforming growth factor β increases steady state levels of type I procollagen and fibronectin messenger RNAs posttranscriptionally in cultured human dermal fibroblasts, *J Clin Invest* 79:1285, 1987.

122. Ramachandran GN: Structure of collagen at the molecular level. In Ramachandran GN, editor: *Treatise on collagen*, vol 1, New York, 1967, Academic Press, p 103.

123. Rao NV, Adams E: Partial reaction of prolyl hydroxylase (Gly-Pro-Ala)n stimulates α-ketoglutarate decarboxylation without prolyl hydroxylation, *J Biol Chem* 253:6327, 1978.

124. Raviola G: The fine structure of the ciliary zonule and ciliary epithelium with special regard to the organization and insertion of the zonular fibrils, *Invest Ophthalmol* 10:851-869, 1971.

125. Reid KBM: Complete amino acid sequences of the three collagen-like regions present in subcomponent C1q of the first component of human complement, *Biochem J* 179:367, 1979.

126. Risteli J, Tryggvason K, Kivirikko KI: A rapid assay for prolyl 3-hydroxylase activity, *Anal Biochem* 84:423, 1978.

127. Roberts AB et al: Transforming growth factor type β: rapid induction of fibrosis and angiogenesis in vivo and stimulation of collagen formation in vitro, *Proc Natl Acad Sci USA* 83:4167, 1986.

128. Rosenbloom J, Harsch M, Jimenez S: Hydroxyproline content determines the denaturation temperature of chick tendon collagen, *Arch Biochem Biophys* 158:478, 1973.

129. Ross R, Bornstein P: The elastic fiber. I. The separation and partial characterization of its macromolecular components, *J Cell Biol* 40:366-381, 1969.

130. Rossi P, de Crombrugghe B: Identification of a cell-specific transcriptional enhancer in the first intron of the mouse α2 (type I) collagen gene. *Proc Natl Acad Sci USA* 84:5590, 1987.

131. Ryynaenen M et al: Human type VII collagen: genetic linkage of the gene (COL7A1) on chromosome 3 to dominant dystrophic epidermolysis bullosa, *Am J Hum Genet* 49:797-803, 1991.

132. Sakai LY, Keene DR. Engvall E: Fibrillin, a new 350 kd glycoprotein, is a component of extracellular microfibrils, *J Cell Biol* 103:2499-2509, 1986.

133. Sakurai Y, Sullivan M, Yamada Y: α1 type IV collagen gene evolved differently from fibrillar collagen genes, *J Biol Chem* 261:6654, 1986.

134. Sangiorgi FO et al: Isolation and partial characterization of the entire human pro α1(II) collagen gene, *Nucleic Acids Res* 13:2207, 1985.

135. Schmid TM, Linsenmayer TF: Type X collagen. In R Mayne, RE Burgeson, editors: *Structure and function of collagen types*, Orlando, Fla, 1987, Academic Press, p 223.

136. Schmidt A, Rossi P, de Crombrugghe B: Transcriptional control of the mouse alpha 2 (1) collagen gene: functional deletion analysis of the promotor and evidence for cell-specific expression, *Mol Cell Biol* 6:347, 1986.

137. Schmidt A, Yamada Y, de Crombrugghe B: DNA sequence comparison of the regulatory signals at the 5' end of the mouse and chick α2 type I collagen genes, *J Biol Chem* 259:7411, 1984.

138. Scott JE, Haigh M: "Small"-proteoglycan: collagen interactions: keratan sulphate proteoglycan associated with rabbit corneal collagen fibrils at the 'a' and 'c' bands, *Biosci Rep* 5:765-774, 1985.

139. Siegel RC: Lysyl oxidase, *Int Rev Connect Tissue Res* 8:73, 1979.

140. Solomon E, Hall V, Kurkinen M: The human α2(IV) collagen gene, COL4A2, is syntenic with the α1(IV) gene, COL4A1, on chromosome 13, *Ann Hum Genet* 51:125, 1987.

141. Solomon E et al: Regional localization of the human α2(I) collagen gene on chromosome 7 by molecular hybridization, *Cytogenet Cell Genet* 35:64, 1983.

142. Strom CM, Eddy RL, Shows TB: Localization of human type II procollagen gene (COL2A1) to chromosome 12, *Somatic Cell Mol Genet* 10:651, 1984.

143. Sunda Raj CV et al: Assignment of the gene for human type I procollagen to chromosome 17 by analysis of cell hybrids and microcell hybrids, *Proc Natl Acad Sci USA* 74:4444, 1977.

144. Thomas JT, Boot-Handford RP, Grant ME: Modulation of the type X collagen gene expression by calcium β-glycerophosphate and levamisole: implications for type X collagen in endochondral bone formation, *J Cell Sci* 95:639-648, 1990.

145. Thomas JT et al: The human collagen X gene: complete primary translated sequence and chromosomal localization, *Biochem J* 280:617-623, 1991.

146. Tuderman L, Kivirikko KI, Prockop DJ: Partial purification and characterization of a neutral protease which cleaves the N-terminal propeptides from procollagen, *Biochemistry* 17:2948, 1978.

147. Tuderman L, Prockop DJ: Procollagen N-proteinase: properties of the enzyme purified from chick embryo tendons, *Eur J Biochem* 125:545, 1982.

148. Turpeenniemi-Hujanen TM, Puistola U, Kivirikko KI: Isolation of lysyl hydroxylase, an enzyme of collagen synthesis, from chick embryos as a homogenous protein, *Biochem J* 189:247, 1980.

149. van der Rest M, Mayne R: Type IX collagen. In R Mayne, RE Burgeson, editors: *Structure and function of collagen types*, Orlando, Fla, 1987, Academic Press, p 195.

150. van der Rest M, Mayne R: Type IX collagen proteoglycan from cartilage is covalently cross-linked to type II collagen, *J Biol Chem* 263:1615, 1988.

151. Vogel KG, Paulsson, Heinegard D: Specific inhibition of type I and type II collagen fibrillogenesis by the small proteoglycan of tendon, *Biochem J* 223:587-597, 1984.

152. Vuorio E, deCrombrugghe B: Collagen genes, *Ann Rev Biochem* 58:990-1043, 1990.

153. Weil D et al: Cloning and chromosomal localization of human genes encoding the three chains of type VI collagen, *Am J Hum Genet* 42:435, 1988.

154. Wight TN, Heinegard KD, Hascall VC: Proteoglycans: structure and function. In Hay ED, editor: *Cell biology of extracellular matrix*, ed 2, New York, 1991, Plenum, pp 45-78.

155. Williamson PR et al: Evidence for pyrroloquinoline-quinone as the carbonyl cofactor in lysyl oxidase by absorption and resonance Raman spectroscopy, *J Biol Chem* 261:16302, 1986.

156. Reference deleted in proofs.

157. Yamada Y, Mudryj M, de Crombrugghe B: A uniquely conserved regulatory signal is found around the translation initiation site in three different collagen genes, *J Biol Chem* 258:14914, 1983.

158. Yamagata M et al: The complete primary structure of type XII collagen shows a chimeric molecule with reiterated fibronectin type III motifs, von Willebrand factor A motifs, a domain homologous to a noncollagenous region of type IX collagen and short collagenous domains with an Arg-Gly-Asp site, *J Cell Biol* 115:209-221, 1991.

159. Zimmerman DR, Ruoslahti E: Multiple domains of the large fibroblast proteoglycan, versican, *EMBO J* 8:2975-2981, 1989.

CHAPTER 3

The Marfan Syndrome

Maurice Godfrey

The Marfan syndrome is a well-known auto-somal dominant disorder in which tall stature and excessive limb and digital length are associated with abnormalities in the skeletal, ocular, and cardiovascular systems. The nature of the basic defect has long been enigmatic, but the two decades since the fourth edition of this work was published have seen great progress in the understanding of the pathogenesis. Indeed, the search for the cause of this disorder culminated in the middle of 1991 with the discovery of mutations in the gene that had been linked to the Marfan syndrome.

The discovery made in 1991 is not an ending but a beginning in the quest to elucidate the biology of the group of proteins that are abnormal in this disorder. This understanding will undoubtedly lead to improved management and a better prognosis. Of immediate benefit, primarily to affected families, will be the availability of techniques for prenatal and presymptomatic diagnosis.

An endeavor of this magnitude is rarely accomplished without invaluable discussions with colleagues. I owe infinite thanks to Dr. Petros Tsipouras for his patience with my endless questions and to Dr. Peter Beighton for his editing and polishing. Dr. Richard Devereux wrote the section concerning cardiovascular manifestations and contributed significantly to the section on cardiovascular management. For this assistance I offer my deepest gratitude. This chapter was originally to be written by my friend and mentor, the late Dr. David W. Hollister. I hope that this work would have met his impeccable standards, and it is to him that I dedicate my efforts.

HISTORICAL NOTE

In 1896[298] Marfan* described the gross skeletal manifestations of the syndrome that bears his name; he termed the condition *dolichostenomelia* (long, thin extremities) (Figs. 3-1 and 3-2). A similar but not identical disorder was named "arachnodactyly" by Achard[1] in 1902; Marfan had used the simile "pattes d'araignée," that is, spider legs. Marfan's patient, Gabrielle P, was 5½ years of age at the time of the original report[298] and 11½ years of age at the time of the follow-up report by Méry and Babonneix.[323] The latter authors commented on Gabrielle's scoliosis, which was studied by the method introduced by Wilhelm Röntgen in the same year that Marfan's report was published. Gabrielle also had fibrous contractures of the fingers, but no ocular or cardiac abnormality was noted. Méry and Babonneix[323] used the denomination "hypercondroplasie," a term also used by Rubin[411] (in its anglicized form). In suggesting the designation "hyperchondroplasia," they had the contrast with achondroplasia specifically in mind. It is possible that Marfan's patient had congenital contractural arachnodactyly[29,218] rather than the disorder that currently bears Marfan's name. It has also been suggested that the condition documented by Achard[1] was yet another autonomous

*Antoine Bernard-Jean Marfan (1858-1942), Parisian professor of pediatrics, did much to establish pediatrics as a specialty in France and elsewhere. He was the author of several widely read textbooks and monographs on pediatric topics and editor of "Le Nourrisson" for many years.

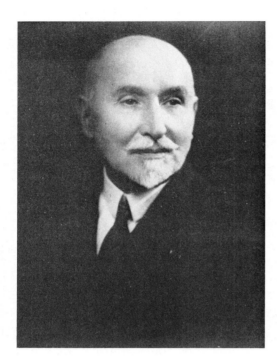

Fig. 3-1. Marfan. (Courtesy Académie de Médecine, Paris.)

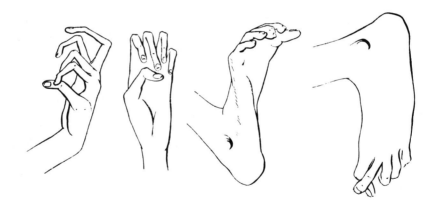

Fig. 3-2. Arachnodactyly in Marfan's case. (From Marfan AB: *Bull Mém Soc Med Hôp Paris* 13:220, 1896.)

entity. In any event, the Marfan eponym is firmly established and best left alone; there is little doubt that any attempt at semantic purity would engender great confusion.

Salle[415] in 1912 reported necropsy observations in a 2½-month-old infant who died of cardiac symptoms and showed generalized dilation of the heart and a patent foramen ovale. Changes in the mitral leaflets were also found. In 1914 Boerger[51,52] first clearly related ectopia lentis to the other manifestations. Vague references to cases of what was cer-

tainly this syndrome can be found in medical reports antedating the definitive descriptions. For instance, Williams,[518] an ophthalmologist in Cincinnati, in 1876 described ectopia lentis in a brother and sister who were exceptionally tall and had been loose-jointed from birth. Inasmuch as both Marfan's patient and Achard's patients seem not to have had the Marfan syndrome, Williams' report was many years ahead of its time.

In 1931 Weve[514] first clearly demonstrated the heritable nature of the syndrome and its transmis-

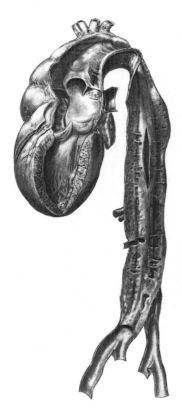

Fig. 3-3. An early reported case of dissecting aneurysm in a patient who in retrospect appears to have had the Marfan syndrome. In 1909 MacCallum reported from The Johns Hopkins Hospital the case of "L.R., Negro, aged 30 . . . slender built." The man had been seen 1 year before death, at which time signs of aortic regurgitation were present. The patient was described in life as having a congenital umbilical hernia. A difference in the radial pulse rates was noted by Dr. Thomas McCrae. Dissecting aneurysm was not suspected, however, by Osler, Rufus Cole, and the other physicians who examined him. There was paralysis of the left recurrent laryngeal nerve. The mother and several brothers had died, as well as the patient's only child, who died at the age of 2 years. No definitely corroboratory features of the family history were recorded, however, and no note of ocular abnormality was made. The ascending aorta, as shown here, resembles that seen in Fig. 3-27. Furthermore, the pronounced dilation in the region of the sinuses of Valsalva suggests the Marfan syndrome. (From MacCallum WG: *Bull Hopkins Hosp* 20:9, 1909.)

sion as a dominant trait. Furthermore, he conceived of this syndrome as a disorder of mesenchymal tissues and accordingly designated it *dystrophia mesodermalis congenita, typus Marfanis.*

Two of the major cardiovascular complications, namely aortic dilation and dissecting aneurysm, were first clearly described in 1943 by Baer, Tau-

ssig, and Oppenheimer[20] and by Etter and Glover,[147] respectively. Again, although earlier reports of the aortic complications can be discovered[65] (Fig. 3-3), these later authors first drew attention to them and opened the way for clearer recognition of the internal medical complications of this syndrome in adults.

It is difficult to imagine a better description of the Marfan syndrome than that given by Bronson and Sutherland[65] in 1918 in a report of a 6-year-old child with an aneurysm of the ascending aorta, which ruptured into the pericardium: "The unusual shape of his head and ears and the looseness of his joints attracted attention early in infancy." An inguinal hernia was repaired surgically when the patient was 2 years of age, and a left diaphragmatic hernia was discovered by radiographic examination. He was always undernourished but was sensitive and mentally advanced for his age, with a quaint way of expressing himself and a "sense of humor of his own." The forehead was high and full, the palate highly arched. The ears were large and without the normal folds of the pinnae. The joints were lax, the limbs were flaillike, and the elbows showed definite subluxation. Lordosis and pigeon breast were present; an increased prominence was evident in the right side of the chest, which showed better expansion than the left side. A pulsating mass was discernible to the right of the sternum. Although no diastolic murmur was mentioned, the left ventricle was found to be hypertrophied at autopsy. Partial coarctation proximal to the left subclavian artery was also present. The authors presented a detailed review of reports made previously; many of these concern reasonably clear instances of the Marfan syndrome.

Gordon[192] and Schwartz[433] have suggested that Abraham Lincoln had the Marfan syndrome.[412] Both based the impression in part on Lincoln's long extremities and on statements of his contemporaries that he was unusually loose-jointed. Nathaniel Hawthorne described him as a "tall, loose-jointed figure." The Washington correspondent of the London "Times" described Lincoln as a "tall, lank, lean man, considerably over six feet in height, with stooping shoulders, long pendulous arms terminating in hands of extraordinary dimensions, which, however, were far exceeded in proportion by his feet." Lincoln's mother, Nancy Hanks, who in the opinion of Gordon[192] had the Marfan syndrome, was of unknown paternity. (Her death is more usually attributed to "milk sickness," hypoglycemia caused by milk from cows that have fed on white snakeroot). On the other hand, Schwartz[433] thought he had evidence that Lincoln inherited the Marfan syndrome from his father; Schwartz also knew a patient named Lincoln with seemingly typical Marfan syndrome who was a descendant of Lincoln's grandfather. Because of the obvious general interest, the conclusions of Gordon and Schwartz found their way into the lay press.* Considerable debate followed, although the question of whether Lincoln had the Marfan syndrome remained unresolved.

In 1991 the announcement of the discovery of the locus of the Marfan syndrome gene prompted the reopening of the question as to whether Abraham Lincoln had the Marfan syndrome. In the light of the availability of new technologies and the belief that the cause of the Marfan syndrome had been found, a request to examine some of Lincoln's tissues was made to the National Museum of Medicine. Approval for such studies was granted, and researchers are now addressing the logistic and technical hurdles inherent in examining small fragments of bone or blood stains. With some luck the issue of Abraham Lincoln and the Marfan syndrome will finally be put to rest by means of these investigations.[318]

No historical survey of the Marfan syndrome would be complete without mention of its most important historian. Dr. Victor McKusick has made massive contributions to the understanding and development of concepts concerning the disorder. These include the cataloging of the early literature and the description of the natural history, especially in relation to the cardiovascular system.[315,317] McKusick was responsible for recognizing pleiotropism and demonstrating the intrafamilial variability of ectopia lentis. He also recognized genetic heterogeneity, mainly with respect to homocystinuria. These contributions are further discussed in the pertinent sections of this chapter.

In 1991 McKusick provided an excellent resume of the Marfan syndrome in the journal "Nature." In particular, he gave overviews of the elucidation of the basic defect and the current status of diagnosis. He also summarized the arguments and ethical issues relating to Abraham Lincoln and the disorder.[318]

By 1972, when the fourth edition of this book was published, the manifestations and natural history of the Marfan syndrome had been well documented. Autosomal dominant inheritance was established, but the questions of phenotypic boundaries and possible heterogeneity remained unresolved. Similarly the pathologic features had been comprehensively studied, although the basic defect was still unknown. The next 20 years witnessed unremitting efforts by numerous researchers to elucidate the basic defect. The race to find the locus of the Marfan syndrome gene and to identify its product intensified, but the cause of this disorder remained elusive until 1990, when a dramatic series of breakthroughs resolved this seemingly intractable problem. (An account of the events leading up to the detection of the fundamental defect in this syndrome is given later in this chapter in the section, Pathology.)

CLINICAL MANIFESTATIONS
General Features

The primary manifestations of the Marfan syndrome involve three major systems: the skeletal system (where the hallmark is excessive length of

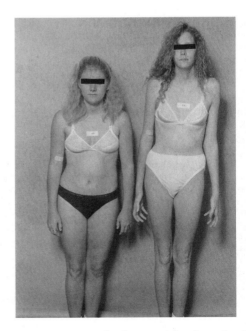

Fig. 3-4. Sisters, one of whom, *right*, has the Marfan syndrome. The affected sister is 13 years of age; her unaffected sib is 15 years of age. (Courtesy Terry Cue and Dr. Bruce McManus, Cardiovascular Registry, The University of Nebraska Medical Center, Omaha.)

Newsweek, June 11, 1962.

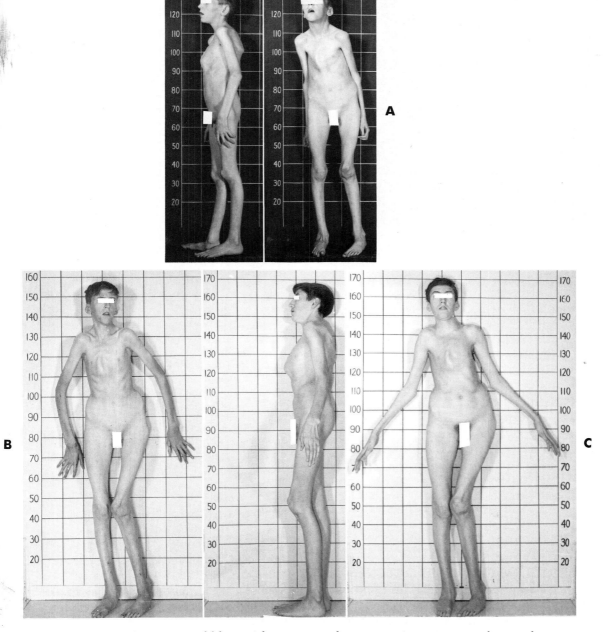

Fig. 3-5. A, Seven-year-old boy with pronounced pectus carinatum, normal mentality, nystagmus, bilateral ectopia lentis, "rocker-bottom" feet, and sparse subcutaneous fat. Photograph taken August 1954. **B,** Same patient as shown in **A.** Photograph taken August 1958. **C,** Same patient as shown in **A** and **B.** Photograph taken November 1960.

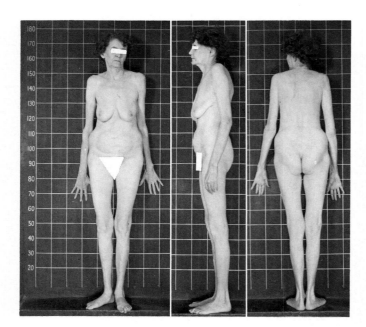

Fig. 3-6. A woman with Marfan syndrome shown at 53 years of age.

the limbs (Fig. 3-4), as well as loose-jointedness, scoliosis, and anterior chest deformity) (Figs. 3-5 and 3-6); the eye (where the hallmark is ectopia lentis, although myopia and retinal detachment also occur); and the cardiovascular system (in particular, a defect in the tunica media of the ascending aorta, which leads to aortic dilation and dissecting aneurysm). Pleiotropic manifestations such as hernia and dural ectasia have also been recognized in other systems. Wide variability from case to case, even in a single family, is the rule, and definitive diagnosis can be difficult. This problem was addressed by a committee of clinical experts, and in 1986 the criteria for the clinical diagnosis of the Marfan syndrome were promulgated in the Berlin nosology[36] (see the box on p. 57).

Skeletal Aspects

Facies and habitus. The bones of the skull and face are affected, with resulting dolichocephaly; highly arched palate; long, narrow face; and prognathism. Craniofacial manifestations of the Marfan syndrome are listed in Table 3-1. (That a palate is highly arched is a subjective statement. Methods for palate measurement are available.[257,367,389,395,438] The gothic palate is not specific to the Marfan syndrome and may be present in isolation or as a component of other disorders

Table 3-1. Craniofacial manifestations of the Marfan syndrome

Manifestation	Frequency (%)
Dolichocephaly	65
High palatal vault	60-75
Long, narrow dental arch	60
Retrognathism	37
Prognathism	30
External ear abnormality	25
Cleft palate	2.5

From Poole AE: *Birth Defects Original Article Series* 25(4):73-81, 1989.

such as myotonic dystrophy or nemaline myopathy.)

Dolichomorphism is the characteristic skeletal abnormality of the Marfan syndrome. The extremities are long, the lower-segment (LS) (pubis-to-sole) measurement is in excess of the upper-segment (US) (pubis-to-vertex) measurement, and the arm span (fingertip-to-fingertip) is in excess of height. In general the more distal bones of the extremities tend to demonstrate this excess length most strikingly, and arachnodactyly is the result. Skeletal proportions are more important than actual height. Affected persons are often extremely

Diagnostic Manifestations of the Marfan Syndrome*

Skeletal

Anterior chest deformity, especially asymmetric pectus excavatum or carinatum
Dolichostenomelia
Arachnodactyly
Vertebral column deformity
  Scoliosis
  Thoracic lordosis or reduced thoracic kyphosis
Tall stature, especially when compared to stature of unaffected first-degree relatives
High, narrowly arched palate and dental crowding
Protrusio acetabuli
Abnormal appendicular joint mobility
  Congenital flexion contractures
  Hypermobility

Ocular

Ectopia lentis[†]
Flat cornea
Elongated globe
Retinal detachment
Myopia

Cardiovascular

Dilation of ascending aorta[†]
Aortic dissection[†]
Aortic regurgitation
Mitral regurgitation resulting from mitral valve prolapse
Calcification of mitral annulus
Mitral valve prolapse
Abdominal aortic aneurysm
Arrhythmia
Endocarditis

Pulmonary

Spontaneous pneumothorax
Apical bleb

Skin and integument

Striae distensae
Inguinal hernia
Other hernia (umbilical, diaphragmatic, or incisional)

Central nervous system

Dural ectasia[†]
Lumbosacral meningocele
Dilated cisterna magna
Learning disability (verbal-performance discrepancy)
Hyperactivity

Genetics: Autosomal dominant inheritance; 25% to 30% of cases are sporadic; paternal-age effect
Requirements for diagnosis in absence of an unequivocally affected first-degree relative: Involvement of at least two systems; at least one major manifestation preferred, depending somewhat on family's phenotype; urine amino acid analysis in absence of pyridoxine supplementation confirms absence of homocystinuria

From Beighton P et al: *Am J Med Genet* 29:581-594, 1988.
*Listed in approximate decreasing order of specificity.
†Major manifestation.

tall: one patient was 6 feet tall at the age of 12 years,[77] and an adult was 7 feet tall.[516] It has been proposed that as indices of arachnodactyly the hand-height ratio should be greater than 11% and the foot-height ratio greater than 15%.[516] Furthermore, it is stated that the length of the fingers, especially the middle finger, should be 1½ times greater than the length of the metacarpal. Great overlap with the normal proportions exists; therefore these indices represent diagnostic indicators

rather than pathognomonic criteria. More significance can be attached to measurements if they are particularly abnormal or if they differ from those in other members of the family.

The ratio of US to LS is an index of some value. The LS is measured from the top of the pubic symphysis to the floor. The US is derived by subtracting this value from the height. As indicated by the illustration provided by Stratz[461] in 1902 (Fig. 3-7), the legs grow faster than the trunk during

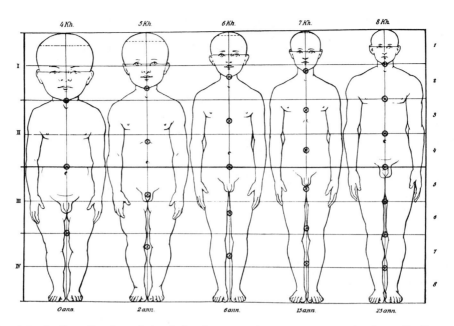

Fig. 3-7. Ordinarily the adult skeletal proportions are not attained until after puberty. There is evidence that the body proportions (as indicated by US/LS ratio) are different now from those at the turn of the century, when this diagram was made, and that the pattern differs in whites and blacks. (From Stratz CH: *Der Körper des Kindes*, Stuttgart, 1902, Ferdinand Enke.)

postnatal life. As a result the midportion of the body moves progressively downward. The US/LS ratio is roughly 0.93 in the normal white adult, having been higher in the prepubertal period (Fig. 3-7). The individual born with the Marfan syndrome tends to have an abnormally low US/LS ratio in infancy. Furthermore, he or she passes more rapidly through the sequence shown in Stratz's drawing, overshoots the mark, and eventually attains a US/LS ratio in the vicinity of 0.85. Growth curves for males and females with the Marfan syndrome are shown in Fig. 3-8.

The dip in the US/LS ratio at the stage of puberty, with subsequent slight rise, is noteworthy,[458] and if puberty is delayed, the dip may be even more striking. In the Marfan syndrome the occurrence of kyphoscoliosis with shortening of the trunk also reduces the segment ratio; in this way both trunk shortening and extremity lengthening are collaborating in producing the low segment ratio. Although the US/LS ratio is widely used in the assessment of skeletal proportions in the Marfan syndrome, Pyeritz et al.[382] have found the accuracy of these measurements to be some-

times questionable. An alternative index based on the ratio of sitting height to sitting length also has been proposed but subsequently abandoned.[319]

Sinclair, Kitchin, and Turner[445] suggested the metacarpal index as an objective indication of arachnodactyly. In the radiograph of the right hand the length (in millimeters) of the second, third, fourth, and fifth metacarpals is measured. At the exact midpoint of each shaft the breadth is also measured, and this value is divided into the length. The figures for the four metacarpals are averaged. The metacarpal index, then, is the average ratio of length to breadth of the second through fifth metacarpals. It is doubtful whether the metacarpal index is any more specific than the US/LS ratio or the ratio of the arm span to height, and the index is now rarely used in the diagnostic evaluation of the Marfan syndrome.

Spine. Spinal malalignment, notably scoliosis or kyphoscoliosis, sometimes with a significant anteroposterior curvature, occurs in 30% to 60% of persons with the Marfan syndrome (Fig. 3-9). This abnormality is variable, but some individuals

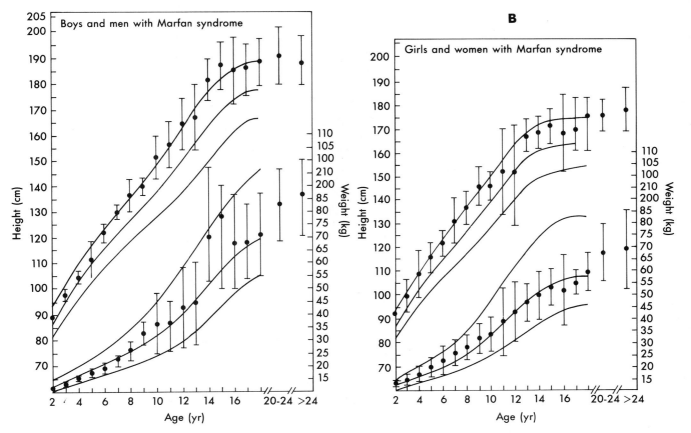

Fig. 3-8. Growth in the Marfan syndrome. Plots of height and weight versus age in, **A,** boys and men and, **B,** girls and women who did not receive treatment with hormones. Both cross-sectional and longitudinal data of approximately 200 white patients were used in construction of these preliminary curves. The points show the mean age for persons grouped in 1-year intervals, and the bars show standard deviation of plus or minus 1. The curved lines show the fifth, fiftieth, and ninety-fifth percentiles of the unaffected population. (From Pyeritz RE. In Emery AH, Rimoin DL, editors: *Principles and practices of medical genetics*, vol 2, New York, 1990, Churchill Livingstone, pp 1047-1063.)

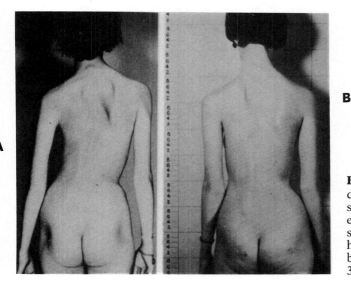

Fig. 3-9. A, Fourteen-year-old girl with the Marfan syndrome and thoracic scoliosis. Prominence of the right scapula and mild right thoracic rib-hump deformity are evident. **B,** Back view of the patient at 17 years of age, showing marked improvement of malalignment that had occurred with management with a Milwaukee brace. (From Robins PR: *J Bone Joint Surg* 57(A):358-368, 1975.)

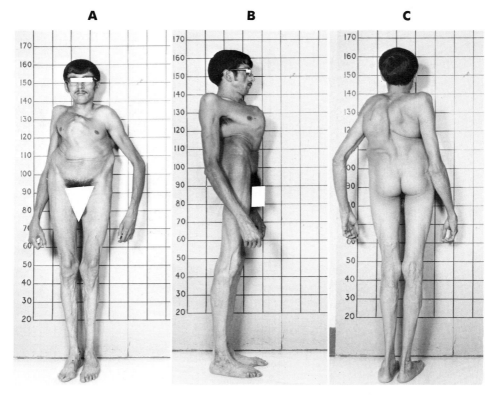

Fig. 3-10. Severe scoliosis in a 29-year-old man with the Marfan syndrome. The man is only 63 inches tall, and a low US/LS value is evident in **A, B,** and **C.** He has bilateral slight upward displacement of the lenses, marked striae distensae of both thighs, bilateral varicosities of the leg veins, and pes planus, with contractures of the toes.

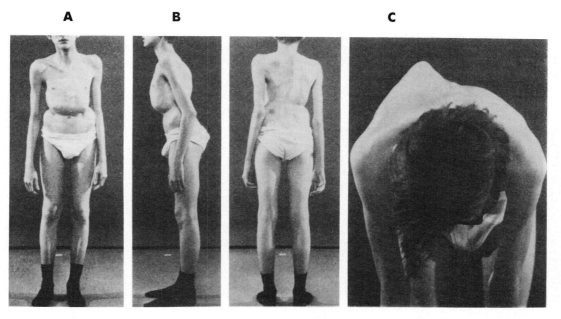

Fig. 3-11. A, A seventeen-year-old boy with Marfan syndrome, scoliosis, and back pain. Previous treatment included use of a Milwaukee brace. **B,** Deformity of the thorax. **C,** Posterior views showing scoliosis and rib-hump deformity. (From Robins PR: *J Bone Joint Surg* 57(A):358-368, 1975.)

are severely affected and the prognosis of scoliosis in the Marfan syndrome has been reported to be worse than that of idiopathic scoliosis.[46,81] In a retrospective study of 45 patients with well-documented Marfan syndrome, 60% had scoliosis with a mean age of onset of 8.8 years.[402] In these persons 48% had double right thoracic–left lumbar curves and 33% had right thoracic spinal malalignment. Birch and Herring[46] reported that in their series of 14 patients with spinal deformities and the Marfan syndrome the scoliosis curve patterns observed are similar to those of idiopathic scoliosis, whereas Robins, Moe, and Winter[402] disagreed, noting that double curves are more common in "Marfan scoliosis" than in idiopathic scoliosis.

Thoracic kyphosis is associated with pulmonary deficiencies, including reduced vital capacity and residual volume[296] (Fig. 3-10). In rare instances hemivertebra is responsible in part for spinal deformity.[291] At times the spinal deformity has been thought to be due to Scheuermann disease.[297] Scoliosis is likely to increase rapidly during the years of maximal vertebral growth, from 11 to 15 years of age. Early recognition of scoliosis is assisted by examining the patient in a "bending forward" position. This maneuver renders asymmetry more obvious because of angulation of the ribs on one side[396] (Fig. 3-11). When the deformity is still slight, much can be accomplished by means of exercise and other measures.

The spinal canal is often enlarged in depth or width, or both.[343] Fishman et al.[161] examined five Marfan patients by means of computed tomography (CT) and observed an enlarged central sacral canal, ectasia of neural foramina, and sacral erosion in each instance. This feature, which is termed "dural ectasia," is now regarded as a valuable diagnostic pointer (Figs. 13-12 to 13-14). An exaggeration of the normally slight concavity of the dorsal aspect of the vertebral bodies, termed "scalloping," has been described in the Marfan syndrome, but this feature is of no pathologic significance.[343,519]

Articular hypermobility. Ligamentous laxity and joint hypermobility are common in the Marfan syndrome. Redundancy and "weakness" of joint capsules, ligaments, tendons, and fasciae are responsible for a large group of manifestations, including pes planus; genu recurvatum; recurrent dislocation of hips,[197] patella,[354] clavicles, mandi-

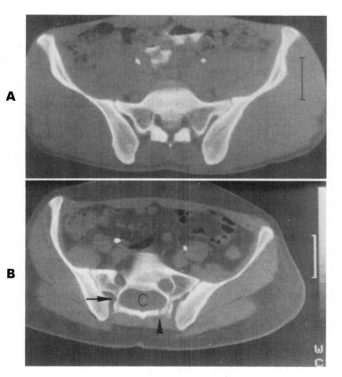

Fig. 3-12. Computed tomogram of the first sacral vertebra (S1) in young men with the Marfan syndrome. **A,** No evidence of dural ectasia in a 26-year-old. **B,** The neural canal, *C,* is widened, and the pedicles, *arrow,* and laminae, *arrowhead,* are thinned in a 30-year-old. The bars indicate 5 cm in both cases. (From Pyeritz RE et al: *Am J Hum Genet* 43:726-732, 1988.)

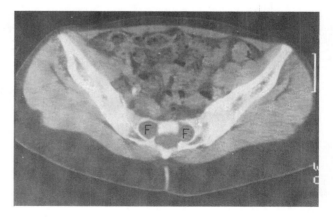

Fig. 3-13. Computed tomogram of the S2-3 vertebral level in a 27-year-old woman with the Marfan syndrome. The neural foramina, *F,* are markedly widened, and the cortex of the pedicles and laminae is eroded. The bar indicates 5 cm. (From Pyeritz RE et al: *Am J Hum Genet* 43:726-732, 1988.)

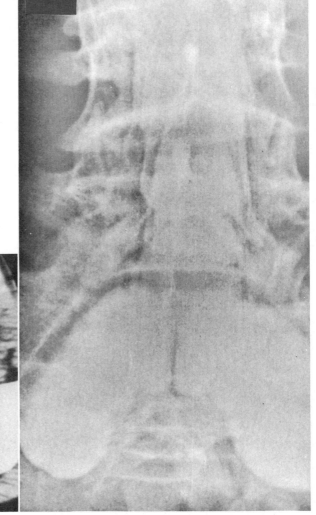

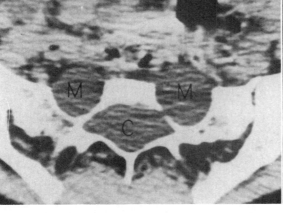

Fig. 3-14. Severe dural ectasia and anterior meningoceles in a 29-year-old woman with the Marfan syndrome. **A,** Computed tomogram of the pelvis at L5 vertebral level, showing marked enlargement of the neural canal, *C,* and two intrapelvic cysts (meningoceles), *M,* with absorbencies characteristic of water, which appear to emanate from the neural foramina. **B,** A metrizamide myelogram showing that the intrapelvic cysts communicate with the subarachnoid space. (From Pyeritz RE et al: *Am J Hum Genet* 43:726-732, 1988.)

ble,[331] and other joints; ganglia; hernias; synovial diverticula; and kyphoscoliosis.

The "flat feet" may be so advanced that the medial malleolus almost literally rests on the floor. Much less commonly a pes cavus deformity is present.[520] The relatively narrow palm of the hand, together with a long thumb and loose-joint-edness, is the basis of the Steinberg thumb sign[454] (Fig. 3-15). (This sign is positive when the thumb opposed across the palm extends well beyond the ulnar margin of the hand.) Feingold[157] found the "thumb sign" positive in 1.1% of normal white children and 2.7% of normal black children. It was negative in children with homocystinuria. A simi-

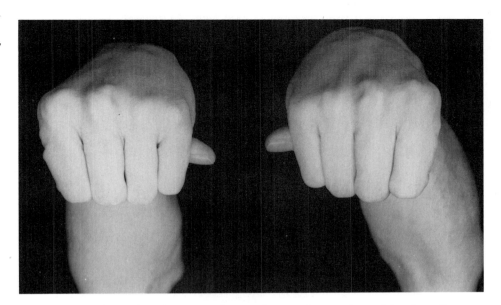

Fig. 3-15. Steinberg thumb sign in the Marfan syndrome. A combination of narrow hand, long digits, and loose-jointedness permits the thumb to extend well beyond the ulnar surface of the hand when held as shown.

lar indicator, the wrist sign,[508] reflects both the thin wrist and the long digits: the thumb and fifth finger, when clasped around the wrist, usually overlap appreciably in a person with the Marfan syndrome (Fig. 3-16).

At times the great toes are elongated out of proportion to the others[8,153,343,484] (Fig. 3-17). This occurrence may be related to the terminal center of ossification, which normally appears somewhat earlier in the metatarsus of the hallux than in that of the other toes. (The long bones of the hands and feet usually grow only or predominantly from one terminus. The first metatarsal has a proximal epiphyseal junction, whereas the epiphysis is distal in the other metatarsals—another point of difference in development of the first and other toes.) Hallux valgus and contractures of the toes (i.e., hammer toes) are frequent. "Spurring" of the heels may be present as a result of excessive length of the os calcis.

Thorax. The ribs participate in the excessive longitudinal growth with formation of pectus excavatum ("funnel chest") (Fig. 3-18, *A*), pectus carinatum ("pigeon breast") (Fig. 3-18, *B*), or less symmetric varieties of thoracic cage deformity. Pectus excavatum is a common defect occurring in eight of every 1000 live births.[424] Approximately

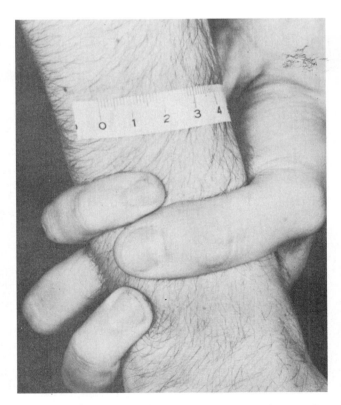

Fig. 3-16. Walker-Murdoch wrist sign in the Marfan syndrome. The combination of thin wrist and long digits results in overlap of the first and fifth fingers when the wrist is grasped as shown.

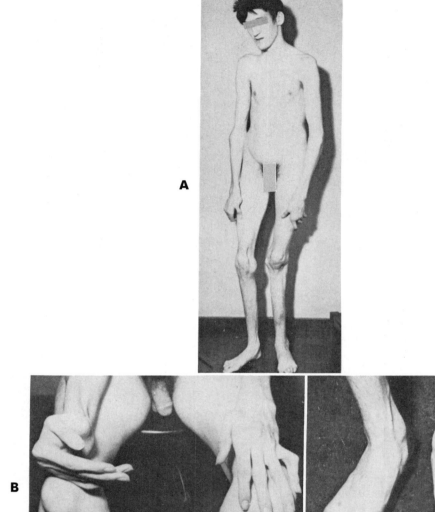

Fig. 3-17. Seventeen-year-old patient who died suddenly at home 18 months after photograph was taken. The patient was moderately crippled by the skeletal abnormality. Pain in the joints, especially in the knees, seemed to be related to the loosejointedness. The patient had ectopia lentis and was referred because of spontaneous retinal detachment. **A,** General view. **B,** Striking arachnodactyly with partial contractures of fingers. **C,** Extraordinary length of the great toes is well demonstrated.

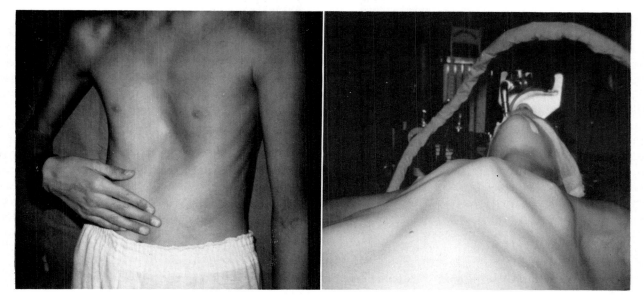

Fig. 3-18. A, Pectus excavatum in a 7-year-old boy. **B,** Pectus carinatum in a 12-year-old girl. (From Ellis DG: *Pediatr Ann* 18:161-165, 1989.)

two thirds of Marfan patients have this chest wall deformity; therefore it is imperative to consider the Marfan syndrome when a child with pectus excavatum is evaluated.[379,424] In fact, in one third of a series of patients reviewed by Arn et al.[16] the diagnosis of Marfan syndrome was made after initial pectus excavatum repair. Arn et al.[16] compared surgical repair for pectus excavatum in 28 patients with the Marfan syndrome and 30 persons with isolated pectus excavatum. They noted recurrence of the abnormality in 11 of 28 patients with the Marfan syndrome and concluded that this problem was associated with initial surgery at a young age and with the specific type of surgical procedure. The condition recurred from 3 months to 5 years after initial repair. By contrast, only two of 30 patients without the Marfan syndrome had a recurrence of pectus excavatum. These investigators also measured the ratio of the "narrowest anteroposterior diameter of the chest" to "maximum transverse diameter" and found that the ratio was smaller in Marfan patients, indicating that the severity of the defect was greater in Marfan patients. The thoracic abnormality can compromise pulmonary function by reducing lung capacity and may be severe enough to restrict exercise. After surgical repair, tolerance to exercise may increase.[190]

Other musculoskeletal features. Sinclair[444] documented complaints of a musculoskeletal nature of sufficient severity to warrant medical attention in 20 of 40 individuals with the Marfan syndrome. Of the 20 patients, seven had low back pain and two of these were at first considered to have ankylosing spondylitis. In five persons there were joint effusions; of these, three had been misdiagnosed as having tuberculosis, one as having rheumatic fever, and one as having rheumatoid arthritis. Hip joint pain was severe in two individuals, and metatarsalgia was prominent in three patients. Precocious osteoarthrosis tends to develop in individuals with joint hypermobility of any cause but is not a conspicuous feature of the Marfan syndrome. Acetabular protrusion[156,263,513] is a fairly common manifestation of the Marfan syndrome and occurs in approximately 50% of patients. This abnormality is often associated with scoliosis and may be more frequent in women and girls.

Muscular underdevelopment and hypotonia are frequent[152,481] but by no means invariable. In some instances, however, these features have been so striking as to suggest a primary disorder of muscle. It is probable that the muscular manifestations in the Marfan syndrome result from the abnormality of bones and joints and from abnormality of the perimysial connective tissue and are not due to primary involvement of the muscle cell itself. This view is supported by the finding of a normal creatinine coefficient, which is an index of total muscle mass.[487]

Pronounced sparsity of subcutaneous fat is a striking feature in most affected persons and is not easily reconciled with a fundamental defect of connective tissue. In children it is possible that the rapid growth accounts for the failure to store fat. One patient who was thin as a child became exceedingly obese in early middle age, in large part as a result of inactivity associated with blindness produced by bilateral retinal detachment.

It has been suggested that bone age in the Marfan syndrome is in advance of chronologic age and that the epiphyses tend to close earlier than normal.[499] In the patients studied by McKusick no marked deviation in bone age was observed, although no systematic controlled observations were undertaken. It is certain, however, that the excess length of the legs is not due to delayed closure of the epiphyses. Indeed, the excess limb length is often demonstrable at birth and throughout childhood and adolescence.

The Eye

Ectopia lentis, almost always bilateral, is the hallmark of ocular involvement in this syndrome[9,225,397,459] (Fig. 3-19). The zonules (suspensory ligaments), when visualized with the slit lamp, are redundant, attenuated, and often broken (Fig. 3-20). The lower ligaments are more likely to be defective. Upward displacement of the lens is the usual finding. Although early reports suggested that Marfan patients had abnormally small, spheric lenses,[160,287,288] more recent observations suggest that most lenses are of normal size and shape.[308] Iridodonesis (i.e., tremor of the iris) is often a tip-off to the presence of dislocation of the lens. Occasionally the edge of the dislocated lens is visible through the undilated pupil, or there may be complete dislocation of the lens into the anterior chamber. To exclude minor subluxation, it is necessary to dilate the pupil fully and perform a slit lamp examination. When complete or almost complete detachment of the lens occurs, the patient can move the lens about voluntarily[113] by changing the position of the head.

A perspective of the relative frequency of the various causes of ectopia lentis can be obtained from the observations of Jarrett,[241] who reviewed

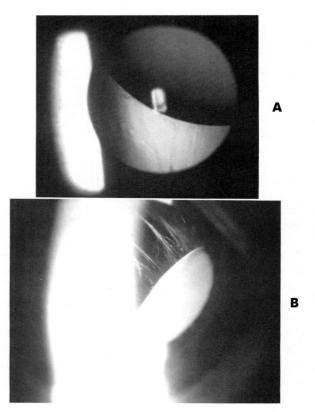

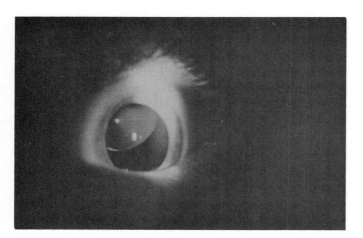

Fig. 3-19. Upward and temporal displacement of the lens in the Marfan syndrome. (Courtesy Dr. Béla Varga, Eger, Hungary.)

Fig. 3-20. Irregular arrangement of broken zonular fibers, which are in part matted on lens surface. (Eyes are from unrelated patients.) **A,** Lens is dislocated temporally upward, and, **B,** lens is dislocated temporally downward. (Courtesy Dr. Irene H. Maumenee. From *Trans Am Ophthalmol Soc* 79:684-733, 1981.)

166 patients with ectopia lentis who were admitted to hospital. These included 24 instances of the Marfan syndrome, two of homocystinuria and two of the Weill-Marchesani syndrome. The most frequent cause of lens dislocation was trauma, which accounted for 85 cases.

At one time it was conventional wisdom that the majority of persons with the Marfan syndrome had ectopia lentis, but it is now accepted that only about 50% to 80% have this abnormality. Indeed, McKusick's demonstration that ectopia lentis could be present in some affected family members and absent in other close relatives was fundamental to his elaboration of the concept of pleiotropism in the disorder. In Maumenee's series,[308] 60.3% of Marfan patients had dislocation of the lenses that occurred in all directions; the most common (77%) was upward, a direction never seen in persons with homocystinuria.[109] Lens dislocation may be progressive, and participation in contact sports is contraindicated in patients with the Marfan syndrome because of increased risks of retinal detachment.[308] The cardiovascular aspects of the disorder represent further reasons for discouraging involvement in contact sports.[329]

Lens surgery is indicated in the case of lens opacities and when the lens is in contact with the corneal epithelium. Imminent complete luxation of the lens is an additional indication. Dislocation of the lens into the vitreous cavity has been well tolerated by some patients for years; in some instances, however, glaucoma has developed.[308]

In a study of visual acuity in a series of 151 Marfan patients, 70.5% of all eyes tested had a Snellen visual acuity of better than 20/40 and 89% were measured at better than 20/200.[308] Myopia is usually present in a high degree. A large globe has been noted almost universally in persons with the Marfan syndrome,[505] as has an increase in corneal diameter. Megalocornea is often impressive to the unaided eye (Fig. 3-21). Marfan patients have flatter corneas than normal,[304,308] and those with ectopia lentis have even flatter corneas than do patients without this feature.[308] The spherophakia may be the result of lack of the normal tension on the lens by the zonules. By gonioscopy von Noorden and Schultz[503] detected changes in the angle of the anterior chamber of the eye, including bridging pectinate strands, iris processes, and irregularity of the iris root (Fig. 3-22). These findings are not specific for the Marfan syndrome, since they have been found in a variety of conditions that may be construed as connective tissue disorders.[72] These include severe idiopathic scoliosis, idiopathic genu varum, Legg-Perthes disease, slipped upper femoral epiphyses, and Osgood-Schlatter disease.[72] When the angle changes are extreme in the Marfan syndrome, they may lead to glaucoma.[70]

Blue sclera have been recorded in the Marfan syndrome,[49] but this is probably a chance concomitant or the end of the normal spectrum of scleral color. Clouding of the cornea occurs occasionally; this is not, however, a primary element of the connective tissue disease but rather a result of the secondary iritis and glaucoma.

Spontaneous retinal detachment[336] occurs in an unusually high incidence and represents an important complication of lens extraction. In a group of Marfan patients, Jarrett[241] found eight eyes in which retinal detachment occurred before lens extraction and only three in which it occurred (all within 3 months) after lens extraction. Maumenee,[308] who studied a series of 160 persons with

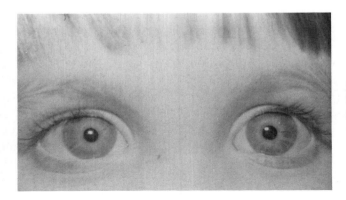

Fig. 3-21. Megalocornea and slight ectopia of pupils. (Courtesy Dr. Irene H. Maumenee. From *Trans Am Ophthalmol Soc* 79:684-733, 1981.)

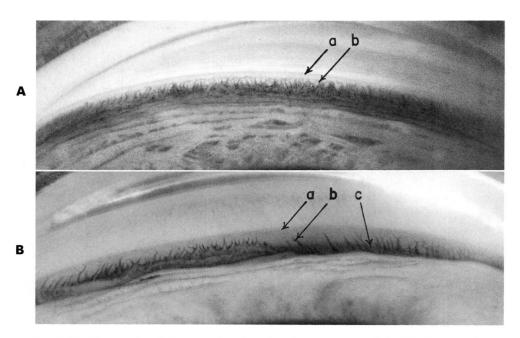

Fig. 3-22. The angle of the anterior chamber in two cases of the Marfan syndrome with ectopia lentis: *a*, Schwalbe's line; *b*, pectinate ligaments; *c*, ciliary body band. **A** and **B,** Pectinate strands as described by von Noorden and Schultz[503] are evident. **B,** Irregular insertion of the peripheral iris can be seen. (Courtesy Dr. Gunter K. von Noorden, Baltimore.)

the Marfan syndrome, commented that the high percentage of patients with retinal detachment in Jarrett's group may indicate that the sample was biased, since hospital admission of these persons was for dislocated lenses. In another series[336] nine of 142 patients with juvenile retinal detachment had the Marfan syndrome. These nine individuals with retinal detachment also had dislocated lenses. Retinal detachment is probably related in part to the myopic eyeball, therefore, indirectly, to the connective tissue defect; that there is a more direct relationship is strongly suspected[234] because of the high incidence of retinal detachment in persons with the Marfan syndrome, even in those with only a moderate degree of myopia. Nevertheless, no spontaneous retinal detachment has been observed in patients with normal axial length.[308] Assessment of the retinal status by fundoscopy in the Marfan syndrome may not be easily accomplished, since it is often difficult to dilate the pupil; the dilator muscle appears to be hypoplastic.[418]

Ectopia lentis per se probably causes relatively little impairment of vision. Conversely, severe myopia, retinal detachment, and the iritis or glaucoma, or both, that may result from the ectopia lentis are often responsible for severe limitations of visual acuity or even for total blindness. Lenticular cataracts may also develop as a consequence of these complications.

Cardiovascular System*

The seminal description of the cardiovascular manifestations of the Marfan syndrome and their natural history was published in 1955 by McKusick.[315] In this and subsequent articles he pointed out that aortic aneurysm in the Marfan syndrome is not congenital but develops progressively in postnatal life, sometimes not until adulthood. He also recognized that aortic dilation usually commenced in the first part of the ascending aorta and that since this region was situated within the radiographic shadow of the heart, it did not show up

---

*This section was written by Richard B. Devereux, MD.

Fig. 3-23. J.S. was born in 1964. The diagnosis of the Marfan syndrome was made at birth by the pediatrician. Right inguinal hernia was detected at 2 weeks of age and was corrected surgically at 3 months of age. Kyphoscoliosis was first noted at 1 year of age. When first seen at the hospital at 20 months of age (after two episodes of congestive heart failure), he demonstrated signs of severe Marfan syndrome: striking arachnodactyly, subluxated lenses, large anterior segments of the eyes, and mitral regurgitation. Cardiac catheterization showed mild tricuspid regurgitation, dilated pulmonary artery and aortic root without regurgitation, and severe mitral regurgitation.

The father and the mother, 33 and 30 years of age, respectively, at the patient's birth, as well as four sibs, were unaffected. The child died March 4, 1968, of heart failure at the age of 4 years. Autopsy (Dr. W.E.B. Hall) showed marked generalized cardiac enlargement, changes in the tricuspid aortic and mitral valves, and a remarkably thin-walled aorta without aneurysm (indeed, of reduced caliber). The tricuspid and mitral valves were thickened and puckered. The mitral orifice was reduced in size, suggesting mitral stenosis. The mitral chordae were thickened. The left atrium was markedly dilated, with thickening of the endocardium. The aortic valve had a peculiar cordlike thickening of the entire margin of one cusp and part of a second.

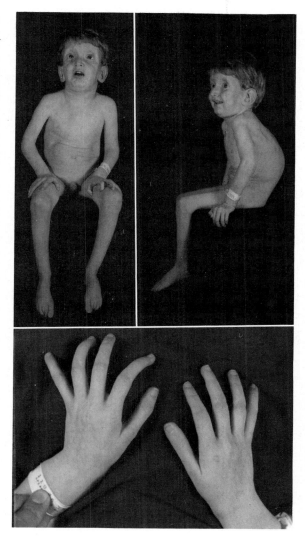

on standard films. For this reason aortic regurgitation consequent on dilation of the aortic root can occur without any recognizable abnormality in the chest radiograph. Therefore echocardiography is a powerful noninvasive technique for surveillance of the main life-threatening complication of the Marfan syndrome.

McKusick recognized that dissection of the aorta occurred against a background of progressive dilation of the aortic root and that this catastrophe did not usually occur before the diameter of the dilated root exceeded 5.5 to 6 cm. He also developed the hypothesis that expansile pulsation, especially the rate of pressure rise in the ascending aorta, is a major factor in the pathogenesis of aortic dissection. The hypothesis developed by McKusick led to the introduction of long-term therapy with beta blockers in the prophylaxis of the disorder.

The underlying abnormality of the tunica media of the great vessels in the Marfan syndrome may result in diffuse dilation of the ascending aorta or pulmonary artery, in dissecting aneurysm, in a combination of dilation and dissection, or in aneurysms of the more distal aorta and its branches. Significant involvement of the pulmonary artery occurs much less commonly than does the corresponding involvement of the aorta. Nevertheless, a clinical picture similar to that of idiopathic dilation of the pulmonary artery[250] may occur, as well as dissecting aneurysm of the pulmonary artery.[12,517]

Table 3-2. Cardiac abnormalities in the Marfan syndrome

Author	No. of patients	Age range (yr)	Mean age (yr)	Mitral study method	Mitral valve prolapse (%)	Mitral valve complication (%)	Aortic dilation (%)	Aortic regurgitation (%)	Dissection (%)
Roman et al.[404]	59	7-66	29	Echocardiography	66	7	63	22	2
Bruno et al.[67]	29	9-53	24	Echocardiography	79	—	79	48	—
Sisk et al.[446]	15	0.1-3.5	1.5	Echocardiography	100	27	100	7	0
Roberts et al.[401]	18	15-52	34	Necropsy	39	11	72	72	17
Freed et al.[170]	11	7-48	29	Echocardiography	64	—	100	—	—
Brown et al.[66]	35	3-61	21	Echocardiography	91	—	60	23	—
Spangler et al.[451]	22	0.1-51	25	Echocardiography	77	0	50	18	14
Pyeritz et al.[383]	166	0.1-22	11	Echocardiography	68	5	—	—	—
Come et al.[96]	61	8-63	29	Echocardiography	57	—	69	23	—
Chan et al.[79]	28	32-72	46	Echocardiography, radiography, auscultation	29	—	64	53	21
Marsalese et al.[302]	84	2-67	27	Echocardiography, catheterization, auscultation	—	4	—	≥55	20
Devereux et al.[126]	129	1-	—	Echocardiography	58	6	76	30	7
Pan et al.[355]	30	4-51	—	Echocardiography	83*	6	73	—	—
Sun et al.[467]	181†	2-87	—	Variable	14	8	80	33	—
Chen et al.[84]	24	0.3-16	5	Echocardiography, catheterization, phonocardiography	67	13	38	—	—
Geva et al.[177]	25	0-16	8	Echocardiography	100*	8	80	20	4
Geva et al.[178]	9	0-1.0	0.5	Echocardiography, catheterization, necropsy	100	67	100	56	—
	86	0-1.0	0.5	Echocardiography, catheterization, necropsy	96	84	86	26	—
Morse et al.[335]	22	0-0.3	—	Echocardiography	73	55	73	—	5
Phornphutkul et al.[362]	36	0-16	7	Catheterization, radiography, auscultation	—	47	28	11	3
Liang et al.[279]	52	5-63	—	Echocardiography	21	—	92	13	—

*Criteria that were used (Morganroth J et al: *Am J Cardiol* 46:1164-1177, 1980) have been shown to have low specificity (Warth DC et al: *J Am Coll Cardiol* 39:422-431, 1977, and Levine RA et al: *Circulation* 75:756-767, 1987).
†Subset of subjects in whom cardiovascular findings were present.

A later development in the understanding of the Marfan syndrome was the appreciation of the frequency and functional significance of mitral valve prolapse and mitral regurgitation. As in many other areas of medicine, knowledge of cardiovascular features of the Marfan syndrome has been advanced by developments in diagnostic methodology and by observations relating to the results of medical and surgical treatment.

Structural cardiovascular abnormalities occur in most patients with the Marfan syndrome (Table 3-2); the most common of these are aortic root dilation, mitral valve prolapse, and aortic regurgitation* (Fig. 3-23). Echocardiography has proven to be a far more sensitive technique for detecting the cardiac manifestations of the Marfan syndrome than either physical examination or chest radiography. For instance, Pyeritz and McKusick[379] reported that 48 of 50 consecutive patients (96%) had abnormal echocardiograms, whereas only 64% had pathologic murmurs or clicks. Similarly Brown et al.[66] found that 34 of 35 Marfan patients (97%) had abnormal echocardiograms, whereas auscultatory or phonocardiographic abnormalities were detected in only 54% of these individuals. Echocardiography was found to be more sensitive than chest radiography in detecting aortic dilation.[96,279] Thus echocardiographic examination has become a requisite part of the evaluation of patients with the Marfan syndrome. Other imaging techniques, including magnetic resonance imaging (MRI),† digital subtraction angiography,[122] CT,[108,450] and transesophageal echocardiography,[2,497] allow noninvasive or semiinvasive identification of abnormalities of the more distal aorta and its branches.

There has been some variability in the reported frequency of the different cardiac manifestations of the Marfan syndrome. In part, this situation reflects differences in the proportions of patients who had been referred to specific institutions because cardiac complications of the Marfan syndrome had already developed. An even more important factor is the age at which specific complications of the Marfan syndrome tend to become manifest. In series of pediatric patients with the Marfan syndrome, mitral valve prolapse and severe mitral regurgitation were the most common cardiac manifestations,* whereas among adults with the Marfan syndrome aortic root dilation, aortic regurgitation, and aortic dissection predominate.† Phornphutkul, Rosenthal, and Nadas[362] studied 36 patients with the Marfan syndrome; in most of these patients (72%) the diagnosis was made before the age of 10 years. These investigators noted that children with the least weight gain had the most severe cardiovascular disease and concluded that retarded growth might suggest extensive cardiac involvement. Although cardiovascular manifestations in childhood are usually more subtle and less severe than those in adults, they still represent the major cause of death in young patients. Five of the individuals in this series died, four as a direct result of cardiac involvement. Death of young patients with the Marfan syndrome is generally attributable to congestive heart failure, infection, or dissection and aortic rupture. In particular, mitral valve dysfunction is a major contributor to morbidity and mortality in these persons, and ventricular dysrhythmia also may be a factor.[84] It is not surprising that severely affected individuals in whom the diagnosis is made early in life are those who are at increased risk for progressive cardiac complications.

Aortic root dilation. To identify aortic root enlargement in Marfan patients, standardized measurements of aortic diameter must be compared with normal values that take into account the effects of age and body size. Nomograms reflecting these values have been developed for echocardiographic investigations[221,406,449] (Figs. 3-24 and 3-25) and can be applied approximately to measurements obtained by MRI. Accurate detection of aortic enlargement requires that diameter measurements be made perpendicularly to the axis of the aorta and its walls, at levels that can be recognized by internal landmarks (the aortic valve annulus, the sinuses of Valsalva, the sinotubular junction, and in the ascending aorta).

In general, enlargement of the aortic root in Marfan patients is most common and most marked at the level of the sinuses of Valsalva. Al-

---

*References 66, 67, 79, 84, 96, 125, 170, 177, 279, 295, 301, 334, 335, 355, 362, 364, 381, 401, 405, 446, 451, and 467.

†References 11, 62, 252, 253, 421, and 450.

---

*References 84, 177, 178, 335, 362, 381, and 446.

†References 66, 67, 79, 96, 170, 301, 401, 405, and 451.

Fig. 3-24. A, Normal confidence limits of 95% for aortic root diameter at the sinuses of Valsalva in relation to body surface area in adults younger than 40 years of age. **B,** Normal confidence limits of 95% for aortic root diameter at the supraaortic ridge in relation to body surface area in adults under 40 years of age. (From Roman MJ et al: *Am J Cardiol* 64:507-512, 1989.)

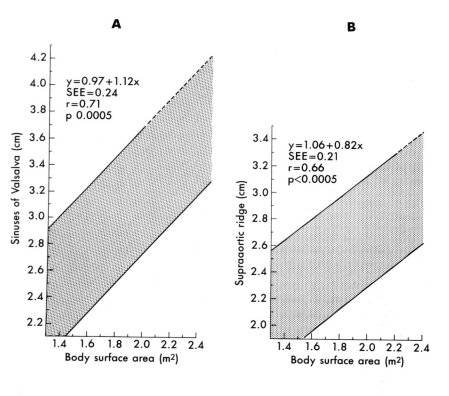

A

$y=0.97+1.12x$
$SEE=0.24$
$r=0.71$
$p\ 0.0005$

B

$y=1.06+0.82x$
$SEE=0.21$
$r=0.66$
$p<0.0005$

Fig. 3-25. A, Normal confidence limits of 95% for aortic root diameter at the sinuses of Valsalva in relation to body surface area in adults 40 years of age and older. **B,** Normal confidence limits of 95% for aortic root diameter at the supraaortic ridge in relation to body surface area in older adults. (From Roman MJ et al: *Am J Cardiol* 64:507-512, 1989.)

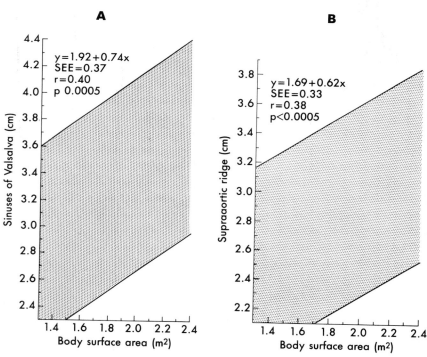

A

$y=1.92+0.74x$
$SEE=0.37$
$r=0.40$
$p\ 0.0005$

B

$y=1.69+0.62x$
$SEE=0.33$
$r=0.38$
$p<0.0005$

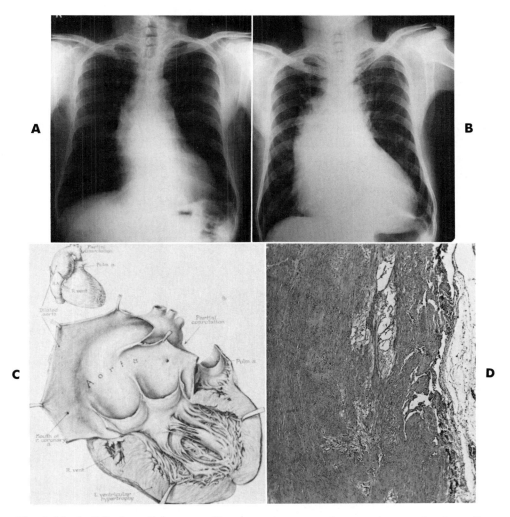

Fig. 3-26. A, Dilation of the ascending aorta is present but not impressive in radiographs made 18 months before patient's death. **B,** Radiograph made 4 months before death in the same patient. **C,** Sketch of the heart and great vessels as visualized at autopsy. Mild coarctation was present. Dilation limited to the ascending aorta and tremendous sacculation of the aortic cusps are conspicuous features. The relatively high position of the coronary ostia is evident. **D,** Histologic section obtained from the ascending aorta in same case. (From McKusick VA: *Circulation* 11:321-342, 1955.)

though the prevalence of aortic root dilation varies among reports, in series where relatively few Marfan patients have been evaluated because of severe preexisting cardiac complications, more than 50% of children (excluding severely affected infants) and approximately 70% to 80% of affected adults have had dilated aortic roots (Fig. 3-26). The age-related increase in prevalence of aortic enlargement observed in cross-sectional studies has been confirmed by the occurrence of progres-

sive aortic dilation during longitudinal follow-up studies of both children[446] and adults.[226] Aortic dilation does not develop in all affected persons, and a small percentage of patients with clear-cut Marfan syndrome maintain normal aortic diameters at least into their sixties. In some Marfan patients with dilation of the sinuses of Valsalva the aortic diameter returns to normal at and above the supraaortic ridge,[404] whereas in others the aortic enlargement extends nearly to the innominate artery or may extend further. Marfan patients who have aortic enlargement limited to the sinuses of Valsalva appear to have a lower prevalence of aortic regurgitation and a more benign short-term clinical course than do persons with more generalized aortic enlargement.[404]

Dilation of distal aortic segments and other arteries. It has long been recognized that the descending thoracic or abdominal aorta, or both, may be dilated in Marfan patients.[269,306,317,480] Isolated descending thoracic or abdominal aortic aneu-

rysms in Marfan patients may dissect,[22,265,496] rupture either freely or into the inferior vena cava,[211,219,238,266,499] or enlarge without dissection or rupture to an extent that surgery is required.* Dilation or dissection of the aortic arch or the distal aorta in Marfan patients is far less commonly encountered in clinical practice or detected by modern imaging methods than are proximal aortic abnormalities. Extensive involvement of multiple aor-

---

*References 116, 212, 233, 269, 330, and 370.

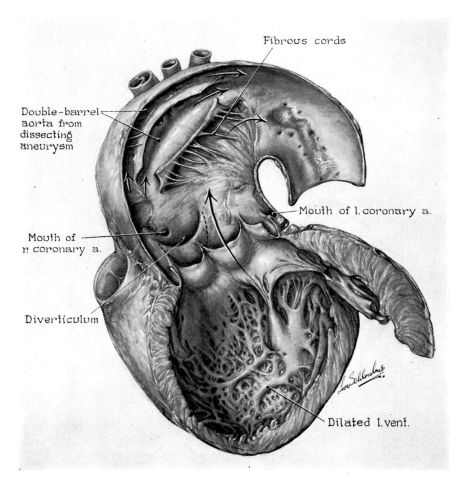

Fig. 3-27. Autopsy specimen. Chronic dissection of the ascending aorta was present. The patient died of heart failure. The drawing demonstrates three structures that might vibrate periodically, with production of a musical murmur. These are the fibrous cords that traverse the false channel, the lip of the inner tube of the double-barrel aorta, and the lip of the "diverticulum" above the sinuses of Valsalva. Why any one of these three structures should be incited in late diastole, with production of the musical murmur, is not clear. (From McKusick VA et al: *Bull Hopkins Hosp* 97:136-176, 1955.)

tic segments occurs in the most severely affected patients.[122,333]

Medium-sized arterial branches of the aorta may be involved in the Marfan syndrome, and aneurysmal dilation of the internal or external carotid arteries or of intracranial branches has been reported.[159,212,224,271,284] Dissection may extend into the carotid artery from the innominate artery or aorta[17,283] but has not been reported to arise locally. Aneurysms of the pulmonary arteries or of a patent ductus arteriosus have also been documented,[134,159,179,337] and dissection limited to the coronary arteries has been described in the Marfan syndrome.[251,314,422] Mild coarctation of the aortic isthmus is common but rarely significant.[141,499] Aneurysmal dilation or dissection of the iliac artery may occur and requires surgical management.[24,162] Ruptures of an aortic sinus of Valsalva into the right side of the heart and of dissecting aortic aneurysms into the right atrium or ventricle have been documented. Varicose veins probably occur more frequently and in more se-

vere form in the Marfan syndrome than ordinarily would be expected.[520]

Aortic dissection. The Marfan syndrome is a leading "cause" of dissecting aneurysm in persons under the age of 40 years. Dissecting aneurysm may occur as the first recognized aortic complication in Marfan patients, but the aneurysm is almost always superimposed on underlying dilation of the aortic root and, commonly, of the ascending aorta as well.[380] Dissection may occur in the first decade of life[525] or may not develop until the seventh decade. Aortic dissection usually becomes evident when the patient has severe midline pain in the front or back of the chest or abdomen, but relatively small dissections in the ascending aorta, which have apparently developed without any pain or discomfort, are often present by the time patients reach surgery for treatment of severe aortic dilation. Most aortic dissections in Marfan patients arise in the aortic root or the proximal ascending aorta and extend distally through a vari-

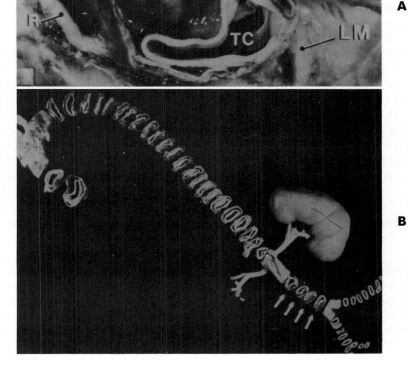

Fig. 3-28. Dissection of the entire aorta in a 33-year-old man who had been asymptomatic until 15 days before death, when he had severe chest pain and an aortogram showed dissection of the entire aorta. **A,** Aorta seen from above showing a large false channel *(FC)* and the true channel. The ostium of the right coronary artery has been completely separated from the true channel *(TC)*. **B,** Cross-section of the aorta. Thrombus is present in the false channel of the abdominal aorta, *arrows.* The aorta is not dilated. (From Roberts WC, Honig HS: *Am Heart J* 104:115-135, 1982.)

able portion of the aorta and its branches (Figs. 3-27 and 3-28), but, as mentioned previously, dissections can also begin in more distal aortic segments.[97,102,107,270,401]

In general the clinical picture of dissecting aneurysm in persons with the Marfan syndrome is little different from that in persons without this syndrome,[111,118,119,121] except that in patients with the Marfan syndrome aortic regurgitation is more likely to be present (as a result of preexisting dilation in the first part of the aorta), the average patient age is about 20 years younger than that for other dissecting aneurysms, and hypertension is usually absent. As in the case of any dissecting aneurysm, the patient may demonstrate inequality of the radial or femoral pulse.[356] Dissection of the coronary arteries in the Marfan syndrome is an established, although rare, complication.[251,314,422]

The occurrence of aortic regurgitation with dissecting aneurysm has been well recognized since 1925, when the study of Resnik and Keefer[393] was published. Mechanisms for the association include deformation of the aortic ring by the intramural hematoma[207] and preexisting dilation of the aortic ring as a result of the same underlying connective tissue defect.

In patients with the Marfan syndrome the sudden development of a murmur, especially a musical, buzzing murmur over the ascending aorta, may be a valuable clue to the presence of dissection.[82,316] The murmur, which may be either systolic or, less commonly, diastolic, appears to be produced by vibrations excited in some of the anomalous structures such as lips, fibrous cords, and narrowed branches of the aortic arch, which are created by the dissection (Fig. 3-29). The quality of the early diastolic murmur created at the aortic valve may be musical[256] and, as in the case of many musical murmurs, may be loud: such murmurs may be audible at a distance from the chest.[20,30] A diastolic murmur loudest at the right sternal border is more frequent in the Marfan syndrome or other conditions causing aortic root enlargement than in rheumatic aortic regurgitation.[216]

Aortic dissection is classified according to its location as revealed by angiography, MRI, or CT scans. DeBakey et al.[118,119] grouped dissections as follows: those arising in the ascending aorta and extending to more distal segments (type I), those limited to the ascending aorta (type II), and those limited to the descending aorta (type III). The separation of proximal from more distal dissections is important because many patients in the latter group do well with long-term medical treatment or exhibit gradual progressive enlargement of involved aortic segments that permits delayed elective surgical repair to be successfully performed.[105,121,183,307,474] An incorrect angiographic diagnosis of dissection of the aorta may be made, however, on the basis of adventitial or venous opacification, which gives an impression of a double lumen, or false channel. Occasionally, false-negative results of aortograms may also be obtained, probably because a limited number of projections may not have included views that would have displayed a small aortic flap.

Aortic regurgitation. Aortic regurgitation is a common and usually progressive complication of the Marfan syndrome (Fig. 3-30). Nevertheless, aortic regurgitation is relatively uncommon in childhood, with reported prevalences of 7% to 20%.[362,446,528] The frequency rises progressively during adult life, ranging from approximately 20% to more than 70% among groups of patients ascertained in different ways and evaluated by a variety of methods (auscultation, echocardiography, cardiac catheterization, and necropsy).

Aortic regurgitation occurs only rarely in Marfan patients with normal-sized aortic roots. This situation is in striking contrast to the general lack of aortic dilation in nonMarfan patients with specific valvular causes of aortic regurgitation.[403] Lima et al.[282] observed a strong positive correlation between aortic root diameter and aortic regurgitation in a series of 83 adult Marfan patients. The mechanism whereby dilation of the aorta in persons with the Marfan syndrome produces aortic regurgitation involves progressive displacement of the points of attachment of the aortic cusp to the aortic wall away from the center of the aorta, as the aorta enlarges. Dilation of the aorta at the level of the supraaortic ridge (also known as the sinotubular junction), where the aortic commissures are supported by the aortic wall, seems to be most important in this process.[115,403] This dilation ultimately leads to inability of the aortic cusps to close adequately, and the resultant regurgitant orifice may become quite large, as shown in Fig. 3-31.

In some Marfan patients the development of

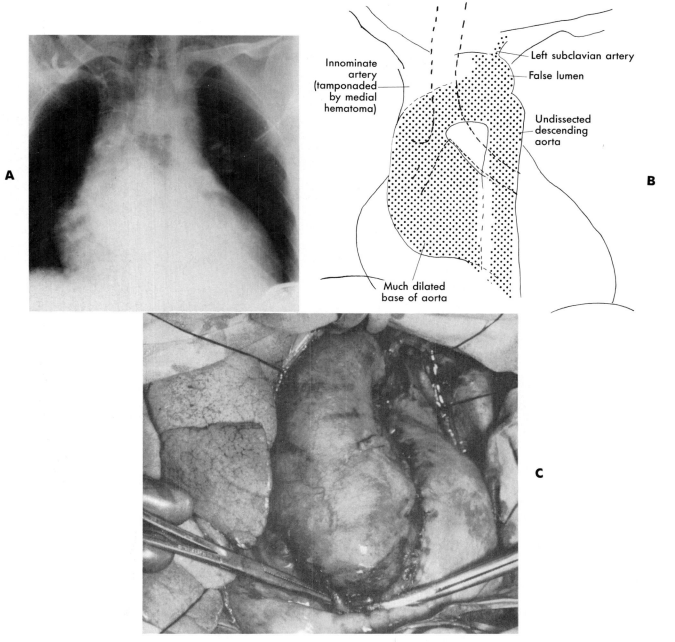

Fig. 3-29. A and **B,** S.C. had ectopia lentis and skeletal proportions of the Marfan syndrome. He died at the age of 37 years during an attempt at surgical repair of the ascending aorta. With the episode of dissection in October 1955, a musical systolic murmur developed over the ascending aorta. This sign, a valuable diagnostic clue in such cases, probably owes its origin to vibration in intimal lip or fibrous bands in the ascending aorta. Angiocardiogram showed striking dilation of the base of the aorta within the shadow of the heart, surprisingly little enlargement of the distal portion of the ascending aorta, failure of opacification of the innominate artery, the lumen of which was tamponaded by a medial dissection, and, finally, pseudocoarctation of the type so typical of the Marfan syndrome. **C,** The gourdlike appearance of the ascending aorta as exposed through a surgical incision in the right interior thorax. A clamp lies under the right coronary artery. Unusually high displacement of this vessel made operation difficult, as did the high extension of the aortic commissures. The patient died during surgery. The mother of this patient died of the cardiac complications of the Marfan syndrome at the age of 40 years. An older sister of the patient had the Marfan syndrome. (From McKusick VA: *Ann Intern Med* 49:556-567, 1958.)

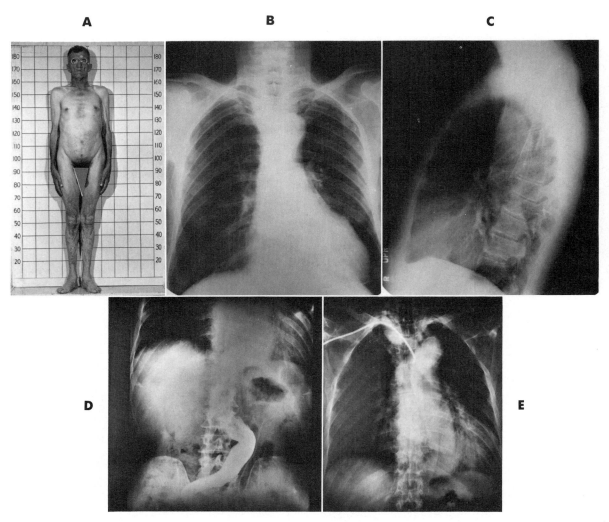

Fig. 3-30. Tortuous aorta in the Marfan syndrome. A white man, born in 1900, had ectopia lentis from birth and was educated until age 16 at the Iowa School for the Blind. Subsequently, after being fitted for spectacles, he was able to attend regular school and was gainfully employed all his life as an electrical engineer. Both parents died in their eighties. No other certain instance of the Marfan syndrome in the family is known. The right eye was enucleated in 1951; several operations for glaucoma were performed on the left eye, and the lens was removed in 1952. In 1955 he had subtotal gastrectomy for peptic ulcer. Fourteen days after operation he had sudden, severe chest pain while sitting on the toilet. In retrospect, this event seems to have been either pulmonary embolism or aortic dissection, probably the former. Hearing was diminished, beginning about 1940.

When first seen by McKusick in 1959, the patient was tall, with mild pectus excavatum, **A,** He had a loud murmur of aortic regurgitation and blood pressure of 136/40 mm Hg. Chest radiographs, **B** and **C,** showed left ventricular enlargement, prominent aortic knob, and apparent aneurysm of descending thoracic aorta *(arrow)*. Retrograde aortogram via femoral artery showed, **D,** a markedly tortuous abdominal aorta without aneurysm. Since the catheter could not be passed further up the aorta, aortography was performed via the brachial artery, with demonstration, **E,** that the apparent aneurysm was a buckled segment of the descending aorta. A suggestive double shadow in the area of the aorta above the diaphragm raised the question of dissection.

The patient died in 1961. "Coronary thrombosis," occurring 4 days before death, was listed as the cause of death.

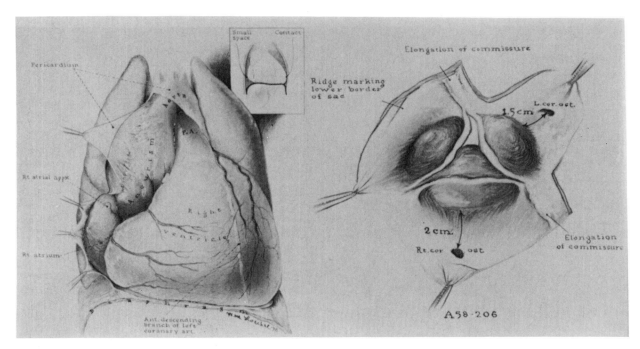

Fig. 3-31. Drawing of heart, great arteries, and lungs, *left*, and aortic valve from above, *right*, in a 36-year-old woman with severe aortic regurgitation and a hugely dilated ascending aorta and heart. The aortic valve cusps protrude excessively toward the left ventricle. Chronic congestive cardiac failure began 2 years before death. (From Roberts WC, Honig HS: *Am Heart J* 104:115-135, 1982.)

aortic regurgitation as a result of aortic dilation seems to accelerate the rate of aortic enlargement.[401] This situation may reflect an increase in hemodynamic stress imposed on the aorta, since the addition of the aortic regurgitant volume to the normal stroke volume leads to increases in the volume, velocity, and kinetic energy of the blood ejected into the aorta with each heart beat.

Mitral valve. Approximately 60% to 70% of persons with the Marfan syndrome exhibit mitral valve prolapse (Fig. 3-32). The mitral cusps and chordae tendineae may be redundant, with resulting mitral regurgitation. Bacterial endocarditis, which most often affects the mitral valve in the Marfan syndrome, may become engrafted on the valvular abnormality.* Murmurs that may be partly musical may result from redundancy of the

chordae tendineae and valve leaflets, with incompetence of atrioventricular valves. In a patient with a musical mitral systolic murmur, autopsy revealed a tear at the insertion of the posterior mitral cusp, which amounted to a partial avulsion of the cusp. Midsystolic clicks also may occur either alone or in association with a late systolic murmur. In some patients with the Marfan syndrome who have mitral prolapse the anatomic distribution of the systolic murmur simulates that of aortic stenosis, and at autopsy a jet lesion of the left atrial wall underlying the aortic ring has been found.[326]

In some affected persons mitral and tricuspid valve regurgitation may be the predominant cardiovascular lesion and can lead to early death.[437,443] Redundancy of the chordae tendineae or distortion and ballooning of leaflet segments or entire atrioventricular valve leaflets may be responsible to a variable extent for the valvular dysfunction. Tricuspid, or even quinquecuspid, mitral valves have been present in some cases. In a de-

_____
*References 61, 94, 130, 220, 303, 352, 372, 502, and 527.

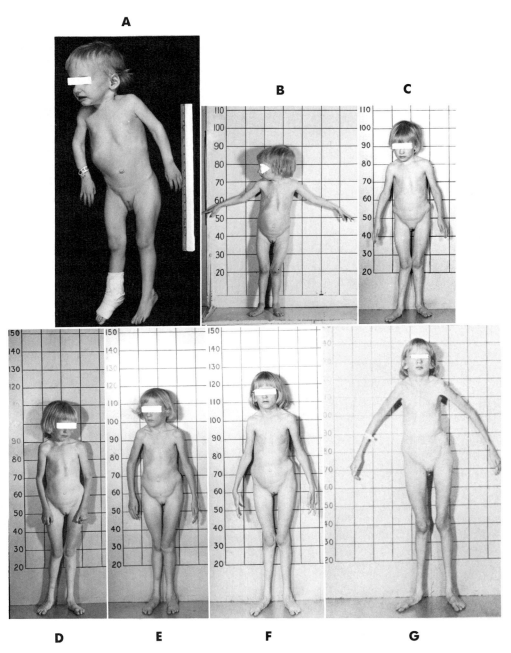

Fig. 3-32. Mitral regurgitation in Marfan syndrome. **A** to **F,** The appearance at 14 months, 2 years, 3 years, 4 years, 5 years, and 6 years of age, respectively. Chest deformity—first, pectus excavatum and, later, predominantly pectus carinatum—is shown. Dolichostenomelia and loose-jointedness were striking. Bilateral ectopia lentis was present. **G,** Appearance at 8½ years of age (September 1967), within a month of her death.

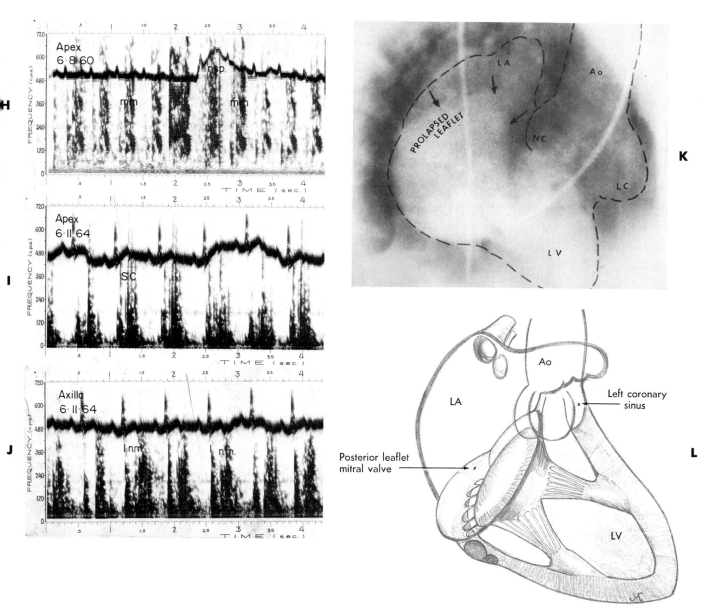

Fig. 3-32, cont'd. H to **J,** Auscultatory findings as demonstrated by spectral phono-cardiograms. At the age of 14 months the patient showed a loud musical late sys-tolic murmur, which was initiated by a click and which extended across the second heart sound, **H.** Later, the findings were predominantly multiple clicks in the latter two thirds of systole, **I,** and, in other areas, a noisy late systolic murmur extending over the second sound, **J.** Selective left ventricular cineangiocardiography, **K,** made of patient at 5 years of age demonstrated prolapsed posterior mitral leaflet and mi-tral regurgitation. The catheter was introduced in retrograde fashion via the femo-ral artery. In the right anterior oblique view, **K,** the sinuses of Valsalva are seen to be markedly dilated. (LA, Left atrium; LV, left ventricle; NC and LC, noncoronary and left coronary sinuses of Valsalva.) (No auscultatory evidence of aortic regurgita-tion had developed.) Toward the end of systole, the posterior leaflet of the mitral valve bulged markedly into the left atrium *(arrows),* and mitral regurgitation was present. The systolic clicks coincided temporally with maximum prolapse of the valve. **L,** A diagram of the normal heart as viewed in the right anterior oblique po-sition. (**K** and **L** from Criley JM et al: *Br Heart J* 28:488-496, 1966.)   *Continued.*

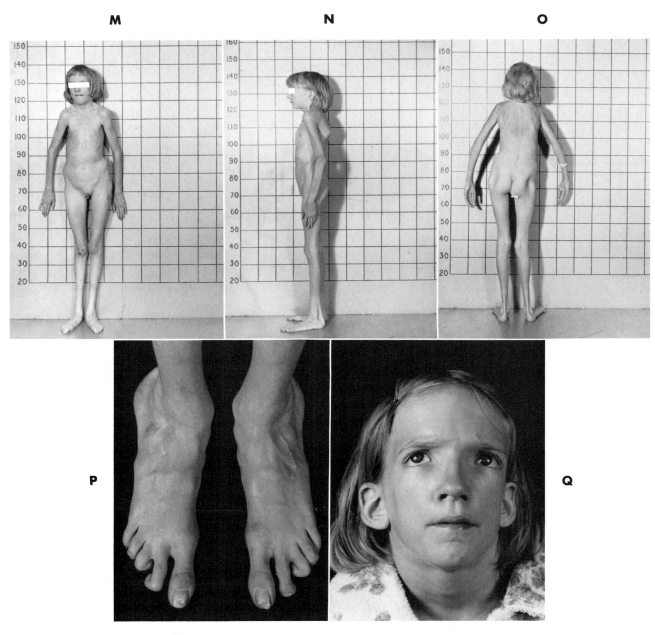

Fig. 3-32, cont'd. M to **Q,** Appearance at 8½ years of age. **M** to **O,** Demonstrated are excessive height, pectus carinatum, scoliosis, narrow, flat feet, and sparsity of subcutaneous fat. **P,** The feet are long, narrow, and everted, with prominent heels and contracted third, fourth, and fifth toes. **Q,** Characteristic Marfan facies. Megalocornea and small, somewhat eccentric pupils are evident.

Between 7 and 8 years of age signs of aortic regurgitation developed, and the patient had episodes of severe chest pain, interpreted as indicating acute dissection of the aorta. Despite therapy with reserpine, rupture of the aorta occurred less than 1 month after these views were photographed.

scription of the appearance of the mitral valve during angiocardiography and at autopsy Grondin, Steinberg, and Edwards[198] noted that "the mitral leaflets were divided into several large serrations which bulged into the left atrium." Interchordal protrusions, essentially herniations, are present between the extensions of the chordae tendineae onto the valve leaflet. Striking mitral regurgitation has been observed in infants with other severe manifestations of the Marfan syndrome.[229]

By the early 1970s it had become clear[49,164,273] that clicks and late systolic murmurs, as well as holosystolic murmurs of more severe mitral regurgitation, were due to retroversion or "prolapse" of a redundant posterior mitral cusp, with a leak from the left ventricle to the atrium in late systole, as was first demonstrated by cineangiocardiography.[435] Barlow et al.[25] found that two of 90 patients with late systolic murmurs and nonejection mid- to late-systolic clicks had the Marfan syndrome. In the general population, however, primary mitral valve prolapse is far more common than mitral valve prolapse resulting from the Marfan syndrome[278,405] (see the section, Differential Diagnosis). In fact, five of the patients with mitral valve prolapse documented by Barlow et al.[25] had a familial basis to their conditions, which was independent of the Marfan syndrome. Hunt and Sloman[235] and Shell et al.[441] described families with many affected persons in several generations; subsequent studies have confirmed the autosomal dominant inheritance of primary mitral valve prolapse.[128,129,460,512]

Echocardiographic findings in individuals with the Marfan syndrome and in those with mitral valve prolapse syndrome are almost indistinguishable. In a minority of Marfan patients, however, Pini et al.[364] found a distinct combination of anatomic and functional abnormalities in which all visualized chordae tendineae of the posterior mitral leaflet arose from the posterior left ventricular wall, either directly or via muscle bundles. This finding contrasted with the normal situation in which the major papillary muscles and the mitral leaflets exhibit immediate prolapse into the left atrium in the first echocardiographic frame in systole. Calcification of the mitral annulus has been demonstrated in a number of instances.*

_____
*References 44, 56, 191, 200, 326, and 480.

Other cardiac involvement. Although no form of congenital heart disease is systematically associated with the Marfan syndrome, numerous examples of what probably represent chance coexistences have been reported. These have included ostium secundum atrial septal defects,[59,264] interventricular septal defects of varied type,[350,409,482] congenital absence of pulmonic valve,[89] and anomalous origin of coronary arteries.[322] Others are mentioned in the next section of this chapter.

Much was written in the older literature about cardiac disability resulting from pectus excavatum* (Fig. 3-33), and as originally proposed by Flesch[163] in 1873, excessive longitudinal growth of the ribs has often been thought to be the causative mechanism. Wachtel, Ravitch, and Grisham[504]

_____
*References 149, 154, 276, 331, 388, and 468.

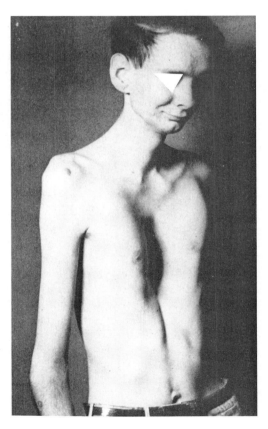

Fig. 3-33. Severe pectus excavatum in the Marfan syndrome. (From McKusick VA: *Circulation* 11:321-342, 1955.)

suggested that pectus excavatum could lead to dyspnea or other cardiac symptoms because of the following factors:

1. Twisting and distortion of the great veins might impede venous return.
2. Restriction of diastolic expansion of the heart between the displaced sternum anteriorly and the space posteriorly might limit delivery of more blood on demand.
3. Impingement on the atria might lead to supraventricular arrhythmias.
4. Respiratory reserve might be decreased as a result of impairment of the intercostal component of respiration.

Despite the plausible mechanisms just listed, it has yet to be demonstrated that cardiac function in persons with the Marfan syndrome is impaired by pectus excavatum. Nevertheless, symptomatic improvement of cardiopulmonary performance after pectus repair has been reported.[424]

Prolongation of the P-R interval of the electrocardiogram is common in the Marfan syndrome in the presence of aortic regurgitation,[20,77,321] and bundle-branch block may also occur. The Wolff-Parkinson-White syndrome also has been observed in affected persons.[23,217,223,243] These conduction abnormalities are of particular interest in view of the occurrence of similar preexcitation in patients with mitral valve prolapse syndrome,[127] which suggests that there might be a common deficiency of electrical insulation between the atria and ventricles in both conditions. A variety of atrial and ventricular arrhythmias have been described in the Marfan syndrome, but these appear to be primarily related to the severity of mitral and aortic valve dysfunction rather than to the condition itself.[84,133,413]

Thrombosis in arteries or veins should always raise the suspicion of homocystinuria rather than the Marfan syndrome. However, bilateral renal vein thrombosis leading to the nephrotic syndrome has been observed in an individual with unequivocal Marfan syndrome who also had aortic dissection from the left subclavian artery to the bifurcation.[7]

Other Manifestations

In addition to the major manifestations involving the three principal systems affected in the Marfan syndrome, the Berlin nosology (see the box on p. 57) lists other features, some fairly common,

some rare, that are components of this disorder. Since the gene in which mutations cause this disorder is expressed in many tissues outside the skeletal, ocular, and cardiovascular systems, it is not unreasonable to predict that a defective protein or protein complex, which is widely distributed, would produce a variety of phenotypic effects. Future studies leading to the understanding of correlations between clinical and pathologic features, as well as the pathophysiologic expression of the faulty gene, should shed light on the pleiotropy of the Marfan syndrome.

Certain congenital malformations occur often enough in the Marfan syndrome to be considered more than coincidental associations. In the cardiovascular system these include coarctation of the aorta,* patent ductus arteriosus,[12,494] anomaly of valvular cuspation, absent pulmonary valve,[89] interatrial defect,[14,140,269,366] and, possibly, pulmonary stenosis[499]; in the skeletal system, spina bifida occulta, hemivertebra, and cleft palate[410,520]; and in the eye, microphakia, hypoplasia, or aplasia of the dilator pupillae muscle, coloboma lentis, and coloboma iridis.[256] Encephalocele occurred in the forehead area in one patient, and internal hydrocephalus has also been reported.[357,385] The occurrence of these abnormalities is difficult to reconcile with a unitary theory of a connective tissue defect, unless it is assumed that the presence of the defective protein during embryogenesis provides an abnormal environment in which these anomalies, which are congenital malformations in the usual sense, occur with increased incidence. In accordance with this not improbable proposition, these particular abnormalities can be regarded as secondary manifestations of the Marfan syndrome.

Dural ectasia. The only "major manifestation" outside the skeletal, ocular and cardiovascular systems, as defined by the Berlin nosology,[35] is the presence of dural ectasia[214,383,455] (Figs. 3-12 to 3-14). Patients are regarded as having dural ectasia when any of the following are present[383]: (1) widening of the neural canal, (2) thinning of the bony cortex of the vertebral bodies and pedicles, (3) dilation of neural foramina, or (4) protrusion of dura outside the neural canal. In a prospective

---

*References 141, 148, 151, 160, 315, 496, and 499.

study Pyeritz et al.[383] examined 57 patients with the Marfan syndrome who had the classic skeletal, ocular, and cardiovascular abnormalities. These persons were compared to age- and sex-matched controls without connective tissue disease who had CT scans during the same period. Thirty-six of the 57 Marfan patients (24 men and 12 women) were diagnosed as having dural ectasia (i.e., 63%). By contrast, none of the controls had dural ectasia. There was no association between ectasia of the dura and other major features of the Marfan syndrome, namely, ectopia lentis, aortic dissection, scoliosis, or joint laxity.[383] Genetic heterogeneity alone could not account for dural ectasia, since an affected pair of first cousins was discordant for this abnormality. In many patients no symptoms are produced, but some persons with prominent dural ectasia have low back pain. This association has not yet been studied systematically.[123] Nevertheless, the presence of dural ectasia represents an important diagnostic criterion. Specialized imaging techniques are necessary for the demonstration of dural ectasia, however, which detracts from its diagnostic value.

In the general population dural ectasia usually results from elevated intrathecal pressure, trauma, or spinal surgery.[325] Dural ectasia also is a rare finding in neurofibromatosis and the Ehlers-Danlos syndrome (EDS).[158,328]

Pulmonary involvement. In view of the significant amount of elastin, hence, microfibrils, in the lungs,[208] it is easy to imagine that abnormalities in the support system of elastin could cause pulmonary abnormalities. The most common pulmonary complication in patients with the Marfan syndrome is spontaneous pneumothorax, which occurs in approximately 5% of affected persons[139,203,286,495,526] (Fig. 3-34). This statistic indicates that the probability of spontaneous pneumothorax is several hundred times more likely in persons with the Marfan syndrome than in the general population.[526] In a large retrospective study Wood et al.[526] examined the records of 100 patients with the Marfan syndrome. The authors admit to a series biased in favor of pulmonary findings, since the records were obtained from hospitals specializing in cardiopulmonary disorders. They found 11 persons with the Marfan syndrome who had histories of spontaneous pneumothorax; 10 were recurrent and six were bilateral. In a retrospective study from a genetics clinic, which is

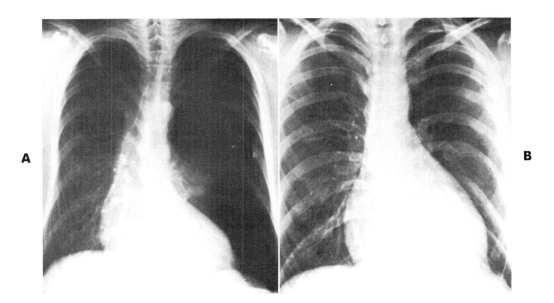

Fig. 3-34. A, Posteroanterior chest radiograph of a 15-year-old boy with the Marfan syndrome on the occasion of his first pneumothorax. **B,** Posteroanterior chest radiograph of the same patient after removal of the chest tube and reexpansion of the left lung. An apical bulla is evident. (From Hall JR et al: *Ann Thorac Surg* 37:500-504, 1984.)

thus seemingly more representative of the entire spectrum of involvement in this disease, Hall et al.[203] found the frequency of spontaneous pneumothorax to be 4.4% (11 of 249 patients over 12 years of age). As found in other investigations, more males than females had this complication, but the severity was independent of gender.

Apical bullae occur in the Marfan syndrome with and without spontaneous pneumothorax, but they undoubtedly cause predisposition to this complication.[203,439,526] Spontaneous pneumothorax is sometimes familial in the absence of evident Marfan syndrome[41,63]; Brock[64] favored the presence of hereditary lung cysts as the anatomic substrate. On statistic study spontaneous pneumothorax occurs most often in tall, slim young men[166,524]; this observation may reflect a pathogenetic link with the Marfan syndrome.

Congenital cystic lung disease is a rare manifestation of the Marfan syndrome[286]; as with some structural cardiac abnormalities, it is possible that the presence of the connective tissue defect during embryogenesis conditions the development of this pulmonary anomaly.

Emphysema may occur in patients with the Marfan syndrome.[54,493] In one group of seven patients, six had evidence of pulmonary dysaeration; two showed compression of the left main bronchus caused by a giant left atrium, with atelectasis of the lung and compensatory emphysema of the right lung; two showed chronic pulmonary emphysema; three had apical bullae bilaterally; and one had pneumothorax. During autopsy studies Bolande and Tucker[54] could not detect on histologic study any changes in the lungs that might lead to emphysema. Increased deposition of elastic fibers in the alveolar septa was interpreted as a response to mechanical stress, since elastin depletion is seen in other, comparable situations in patients without the Marfan syndrome. It was suggested that flaccidity of the walls of the respiratory and terminal bronchioles may cause predisposition to collapse during expiration and result in air trapping and emphysema. Neimann et al.[342] described a severely affected infant who died at 10 weeks of age of severe pulmonary emphysema. Dominguez, Weisgrau, and Santamaria[135] reported four sporadic patients with the Marfan syndrome who came to medical attention in infancy with a constellation of respiratory abnormalities, including tracheobronchomalacia, repeated pneu-

monia, atelectasis, cor pulmonale, and emphysema.

Pulmonary function in the Marfan syndrome was studied by Fuleihan, Suh, and Shepard[173] and by Chisholm, Cheriack, and Carton.[90] The latter workers concluded that "elasticity-determining tissues of the lung are not primarily affected by the Marfan lesion." Streeten, Murphy, and Pyeritz[465] observed that when persons with the Marfan syndrome and unaffected controls were matched for sitting height rather than standing height, there was no observable difference in pulmonary function. As would be expected, thoracic cage abnormalities had an adverse effect on pulmonary function both in persons with the Marfan syndrome and in controls with the same physical abnormalities. It is evident that the underlying defect has little impact, other than the increased risk of spontaneous pneumothorax, on "static lung function" in persons with the Marfan syndrome.[465]

On rare occasions severe kyphoscoliosis in the Marfan syndrome may precipitate or make a major contribution to cardiopulmonary failure. The pathogenesis of this complication is the same as in cardiorespiratory failure resulting from kyphoscoliosis of other cause.[40,210]

Hernias. Inguinal, femoral, and incisional hernias occur commonly in the Marfan syndrome. Diaphragmatic hernias were present in some patients known to McKusick and in others reported in the literature.[256,466] Hydrocele is occasionally encountered. Hernias are presumably a manifestation of the underlying connective tissue defect, and as such, they are of considerable diagnostic importance. In view of the preponderance of hernias in men, the presence of hernias in women suspected of having the Marfan syndrome has special diagnostic significance.

Cutaneous striae. Cutaneous striae in the pectoral and deltoid areas and radially oriented around the breasts and over the thighs are frequently found in the Marfan syndrome[246,289,332,425] (Figs. 3-35 and 3-36). These striae, which are otherwise known as striae atrophica or distensae, are observable in patients in their teens and cannot be attributed to weight loss. In a patient with the Marfan syndrome who had nephrotic syndrome,[7] subcutaneous edema greatly exaggerated the striae. Subtle striae may be difficult to discern,

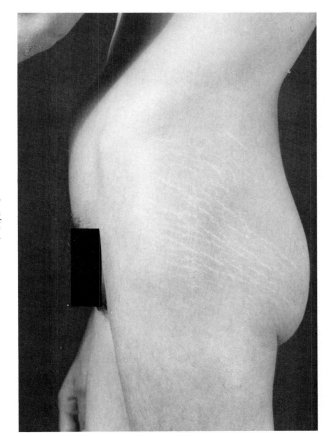

Fig. 3-35. Striae distensae. A girl born in 1951 had severe skeletal, ocular, and cardiac features of the Marfan syndrome. The patient was 16 years of age at the time of this photograph, which demonstrates striae of the lateral buttock area.

but in appropriate circumstances their presence should be sought, since they can be a useful diagnostic indicator. Indeed, recognition of the presence of striae is of considerable importance in the diagnosis of doubtful cases.

Miscellaneous features. *Miescher elastoma,* or *elastoma intrapapillare perforans verruciformis,* is a rare skin lesion that may be associated with the Marfan syndrome.[202] The elastoma occurs particularly on the neck and becomes evident as small reddish nodules or papules. Histologic studies reveal cysts occupied by whorls of material that have the tinctorial characteristics of elastic fibers and that seem to have erupted into the epidermis from the upper corium. In addition to Miescher elastoma's infrequent occurrence in the Marfan syndrome, it also is encountered occasionally in EDS[13] and osteogenesis imperfecta.[391]

Hematologic abnormalities are unusual in the Marfan syndrome. Estes, Carey, and Desai[146] described a family with apparently typical Marfan

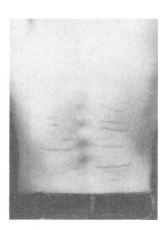

Fig. 3-36. Transverse striae distensae in the lumbar area.

syndrome in seven members. Five of the seven had easy bruising, an increase in the level of circulating immature granulocytes, an increase in leukocyte alkaline phosphatase activity, giant platelets, and functional platelet abnormalities. It is possible that these hematologic features represent chance concomitants in this family, since the majority of persons with the Marfan syndrome have no problems with bleeding.

Mental retardation, contrary to previous emphasis,[117,287,357,429] is not a component of the Marfan syndrome. Affected persons are usually as bright as their sibs, but their innate intelligence is sometimes not fully realized because of the limitation of opportunities imposed by severe visual impairment and other physical handicaps. The occurrence of mental retardation as a conspicuous feature of homocystinuria, which in several other respects simulates the Marfan syndrome, may be another reason why mental retardation was initially thought to be a feature of the Marfan syndrome. A number of reports[4,76,91,473] have suggested a possible link between the Marfan syndrome and epilepsy caused by abnormalities of the brain resulting from the underlying connective tissue defect. The prevalence of mental retardation in these patients makes the diagnosis of Marfan syndrome suspect.

The *voice* in patients with the Marfan syndrome is sometimes rather high-pitched, with a timbre sufficiently characteristic that one author[60] thought he could recognize affected persons over the telephone.

Congenital cystic kidneys have been documented in a person with arachnodactyly,[57] but it is uncertain whether the genuine Marfan syndrome was actually present in this individual.

Deafness occurs in a small proportion of affected persons, but it is uncertain whether hearing loss is a specific manifestation of the Marfan syndrome.[384] The actual mechanism of the deafness is unknown, although Everberg[150] concluded that deafness is an integral feature and that it is of the perceptive type.

Other features that have been observed in persons with the Marfan syndrome include isolated instances of biliary tract problems,[324] recurrent nephrolithiasis and bilateral medullary sponge kidney,[430] rheumatoid arthritis,[3] neurofibromatosis,[98,275] penicillin-induced esophageal ulceration,[196] Wilms tumor,[347] and neuropsychiatric dysfunction.[274,407,498] Their causal relationship, if any, with the underlying defect in this disease is not clearly understood, and they are probably unrelated random events.

Prognosis

Life expectancy in patients with the Marfan syndrome, which is generally reduced because of the cardiovascular complications, can be significantly prolonged by well-managed medical treatment. Indeed, some patients with the Marfan syndrome live long, active, and productive lives.

Among 16 deceased affected members of a large family, Bowers[60] found the average age at death to be 43 years in the men and 46 years in the women; one individual survived to 73 years of age and another died at 9 years of age. In a comprehensive study of 72 deceased patients, Murdoch et al.[339] showed that the average age at death was 32 years. Cardiac problems led to 52 of the 56 deaths of known cause; aortic dilation and its complications accounted for about 80% of these deaths.

Survivorship curves based on experience with 257 cases of the Marfan syndrome diagnosed on the basis of stringent criteria are shown in Fig. 3-37. The more favorable prognosis is in women. When sporadic and familial cases were considered separately, survivorship was found to be better in persons with affected relatives. This observation probably stems from an ascertainment bias. It must be emphasized that the findings of Bowers[60] and of Murdoch et al.[339] antedated the modern era of diagnosis and treatment and that the prognosis for patients receiving adequate treatment has greatly improved.

Marfan Syndrome in Infancy and Early Childhood

Although infants and young children were among the initial patients in whom the Marfan syndrome was documented, recognition of the disorder in early life is not always an easy matter.

Geva et al.[178] have documented extensive cardiovascular abnormalities in nine affected infants. The cardiovascular features in these infants and in 86 similar cases from the literature are summarized in the box on p. 89. These data suggest that involvement of the mitral and tricuspid valves is significant in infants with the Marfan syndrome, although aortic regurgitation is infrequent.

In an extensive study Morse et al.[335] described 22 infants in whom the Marfan syndrome had been diagnosed within the first 3 months of life,

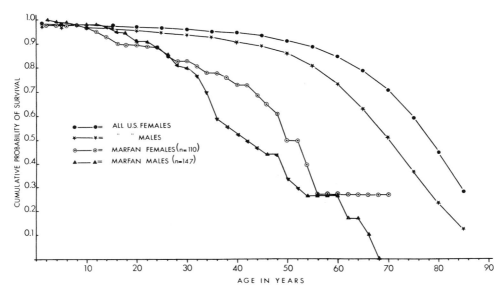

Fig. 3-37. Survivorship in the Marfan syndrome analyzed by the life-table method. With modern diagnosis and management, the prognosis in the Marfan syndrome has greatly improved since 1972, when these tables were promulgated. (From Murdoch JL et al: *New Engl J Med* 286:804-808, 1972.)

Summary of Cardiovascular Features in 95 Infants with the Marfan Syndrome

Male-to-female ratio: 2:3
Positive family history: 18/68 (26%)
Mean age at diagnosis: 3.2 mo (range, birth to 12 mo)
Mitral valve
  Mitral valve prolapse: 73/76 (96%)
  Mitral regurgitation: 64/76 (84%)
Aorta
  Aortic root dilation: 71/81 (88%)
  Aortic regurgitation: 17/60 (28%)
Tricuspid valve
  Tricuspid valve prolapse: 28/51 (55%)
  Tricuspid regurgitation: 18/60 (30%)
Pulmonary root
  Pulmonary root dilation: 12/50 (24%)
Congestive heart failure: 39/53 (74%)
Surgical intervention: 11/53 (21%)
Mortality rate: 49/72 (68%)
Mean age at death: 15.7 mo (range, birth to 14 yr)

Adapted from Geva et al: *Am J Cardiol* 65:1230-1237, 1990.

and in the literature search these authors identified 32 additional infants with the Marfan syndrome. The frequency of different manifestations in the patients is shown in Table 3-3. The most common skeletal findings included arachnodactyly, characteristic facies, highly arched palate, hyperextensible joints, flexion contractures, pes planus, and sternothoracic abnormalities. About 60% of these infants had dislocated lenses, and the more severely affected had pronounced megalocornea. Before 2 months of age none of them had ectopia lentis, but lens dislocation was subsequently observed in five of these patients. Cardiovascular evaluation demonstrated both mitral valve prolapse and aortic root dilation in several infants; the more severely affected had both abnormalities, whereas the less severely affected had mitral valve prolapse alone.

The authors suggested that these infants had a distinct infantile or neonatal form of the Marfan syndrome, which might be an autonomous entity. In this context it has been pointed out that the family history is almost always negative in the severely affected infants.*

Decreased expression of the gene encoding

*References 5, 68, 177, 199, 236, 240, 335, and 362.

Table 3-3. Clinical and echocardiographic findings in infantile Marfan syndrome

Finding	Frequency in 22 patients (%)	Frequency in literature (%)	Combined frequency (%)
Skeletal*			
Arachnodactyly	19/22 (86)	28/32 (88)	47/54 (87)
Joint laxity	15/22 (68)	17/32 (48)	32/54 (59)
Flexion contractures	14/22 (64)	15/32 (47)	29/54 (54)
Joint dislocations	8/22 (36)	—	8/22 (36)
Pes planus	7/22 (32)	1/26 (4)	8/48 (17)
Dolichocephaly	14/22 (64)	6/25 (24)	20/47 (43)
Distinctive facies	15/22 (68)	3/25 (12)	18/47 (38)
Large, floppy ears	9/22 (41)	3/25 (12)	12/47 (26)
High-arched palate	11/22 (50)	6/25 (24)	17/47 (36)
Micrognathia	12/22 (55)	2/25 (8)	14/47 (30)
Scoliosis	7/22 (32)	2/25 (8)	9/47 (19)
Pectus deformity	12/22 (55)	14/32 (31)	26/54 (48)
Ocular			
Iridodenesis	10/22 (46)	5/13 (38)	15/35 (43)
Ectopia lentis	13/22 (59)	12/18 (55)	25/40 (63)
Megalocornea	9/22 (41)	1/11 (9)	10/33 (30)
Myopia	12/22 (55)	2/11 (18)	14/33 (42)
Cardiovascular			
Murmur	10/22 (45)	17/30 (57)	27/52 (52)
Mitral valve prolapse†	16/22 (73)‡	16/17 (94)	32/39 (82)
Aortic root dilation†	16/22 (73)‡	14/17 (82)	32/39 (82)

From Morse RP et al: *Pediatrics* 86:888-895, 1990.
*Joint laxity in order of most frequent occurrence: digits, wrists, and ankles. Flexion contractures in order of most frequent occurrence: elbows, knees, and digits. Joint dislocations most commonly involved knees and hips. Distinctive facies with deep-set eyes, malar hypoplasia, and an appearance like that of "an old man" were described.
†Echocardiographic determination from Morse RP et al: *Pediatrics* 86:888-895, 1990.
‡Finding by echocardiography or cardiac catheterization, from the literature.

decorin has been recognized in an infant with "lethal" Marfan syndrome,[371] and preliminary immunohistochemical analyses have demonstrated a microfibril abnormality in the infantile form, which is apparently different from that seen in classic Marfan syndrome.[185] The question arises, is infantile Marfan syndrome solely a descriptive term emphasizing early diagnosis, or does it define a similar but rare and potentially lethal autonomous entity? McKusick[319] holds the firm opinion that these sporadic infants represent severely affected new mutants for the conventional form of the disorder. The eventual identification of the gene mutations causing this form of the Marfan syndrome will facilitate resolution of this dilemma.

PREVALENCE AND INHERITANCE

The Marfan syndrome has long been known to be inherited as an autosomal dominant trait, and numerous pedigrees on record exhibit this pattern of inheritance. The autosomal dominance is clearly shown in Fig. 3-38, which portrays one of the largest known families with a well-documented history of the Marfan syndrome.[75]

The Marfan syndrome is relatively common; its frequency is about 1 per 10,000 in the United States. The sexes are equally affected.[294,384] It has been reported in virtually every European country and in blacks,* Chinese,[45,80,213,280,467] Japanese,[346,447,492] Hindus,[42] American Indians,[180] and Jews.[254,294] The incidence of the Marfan syndrome in American blacks is probably essentially the same as in whites, and there is no evidence of particular ethnic predilection. In this context, contrary to what is true of recessive disorders, variation in ethnic frequency would not be expected in

_____
*References 95, 138, 174, 315, 401, and 505.

Table 3-4. Parental age and birth order in 23 sporadic cases of the Marfan syndrome

	Father's age (yr)		Mother's age (yr)		Birth order	
	Mean	**SD**	**Mean**	**SD**	**Mean**	**SD**
Sporadic cases	36.61	9.06	29.30	5.36	3.17	2.48
General population	29.85	6.95	26.54	6.07	2.64	1.73

SD, Standard deviation.

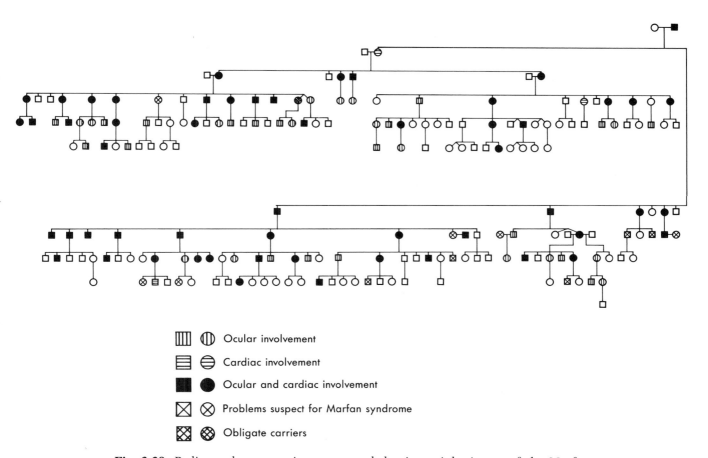

▯▯▯ ⬭ Ocular involvement

▤ ⊖ Cardiac involvement

■ ● Ocular and cardiac involvement

⊠ ⊗ Problems suspect for Marfan syndrome

⧆ ⊗ Obligate carriers

Fig. 3-38. Pedigree demonstrating autosomal dominant inheritance of the Marfan syndrome in one of the largest families known. The family spans six generations and has more than 200 members. (Courtesy Ronald Cadle and Dr. Brian Hall, University of Kentucky, Lexington, Ky, and Drs. Harry C. Dietz and Reed E. Pyeritz, Johns Hopkins University, Baltimore.)

a detrimental mendelian dominant trait such as the Marfan syndrome.

The Marfan syndrome is one of the conditions in which the paternal-age effect on mutation has been demonstrated. The average age of fathers of persons with sporadic "new mutation" cases is about 7 years greater than the mean age of fathers generally[338] (Table 3-4). For example, the fathers of four patients with sporadic cases were 73, 69, 63, and 42 years of age at the time of the patients' births.

Once linkage to chromosome 15 was established and the gene product, fibrillin, was identified, the question of genetic heterogeneity could be formally tested. More than 30 affected families have been assessed in independent studies by means of specific fibrillin probes, but no evidence for genetic heterogeneity has been found in this series.[131,272,491] (An exception is mentioned in the following paragraph.) The combined logarithm of the odds score of these studies was more than 30, with a recombination fraction of zero. This means that the probability is greater than 10^{30} that these findings are *not* due to chance.

A single report[53] has been made of a large affected French family in which the condition is not linked to the locus on chromosome 15. The affected members of this kindred have the characteristic skeletal and cardiovascular manifestations, but they lack ocular abnormalities; the phenotype is otherwise similar to that of the classic Marfan syndrome. The authors have concluded that a second Marfan locus exists and remains unmapped.

There is some evidence for the existence of a severe autosomal recessive form of the Marfan syndrome.[83,171,431] Findings in affected sibs of a first-cousin mating[83] included elongated facies, corneal opacities, highly arched palate, loose skin and joints, arachnodactyly, hernia, pectus deformity, ectopia lentis, megalocornea, mitral valve prolapse, mitral insufficiency, and aortic root dilation. Both children died at 2½ years of age, one during open heart surgery, the other of cardiac

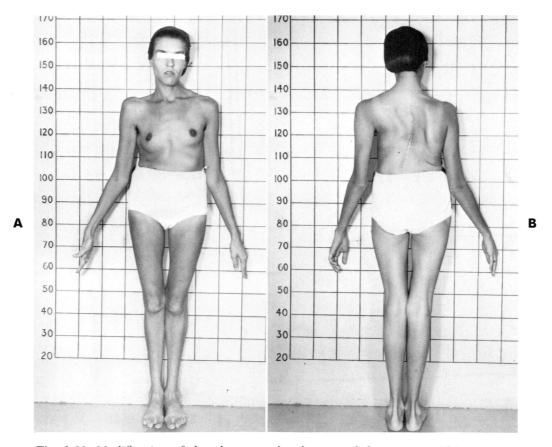

Fig. 3-39. Modification of the phenotype by the rest of the genome. This patient, born in 1945, has bilateral upward displacement of the lenses and severe scoliosis, with major thoracic convexity to the right, for which spinal fusion was performed at the age of 10 years. All joints are moderately hyperextensible. The father and mother were 37 and 35 years of age, respectively, at her birth. Her abnormality was thought to be the result of a fresh mutation. That this patient was only 64 inches tall is in part because of the short stature of her parents. The father was only 61 inches tall. **A,** Front view; **B,** posterior view. The right genu valgum and the scar of the spinal fusion are evident.

failure. The consanguinity of their unaffected parents could be construed as suggestive of autosomal recessive inheritance, but at present this concept is highly speculative.

Approximately 30% of all Marfan cases are sporadic and apparently due to new dominant mutations. It has often been claimed that sporadic cases are more severe than cases that occur in a familial setting, but this situation probably reflects biased ascertainment. Indeed, a proportion of sporadic cases become familial when the affected individual reaches adulthood and reproduces. Again, however, autosomal recessive inheritance in the severe sporadic cases cannot be entirely discounted. Monozygotic twins and triplets with the Marfan syndrome have been reported.

Nonpenetrance can cause difficulties in the genetic assessment of affected families, although skipping of generations has never been observed in any thoroughly studied pedigree.[215] Nevertheless, variation in phenotypic expression or partial submersion of the clinical manifestations, depending apparently on the rest of the genetic milieu in which the mutant gene is operating, has been observed frequently.[315] For instance, when the mutation occurs in a family with an unusually pyknic physique, the affected person's habitus may be comparatively normal, although ocular and cardiac abnormalities are still present (Fig. 3-39). This process of phenotypic modification by other alleles or genes is known as epistasis. McKusick cited the instance of a pedigree in which a woman with the Marfan syndrome married twice. By the first husband, a "nonMarfan" but tall man, there were two children; one died in infancy and one had a severe form of the Marfan syndrome. By the second husband, "a small, square-built man," one child was normal and a second had only mild skeletal and cardiac manifestations. The availability of transgenic animals that display mutations of the gene causing the Marfan syndrome on different genetic backgrounds will help unravel the mechanisms and consequences of the interaction of genes and alleles at the same and different loci.

Prenatal Diagnosis

The first reported attempt at prenatal diagnosis in the Marfan syndrome was undertaken by means of ultrasonic techniques.[260] In an "at-risk" pregnancy, diagnosis was established at 24 weeks' gestation by demonstration of abnormal skeletal length. After termination of the pregnancy the aborted fetus was found to have a typical marfanoid habitus and degenerative changes in the aorta. In a second pregnant patient, who sought medical advice at 24 weeks' gestation, fetal skeletal length was found on ultrasonic investigations to be within normal limits. The pregnancy proceeded, and an apparently normal infant was delivered. At 21 months of age, however, the infant's US/LS and arm span-to-height ratios were found to be abnormal, although no eye or cardiac abnormalities were detected at that time. It is clear that at present an accurate prenatal diagnosis cannot be obtained by diagnostic imaging techniques.

The recognition of genetic linkage has made prenatal and presymptomatic diagnosis potentially feasible in families with more than one affected individual. This process involves gene tracking in the kindred by use of restriction fragment length polymorphisms and Southern blotting with variable number dinucleotide repeat techniques. These methodologies have already been used for prenatal diagnosis in two cases of familial Marfan syndrome,[188] and undoubtedly others will follow. It is of practical importance that not all affected families will be "informative," but as additional probes become available, the likelihood of informativity will increase. This approach will not be applicable to the sporadic individual, but identification of the molecular defect and the development of gene-specific probes will ultimately resolve this difficulty.

DIFFERENTIAL DIAGNOSIS

The diagnosis of the Marfan syndrome can be a difficult matter; for every person in whom a firm diagnosis can be reached, several others with partial features of the condition are likely to be encountered.[182,239,500] This point is far from being merely academic, since the establishment of a positive diagnosis has serious implications; these include curtailment of life-style, high risk of life-threatening complications, and possible limitation of life span. In addition, lifelong prophylactic therapy with beta blockers may be initiated once the diagnosis is confirmed.

The concept of the *m*itral valve, *a*ortic, *s*keletal, and *s*kin involvement *(MASS)* phenotype, which was developed by Glesby and Pyeritz,[182] represents a useful approach to this difficult problem. This acronym is derived from the involvement present in many patients who have features that do not add up to the classic Marfan syndrome. The acronym has the advantage of making it possible to avoid attaching the label "Marfan syndrome," with all the prognostic, therapeutic, and psychologic implications that this diagnosis carries, to a doubtful case.

Difficulty with diagnostic precision, which frequently arises in the practice of medical genetics, was one of the driving forces behind the formula-

---

Conditions that Share Clinical Features with the Marfan Syndrome

Skeletal

Homocystinuria
Congenital contractural arachnodactyly
Osteogenesis imperfecta
Mitral valve prolapse syndrome
Pseudoxanthoma elasticum
Klinefelter syndrome (47, XXY)
Trisomy 8 (47, XX or XY, +8)
Goodman camptodactyly syndrome B
Stickler syndrome
Syndrome of nerve deafness, eye anomalies, and marfanoid habitus
Nemaline myopathy
Syndrome of pigmentary degeneration, cataract, microcephaly, and arachnodactyly
Myotonic dystrophy
Multiple endocrine adenomatosis, type III
Fragilitas oculi
Achard syndrome

Ocular

Homocystinuria
Familial ectopia lentis
Weill-Marchesani syndrome
Ehlers-Danlos syndrome, type VI
Stickler syndrome

Cardiovascular

Syphilitic aortitis
Ehlers-Danlos syndromes
Familial bicuspid aortic valve
Mitral valve prolapse syndrome
Osteogenesis imperfecta
Erdheim cystic medial necrosis
Relapsing polychondritis
Ankylosing spondylitis
Reiter syndrome

From Pyeritz RE, Murphy EA, McKusick VA: *Birth Defects, Original Articles Series* 15(5B):155-178, 1979.

---

tion of diagnostic criteria for the Marfan syndrome as promulgated in the Berlin nosology.[35] Although the criteria are helpful, they are imprecise, and numerous doubtful or partial cases (formes fruste) may still remain undiagnosed. Conditions that may engender diagnostic confusion are listed in the box on this page. The discovery of fibrillin and the identification of the locus of the Marfan gene will eventually be extremely useful in the diagnostic process, but today their role is limited.

Habitus

The excessive height and long limb length in persons with the Marfan syndrome can be simulated by unusually tall, asthenic individuals with normal health: the Dinka people of the Upper Nile and the Watusi of Central Africa are notable examples. Delayed puberty may be accompanied by marfanoid body proportions, and the gracile habitus of many persons with atrial septal defect often leads to a mistaken diagnosis of the Marfan syndrome. The high frequency of chest wall deformity in patients with congenital malformations of the heart[309] may further increase the confusion with the Marfan syndrome. Other conditions with features that resemble those of the Marfan syndrome are the Klinefelter syndrome, the fragile-X syndrome, familial aortic dissection, and various unclassifiable forms of EDS. Gigantism caused by excessive anterior pituitary activity is also sometimes confused with the Marfan syndrome, although differentiation is not difficult. It is of practical importance that arachnodactyly, or excessive length of the digits, is far from being specific for the Marfan syndrome. Indeed, arachnodactyly can occur in otherwise normal individuals and as a component of a number of genetic syndromes.

Ectopia Lentis

Ectopia lentis is a major manifestation of the Marfan syndrome, but it also occurs in isolation in the form of an autosomal recessive trait[344] and in conjunction with aniridia.[114] Dislocated lenses also are seen in persons with other ocular[206,242,344] and systemic[32,448] disorders. In addition, dislocated lenses are a component of the Weill-Marchesani syndrome, in which shortening of the limbs and digits contrasts with the characteristic lengthening in the Marfan syndrome (see Chapter 5) and homocystinuria (see Chapter 4). Linkage studies[491] in two families with dominantly inherited ectopia lentis have documented cosegregation of the phenotype with the fibrillin gene on chromosome 15.

Mitral Valve Prolapse

Prolapse of the mitral valve, which is detected on auscultation and confirmed by means of echocardiography or similar techniques,[360] is the most common cardiac abnormality.[85,86,124] This condition is generally considered benign,[34,85,86,124,299] and women and girls are much more often affected than men and boys.[299] Many individuals with mitral valve prolapse have a marfanoid habitus* and this factor, together with the autosomal dominant transmission of the valvular defect,[124] necessitates careful differentiation from the Marfan syndrome.[182] Comparisons of phenotypic features of the Marfan syndrome with those of mitral valve prolapse syndrome are shown in Tables 3-5 to 3-7. Only about 0.25% of all individuals

_____

*References 34, 55, 124, 405, 416, and 432.

Table 3-5. Prevalence of skeletal abnormalities in persons with Marfan syndrome, in persons with mitral valve prolapse, and in control subjects

Abnormality	Marfan syndrome (n = 59)			Mitral valve prolapse (n = 53)			Normal (n = 59)		
	No.	Percent	p value*	No.	Percent	p value†	No.	Percent	p value‡
Arachnodactyly	45	76	<0.0001	5	9	NS	0		<0.0001
Abnormal segment ratio	38	66	<0.0001	1	2	NS	4	7	<0.0001
Pectus excavatum	29	49	NS	23	43	<0.0005	7	12	<0.0001
Pectus carinatum	14	24	<0.0005	0		NS	1	2	<0.001
Scoliosis	36	61	<0.0001	11	21	NS	10	17	<0.0001
Straight back	4	7	NS	7	13	<0.05	0		NS
Arm span 3 or more inches greater than height	16	28	NS (0.06)	6	12	NS	4	7	<0.01

From Roman MJ et al: _Am J Cardiol_ 63:317-321, 1989.
*Marfan syndrome versus mitral valve prolapse.
†Mitral valve prolapse versus normal.
‡Marfan syndrome versus normal.
_NS_, Not significant.

Table 3-6. Prevalence of auscultatory findings in persons with Marfan syndrome, in persons with mitral valve prolapse, and in control subjects

Finding	Marfan syndrome (n = 59)		Mitral valve prolapse (n = 59)		Normal (n = 59)	
	No.	Percent	No.	Percent	No.	Percent
Silent or midsystolic murmur	20	34	15	25	59	100
Midsystolic click	8	14	13	22		0
Late systolic click	7	12	12	20		0
Midsystolic click/late systolic murmur	12	20	15	25		0
Holosystolic murmur	1	2	4	7		
Midsystolic click, late systolic murmur, or early diastolic murmur	1	2		0		
Midsystolic click and early diastolic murmur	2	3		0		0
Early diastolic murmur	8	14		0		0

From Roman MJ et al: _Am J Cardiol_ 63:317-321, 1989.

Table 3-7. Echocardiographic measurements in persons with Marfan syndrome, in persons with mitral valve prolapse, and in control subjects

Measurement	Marfan syndrome (n = 59)		Mitral valve prolapse (n = 53)		Normal (n = 59)	
		p value*		p value†		p value‡
Aortic dimensions (cm)						
Annulus	2.8 ± 0.4	<0.0005	2.4 ± 0.3	NS	2.4 ± 0.4	<0.005
Sinuses of Valsalva	4.1 ± 0.9	<0.0005	3.1 ± 0.5	NS	3.0 ± 0.4	<0.0005
Supraaortic ridge	3.5 ± 1.0	<0.0005	2.7 ± 0.5	NS	2.5 ± 0.4	<0.0005
Proximal ascending aorta	3.5 ± 1.0	<0.0005	2.7 ± 0.5	NS	2.5 ± 0.4	<0.0005
Left ventricular end-diastolic dimensions (cm)	5.3 ± 0.8	NS	5.1 ± 0.7	NS	5.1 ± 0.6	NS
Left ventricular mass (g)	155 ± 69	<0.005	127 ± 54	NS	119 ± 46	<0.005
Fractional shortening (%)	35 ± 5	NS	34 ± 6	NS	33 ± 4	NS
Left atrial dimension (cm)	2.7 ± 0.6	NS	3.0 ± 0.9	NS	3.0 ± 0.5	<0.05

From Roman MJ et al: *Am J Cardiol* 63:317-321, 1989.
Multivariate analysis of variance, $p < 0.00005$.
*Marfan syndrome versus mitral valve prolapse.
†Mitral valve prolapse versus normal.
‡Marfan syndrome versus normal.
NS, Not significant.

with mitral valve prolapse have the classic Marfan syndrome.[405] Investigations of the fibrillin genes and their chromosomal loci may permit resolution of the problem of the interrelationship between the mitral valve prolapse syndrome and the Marfan syndrome.

Annuloaortic Ectasia

There have been many reports of pathologic features of Erdheim cystic medial necrosis in patients with aortic dilation and dissection in the absence of skeletal and ocular features of the Marfan syndrome.[142,427,506] This condition, known as annuloaortic ectasia, may be transmitted as an autosomal dominant trait,* and because its natural history resembles that of the Marfan syndrome, there is potential for diagnostic confusion. Unlike in persons with the Marfan syndrome, in whom the mean age at the occurrence of dissecting aneurysm of the aorta is 30 years, dissecting aneurysms in persons with annuloaortic ectasia most frequently occur between the ages of 40 and 70 years (mean age is 50 years). It is significant, however, that aortic dissections have also been ob-

served in infants.[143,227,302,403] As in the Marfan syndrome, the aortic valve may be bicuspid and incompetent in annuloaortic ectasia. On clinical examination the major distinction between these conditions is the absence of skeletal and ocular involvement in the latter disorder. Immunohistochemical analyses of tissue obtained from individuals with annuloaortic ectasia, performed by use of antibodies to fibrillin, have detected no abnormalities.[184,348] Pathologic examination has suggested a less severe disruption of the elastic lammelae of the aorta in annuloaortic ectasia than in the Marfan syndrome.[359,420,486] Nevertheless, the identification of the pathogenetic mechanism must await the molecular and biochemical analyses of the fibrillins and other connective tissue proteins.

Congenital Contractural Arachnodactyly

In 1971 Beals and Hecht[29] described two kindreds with an autosomal dominant disorder of connective tissue. Epstein et al.[144] had documented a similar family a few years earlier. These patients had multiple joint contractures, arachnodactyly, dolichostenomelia, kyphoscoliosis, and "crumpled" external ears. The authors termed this condition "congenital contractural arachnodactyly

---

*References 47, 143, 205, 209, 227, 320, 348, 419, 483, and 509.

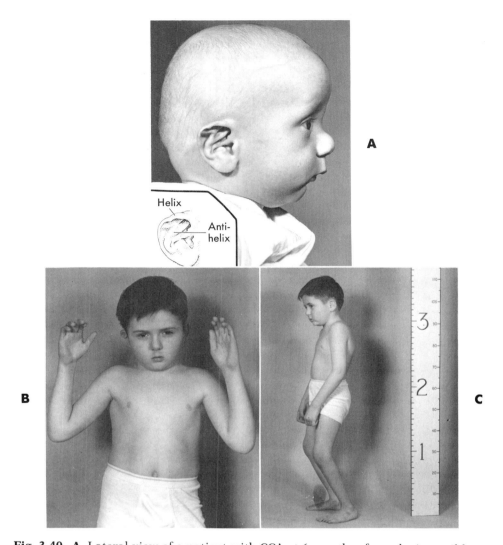

Helix

Anti-
helix

Fig. 3-40. A, Lateral view of a patient with CCA at 6 months of age depicts mild retrognathia, oval-shaped head, and the crumpled appearance of the antihelix with flattening of the helix and partial obliteration of the concha. **B,** Anteroposterior photograph of the patient at 4 years of age illustrates the maximum extension of the fingers. **C,** Lateral view of patient at 6 years of age demonstrates flexion contractures of the knees, elbows, fingers, and toes. Mild retrognathia is present, and the antihelix of the ear is crumpled in appearance. Also evident is the adducted position of the thumb. (From Beals RK, Hecht F: *J Bone Joint Surg* 53[A]:987-993, 1971.)

(CCA)" (Fig. 3-40) and identified in the literature a number of persons with the same condition. They suggested that Marfan's original patient, Gabrielle, had this disorder. At 5 years of age she had contractures of the elbows, fingers, knees, and toes and had long, narrow fingers and toes.[298] Her case was later followed up by Méry and Babonneix,[323] and scoliosis was noted. Neither report mentioned any cardiac or ocular abnormality.

As with the Marfan syndrome, CCA does not have any special gender, geographic, or ethnic predilection.* Sporadic patients, who presumably represent new dominant mutations, have been described.[48,285,292] The phenotypic boundaries are not clearly defined, and a number of disorders

---

*References 48, 165, 228, 327, 453, 485, and 501.

Table 3-8. Frequency of clinical features in congenital contractural arachnodactyly

Clinical feature	Frequency (%)
Craniofacial	
Unusual shape of head	30.0
Micrognathia	23.4
High-arched palate	28.3
Crumpled ear	65.6
Extremities	
Limited extension	
Elbows	84.4
Knees	79.0
Hips	29.0
Camptodactyly	89.1
Arachnodactyly	85.9
Adducted thumbs	48.9
Kyphosis, scoliosis, or both	50.0
Clubfoot deformity	37.3
Bowed long bones	25.0
Hypoplastic muscles	60.0
Other	
Heart defect	14.7
Osteoporosis	5.7
Spontaneous improvements of contractures with time	93.7

Modified from Ramos Arroyo MA et al: *Clin Genet* 27:570-581, 1985.

that are similar to but not identical with CCA have also been reported.[358] The overlap with the Marfan syndrome is such that both CCA and Marfan patients have been documented in the same kindred.[26] A summary of the frequency of clinical features in persons with CCA is shown in Table 3-8.

The joint contractures are most obvious in the digits and most severe in the hand. On clinical examination the most important feature of CCA is progressive scoliosis, which has been observed in many patients. Like the Marfan syndrome, CCA is not associated with mental retardation.[29] Persons with CCA do not usually have the cardiovascular features of the Marfan syndrome, although some congenital heart anomalies have been observed.[285] Since cardiac problems are not a prominent feature of CCA, the prognosis is better than in the Marfan syndrome. Ectopia lentis has been docu-

mented in a boy with CCA who also had aortic root dilation,[27] but eye involvement is distinctly uncommon in the disorder.

The "marfanoid" appearance of patients with CCA has generated a great deal of confusion in the differential diagnosis of these two conditions. Indeed, in the past CCA was often considered a pleiotropic manifestation of the Marfan syndrome.[375] The reason for this similarity became evident when the gene that causes CCA was identified.[272] The search for the Marfan syndrome gene resulted in the fortuitous discovery of a second fibrillin-like gene that was localized to chromosome 5 and linked to the phenotype in three large families with CCA.[272,491] Formal proof of this association awaits identification of mutations in this gene in patients with CCA.

Homocystinuria

Homocystinuria closely resembles the Marfan syndrome; indeed, it was first delineated in institutionalized persons who were regarded as having the Marfan syndrome and mental retardation. McKusick pointed out the main differentiating features, which are given in Table 3-9.

A full account of homocystinuria is given in Chapter 4.

Klinefelter Syndrome

Men with Klinefelter syndrome are often lanky and thin and have body proportions that resemble those of persons with the Marfan syndrome. These men lack the cardiac and ocular features, however, and they do not meet the diagnostic criteria in the Berlin nosology. Small testes and supernumerary X chromosomes further distinguish these individuals.

Stickler Syndrome

The Stickler syndrome was first described in 1965[456] as an autosomal dominant disorder that affected the skeleton and eye.* Sensorineural hearing loss was documented in subsequent reports.[281,457] The skeletal abnormalities include bony enlargements of joints, which may be evident at birth, and a marfanoid habitus. Mandibular hypoplasia, cleft palate, bifid uvula, highly arched palate, and abnormal teeth have also been

---

*References 37, 43, 78, 222, 434, and 452.

Table 3-9. Main differentiating features in homocystinuria and the Marfan syndrome

Feature	Marfan syndrome	Homocystinuria
Major cardiovascular involvement	Aortic	Thrombolic
Ectopia lentis	Present at birth; lenses predominantly dislocated upward	Develops in later years; lenses predominantly dislocated downward
Mental retardation	Absent	Variable

reported.[222,281] Thus infants who have had a diagnosis of the Pierre-Robin anomaly warrant evaluation for the Stickler syndrome.[353] The frequency of mitral valve prolapse in patients with the Stickler syndrome is almost 50%.[281] Progressive degenerative arthropathy, which predominantly involves the weight-bearing joints, develops during adulthood. Articular hypermobility, which is maximal in the hips and fingers, may also be present.

Ophthalmic complications are the most important feature of the Stickler syndrome, and loss of vision is a major problem.[222] Affected persons have severe myopia that is progressive and often is associated with chorioretinal degeneration and retinal detachment.[43,479] Diagnostic precision is crucial for appropriate management of these potentially serious ophthalmic complications.[434]

Disorders that enter into the differential diagnosis of the Stickler syndrome include Marshall and Weissenbacher-Zweymuller syndromes (now thought to be the same entities as the Stickler syndrome), Kneist dysplasia, multiple epiphyseal dysplasia, spondyloepiphyseal dysplasia congenita, and Wagner syndrome.[341,479] Genetic counseling follows conventional guidelines for any autosomal dominant disorder in which phenotypic expression is variable.

Genetic linkage studies have documented cosegregation of the gene encoding type II collagen with the Stickler syndrome in some[167,169,258,369] but not all[172,258] families. A premature stop codon in one procollagen allele has been found in all affected members of a kindred with the condition.[6] It can be anticipated that other collagens or connective tissue proteins that are involved in the pathophysiologic features of the Stickler syndrome will be identified in the future. The Stickler syndrome is also discussed in Chapter 14, p. 605.

Marfanoid Hypermobility Syndrome

The marfanoid hypermobility syndrome was delineated by Walker, Beighton, and Murdoch[507] in a young man with a marfanoid habitus, gross articular laxity, and dermal extensibility who had no ocular or cardiac abnormalities (Fig. 3-41). Similar examples can be identified in the literature.[239] The genetic basis of this disorder is uncertain, and whether it is an autonomous entity separate from the Marfan syndrome is in doubt.[36] In this context it is significant that the prototypic patient[507] subsequently died of rupture of the aorta after progressive dilation of the aortic root with aortic regurgitation.[319]

PATHOLOGY
Cardiovascular Features

More than 90% of deaths in the Marfan syndrome are due to cardiovascular involvement, and many studies of the cardiovascular complications may be found in the literature. Roberts and Honig[401] reviewed necropsy findings in 151 previously published cases and in 18 personally studied patients. These authors separated the patients into three groups based on the observed cardiovascular lesions. Group 1 had fusiform aneurysms of the ascending aorta; group 2 had aortic dissection; and group 3 had the primary cardiovascular findings of mitral regurgitation, floppy mitral leaflets, and dilated mitral annuli. A fourth "miscellaneous" group was needed to include some patients who did not fit into group 1, 2, or 3. These findings, including the observations from a review of the literature, are summarized in Table 3-10.

Gross pathologic findings in the heart and major blood vessels in the Marfan syndrome have been well described (Figs. 3-42 and 3-43). Aneurysms are fairly common, usually in the ascending

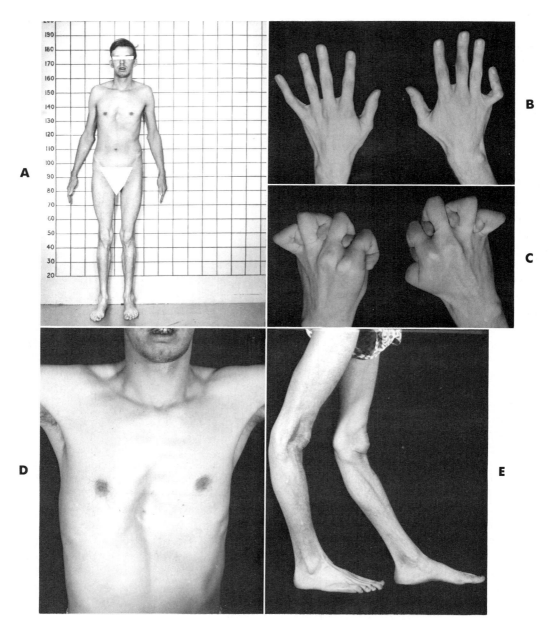

Fig. 3-41. Marfanoid hypermobility syndrome. This 27-year-old man was the youngest of eight children and the only sib with the features demonstrated here. The father and mother were likewise healthy. They were not consanguineous and were 40 and 41 years of age, respectively, at the time of his birth. Extreme articular laxity, with ability to dislocate the sternoclavicular joints, had been present all his life. He was myopic. **A,** His US/LS value was 0.92. **B,** Pronounced pectus excavatum, mild lower thoracic scoliosis, and, **C,** arachnodactyly with camptodactyly were present. Steinberg's thumb sign was positive. **D,** He showed extreme loose-jointedness in the fingers. **E,** Genu recurvatum. He also showed hyperextensibility of the skin with numerous horizontal striae distensae over the lower back. A loud mid-systolic click was audible over the entire precordium.

Table 3-10. Cardiovascular abnormalities observed on necropsy in 169 patients with the Marfan syndrome

Feature	Frequency (number and %)	Age range (mo, yr)	Mean age (yr)	Aortic regurgitation (number and %)
Fusiform ascending aortic aneurysm	66 (39)	7 mo-62 yr	29	53/55 (96)
Aortic dissection	60 (36)	13 yr-52 yr	28	3/30 (10)
Mitral regurgitation without other cardiovascular involvement	35 (21)	2 mo-65 yr	13	1/33 (3)
Other	8	Stillborn-35 yr	—	0

Adapted from Roberts WC, Honig HS: *Am Heart J* 104:115-135, 1982.

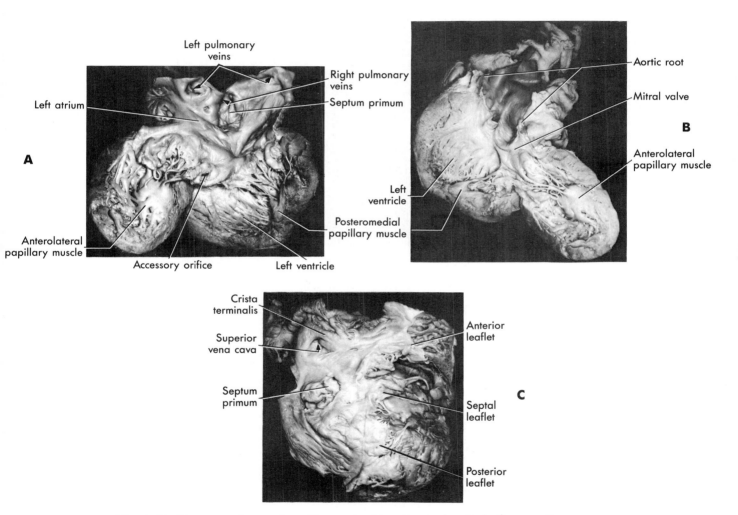

Fig. 3-42. Heart specimen of an 11-month-old patient who died of congestive cardiac failure. **A,** Left ventricular view. Thickened, redundant valve leaflets herniate toward the left atrium, giving rise to the "hemorrhoidal" appearance of the valve. The chordae tendineae are thickened, elongated, and redundant. Note the accessory orifice in the anterior leaflet of the mitral valve. The left atrium is markedly dilated, and the septum primum is redundant. The left ventricle is enlarged and hypertrophied with a prominent anterolateral papillary muscle, compared to the posteromedial papillary muscle. **B,** Left ventricular view showing a markedly dilated aortic root at the sinuses of Valsalva. The ascending aortic diameter tapers distally. **C,** Right ventricular view. The anterior leaflet, septal leaflet, and posterior leaflet of the tricuspid valve are thickened and redundant and protrude toward the markedly dilated right atrium. The chordae tendineae are elongated, and redundancy of septum primum is evident. (From Geva T et al: *Am J Cardiol* 65:1230-1237, 1990.)

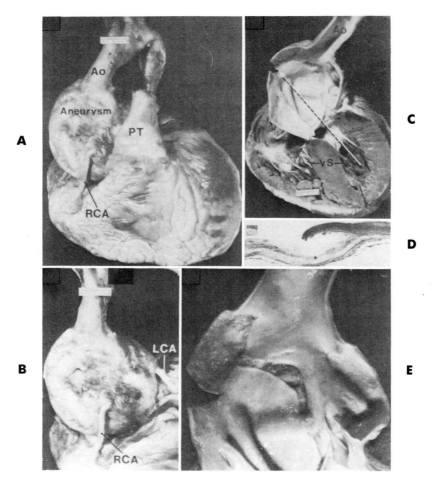

Fig. 3-43. Rupture of an ascending aortic aneurysm in a 38-year-old black man with the Marfan syndrome. The patient was known to have a murmur of aortic regurgitation (aortic pressure, 115/55 mm Hg), but there was no evidence of congestive heart failure. He died suddenly at home, and at necropsy the pericardial space was filled with blood and a tear was present in a large aneurysm involving all three sinuses of Valsalva and the proximal tubular portion of ascending aorta. **A,** View of heart shows the size of the aneurysm in comparison with the sizes of other structures. **B,** A closer view of the large aneurysm with the coronary arteries arising from it. **C,** The anterior half of the heart and aorta have now been removed. The dashed line depicts the direction of the blood ejected from the left ventricle. The arrow points to the rupture site in the wall of the aneurysm. The right lateral wall is the site of the rupture. **D,** Close-up of the interior lining of aortic aneurysm at the site of rupture. Several healed incomplete tears are present in the wall of the aneurysm, and these have been confused with aortic dissections. **E,** Photomicrograph through one of the aortic tears showing massive degeneration of elastic fibers. *Ao,* Aorta; *LCA,* left coronary artery; *PT,* pulmonary truck; *RCA,* right coronary artery; *VS,* ventricular septum. (From Roberts WC: *Cardiovasc Clin* 10:407-453, 1979.)

aorta. Aortic dissection is also frequent. The dissections are characterized by separation of the medial layers of the wall of the aorta parallel to the direction of blood flow.[399] Dissection frequently involves the descending thoracic and abdominal aorta, extending from the ascending aorta. At times, what appears to be dissection of the ascending aorta is probably direct "through-and-through" rupture of an aortic aneurysm.[401] Aortic dissection is associated with bicuspidity of the aortic valve both in patients with the Marfan syndrome and in persons without the syndrome. Left ventricular hypertrophy is present in the majority of patients with the Marfan syndrome who have aortic dissections and is probably a sign of the presence of significant aortic regurgitation, which is due to aortic dilation that predisposes to aortic dissection.[123,398,399,401]

Abnormalities of the cardiac valves are frequent in the Marfan syndrome. Indeed, although rupture or dissection of an aneurysm is an obvious and dramatic cause of death, the major consequence of aortic aneurysm in Marfan patients is aortic regurgitation. In the review of Roberts and Honig[401] the authors noted cardiac valve changes, which included thinned and stretched aortic valve cusps, thickened margins of aortic valve cusps, endocarditis of the mitral valve, calcification of the mitral annulus and leaflets, dilated mitral valve annulus, floppy mitral leaflets, and ruptured and elongated mitral chordae tendineae. Dilation of the sinuses of Valsalva is a normal phenomenon of aging that is common in hypertensive individuals, but premature dilation of the sinuses may also occur in the Marfan syndrome.[398,400] Autopsy examination of a 2-day-old child with infantile Marfan syndrome, who died of congestive heart failure, revealed an enlarged heart, wrinkled aortic intima, and elongated mitral and tricuspid leaflets.[401]

Histologic changes in the tunica media of the great vessels and in the heart valves are well documented in the Marfan syndrome, but it must be emphasized that these changes are far from specific. Medial thinning caused by tears of the aortic wall after aneurysm rupture is a frequent finding, and healed nontransmural tears often can be seen in some of the same tissue sections.[401] The aortic wall at the site of tears is thin. Schlatmann and Becker[427] described an abrupt laceration in the media of both incomplete and complete aortic an-

eurysms. A channel (false lumen) representing the dissection is formed from the tear in patients with complete dissections. If the false lumen connects to the true lumen distally, the chronic dissection may exist for a long time.

Limited ultrastructural analyses have been performed in cardiovascular tissues of Marfan patients. Renteria et al.[392] recorded alteration of collagen fibrils in the leaflets and chordae tendineae in floppy mitral valves. Fragmented elastic fibers, granular cells, and cystic spaces were also described. Patterns of fine filaments and electron-dense spheres representing acid mucopolysaccharides have been observed.[392,470] Changes in elastin, described as "moth-eaten" atrophy, are common ultrastructural features.[470] Interestingly, no apparent electron microscopic abnormalities of elastin-associated microfibrils have been observed in aortic tissue of affected persons.[230,515]

The most common histologic manifestation seen in persons with the Marfan syndrome is the so-called cystic medial necrosis. The term was coined by Erdheim,[145] who recognized its specific inaccuracy. "Massive degeneration of elastic fibers" has been proposed as a more accurate description.[401] Nevertheless, the descriptive designation "cystic medial necrosis" is used by pathologists to describe characteristic medial changes, since it reflects the severity of destruction of tissue architecture.

A typical pattern of medial degeneration with "cystic medial necrosis" in a Marfan patient is compared to a normal control in Fig. 3-44. The short, irregular, fragmented elastic fibers are readily apparent in the section obtained from the aneurysmal aorta. Collagen fibrils and mucoid material fill the space once occupied by elastic fibers. Virtually all aortic aneurysms in persons with the Marfan syndrome display severe medial degeneration, but these changes are much less marked in aortic dissection in patients who do not have the Marfan syndrome.[401,417,472] Takebayashi, Kubota, and Takagi[470] and Saruk and Eisenstein[417] recorded capillary invasion from the vasa vasorum into the "cystic" lesion. Roberts and Honig[401] commented that aortic aneurysms have not been described in neonates with the Marfan syndrome, and these authors postulated that although the genetic abnormality of connective tissue is present at birth, the formation of the aneurysm is due to intraaortic pressure on a defective

A   B

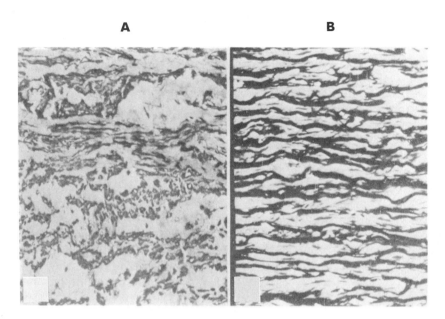

Fig. 3-44. Photomicrograph of segment of dilated ascending aorta, **A,** compared with control, **B,** in a 35-year-old woman with the Marfan syndrome. Histologic study of the wall of the aortic aneurysm showed virtual absence of elastic fibers (compared with normal, **B**), and increased mucoid material. (Movat stains; each original magnification × 330.) (From Roberts WC, Honig HS: *Am Heart J* 104:115-135, 1982.)

aortic wall.[401,427] Electron microscopic examination of cystic medial degeneration shows areas with many smooth-muscle cells but with little elastic tissue. Adjacent areas may have few cells but significant amounts of ill-defined extracellular material.[417] Most interestingly, Saruk and Eisenstein[417] found clusters of microfibrils without amorphous elastin. This observation has been confirmed by immunohistochemical studies in abdominal aortic aneurysms and atherosclerotic lesions in patients without the Marfan syndrome.[28] It has long been thought that this process may be an abortive attempt at repair.[417] Medial degenerative changes also have been observed in arteries from peripheral organs,[471] in coronary arteries,[31] and in pulmonary arteries.[134]

Most of the vascular abnormalities observed in the Marfan syndrome are not specific to the disease. Indeed, medial degeneration is a normal phenomenon of aging,[426] and premature or severe medial degeneration is seen in aortic aneurysms in persons without the Marfan syndrome.[302] Such aneurysms include annuloaortic ectasia[320,348,509] and those associated with bicuspid aortic valves[140] or systemic hypertension.[417]

Ocular Features

A number of studies have been concerned with the pathologic features of the eye in the Marfan syndrome.* The first and definitive histopathologic description was published in 1941 by Dvorak-Theobald.[138] She examined an eye removed at autopsy from a 27-month-old child with the Marfan syndrome. Her findings included a striking megaloglobus, displaced lenses, increased distance from the limbus to the insertion of each rectus muscle, incomplete separation between the iris and trabeculum, undeveloped pupil dilator and ciliary muscles, stretched retina with absence of pigment epithelium in places, thin choroid, and wavy zonular fibers. These observations have been confirmed in other patients.[71,386,390]

In scanning electron microscopic investigations of eyes obtained from two Marfan patients in whom ectopia lentis was not manifest, Ramsey et al.[386] observed a lack of widespread separation of the zonular fibers into a fan of filaments. The filaments became attenuated toward the lens capsule.

———

*References 138, 155, 308, 386, 436, 464, and 505.

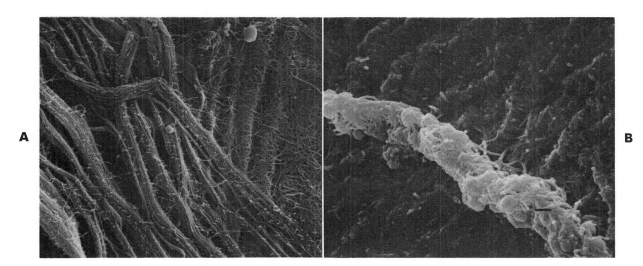

Fig. 3-45. Zonules from comparable posterior-equatorial regions of human lenses. **A,** Normal lens contains numerous well-organized zonules composed of parallel fibrils *(arrow).* **B,** Lens from patient with the Marfan syndrome displays one malformed zonule composed of irregular aggregates *(arrow).* (From Farnsworth PN et al: *Arch Ophthalmol* 95:1601-1606, 1977.)

These abnormalities were not visible by light microscopy. Scanning electron microscopic examination of the lens in a Marfan patient with subluxated lenses revealed a few malformed zonules, larger lens fibrils than normally seen, and an apparent decrease in zonular elasticity when compared to normal[155] (Fig. 3-45). Setälä, Ruusuvaara, and Karjalainen[436] examined the corneal endothelium in 41 patients with the Marfan syndrome. Fifteen had dislocated lenses, whereas 26 had no lens subluxation. In the former subgroup guttata formation was present in most instances, whereas little guttata formation was seen in the latter subgroup. These authors concluded that persons with more prominent ocular manifestations have more significant endothelial abnormalities. Immunohistochemical analyses of zonular fibers have demonstrated apparent fibrillin abnormalities.[464]

BASIC DEFECT

In 1956 Dr. McKusick, writing presciently in the first edition of this book, stated, "What the suspensory ligament of the lens has in common with the tunica media of the aorta is obscure. If this common factor were known, the basic defect of the Marfan syndrome might be understood." Although it was predicted that the Marfan syndrome would be among the first of the heritable disorders of connective tissue in which the underlying defect was identified, this proved not to be the case. Indeed, before the recent dramatic breakthroughs, the origin of the condition remained enigmatic, despite the efforts of numerous researchers.

The quest for the basic defect causing the Marfan syndrome continued unabated during the decades following McKusick's statement. Early reports suggested abnormalities in serum seromucoid,[18] hyaluronic acid,[15,268] beta glucuronic acid,[340] collagen,[58,73,267,423] and elastin.* More recently, linkage studies excluded the collagen types I, II, III, and VI[112,168,351,489] and, to a limited degree, elastin.[248,408] The way in which the underlying biomolecular abnormalities in the Marfan syndrome were finally elucidated is outlined in this section.

Immunohistochemical Studies

In the early 1980s in the Los Angeles laboratory of David Hollister, a monoclonal antibody that

---

*References 120,201,359,365,471,and 492.

produced a striking pattern when used to stain the immunizing tissue, amniotic membranes, was serendipitously developed.[231] Characterization of this antigen demonstrated a protein of about 350 kd molecular weight that was immunoreactive in the dermal-epidermal junction and basement membrane of skin. Subsequent analyses of this microfibrillar protein, termed *fibrillin,* showed a ubiquitous distribution, including the suspensory ligament of the lens and aortic media.[414] In light of McKusick's remarks concerning the potential importance of a common factor in these tissues, studies of Marfan patients by means of this new antibody to microfibrillar fibers were undertaken.

Microfibrils are fibers 10 to 12 nm in diameter that, when visualized by electron microscopy, appear as linear bundles. Microfibrillar fibers are a widely distributed and pleiomorphic fiber system in human tissues.[237,290] They are believed to form the scaffolding for the deposition of elastin during elastogenesis,[92,93,189] and in many tissues these fibers become incorporated into the elastic structures. Although always found in elastic tissues, microfibrils are much more widely distributed than elastin. They have been observed by means of immunolocalization in skin, tendon, cartilage, muscle, kidney, perichondrium, periosteum, blood vessels, pleura, dura mater, and ciliary zonules of the lens.* The distribution of microfibrils clearly encompasses all tissues in which phenotypic effects are observed in the Marfan syndrome.

Fibrillin is one of the most extensively characterized of the microfibrillar proteins. Amniotic membrane digests have allowed the isolation of three pepsin-resistant fragments.[295] One fragment was shown to contain the domain that was reactive with the monoclonal antibody used in the immunohistochemical studies of the Marfan syndrome and other disorders. The molecular weight of two constituent peptides is equal to about half the weight of the intact molecule, which suggests a stable secondary structure resulting from intrachain disulfide bonding.[414] Nevertheless, the relationship among the peptides or between them and elastin or other microfibrillar entities is not known.

To assess putative changes in microfibrillar fi-

bers in patients with the Marfan syndrome, a large single-blind study was initiated.[232] In this study of 65 persons, 27 of whom had been diagnosed as having unequivocal Marfan syndrome, almost 90% showed abnormalities in the distribution of microfibrils in skin and their production in dermal fibroblasts.

These analyses were based on the immunoreactive pattern as assessed by indirect immunofluorescence of 15-μm sections of skin and by hyperconfluent minicultures of skin fibroblasts. The patterns observed in a person with the Marfan syndrome and an age-matched control are shown in Figs. 3-46 and 3-47. The characteristic and reproducible immunostaining pattern seen in cryosections of normal human skin when stained with antibodies to fibrillin is depicted in Fig. 3-46, *A* and *B.* The dermal-epidermal junction is a brightly stained meshwork with a nearly continuous fluorescent band at the basement membrane. Intensely fluorescent large fibers are seen in the reticular dermis. These are elastin profiles that appear surrounded by immunostainable fibrillin fibers. Similarly prepared specimens obtained from an age- and sex-matched patient with the Marfan syndrome is shown in Fig. 3-46, *C* and *D.* The apparent amount of immunofluorescence at the dermal-epidermal junction, the basement membrane, and the surrounding elastin profiles is clearly decreased when compared to that in the control. Analyses of microfibril production as assayed by immunofluorescence with the use of antibodies directed against fibrillin yielded similar results. Fig. 3-47, *A* shows the immunofluorescence pattern of microfibrillar fibers accumulating in hyperconfluent fibroblast cultures of specimens obtained from a normal individual. When the pattern in specimens obtained from an age- and sex-matched patient with the Marfan syndrome is compared (Fig. 3-47, *B*), a significant diminution of immunoreactive material is observed.

This observation of diminished immunofluorescence of microfibrillar fibers as assayed by means of antibodies to the protein fibrillin suggested an etiologic involvement of microfibrils, perhaps fibrillin, in the pathogenesis of the Marfan syndrome.

Three patterns of immunofluorescence were found.[186,232] Apparent diminished amounts of microfibrils in both skin sections and dermal fibroblasts were observed in about 70% of the Marfan

---

*References 100, 255, 387, 414, 462, and 463.

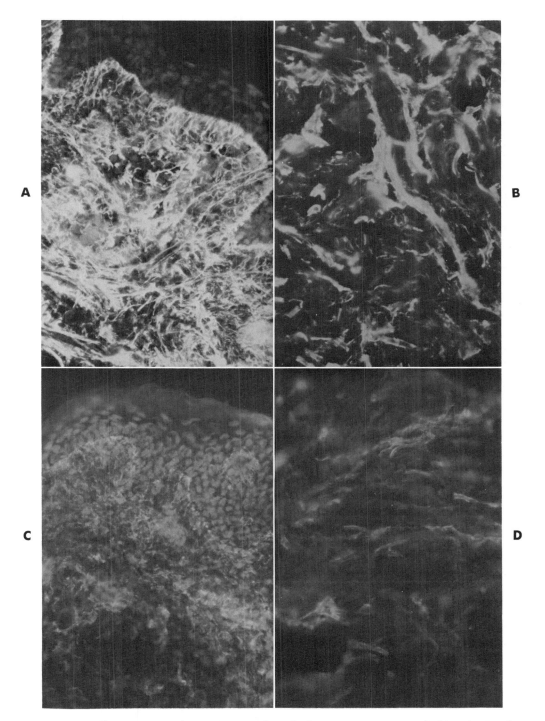

Fig. 3-46. Fluorescence photomicrographs of 15 μm cryosections of skin obtained from a healthy 32-year-old man and a 37-year-old man with the Marfan syndrome (original magnification × 375). Sections were incubated with murine monoclonal antibody against fibrillin, and bound antibody was visualized with goat antimouse IgG antiserum conjugated with phycoerythrin. Nuclei were visualized with propidium iodide. **A** and **B,** The papillary and reticular dermis, respectively, from the normal subject. Brightly stained fibers extend from the dermal-epidermal junction into a complex meshwork in the papillary dermis, **A.** In the reticular dermis, **B,** prominent fluorescence is associated with large, undulating fibers. **C** and **D,** The papillary and reticular dermis, respectively, from the patient with the Marfan syndrome. The papillary dermis, **C,** displays markedly decreased fluorescence staining, and there is little microfibrillar fluorescence associated with elastic fibers in the reticular dermis, **D.** (From Hollister DW et al: *New Engl J Med* 323:152-159, 1990.)

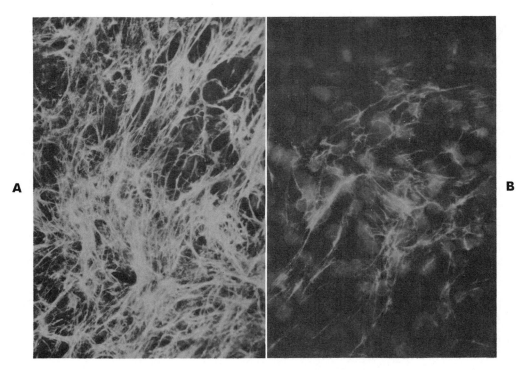

Fig. 3-47. Hyperconfluent multilayers of dermal fibroblasts from a normal subject, **A,** and from an individual with the Marfan syndrome, **B** (original magnification × 375). The normal fibroblasts, **A,** show a prominent meshwork of fibrous material in a 48-hour culture assay. In contrast, fibroblasts of the patient with the Marfan syndrome, **B,** show a sharply decreased amount of immunostainable fibrous meshwork. (From Hollister DW et al: *New Engl J Med* 323:152-159, 1990.)

patients. Approximately 25% of Marfan patients had normal-appearing skin sections but decreased accumulation of immunoreactive material in hyperconfluent fibroblast cultures. The converse, namely, normal accumulation in *in vitro* fibroblast cultures but decreased fluorescence in skin cryosections, was rarely seen (less than 5%). The clinical significance of or relationship to phenotypic manifestations of these varying fluorescence patterns, if any, remains unclear.

Patients with other connective tissue disorders were studied by means of these same assays. About 25% of these patients demonstrated diminished microfibrillar staining when examined by means of skin section or fibroblast culture. With the exception of one person with homocystinuria, however, on clinical examination none of these patients could be confused with persons who have the Marfan syndrome.[232]

These studies were extended to determine whether the apparent diminution of immunoreactive fibers would segregate with the Marfan phenotype in families.[186] Nine Marfan kindreds were studied by means of the antibodies to fibrillin. In every instance microfibrillar abnormalities were seen only in Marfan patients, and the abnormalities segregated with the Marfan phenotype in affected families. Further, the identical immunofluorescence patterns segregated within each kindred.

In the final phase of this section of the investigation a unique patient, a girl described as having unilateral Marfan syndrome, was studied[69] (Fig. 3-48). Skin biopsy specimens were taken from both upper arms and both thighs and examined for fibrillin immunofluorescence. This patient had a 3.5-cm difference in lower limb length (left leg longer), a 4-cm difference in upper limb length (left arm longer), aortic dilation of 28 mm (normal at her age, 12 to 18 mm), and subluxated lens in her left eye only.

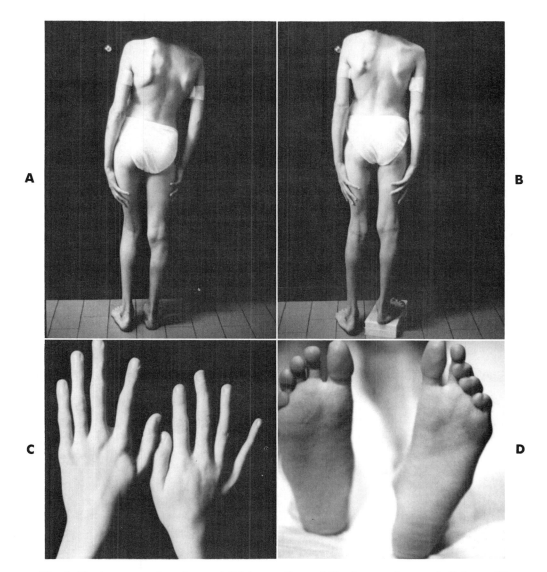

Fig. 3-48. An unusual patient exhibiting unilateral Marfan syndrome. **A,** It is readily apparent that her left arm and left leg are longer than the limbs on the right. **B,** When the right leg is placed on a 4-cm block to level the pelvis, the left leg is clearly longer than the right and slight scoliosis is observed to be more prominent on the left. **C** and **D,** The left hand and fingers and left foot are longer than their respective right counterparts. (This patient was initially reported by Burgio RG et al: *Am J Med Genet* 30:905-909, 1988.)

Immunofluorescence results[187] showed decreased staining of microfibrils in skin sections and dermal fibroblasts derived only from the left side. Skin and fibroblasts from the right side of the body were similar to those of normal age-matched controls.[187] These findings were consistent with the Marfan phenotype being more pronounced on the left side of her body. These studies were the first piece of evidence that abnormalities of microfibrils and, more precisely, fibrillin were the cause of the Marfan syndrome.

Biochemical Studies

The next series of experiments to further suggest fibrillin abnormalities in the Marfan syndrome were carried out by examining the synthesis and secretion of fibrillin from fibroblasts of Marfan patients.[313] In these studies intrinsic labeling of cysteine-rich fibrillin with ^{35}S cysteine was used. Four subgroups of Marfan patients were demonstrated. In the first group the overall synthesis of fibrillin was decreased. In the second group fibrillin was not secreted normally. The third group of patients appeared to have both normal synthesis and normal secretion but defective microfibril formation in the matrix. In the fourth group of patients no abnormalities were found. The correlation of these subgroups to the subgroups identified by means of immunohistochemical techniques is not known. Consistent with the immunohistochemical findings, however, no differences were observed between affected members of the same kinship. Further, no abnormalities in control individuals were noted.

Mapping of Marfan Syndrome Locus

In an independent but simultaneous approach to the identification of a chromosomal region linked to the Marfan syndrome a consortium of laboratories was organized by Dr. Petros Tsipouras.[488] This group began the painstaking task of searching for a chromosomal region linked to the Marfan syndrome by systematically excluding areas of the genome.

Since the most logical candidates, the fibrillar collagens and elastin, had already been excluded, an exclusion map was established by means of anonymous probes. More than 90% of the human genome was eliminated as a possible locus for the Marfan syndrome gene.[50] The map did not exclude the majority of chromosome 15; therefore probes for this chromosome were used in several family studies. Kainulainen et al.[247] were the first to show that the Marfan syndrome was linked to the long arm of chromosome 15. Subsequently analyses in two other laboratories confirmed the linkage and refined the location with more precise boundaries.[132,490]

Fibrillin Defects

Working independently, Godfrey, Lee, Ramirez, Hauster, Maslen, and Sakai searched for the gene encoding fibrillin so that the formal proof of causal relationship could be assessed. The gene was successfully isolated by use of degenerate oligonucleotides derived from peptide sequences, both in polymerase chain reaction (PCR)–based approaches[272] and by means of direct complementary DNA (cDNA) library screening techniques.[305]

The locus of the newfound fibrillin gene was shown to be in the same region of chromosome 15 that recently had been linked to the Marfan syndrome.[272] The next step was linkage analyses with polymorphic markers of the fibrillin gene. In a series of studies[131,272,491] fibrillin has now been linked to the Marfan syndrome with a fibrillin logarithm of the odds score of more than 30 at a recombination fraction of 0. This means that the chances that defects in fibrillin are the cause of this disorder are more than 10^{30} to 1. In light of the phenotypic diversity in the Marfan syndrome, the possibility of genetic heterogeneity remained (i.e., that more than one gene may be responsible for the same clinical phenotype). Therefore studies of numerous families from diverse populations were carried out.[249,491] In all informative families, linkage of the Marfan syndrome with fibrillin or nearby random probes was absolute. There has been only one exception to this finding. A large French pedigree with, according to the authors,[53] typical skeletal and cardiovascular features but no ocular abnormalities does not link to the fibrillin gene on chromosome 15. The significance of the findings in this family remains to be explained.

The results in all but the French family were indicative of a causal relationship between fibrillin and the Marfan syndrome. Absolute formal proof had to await the discovery of a mutation in the fibrillin gene. This discovery was achieved when Dietz et al.[131] demonstrated a *de novo* missense mutation in the fibrillin gene in one allele in each of two sporadic patients with similar phenotypic features of the Marfan syndrome. Sequencing of reverse transcribed RNA revealed a guanine-to-cytosine transversion, which resulted in an arginine-to-proline substitution (Figs. 3-49 and 3-50). The substitution of proline, a nonpolar amino acid, for a basic amino acid may cause a disruption in the secondary structure of the protein. Screening of a random population of individuals who did not have the Marfan syndrome revealed that this was not a normally occurring polymorphism. The first patient in whom the mutation was found had previously been shown to have abnormalities in fibrillin in both skin and fibroblast culture studies by use of the chemical techniques of Hollister et al.[232] In both instances it was demonstrated that the unaffected parents did not have the mutated allele.

Related Disorders

Unexpectedly but serendipitously the search undertaken by Lee et al.[272] for the fibrillin gene turned up two additional fibrillin-like genes. Their locations to chromosomes 5 and 17 did not make them candidates for the Marfan syndrome, given the previous linkage of this disorder to chromosome 15 by random markers. Nevertheless, their involvement in other phenotypically similar disorders warranted consideration.

One of the first candidates approached was CCA, or Beals syndrome, which was first described by Epstein et al.[144] Beals and Hecht[29] had suggested (see the section, Historical Survey) that Marfan's original patient did not have what is now known as the Marfan syndrome but rather, had CCA. Studies[272,491] of three large CCA pedigrees demonstrated linkage to the fibrillinlike gene on chromosome 5. As with the Marfan syndrome, formal proof must await the identification of mutations.

Continuing in this vein, Tsipouras et al.[491] examined three other disorders in which the clinical phenotype overlaps that of the Marfan syndrome. They showed that dominantly inherited ectopia lentis is also linked to the fibrillin gene on chromosome 15, whereas annuloaortic ectasia is not linked to the fibrillin genes on chromosomes 5 and 15. Mitral valve prolapse syndrome is not linked to the fibrillin gene on chromosome 5, but polymorphic markers of the fibrillin gene on chromosome 15 were not informative in the families investigated. Studies of the fibrillin gene on chromosome 17 and other microfibril-encoding genes have yet to be performed.

The sequence of events leading to the final proof that mutations in the fibrillin gene are the cause of the Marfan syndrome represents one of the most elegant examples of the candidate-gene approach to the identification of the cause of a particular disorder.

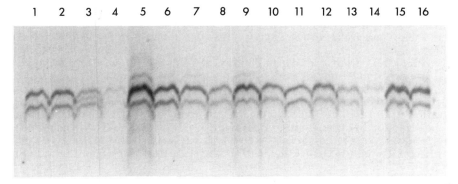

Fig. 3-49. Single-strand confirmation polymorphism analysis of PCR-amplified fibrillin cDNA from two normal individuals (lanes 6 and 11) and 14 patients with isolated Marfan syndrome (lanes 1 to 5, 7 to 10, and 12 to 16). There is an anomalously migrating fragment in lane 3. The bands immediately above and below this position are seen in all individuals tested. Additional bands are occasionally observed in lanes with higher DNA concentrations. (From Dietz H et al: *Nature* 352:337-339, 1991.)

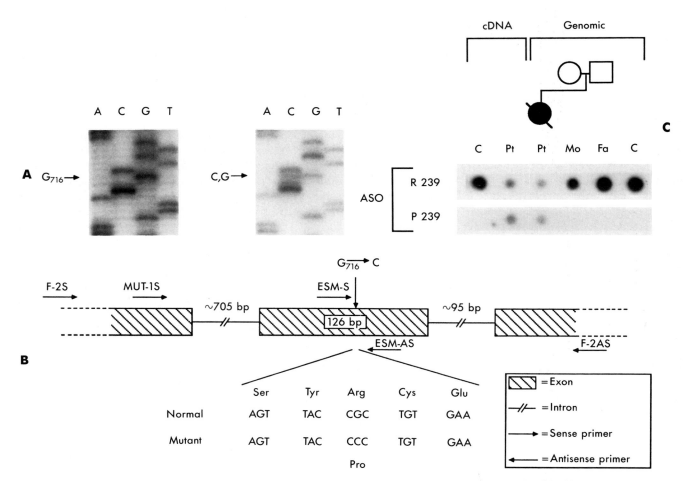

Fig. 3-50. Localization and characterization of the missense mutation in the fibrillin gene in the patient whose cDNA analysis is shown in lane 3 in Fig. 3-49, and identification of intron-exon boundaries in the region. **A,** Direct sequence of PCR-amplified fibrillin cDNA from, *left,* normal control subject and, *right,* patient showing a G-to-C transversion in one of the patient's alleles. **B,** Schematic representation of the fibrillin gene in the region of the mutation. Relative positions of PCR primers are demonstrated in relation to intron-exon boundaries, the point of mutation, and each other. **C,** Dot blot of PCR-amplified cDNA and genomic DNA from control subjects, patient, and her mother and father hybridized to ^{32}P-labeled allele-specific oligonucleotides. Control and parents hybridized only with the normally occurring allele, whereas the patient hybridizes with both the normal allele and the mutant allele. *ASO,* Allele-specific oligonucleotides; *C,* control subjects; *Fa,* father; *Mo,* mother; *P239,* proline at position 239 (mutation); *R239,* arginine at position 239 (normal). (From Dietz H et al: *Nature* 352:337-339, 1991.)

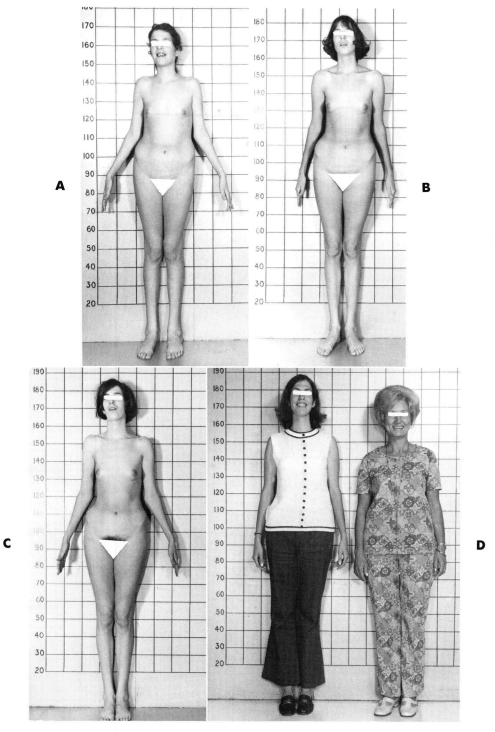

Fig. 3-51. Control of excessive height in the Marfan syndrome by means of estrogen therapy. **A,** Age, 9⁷/₁₂ years; **B,** age, 12²/₁₂ years; **C,** age, 13⁸/₁₂ years; **D,** age, 15¹¹/₁₂ years, with a normal adult. *Continued.*

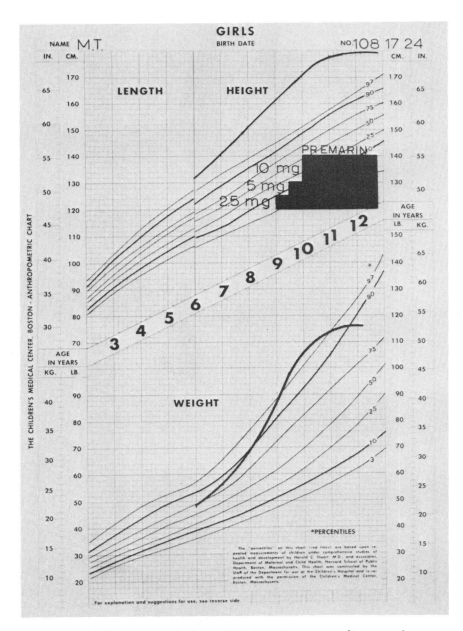

Fig. 3-51, cont'd. E, Growth chart. (For **A** to **D** see preceding page.)

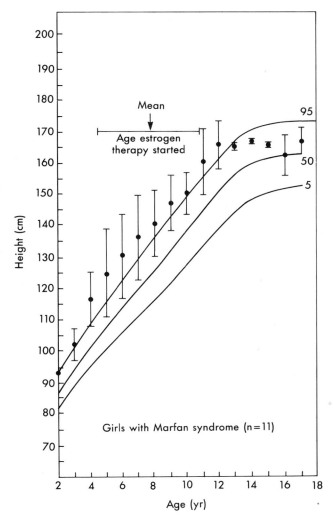

Fig. 3-52. Hormonal modulation of height in girls affected by the Marfan syndrome. In all cases treatment with ethinyl estradiol (0.05 mg/10 kg daily) and conjugated estrogen (Premarin, 10 mg on days 25 to 28 of each menstrual cycle) was begun before menarche. Therapy was continued until the time menarche was likely to have occurred naturally or until bone maturation was well advanced, whichever occurred first. Comparison with Fig. 3-51, **E**, shows early cessation of growth and reduction in height of the girls who received treatment. (From Pyeritz RE. In Emery AH, Rimoin DL, editors: *Principles and practices of medical genetics*, vol 2, New York, 1990, Churchill Livingstone, pp 1047-1063.)

MANAGEMENT

The clinical management of patients with the Marfan syndrome requires a coordinated effort from practitioners in a variety of specialities, and many believe that this approach is best accom-

plished in a multidisciplinary clinic. Equally, this clinical environment is optimal for diagnostic confirmation or negation in doubtful cases.

Skeletal Complications

Scoliosis sometimes causes orthopedic problems in the Marfan syndrome.[379,500] Onset is occasionally in early childhood but usually in puberty, when its progression may be rapid. It is recommended that patients with progressive spinal malalignment be evaluated twice a year.[377,379] Radiographic confirmation of the progression should be obtained at each visit, and mechanical bracing warrants consideration when curvature is greater than 20 degrees.[377,379] Some studies report limited success in treatment by bracing.[46,259] Operative approaches, which have yielded good results, include segmental fixation, fusion with a Harrington rod, and, occasionally, bone grafting for stabilization.*

Estrogen therapy has been given to girls with the Marfan syndrome to induce puberty and promote epiphyseal closure, thus reducing final height[377] (Fig. 3-51). The progression of scoliosis, which often accelerates at puberty, may also be slowed by this treatment, although this result remains unproven. In this therapeutic regime progesterone, to prevent excessive bleeding, is added for 5 days during each cycle.[377] Treatment should begin before 11 years of age, and therapy in girls as young as 5 years of age has been well tolerated.[259,379] Although final adult height has been reduced by means of hormonal therapy in girls (Fig. 3-52), data are not yet conclusive concerning the effects in minimizing the progression of spinal deformities.[259,377]

Chest abnormalities, notably, pectus excavatum or carinatum, are present in more than two thirds of persons with the Marfan syndrome.† Surgical measures are not usually warranted, and surgery for cosmetic effect at the patient's insistence is generally the only acceptable reason to perform operations of this type. Recurrence of the sternal abnormality has been observed in a significant number of patients in whom repair was performed at an early age,[16] and delay of surgery until skeletal maturity is the optimal course.[16,424] The successful coupling of operation of an aortic aneu-

---

*References 46, 259, 476, 521, 522, and 523.
†References 16, 190, 204, 349, 424, and 511.

rysm with that for pectus excavatum has been reported.[16]

Pes planus and its associated deformities frequently cause symptoms in the average patient, and hammertoes may require surgical measures. Protrusio acetabulae is common in affected adults,[156,263,513] but orthopedic intervention usually is not necessary. Other orthopedic complications such as recurrent joint dislocations and subluxations are managed according to established orthopedic principles.

Cardiovascular Management

Cardiovascular manifestations are the most significant cause of morbidity and mortality in Marfan patients, and management revolves around prevention of complications and their correction when they occur. Death in adult patients with the Marfan syndrome is most commonly due to aortic root disease, in which progressive dilation results in either aortic regurgitation or aortic dissection and rupture. The cardiologic examination schedule depends on the severity of the cardiovascular complications; in persons with mild features, such as mitral valve prolapse and minimal aortic dilation, annual evaluation is sufficient. If aortic dilation and regurgitation are severe, however, more frequent follow-up is needed. In any event, yearly echocardiography is warranted in all affected individuals. Computed tomography and MRI are additional tools that have a role in the evaluation of the aorta in the Marfan syndrome.

It is of great importance that undue physical activity of Marfan patients be curtailed. It is reasonable, however, that affected children be allowed to play and socialize with their peers. As children grow older, counseling concerning their daily lives is necessary, and their interests should be directed toward appropriate activities. Contact sports, isometric exercise, scuba diving, and competitive athletics should all be proscribed for these persons. Alternative activities that are recommended include walking, noncompetitive swimming, and bicycle riding.

A direct relationship has been observed between aortic root dimension and complications of the Marfan syndrome. Thus, Pyeritz et al.[380] reported that aortic regurgitation was virtually nonexistent in Marfan patients whose aortic root dimension was 3.6 cm or less but occurred uniformly in persons with an aortic root dimension of 6 cm or greater. Patients in whom aortic dilation extended into the ascending aorta were more likely to have aortic regurgitation and appeared to be at greater short-term risk of progressive dilation necessitating surgery than were Marfan patients in whom aortic dilation was limited to the sinuses of Valsalva.[405] McFarland et al.[312] were the first to suggest that propranolol, the prototypic beta-adrenoreceptor blocker, should be included among agents used for the medical treatment of dissecting aortic aneurysms. Its mode of action, blocking beta receptors, prevents the effects of both sympathetic nervous system discharge and circulating catecholamines. Since the publication of an abstract by Pyeritz[373] in 1983, the use of beta blockade in patients with the Marfan syndrome has become almost ubiquitous. Pyeritz[374,376] demonstrated that propranolol therapy results in a reduction in the rate of dilation of the aorta in affected children and adults. Follow-up of these patients, for a decade in some instances, continued to show the efficacy of beta blockade, but subsequent data indicated that protection from aortic dissection is not indefinite.[378] Some physicians limit beta-blocker therapy to persons with dilated aortic roots or to the period before and after aortic surgery.[301] Atenolol, a longer-acting, more cardioselective beta blocker, has now largely replaced propranolol as the beta blocker of choice. Alpert et al.[10] undertook a 12-month study of 15 patients receiving 2 mg/kg/day of atenolol in 12 hourly doses. Average decreases of 12% in resting heart rate, 15% in exercise heart rate, 6% in systolic blood pressure, and 12% in exercise systolic blood pressure were observed. Further follow-up of these patients will be necessary to evaluate the long-term effects of this therapeutic regime on aortic dilation. Pharmacokinetic studies have shown that the Marfan patients need twice the dosage of atenolol to achieve the same effect as that achieved in control individuals.[244] The mechanism of this difference is not known.[363] A treatment schedule beginning with atenolol 25 mg or nadolol 20 to 40 mg (depending on body size) and followed by an increase in the dosage to reduce blood pressure to the lower part of the normal range for age and to reduce the heart rate (beats per min) into the 50s, or even into the high 40s in selected patients, is recommended.[123]

One limitation of the preceding therapeutic approach to preventive management is that many patients cannot tolerate fully effective doses of beta blockers because of a variety of side effects, including fatigue, exacerbation of depression or asthma, and the occasional induction of intractable diarrhea. Approximately 10% of Marfan patients have at least mild degrees of one or more of these side effects.[123] In addition, beta-adrenoreceptor blockade is not safe in diabetics receiving treatment who are at risk for episodes of treatment-induced hypoglycemia. Alternative therapy

in these situations includes the use of long-acting forms of verapamil (a calcium-channel inhibitor), which may be taken once or twice daily. Verapamil also decreases arterial pressure, heart rate, and the rate of pressure rise in the aorta; if this therapeutic agent cannot be tolerated (because of constipation, atrioventricular heart block, edema, or gastrointestinal upset) the combination of an angiotensin-converting enzyme inhibitor with low-dose beta blockade may be effective.

As patients age, hemodynamic forces exert in-

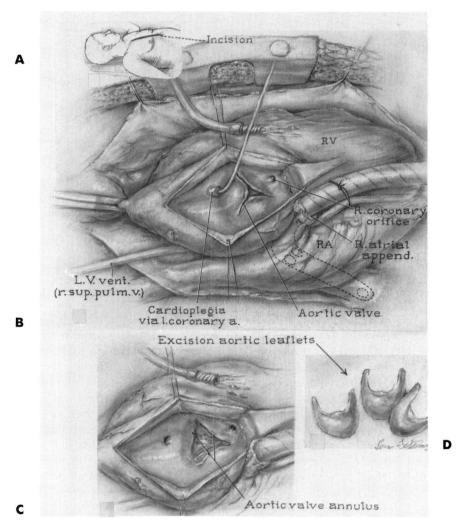

Fig. 3-53. A to **H,** Standard composite graft repair as adapted from Bentall and DeBono.[39] **E,** Mattress sutures are placed below annulus if coronary ostia are low. **I,** Aorta is completely transected to facilitate distal end-to-end anastomosis. A "no-wrap" technique is used; redundant aneurysm wall is tacked loosely over composite graft. *LV,* Left ventricle; *RA,* right atrium; *RV,* right ventricle. (From Gott VL et al: *Ann Thorac Surg* 52:38-45, 1991.)

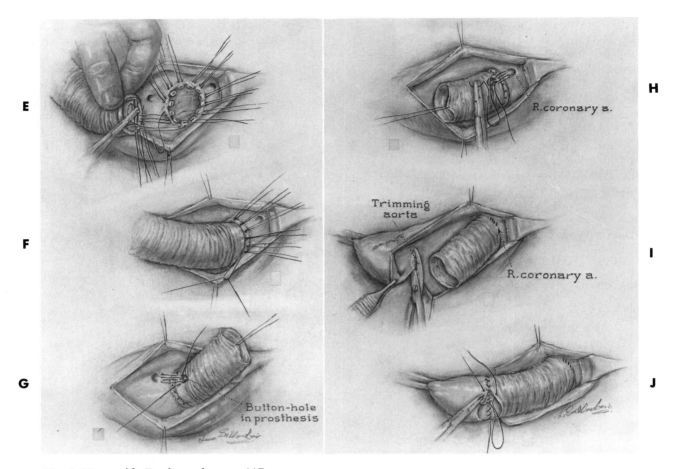

Fig. 3-53, cont'd. For legend see p. 117.

creased pressure on the aorta and cardiac valves. For this reason, although beta blockade may reduce the rate of aortic dilation, a large proportion of individuals with the Marfan syndrome still require cardiovascular surgery. The development of improved surgical techniques for repair of the dilated or dissected aortic root with simultaneous replacement of the aortic valve[38,74] has been of great importance. Gallotti and Ross[176] reported 50 Marfan patients who had surgery at the National Heart Hospital in London, 46 of whom required repair of dilated or dissected aortic roots, or both, and 48 of whom had aortic valve replacement. Operative mortality was 12% (6 of 50), and subsequent mortality in 43 patients who could be followed up for a mean time of 3.5 years was 16%. In a series of 100 Marfan patients in whom graft replacement of aortic aneurysms was undertaken,

Gott et al.[195] reported a 5-year survival rate of 92.6% and a 10-year survival rate of more than 75%. Their data indicate that elective repair is preferable to emergency repair and that greater surgical experience and improved techniques increase long-term survival. They recommended repair of aneurysms that are 6 cm in diameter or larger, even in patients who have no overt cardiac compromise. A modified Bentall procedure[39] (Fig. 3-53) with a variety of composite grafts is used. The last 51 patients in this series received a St. Jude medical composite graft. After surgery affected individuals are placed on a maintenance regimen of warfarin sodium and beta blockade. In addition to staged aortic replacement as illustrated in Fig. 3-54, another procedure, termed "the elephant trunk operation," has been used in the replacement of the ascending and distal aorta.[108]

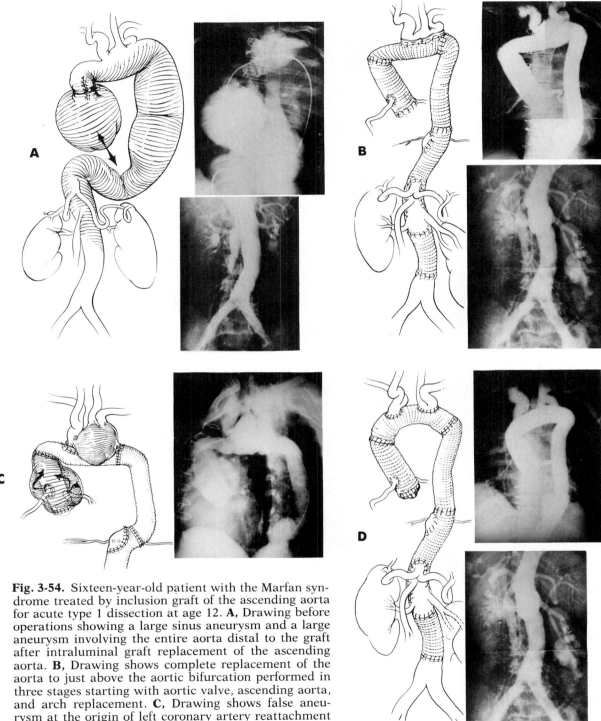

Fig. 3-54. Sixteen-year-old patient with the Marfan syndrome treated by inclusion graft of the ascending aorta for acute type 1 dissection at age 12. **A,** Drawing before operations showing a large sinus aneurysm and a large aneurysm involving the entire aorta distal to the graft after intraluminal graft replacement of the ascending aorta. **B,** Drawing shows complete replacement of the aorta to just above the aortic bifurcation performed in three stages starting with aortic valve, ascending aorta, and arch replacement. **C,** Drawing shows false aneurysm at the origin of left coronary artery reattachment and aneurysmal enlargement of island of aortic arch used to reattach the brachiocephalic arteries. **D,** Drawing made after the third operation showing final satisfactory reconstruction. (From Crawford ES et al: *Ann Surg* 211:521-537, 1990.)

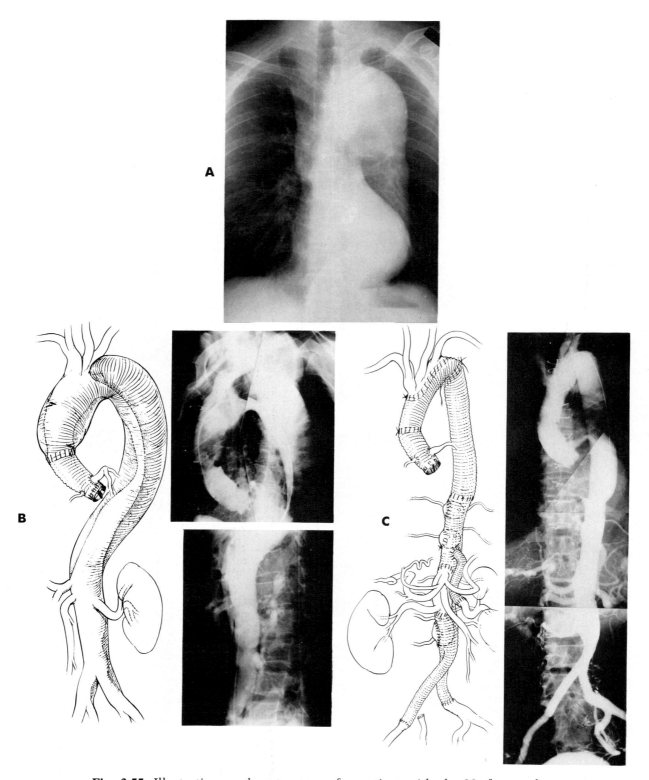

Fig. 3-55. Illustrations and aortograms of a patient with the Marfan syndrome showing total aortic involvement by chronic aortic dissecting aneurysm 4 years after composite valve graft replacement of the aortic valve and ascending aorta performed at the time of aortic dissection. **A,** Plain radiograph of the chest showing the size and extent of the aneurysm. **B,** Drawing shows location and extent of the old graft and aneurysm. **C,** Drawing shows complete aortic and iliac artery replacement in two stages using the elephant trunk technique. (From Crawford ES et al: *Ann Surg* 211:521-537, 1990.)

The result of such an operation in a Marfan patient is shown in Fig. 3-55.

The occurrence of dissection before surgery or the presence of aneurysms in multiple aortic segments is associated with an unfavorable postoperative prognosis. Crawford and Coselli,[103] Crawford et al.,[108] and Svensson et al.[469] reported a 10-year survival rate of 56% in 155 Marfan patients who had 280 operations. Taniguchi et al.[475] reported an 8-year survival of 37% in 20 patients with evidence of the Marfan syndrome. These results suggest that it is particularly important to perform elective aortic surgery before dissection supervenes and to follow up carefully by means of regular echocardiography, MRI, or CT those patients who have involvement of aortic segments that have not been grafted in initial surgical procedures.

Postoperative continuation of hypotensive medication and restriction of exercise is still necessary, since Marfan patients remain vulnerable to dissection of more distal segments of the aorta. Complications after aortic surgery include failure of the repair itself, such as development of paragraft false aneurysms[245] or partial dehiscence of a coronary artery from the graft,[394] and the occurrence of progressive enlargement or dissection in other aortic segments or of mitral valve degeneration. As surgeons develop greater experience in the performance of cardiac surgery in patients with the Marfan syndrome* and since surgery now is often undertaken electively at an early stage in the natural history of the disorder, it is likely that both the operative and late postoperative mortality will decrease significantly.

Replacement of the aortic or mitral valves is a frequent procedure in Marfan patients.[103,106,195,262] In children with mitral regurgitation, reconstruction of the mitral valve rather than its replacement is often feasible.[88,442] Some surgical experts consider that aortic graft and mitral valve replacement should be undertaken simultaneously rather than as staged procedures.[103] A transaortic approach for mitral valve replacement has been developed by Crawford and Coselli.[103] Higashida et al.[224] have successfully treated a carotid aneurysm in a Marfan patient with balloon embolization.

Because of the exceptional difficulty that may be encountered in curing bacterial infection of aortic composite grafts,[194,311] it has been recommended that intravenous antibiotics be administered to prevent endocarditis arising from bacterial seeding during major dental procedures or other high-risk operations.[126] Success has been achieved in replacing infected composite grafts either with aortic heterografts[193] or with another composite graft that is wrapped with a portion of the omentum drawn through a surgically constructed diaphragmatic hernia to surround the new graft with healthy tissue.[99] Techniques have also been reported for replacement of artificial aortic valves without the need to remove the aortic graft component of a composite graft.[440]

Ocular Complications

Regular ophthalmic evaluation is an important aspect of management in the care of patients with the Marfan syndrome. Improvement of impaired visual acuity resulting from myopia is achieved by conventional means, and contact lenses are well tolerated.[308,345]

The most common complications in the eyes result from lens dislocation. Although not indicated in the routine management of ectopia lentis, surgical removal of the lens should be considered if satisfactory visual acuity cannot be reached by means of standard aphakic and phakic refraction.[33,361] Behki, Noel, and Clarke[33] have used limbal lensectomy in nine children with the Marfan syndrome and ectopia lentis (15 eyes); complications were minimal and improvement in visual acuity was significant. The authors noted that early lensectomy may prevent amblyopia, which would preclude successful visual rehabilitation if surgery were performed at a later date. An alternative to surgery that has been attempted with some success is neodymium laser treatment.[477] This procedure attempts to move the displaced lens out of the visual axis. In a series of seven patients (nine eyes) visual acuity was improved in eight eyes. Complications, however, necessitated the removal of the lens in two of the eyes.

Acute glaucoma is uncommon in the Marfan syndrome,[101,110,308] but successful management by means of lens removal has been documented.

Psychologic Aspects

Although most psychiatric problems that have been reported in persons with the Marfan syn-

---

*References 19, 38, 102, 104, 107, 136, 175, 261, 301, 368, and 475.

drome are probably incidental,[274] psychologic problems can certainly be generated by the diagnosis of the Marfan syndrome. Most persons with this disorder cope well with their particular disability, but the lifelong stigmata and the exclusion from participation in sports, especially for boys, may necessitate psychologic counseling as part of the complete management.

In a psychosocial study[87] of patients and their relatives, shock and resentment on diagnosis was compounded by guilt in affected persons who already had children. Women were more distressed than men, and spouses who did not have the Marfan syndrome were angrier if diagnosis was made after the birth of children with the syndrome. Education of sibs without the syndrome and of teachers was important in an effort to decrease the teasing that children with the Marfan syndrome sometimes have to endure. The dual risk for women with this disorder, of endangering their lives, if pregnant, and of transmitting the defect to progeny, was cause for concern and depression. Schneider et al.[428] found normal psychosocial adaptation in the 22 patients, although these individuals perceived that the quality of life without the disorder would be better.

Pregnancy

Women with the Marfan syndrome require counseling not only about the genetic risk to their progeny but also concerning the considerable risks inherent in pregnancy in the Marfan syndrome.[35] In general, individuals with the Marfan syndrome who have aortic root dilation or a valvular disease are at greatest risk, whereas those with minimal cardiac involvement tolerate pregnancy well. Pyeritz[372] reviewed the pregnancies of 26 women with the Marfan syndrome and a comparable number of normal controls. He found no difference in the incidence of complications of pregnancy in these two groups, although the spontaneous abortion rate was higher in the women with the Marfan syndrome. Pyeritz recommended that an aortic diameter of more than 40 mm, as measured by means of echocardiography, or any evidence of cardiac decompensation be regarded as a contraindication to pregnancy. The continued use of propranolol during pregnancy and the potential effect of this drug on the fetus continue to be subjects of debate.[181,478] Management of labor and delivery is aimed at reducing cardiovascular stress by means of uninduced labor, minimal anesthesia, and vaginal delivery.[372]

Athletics

Although patients with the Marfan syndrome are at considerable risk if they participate in competitive athletics, the majority of sudden deaths in all young athletes are not due to the Marfan syndrome but rather to other cardiovascular disorders.[329] The most common of these are hypertrophic cardiomyopathy, cardiac conduction defects, and coronary insufficiency.[137,300,329]

The Marfan syndrome is the most common cause of aortic dissection and rupture in the young. Indeed, there have been a number of reports of sudden death resulting from aortic rupture in young athletes in whom the diagnosis of the Marfan syndrome was subsequently made.[21,293,300] When examining the "tall, slender athlete,"[310] the physician must keep in mind the possibility and the clinical criteria of the Marfan syndrome. In view of the importance of recognizing the Marfan syndrome, Driscoll[137] suggested that comprehensive, unhurried clinical evaluation of all athletes should be performed in a suitable examining room with the availability of appropriate equipment, not in a gymnasium or a locker room. Persons with the unequivocal diagnosis of the Marfan syndrome should be counseled about an appropriate life-style and referred for genetic, cardiologic, ophthalmic, and other relevant evaluation. For the sake of balanced psychosocial development, it is reasonable for children with the Marfan syndrome to participate in some competitive sports such as Little League baseball. Equally, most adults can involve themselves in aerobic, noncompetitive exercise.

The National Marfan Foundation of the United States and similar lay groups in other countries provide valuable support for persons with the Marfan syndrome and their families. Among other activities these organizations promote personal interaction and coordinate the dissemination of information to interested persons. These organizations continue to extend the range and scope of their activities, and the importance of their role in the overall management of the Marfan syndrome cannot be overemphasized.

SUMMARY

The cardinal manifestations of the Marfan syndrome are skeletal, ocular, and aortic. Dolichostenomelia (long, thin extremities) and redundant ligaments and joint capsules characterize the skeletal changes. Ectopia lentis is the hallmark of the disorder in the eye. In the aorta progressive dilation of the root may cause valvular insufficiency and lead to dissection and rupture of the aortic wall.

The only obvious histopathologic changes are those in the aorta, where degeneration of the elastic lamellae is evident. The basic defect involves fibrillin, a microfibrillar protein, which is widely distributed in connective tissues and often associated with elastin.

Autosomal dominant inheritance is well established but in some families phenotypic expression can be variable. The gene for the Marfan syndrome is situated on the long arm of chromosome 15. Studies in 30 affected families have revealed linkage between the phenotype, fibrillin, and this locus. There is evidence for intragenic heterogeneity, but with the exception of a single large French family, there is no evidence for nonallelic heterogeneity.

Considerable advances in the management of the Marfan syndrome have been made during the past 20 years. These include long-term prophylactic therapy with beta-blocking agents to minimize the deleterious effects of expansile pulsation of the aorta and increasingly sophisticated surgical procedures for correction of aortic and valvular problems.

The nature of the relationship between the classic Marfan syndrome and a number of Marfan-like disorders largely remains to be determined. A condition of this type, CCA (Beals syndrome), has been found to be linked to a member of the fibrillin gene family situated on chromosome 5.

REFERENCES

1. Achard C: Arachnodactylie, *Bull Mem Soc Méd Hôp* 19:834, 1902.
2. Adachi H et al: Emergency surgical intervention of acute aortic dissection with the rapid diagnosis by transesophageal echocardiography, *Circulation* 84(suppl III):14-19, 1991.
3. Aelion JA, Wolfe SE, Kaplan SB: Concomitant rheumatoid arthritis and Marfan's syndrome (letter), *Arthritis Rheum* 30:1073-1074, 1987.
4. Agarwal T et al: Marfan's syndrome associated with epilepsy and mental deficiency, *J Assoc Physicians India* 34:594-595, 1986.
5. Agarwala BN: A long, thin infant with congestive heart failure, *Hosp Pract (Off)* 22:190-196, 1987.
6. Ahmad NN et al: Stop codon in the procollagen II gene (COL2A1) in a family with the Stickler syndrome (arthroophthalmopathy), *Proc Natl Acad Sci USA* 88:6624-6627, 1991.
7. Alarcón-Segovia D et al: Bilateral renal vein thrombosis and nephrotic syndrome in a patient with the Marfan syndrome, *Dis Chest* 54:153-156, 1968.
8. Albanese A: Sulla dolichostenomelia, *Arch Ortop* 47:539-575, 1931.
9. Allen RA et al: Ocular manifestations of the Marfan syndrome, *Trans Am Acad Ophthalmol Otolaryngol* 71:18-38, 1967.
10. Alpert B et al: Hemodynamic responses to dynamic exercise in adolescents and young adults with the Marfan syndrome, *Am J Med Genet* 32:245, 1989.
11. Amparo EG et al: Aortic dissection: magnetic resonance imaging, *Radiology* 155:399-406, 1985.
12. Anderson M, Pratt-Thomas HR: Marfan's syndrome, *Am Heart J* 46:911-917, 1953.
13. Anning ST: Elastoma intrapapillare perforans verruciforme (Miescher), *Proc R Soc Med (Sect Derm)* 51:932, 1958.
14. Apert E: Les formes frustes du syndrome dolichostenomelique de Marfan, *Nourrisson* 26:1-12, 1938.
15. Appel A, Horwitz A, Dorfman A: Cell-free synthesis of hyaluronic acid in Marfan syndrome, *J Biol Chem* 254(23):12199-12203, 1979.
16. Arn PH et al: Outcome of pectus excavatum in patients with Marfan syndrome and in the general population, *J Pediatr* 115:954-958, 1989.
17. Austin MG, Schaefer RF: Marfan's syndrome with unusual blood vessel manifestations: primary medionecrosis dissection of right innominate, right carotid, and left carotid arteries, *Arch Pathol* 64:205-209, 1957.
18. Bacchus H: A quantitative abnormality in serum mucoproteins in the Marfan syndrome, *Am J Med* 25:744-748, 1958.
19. Bachet J et al: Repeated surgery for recurrent dissection of the aorta, *Eur J Cardiothorac Surg* 4:238-244, 1990.
20. Baer RW, Taussig HB, Oppenheimer EH: Congenital aneurysmal dilation of the aorta associated with arachnodactyly, *Bull Hopkins Hosp* 72:309-331, 1943.
21. Bain MA, Zumwalt RE, van der Bel-Kahn J: Marfan syndrome presenting as aortic rupture in a young athlete: sudden unexpected death, *Am J Forensic Med Pathol* 8:334-337, 1987.
22. Baker CB, Wilson TK, Woods JM: Marfan's syndrome; a successful aortic homograft for a dissecting aneurysm of the thoracic aorta, *Can J Surg* 1:371-375, 1958.
23. Banerjee AK: Marfan's syndrome associated with Wolff-Parkinson-White syndrome type B, *Jpn Heart J* 29:377-380, 1988.
24. Barker SG, Burnand KG: Retrograde iliac artery dissection in Marfan's syndrome. A case report, *J Cardiovasc Surg (Torino)* 30:953-954, 1989.
25. Barlow JB et al: Late systolic murmurs and non-ejection ("mid-late") systolic clicks: an analysis of 90 patients, *Br Heart J* 30:203-218, 1968.
26. Bass HN et al: Congenital contractural arachnodactyly, keratoconus, and probable Marfan syndrome in the same pedigree, *J Pediatr* 98:591-594, 1981.

27. Bawle E, Quigg MH: Ectopia lentis and aortic root dilatation in congenital contractural arachnodactyly, *Am J Med Genet* 42:19-21, 1992.

28. Baxter BT et al: Elastin and microfibrillar proteins in abdominal aortic aneurysm, *Clin Res* 39:118A, 1991.

29. Beals RK, Hecht F: Congenital contractural arachnodactyly, a heritable disorder of connective tissue, *J Bone Joint Surg* 53(A):987-993, 1971.

30. Bean WB: Precordial noises heard at a distance from the chest. In *Monographs in medicine*, Baltimore, 1952, Williams & Wilkins, p 22.

31. Becker AE, van Mantgem J-P: The coronary arteries in Marfan's syndrome: a morphologic study, *Am J Cardiol* 36:315-321, 1975.

32. Beemer FA, Deileman JW: Combined deficiency of xanthene oxidase and sulfite oxidase; ophthalmological findings in a 3-week-old girl, *Metab Pediatr Syst Ophthalmol* 4:49, 1980.

33. Behki R, Noel LP, Clarke WN: Limbal lensectomy in the management of ectopia lentis in children, *Arch Ophthalmol* 108:809-811, 1990.

34. Beighton P: Mitral valve prolapse and a marfanoid habitus, *Br Med J* 284:920, 1982.

35. Beighton P: Pregnancy in the Marfan syndrome, *Br Med J* 285:464, 1982.

36. Beighton P et al: International nosology of heritable disorders of connective tissue, Berlin, 1986, *Am J Med Genet* 29:581-594, 1988.

37. Bennett JT, McMurray SW: Stickler syndrome, *J Pediatr Orthop* 10:760-763, 1990.

38. Bentall HH: Operation for ascending aortic aneurysm and aortic regurgitation: pathological influence on survival, *Jpn J Surg* 17:425-430, 1987.

39. Bentall HH, DeBono AA: A technique for complete replacement of the ascending aorta, *Thorax* 23:338-339, 1968.

40. Bergofsky EH, Turino GM, Fishman AP: Cardiorespiratory failure in kyphoscoliosis, *Medicine* 38:263-317, 1959.

41. Berlin R: Familial occurrence of pneumothorax simplex, *Acta Med Scand* 137:268-275, 1950.

42. Bhat PK: Bilateral ectopia lentis with arachnodactyly: Marfan's syndrome with report of case and review of literature, *Antiseptic* 43:651, 1946.

43. Billington BM, Leaver PK, McLeod D: Management of retinal detachment in the Wagner-Stickler syndrome, *Trans Ophthalmol Soc UK* 104:875-879, 1985.

44. Bingle J: Marfan's syndrome, *Br Med J* 1:629-630, 1957.

45. Bing-xin L, Guo-xiang P, Wen-shu M: Marfan syndrome in Chinese, *Chin Med J* 99:829-831, 1986.

46. Birch JG, Herring JA: Spinal deformity in Marfan syndrome, *J Pediatr Orthop* 7:546-552, 1987.

47. Bixler D, Antley RM: Familial aortic dissection with anomalies: a new connective tissue syndrome, *Birth Defects* 12(5):229-234, 1976.

48. Bjerkreim I, Skogland LB, Trygstad O: Congenital contractural arachnodactyly, *Acta Orthop Scand* 47:250-253, 1976.

49. Black HH, Landay LH: Marfan's syndrome: report of five cases in one family, *Am J Dis Child* 89:414-420, 1955.

50. Blanton SH et al: An exclusion map of Marfan syndrome, *J Med Genet* 27:73-77, 1990.

51. Boerger F: Ueber zwei Fälle von Arachnodaktylie, *Monatsschr Kinderheilkd* 12:161-184, 1914.

52. Boerger F: Ueber zwei Fälle von Arachnodaktylie, *Monatsschr Kinderheilkd* 13:335, 1914.

53. Boileau C et al: Genetic heterogeneity reveals a second locus for Marfan syndrome (MAS2), *Am J Hum Genet* 49(suppl):336, 1991 (abstract).

54. Bolande RP, Tucker AS: Pulmonary emphysema and other cardio-respiratory lesions as part of the Marfan abiotrophy, *Pediatrics* 33:356-366, 1964.

55. Bon Tempo CP et al: Radiographic appearance of the thorax in systolic click–late systolic murmur syndrome, *Am J Cardiol* 36:27-31, 1975.

56. Boone JA, Clowes GH Jr: Calcified annulus fibrosus with mitral insufficiency in the Marfan syndrome, with prosthetic replacement of the mitral valve, *South Med J* 62:682-690, 1969.

57. Booth CC, Louchbridge LW, Turner MD: Arachnodactyly with congenital lesions of the urinary tract, *Br Med J* 2:80-83, 1957.

58. Boucek RJ et al: The Marfan syndrome: a deficiency in chemically stable collagen cross-links, *New Engl J Med* 305(17):988-991, 1981.

59. Bowden DH, Favara BE, Donahoe JL: Marfan's syndrome: accelerated course in childhood associated with lesions of mitral valve and pulmonary artery, *Am Heart J* 69:96-99, 1965.

60. Bowers D: Unpublished observations, 1972.

61. Bowers D, Lim DW: Subacute bacterial endocarditis and Marfan's syndrome, *Can Med Assoc J* 86:455-458, 1962.

62. Boxer RA et al: Evaluation of the aorta in the Marfan syndrome by magnetic resonance imaging, *Am Heart J* 111:1001-1002, 1986.

63. Boyd DHA: Familial spontaneous pneumothorax, *Scott Med J* 2:220-221, 1957.

64. Brock RC: Recurrent and spontaneous pneumothorax, *Thorax* 3:88-111, 1948.

65. Bronson E, Sutherland GA: Ruptured aortic aneurysms in childhood, *Br J Child Dis* 15:241, 1918.

66. Brown OR et al: Aortic root dilatation and mitral valve prolapse in Marfan's syndrome: an echocardiographic study, *Circulation* 52:651-657, 1975.

67. Bruno L et al: Cardiac, skeletal, and ocular abnormalities in patients with Marfan's syndrome and in their relatives; comparison with the cardiac abnormalities in patients with kyphoscoliosis, *Br Heart J* 51:220-230, 1984.

68. Buchanan R, Wyatt GP: Marfan's syndrome presenting as an intrapartum death, *Arch Dis Child* 60:1074-1076, 1985.

69. Burgio RG et al: Asymmetric Marfan syndrome, *Am J Med Genet* 30:905-909, 1988.

70. Burian HM: Chamber angle studies in developmental glaucoma: Marfan syndrome and high myopia, *J Missouri Med Assoc* 55:1088-1090, 1958.

71. Burian HM, Allen L: Histologic study of the chamber angle of patients with Marfan's syndrome, *Arch Ophthalmol* 65:323-333, 1961.

72. Burian HM, von Noorden GK, Ponseti IV: Chamber angle anomalies in systemic connective tissue disorders, *Arch Ophthalmol* 64:671-680, 1960.

73. Byers PH et al: Marfan syndrome: abnormal alpha 2 chain in type I collagen, *Proc Natl Acad Sci USA* 78:7745-7749, 1981.

74. Cabrol C et al: Long-term result with total replacement of the ascending aorta and reimplantation of the coronary arteries, *J Thorac Cardiovasc Surg* 91:17-25, 1986.

75. Cadle RG et al: Marfan syndrome: a study of clinical variability in the largest known Marfan kindred, *Am J Med Genet* 32:239, 1989.

76. Capocchi G et al: A unique association of Marfan syndrome with craniofacial hypoplasia, oligophrenia, and severe microphthalmia, *Ital J Neurol Sci* 9:397-400, 1988.

77. Case records of the Massachusettes General Hospital, *New Engl J Med* 243:346-350, 1950.

78. Chambers HG, Bucknell AL: Intraarticular lipoma in Stickler syndrome, *Orthopedics* 13:565-567, 1990.

79. Chan KL et al: Marfan syndrome diagnosed in patients 32 years of age or older, *Mayo Clin Proc* 62:589-594, 1987.

80. Chang CE: Marfan's syndrome: review of literature and report of one case, *Chin Med J* 69:433-439, 1951.

81. Chaouch H et al: Cardiovascular manifestations of Marfan syndrome: apropos of 15 cases, *Tunis Med* 68:193-197, 1990.

82. Chapman DW et al: Annulo-aortic ectasia with cystic medial necrosis: diagnosis and surgical treatment, *Am J Cardiol* 16:679-687, 1965.

83. Chemke J et al: Homozygosity for autosomal dominant Marfan syndrome, *J Med Genet* 21:173-177, 1984.

84. Chen S et al: Ventricular dysrhythmias in children with Marfan's syndrome, *Am J Dis Child* 139:273-276, 1985.

85. Cheng TO: Mitral valve prolapse, *Disease-A-Month* 33(9):486-534, 1987.

86. Cheng TO, Barlow JB: Mitral leaflet billowing and prolapse: its prevalence around the world, *Angiology* 40:77-87, 1989.

87. Child A, Hicks J: Psychosocial aspects of Marfan syndrome, *Am J Med Genet* 32:249, 1989.

88. Child JS, Perloff JK, Kaplan S: The heart of the matter: cardiovascular involvement in Marfan's syndrome (editorial), *J Am Coll Cardiol* 14:429-431, 1989.

89. Childers RW, McCrea PC: Absence of the pulmonary valve: a case occurring in the Marfan syndrome, *Circulation* 29(suppl):598-603, 1964.

90. Chisholm JC, Cheriack NS, Carton RW: Results of pulmonary function testing in 5 persons with the Marfan syndrome, *J Lab Clin Med* 71:25-28, 1968.

91. Chu NS: Marfan's syndrome and epilepsy: report of two cases and review of the literature, *Epilepsia* 24:49-55, 1983.

92. Cleary EG: The microfibrillar component of the elastic fibers: morphology and biochemistry. In Uitto J, Perejda AJ, editors: *Connective tissue disease: molecular pathology of the extracellular matrix*, New York, 1987, Marcel Dekker, pp 55-81.

93. Cleary EG, Gibson MA: Elastin-associated microfibrils and microfibrillar proteins, *Int Rev Connect Tissue Res* 10:97-209, 1983.

94. Cohen DN, Kaye D: Staphylococcal endocarditis in narcotic addict with Marfan's syndrome, *New York J Med* 67:2362-2367, 1967.

95. Cohen PR, Schneiderman P: Clinical manifestations of the Marfan syndrome, *Int J Dermatol* 28:291-299, 1989.

96. Come PC et al: Echocardiographic assessment of cardiovascular abnormalities in the Marfan syndrome: comparison with clinical findings and with roentgenographic estimation of aortic root size, *Am J Med* 74:465-474, 1983.

97. Cooke JP, Safford RE: Progress in the diagnosis and management of aortic dissection, *Mayo Clin Proc* 61:147-153, 1986.

98. Copeland T, Tiwary CM, Coker S: Coexistence of neurofibromatosis and Marfan's syndrome, *South Med J* 79:489-492, 1986.

99. Coselli JS: Personal communication, 1992.

100. Cotta-Pereira G, Rodrigo FG, Bittencourt-Sampaio S: Oxytalan, elaunin, and elastic fibers in human skin, *J Invest Dermatol* 66:143-148, 1976.

101. Crandall AS: Developmental ocular abnormalities and glaucoma, *Int Ophthalmol Clin* 24:73-86, 1984.

102. Crawford ES: Marfan's syndrome: broad spectral surgical treatment cardiovascular manifestations, *Ann Surg* 198:487-505, 1983.

103. Crawford ES, Coselli JS: Marfan's syndrome: combined composite valve graft replacement of the aortic root and transaortic mitral valve replacement, *Ann Thorac Surg* 45:296-302, 1988.

104. Crawford ES, Crawford JL: Marfan's syndrome. In *Diseases of the aorta*, Baltimore, 1984, Williams & Wilkins, pp 215-248.

105. Crawford ES, Crawford JL: *Diseases of the aorta*, Baltimore, 1984, Williams & Wilkins.

106. Crawford ES et al: Total aortic replacement for chronic aortic dissection occurring in patients with and without Marfan's syndrome, *Ann Surg* 199:358-362, 1984.

107. Crawford ES et al: Redo operations for recurrent aneurysmal disease of the ascending aorta and transverse aortic arch, *Ann Thorac Surg* 40:439-455, 1985.

108. Crawford ES et al: Diffuse aneurysmal disease (chronic aortic dissection, Marfan, and mega aorta syndromes) and multiple aneurysm: treatment by subtotal and total aortic replacement emphasizing the elephant trunk operation, *Ann Surg* 211:521-537, 1990.

109. Cross HE, Jensen AD: Ocular manifestations in the Marfan syndrome and homocystinuria, *Am J Ophthalmol* 75:405-420, 1973.

110. Croxatto JO, Lombardi A, Malbran ES: Inflamed eye in Marfan's syndrome with posteriorly luxated lens, *Ophthalmologica* 193:23-26, 1986.

111. Daily PO et al: Management of acute aortic dissections, *Ann Thorac Surg* 10:237-247, 1970.

112. Dalgleish R, Hawkins JR, Keston M: Exclusion of the alpha 2(I) and alpha 1(III) collagen genes as the mutant loci in a Marfan syndrome family, *J Med Genet* 24:148-151, 1987.

113. Das Gupta BK, Basu RK: Bilateral dislocation of the lens under voluntary control in Marfan syndrome with cardiovascular anomaly, *Br J Ophthalmol* 39:566-568, 1955.

114. David R, MacBeath L, Jenkins T: Aniridia associated with microcornea and subluxated lenses, *Br J Ophthalmol* 62:118-121, 1978.

115. Davies MJ: *Pathology of Cardiac Valves*, London, 1980, Butterworths, pp 59-131.

116. Davis JH, Benson JW, Miller RC: Thoracoabdominal aneurysm involving celiac, superior mesenteric and renal arteries: report of a case successfully treated by resection and nylon-graft replacement, *Arch Surg* 75:871-876, 1957.

117. Dax EC: Arachnodactyly, *J Ment Sci* 87:434-438, 1941.

118. DeBakey ME et al: Surgical management of dissecting aneurysms of the aorta, *J Thorac Cardiovasc Surg* 49:130-149, 1965.

119. DeBakey ME et al: Dissection and dissecting aneurysm of the aorta: twenty-year follow-up of five hundred twenty seven patients treated surgically, *Surgery* 92:1118-1134, 1982.

120. Derouette S et al: Studies on elastic tissue of aorta in aortic dissections and Marfan syndrome, *Pathol Biol (Paris)* 29:539-547, 1981.

121. DeSanctis RW et al: Aortic dissection, *New Engl J Med* 317:1060-1067, 1987.

122. Detrano R et al: Intravenous digital subtraction aortography in the preoperative and postoperative evaluation of Marfan's aortic disease, *Chest* 88:249-253, 1985.

123. Devereux RB: Personal communication, 1992.

124. Devereux RB, Brown WT: Genetics of mitral valve prolapse, *Prog Med Genet* 5:139-161, 1983.

125. Devereux RB, Kramer-Fox R, Roman MJ: Unpublished data, 1992.

126. Devereux RB, Pyeritz RE, Gott VL: Endocarditis prophylaxis for people with the Marfan syndrome who have had cardiac surgery, *Connective Issues* 10(4):3, 1991.

127. Devereux RB et al: Mitral valve prolapse, *Circulation* 54:3-14, 1976.

128. Devereux RB et al: Inheritance of mitral valve prolapse: effect of age and sex on gene expression, *Ann Intern Med* 97:826-832, 1982.

129. Devereux RB et al: Diagnosis and classification of severity of mitral valve prolapse: methodologic, biologic, and prognostic considerations, *Am Heart J* 113:1265-1280, 1987.

130. Di Matteo J et al: Anéurysmes multiples de la valve mitrale. Endocardite bactérienne et syndrome de Marfan, *Coeur Med Intern* 10:519-524, 1971.

131. Dietz HC et al: Marfan syndrome caused by a recurrent de novo missense mutation in the fibrillin gene, *Nature* 352:337-339, 1991.

132. Dietz HC et al: The Marfan syndrome locus: confirmation of assignment to chromosome 15 and identification of tightly linked markers at 15q15-q21.3, *Genomics* 9:355-361, 1991.

133. Dietzman RH et al: Mitral insufficiency in Marfan's syndrome: a case of surgical correction, *Dis Chest* 51:650-653, 1967.

134. Disler LJ, Manga P, Barlow JB: Pulmonary arterial aneurysms in Marfan's syndrome, *Int J Cardiol* 21:79-82, 1988.

135. Dominguez R, Weisgrau RA, Santamaria M: Pulmonary hyperinflation and emphysema in infants with the Marfan syndrome, *Pediatr Radiol* 17:365-369, 1987.

136. Donaldson RM, Ross DN: Composite graft replacement for the treatment of aneurysms of the ascending aorta associated with aortic valvular disease, *Circulation* 66(suppl I):116-121, 1982.

137. Driscoll DJ: Cardiovascular evaluation of the child and adolescent before participation in sports, *Mayo Clin Proc* 60:867-873, 1985.

138. Dvorak-Theobald G: Histologic eye findings in arachnodactyly, *Am J Ophthalmol* 24:1132-1137, 1941.

139. Dwyer EM Jr, Troncale F: Spontaneous pneumothorax and pulmonary disease in the Marfan syndrome: report of two cases and review of the literature, *Ann Intern Med* 62:1285-1292, 1965.

140. Edwards WD, Leaf DS, Edwards JE: Dissecting aortic aneurysm associated with congenital bicuspid aortic valve, *Circulation* 57:1022-1025, 1978.

141. Eldridge R: Coarctation in the Marfan syndrome, *Arch Intern Med* 113:342-349, 1964.

142. Ellis PR, Cooley DA, DeBakey ME: Clinical considerations and surgical treatment of annulo-aortic ectasia, *J Thorac Cardiovasc Surg* 42:363-370, 1961.

143. Emanuel R et al: Formes frustes of Marfan's syndrome presenting with severe aortic regurgitation: clinicogenetic study of 18 families, *Br Heart J* 39:190-197, 1977.

144. Epstein CJ et al: Hereditary dysplasia of bone with kyphoscoliosis, contractures, and abnormally shaped ears, *J Pediatr* 73:379-386, 1968.

145. Erdheim J: Medionecrosis aortae idiopathica cystica, *Virchows Arch (A)* 276:187-229, 1930.

146. Estes JW, Carey RJ, Desai RG: Marfan's syndrome: hematological abnormalities in a family, *Arch Intern Med* 116:889-893, 1965.

147. Etter LE, Glover LP: Arachnodactyly complicated by dislocated lens and death from rupture of dissecting aneurysm of the aorta, *JAMA* 123:88, 1943.

148. Evans PA: A hereditary tendency to hernia, *Lancet* 2:293, 1942.

149. Evans W: The heart in sternal depression, *Br Heart J* 8:162-170, 1946.

150. Everberg G: Marfan's syndrome associated with hearing defect: report of a case in one of a pair of twins, *Acta Paediatr* 48:70-76, 1959.

151. Fabré J, Veyrat R, Jeanneret O: Syndrome de Marfan avec aneurysme et coarctation de l'aorte: étude anatomo-clinique, *Schweiz Med Wochenschr* 87:49-53, 1957.

152. Fahey JJ: Muscular and skeletal changes in arachnodactyly, *Arch Surg* 39:741-760, 1939.

153. Fairbank TJ, Wynne-Davis R: *Fairbank's atlas of general affections of the skeleton*, Edinburgh, 1976, Churchill Livingstone, pp 152-155.

154. Faivre G et al: Le coeur des dépressions sternales congénitales, *Arch Mal Coeur* 47:322-332, 1954.

155. Farnsworth PN et al: Ultrastructural abnormalities in a Marfan's syndrome lens, *Arch Ophthalmol* 95:1601-1606, 1977.

156. Fast A et al: Protrusio acetabuli in Marfan's syndrome: report on two patients, *J Rheumatol* 11:549-551, 1984.

157. Feingold M: The "thumb sign" in children, *Clin Pediatr* 7:423-424, 1968.

158. Feldman F: Tuberous sclerosis, neurofibromatosis, and fibrous dysplasia. In Resnick D, Niwayama G, editors: *Diagnosis of bone and joint disorders*, ed 2, Philadelphia, 1988, WB Saunders, pp 4033-4072.

159. Finney HL, Roberts TS, Anderson RE: Giant intracranial aneurysm associated with Marfan syndrome, *J Neurosurg* 45:342-347, 1976.

160. Fischl AA, Ruthberg J: Clinical implications of Marfan's syndrome, *JAMA* 146:704-707, 1951.

161. Fishman EK et al: Sacral abnormalities in Marfan syndrome, *J Comput Assist Tomogr* 7:851-856, 1983.

162. Flanagan PV, Geoghegan J, Egan TJ: Iliac artery aneurysm in Marfan's syndrome, *Eur J Vasc Surg* 4:323-324, 1990.

163. Flesch M: Ueber eine seltene Missbildung des Thorax, *Virchows Arch (A)* 57:289, 1873.

164. Fontana ME et al: The varying clinical spectrum of the systolic click—late systolic murmur syndrome: a postural auscultatory phenomenon, *Circulation* 41:807-816, 1970.

165. Forbes D, Hagan R: Congenital contractural arachnodactyly, *Med J Aust* 1:128, 1983.

166. Forgacs P: Stature in simple pneumothorax, *Guy's Hosp Rep* 118:199-204, 1969.
167. Francomano CA et al: The Stickler syndrome: evidence for close linkage to the structural gene for type II collagen, *Genomics* 1:293-296, 1987.
168. Francomano CA et al: Marfan syndrome: exclusion of genetic linkage to three major collagen genes, *Am J Med Genet* 29:457-462, 1988.
169. Francomano CA et al: The Stickler syndrome is closely linked to COL2A1, the structural gene for type II collagen, *Pathol Immunopathol Res* 7:104-106, 1988.
170. Freed C, Schiller NB: Echocardiographic findings in Marfan's syndrome, *West J Med* 126:87-90, 1977.
171. Fried K, Krakowsky D: Probable autosomal recessive Marfan syndrome, *J Med Genet* 14:359-361, 1977.
172. Fryer AE et al: Exclusion of COL2A1 as a candidate gene in a family with Wagner-Stickler syndrome, *J Med Genet* 27:91-93, 1990.
173. Fuleihan FJ, Suh SK, Shepard RH: Some aspects of pulmonary function in the Marfan syndrome, *Bull Hopkins Hosp* 113:320-329, 1963.
174. Futcher PH, Southworth H: Arachnodactyly and its medical complications, *Arch Intern Med* 61:693-703, 1938.
175. Galbraith TA: Personal communication, 1992.
176. Gallotti R, Ross DN: The Marfan syndrome: surgical technique and follow-up of 50 patients, *Ann Thorac Surg* 29:428-433, 1980.
177. Geva T, Hegesh J, Frand M: The clinical course and echocardiographic features of Marfan's syndrome in childhood, *Am J Dis Child* 141:1179-1182, 1987.
178. Geva T et al: Two-dimensional and Doppler echocardiographic and pathologic characteristics of the infantile Marfan syndrome, *Am J Cardiol* 65:1230-1237, 1990.
179. Gillan JE et al: Spontaneous dissecting aneurysm of the ductus arteriosus in an infant with Marfan syndrome, *J Pediatr* 105:952-955, 1984.
180. Gilston RJ: Marfan's syndrome, *Med Ann DC* 24:127-129, 1955.
181. Gladstone GR, Hordof A, Gersony WM: Propranolol administration during pregnancy: effects on the fetus, *J Pediatr* 86:962-964, 1975.
182. Glesby MJ, Pyeritz RE: Association of mitral valve prolapse and systemic abnormalities of connective tissue: a phenotypic continuum, *JAMA* 262:523-528, 1989.
183. Glower DD et al: Comparison of medical and surgical therapy for uncomplicated descending aortic dissection, *Circulation* 82(suppl IV):39-46, 1990.
184. Godfrey M, Bixler D: Unpublished data, 1991.
185. Godfrey M, Raghunath M: Manuscript in preparation, 1992.
186. Godfrey M et al: Cosegregation of elastin-associated microfibrillar abnormalities with the Marfan phenotype in families, *Am J Hum Genet* 46:652-660, 1990.
187. Godfrey M et al: Unilateral microfibrillar abnormalities in a case of asymmetric Marfan syndrome, *Am J Hum Genet* 46:661-671, 1990.
188. Godfrey M et al: Fibrillin mutation and prenatal diagnosis in a family with the Marfan syndrome. Submitted to the 42nd Annual Meeting of the American Society of Human Genetics, Nov 1992.
189. Godfrey M et al: Elastin and fibrillin mRNA and protein levels in the ontogeny of normal human aorta, *Connect Tissue Res*, 1992 (in press).
190. Golladay ES, Char F, Mollitt DL: Children with Marfan's syndrome and pectus excavatum, *South Med J* 78:1319-1323, 1985.
191. Goodman HB, Dorney ER: Marfan's syndrome with massive calcification of the mitral annulus at age twenty-six, *Am J Cardiol* 24:426-431, 1969.
192. Gordon AM: Abraham Lincoln: a medical appraisal, *J Ky Med Assoc* 60:249-253, 1962.
193. Gott VL: Personal communication, 1992.
194. Gott VL et al: Surgical treatment of aneurysms of the ascending aorta in the Marfan syndrome: results of composite-graft repair in 50 patients, *New Engl J Med* 314:1070-1074, 1986.
195. Gott VL et al: Composite graft repair of Marfan aneurysm of the ascending aorta: results in 100 patients, *Ann Thorac Surg* 52:38-45, 1991.
196. Gould PC, Bartolomeo RS, Sklarek HM: Esophageal ulceration associated with oral penicillin in Marfan's syndrome (letter), *New York J Med* 85:199-200, 1985.
197. Green H, Emerson PW: Arachnodactylia, *Arch Pediatr* 60:299-312, 1943.
198. Grondin CM, Steinberg CL, Edwards JE: Dissecting aneurysm complicating Marfan's syndrome (arachnodactyly) in a mother and son, *Am Heart J* 77:301-306, 1969.
199. Gross DM et al: Severe perinatal Marfan syndrome, *Pediatrics* 84:83-89, 1989.
200. Grossman M, Knott AP Jr, Jacoby WJ Jr: Calcified annulus fibrosus with mitral insufficiency in the Marfan syndrome, *Arch Intern Med* 121:561-563, 1968.
201. Gunja-Smith Z, Boucek RJ: Desmosines in human urine: amounts in early development and in Marfan's syndrome, *Biochem J* 193:915-918, 1981.
202. Haber H: Miescher's elastoma (elastoma intrapapillare perforans verruciforme), *Br J Dermatol* 71:85-96, 1959.
203. Hall JR et al: Pneumothorax in the Marfan syndrome: prevalence and therapy, *Ann Thorac Surg* 37:500-504, 1984.
204. Haller JA Jr, Kramer SS, Lietman SA: Use of CT scans in selection of patients for pectus excavatum surgery: a preliminary report, *J Pediatr Surg* 22:904-906, 1987.
205. Halme T et al: Elastin and collagen in the aortic wall: changes in the Marfan syndrome and annuloaortic ectasia, *Exp Mol Pathol* 43:1-12, 1985.
206. Halpern BL, Sugar A: Retinitis pigmentosa associated with bilateral ectopia lentis, *Ann Ophthalmol* 13:823-824, 1981.
207. Hamman L, Apperly FL: Spontaneous rupture of the aorta with aortic insufficiency, *Int Clin* 4:251-272, 1933.
208. Hance AJ, Crystal RG: The connective tissue of lung, *Am Rev Respir Dis* 112:657-711, 1975.
209. Hanley WB, Jones NB: Familial dissecting aortic aneurysms: a report of three cases within two generations, *Br Heart J* 29:852-858, 1967.
210. Hanley T et al: Heart failure of the hunchback, *Q J Med* 28:155-171, 1958.
211. Hardin CA: Ruptured abdominal aneurysm occurring in Marfan's syndrome: attempted repair with the use of a nylon prothesis, *New Engl J Med* 260:821-822, 1959.
212. Hardin CA: Successful resection of carotid and abdominal aneurysm in two retarded patients with Marfan's syndrome, *New Engl J Med* 267:141-142, 1962.

213. Haridas G: Arachnodactylia in a Chinese infant, *Arch Dis Child* 16:257, 1941.

214. Harkens KL, el Khoury GY: Intrasacral meningocele in a patient with Marfan syndrome: case report, *Spine* 15:610-612, 1990.

215. Harrison J, Klainer MJ: Arachnodactyly: its occurrence in several members of one family, *New Engl J Med* 220:621-623, 1939.

216. Harvey WP, Corrado MA, Perloff JK: "Right-sided" murmurs of aortic insufficiency, *Am J Med Sci* 245:533-543, 1963.

217. Hazenberg HJ, Tietge FC: Amiodarone-induced hyperthyroidism in a patient with Marfan's syndrome and Wolff-Parkinson-White syndrome, *Clin Nucl Med* 10:341-343, 1985.

218. Hecht F, Beals RK: "New" syndrome of congenital contractural arachnodactyly originally described by Marfan in 1896, *Pediatrics* 49:574-579, 1972.

219. Heitzman EJ, Bryant RB: The Marfan syndrome, gigantism and ruptured abdominal aneurysm, *New York J Med* 64:436-440, 1964.

220. Heldrich FJ Jr, Wright CE: Marfan's syndrome: diagnosis in the neonate, *Am J Dis Child* 114:419-423, 1967.

221. Henry WL, Gardin JM, Ware JH: Echocardiographic measurements in normal subjects from infancy to old age, *Circulation* 62:1054-1061, 1980.

222. Herrmann J et al: The Stickler syndrome (hereditary arthroophthalmopathy), *Birth Defects* 11:76-103, 1975.

223. Hiejima K et al: Two cases of Marfan's syndrome associated respectively with subacute bacterial endocarditis and the Wolff-Parkinson-White syndrome, *Jpn Heart J* 9:208-218, 1968.

224. Higashida RT et al: Cavernous carotid artery aneurysm associated with Marfan's syndrome: treatment by balloon embolization therapy, *Neurosurgery* 22:297-300, 1988.

225. Hindle NW, Crawford JS: Dislocation of the lens in Marfan's syndrome: its effect and treatment, *Can J Ophthalmol* 4:128-135, 1969.

226. Hirata K et al: The Marfan syndrome: rate of aortic root dilatation, *Circulation* 80(suppl II):529, 1989.

227. Hirst AE Jr, Johns VJ Jr, Kime SW Jr: Dissecting aneurysm of the aorta: a review of 505 cases, *Medicine* 37:217-279, 1958.

228. Ho N-K, Khoo T-K: Congenital contractural arachnodactyly, *Am J Dis Child* 133:639-640, 1979.

229. Hohn AR, Webb HM: Cardiac studies of infant twins with Marfan's syndrome, *Am J Dis Child* 122:526-528, 1971.

230. Hollister DW, Keene DR, Godfrey M: Unpublished observations, 1989.

231. Hollister DW, Sakai LY, Burgeson RE: Identification of novel human basement membrane zone components by monoclonal antibodies. In Fleischmajer R, Olsen BR, Kühn K, editors: *Biology, chemistry, and pathology of collagen*, New York, 1985, New York Academy of Sciences, pp 449-452.

232. Hollister DW et al: Immunohistologic abnormalities of the microfibrillar-fiber system in the Marfan syndrome, *New Engl J Med* 323:152-159, 1990.

233. Huang PJ et al: Abdominal aortic aneurysm in Marfan's syndrome: a case report, *J Formosan Med Assoc* 82:868-873, 1983.

234. Hudson JR: Marfan's syndrome with retinal detachment, *Br J Ophthalmol* 35:244-245, 1951.

235. Hunt D, Sloman G: Prolapse of the posterior leaflet of the mitral valve occurring in eleven members of a family, *Am Heart J* 78:149-153, 1969.

236. Imaizumi K et al: Three cases with infantile Marfan syndrome, *Am J Hum Genet* 49(suppl):142, 1991.

237. Inoue S, Leblond CP: The microfibrils of connective tissue. I. Ultrastructure, *Am J Anat* 176:121-138, 1986.

238. Irwin JW, Hancock DM, Sharp JR: Ruptured abdominal aortic aneurysm in Marfan's syndrome, *Br Med J* 1:1293-1294, 1964.

239. Jaffer Z, Beighton P: Arachnodactyly, joint laxity, and spondylolisthesis, *J Clin Dysmorphol* 1:14-18, 1983.

240. Jalaguier J et al: Fatal Marfan syndrome in the neonatal period, *J Genet Hum* 33:435-444, 1985.

241. Jarrett WH II: Dislocation of the lens: a study of 166 hospitalized cases, *Arch Ophthalmol* 78:289-296, 1967.

242. Jensen AD: Heritable ectopia lentis. In Goldberg MF, editor: *Genetic and metabolic eye disease*, Boston, 1974, Little, Brown.

243. Johnson CD: The Wolff-Parkinson-White syndrome associated with Marfan's syndrome, *Bol Asoc Med P Rico* 81:361-364, 1989.

244. Johnson KE et al: Rapid elimination of atenolol in adolescents with the Marfan syndrome, *Am J Med Genet* 32:245-246, 1989.

245. Josephson RA et al: Systolic expansion of the aortic root: an echocardiographic and angiographic sign of aortic composite graft dehiscence, *Cathet Cardiovasc Diagn* 14:105-107, 1988.

246. Kachele GE: The embryogenesis of ectopia lentis, *Arch Ophthalmol* 64:135-139, 1960.

247. Kainulainen K et al: Location on chromosome 15 of the gene defect causing Marfan syndrome, *New Engl J Med* 323:935-939, 1990.

248. Kainulainen K et al: Marfan syndrome: exclusion of genetic linkage to five genes coding for connective tissue components in the long arm of chromosome 2, *Hum Genet* 84:233-236, 1990.

249. Kainulainen K et al: Marfan syndrome: no evidence for heterogeneity in different populations, and more precise mapping of the gene, *Am J Hum Genet* 49:662-667, 1991.

250. Kaplan BM et al: Idiopathic congenital dilatation of the pulmonary artery, *J Lab Clin Med* 41:697-707, 1953.

251. Kaufman G, Engelbrecht WJ: Hemorrhagic intramedial dissection of coronary artery with cyctic medial necrosis, *Am J Cardiol* 24:409-413, 1969.

252. Kersting Sommerhoff BA et al: MR imaging of the thoracic aorta in Marfan patients, *J Comput Assist Tomogr* 11:633-639, 1987.

253. Kessler G et al: Preoperative magnetic resonance imaging in Marfan syndrome, *Isr J Med Sci* 26:278-280, 1990.

254. Kesten Y: *Diary of a heart patient*, New York, 1968, McGraw-Hill.

255. Kewley MA, Steven FS, Williams G: Preparation of a specific antiserum towards the microfibrillar protein of elastic tissues, *Immunology* 32:483-489, 1977.

256. Knight AM Jr: The Marfan syndrome, *J Med Assoc Ga* 46:413, 1957.

257. Knott VB, Johnson R: Height and shape of the palate in girls: a longitudinal study, *Arch Oral Biol* 15:849-860, 1970.

258. Knowlton RG et al: Genetic linkage analysis of hereditary arthro-ophthalmopathy (Stickler syndrome) and the type II procollagen gene, *Am J Hum Genet* 45:681-688, 1989.

259. Knudtzon J, Aarskog D: Estrogen treatment of excessively tall girls with Marfan syndrome, *Acta Paediatr Scand* 77:537-541, 1988.

260. Koenigsberg M et al: Fetal Marfan syndrome: prenatal ultrasound diagnosis with pathological confirmation of skeletal and aortic lesions, *Prenat Diagn* 1:241-247, 1981.

261. Kouchoukos NT, Karp RB, Lell WA: Replacement of the ascending aorta and aortic valve with a composite graft: results in 25 patients, *Ann Thorac Surg* 24:140-148, 1977.

262. Kouchoukos NT, Marshall WG Jr, Wedige Stecher TA: Eleven-year experience with composite graft replacement of the ascending aorta and aortic valve, *J Thorac Cardiovasc Surg* 92:691-705, 1986.

263. Kuhlman JE et al: Acetabular protrusion in the Marfan syndrome, *Radiology* 164:415-417, 1987.

264. Kumar V, Berenson GS: The Marfan syndrome: report of an interesting case with unusual anatomic findings, *J La Med Soc* 118:511-517, 1966.

265. Kunz R, Valentine R: Marfan's syndrome presenting as a type 3 aortic dissection, *Chest* 88:463-465, 1985.

266. Lafferty K et al: Ruptured abdominal aortic aneurysm in Marfan's syndrome, *Postgrad Med J* 63:685-687, 1987.

267. Laitinen O et al: Collagen metabolism of the skin in Marfan's syndrome, *Clin Chim Acta* 21:321-326, 1968.

268. Lamberg SI, Dorfman A: Synthesis and degradation of hyaluronic acid in the cultured fibroblasts of Marfan's disease, *J Clin Invest* 52:2428-2433, 1973.

269. Langeron T et al: Maladie de Marfan et aneurysme abdominal, *Bull Soc Méd Hôp Paris* 70:374-376, 1954.

270. Larson EW, Edwards WD: Risk factors for aortic dissection: a necropsy study of 161 cases, *Am J Cardiol* 53:849-855, 1984.

271. Latter DA et al: Internal carotid artery aneurysm and Marfan's syndrome, *Can J Surg* 32:463-466, 1989.

272. Lee B et al: Linkage of Marfan syndrome and a phenotypically related disorder to two different fibrillin genes, *Nature* 352:330-334, 1991.

273. Lenchman RD, Franceschi AD, Zamalloa O: Late systolic murmur and clicks associated with abnormal mitral valve ring, *Am J Cardiol* 23:679-683, 1969.

274. Leone JC, Swigar ME: Marfan's syndrome and neuropsychiatric symptoms: case report and literature review, *Compr Psychiatry* 27:247-250, 1986.

275. Leramo OB, Fraser H, Morgan OS: Sporadic concurrence of von Recklinghausen's neurofibromatosis and Marfan syndrome, *West Indian Med J* 34:131-133, 1985.

276. Lester CW: The surgical treatment of funnel chest, *Ann Surg* 123:1003-1022, 1946.

277. Levine RA et al: The relationship of mitral annular shape to the diagnosis of mitral valve prolapse, *Circulation* 75:756-767, 1987.

278. Levy D, Savage D: Prevalence and clinical features of mitral valve prolapse, *Am Heart J* 113:1281-1290, 1987.

279. Liang GF et al: Echocardiographic study of Marfan's syndrome, *Acta Acad Med Wuhan* 4:163-169, 1984.

280. Liang ST: Marfan syndrome, recurrent preterm labour and grandmultiparity, *Aust NZ J Obstet Gynaecol* 25:288-289, 1985.

281. Liberfarb RM, Goldblatt A: Prevalence of mitral-valve prolapse in the Stickler syndrome, *Am J Med Genet* 24:387-392, 1986.

282. Lima SD et al: Relation of mitral valve prolapse to left ventricular size in Marfan's syndrome, *Am J Cardiol* 55:739-743, 1985.

283. Lindeboom GA, Bouwer WF: Dissecting aneurysm (and renal cortical necrosis) associated with arachnodactyly (Marfan's disease), *Cardiologia* 15:12-20, 1949.

284. Lindeboom GA, Westerveld-Brandon ER: Dilatation of the aorta in arachnodactyly, *Cardiologia* 17:217-222, 1950.

285. Lipson EH, Viseskul C, Herrmann J: The clinical spectrum of congenital contractural arachnodactyly: a case with congenital heart disease, *Z Kinderheilk* 118:1-8, 1974.

286. Lipton RA, Greenwald RA, Seriff NS: Pneumothorax and bilateral honeycombed lung in Marfan syndrome: report of a case and review of the pulmonary abnormalities in this disorder, *Am Rev Resp Dis* 104:924-928, 1971.

287. Lloyd RI: Arachnodactyly, *Arch Ophthalmol* 13:744-750, 1935.

288. Lloyd RI: Clinical course of the ocular complications of Marfan's syndrome, *Arch Ophthalmol* 40:558-569, 1948.

289. Loveman AB, Gordon AM, Fliegelman MT: Marfan's syndrome: some cutaneous aspects, *Arch Dermatol* 87:428-435, 1963.

290. Low FN: Microfibrils: fine filamentous components of the tissue space, *Anat Rec* 142:131-137, 1962.

291. Lowe RC: Polycythemia vera (erythremia): arachnodactyly with congenital defect of vertebral column, and familial muscular dystrophy in Negroes; case reports, *Tri-State Med J* 13:2679, 1941.

292. Lowry RB, Guichon VC: Congenital contractural arachnodactyly: a syndrome simulating Marfan's syndrome, *Can Med Assoc J* 107:531-533, 1972.

293. Luckstead EF: Sudden death in sports, *Pediatr Clin North Am* 29:1355-1362, 1982.

294. Lutman FC, Neel JV: Inheritance of arachnodactyly, ectopia lentis and other congenital anomalies (Marfan's syndrome) in the E. family, *Arch Ophthalmol* 41:273-305, 1949.

295. Maddox BK et al: Connective tissue microfibrils: isolation and characterization of three large pepsin-resistant domains of fibrillin, *J Biol Chem* 264:21381-21385, 1989.

296. Magid D, Pyeritz RE, Fishman EK: Musculoskeletal manifestations of the Marfan syndrome: radiologic features, *Am J Roentgenol* 155:99-104, 1990.

297. Mamou H, Herault P: Maladie de Marfan et maladie de Scheuermann, *Sem Hôp Paris* 27:3071, 1951.

298. Marfan AB: Un cas de déformation congénitale des quatre membres plus prononcée aux extrémités characterisée par l'allongement des os avec un certain degré d'amincis-sement, *Bull Mem Soc Méd Hôp Paris* 13:220-226, 1896.

299. Markiewicz W et al: Mitral valve prolapse in one hundred presumably healthy young females, *Circulation* 53:464-473, 1976.

300. Maron BJ et al: Sudden death in young athletes, *Circulation* 62:218-229, 1980.

301. Marsalese DL et al: Marfan's syndrome: natural history and long-term follow-up of cardiovascular involvement, *J Am Coll Cardiol* 14:422-428, 1989.

302. Marsalese DL et al: Cystic medial necrosis of the aorta in patients without Marfan's syndrome: surgical outcome and long-term follow-up, *J Am Coll Cardiol* 16:68-73, 1990.

303. Martin R: *Lehrbuch der Anthropologie*, Jena, 1928, Gustav Fischer.

304. Mash AJ, Hegmann JP, Spivey BE: Genetic analysis of indices of corneal power and corneal astigmatism in human populations with varying incidences of strabismus, *Invest Ophthalmol* 14:826-832, 1975.

305. Maslen CL et al: Partial sequence of a candidate gene for the Marfan syndrome, *Nature* 352:334-337, 1991.

306. Massumi RA, Lowe EW, Misanik LF: Multiple aortic aneurysms (thoracic and abdominal) in twins with Marfan's syndrome: fatal rupture during pregnancy, *J Thorac Cardiovasc Surg* 53:223-230, 1967.

307. Masuda Y et al: Prognosis of patients with medically treated aortic dissections, *Circulation* 84(suppl III):7-13, 1991.

308. Maumenee IH: The eye in the Marfan syndrome, *Trans Am Ophthalmol Soc* 79:684-733, 1981.

309. Maxwell GM: Chest deformity in children with congenital heart disease, *Am Heart J* 54:368-375, 1957.

310. McClain LG: The tall athlete and Marfan syndrome: need for clinical differentiation, *J Adolesc Health Care* 10:564-566, 1989.

311. McDonald GR et al: Surgical management of patients with the Marfan syndrome and dilatation of the ascending aorta, *J Thorac Cardiovasc Surg* 81:180-186, 1981.

312. McFarland J et al: Medical treatment of dissecting aortic aneurysms, *New Engl J Med* 286:115-119, 1972.

313. McGookey-Milewicz D: Marfan syndrome: defective synthesis, secretion, and extracellular matrix formation of fibrillin by cultured dermal fibroblasts, *J Clin Invest* 89:79-86, 1992.

314. McKeown F: Dissecting aneurysm of the coronary artery in arachnodactyly, *Br Heart J* 22:434-436, 1960.

315. McKusick VA: The cardiovascular aspects of Marfan's syndrome, *Circulation* 11:321-342, 1955.

316. McKusick VA: *Cardiovascular sound in health and disease*, Baltimore, 1958, Williams & Wilkins.

317. McKusick VA: The genetic aspects of cardiovascular diseases, *Ann Intern Med* 49:556-567, 1958.

318. McKusick VA: The defect in Marfan syndrome, *Nature* 352:279-281, 1991.

319. McKusick VA: Personal communication, 1992.

320. McManus BM et al: Familial aortic dissection in absence of ascending aortic aneurysms: a lethal syndrome associated with precocious systemic hypertension, *Am J Cardiovasc Pathol* 1(1):55-67, 1986.

321. Meilman E, Urivetsky MM, Rapoport CM: Urinary hydroxyproline peptides, *J Clin Invest* 42:40-50, 1963.

322. Menon VK, Alurkar VM, Durairaj M: Anomalous origin of the coronary artery in Marfan's syndrome, *Indian Heart J* 35:176-177, 1983.

323. Méry H, Babonneix L: Un cas de déformation congénitale des quatre membres: hyperchondroplasie, *Bull Mém Soc Méd Hôp Paris* 19:671, 1902.

324. Merza AP, Raiser MW: Biliary tract manifestations of the Marfan syndrome, *Am J Gastroenterol* 82:779-782, 1987.

325. Meschan I, Colin CG: Computed tomography of the spine. In Meschan I, Farrer-Meschan RM, editors: *Roentgen signs in diagnostic imaging, vol 3. Spine and central nervous system*, Philadelphia, 1985, WB Saunders.

326. Miller R Jr, Pearson RJ Jr: Mitral insufficiency simulating aortic stenosis: report of an unusual manifestation of Marfan's syndrome, *New Engl J Med* 260:1210-1213, 1959.

327. Mirise RT, Shear S: Congenital contractural arachnodactyly: description of a new kindred, *Arthritis Rheum* 22:542-546, 1979.

328. Mitchell GE, Lourie H, Berne AS: The various causes of scalloped vertebrae with notes on their pathogenesis, *Radiology* 89:67-74, 1967.

329. Mitchell JH, Maron BJ, Epstein SE: 16th Bethesda conference: cardiovascular abnormalities in the athlete: recommendations regarding eligibility for competition, *J Am Coll Cardiol* 6:1186-1232, 1985.

330. Mohr R, Adar R, Rubinstein Z: Multiple aortic aneurysms in Marfan's syndrome: case report and review of the literature, *J Cardiovasc Surg (Torino)* 25:566-570, 1984.

331. Moore HC: Marfan syndrome, dissecting aneurysm of the aorta, and pregnancy, *J Clin Pathol* 18:277-281, 1965.

332. Moretti G et al: La Peau dans le syndrome de Marfan, *Presse Med* 72:2985-2990, 1964.

333. Morganroth J et al: Two dimensional echocardiography in mitral, aortic, and tricuspid valve prolapse: the clinical problem, cardiac nuclear imaging considerations, and a proposed standard for diagnosis, *Am J Cardiol* 46:1164-1177, 1980.

334. Morrison JC et al: Structural proteins of the neonatal and adult lamina cribrosa, *Arch Ophthalmol* 107:1220-1224, 1989.

335. Morse RP et al: Diagnosis and management of infantile Marfan syndrome, *Pediatrics* 86:888-895, 1990.

336. Muinos A, Sellyei L: Juvenile retinal detachment at the Barraquer clinic, *Mod Probl Ophthalmol* 8:284-293, 1969.

337. Muller NL et al: Ductus arteriosus aneurysm in Marfan syndrome, *Can Assoc Radiol J* 37:195-197, 1988.

338. Murdoch JL, Walker BA, McKusick VA: Parental age effects on the occurrence of new mutations for the Marfan syndrome, *Ann Hum Genet* 35:331-336, 1972.

339. Murdoch JL et al: Life expectancy and causes of death in the Marfan syndrome, *New Engl J Med* 286:804-808, 1972.

340. Nakashima Y: Reduced activity of serum beta-glucuronidase in Marfan syndrome, *Angiology* 37:576-580, 1986.

341. Neetens A: Kniest (Wagner-Stickler Variant) and Goldmann-Favre disease in one sibship, *Bull Soc Belge Ophthalmol* 223:27-32, 1987.

342. Neimann N et al: Maladie de Marfan chez un nouveau-né avec atteintes polyviscerales, *Ann Pediatr* 15:619-624, 1968.

343. Nelson JD: The Marfan syndrome, with special reference to congenital enlargement of the spinal canal, *Br J Radiol* 31:561-564, 1958.

344. Nelson LB, Maumenee IH: Ectopia Lentis. In Renie WA, editor: *Goldberg's genetic and metabolic eye disease*, ed 2, Boston, 1986, Little, Brown.

345. Nelson LB, Szmyd SM: Aphakic correction in ectopia lentis, *Ann Ophthalmol* 17:445-447, 1985.

346. Nemoto H, Yanai N: Marfan's syndrome, a hereditary enzymopenia (letter), *Jpn J Hum Genet* 5:199, 1961.

347. Newbold SG et al: Stage III Wilms' tumor of a solitary kidney in a patient with Marfan's syndrome: a 5-yr survival, *J Pediatr Surg* 17:841-842, 1982.

348. Nicod P et al: Familial aortic dissecting aneurysm, *J Am Coll Cardiol* 13:811-819, 1989.

349. Obarski TP, Schiavone WA: Thoracic cage deformities in the early diagnosis of the Marfan syndrome and cardiovascular disease, *J Am Osteopath Assoc* 90:446-450, 1990.

350. O'Doherty NJ: Neonatal Marfan's syndrome, with malformation of the urinary tract, *Proc R Soc Med* 59:483, 1966.

351. Ogilvie DJ et al: Segregation of all four major fibrillar collagen genes in the Marfan syndrome, *Am J Hum Genet* 41:1071-1082, 1987.

352. Olcott CT: Arachnodactyly (Marfan's syndrome) with severe anemia, *Am J Dis Child* 60:660-668, 1940.

353. Opitz JM et al: The Stickler syndrome, *New Engl J Med* 286:546-547, 1972.

354. Ormond AW: The etiology of arachnodactyly, *Guy's Hosp Rep* 80:68-81, 1930.

355. Pan CW et al: Echocardiographic study of cardiac abnormalities in families of patients with Marfan's syndrome, *J Am Coll Cardiol* 6:1016-1020, 1985.

356. Pappas BG, Mason D, Denton C: Marfan's syndrome: a report of three patients with aneurysms of the aorta, *Am J Med* 23:426-433, 1957.

357. Pasachoff HD, Madonick MJ, Drayer C: Arachnodactyly in four siblings with pneumoencephalographic observations of two, *Am J Dis Child* 67:201-204, 1944.

358. Passarge E: A syndrome resembling congenital contractural arachnodactyly, *Birth Defects* 11:53-56, 1975.

359. Perejda AJ et al: Marfan's syndrome: structural, biochemical, and mechanical studies of the aortic media, *J Lab Clin Med* 106:376-383, 1985.

360. Perloff JK, Child JS, Edwards JE: New guidelines for the clinical diagnosis of mitral valve prolapse, *Am J Cardiol* 57:1124-1129, 1986.

361. Peyman GA et al: Management of subluxated and dislocated lenses with the vitreophage, *Br J Ophthalmol* 63:771-778, 1979.

362. Phornphutkul C, Rosenthal A, Nadas AS: Cardiac manifestations of Marfan syndrome in infancy and childhood, *Circulation* 47:587-596, 1973.

363. Pieper JA et al: Mechanisms responsible for altered pharmacokinetics of atenolol in adolescents with the Marfan syndrome, *Am J Med Genet* 32:246, 1989.

364. Pini R et al: Mitral valve dimensions and motion in Marfan patients with and without mitral valve prolapse: comparison to primary mitral valve prolapse and normal subjects, *Circulation* 80:915-924, 1989.

365. Pinkus H, Keech MK, Mehregan AH: Histopathology of striae distensae, with special reference to striae and wound healing in the Marfan syndrome, *J Invest Dermatol* 46:283-292, 1966.

366. Piper RK, Irvine-Jones E: Arachnodactylia and its association with congenital heart disease: report of a case and review of the literature, *Am J Dis Child* 31:832-839, 1926.

367. Poole AE: Craniofacial aspects of the Marfan syndrome, *Birth Defects* 25:73-81, 1989.

368. Pressler V, McNamara JJ: Aneurysm of the thoracic aorta: review of 260 cases, *J Thorac Cardiovasc Surg* 89:50-54, 1985.

369. Priestley L, Kumar D, Sykes B: Amplification of the COL2A1 3' variable region used for segregation analysis in a family with the Stickler syndrome, *Hum Genet* 85:525-526, 1990.

370. Pruzinsky MS et al: Isolated descending thoracic aortic aneurysm in Marfan's syndrome, *Am J Cardiol* 61:1159-1160, 1988.

371. Pulkkinen L et al: Deficient expression of the gene coding for decorin in a lethal form of Marfan syndrome, *J Biol Chem* 265:17780-17785, 1990.

372. Pyeritz RE: Maternal and fetal complications of pregnancy in the Marfan syndrome, *Am J Med* 71:784-790, 1981.

373. Pyeritz RE: Propranolol retards aortic root dilatation in the Marfan syndrome, *Circulation* 68(suppl III):365, 1983.

374. Pyeritz RE: Protection of the aortic root by propranolol in Marfan syndrome, *J Med Genet* 23:469, 1986.

375. Pyeritz RE: Arthrogryposis in Marfan syndrome: an explanation for congenital contractural arachnodactyly, *Am J Med Genet* 25:725-726, 1986.

376. Pyeritz RE: Effectiveness of beta-adrenergic blockade in the Marfan syndrome: experience over 10 years, *Am J Med Genet* 32:245, 1989.

377. Pyeritz RE: Marfan syndrome. In Emery AEH, Rimoin DL, editors: *Principles and practice of medical genetics*, ed 2, New York, 1990, Churchill Livingstone, pp 1047-1063.

378. Pyeritz RE: Predictors of dissection of the ascending aorta in Marfan syndrome, *Circulation* 84(suppl II):351, 1991.

379. Pyeritz RE, McKusick VA: Current concepts: the Marfan syndrome: diagnosis and management, *New Engl J Med* 300:772-777, 1979.

380. Pyeritz RE, Reider R, Fortuin NJ: Aortic complications in adult Marfan syndrome are associated with aortic root diameter, *Clin Res* 29:315A, 1981.

381. Pyeritz RE, Wappel MA: Mitral valve dysfunction in the Marfan syndrome: clinical and echocardiographic study of prevalence and natural history, *Am J Med* 74:797-807, 1983.

382. Pyeritz RE et al: Growth and anthropometrics in the Marfan syndrome, *Prog Clin Biol Res* 200:355-366, 1985.

383. Pyeritz RE et al: Dural ectasia is a common feature of the Marfan syndrome, *Am J Hum Genet* 43:726-732, 1988.

384. Rados A: Marfan's syndrome, *Arch Ophthalmol* 27:477-538, 1942.

385. Rambar AC, Denenholz EJ: Arachnodactyly, *J Pediatr* 15:844-852, 1939.

386. Ramsey MS et al: The Marfan syndrome: a histopathologic study of ocular findings, *Am J Ophthalmol* 76:102-116, 1973.

387. Raviola G: The fine structure of the ciliary zonule and ciliary epithelium, with special regard to the organization and insertion of the zonular fibrils, *Invest Ophthalmol* 10:851-869, 1971.

388. Ravitch M: Pectus excavatum and heart failure, *Surgery* 30:178-194, 1951.

389. Redman RS, Shapiro BL, Gorlin RJ: Measurement of normal and reportedly malformed palatal vaults. II. Normal juvenile measurements, *J Dent Res* 45:266-269, 1966.

390. Reeh MJ, Lehman WL: Marfan's syndrome (arachnodac-

tyly) with ectopia lentis, *Trans Am Acad Ophthalmol* 58:212-216, 1954.

391. Relias A et al: Lutz-Miescher elastosis perpiginosa and osteogenesis imperfecta, *Ann Dermatol Syphiligr* 95:491-504, 1968.

392. Renteria VG et al: Intracellular collagen fibrils in prolapsed ("floppy") human atrioventricular valves, *Lab Invest* 35:439-443, 1976.

393. Resnik WH, Keefer CS: Dissecting aneurysm with signs of aortic insufficiency, *JAMA* 85:422-424, 1925.

394. Rice MJ, McDonald RW, Reller MD: Diagnosis of coronary artery dehiscence and pseudoaneurysm formation in postoperative Marfan patient by color flow Doppler echocardiography, *J Clin Ultrasound* 17:359-365, 1989.

395. Riquelme A, Green LJ: Palatal width, height, and length in human twins, *Am J Orthod* 40:71-79, 1970.

396. Risser JC: Clinical evaluation of scoliosis, *JAMA* 164:134-136, 1957.

397. Rizzuti AB: Complications in the surgical management of the displaced lens, *Int Ophthalmol Clin* 5:3-54, 1965.

398. Roberts WC: Congenital cardiovascular abnormalities usually "silent" until adulthood: morphologic features of the floppy mitral valve, valvular aortic stenosis, discrete subvalvular aortic stenosis, hypertrophic cardiomyopathy, sinus of Valsalva aneurysm, and the Marfan syndrome, *Cardiovasc Clin* 10:407-453, 1979.

399. Roberts WC: Aortic dissection: anatomy, consequences, and causes, *Am Heart J* 101:195-214, 1981.

400. Roberts WC, Dangel JC, Bulkley BH: Nonrheumatic valvular cardiac disease: a clinicopathologic survey of 27 different conditions causing valvular dysfunction, *Cardiovasc Clin* 5:333-446, 1973.

401. Roberts WC, Honig HS: The spectrum of cardiovascular disease in the Marfan syndrome: a clinico-morphologic study of 18 necropsy patients and comparison to 151 previously reported necropsy patients, *Am Heart J* 104:115-135, 1982.

402. Robins PR, Moe JH, Winter RB: Scoliosis in Marfan's syndrome, *J Bone Joint Surg (Am)* 57(A):358-368, 1975.

403. Roman MJ et al: Aortic root dilatation as a cause of isolated, severe aortic regurgitation: prevalence, clinical and echocardiographic patterns, and relation to left ventricular hypertrophy and function, *Ann Intern Med* 106:800-808, 1987.

404. Roman MJ et al: Aortic root dilatation in the Marfan syndrome: patterns, familiarity, and short-term clinical courses, *J Am Coll Cardiol* 11:74A, 1988.

405. Roman MJ et al: Comparison of cardiovascular and skeletal features of primary mitral valve prolapse and Marfan syndrome, *Am J Cardiol* 63:317-321, 1989.

406. Roman MJ et al: Two-dimensional echocardiographic aortic root dimensions in normal children and adults, *Am J Cardiol* 64:507-512, 1989.

407. Romano J, Linares RL: Marfan's syndrome and schizophrenia: a case report (letter), *Arch Gen Psychiatry* 44:190-192, 1987.

408. Rosenbloom J: Elastin: relation of protein and gene structure to disease, *Lab Invest* 51:605-623, 1984.

409. Ross JK, Gerbode F: The Marfan syndrome associated with an unusual interventricular septal defect, *J Thorac Surg* 39:746-750, 1960.

410. Ross LJ: Arachnodactyly: review of recent literature and report of case with cleft palate, *Am J Dis Child* 78:417-436, 1949.

411. Rubin P: *Dynamic classification of bone dysplasias*, St Louis, 1964, Mosby–Year Book, pp 207-212.

412. Russell F: An inquiry into the health of Mr. Lincoln, *Del Med J* 36:103-106, 1964.

413. Sahadevan MG, Raman PT, Hoon RS: Chronic atrial flutter in a case of Marfan's syndrome, *Am J Med* 47:965-966, 1969.

414. Sakai LY, Keene DR, Engvall E: Fibrillin, a new 350-kD glycoprotein, is a component of extracellular microfibrils, *J Cell Biol* 103:2499-2509, 1986.

415. Salle V: Ueber einen Fall von angeborener abnormen Grosse der Extremitaten mit einen an Akronemegalia erinnerden Symptomenkomplex, *Jahrb Kinderheilk* 75:540-550, 1912.

416. Salomon J, Shah PM, Heinle RA: Thoracic skeletal abnormalities in idiopathic mitral valve prolapse, *Am J Cardiol* 36:32-36, 1975.

417. Saruk M, Eisenstein R: Aortic lesion in Marfan syndrome: the ultrastructure of cystic medial degeneration, *Arch Pathol Lab Med* 101:74-77, 1977.

418. Sautter H: Aplasie des dilatator pupillae beim Marfanschen symptomenkomplex, *Klin Monatsbl Augenheilkd* 114:449-453, 1949.

419. Savunen T: Cardiovascular abnormalities in the relatives of patients operated upon for annulo-aortic ectasia: a clinical and echocardiographic study of 40 families, *Eur J Cardiothorac Surg* 1:3-10, 1987.

420. Savunen T, Aho HJ: Annulo-aortic ectasia: light and electron microscopic changes in aortic media, *Virchows Arch (A)* 407:279-288, 1985.

421. Schaefer S et al: Nuclear magnetic resonance imaging in Marfan's syndrome, *J Am Coll Cardiol* 9:70-74, 1987.

422. Schatz IJ, Yaworsky RG, Fine G: Myocardial infarction and unusual myocardial degeneration in Marfan's syndrome, with dissection of the right coronary artery and aorta, *Am J Cardiol* 12:553-560, 1963.

423. Scheck M et al: Aortic aneurysm in Marfan's syndrome: changes in the ultrastructure and composition of collagen, *J Anat* 129(3):645-657, 1979.

424. Scherer LR et al: Surgical management of children and young adults with Marfan syndrome and pectus excavatum, *J Pediatr Surg* 23:1169-1172, 1988.

425. Schilling V: Striae distensae als hypophysäres symptom bei basophilem vorderlappenadenom (Cushingschem syndrom) und bei arachnodaktylie (Marfanschem symptomenkomplex) mit hypophysentumor, *Med Welt* 10:183,219,259, 1936.

426. Schlatmann TJM, Becker AE: Histologic changes in the normal aging aorta: implications for dissecting aortic aneurysm, *Am J Cardiol* 39:13-20, 1977.

427. Schlatmann TJM, Becker AE: Pathogenesis of dissecting aneurysm of aorta, *Am J Cardiol* 39:21-26, 1977.

428. Schneider MB et al: Marfan syndrome in adolescents and young adults: psychosocial functioning and knowledge, *J Dev Behav Pediatr* 11:122-127, 1990.

429. Schneider WF: Arachnodactyly: unusual complication following skull injury, *J Pediatr* 27:583-588, 1945.

430. Schoeneman MJ et al: Marfan syndrome and medullary sponge kidney: case report and speculation on pathogenesis, *Int J Pediatr Nephrol* 5:103-104, 1984.

431. Schollin J, Bjarke B, Gustavson KH: Probable homozygotic form of the Marfan syndrome in a newborn child, *Acta Paediatr Scand* 77:452-456, 1988.

432. Schutte JE et al: Distinctive anthropometric characteristics of women with mitral valve prolapse, *Am J Cardiol* 71:533-538, 1981.

433. Schwartz H: Abraham Lincoln and the Marfan syndrome, *JAMA* 187:473-479, 1964.

434. Seery CM et al: Distinctive cataract in Stickler syndrome, *Am J Ophthalmol* 110:143-148, 1990.

435. Segal B, Kasparian H, Likoff W: Mitral regurgitation in a patient with the Marfan syndrome, *Dis Chest* 41:457-462, 1962.

436. Setälä K, Ruusuvaara P, Karjalainen K: Corneal endothelium in Marfan syndrome: a clinical and specular microscopic study, *Acta Ophthalmol* 66:334-340, 1988.

437. Shankar KR, Hultgren MK, Lauer RM: Lethal tricuspid and mitral regurgitation in Marfan's syndrome, *Am J Cardiol* 20:122-127, 1967.

438. Shapiro BL, Redman RS, Gorlin RJ: Measurements of normal and reportedly malformed palatal vaults. I. Normal adult measurements, *J Dent Res* 42:1039, 1963.

439. Sharma BK, Talukdar B, Kapoor R: Cystic lung in Marfan's syndrome, *Thorax* 44:978-979, 1989.

440. Shawkat S, Sarangi PP, Firmin RK: A technique for replacing a prosthetic aortic valve after total aortic root replacement, *Br Heart J* 63:260-261, 1990.

441. Shell WE et al: The familial occurrence of the syndrome of mid-late systolic click and late systolic murmur, *Circulation* 39:327-337, 1969.

442. Shumway SJ, Gott VL, Reitz BA: A "designer" annuloplasty ring for patients with massive mitral annular dilatation, *Ann Thorac Surg* 46:695-696, 1988.

443. Simpson JW, Nora JJ, McNamara DG: Marfan's syndrome and mitral valve disease-acute surgical emergencies, *Am Heart J* 77:96-99, 1969.

444. Sinclair RJG: The Marfan syndrome, *Bull Rheum Dis* 8:153-154, 1958.

445. Sinclair RJG, Kitchin AH, Turner RWD: The Marfan syndrome, *Q J Med* 29:19-46, 1960.

446. Sisk HE, Zahka KG, Pyeritz RE: The Marfan syndrome in early childhood: analysis of 15 patients diagnosed at less than 4 years of age, *Am J Cardiol* 52:353-358, 1983.

447. Sjoerdsma A et al: Increased excretion of hydroxyproline in Marfan's syndrome, *Lancet* 2:994, 1958.

448. Smith TH, Holland MG, Woody NC: Ocular manifestations of familial hyperlysinemia, *Trans Am Acad Ophthalmol Otolaryngol* 75:355-360, 1971.

449. Snider AR et al: Two-dimensional echocardiographic determination of aortic and pulmonary artery sizes from infancy to adulthood in normal subjects, *Am J Cardiol* 53:218-229, 1984.

450. Soulen RL et al: Marfan syndrome: evaluation with MR imaging versus CT, *Radiology* 165:697-701, 1987.

451. Spangler RD et al: Echocardiography in Marfan's syndrome, *Chest* 69:72-78, 1976.

452. Spranger J: Pattern recognition in bone dysplasias. In Papadatos CJ, Bartsocas CS, editors: *Endocrine genetics and genetics of growth*, 1985, Alan R Liss.

453. Steg NL: Congenital contractural arachnodactyly in a Black family, *Birth Defects* 11:57-62, 1975.

454. Steinberg I: A simple screening test for the Marfan syndrome, *Am J Roentgenol* 97:118-124, 1966.

455. Stern WE: Dural ectasia and the Marfan syndrome, *J Neurosurg* 69:221-227, 1988.

456. Stickler GB et al: Hereditary progressive arthro-ophthalmopathy, *Mayo Clin Proc* 40:433-455, 1965.

457. Stickler GB, Pugh DG: Hereditary progressive arthro-ophthalmopathy. II. Additional observations on vertebral abnormalities, a hearing defect, and a report of a similar case, *Mayo Clin Proc* 42:495-500, 1967.

458. Stolz HR, Stolz LM: *Somatic development of adolescent boys: a study of the growth of boys during the second decade of life*, New York, 1951, Macmillan.

459. Straatsma BR, Christensen RE, Pettit TH: Lens subluxation and surgical aphakia treated with photocoagulation of the iris, *Doc Ophthalmol* 26:664-678, 1969.

460. Strahan NV et al: Inheritance of the mitral valve prolapse syndrome: discussion of a three-dimensional penetrance model, *Am J Med* 74:967-972, 1983.

461. Stratz CH: *Der Körper des Kindes*, Stuttgart, 1902, Ferdinand Enke.

462. Streeten BW, Licari PA: The zonules and the elastic microfibrillar system in the ciliary body, *Invest Ophthalmol Vis Sci* 24:667-681, 1983.

463. Streeten BW et al: Immunohistochemical comparison of ocular zonules and the microfibrils of elastic tissue, *Invest Ophthalmol Vis Sci* 21:130-135, 1981.

464. Streeten BW et al: The ocular zonule in Marfan's syndrome, *Invest Ophthalmol Vis Sci* 31(suppl):102, 1991.

465. Streeten EA, Murphy EA, Pyeritz RE: Pulmonary function in the Marfan syndrome, Chest 91:408-412, 1987.

466. Subirats-i-Bayego E et al: Marfan syndrome and diaphragmatic hernia (letter), *Med Clin (Barc)* 81:597, 1983.

467. Sun QB et al: Marfan syndrome in China: a collective review of 564 cases among 98 families, *Am Heart J* 120:934-948, 1990.

468. Sutton GEF: Cardiac anomalies associated with funnel chest, *Bristol Med Clin J* 64:45-48, 1947.

469. Svensson LG et al: Impact of cardiovascular operation on survival in the Marfan patient, *Circulation* 80:233-242, 1989.

470. Takebayashi S, Kubota I, Takagi T: Ultrastructural and histochemical studies of vascular lesions in Marfan's syndrome, with report of 4 autopsy cases, *Acta Pathol Jpn* 23:847-866, 1973.

471. Takebayashi S et al: "Osmiophilic elastolysis" of peripheral organ arteries in patients with Marfan's syndrome, *Acta Pathol Jpn* 38:1433-1443, 1988.

472. Takeichi S: An autopsy case of Marfan syndrome with histochemical studies on the cardiovascular system, *Tokushima J Exp Med* 31:33-39, 1984.

473. Taly AB, Nagaraj D, Vasanth A: Association of Marfan's syndrome and epilepsy (letter), *J Assoc Physicians India* 35:247, 1987.

474. Tanaka K et al: Medical vs surgical treatment of acute aortic dissection in an intensive care unit, *Jpn Circ J* 55:815-820, 1991.

475. Taniguchi K et al: Long-term survival and complications after composite graft replacement for ascending aortic aneurysm associated with aortic regurgitation, *Circulation* 84 (suppl III):31-39, 1991.

476. Taylor LJ: Severe spondylolisthesis and scoliosis in association with Marfan's syndrome: case report and review of the literature, *Clin Orthop* 221:207-211, 1987.

477. Tchah HW et al: Neodymium:YAG laser zonulysis for treatment of lens subluxation, *Ophthalmology* 96:230-235, 1989.

478. Tcherdakoff PH et al: Propranolol in hypertension during pregnancy, *Br Med J* 2:670, 1978.

479. Temple IK: Stickler's syndrome, *J Med Genet* 26:119-126, 1989.

480. Thomas J et al: Marfan syndrome: a report of three cases with aneurysm of the aorta, *Am J Med* 12:613-618, 1952.

481. Thursfield H: Arachnodactyly, *St Bartholomew's Hosp Rep* 53:35, 1917.

482. Tolbert LE Jr, Birchall RB: Marfan's syndrome with interventricular septal defect found at autopsy, *Oschner Clin Rep* 2:48, 1956.

483. Toyama M, Amano A, Kameda T: Familial aortic dissection: a report of rare family cluster, *Br Heart J* 61:204-207, 1989.

484. Traub E: Epiphyseal necrosis in pituitary gigantism, *Arch Dis Child* 14:203-216, 1939.

485. Travis RC, Shaw DG: Congenital contractural arachnodactyly, *Br J Radiol* 58:1115-1117, 1985.

486. Trotte SE, Olsen EGJ: Marfan's disease and Erdheim's cystic medionecrosis: a study of their pathology, *Eur Heart J* 12:83-87, 1991.

487. Trüb CLP: Aortenwanderkrankung (medianecrosis aortae idiopathica), aortenzerreissung und arbeitsunfall, *Mschr Unfallheilk* 54:321, 1951.

488. Tsipouras P: A workshop on Marfan syndrome, 10 June 1989, Farmington, CT, USA, *J Med Genet* 27:139-140, 1990.

489. Tsipouras P et al: Marfan syndrome: exclusion of genetic linkage to the COL1A2 gene, *Clin Genet* 30:428-432, 1986.

490. Tsipouras P et al: Marfan syndrome is closely linked to a marker on chromosome 15q1.55q2.1, *Proc Natl Acad Sci USA* 88:4486-4488, 1991.

491. Tsipouras P et al: Linkage analysis demonstrates that Marfan syndrome, dominant ectopia lentis, and congenital contractural arachnodactyly are linked to the fibrillin genes on chromosomes 15 and 5, *New Engl J Med* 326:905-909, 1992.

492. Tsuji T: Marfan syndrome: demonstration of abnormal elastic fibers in skin, *J Cutan Pathol* 13:144-153, 1986.

493. Tucker AS, Bolande RP: Pulmonary dysaeration in Marfan's syndrome, *Ann Radiol* 7:450-458, 1964.

494. Tung HL, Liebow AA: Marfan's syndrome: observations at necropsy, with special reference to medio-necrosis of the great vessels, *Lab Invest* 1:382-406, 1952.

495. Turner JA, Stanley NN: Fragile lung in the Marfan syndrome, *Thorax* 31:771-775, 1976.

496. Uyeyama H, Kondo B, Kamins M: Arachnodactylia and cardiovascular disease, *Am Heart J* 34:580-591, 1947.

497. Vallal RS et al: Usefulness of transesophageal echocardiography in assessment of aortic dissection, *Circulation* 84:1903, 1991.

498. van Bavel LP et al: Delusions in Marfan syndrome (letter), *J Clin Psychiatry* 50:473, 1989.

499. Van Buchem FSP: Cardiovascular disease in arachnodactyly, *Acta Med Scand* 161:197-205, 1958.

500. Viljoen D, Beighton P: Marfan syndrome: a diagnostic dilemma, *Clin Genet* 37:417-422, 1990.

501. Viljoen D, Ramesar R, Behari D: Beals syndrome: clinical and molecular investigations in a kindred of Indian descent, *Clin Genet* 39:181-188, 1991.

502. Vivas-Salas E, Sanson RE: Sindrome d Marfan, sin cardiopatia congenita y con endocarditis lenta conformada por la autopsia, *Arch Inst Cardiol Mex* 18:217-230, 1948.

503. von Noorden GK, Schultz RO: A gonioscopic study of the chamber angle in Marfan's syndrome, *Arch Ophthalmol* 64:929-934, 1960.

504. Wachtel FW, Ravitch MM, Grisham A: The relation of pectus excavatum to heart disease, *Am Heart J* 52:121-137, 1956.

505. Wachtel JG: The ocular pathology of Marfan's syndrome, including a clinicopathological correlation and an explanation of ectopia lentis, *Arch Ophthalmol* 76:513-522, 1966.

506. Wagenvoort CA, Neufeld HN, Edwards JE: Cardiovascular system in Marfan's syndrome and in idiopathic dilatation of the ascending aorta, *Am J Cardiol* 9:496-507, 1962.

507. Walker BA, Beigthon PH, Murdoch JL: The marfanoid hypermobility syndrome, *Ann Intern Med* 71:349-352, 1969.

508. Walker BA, Murdoch JL: The wrist sign: a useful physical finding in the Marfan syndrome, *Arch Intern Med* 126:276-277, 1970.

509. Warnes CA, Kirkman PM, Roberts WC: Aortic dissection in more than one family member, *Am J Cardiol* 55:236-238, 1985.

510. Warth DC et al: Prevalence of mitral valve prolapse in normal children, *J Am Coll Cardiol* 39:422-431, 1977.

511. Waters P et al: Scoliosis in children with pectus excavatum and pectus carinatum, *J Pediatr Orthop* 9:551-556, 1989.

512. Weiss AN et al: Echocardiographic detection of mitral valve prolapse: exclusion of false positive diagnosis and determination of inheritance, *Circulation* 52:1091-1096, 1975.

513. Wenger DR et al: Protrusio acetabuli in Marfan's syndrome, *Clin Orthop Rel Res* 147:134-138, 1980.

514. Weve H: Ueber Arachnodaktylie (Dystrophia mesodermalis congenita, typus Marfanis), *Arch F Ophth* 104:1-46, 1931.

515. White JF et al: An immuno-electron microscopic study of the elastic tissue defects in thoracic aortic dissecting aneurysms, Pan Pacific Connective Tissue Societies Symposium, Cairns, Australia, Nov 1989.

516. Whitfield AGW, Arnott WM, Stafford JS: "Myocarditis" and aortic hypoplasia in arachnodactylia, *Lancet* 1:1387-1391, 1951.

517. Wilkinson KD: Aneurysmal dilatation of the pulmonary artery, *Br Heart J* 2:255-259, 1940.

518. Williams E: Rare cases, with practical remarks, *Trans Am Ophthalmol Soc* 2:291-301, 1879.

519. Wilner HI, Finby N: Skeletal manifestations in the Marfan syndrome, *JAMA* 187:490-495, 1964.

520. Wilson R: Marfan's syndrome: description of a family, *Am J Med* 23:434-444, 1957.

521. Winter RB: Severe spondylolisthesis in Marfan's syndrome: report of two cases, *J Pediatr Orthop* 2:51-55, 1982.

522. Winter RB: Thoracic lordoscoliosis in Marfan's syndrome: report of two patients with surgical correction using rods and sublaminar wires, *Spine* 15:233-235, 1990.

523. Winter RB, Anderson MB: Spinal arthrodesis for spinal deformity using posterior instrumentation and sublaminar wiring: a preliminary report of 100 consecutive cases, *Int Orthop* 9:239-245, 1985.

524. Withers JN et al: Spontaneous pneumothorax: suggested etiology and comparison of treatment methods, *Am J Surg* 108:772-776, 1964.

525. Wong FL, Friedman S, Yakovac W: Cardiac complications of Marfan's syndrome in a child: report of a case with rapidly pregressive course terminating with rupture of dissecting aneurysm, *Am J Dis Child* 107:404-409, 1964.

526. Wood JR et al: Pulmonary disease in patients with Marfan syndrome, *Thorax* 39:780-784, 1984.

527. Wunsch CM, Steinmetz EF, Fisch C: Marfan's syndrome and subacute bacterial endocarditis, *Am J Cardiol* 15:102-106, 1965.

528. Yasuura K et al: A case report of surgical treatment of Marfan's syndrome with mitral annular calcification at a young age, *Kokyu To Junkan* 35:1321-1324, 1987.

Homocystinuria

Reed E. Pyeritz

A number of inborn errors of metabolism result in elevated plasma levels of sulfurated amino acids such as methionine and homocysteine. Deficiency of the cytosolic enzyme cystathionine β-synthase (CBS) produces a phenotype that is largely but not exclusively due to abnormalities of the extracellular matrix (ECM). This phenotype, commonly referred to by the generic term homocystinuria, *is considered in this chapter. Homocystinuria is classified as a secondary disorder of connective tissue because the ECM has no intrinsic defect; rather, the biochemical, histologic, and functional abnormalities result from an extrinsic cause acting on the various components of the ECM.[6]**

Homocystinuria did not appear in the earliest editions of this book because the phenotype was not recognized as a separate entity and the manifestations in the ECM were not described until the early 1960s. Before that time most patients either were thought to have an unclassified form of mental retardation or were misdiagnosed as having Marfan syndrome. Although heightened clinical awareness of the phenotype and newborn screening programs have greatly improved diagnostic accuracy, still a disturbing number of affected children and adults are ascertained only after irreversible organ system damage has occurred. This is not to say that all the deleterious manifestations of the disorder can be prevented completely, but even in the cases most resistant to therapy the clinical problems can be ameliorated; although no ther-

apy will reverse established organ and tissue damage, the earlier preventive measures are introduced, the better the outcome.[77]

Over the past quarter-century considerable progress has been made in understanding the phenotype, natural history, and basic defect of CBS deficiency, and a concise review of this knowledge forms the bulk of this chapter.* What remains as the greatest challenge is to understand the pathophysiology of homocystinuria. In other words, how is the fundamental defect—a gene mutation causing partial or complete absence of CBS activity—translated into the clinical phenotype? Only when the pathogenetic mechanisms are known can truly effective therapy be designed and evaluated. This is just as true for somatic cell gene therapy as it is for more mundane methods such as vitamin supplementation and dietary restrictions.

Another substantial challenge is to understand how minor degrees of homocystinemia, such as may occur chronically or episodically in people who are heterozygotes for CBS deficiency, cause predisposition to common maladies such as arteriovascular disease, osteoporosis, or psychopathy. Although not a major focus of this chapter, recent investigations along these lines are discussed.

✦ HISTORICAL NOTE

During the early 1960s Carson and Neill,[15] Carson et al.,[16] and Gibson, Carson, and Neill,[34] using urine chromatography, screened institutionalized

---

*The causes of homocysteinemia and homocystinuria aside from deficiency of CBS are reviewed in references 72 and 73.

*For details and extensive bibliographies, refer to Mudd, Levy, and Skovby.[72,73]

persons with mental retardation in Northern Ireland. Several specimens contained homocystine, an amino acid normally not present in urine. Furthermore, the patients who provided these abnormal samples had the unusual ocular problem of ectopia lentis. Simultaneously and independently Gerritsen, Vaughn, and Waisman[31] and Gerritsen and Waisman[32,33] in Madison, Wisconsin, found the same metabolic defect in an infant with "cerebral palsy." The occurrence of thromboembolic complications soon became evident.[34]

In 1964 Professor Charles E. Dent of London, a collaborator of Carson,[15] visited the Johns Hopkins Hospital in Baltimore as the Thayer lecturer and discussed inborn errors of metabolism, including the new information on homocystinuria. The skeletal and ocular manifestations of the Irish patients were suggestive of Marfan syndrome, and proneness to thromboembolism brought to McKusick's mind several of his patients from the medical genetics clinic of the Johns Hopkins Hospital. In particular, he recalled three sibs (described in detail as Family 1, pp. 161 to 165) who had been diagnosed as having Marfan syndrome but had below average intelligence and apparently unaffected parents. McKusick immediately arranged to obtain a urine specimen from the youngest and only surviving sib. The urine test result was positive for the cyanide-nitroprusside reaction, which at that time was routinely used to screen for cystinuria but which could indicate the presence of any di-sulfides. Before Professor Dent returned home, he knew that homocystinuria occurred on both sides of the Atlantic. McKusick, his curiosity piqued, organized a systematic survey of "Marfan" patients in the Moore Clinic and turned up a few more pedigrees and patients with homocystinuria, whose clinical characteristics were detailed in the fourth edition of this text and elsewhere.[91,94,95] Neil Schimke, then a postdoctoral fellow in medical genetics, and McKusick organized a project to screen patients from around the country with ectopia lentis. Urine was collected by cooperating ophthalmologists and mailed to the Johns Hopkins Hospital; 14 of 442 patients (3%) with nontraumatic ectopia lentis had positive results in the cyanide-nitroprusside test.[95] This survey demonstrated that mental retardation is not an invariable feature of homocystinuria.

Mudd et al.,[74] from their previous studies of methionine metabolism, suspected that the defect in homocystinuria might be in the enzymatic condensation of homocysteine and serine that forms cystathionine. Their suspicions were confirmed by demonstration of deficiency of cystathionine β-synthase activity in liver. Uhlendorf and Mudd[111] made the important observation that enzymatic diagnosis of homocystinuria can be made by the use of fibroblasts cultured from biopsy specimens of skin. Barber and Spaeth[4] demonstrated that some patients with homocystinuria respond to vitamin B_6 supplementation (oral pyridoxine), which clears the urine of homocystine. During the 1970s and 1980s the laboratories of Mudd, Gaull,[27,61] and, especially, Rosenberg[28,54,96,99-101] led the studies of CBS that provided both a biochemical explanation for differential pharmacologic response to pyridoxine and proof of even more extensive genetic heterogeneity.

In 1986 the CBS gene was cloned by the Rosenberg group (Kraus et al.[58]) and mapped to human chromosome 21q.[78] The 2500-kilobase (kb) complementary DNA (cDNA) was first successfully used to identify specific mutations in 1991.[37,57]

CLINICAL MANIFESTATIONS AND NATURAL HISTORY

More so than phenylketonuria and many other Garrodian inborn errors of metabolism, homocystinuria is a paradigm of the three principles of clinical genetics, pleiotropism, variability, and genetic heterogeneity. Pleiotropism is evident from the abundance and variety of organ and tissue manifestations. Four organ systems are most severely affected and draw much of the clinical attention: the central nervous system, the skeleton, the eye, and the vasculature. Qualitative and quantitative differences in expression of the phenotype are in large measure due to genetic heterogeneity, but sufficient intrafamilial variability occurs to indicate that other factors are at work. Finally, the molecular genetic investigations that are now becoming routine prove how rich a diversity of mutations in CBS produce this disease.

The following review of the phenotype is based in part on the descriptions of cases in the literature and in part on a review of more than 120 cases evaluated in the medical genetics clinic of the Johns Hopkins Hospital over the past 25 years. The single most important source is an international survey coordinated by Mudd et al.,[77] which compiled data on 629 patients, including most of the Johns Hopkins Hospital patients.

Table 4-1. Mental capacity in patients with homocystinuria

Patients	Mental capacity (% of patients)			
	Grossly retarded	**Mildly retarded**	**Average or above with learning disability**	**Average or above**
All B_6 categories	22	39	6	33
B_6-responsive	5	33	11	51
B_6-nonresponsive	38	47	4	11

Adapted from Mudd SH et al: *Am J Hum Genet* 36:1-31, 1985.
Patients were those not discovered by newborn screening. Ratings of mental capacity were available for the following numbers of patients: all B_6 categories, 283; B_6-responsive, 116; B_6-nonresponsive, 73.

Central Nervous System

The central nervous system manifestations include those directly caused by the metabolic defect, such as mental retardation and psychiatric disturbances; those resulting from vascular problems such as stroke; and those that could arise from either mechanism, such as seizures and extrapyramidal signs.

A decrease in intellectual capacity and achievement occurs in most patients with homocystinuria. The most severe retardation occurs in pyridoxine-unresponsive patients who were never treated by diet, whereas pyridoxine-responsive patients treated from infancy have the best performance on intelligence tests.[77] There is a statistically significant difference of about 22 intelligence quotient (IQ) points between pyridoxine-responsive and pyridoxine-unresponsive patients (Fig. 4-1). The spread in IQ scores is large (10 to 138), but the scores of sibs are usually closely clustered. In the early Johns Hopkins Hospital series of 83 cases, 41 patients had average intelligence or higher. One subject held a doctoral degree and was a university instructor, and several others had completed college. Table 4-1 shows the frequencies of general classes of intellectual capacity among patients with homocystinuria *not* detected by newborn screening.

It is unlikely that intracranial thrombosis has much effect on baseline intelligence, since IQ scores vary little over time, and retardation, when present, usually dates from childhood in patients who receive neither dietary nor vitamin therapy.[77] The young woman described in Family 10 (p. 173) is an exception; her intellect was clearly affected by a stroke. Clinically evident cerebrovascular disease is uncommon in childhood. However, the ac-

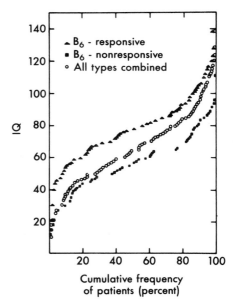

Fig. 4-1. Distribution of IQs among patients with homocystinuria not detected by newborn screening. The curves are based on the following numbers of patients with reported IQs: all B_6 categories, 284; B_6-responders, 107; B_6-nonresponders, 115. For any specified IQ value, the curves show the total percent of each category of patients with IQs equal to or less than the specified value. (From Mudd et al: *Am J Hum Genet*, 36:1-31, 1985.)

tual pathogenesis of the intellectual defect is unclear. Hypotheses include a direct toxic effect of homocysteine and deficiency of cystine. Learning problems often occur in patients with Marfan syndrome, although intelligence is seemingly unaffected.[45]

Seizures, usually of the grand mal type, occur

in one fifth of untreated patients, and electroencephalogram (EEG) abnormalities may be present even in the absence of overt seizures.[72] Seizures tend to occur earlier in untreated, pyridoxine-unresponsive patients. In anecdotal experience dietary or vitamin therapy has had limited success in preventing seizures once these had become established.[72]

Most neurologic signs can be traced to ischemic events, but some patients have extrapyramidal signs of unclear cause, such as dystonia.[72]

Patients with a variety of psychiatric disturbances have been described. Schizophrenia was mentioned in early reports; indeed, the first Johns Hopkins Hospital patient was thought to be so affected.[106] However, the first (and only) systematic survey of psychopathologic conditions, which involved 63 patients and included the patient just mentioned (Family 1, Case 3 [p. 162]) showed no evidence of schizophrenia.[1] More important, in about half the cases the patients did have psychiatric abnormalities, including personality disorders in 19%, chronic behavioral disturbances in 17%, episodic depression in 10%, and obsessive-compulsive disorder in 5%. Personality disorders occurred in patients of all IQs, whereas behavioral and compulsive disorders were more common in patients with lower IQs.

Intracranial venous and arterial thromboses create a variety of clinical pictures in young children with homocystinuria. This metabolic error must be kept in mind in connection with acute hemiplegia of infancy and childhood.[17] Intracranial venous thrombosis can lead to a characteristic picture of headache, neck stiffness, and bloody cerebrospinal fluid. Poliomyelitis may be mistakenly diagnosed in cases of acute paraplegia; indeed, meningoencephalitis may be mistakenly diagnosed in cases of intracranial venous thrombosis.[25] Young children with unsuspected homocystinuria were frequently thrown into that meaningless diagnostic hodgepodge, "cerebral palsy." One patient had marked spasticity and died at 1 year of age; autopsy showed cystic degeneration of the brain.[18] One case of "temporal lobe agenesis" appears from the description to have represented homocystinuria; both the patient, who died at 20 years of age, and his brother were thought to have Marfan syndrome.[88]

The brain shows focal necrosis and gliosis. Chou and Waisman[18] described severe spongy degeneration of the brain with micropolygyria and hypo-plasia of the corpus callosum in an unaffected child who died at 1 year of age.

Thrombosis of the carotid arteries has been known to occur in a number of instances, for example, in an 18-year-old boy (Family 1, Case 1 [p. 161]) and in a 12-year-old girl of another family (Family 14 in the fourth edition of this book). In both instances the evidence is clear that cerebral arteriograms accelerated the thrombotic process and led to death soon after. In the 18-year-old, both internal carotid arteries were completely occluded but the stenosis and occlusion occurred episodically because fresh thrombus, canalizing thrombus, and organized thrombus of several vintages were present, showing new internal elastic lamellae (see Fig. 4-11). Intracranial thrombosis leading to death occurred in an 8-year-old boy of Irish extraction whose case was the subject of a clinicopathologic conference at the Massachusetts General Hospital in 1933. Homocystinuria was established retrospectively by Shih and Efron[98] by demonstration of the disorder in living members of the kindred. The histopathologic findings were reviewed by McCully,[66] who used them as the point of departure for his studies of the role of homocysteine in ordinary arteriosclerosis.[67,68]

Skeletal Features

Osteoporosis, tendency to fracture, scoliosis, deformity of the anterior chest, kyphoscoliosis, excessive length of the bones of the limbs, which results in tall stature, enlarged ossification centers, a "buried spicule" type of epiphyseal-metaphyseal change, and a modest degree of limitation of joint mobility are all found to varying degrees in patients with homocystinuria. The hands of patients with homocystinuria tend to have a "tight feel" of restricted joint mobility in the fingers, in contrast to the loose-jointed hands of the patient with Marfan syndrome.

Excessive height and a reduced upper-segment (US) to lower-segment (LS) ratio (US/LS) are usual findings in homocystinuria and are points of similarity with Marfan syndrome (Fig. 4-2, A and B). Platyspondyly and, particularly, scoliosis reduce the height to some extent and exaggerate the reduction in the US/LS value.

The radiographic features of 26 patients who varied from 6 to 45 years of age, have been reported,[70] and examples are reproduced in this chapter. The findings were consistent with surveys of others.[62,103] In 25 of 26 patients the vertebral

A   **B**   **C**

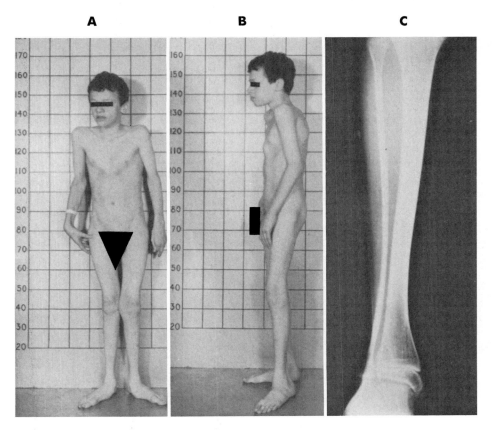

Fig. 4-2. Homocystinuria in a 12-year-old boy. **A** and **B,** Pectus carinatum, left genu valgum, and "rocker-bottom" feet are evident. **C,** Radiograph of right leg, showing that the tibia and fibula are slender and mildly bowed.

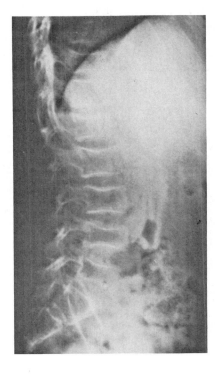

Fig. 4-3. Osteoporosis of the lumbar spine in a 22-year-old woman with homocystinuria.

bodies were osteoporotic, and in 19 the porosis was associated with concavity of the vertebral end plates (Fig. 4-3). Scoliosis was noted in 17 patients, and exaggerated thoracic kyphosis in five. Two patients had spondylolisthesis. It is likely that degeneration of the intervertebral disks was a feature in some cases. Chronic back pain was a major problem in some. In most patients the long bones of the limbs were also osteoporotic, and in many they were unusually long and thin (Fig. 4-2, C). In eight of 18 patients measured, the metacarpal index exceeded 8.5, a quasiobjective criterion of arachnodactyly. Nine of 23 patients showed varus deformity of the proximal humerus (Fig. 4-4), which is an unusual finding in normal persons and which in patients with homocystinuria may be related to round-shoulderedness. Flaring of the distal femur and large distal femoral epiphyses are exaggerated by the general thinness of the thighs and legs. As a consequence, large, knobbly knees are commonly noted.

Some of the most distinctive changes occur in

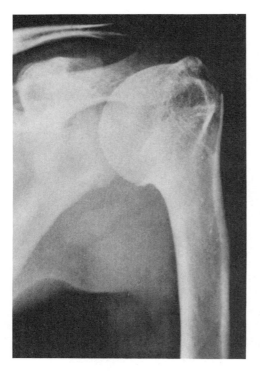

Fig. 4-4. Varus deformity of the proximal humerus in an 18-year-old man with homocystinuria.

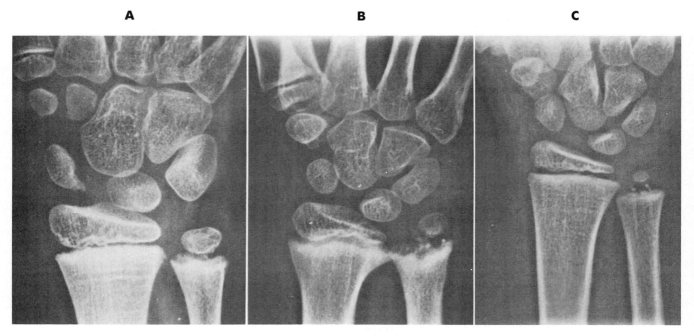

Fig. 4-5. Radiographs of the wrist in three patients with untreated homocystinuria. **A,** A 6-year-old boy, showing enlarged hamate and capitate bones, calcific spicules in both the radial and ulnar epiphyses, and buried spicules within the radial metaphysis. The ulnar epiphysis is slightly widened, with cupping of the end of the metaphysis. **B,** An 8-year-old girl, showing widening of the epiphyses, especially the ulnar, and multiple calcified dots in the ulnar epiphysis. The ulnar metaphysis is cupped, and both metaphyses, especially the radial, contain buried spicules. **C,** A 9-year-old boy, showing retarded ossification of all bones, particularly of the lunate. The ulnar epiphysis is widened and contains conspicuous spicules and dots. Particularly striking buried spicules are evident in the radial and ulnar metaphyses.

the wrists (Fig. 4-5), particularly in children. In all of 12 children studied, the distal radial and ulnar physes contained focal calcifications, which were sometimes punctate but more often were in the form of narrow spicules. Moreover, striking longitudinal linear radiodensities were present in the distal radius and ulna of most of the patients, both adults and children. These densities, which have been found consistently,[29,47] represent physeal spicules that become buried in the metaphyseal bone with growth. All these patients were studied before therapy, dietary or other, had been given. The carpal bones were selectively enlarged and malformed in eight patients: the capitate and hamate bones in three, the capitate and triquetral bones in one, the capitate bone alone in three, and the triquetral bone alone in two. Like the knees, the wrists tend to be enlarged on clinical examination. In six children development of the lunate bones was retarded.

Among 15 prepubertal patients, skeletal maturation exceeded chronologic age by more than two standard deviations in four patients, was retarded in one, and was normal in 10.

In six of 24 patients the skulls were abnormally small with abnormally thick calvaria, and in four patients, unusually large paranasal sinuses (Fig. 4-6; see Fig. 4-21, *H*) were demonstrated. These six

patients were mentally retarded, as were at least six of the 18 patients whose skull radiographs were judged to be normal.

Clinically the skeletal manifestations are reminiscent of Marfan syndrome. Anterior chest deformity is common and can be either a pectus carinatum or pectus excavatum; however, the asymmetric defect typical of patients with Marfan syndrome is uncommon in patients with homocystinuria. Vertebral column deformity is common, but scoliosis and abnormal kyphosis predominate, as compared to the reduction or reversal of thoracic kyphosis typical of Marfan syndrome. As noted previously, joint mobility is usually restricted in patients with homocystinuria; one reflection of this tendency is that the "thumb sign" often present in patients with Marfan syndrome is seldom present. A high, narrow palate similar to that in persons with Marfan syndrome is present in many patients with homocystinuria. The teeth are often crowded and irregularly aligned. Early eruption of teeth has been noted in a number of cases. Mandibular prognathism occurs as an expression of the generalized overgrowth.

Osteoporosis appears early in life in untreated patients (Fig. 4-7). The spine is most commonly affected, and involvement is more severe in pyridoxine-unresponsive patients. Vertebral collapse may

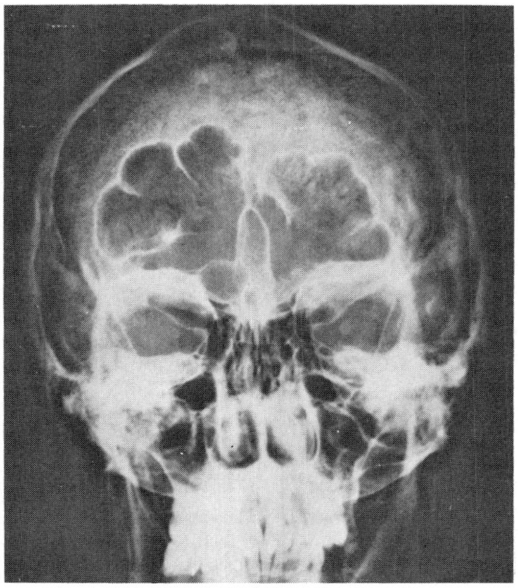

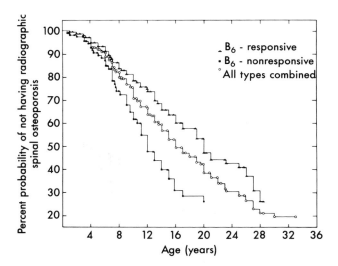

Fig. 4-7. Time-to-event graph of radiologic spinal osteoporosis in patients with untreated homocystinuria. The curves are based on only those patients who were reported either to have or not to have osteoporosis on the basis of a lateral radiograph of the spine. Numbers of patients are as follows: B_6-responsive, 154; B_6-nonresponsive, 137; all types, 364. (From Mudd et al: *Am J Hum Genet* 36:1-31, 1985.)

Fig. 4-6. Skull radiograph of a 26-year-old woman with homocystinuria, showing a small head and large paranasal sinuses.

A

B

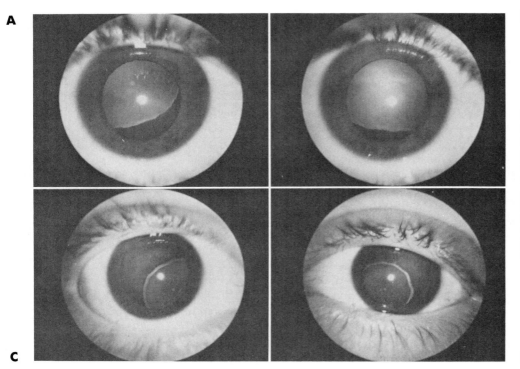

Fig. 4-8. Comparison of the ectopia lentis in the Marfan syndrome and in homocystinuria. **A** and **B,** A 15-year-old boy with typical skeletal features of the Marfan syndrome and no homocystinuria. The lenses are displaced upward. **C** and **D,** A 14-year-old girl with homocystinuria; her lenses are displaced downward.

C

D

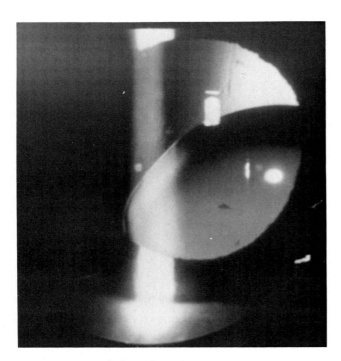

Fig. 4-9. View of the inferiorly displaced lens in a 16-year-old girl with homocystinuria. Ruptured zonules are matted on the lens. (Courtesy Irene H. Maumenee, MD.)

contribute to kyphoscoliosis and back pain. Fractures of long bones probably occur more easily than in the general population.

The Eye

Ocular features include myopia, ectopia lentis, glaucoma with or without pupillary entrapment of the dislocated lens, buphthalmos, staphyloma, retinal detachment, and optic atrophy.

Ectopia lentis is the ocular hallmark of homocystinuria. A notable distinction is that the lens tends to be dislocated upward in patients with Marfan syndrome but downward in those with homocystinuria[23] (Fig. 4-8). The major reason for this difference resides with the zonules. In homocystinuria they break and the lens falls of its own weight (Fig. 4-9), whereas in Marfan syndrome the zonules stretch and, although more susceptible than usual to traumatic rupture, tend to tug the lens away from the inferior limbus of the iris. Henkind and Ashton[43] showed that on histologic examination the zonular fibers in homocystinuric eyes "recoiled to the surface of the ciliary body, where they lay matted and retracted into a feltwork that fused with a greatly thickened ciliary

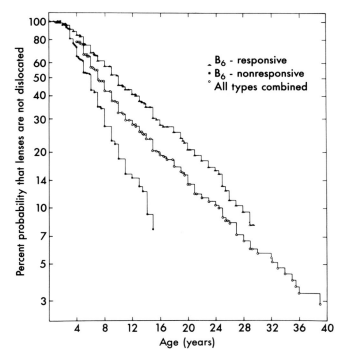

Fig. 4-10. Time-to-event graph of lens dislocation in untreated patients. Patients were removed from the at-risk groups upon commencement of any therapy. Probabilities were calculated according to the Kaplan-Meier method and are plotted on a logarithmic scale. Only first and last time points for a given probability are plotted. Numbers of patients are as follows: B_6-responsive, 231; B_6-nonresponsive, 231; all types, 628. Each curve is discontinued when the number of patients remaining at risk decreases to 10. (From Mudd et al: *Am J Hum Genet*, 36:1-31, 1985.)

epithelium." Electron microscopy showed a disorganized, granular appearance of the fibers.

The lens is rarely dislocated in infants with homocystinuria detected through newborn screening. Fig. 4-10 shows the age of onset of this feature. Dislocation is noted earlier in patients with pyridoxine-unresponsive disease than in pyridoxine-responders. Most untreated patients with homocystinuria have demonstrable ectopia lentis by 10 years of age. Effective treatment does seem to prevent dislocation.

As in the Marfan syndrome, most patients with homocystinuria are myopic. Causes include an excessively long globe and spherophakia resulting from lack of the normal tension on the lens by the zonules. The myopia, which is progressive, antedates ectopia lentis.

Glaucoma, a frequent ocular complication of homocystinuria, is never present without ectopia lentis. Glaucoma often develops acutely from pupillary entrapment of the dislocated lens, but it can develop in the absence of entrapment. The abnormally spheric lens seems to act like the ball of a ball valve in these cases. In younger children buphthalmos, a generalized bulging of the globe, can result. Buphthalmos and staphyloma, a localized bulging of the globe, are probably particularly likely to occur in patients with homocystinuria and occur at lower pressures than in the normal eye because of the presumably weakened state of the sclera.

Detachment of the retina is a complication of lens surgery in patients with homocystinuria,[48] as it is in patients with Marfan syndrome.[65] In distinction to Marfan syndrome, in a significant proportion of cases of homocystinuria retinal detachment also occurs spontaneously. Whereas the long myopic globe may be a causative factor, defective extracellular matrix (ECM) that fixes the retina to the sclera is probably another effect of the metabolic defect.

Optic atrophy may result from both glaucoma and arterial occlusion.[121]

Cardiovascular System

McKusick suspected that in some persons with homocystinuria, thrombosis occurs in essentially every artery and vein of the body (Fig. 4-11). Thrombophlebitis with or without pulmonary embolism, coronary artery occlusion, renal arterial stenosis with hypertension, and intracranial venous and arterial thromboses are the problems of major clinical import. Mudd et al.[77] recorded 253 episodes of vascular occlusion or embolism in 158 patients, whereas 471 patients had no recognized vascular complications. Half of the first vascular events occurred by the time patients were 28 years of age (Fig. 4-12).

Among the Johns Hopkins Hospital patients fatal coronary occlusion occurred in several adolescents, and other such early deaths from myocardial infarction have been reported.[13] The histopathologic changes in elastic and muscular arteries include evidence of partial luminal obstruction, apparently caused by episodic thrombosis followed by fibroelastic organization. The tunica media of these vessels shows thinning of muscular elements and disarray of the elastic laminae that become separated by a ground substance

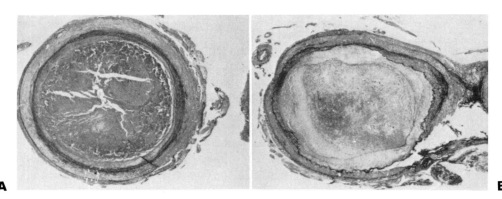

Fig. 4-11. Thrombosis of the carotid arteries in an 18-year-old man with untreated homocystinuria (Case 1, Family 1, described on p. 161). **A,** Right carotid artery. **B,** Left carotid artery.

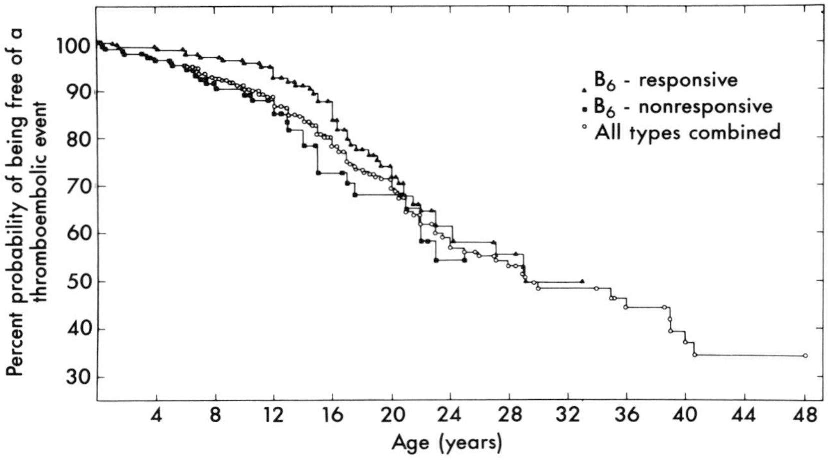

Fig. 4-12. Time-to-event graph of first thromboembolic event in untreated patients. Methods are as described in Fig. 4-10. Numbers of patients are as follows: B_6-responsive, 231; B_6-nonresponsive, 231; all types, 627. Each curve is discontinued when the number of patients remaining at risk decreases to 10. (From Mudd et al: *Am J Hum Genet* 36:1-31, 1985.)

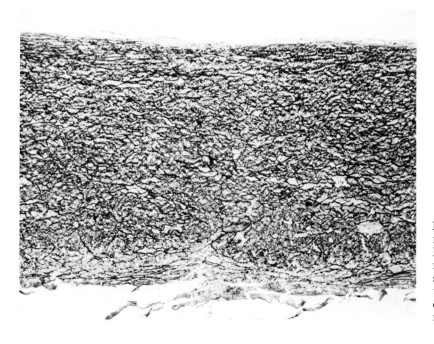

Fig. 4-13. Section of aorta in an 18-year-old man with untreated homocystinuria (Case 1, Family 1, described on p. 161). Disarray and minor fragmentation of elastic fibers and some clear areas, which would stain as proteoglycan, are evident. The impression is one of mild "cystic medial necrosis," itself a misnomer.

whose exact biochemical nature has not been determined (Fig. 4-13).

During autopsy the aorta has shown streaked intimal thickening. Thrombosis of the terminal aorta occurred in a 28-year-old man, and a 6½-year-old girl had exploratory thoracotomy for coarctation of the aorta. The occlusion in the latter patient was described as proximal to the left subclavian artery and not amenable to surgical repair. Although it is possible that two rare abnormalities, one a congenital malformation and the other an inborn error of metabolism, were present in this patient, homocystinuria alone might be responsible for the aortic occlusion.

Dilation and dissection of the aorta have not been found in most persons with homocystinuria. However, as patients live longer as a result of specific therapy and improved medical care in general, it will be of interest to determine whether the aorta is at increased risk for either abnormality.[2] On histologic examination patchy disruption of the elastic laminae of the aortic tunica media has been found.[95] In one case peculiar transverse intimal striations were noted in the descending aorta overlying areas of disruption of medial elastic fibers.

Heart failure has most often been due to cor

pulmonale resulting from thromboembolism of the pulmonary arterial tree and abetted by ischemic heart disease. Atrial fibrillation can occur as a consequence of either ischemic heart disease or pulmonary embolism. Fibroelastic thickening of the endocardium of the left atrium has been found in most cases.

Acute gangrene of the leg, which necessitated amputation, was described in an 18-year-old boy.[72] Plain radiographs showed calcification of the femoral artery in two patients and of the abdominal aorta in one young patient seen by the author. Contrast radiography performed in a 13-year-old girl (before the dangers of the procedure were realized) showed corrugation of the wall of the iliac arteries (Fig. 4-14), thought to be due to striations of the type observed in the aorta. Thrombosis of the inferior vena cava and of the portal and mesenteric veins occurred in patients followed up in the Johns Hopkins Hospital clinic (Fig. 4-15). For example, one 8-year-old boy was without pulses in all four limbs and had occlusion of the inferior vena cava; he was still alive at 20 years of age. Thrombophlebitis, particularly in the legs, is a frequent occurrence, even in the first decade of life, and pulmonary embolism often ensues (Fig. 4-16). "Varicose ulcers" of the leg are a fre-

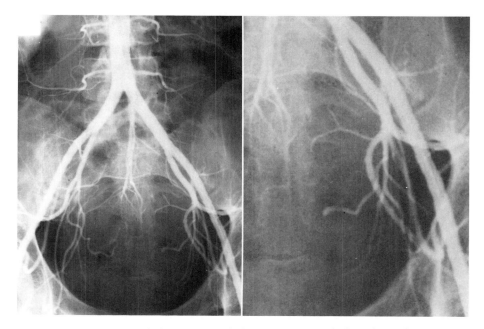

Fig. 4-14. Corrugation of the intima of iliac arteries and their branches in an 11-year-old girl who had multiple venous and peripheral arterial thromboses.

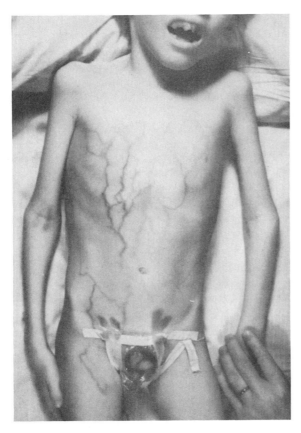

Fig. 4-15. Collateral venous pattern indicative of thrombosis of the inferior vena cava in a 7-year-old boy with untreated pyridoxine-responsive homocystinuria (Case 13, p. 169).

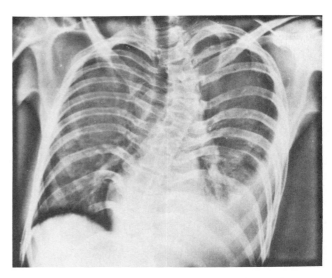

Fig. 4-16. Left pleural reaction caused by pulmonary embolism in an 18-year-old boy with untreated homocystinuria.

quent problem. It is likely that arteriolar thrombosis contributes to the development of these ulcers and to their refractoriness to treatment.

It was repeatedly observed in the early Johns Hopkins Hospital series and noted in several published cases that vascular thrombosis is likely to follow surgical procedures. A variety of factors have contributed to a reduction in this complication: fewer vascular cannulations, decreased immobility postoperatively, use of antiplatelet agents, and dietary and vitamin therapy. In the international survey, 11 instances of thrombosis that occurred after 345 ophthalmologic procedures and 14 instances that occurred after 241 other surgical procedures were recorded.[77]

Gastrointestinal bleeding of uncertain cause has occurred in some patients with homocystinuria. In one case (described in the fourth edition of this text), contrast radiography of the lumen showed small, wedge-shaped ulcerations of the gastric mucosa consistent with focal infarctions. Massive and fatal intestinal infarction caused by mesenteric artery occlusion occurred in one patient in the early Johns Hopkins Hospital series.

The Skin

Cutaneous features include malar flushing, wide pores of the facial skin, cutis marmorata, curious longitudinal creases of the fingers, thin and focally even papyraceous skin, light-colored hair, and changes secondary to vascular thrombosis, such as ulcers of the ankles and varicose veins.

In patients with homocystinuria the skin of the face is often coarse and wide-pored (see Fig. 4-21, *F*). Skin elsewhere, on both the trunk and the limbs, often shows cutis marmorata (livedo reticularis). The skin is generally thin, with the venous pattern showing through clearly, and in some areas it may be papyraceous, resembling that of patients after prolonged therapy with penicillamine. (The structural similarity of penicillamine and homocysteine and the documented effects of penicillamine on connective tissue[39,80] make the analogy more than merely descriptive.) Fine telangiectases are often noted around scars.[84]

The hair is often coarse and almost always of light color in patients with homocystinuria. The latter feature is impressive in comparison with the hair of unaffected sibs, and its darkening as a result of restricted methionine intake and vitamin B₆ therapy confirms that light hair is a genuine manifestation of homocystinuria. Premature graying of the hair, even in teenagers, is also a feature of homocystinuria and also responds to therapy with a low-methionine diet and vitamin B₆ supplementation.

Eczema seems to be unusually frequent in patients with homocystinuria.

Miscellaneous Features

Fatty changes have been observed in the liver at autopsy, as have hepatomegaly and disturbance of liver function during life. Pancreatitis has been reported[21] but is uncommon.

Many patients have been said to have asthma. Although multiple pulmonary emboli are a likely explanation in some instances, the frequency of true bronchial asthma may be increased in patients with homocystinuria. Pneumothorax has been observed in asthmatic homocystinuric patients[20] (fourth edition of this text), and it is probable that occurrence is facilitated by the intrinsic connective tissue changes. Pneumothorax occurs in about 5% of patients with Marfan syndrome, usually as a result of rupture of an apical bleb.[38]

LIFE EXPECTANCY

Death has been reported in patients as young as 1 year of age and throughout childhood and adolescence. Nevertheless, the extremely dismal prognosis suggested by the Johns Hopkins Hospital series two decades ago—a median survival of 20 years—has not been confirmed by more extensive experience. In the international survey, only 20% of pyridoxine-unresponsive patients were dead by age 20 years, whereas only 5% of pyridoxine-responsive patients had succumbed at the same age (Fig. 4-17). The discrepancy with the earlier survey can be explained in part by the effect of treatment and, probably, in part by the bias of ascertainment of more severely affected patients in early stages of the investigation. The cause of death in 42 of 59 patients was clearly a thromboembolic event.[77]

GENETIC ASPECTS
Family and Biochemical Studies

Like most other Garrodian inborn errors of metabolism, homocystinuria is inherited as an autosomal recessive trait. The evidence consists of the following facts: both males and females are affected; brothers and sisters with normal parents

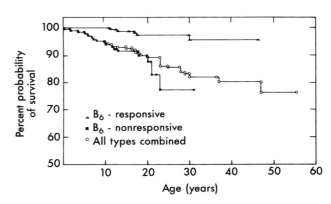

Fig. 4-17. Mortality in homocystinuria: time-to-death curves. Patients were not removed from the at-risk groups upon initiation of therapy. Otherwise, the statistical methods are as described in Fig. 4-10. Numbers of patients are as follows: B₆-responsive, 231; B₆-nonresponsive, 231; all types, 629. (From Mudd et al: *Am J Hum Genet* 36:1-31, 1985.)

are observed; parental consanguinity has an increased frequency; and both parents of affected persons, although normal on clinical examination, show about half the normal level of hepatic CBS activity.

Early studies of obligate heterozygotes relied on CBS assay of tissue from a liver biopsy specimen. The enzyme activity of fibroblasts grown from heterozygotes initially showed too much overlap with that of fibroblasts from normal homozygotes to be depended on. However, in phytohemagglutinin-stimulated blood lymphocytes, heterozygotes can be identified by an intermediate level of enzyme activity, and this technique facilitated early biochemical and family investigations. Subsequently assay methods have been refined, so virtually any cell or tissue that normally expresses CBS activity can be used for heterozygote detection.[72] In the future, however, in families with an affected patient it is likely that heterozygotes will be detected by direct assay of CBS mutations. This approach is impractical if the mutation is not known, and since genetic heterogeneity is extensive, screening either the general population or specific groups (such as people with vascular disease) for heterozygosity will continue to be performed by other methods (discussed later in this chapter).

Population Aspects

The ethnic distribution of homocystinuria is wide. Because the condition was first described in Northern Ireland and a number of Irish kindreds were among the first to be evaluated at the Johns Hopkins Hospital, McKusick suggested that the frequency of the homocystinuria gene might be somewhat higher in Americans of Irish extraction than in other Americans. However, the frequency was not likely to be more than a few times higher: certainly there was no concentration of the gene in the Irish comparable to that of the Tay-Sachs gene in Ashkenazim.

The preceding evidence, particularly the finding of CBS activity in parents intermediate to that in their affected children and in the normal range, is adequate evidence for recessive inheritance. Nevertheless, McKusick performed segregation analysis as a check on randomness or completeness of ascertainment, or distortion of segregation.

As can be seen in Table 4-2, the number of affected persons, on the assumption of either complete ascertainment or random ascertainment of affected sibships, exceeded that expected by more than three standard deviations. Although inaccurate diagnosis in presumed affected sibs of living patients was possible, it was considered more likely that the probability of ascertainment in this study was related to the number of sibs affected. When the correction appropriate for random ascertainment of affected individuals was used—subtracting one affected for each sibship (N) from both the affected group (R) and the total group of sibs (I)—the proportion of affected sibs closely approached the expected 25%.

Incomplete single ascertainment, that is, random ascertainment of affected individuals, means that whereas the chance of ascertaining any particular affected person is low, a given sibship has a probability of entering the series, which is directly proportional to the number of sibs affected. For example, a three-sib family with all three sibs affected has a probability of being included in the sample three times greater than that of a three-sib family with only one sib affected. In retrospect, it is plausible that this situation would have obtained in this series because such a large proportion of the families were ascertained through eye clinics.

Nine of the 83 affected persons in McKusick's original series (seven males and two females) in eight kindreds had a total of 17 children. None of the 17 children had homocystinuria, as predicted by the recessive hypothesis; however, they represent a series of obligatory heterozygotes for study

Table 4-2. Segregation analysis of sibships with homocystinuria

Sibship size	Number of sibships	Number of sibs affected	Number of sibs affected Expected	Variance
1	5	5	5.0	0
2	13	18	14.9	1.6
3	7	12	9.1	1.8
4	10	22	14.6	4.2
5	1	3	1.6	0.5
6	3	7	4.9	2.3
7	4	10	8.1	3.9
8	2	4	4.4	2.3
9	0	0	0	
10	1	1	2.6	1.6
11	0	0	0	
12	1	1	3.6	2.4
Totals	47	83	68.9	20.7 (SD = 4.6)

Deviation of observed from expected: $\dfrac{83 - 68.9}{4.6} = 3.1$ SD

The method assumes random ascertainment of sibships. Because of the large deviation from expected, this assumption was likely invalid.

SD, Standard deviation.

of possible manifestations. In estimating the fitness of a given genotype, selection of the appropriate comparison group is usually a problem. It is clear, however, that the average reproductive fitness of the *untreated* homocystinuric homozygote is severely reduced; fitness is probably between 0.01 and 0.1, the normal value being 1.0. The reduced reproductive fitness is apparently due mainly to reduced survivorship (Fig. 4-7).

Effects of Homocystinuria on Pregnancy

Although no systematic survey has been made of the patients seen at the Johns Hopkins genetics clinic, there has been no suspicion of a teratogenic effect of homocystinemia.[59] The international survey collected the data shown in Table 4-3. The high rate of fetal loss among pyridoxine-responsive women is misleading; 20 of the 25 losses occurred among just three women.[77]

Recently homocystinemia was suggested to be a cause of neural tube defects[108] and a potential cause of intrauterine growth retardation.[12] These concerns were raised because of the relatively high frequency of heterozygotes for CBS deficiency

Table 4-3. Outcomes of pregnancies in women with homocystinuria

	B₆-responsive		B₆-nonresponsive	Intermediate response	Response unknown
	Therapy during pregnancy			**Therapy during pregnancy**	
	None	**B₆**	**Folate, aspirin, and dipyridamole**	**None**	**None**
Full-term, normal child	25	18	1	5	11*
Child with abnormality	2†	1‡	. . .	. . .	. . .
Premature birth	. . .	1§	. . .	1‖	. . .
Stillborn	5	2	. . .	. . .	1#
Spontaneous abortion	19	4	. . .	3	. . .
Ectopic pregnancy	1	1	1	. . .	. . .
Total	52	27	2	9	12

Adapted from Mudd SH et al: *Am J Hum Genet* 36:1-31, 1985.
*Includes one patient who was not specified as either treated or not treated.
†One child with coloboma of iris, otherwise normal at age 4; one child with fused sagittal suture and mental retardation.
‡One child with trisomy 21.
§Normal child delivered at 33 weeks gestation.
‖Died of hyaline membrane disease.
#Hydrocephalic child, stillborn as a result of a decompression procedure performed to permit delivery.

and the potential for heterozygotes to have episodic homocystinemia. In response investigators in Dublin studied 34 pregnancies among eight obligate CBS heterozygotes.[12] Four of the pregnancies ended in spontaneous abortion, and three of the live-born infants died perinatally: one premature infant was stillborn; one had spina bifida; and one, born at 31 weeks gestational age, died of prematurity. The mean birth weight of the survivors was not different from average. The investigators then examined fasting plasma-homocysteine levels in women who had delivered low–birth-weight infants at term and found no difference in the mean level from women who delivered babies with birth weights above the 90th percentile for gestational age. Whether there is an increased perinatal risk of homocystinemia for offspring of CBS heterozygotes remains an open question. If the effect were strong, however, it probably would have been noted among the offspring of women with marked CBS deficiency.

DIAGNOSIS

When most of the phenotypic manifestations are present in a patient, the diagnosis can be made with virtual certainty on clinical grounds alone. Table 4-4 shows the clinical feature(s) that brought patients to diagnosis. Obviously, presence of a similarly affected sib and unaffected parents reinforces the bedside impression. Uncertainties arise when the suspected case is the first in a family, when the phenotype is mild, and when the proband is young. Confusion with Marfan syndrome persists, especially in young, tall children with ectopia lentis and intelligence within the broad range of average. When such a child has a dilated aorta, intact zonules, and joint hypermobility, the diagnosis clearly is not homocystinuria. Except for such an unambiguous case, however, biochemical testing to examine for homocystinuria should always be performed.

The specific diagnosis is made by demonstration of the typical pattern of amino acid disturbances in the blood: elevated methionine and homocysteine levels and abnormally low cysteine levels. The cyanide-nitroprusside reaction is a useful screening tool in the clinic, but the reagents are rarely available except in biochemical genetics laboratories, and quantitative amino acid analyses are relatively rapid and inexpensive. The cyanide-nitroprusside test result is positive whenever disulfides are present in the urine, including cystinuria, β-mercaptolactae-cysteinuria, and homocystinuria caused by defects in other than CBS. Thus a positive result requires confirmation by amino acid analysis. A false-negative result can

Table 4-4. Clinical manifestations leading to a diagnosis of homocystinuria

Clinical feature	Sole cause (% of patients)	Contributory cause* (% of patients)	Total impact (% of patients)
Ectopia lentis	20.6	65.0	85.6
Mental retardation	4.0	51.7	55.7
Developmental retardation	1.5	21.0	22.5
Early thromboembolic disorder	1.1	15.0	16.1
Marfanoid characteristics	0.9	36.0	36.9
Bony abnormality	0.2	23.3	23.5
Seizures	0.2	3.0	3.2
Behavioral or psychiatric disorder	0	2.8	2.8
Other†	0.4	10.6	11.0

Adapted from Mudd SH et al: *Am J Hum Genet* 36:1-31, 1985.
NOTE: Based on data for 472 patients not ascertained as a result of screening of newborns or screening of all sibs of a proband.
*Includes all patients with the specified feature, as well as at least one other, reported as leading to investigation for homocystinuria.
†Includes a variety of manifestations, none of which was a cause in as many as 2% of the population.

occur in a pyridoxine-responsive patient who requires little vitamin intake to markedly reduce the metabolic block. In some patients, as little pyridoxine as is contained in a single multiple vitamin tablet will prevent detection.[72]

In the analysis of urine or blood for homocystinuria, particular attention is paid to three amino acids. One of these, cysteine, was the first amino acid to be identified, in 1810; another, methionine, was the last, in 1922.[102]

Samples to be used for plasma amino acid analysis must be handled properly to avoid inaccurate results. The type and amount of anticoagulant can be important.[102] Too much heparin can hemolyze erythrocytes, which produces, among other artifacts, a decrease in cystine. Sodium metabisulfite preservative in some heparin preparations can alter cystine and homocystine measurements.[82] Ethylenediamine tetraacetic acid (EDTA) anticoagulant, although not perfect, causes fewer problems. Many biochemical genetics laboratories, however, prefer that specimens be collected in heparin.

Plasma proteins form associations with certain amino acids and artificially lower the measured concentrations if the sample is not deproteinized promptly and effectively.[102] Venous samples drawn into glass tubes containing anticoagulant should be placed immediately in ice-cold water and transported to the laboratory within 1 hour. If the specimen must be shipped, it should be centrifuged to remove both the cells and the buffy coat. The plasma should then be deproteinized immedi-

ately and shipped on wet ice for analysis within 48 hours. If analysis is to be delayed, the deproteinized plasma should be frozen, preferably at −70° C in a glass tube.

Ion-exchange chromatography of urine or plasma reveals the disulfide homocystine in virtually any patient with untreated CBS deficiency; because more than trace amounts (normal range for children and adults is less than 30 nmol/ml and less than 5 nmol/ml in urine and plasma, respectively[97]) are abnormal, most treated patients also have an abnormal chromatogram, especially if they receive an oral methionine challenge. Usually a variety of other disulfides are also present, including cysteine-homocysteine and S-adenosyl homocysteine; they are rarely quantified, but their presence should be noted by the laboratory. The other biochemical causes of homocystinuria (see the box on p. 153) also result in elevated levels of plasma homocystine but can usually be distinguished from CBS deficiency by the pattern of other amino acids. The combination of elevated methionine level and low cystine level is highly consistent with CBS deficiency.

Assay of CBS activity in hepatocytes is most informative because in a few cases deficiency is more pronounced in the liver than in more accessible tissues.[72,73] However, cultured dermal fibroblasts and T-lymphocytes are more convenient tissues for analysis. Few laboratories maintain the CBS assay for clinical use.

In 1989, 21 states in the United States included

Causes of Homocystinuria and Homocystinemia

Inborn errors of metabolism and transport

Cystathionine β-synthase deficiency (also results in hypermethioninemia)

5- and 10-Methylenetetrahydrofolate reductase deficiency

Impaired conversion of cobalamin to both methylcobalamin and adenosylcobalamin (also results in methylmalonic aciduria) or to methylcobalamin alone (no methylmalonic aciduria)

Impaired absorption of vitamin B_{12}

Dietary deficiencies

Folate deficiency

Vitamin B_{12} deficiency (dietary or absorptive)

Drug treatments

6-Azauridine triacetate administration

Isonicotinic acid hydrazide administration

Artifactual

Bacterial metabolsm of cystathionine in nonsterile urine specimens

testing for hypermethioninemia as part of their routine screening of newborns. The usual assay is a semiquantitative bacterial method with a lower limit of sensitivity of 100 μM, which is three times the normal newborn plasma concentration. As a result, infants with mild CBS deficiency, especially those with a pyridoxine-responsive defect who have high levels of vitamins still present from the mother's circulation, and, to a lesser extent, those with a pyridoxine-unresponsive defect who have received little oral protein, may escape detection.[72] As further reductions are made in the protein content of infant formulas and as newborn screening occurs closer to birth, an increasing proportion of affected patients will be missed during screening, and therapy will be delayed. When last surveyed, pyridoxine-unresponsive patients outnumbered responders 6 to 1 in newborn screening, whereas in an older population the two classes were nearly equal.[72, 73]

INCIDENCE AND PREVALENCE

McKusick originally suspected that homocystinuria might have a frequency of about 1 in 30,000 births and that it might compete with ga-

lactosemia for second position in frequency, next to phenylketonuria, among specifically identified inborn errors of metabolism that lead to mental retardation. However, reports from the first newborn screening programs yielded a much lower incidence of about 1 in 200,000 births.[72] The most recent data from the United States confirmed this result, with nine patients detected among 1,350,443 screened.* The test that is used measures the methionine level by use of a Guthrie type of bacterial assay.

Although incidence data are best derived from newborn screening programs, the true incidence is underestimated. Possible causes of homocystinuria being missed in the newborn screening programs are numerous. Mudd, Levy, and Skovby[72] found one infant who had normal methionine levels at 4 days of age and elevated methionine levels at 4 weeks; two others had elevated methionine levels on both occasions. The first infant responded to both pyridoxine supplementation and a low-methionine diet. The other two were nonresponders to pyridoxine. Low protein (hence, methionine) intake, deficient levels of vitamin B_{12} or folic acid, low betaine or choline intake, high vitamin B_6 intake, or some combination of these, might result in falsely abnormal tests for homocystinuria in the newborn period.

If patients with homocystinuria have a reproductive fitness of 0, that is, if none reproduce, and heterozygotes have a fitness of 1 (the population average), the mutation rate (μ) is equal to the frequency of homozygotes. One in 200,000 would be a lower mutation rate than has been calculated for most other traits in humans. When it is estimated that the fitness of patients with homocystinuria is 10% of that of the general population, the estimate of the mutation rate becomes even lower. These considerations suggest that 1 in 200,000 is too low an estimate of the frequency of homocystinuria.

An educated guess about the frequency of homocystinuria is provided by the following mutation rate formula, assuming fitness of 0.1 and average mutation rate of 2×10^{-5}:

$$\mu = q^2 (1 - f)$$
$$q^2 = (2 \times 10^{-5})/0.9 \approx 1/45,000$$

This estimate for the mutation rate takes no account of more recent experience, which has identi-

---

*Data compiled for 1989 by the Council of Regional Genetics Networks.

fied numerous factors that determine the rate at a specific locus.

Special factors, such as founder effect and random genetic drift, based on small population size at some stage in its history, could account for an increase in the frequency in particular groups. There is no evidence for or against a heterozygote advantage, and in view of the seemingly low frequency of homocystinuria, a general advantage of heterozygotes is unlikely. Indeed, as discussed later, substantial evidence suggests the existence of a heterozygote disadvantage.

Accurate prevalence data are lacking. Spaeth and Barber[105] found that homocystinuria had a frequency of about 0.02% (1 in 5000) among institutionalized mentally retarded persons in the United States. In an apparently comparable population of institutionalized persons with mental retardation in Northern Ireland, Carson et al.[16] found a frequency of 0.3% (15 in 5000). Between 3% and 5% of persons with nontraumatic ectopia lentis had positive test results when their urine was screened by use of the cyanide-nitroprusside method.[95] The best estimate of prevalence in the general population is obtained by correcting incidence by use of the life-table analysis shown in Fig. 4-17.

BASIC DEFECT
Cystathionine β-Synthase

As previously noted, the usual pattern of amino acids in the plasma of a patient with this disorder consists of the following: presence of homocystine, elevation of the level of methionine, and reduction of the level of cystine. Examination of the metabolic cycle for sulfurated amino acids (Fig. 4-18) suggested the nature of the basic defect to Mudd.[73] Mudd and his colleagues obtained liver tissue from a patient and documented deficiency of the enzyme that catalyzes condensation of homocysteine and serine to form cystathionine, cystathionine β-synthase. Normally this enzyme is not present in some tissues, including erythrocytes and platelets. Cultured dermal fibroblasts, stimulated T-lymphocytes, cultured lymphoblasts, amniocytes, and chorionic villi all express CBS.[7]

The holoenzyme consists of two identical subunits (each 63 kd) and one pyridoxal 5′-phosphate cofactor.[37] The primary structure can be derived from the cDNA. No studies of higher-order structure have been reported.

The CBS locus maps to 21q22.3, which is in the region most strongly associated with the Down syndrome phenotype. Activity of CBS is often ele-

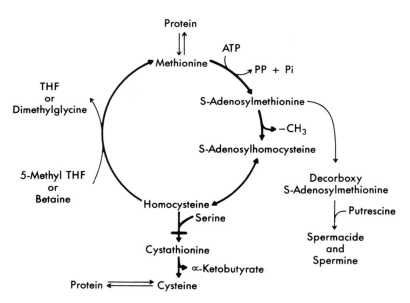

Fig. 4-18. Metabolic pathways of transsulfuration, abbreviated forms. The conversion of homocysteine to methionine is catalyzed by either of two enzymes, whose cofactors are indicated. The metabolic block due to CBS deficiency is indicated by the horizontal bar. ATP, Adenosine triphosphate; PP, pyrophosphate; PI, inorganic phosphate; THF, tetrahydrofolate. (Adapted from Valle D et al: *Johns Hopkins Med J* 146:110-117, 1980.)

vated in patients with trisomy 21, presumably because of gene dosage, but causes no known clinical problems.

Patients with Homocystinuria

The extensive biochemical studies of mutant CBS both *in vivo* and *in vitro* are detailed in the reviews of Mudd, Levy, and Skovby.[72,73] By way of summary the following points deserve particular emphasis.

First, the residual activity present in tissues and cells obtained from patients with homocystinuria varies widely, from undetectable to about 10%. Residual activities of affected sibs show much less variation than do activities among different families.

Second, mutant enzymes differ considerably in biochemical characteristics, including affinity for substrates and the pyridoxal 5′-phosphate cofactor, enhancement in activity in response to supraphysiologic cofactor (from none to normalization), and sensitivity to heat.

Third, most patients have detectable cross-reacting material (CRM) in that antibodies directed against normal CBS detect protein even in the absence of CBS activity; some patients are CRM-negative, which correlates with the absence of messenger RNA (mRNA) for CBS.

Fourth, most patients synthesize CBS subunits that are indistinguishable from normal on gel electrophoresis; a few patients synthesize subunits of aberrant size or no subunits at all.

Fifth, *in vivo* and *in vitro* responsiveness to supraphysiologic concentrations of pyridoxine breed true within a sibship.[77] Most but not all patients who respond on clinical examination to pyridoxine supplementation have some residual CBS activity, but the levels of stimulated activity differ widely. Most but not all patients who do *not* respond on clinical examination to pyridoxine supplementation have undetectable residual CBS activity. *In vitro* responsiveness to pyridoxine does not necessarily predict clinical benefit.

By 1991 the first reports of molecular defects in CBS were emerging. Shih and colleagues found that one of the mutant alleles in two unrelated patients contained a G→A transition resulting in substitution of serine for glycine at residue 307.[37] When this allele was expressed in *Escheria coli*, a peptide of normal mobility on western blot analysis was synthesized but the peptide lacked CBS activity. Kozich and Kraus[57] have used the bacterial

expression system to screen for mutations; loss of CBS activity when a portion of the nucleotide sequence obtained from a patient is inserted suggests that a mutation is present in that region. These authors have identified several point mutations using this approach.

Heterozygotes

As expected in cases of autosomal recessive inheritance, obligate heterozygotes have reduced levels of CBS activity in all tissues. Interestingly, activity levels are generally less than 50% of control values.[72] This phenomenon might be explainable when the dimeric molecular structure of the holoenzyme is recalled. If 50% of the subunits being produced are mutant and dysfunctional, only 25% of dimers will consist of two nonmutant subunits. This effect, well documented in other disorders, including osteogenesis imperfecta and Ehlers-Danlos syndrome type IV (see Chapters 6 and 8), has been termed "protein suicide" and a "dominant-negative effect," but a preferable term might be "poison peptide."[96a]

PATHOGENESIS

The mechanisms by which the pathologic consequences of CBS deficiency develop remain largely unclear. The increasing likelihood that heterozygotes for CBS deficiency manifest susceptibility to vascular disease is a major stimulus to the investigation of the pathogenesis of the relatively much less common recessive syndrome of homocystinuria.

As with most inborn errors of metabolism, two main alternatives exist as to the origin of pathologic changes. On one hand, deficiency of substances distal to the block may result in pathologic manifestations; on the other hand, substances accumulating proximal to the block may have toxic effects. The two possibilities, of course, are not mutually exclusive.

Metabolic Consequences of CBS Deficiency

Under conditions of fast, patients with homocystinuria caused by CBS deficiency have elevated plasma levels of methionine and homocyst(e)ine. Because methionine is efficiently resorbed by the kidney, it is not excreted and its levels in cerebrospinal fluid mirror those in plasma.

Homocysteine *in vivo* exists in numerous forms, including the reduced amino acid, which is rarely present in samples removed from the body; oxidation to disulfides occurs rapidly after death and in deproteinized plasma samples. When the *in vivo* concentration of homocysteine is normal, the predominant form found in plasma specimens is cysteine-homocysteine disulfide.[115] As the homocysteine concentration increases, other disulfides emerge, including homocystine. At any *in vivo* concentration homocysteine is predominantly bound to plasma proteins, with only 20% to 25% free.[3,87,120] Intracellular glutathione maintains a predominance of homocysteine (i.e., the metabolically active moiety) over homocystine and other disulfides.

When transulfuration homeostasis is intact, the levels of various reduced sulfhydral groups and occupancy of protein binding sites are relatively constant. In any of the enzymatic deficiencies that interrupt these pathways and produce elevation of homocysteine level, the patient has considerable deviation from normal metabolic balance in the fasting state and marked variation in levels of different disulfides and active sulfhydral groups in response to stresses such as a protein load or vitamin deficiency. Thus, because of genetic heterogeneity among CBS deficient patients, it is not realistic to speak of a "typical" metabolic profile.

Because homocyst(e)ine is so effectively excreted by the kidney, patients with even complete CBS deficiency do not accumulate sulfate. The relative amounts of methionine and homocyst(e)ine vary among patients, at least in part because of activity of alternative pathways of homocysteine metabolism, especially remethylation to methionine. The existence of these pathways suggests one form of treatment of CBS deficiency, that of stimulating homocysteine methylation by supplementation with betaine.[104,114,119]

Cystathionine concentration is markedly reduced in homocystinuria, and levels of cyst(e)ine are reduced to variable degrees. In the patient with CBS deficiency, cleavage of cystathionine is not the only source of cysteine; dietary protein intake can maintain metabolic needs, provided that the methionine content is controlled (see the case described in Family 11, p. 174).

Potential Deficiencies of Precursors

Cystathionine is normally found in brain tissue in relatively abundant amounts and is absent from or markedly reduced in the brain of the patient with homocystinuria. In fact, cystathionine concentration is normally higher in the brain than in other tissues and higher in the brain of man than in those of other species. Cystathionine synthetase is normally present in the brain but was absent in one case of homocystinuria.[71a] Whether the deficiency of cystathionine is itself responsible for the mental retardation and psychic changes in patients with homocystinuria is unknown.

Preliminary studies of patients with homocystinuria using methionine labeled with ^{35}S, suggested that little if any radioactivity appears in cystine.[11] Absence of cystathionine synthetase might make the affected person dependent on absorbable dietary cystine for protein synthesis. However, the disulfide cystine is relatively insoluble and therefore not well absorbed. During periods of rapid growth dietary cystine might be insufficient for anabolic requirements. It has been suggested that affected infants receiving cow's milk in the first weeks of life may be less adequately nourished than those breast fed, since cow's milk is a much poorer source of cystine.[16]

Are the changes in connective tissue elements of the eyes, skeleton, and arteries due to a relative deficiency of cysteine and cystine? Since the fibrillar collagens have relatively few sulfur-containing amino acids, a deficiency in an amino acid–building block for collagen is not likely to be responsible for the connective tissue changes. On the other hand, because glutathione contains cysteine, is it possible that glutathione-dependent reactions are retarded and that a resultant excess of free radicals has deleterious effects on the ECM? This point is explored later in this chapter.

In the fourth edition of this book McKusick speculated that the cause of ectopia lentis might reside with the lens itself, potentially as a consequence of cystine deficiency. Normally, rapid increases in β-crystallin of the lens, which has a high cystine content, occurs in early embryonic growth. Furthermore, the lens becomes isolated early in embryonic life and depends on its own enzymes for synthesis of necessary protein constituents. However, clinical and pathologic examination of eyes in patients with homocystinuria strongly suggests that the ectopia lentis results from rupture of the zonules.

An intriguing possible consequence of cysteine deficiency involves the protein fibrillin (see p. 158).

Potential Toxic Effects of Homocysteine and Its Disulfides

At levels found in patients with homocystinuria caused by CBS deficiency, methionine is not known to have toxic effects in humans. However, evidence for a direct role of homocysteine in the pathogenesis of many clinical manifestations is substantial, if largely circumstantial. For example, patients with homocystinuria resulting from causes other than CBS deficiency (see the box on p. 153) may have, in the absence of hypermethioninemia, pathologic vascular and connective tissue disease similar to that of CBS deficiency.[5,66] The mechanisms through which homocysteine acts may be quite varied.

Homocysteine bears structural and chemical resemblance to penicillamine, a drug used to chelate copper in Wilson disease and to treat rheumatoid arthritis. Penicillamine interferes with cross-linking of collagen[39,80] and, when taken by a pregnant woman, can produce congenital cutis laxa in her fetus (see Chapter 7). Could homocysteine disrupt cross-linking of fibrillar collagen in an analogous way? Harris and Sjoerdsma[42] demonstrated a decrease in cross-linking of collagen in skin obtained from patients with homocystinuria. Specifically, these authors found an excess of alpha, or monomer, collagen relative to the amount of beta, or dimer, collagen. This line of investigation does not seem to have been pursued. Osteoporosis could also be due to a secondary defect in types I and III collagen.

Over the years it has been suggested that homocysteine interferes with platelet function, endothelial cell function, soluble components of hemostasis, and free-radical metabolism.

Vascular and Hemostatic Pathology

The notion that platelet function is abnormal in patients with homocystinuria first arose in 1964[69] and has had numerous proponents and detractors over the years. Some found increased platelet adhesiveness[19,69] and aggregation,[19] whereas McKusick and his colleagues demonstrated in their early series of patients no abnormality of platelet adhesiveness. Contrasting results arose in part from different assay methods.[72] A direct effect of homocysteine on platelet prostaglandin metabolism was demonstrated *in vitro*.[35] In particular, synthesis of thromboxane A_2, which promotes aggregation, increased.

Chronic infusion of homocysteine into baboons damaged arterial endothelial surfaces.[40,41] This work suggested a direct toxic effect of homocysteine and also led to the hypothesis that platelets aggregated at the site of endothelial desquamation and caused predisposition to thromboses. Studies

of cultured endothelial cells have subsequently shown that homocysteine produced cell lysis;[113] however, the reaction required copper, and lysis was mediated through production of hydrogen peroxide.[107] Thus homocysteine in the absence of copper was not toxic to endothelial cells *in vitro*. It remains unclear what mechanisms are operating *in vivo* in the baboons and other animals in whom arterial damage develops when they are exposed to experimental homocysteinemia.

Endothelial damage could provide a nidus for platelet aggregation on the exposed ECM. If the damage is extensive, an increase in platelet consumption is likely to occur, reflected in a shortened platelet life span. Decreased platelet survival in patients with homocystinuria was reported by Harker et al.[40] in 1974. When pyridoxine-responsive patients were treated with vitamin B_6 therapy, the mean survival of platelets normalized. However, these results could not be replicated in a patient sample containing two of these patients.[109] Subsequently Hill-Zobel et al.[44] at the Johns Hopkins Hospital undertook studies using the radioisotope [111]Indium in labeling and made a variety of kinetic assumptions to show that, regardless of the kinetic model, platelet survival was not abnormal (Fig. 4-19).

Activated factor V obtained from endothelial cells stimulates, through factor X, generation of thrombin. Homocysteine was shown to increase factor V activity in cultured human endothelial cells.[89] Abnormalities of factors VII and XII and

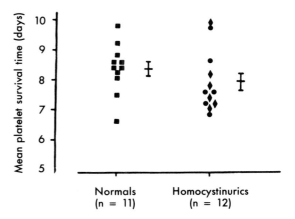

Fig. 4-19. Mean platelet survival time in normal volunteers *(squares)*, in patients with homocystinuria who are taking pyridoxine *(circles)*, and in patients not taking pyridoxine *(diamonds)*. Bars indicate standard error of mean. (Adapted from Hill-Zobel RL et al: *New Engl J Med* 307:781-786, 1982.)

abnormalities of antithrombin III have all been reported in patients with homocystinuria, but the validity and importance of these findings are unclear.[81]

A unified theory of thrombosis, atherogenesis, and venoocclusive events has not emerged, despite considerable experimental work over nearly three decades. It is quite possible that a number of factors contribute and that the importance of individual factors varies among patients or even in the same patient over time. Needless to say, this ignorance has hindered attempts to develop effective prophylactic therapy for the life-threatening complications of CBS deficiency and other causes of homocysteinemia. One avenue that has received insufficient attention in patients with homocystinuria is the role of free radicals.[23] At least three mechanisms exist through which oxygen radicals could be generated excessively in patients with homocystinuria. The first is suggested by the *in vitro* work in which homocysteine and copper produced hydrogen peroxide.[107] The second is the possible oxidation of glutathione by homocysteine; deficient intracellular glutathione in the reduced form is associated with increased free-radical levels. Third, extracellular ceruloplasmin plays an important role in oxidizing Fe_2 to Fe_3; Fe_2 stimulates free-radical generation through interaction with hydrogen peroxide. Could homocysteine in supraphysiologic levels not only bind to but also inhibit the activity of ceruloplasmin?

Microfibrils and Fibrillin

Microfibrils of the ECM are ubiquitous, 10- to 14-nm rods that were first described as a component of elastic fibers.[90] Microfibrils are the suprastructure upon which elastin is deposited; accordingly, nascent elastic fibers contain proportionately more microfibrils than do mature fibers. Microfibrils also occur unassociated with elastin in many tissues. For example, at the epidermal-dermal junction the microfibrils have long been called *oxytalin* by dermatologists. Deeper in the superficial dermis some amorphous elastin is associated with the microfibrils, where they have been termed *elaunin*. Of special note with respect to CBS deficiency and Marfan syndrome are the ocular zonules, whose primary (and perhaps sole) component is microfibrils. In addition, microfibrils are present in the perichondrium and periosteum and, of course, are integral components of the tunica media of elastic arteries.

The principal constituent of microfibrils is fibrillin, a 350-ka glycoprotein first described by Sakai, Keene, and Engvall.[91] The biochemical and immunohistopathologic features of fibrillin and microfibrils[46] are reviewed in Chapter 3. Of particular importance is the primary structure of fibrillin, elucidated both by protein sequencing[63] and by analysis of a partial cDNA.[60,64] Fibrillin is extraordinarily rich in cysteine residues, especially repeated motifs containing six cysteines, which mimic those found in epidermal growth factor, transforming growth factor β-receptor, and several other human proteins.[64,93] All the functions of these epidermal growth factor–like motifs in fibrillin are not known, but the cysteine residues are unquestionably involved in intrachain disulfide bonding.[24,92]

It is the reasoned speculation of this author that important aspects of the pathogenesis of homocystinuria intimately involve fibrillin. Deficiency of cysteine during periods when synthesis of microfibrils is normally high (potentially, early in embryogenesis and, certainly, later in fetal life and in childhood) could produce quantitative and qualitative defects in microfibrils. Elevated levels of homocysteine could interfere with cross-linking of fibrillin when microfibrils are being formed, leading to thin skin, excessive growth of long bones, and taut periarticular structures. It is also possible that fibrillin is a constituent of the ECM across which neurons migrate and that the abnormal cortical microanatomy and connections associated with homocystinuria result from secondary changes in fibrillin. It is clear that deterioration of ocular zonules could occur because of exposure to homocysteine, which could either disrupt existing cross-links or interfere with additions of nascent fibrillin to zonules during growth.

Thrombomodulin contains epidermal growth factor–like repeats.[26] Interference with the function of this endothelial protein, such as circulating homocysteine binding to crucial cysteine residues, would cause diminished inhibition of coagulation.

Susceptibility of Heterozygotes to Vascular Disease

Substantial evidence has been marshalled in favor of the notion that heterozygotes for several inborn errors of transsulfuration are at increased risk of occlusive vascular disease. Because the prevalence of heterozygosity for mutations at the CBS locus alone is in the 0.5% to 1.5% range, the pathogenesis of a considerable proportion of early-onset strokes and myocardial infarctions might be explained on this basis.

The early studies of McCully and Ragsdale[67] and McCully and Wilson[68] stimulated this line of investigation. The first evidence was generated by Wilcken and Wilcken[118] in Australia, when they screened patients with known coronary artery disease for plasma homocysteine-cysteine concentration after a methionine load. Significantly more of the patients had elevated levels of the disulfide than did appropriate controls. The elevations were in the range seen in obligate heterozygotes for CBS deficiency. A few years later Mudd et al.[76] coordinated a retrospective survey of parents (obligate heterozygotes) and grandparents (50% of whom are heterozygotes) of patients with CBS deficiency. The results did not support the hypothesis of an increased susceptibility in heterozygotes because the rate of strokes and heart attacks was not elevated. However, despite the extensiveness of the survey, its power was insufficient to exclude the susceptibility theory. Subsequently Wilcken, Reddy, and Gupta[116] repeated their study of coronary artery disease but excluded obese patients, who were overrepresented in the original investigations and received excessive methionine loads. In this second study no patients had homocysteine-cysteine concentrations consistent with CBS heterozygosity.

Despite this inauspicious start, investigation of the susceptibility hypothesis has continued, especially among Dutch persons. Boers et al.[8-10] used the approach of Wilcken and Wilcken[118] and found increased mixed disulfide plasma levels in significantly more young patients with peripheral and cerebral vascular disease than in controls, whereas the prevalence was not increased in patients with coronary artery disease. Several studies in other countries confirmed these results and also demonstrated homocystinemia in young patients with coronary artery disease.[51,79] These investigations left unanswered several important questions. Were the elevated concentrations of mixed disulfide due to other factors, such as low folate or pyridoxine levels[50] in patients who were not CBS heterozygotes? What was the clinical relevance of a test that administered far more methionine than patients routinely ingest? Were the patients with elevated homocyst(e)ine levels truly CBS heterozygotes?

These issues have not been fully addressed, but investigations continue. Segregation analysis of response to oral methionine challenge was con-

ducted among near relatives of patients with coronary artery disease who had homocystinemia.[30] Half the probands had evidence of familial homocystinemia. Kang et al.[52] have described a mutant allele encoding a variant of methylenetetrahydrofolate reductase that results in homocystinemia. They have shown that this "mild" variant of the severe disease (see Table 4-1) is increased in patients with coronary artery disease.[53] Thus it is likely that the methionine challenge protocol is detecting homocystinemia that results from causes other than CBS deficiency. The way in which this notion of heterozygote susceptibility relates to biochemistry, clinical practice, and public health care should prove an extremely challenging and intriguing issue in the coming decade.

MANAGEMENT OF CBS DEFICIENCY

Therapy for the metabolic defect has taken the following approaches, which can be combined as necessary to keep plasma amino acid concentrations as normal as possible: restriction of dietary methionine, supplementation with pyridoxine and folate, and supplementation with betaine. Ideally therapy should be started in the neonatal period and certainly before irreversible clinical sequelae occur. This is the goal of newborn screening programs. Screening for homocystinuria is not widespread in the United States or elsewhere, and a proportion of patients are missed by current methods.

All patients need routine monitoring of their clinical status and therapy, as well as counseling directed at specific problems.

Dietary Therapy

The rationale of a diet low in methionine is the same as for a low-phenylalanine diet in phenylketonuria: the accumulated metabolites proximal to the site of enzyme block (Fig. 4-18) are toxic and can be reduced by restriction of input to the relevant metabolic pathway. Since cystine becomes an essential amino acid in the patient with homocystinuria, supplementation of the low-methionine diet with cystine seems logical.

Several commercially available diets lacking methionine are available. Nutritional requirements for methionine are titrated with milk or other food. When started in infancy, the diet is well tolerated, although many patients, as they grow into childhood and adolescence, succumb to the temptations of expanding their nutritional intake. The diet is not well tolerated by patients

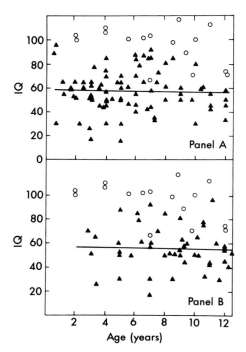

Fig. 4-20. Effect of early treatment on IQ of B_6-responsive patients. Pyridoxine-nonresponsive patients ascertained by newborn screening and treated with methionine restriction from early ages are each represented by an open circle. The same patients are plotted in both panels, *A* and *B*. The ages are those at which the IQs were measured. The comparison populations consist of B_6-nonresponsive patients with homocystinuria not ascertained by newborn screening, represented by a closed triangle. *Panel A,* Age at ascertainment. *Panel B,* Age at last follow-up. The lines show the regression equations calculated for the IQs of the comparison population. (From Mudd et al: *Am J Hum Genet* 36:1-31, 1985.)

who are diagnosed in childhood or later. The patient described in Family 11 at the end of this chapter illustrates the intricacies of dietary management.

The clearest evidence of the effect of dietary therapy emerged from the findings of an international survey published in 1985.[77] Patients who received treatment from infancy (who were usually unresponsive to pyridoxine) had considerably better intelligence, averaging in the normal range, than did untreated patients (Fig. 4-20). Persistent therapy seemed to have reduced the incidence of ectopia lentis and seizures; patients were generally still too young to provide data related to prevention of vascular complications and osteoporo-

sis. Clearly there is a need for a reevaluation of the natural history of these patients and the many additional patients placed on various therapies during the past 10 years.

Pyridoxine and folate supplementation. Any patient meeting the diagnostic criteria for CBS deficiency needs to be examined carefully for responsiveness to pharmacologic doses of pyridoxine. Therapy should be initiated at a high dose (500 mg/day for a child) and should be continued for several weeks before the result is assessed by the screening of urine and the measurement of plasma amino acid levels. If little response is noted, the dose can be increased to 1000 mg/day and the trial repeated. There is little risk of development of peripheral neuropathy or liver dysfunction at this dose in children and adults, but the tolerable limit in infants has not been established. If the patient responds, the dose of pyridoxine can be titrated downward, although it is better to err on the high side to offer protection from dietary and other metabolic stresses.

Adequate serum and erythrocyte folate levels are necessary before the pyridoxine challenge is conducted. Even in pyridoxine-nonresponders, folic acid in pharmacologic doses reduces plasma homocyst(e)ine levels, probably by stimulating remethylation to methionine.[14,71] Moreover, pyridoxine therapy alone reduces serum folate levels even further.[117] Usually 1 mg/day of folate is sufficient, although up to 10 mg/day is administered in some instances.

Documented pyridoxine-nonresponders receive both folate and pyridoxine on the basis of preliminary data showing deficiencies of both vitamins in patients with homocystinuria.

For pyridoxine-responsive patients detected after infancy, some evidence from the international survey suggests that initiating pyridoxine supplementation retards the development of thromboembolic complications and ectopia lentis.[77] Anecdotal reports of improvement in both intellectual performance and seizures also exist.[75]

Betaine and choline supplementation. Trying to reduce homocystinemia by forcing this compound to be remethylated to methionine is not a new concept. Both choline[83] and betaine[55,56] were suggested as dietary supplements for this purpose more than 20 years ago. Betaine has been subjected to several clinical trials.[104,114,119] Whether this agent should be added to routine therapy for pyridoxine-responsiveness in patients has not been formally assessed, but this approach would be reasonable in patients who fall into the "intermediate-response" range.[77]

Medical Management

The many uncertainties about pathogenesis in CBS deficiency should indicate that prophylactic, nonmetabolic therapies have little firm rationale. Many investigators and clinicians feel driven to try to prevent thromboembolic episodes and have focused on agents that interfere with platelet aggregation, such as aspirin and dipyridamole. Since defects in coagulation do not seem to be involved, there seems to be little role for long-term therapy with warfarin analogues or heparin. The latter drug carries the additional potential for increasing the severity of osteoporosis. However patients with homocystinuria who have venous occlusion should be treated in accordance with standard regimens, including anticoagulation therapy.

The patient with homocystinuria has good reason to modulate to the greatest extent possible all known risk factors for atherosclerosis and osteoporosis. Whether estrogen should be prescribed for postmenopausal women with CBS deficiency is unclear; the benefit in terms of reducing the risk of osteoporosis and atherosclerosis might be balanced by the risk of thromboembolism.

All patients and their near relatives should be offered genetic counseling as a routine part of medical management. Prenatal diagnosis is available for parents; couples at risk nearly always come to attention through the birth of an affected child.

ILLUSTRATIVE CASES

To illustrate the clinical features and natural history of homocystinuria, McKusick published an account of 38 cases in 20 families in 1972, and the interested reader is referred to the fourth edition of this book. These were the first 20 families ascertained in his department until 1965, mainly through a urine screening program of patients with presumed Marfan syndrome or nontraumatic ectopia lentis, or both, who were seen at the Johns Hopkins Hospital and at many eye clinics in the United States. Some of the most instructive of these cases are reprinted in this chapter as written by Dr. McKusick, with only slight editorial alter-

ations and, when possible, clinical follow-up. Several additional cases from more recent experience in the clinic are also described.

Family 1

CASE 1*

An 18-year-old male was in good health until 10 days before death. Ectopia lentis was present, and mild mental retardation was evident from his school record. After physical exertion he had the onset of weakness and numbness of the right arm and leg. Examination at that time showed a blood pressure of 180/120 mmHg; no abnormal neurologic signs were detected. One week later he was admitted to the hospital for investigation of hypertension.

Physical examination showed a healthy-appearing, normally developed, and well-nourished young man. The blood pressure was 180/110 mmHg in both arms. Bilateral subluxation of the lenses was detected. A grade II systolic murmur was heard at the left sternal border and was not transmitted into the neck. Wide variability in intensity and some variability in quality of this murmur were noted. Pulsation was thought to be diminished in the left common carotid artery and both femoral arteries, and a loud bruit was audible over the bifurcation of the abdominal aorta and both femoral triangles. No pulses were palpable in the feet. The only abnormal neurologic finding was weakness of the right trapezius muscle.

On the day after admission to the hospital, the patient had the sudden onset of weakness of the right arm and hand. This progressed to involve the right side of the face, and the Babinski sign was positive on the right. Retrograde aortography demonstrated no abnormality of the major branches of the aortic arch. The right hemiparesis increased, and the patient became unresponsive to all except painful stimuli. Ophthalmodynamometry showed marked depression of arterial pressure in the left eye. A left common carotid arteriogram revealed obstruction of the internal carotid artery immediately above the bifurcation. Cyanotic discoloration and lack of pulsations in the right upper extremity were evident.

Surgical exploration of the left common carotid artery was performed on the fourth hospital day. A thrombus was removed from the left internal carotid for a distance of about 3 cm beyond the bifurcation, but adequate backflow was not achieved. The patient died about 24 hours after operation.

Post mortem examination showed that both internal carotid arteries were completely occluded proximal to the circle of Willis. On the left the thrombosis was old and organized, and on the right evidence of both old

*The *Case* designation refers to the number in the fourth edition of this book.

and recent thrombosis was present. Both femoral arteries and the right brachial and the right coronary artery ostia were partly occluded. The aorta showed only scattered atheromata, and no aneurysm was found in any vessel. On histologic examination all large vessels showed peculiar disorganization of the medial elastic fibers but no medial necrosis. There was marked endocardial elastosis of the left atrium. The right kidney weighed 150 g and the left kidney, 230 g. Hypertrophy of the left ventricle suggested long-standing hypertension.

Comment. The hypertension is adequately accounted for by the smallness of the right kidney.

CASE 2

The 20-year-old sister of the patient described in Case 1 was examined after her brother's death. She was a nervous, emotionally unstable girl. She described breathlessness and "jabby" sensations around the left breast at about the time of menstruation and claimed that she felt tired all the time. She had suffered three fractures. Her academic record in school was poor, but she completed high school at 19 years and 9 months of age. Bilateral lens extraction was performed when she was 17 years of age. Her blood pressure was 120/70 mmHg. She was 166 cm tall, with a US/LS of 1.01 (Fig. 4-21). Except for bilateral surgical aphakia and tachycardia, no abnormality was detected on physical examination. During a subsequent examination the patient complained of an ache below the left breast that occurred intermittently during exercise and at rest. The heart rate was 100 beats/min. Third and fourth heart sound gallops were easily heard at the apex. A short, musical early diastolic murmur was audible in the third left interspace close to the sternum.

An electrocardiogram showed changes interpreted as left ventricular hypertrophy and an old posterior myocardial infarction.

Six months after the first examination chest pain suddenly developed in the patient, and she was dead on arrival at the hospital.

On post mortem examination all major coronary arteries showed moderately severe atherosclerosis. Old scarring was present in the anterior part of the interventricular septum and the anterior wall of the left ventricle. Close histologic study of the coronary arteries showed the same type of change as that seen in Case 1.

Comment. If the patient had the same type of change in the left atrial endocardium as did her brother, the mitral opening snap may be no surprise. The origin of the presumed early diastolic murmur in Erb's area is not clear.

CASE 3

The only surviving affected sib of the patients in Cases 1 and 2 was born in 1940. In 1961 she had hematemesis for which investigations uncovered no satis-

factory explanation. She had always stuttered, but this problem became more pronounced after hematemesis. Because of backache, intravenous pyelography was performed in 1956 and 1958, with demonstration of a bifid collecting system on the left. She also complained of ache in the left arm, which was unrelated to exertion. Weakness in the left leg and pain in both legs were likewise noted.

Examination in 1962 showed height of 163 cm with a US/LS of 0.94 (Fig. 4-21). The lenses had been removed. All deep tendon reflexes were hyperactive, especially in the left leg, where ankle clonus was demonstrated, and the Babinski sign was positive.

Because of increasing nervousness and peculiar behavior, psychiatric care was required and improvement was apparent. Pain in the region of the left breast was a frequent complaint. A fracture of the left wrist occurred with adequate trauma and healed satisfactorily. On another occasion fracture of the coccyx resulted from slipping on the ice. Bilateral partial detachment of the retina was detected in 1964.

Her left leg became cyanotic if she crossed her legs for any length of time, and it became stiff if she was nervous or walked a long distance. Occasionally she had numbness without tingling, beginning in the fingers of the left hand and slowly progressing to involve her face. The episodes lasted about 10 minutes. She had difficulty in picking up small objects with the left hand.

Blood pressure, normal during the early part of the period of observation, was about 155/100 mmHg in both arms. Furthermore, pulse rates were weak in the left carotid, radial, femoral, dorsalis pedis, and posterior tibial arteries. A faint early or middiastolic murmur was audible at the apex. The left leg was weak, and she walked with a limp. The toenails were smaller on the left foot than on the right, and the left thumbnail was somewhat smaller than the right one. Hypalgesia of the entire left side was inconsistently present.

Laboratory evaluation revealed normal values for the following: hematologic indices; fasting and postprandial glucose, serum cholesterol, total serum lipid, and serum electrolyte levels; liver function; urinalysis; protein-bound iodine and serum protein levels; and electrocardiogram (ECG). The EEG was abnormal, demonstrating diffuse disorganization without localization or lateralization. There were no seizure potentials. Intermittent photic stimulation did not cause activation. Hyperventilation gave rise only to a minimal increase in slowing, not to abnormal discharges. The EEG pattern was essentially unchanged 2 hours after a methionine load.

Coagulation studies were performed both before and 90 minutes after an oral methionine load. They showed clotting times (in minutes) of 11.13 and 9.12 (glass) and were essentially unchanged in silicone. Prothrombin times were 25 and 23 seconds and bleeding times were 2½ and 4½ minutes, before and after methionine ad-

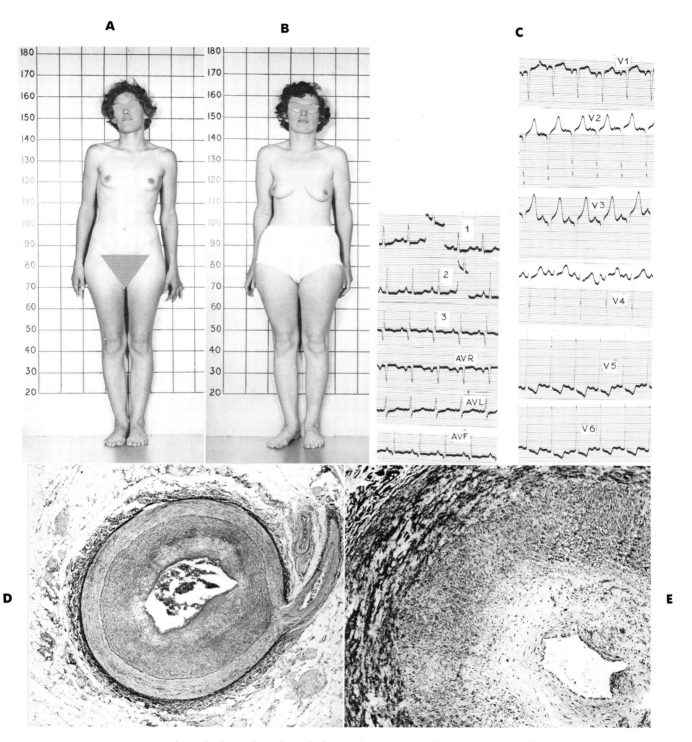

Fig. 4-21. Selected clinical and pathologic data on Family 1, including three affected sibs. **A,** Body habitus of the patient described in Case 2 at 20 years of age. **B,** Body habitus of the patient described in Case 3 at 22 years of age. **C,** Electrocardiogram of the patient described in Case 2 at 20 years of age, indicating an old posterior myocardial infarction. **D** and **E,** Coronary arteries of the patient described in Case 2 are shown. The media is markedly thickened, but a branch is spared. Pools of proteoglycan interspersed in the media are evident. *Continued.*

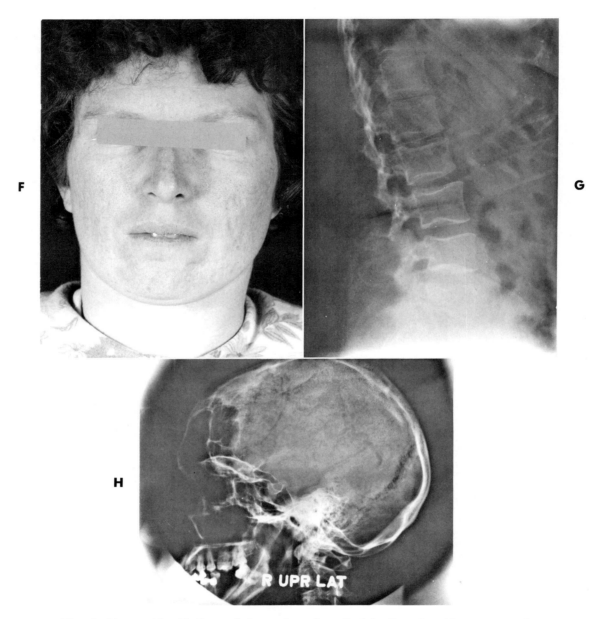

Fig. 4–21, cont'd.. **F,** Face of the patient described in Case 3; wide pores can be seen. **G,** Spine of the patient described in Case 3, showing osteoporosis. **H,** Skull of the patient described in Case 3, showing osteoporosis and large sinuses. Figs. 4-11 and 4-13 show additional features of this family.

ministration, respectively. Platelet counts were 250,000/mm^3 and 183,000/mm^3, and partial thromboplastin times were 75 and 85 seconds. Fibrinogen level was 210 mg/cl and did not change. Euglobulin clot lysis time was normal both before and after methionine administration. None of these values or changes therein were significant. Platelet adhesiveness was considered within normal limits. Clotting, prothrombin, and partial thromboplastin times together with fibrinogen levels and platelet counts were essentially normal. Platelet survival was also normal.[109]

Chest radiographs were normal, except for some scoliosis of the thoracic spine. Skeletal radiographs demonstrated generalized osteoporosis with early "codfish" changes in the lumbar vertebrae. Rarefaction of the skull bones was evident, and the frontal and ethmoidal sinuses were unusually large.

By 32 years of age the patient had been married since 1966 but had remained childless through the use of an intrauterine contraceptive device. Oral contraceptives were avoided because of probable aggravating effects on the thrombotic tendency. The patient responded incompletely to low-methionine diet therapy, which she found difficult to follow, and was a vitamin B$_6$ nonresponder. She was incapacitated by psychiatric disturbances, including many complaints that were thought to be hypochondriacal, and stuttered badly.

Follow-up. In 1974 she was rechallenged with pyridoxine therapy and was found to respond with clearing of homocystine from the urine. Pyridoxine and folate therapies were initiated. At 41 years of age a worsening of left-sided weakness and paresthesiae occurred, but her symptoms resolved within 24 hours, and she was thought to have had a transient ischemic episode. When the patient was 45 years of age, depression was well controlled with desipramine and hypertension was adequately treated with a diuretic and methyldopa. Her principal complaints were of joint stiffness and low back pain. She faithfully took 100 mg pyridoxine daily and 2 mg folic acid twice a week. The joints of her hands and her elbows and knees had diminished extension but no inflammation. Physical examination showed persistence of the mild left hemiparesis. The result of an echocardiogram was normal, and electrocardiography showed only nonspecific ST segment and T wave changes.

Comment. This patient was reported as an example of "schizophrenia" associated with homocystinuria.[106] Her psychiatric disturbance, so prominent in McKusick's description, seems to have improved markedly once she was shown to respond metabolically to pyridoxine. When next given a thorough psychiatric examination, at 40 years of age, she was found to have no evidence of psychopathy; endogenous depression responded to pharmacologic therapy.[1] Her full-scale IQ (Weschler Adult Intelligence Scale) was 77, with verbal and performance scores of 84 and 70, respectively.

Family 2

CASES 4 AND 5

A girl born in 1953 first came to specific medical attention in 1959 because of a heart murmur. Chest radiographs obtained in 1960 showed dilation of the pulmonary artery (Fig. 4-22, *F* and *G*). At that time the diagnosis of Marfan syndrome was suggested because of striking skeletal features (Fig. 4-22, *A* to *E*). Right heart catheterization, performed without complication in 1964, showed normal pressures and no evidence of intracardiac shunt.

The patient had worn spectacles for high-grade myopia since 1960. Repeated eye examinations in 1965 after the diagnosis of homocystinuria was established revealed minimal but definite dislocation of the lenses.

Spinal curvature developed in adolescence. Loose-jointedness was never conspicuous. The fifth fingers of both hands could not be fully extended.

The parents observed her "high coloration" and a tendency to become unusually flushed during exertion in hot weather. The hair and complexion were appreciably lighter than those of both parents and the surviving unaffected sib. Orthodontal correction of malaligned front teeth was necessary. Despite numerous traumata, she sustained no fracture. Menarche occurred at 11 years of age.

The patient's learning ability was definitely retarded. Coordination of brain and body seemed poor. She never learned, for example, to use scissors. She learned by rote reasonably well, and reading and spelling were adequate. In school she had difficulties with social studies and arithmetic.

In 1965 examination of the patient at 11 years and 6 months of age revealed that she was 176 cm in height with a US/LS of 0.72 and a mild upper malar flush. The palate was abnormally high. The hands and feet were cold, but the pulse rates were normal. The hands had a "tight feel," indicating probable reduced joint mobility; both fifth fingers were mildly incurved and could not be fully extended. Pectus excavatum was striking, and considerable scoliosis was present.

The parents were not related, and the ancestry of both originated in the British Isles. The mother had had three pregnancies. (1) A boy born in 1950 died in 1964. He had "cerebral palsy" and never learned to walk, although he could sit. At birth a large omphalocele requiring surgical repair was present. Autopsy results showed "fatty metamorphosis of the liver." It is suspected that he had homocystinuria (Case 5 of this series) and that intracranial thromboses were responsible for the neurologic dysfunction. (2) A girl born in 1952 was normal in every respect. (3) The proband was born in 1953.

At 18 years of age the proband was 185 cm tall. She was shown to be a vitamin B$_6$ responder. She had a decrease in nervousness and other apparent subjective im-

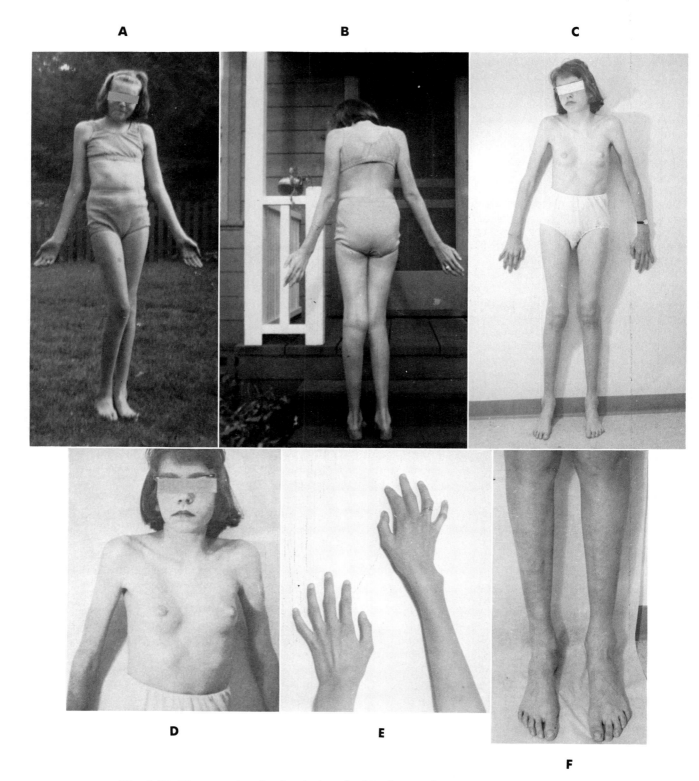

Fig. 4-22. Homocystinuria simulating the Marfan syndrome in Family 2, Case 4. **A** and **B,** Marfanlike skeletal features in the patient at 9 years of age. **C,** The patient at 11½ years of age and height of 173.99 cm (greater than 95th percentile). **D,** Pectus excavatum. **E,** Hands, showing contracture of the fifth fingers. **F,** Long, narrow feet.

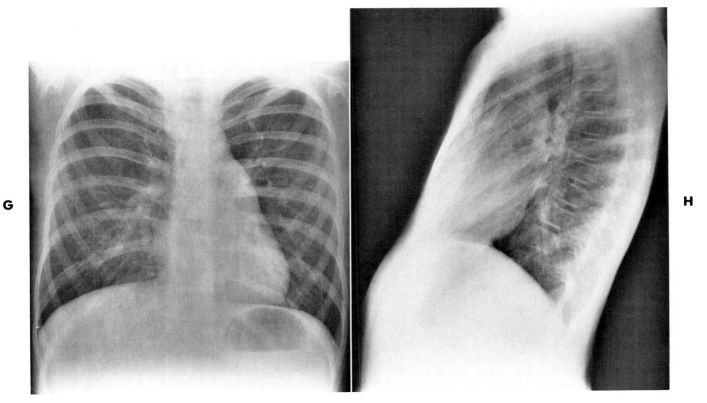

G

H

Fig. 4-22, cont'd. G and **H,** Radiographs of the chest at 7 years of age; dilation of the main pulmonary artery and reduced anteroposterior dimension are evident.

provement after receiving pyridoxine. She completed high school in June 1972, and took special training in nursery school teaching beginning in the fall of 1972.

Follow-up. When last contacted, she was 31 years of age, married, and without medical problems. She claimed to take folic acid and pyridoxine faithfully.

Family 3

CASES 9 AND 10

A boy born in 1942 and his sister, born in 1943, were first examined in 1954, when they sought treatment for ectopia lentis. At that time Marfan syndrome was diagnosed. The skeletal features were more suggestive in the brother than in the sister (Fig. 4-23).

Weakness in the left leg developed in the brother in 1951, and the diagnosis of poliomyelitis was suggested. Function returned to normal in the following few years. In 1957 he sustained a fracture of the right tibia and fibula, which required open reduction with application of a plate. A few weeks later, admission to a hospital was necessitated by the development of acute respiratory symptoms. Radiographic studies showed a "segmental type of pneumonia" with pleural effusion on the right. (Pulmonary embolism seems likely.)

Ectopia lentis was first noted in the brother at 6 years of age; he wore spectacles from that age, but no surgery was performed. Despite school absences resulting from the neurologic problems in 1951 and the fracture and its complications, the patient graduated from a state teacher's college in 1965 and planned to teach at the high school level. He was active in intramural athletics. He was always of nervous inclination. In 1972, at 31 years of age, he worked as a draftsman and was reasonably well.

Examination in 1965 showed a height of 183 cm and a US/LS of 0.84. The feet and hands were long, and he wore a size 12 D shoe. He had high color of the cheeks and coarse, wide-pored facial skin. Pectus excavatum was present. Deep tendon reflexes were hyperactive but symmetric. The IQ was estimated to be between 105 and 110. Platelets were normal in number, morphology, and adhesiveness.

His sister was noted to have ectopia lentis at 3 years

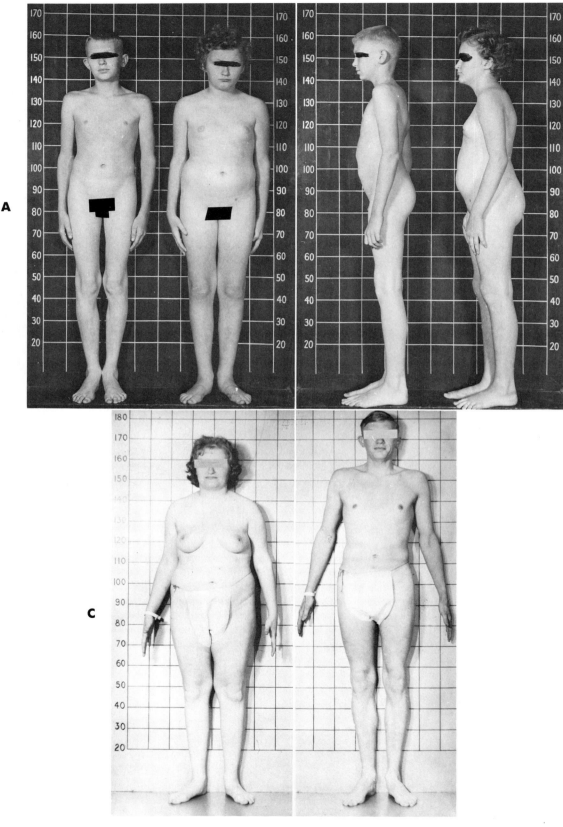

Fig. 4-23. Homocystinuria in a brother and sister, Family 3, Cases 9 and 10. **A** and **B,** The boy at 13½ years of age and the girl at 10¾ years of age; long, everted feet, mild scoliosis, and pectus excavatum are evident. **C,** The sister at 22 years of age and her brother at 25 years of age.

of age. At 11 years of age the right lens was removed. The lenses were described as somewhat globular and dislocated downward and nasally. She did poorly in school and at 21 years of age had not yet succeeded in completing requirements for graduation from high school. Menarche occurred at 11 years of age. At 29 years of age she had hypertension and frequent head-aches and was becoming obese, in part because of inactivity. Therapeutic abortion for an unwanted pregnancy and tubal ligation were tolerated without apparent ill effects in the way of thrombotic episodes.

Examination in 1965 showed a height of 165 cm with a US/LS of 0.88. As indicated by the measurements and by photographs (Fig. 4-23), her body habitus was much less suggestive of Marfan syndrome than was the brother's. The patient's feet "toed out" and were flat and everted. An ejection pulmonary systolic murmur was present when she was recumbent. The IQ was estimated to be about 80.

The parents were not related. The father and mother were 173 and 168 cm tall, respectively. The father was Dutch and the mother, German. A third sib, a girl born in 1947, was normal.

These sibs were vitamin B_6 responders. Biochemical data on the woman were presented by Mudd, Levy, and Skovby.[72]

Follow-up. At 41 years of age the brother had acute glaucoma because of lens entrapment; lens extraction cured the elevated pressure. He also required cholecystectomy for treatment of gallstones. At 47 years of age he completed a doctorate in education and was a college administrator. He was married and had a healthy child.

The sister was also well; her blood pressure was better controlled after weight reduction.

Family 4

CASE 11

A boy born in 1940 had normal birth and development and finished two years of college, being forced to stop because of failing vision. In 1961 and 1963 lenses were extracted without complication. At 17 years of age recurrent thrombophlebitis and varicosities in the left leg developed in the patient. Traumatic fracture of the right femur had been sustained. He had his own insurance business.

The parents, of English-Irish-German extraction, were well and were not known to be related. Of their seven children, three (the patients in Cases 8, 9, and 10) had homocystinuria.

Examination showed normal blood pressure, prominent malar flush with coarse, wide-pored skin of the face, fine blond hair, and moderately high palate. The patient's height was 180 cm and the US/LS was about 1.0. The left leg showed stasis dermatitis and venous varicosities. The left foot was red-blue on dependency,

with thick nails. All pulse rates were adequate, and no arterial bruits were heard. Intelligence was apparently normal, and he had a pleasing personality.

Radiographic studies showed calcification of the left femoral artery (or vein, or both) over an extended segment and generalized osteoporosis.

1972. This patient had been on warfarin therapy for more than 13 years after an episode of phlebitis at age 17. He had discontinued the anticoagulant therapy about 18 months previously and since then had taken vitamin B_6, to which he responded. Varicose veins that were operated on several years previously had recurred. He was successfully employed as an accountant.

CASE 12

A sister of the patient described in Case 11, born in 1942, quit school in grade 11, presumably because of visual difficulties. Upper canine teeth were removed because of crowding. She married and had one child.

Examination in 1965 showed normal blood pressure, a height of 173 cm, a US/LS of about 1, thin blond hair, high color of the cheeks, bilateral dislocation of the lenses with iridodonesis, and highly arched palate. She probably had mild retardation, and radiographic examination revealed generalized osteoporosis.

1972. In 1969, results of examination and testing of her son, then 7 years of age, were normal. In 1970 she completed her second pregnancy, delivering a dead hydrocephalic fetus.

CASE 13

A brother of the preceding two patients was born in 1945. He had ectopic lenses, which were removed in 1952 and 1953. In 1965 he was hospitalized for treatment of thrombophlebitis in the legs. While hospitalized, he had onset of clonic movements in both legs, which spread to involve the arms and trunk and continued for several hours. The focal seizures were thought to be due to sagittal sinus thrombosis. Bruits were heard over both femoral arteries and were louder on the right. In 1966 his height was 189 cm and span, 194 cm.

1972. The patient worked regularly. Because of a chronic ulceration at the ankles, vein stripping was performed. Grand mal seizures, which were well controlled with medication, had their onset at this time.

Family 5

CASE 15

Homocystinuria in a girl born in 1953 was ascertained through a urine screening of patients with ectopia lentis. Birth weight was 3.4 kg and except for vomiting in the neonatal period, no abnormality was noted early in life. She was always irritable, and in hot weather her face became beet red. She was noted to have myopic astigmatism from about 4 years of age. Although she was seen by several competent ophthalmologists, ectopia lentis was not detected until 1964, which suggests that the dislocation had been progressive. Several teeth were removed because of crowding.

Examination in 1965 showed crowded teeth, venous flush of the face when recumbent, dry skin, and thick nails. The lenses were dislocated downward bilaterally. She walked with exaggerated lumbar lordosis attributable to spondylolisthesis. Her height was 137 cm and the US/LS was 0.76. The IQ was estimated to be less than 70 at age 12.

In 1966 grand mal seizures developed and were controlled by a regimen of phenytoin, 50 mg three times daily. She had recurrent bronchial asthma and atopic dermatitis. In 1967 a diet restricted in methionine and supplemented with cystine was instituted and resulted in decreased urinary homocystine. Beginning in 1968, she was maintained on an unrestricted diet supplemented with 250 mg of pyridoxine twice daily. In 1969 she complained of fatigue, weakness, and pallor. She was found to have macrocytic anemia with hemoglobin of 8 to 9 g/dl, a low plasma folate level, and normal plasma vitamin B_{12} activity. Urinary methylmalonate was absent, and a Schilling test showed adequate vitamin B_{12} absorption and excretion (24%). A regimen of oral folic acid, 40 mg per day for 6 days and then 5 mg per day, produced a reticulocyte response and correction of the anemia. Several trials of pyridoxine, folate, and vitamin B_{12} therapy demonstrated that full correction of the homocystinuria by pyridoxine therapy necessitated administration of both folate and vitamin B_{12} in pharmacologic dosages.

Radiographs showed generalized demineralization of the lumbar vertebrae with some flattening of the vertebral bodies. Calcification was evident in the lateral occipital ligaments. Spina bifida occulta and spondylolisthesis were present in the lumbar spine. The EEG was considered abnormal because of an unusual amount of slow activity and bioccipital slowing; sharp wave activity was more evident on the left side.

The parents, both Russian Jews, were not known to be related. Both were in good health. The mother and maternal grandfather had type 1 neurofibromatosis. The mother was 150 cm tall, and the father, 165 cm. A brother of the proband was unusually intelligent at 16 years of age.

Follow-up. She was married, contemplating pregnancy, and physically well at the age of 33 years.

Family 6

CASE 12

A boy was born in 1956, crawled at 7 months of age, walked at 17 months, and talked at 2 years and 6 months. He always seemed backward mentally. The mother noted dislocation of his left lens when he was 5 years of age. Both lenses were extracted in 1961. At 3 or

4 months of age he had left-sided seizures. At 7 years of age, six teeth were extracted to relieve crowding. On several occasions the mother was told he had a heart murmur. He did poorly in school.

Examination in 1965 showed a slender, blond-haired, boy with obvious mental retardation. The skin was pale and unusually transparent but showed no flushing or livedo reticularis. The front teeth were prominent. Other findings included "pigeon breast," systolic ejection pulmonary murmur, and genu valgum.

The parents, of English and Irish extraction, were healthy and were not related. This boy and the boy described in Case 13 were the only children.

Follow-up. At age 12 his verbal IQ was 63, performance IQ, 61, and full-scale IQ (Weschler Intelligence Scale for Children [WISC]), 59. An EEG showed excessive posterior slowing but no specific changes. The plasma homocystine level was markedly reduced when methionine intake was restricted, but he did not tolerate dietary treatment. His biochemical response to pyridoxine was equivocal, and he did not take vitamin supplements for most of adolescence. He had repeated bouts of venous thrombosis in his legs, and it is likely that he had several pulmonary emboli; treatment was chronic warfarin anticoagulation therapy. At age 24 he received pyridoxine therapy, 500 mg twice a day, and marked reduction in plasma homocystine and methionine levels occurred. Platelet survival was normal.[44] Anticoagulation therapy was discontinued when the patient was 26 years of age, after being free of thromboses for several years, and empiric therapy with sulfinpyrazone was begun, to reduce the risk of platelet thrombi. Pulmonary embolism recurred at age 29, and full anticoagulation therapy was reinstituted. His mother reported that he had been noncompliant with his medication regimens, including pyridoxine supplementation. An echocardiogram was normal and his ECG showed right bundle-branch block without ischemia. The patient's condition was stable on clinical examination at the age of 31 years. Detailed ophthalmologic examination showed band keratopathy, marginal corneal dystrophy, a blurred disc margin, and cotton wool spots of one retina (courtesy of Dr. I. H. Maumenee).

CASE 20

The brother of the patient described in Case 12 was born in 1957; pneumonia developed at 11 months of age, and shortly thereafter the patient began to have seizures and left-sided paresis. Seizures were reasonably well controlled with phenobarbital, and by 19 months of age he was walking. Severe seizures developed in the patient at 4 years of age, with a period of coma and right-sided paresis. About the same time, aseptic necrosis of the right femoral head, necessitating traction for 14 months, was discovered. Bilateral lens extractions were performed at 5 years of age. By 6 years of age he was able to play actively with little evident incapacity. At 7 years of age he again had pneumonia, with uneventful recovery. About 4 months later, his right leg became blue and swollen. About 3 weeks after this event the same phenomenon occurred in the left leg. He also had prolapse of the rectum, and the physician told the mother that her son had a "clot in the bowels." The veins of the anterior abdominal wall became prominent. In March 1965, fever leading to coma developed. The right arm became blue and swollen.

Examination in 1965 showed an emaciated boy who responded only to painful stimuli. The only satisfactory pulse was in the left radial artery; others were absent or only weakly palpable. The front teeth were protruding, and malocclusion and high palate were present. The hair was blond and the skin, transparent (Fig. 4-15). Prominent venous collateral on the anterior surface of the trunk filled from below, becoming particularly prominent when he cried. All four extremities were cold. Deep tendon reflexes were unobtainable. Little change occurred during the next 7 years.

Both brothers showed generalized osteoporosis of moderately severe degree, and their skulls had a granular or finely reticular appearance.

Follow-up. His neurologic status failed to improve, and seizure activity was difficult to control. He remained on pyridoxine and folate therapy. Platelet survival was normal.[44] At 33 years of age he remained bedridden, with his mother as full-time caretaker.

Family 7

CASE 27

A man, born in 1920, had a history of visual difficulties from the age of about 20 years, and subluxated lenses were detected at age 25. In 1964 the right lens was found to be dislocated infranasally and the left lens, nasally. The fundi were normal. The left lens was extracted in 1964. At that time blood pressure, ECG, and chest radiographs were normal.

This man received a Bachelor of Science degree in chemistry before World War II and a Bachelor of Science degree in chemical technology after World War II. He worked as a food technologist. During the war he served as a captain in an airborne division in France. In 1942 he fractured a tibia during a parachute jump. Shortly after an automobile accident in 1944 he noticed swelling behind the knees, and possible inferior vena caval thrombosis was subsequently diagnosed. Venous stripping was performed bilaterally in 1954. The patient, who was 188 cm tall and wore a size 12 B shoe, was of Scottish-English-Irish descent. Three male sibs were well. He had five children, all well.

Follow-up. In the late 1960s he was found to respond to vitamin B$_6$ therapy and was subsequently compliant with oral folate and pyridoxine therapy. The left lens was extracted in 1964. In 1971 he had detachment of the right retina, which was promptly treated surgically with good results. He smoked cigarettes for more than 30 years and by age 61 was breathless on mild exertion. At the age of 56 years and thereafter he took one aspirin tablet per day to inhibit platelet function, and he had no further clinical episodes of thrombosis.

On examination at age 61 he was normotensive. He had auscultatory and radiographic signs of emphysema. The legs showed evidence of vein stripping but no active vascular disease. An exercise tolerance test was stopped after 12 minutes because of dyspnea, but no evidence of cardiac ischemia emerged. The aortic root was mildly dilated and was the only echocardiographic abnormality. After the discontinuation of aspirin for several weeks, platelet survival was normal.[44] Urine and plasma amino acid levels were normal. Radiography of the spine showed osteoporosis and anterior wedging of the seventh thoracic vertebra (T7).

Family 8*

This pedigree was ascertained through a 26-year-old man, the oldest of eight sibs, when he developed acute glaucoma as a result of pupillary block. He was then a graduate student in psychology. Ectopia lentis had first been recognized when the patient was 24 years of age, and a diagnosis of Marfan syndrome was made. In childhood he had asthma precipitated by situational factors, beginning at the age of 18 months and continuing until late adolescence. Anterior chest deformity had abrupt onset at the age of 11 or 12 years and was attributed to asthma. He had no recognized fractures or vascular problems.

After extraction of his lenses metabolic studies were performed and homocystinuria, homocystinemia, and hypermethioninemia were demonstrated. All these abnormalities resolved after oral pyridoxine supplementation.

He was well on clinical examination in his late 40s, worked as an academic psychologist, and had several healthy children.

Two sisters were found to have homocystinuria. Both had high-grade myopia but no evidence of lens subluxation on detailed examination. The only peculiarity found was mild generalized osteoporosis and gracile limb bones. Full-scale IQ was measured at 128 in one sib and at 138 in the other. They both received pyridoxine and folate therapy and were found to be well on clinical examination.

Comment. This kindred had perhaps the most benign course in the Johns Hopkins Hospital series;

---

*This family was described initially on p. 245 of the fourth edition of this book.

obviously, persons with milder variants of CBS deficiency must exist but are less likely to come to attention. The "normal" diet these sibs consumed throughout life was evidently rich enough in folic acid and pyridoxine to modulate the phenotype substantially.

Family 9*

A 7-year-old boy was referred to the genetic clinic for evaluation of homocystinuria. He was the 2800-g, full-term infant son of a 24-year-old prima gravida woman who had an uneventful pregnancy. His neonatal course was complicated by recurrent episodes of vomiting and diarrhea, which were thought to be due to milk allergy and which subsided coincident with change to a soy-based formula. Developmental milestones were delayed: he sat unsupported at 12 months of age, walked at age 18 to 20 months, and spoke only a few single words at 24 months. His IQ (Stanford Binet Intelligence Scale) at 3 years of age was 66, and he was enrolled in a special education school, where he made gradual progress. Also when he was 3 years of age, his mother noticed that "the blue of his eye was shaky" and that he held everything close to his eyes. At age 4 he was seen by an ophthalmologist, who prescribed spectacles for the treatment of myopia and by a developmental neurologist, who documented moderate mental retardation. At 5 years of age he was found to have thoracolumbar scoliosis and flat feet, the latter surgically corrected at age 6. He had recurrent episodes of "asthma," which were treated with bronchodilators.

Two days before the patient's referral, pain and scleral erythema developed in the left eye. He was seen at the Wilmer Eye Institute. His right ocular lens was found to be inferonasally dislocated, and the left lens was floating in the anterior chamber, causing acute pupillary-block glaucoma. His urine was strongly positive for the cyanide-nitroprusside reaction.

His parents were unrelated and of German-Finnish and American Indian background. His father's height was 183 cm, and his mother's, 165 cm.

On examination he was a thin, blond, fair-skinned boy with a height of 134 cm (greater than 97th percentile), a weight of 29.8 kg (95th percentile) and a head circumference of 52 cm (50th percentile). His arm span was 143 cm, and the US/LS value was 0.91 (normal for age, 1.0 to 1.1). Iridodonesis was present bilaterally, and the left ocular lens was visible in the anterior chamber. Thoracolumbar scoliosis was present. The limbs were long, and bilateral knock-knees and flat feet were observed. No joint contractures were present. Except for the finding of moderate mental retardation, neurologic examination was normal.

Skeletal radiographs showed moderate diffuse os-

---

*Description of this family is adapted from the *Johns Hopkins Medical Journal*,[112] with permission.

teoporosis. Radiographs of the wrists showed multiple small calcifications in the cartilaginous epiphyseal plates of the radius and ulna. These "buried spicules" were vertically oriented and appeared to extend into the metaphyses. The capitate bones were large and wide; the lunates were small. The moderate thoracolumbar scoliosis was demonstrated. Assay of fasting amino acids showed striking increases in levels of methionine (161 μM; normal, 5 to 49 μM) and homocystine (97 μM; normal, less than 5 μM) and a subnormal cystine level (16 μM; normal, 44 to 96 μM). Additionally several unusual peaks were present on the amino acid chromatogram, one of which corresponded to the mixed disulfide of homocysteine-cysteine. The urine cyanide-nitroprusside test result was strongly positive. Cystathionine β-synthase activity was undetectable in extracts of his cultured skin fibroblasts assayed at both low and high pyridoxine concentrations.

Follow-up. Treatment with oral pyridoxine HCl, 500 mg/day for 4 weeks, supplemented with folic acid 5 mg/day for the last 2 weeks, resulted in no significant change in plasma amino acid levels. He was then placed on a regimen of dipyridamol (100 mg/day) and aspirin (600 mg/day), and extraction of the left ocular lens was successful. Both his physicians and his mother felt that maintenance of a low-methionine diet would be impossible. He subsequently ate *ad libitum* and took 300 mg of aspirin per day. He had scoliosis surgery at age 13 and shortly thereafter had thrombosis of the femoral vein, which was treated with anticoagulation therapy. Therapy with oral betaine was begun; a 3- to 4-fold reduction of the plasma homocystine level resulted, but the level remained greater than 20 μM. Compliance with prescribed medications was always intermittent. At age 16 the boy's IQ was 40 (full scale, WISC-R [Revised]), with a verbal scale of 50 and a performance scale of 45.

He had recurrent episodes of deep venous thrombosis, despite long-term anticoagulation therapy with warfarin. At age 21 he lived at home and was not employed.

When the patient just described was diagnosed, his 5-year-old brother was examined. His mother, a 26-year-old woman, had a full-term pregnancy that was unremarkable. The neonatal period was complicated only by occasional vomiting. Because his older sib was thought to have "milk allergy," the younger brother was placed on a soy formula at 3 weeks of age and continued to take this formula until he was 2 years of age. Developmental milestones were not recalled exactly, but the family considered this child "normal" and clearly more intelligent than his elder brother. He attended regular school but had increasing difficulty with hyperactivity from the age of 5 years.

He was a fair-skinned, healthy-appearing boy whose height was 117.5 cm (80th percentile); weight, 22.0 kg (80th percentile); and head circumference, 50.8 cm (40th percentile). His arm span was 122.5 cm and the

US/LS value was 0.99 (normal, 1.1 to 1.2). Ocular examination results were completely normal. The spine was straight, there were no joint contractures, and the neurologic examination result was normal.

Radiographs of the chest and spine were unremarkable. Radiographs of the wrist showed changes similar to those of his brother. The result of the cyanide-nitroprusside test of his urine was strongly positive, and excessive amounts of methionine and homocystine were demonstrated in his urine by high voltage electrophoresis. Plasma amino acids were all normal, except for elevated levels of methionine (578 μM) and homocystine (82 μM) and a reduced cystine level (14 μM). Trial of oral pyridoxine therapy failed to change his amino acids significantly.

Follow-up. At 7 years of age his full-scale IQ was 82, and he attended a regular first-grade class at school. He required stimulant medication for treatment of hyperactivity and entered a special education program. Betaine therapy was begun when he was 14 years of age, and he continued to ingest an unrestricted diet and 300 mg aspirin daily.

He complained of headache and blurred vision at 17 years of age. Fundoscopic examination showed blurred disc margins and a magnetic resonance imaging scan of the brain showed thrombosis of the sagittal sinus. The symptoms resolved after anticoagulation therapy produced improvement in the venous occlusion. At age 19 he was attempting to complete high school.

Comment. The phenotypic differences between these two brothers, so evident in childhood, have become less striking over time. The older sib had the more severe skeletal, ocular, intellectual, and vascular difficulties, although the sagittal sinus thrombosis in the younger boy was a serious complication. Management in both cases has been similar, although problems with compliance (in part the result of a difficult social situation and their limited intellectual capabilities) have contributed to both acute events and differences in their clinical courses.

Family 10*

An 18-year-old woman was referred to the genetics clinic in 1971 because of dislocated lenses. She was the only child of healthy parents of German ancestry who were unrelated. Pregnancy, delivery, and growth and intellectual development were normal by all reports. She began to wear eyeglasses at 10 years of age because of moderately severe myopia. A cataract was detected at age 14. At age 17 years of age during a physical education class she complained of sudden, severe headache and rapidly became aphasic and then comatose. She was admitted to a local hospital, where a dense right

*Description of this family is adapted from the *Johns Hopkins Medical Journal*,[112] with permission.

hemiparesis and bilateral downwardly dislocated lenses were noted. Her neurologic status improved somewhat, and a cerebral arteriogram was attempted. Injection of contrast medium into the left carotid artery was performed with difficulty; the study was of poor quality, and her neurologic status deteriorated immediately thereafter. The left carotid artery was surgically explored and found to be "hypoplastic." A shunt around the constricted segment could not be completed because the intracranial internal carotid artery was involved and could not be exposed.

She remained hemiparetic and dysphasic but was able to perform chores at home. When she was 18 years of age, a routine ophthalmologic examination again showed ectopia lentis with fragmentation of the zonules. On a urinary metabolic screen, the cyanide-nitroprusside test result was strongly positive and urine amino acid determination showed large amounts of homocystine and methionine. Treatment with oral pyridoxine, 50 mg twice daily, resulted in complete clearing of homocystine and methionine from the urine. Cystathionine β-synthase activity in her cultured skin fibroblasts was 1.4% of the mean normal control activity.

Her condition was followed up annually in the genetics clinic, and supplemental pyridoxine and folic acid therapy was maintained. At age 27 she was 165 cm tall and weighed 76 kg. She had an obvious right hemiparesis and spoke with an expressive dysphasia. The eyes showed striking iridodonesis and downward dislocation of the lenses. The palate was broad. No anterior chest deformity and minimal thoracolumbar scoliosis were present. The only abnormal finding, aside from the neurologic abnormalities, was absence of the left carotid pulse rate. An ECG was normal. Chest radiograph showed mild osteoporosis and scoliosis. Chromatography of the urine showed neither homocystine nor methionine.

Follow-up. A grand mal seizure occurred when she was 31 years of age, and long-term phenytoin therapy was begun. At age 37 she was clinically stable. Her lenses were completely dislocated inferiorly, but she had never had glaucoma. She lived with her parents and was unemployed. The dense right hemiparesis and dysphasia were her major handicaps.

Comment. A disastrous cerebral infarction was this young woman's first and only vascular complication of homocystinuria. Since beginning pyridoxine therapy, she has had no complications other than a seizure and on biochemical examination has remained "normal" under ordinary dietary stress. As in most pyridoxine-responsive patients, residual cystathionine β-synthase activity is detectable in her cultured skin fibroblasts.

The tragedy of delayed detection of this easily treatable inborn error of metabolism is obvious. Stroke in a young person, particularly in one with ectopia lentis, should suggest homocystinuria. Had newborn screening for hypermethioninemia been available at the time of her birth, her condition might have been detected. However, given her mild early course and residual CBS activity, her case may have been one of the "false-negatives" that probably occur relatively often with current methods of screening.

Family 11*

A 24-month-old girl was initially referred for evaluation of an elevated blood methionine concentration detected when she was 3 weeks of age. She was the 3630-g baby of a 30-year-old woman whose full-term pregnancy was complicated by placenta previa. The infant was breast fed and had an uneventful neonatal course. Because she was born in a hospital where no neonatal screening for homocystinuria was available, hypermethioninemia was not detected until she was 3 weeks of age, when at the time of the first visit to her pediatrician another blood sample to be used for neonatal screening was obtained. The Maryland State Laboratory found the blood methionine concentration in this sample to be nearly 800 μM, by use of a Guthrie bacterial-inhibition assay. A repeat sample taken when she was 39 days of age confirmed this abnormality, and the infant was referred to the genetics clinic for further evaluation.

*Description of this family is adapted from the *Johns Hopkins Medical Journal*,[112] with permission.

Her parents were of Irish ancestry and were related; the paternal great-great-great grandmother and the maternal great-great-grandfather were brother and sister.

On examination she was a fair, well-nourished infant with dark brown hair. Her length (55 cm), weight (4350 g) and head circumference (38 cm) were all between the 40th and 60th percentiles. Her span was equal to her height. Her skin was of normal texture, and her head, ears, nose, and throat were normal. Results of ophthalmologic examination, including slit-lamp appraisal, were normal. Her spine was straight, and her limbs had a full range of motion. No other abnormalities were found.

Laboratory studies on her first visit included normal liver function tests and tests of fasting plasma amino acid levels, which showed a 20-fold elevation in the level of plasma methionine (1026 μM), detectable homocystine, and a subnormal cystine level. The mixed disulfide of homocysteine and cysteine was present. The urine cyanide-nitroprusside test result was weakly positive, and large quantities of methionine and homocystine were demonstrable on electrophoresis. A tentative diagnosis of cystathionine β-synthase deficiency was made and later confirmed by direct assay of the enzyme in her cultured skin fibroblasts.

Her biochemical status and growth during the first 4 months of life are shown in Fig. 4-24. Pyridoxine therapy (250 mg orally twice a day) was started when she was 56 days of age and did not result in a significant

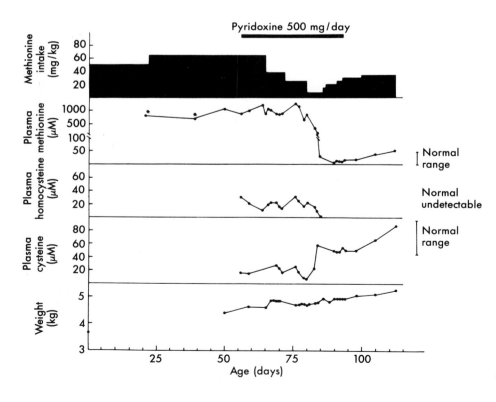

Fig. 4-24. Biochemical and growth data of the pyridoxine-unresponsive girl in Family 11. Methionine intake for the first 65 days of life was estimated from the mother's history and estimated average daily intakes of breast-fed infants. *Asterisk* (*) indicates values calculated from Maryland State Laboratory screening test results. (Adapted from Valle et al: *Johns Hopkins Med J* 146:110-117, 1980.)

change in plasma amino acid levels during the next 10 days. Serum folate concentrations during this time were 4.7 and 9.3 ng/ml (deficient values are less than 3 ng/ml). At age 65 days she was started on a methionine-restricted diet using Mead Johnson product 3200K. The estimated methionine intake on this formula ranged from 25 to 38 mg/kg body weight. Over the next 15 days, however, there was no significant change in plasma amino acid levels. Therefore at age 80 days her diet was changed to a formula prepared by mixing protein-free Mead Johnson product 80056 and Methionaid (Milner Labs). The latter is a nearly methionine-free mixture of L-amino acids and vitamins. This formula supplied an estimated 8 mg/kg/day of methionine, 120 calories/kg/day, and 2 g of Methionaid protein/kg/day. With the patient on this diet there was a rapid decline in plasma methionine to low normal levels, disappearance of detectable plasma homocystine, increase in plasma cystine concentrations, and appropriate daily weight gain. Because plasma methionine values fell to subnormal levels, small amounts of natural protein (provided in the form of cow's whole milk) were added to increase gradually methionine intake as indicated in Fig. 4-24.

After the age of 4 months, she grew normally. Her weight at age 24 months was 12.35 kg (60th percentile), her height 89 cm (75th percentile) and her head circumference 48.5 cm (50th percentile). The result of her ophthalmologic examination, including slit-lamp appraisal, was normal. The result of the remainder of her physical examination, including joint range of motion and neurologic examination, was within normal limits. Formal psychologic testing at age 24 months showed her to be functioning at the 16- to 26-month level.

The major portion of her diet continued to be a formula made by mixing 80056, Methionaid, and cow's whole milk. She also ate measured amounts of fruits and vegetables. Her methionine intake was maintained at approximately 10.5 mg/kg/day, and her protein intake, at 1.7 g/kg/day.

When she was between 6 and 28 months of age, 41 plasma amino acid determinations were performed at 2-week intervals. Her plasma methionine concentrations ranged from 15 to 138 μM with a mean standard deviation $\pm$ 1 of 53 $\pm$ 25 μM. Plasma homocystine was undetectable in 30 of the 41 samples, and in the remainder the level ranged from 1 to 8 μM. Plasma cystine concentration averaged 52 $\pm$ 18 μM. The levels of the remainder of her plasma amino acids were generally in the normal range except for those of serine, threonine, alanine, glycine, and tyrosine, which averaged between 10% and 20% over the normal range. She was normal on clinical examination.

Follow-up. Compliance with the methionine-restricted diet was generally good, primarily because of the careful attention and cooperation of her parents. Betaine therapy, 200 mg daily, was started when she was 10 years of age but was discontinued after 2 years because of its disagreeable taste.

At age 13 she was a superior student in the eighth grade. She had normal ophthalmologic examination results that included neither myopia nor ectopia lentis. There had been no suggestion of seizures or thromboembolic events. Her physical examination showed a height in the range of the 25th to 50th percentiles, a reduced US/LS of 0.83, no anterior chest deformity, mild scoliosis, and a normal neurologic status.

Comment. The reasons for initial difficulties in the dietary management of this patient's condition with 3200K and the ease with which her condition was controlled with Methionaid are not clear but may relate to differences in the cystine and methionine content of these two formulas. Methionaid has a much lower methionine content than 3200K (3.2 mg/g protein versus 11.4 mg/g protein) and a much higher cystine content (58.6 mg/g protein versus 11.4 mg/g protein). In patients with CBS deficiency, particularly those with no residual enzyme activity, cystine becomes an essential amino acid. The dependency of these patients on dietary cystine may be especially prominent in infancy, since even a normal neonate with an intact transulfuration pathway may require some dietary cystine. In retrospect, the failure to establish dietary control with 3200K formula may have been due to cystine deficiency, since weight gain was poor and plasma cystine concentrations were subnormal (see days 65 to 76, Fig. 4-24). After the change to Methionaid formula, in addition to the reduction in methionine intake, there was an increase in cystine intake from 23 to 158 mg/kg/day. After this change there was improved weight gain, a fall in methionine level, and a rise in cystine level. After a normal growth rate was established, the amount of methionine tolerated by the patient increased to levels previously intolerable (e.g., compare methionine intake on days 70 to 75 and days 90 to 100).

During childhood the dietary therapy was effective in maintaining plasma concentrations of methionine, homocysteine, and cystine in only mildly abnormal ranges and in promoting adequate physical growth. She has had none of the clinical problems associated with homocystinuria, which is encouraging. Longer-term observation will be required, however, to determine if good dietary control is effective in preventing complications over a lifetime. Other investigators have had similarly encouraging results in isolated cases of patients who received dietary therapy for as long as 7 years.

REFERENCES

1. Abbott MH et al: Psychiatric manifestations of homocystinuria due to cystathionine beta-synthase deficiency, *Am J Med Genet* 26:959-969, 1987.
2. Almgren B et al: Abdominal aortic aneurysm in homocystinuria, *Acta Chir Scand* 144:545-546, 1978.

3. Araki A, Sako Y: Determination of free and total homocysteine in human plasma by high-performance liquid chromatography with fluorescence detection, *J Chromatogr* 422:43-52, 1987.

4. Barber GW, Spaeth GL: The successful treatment of homocystinuria with pyridoxine, *J Pediatr* 75:463-478, 1969.

5. Baumgartner R et al: Vascular lesions in two patients with congenital homocystinuria due to different defects of remethylation, *J Inherit Metab Dis* 3:101-, 1980.

6. Beighton P et al: International nosology of heritable disorders of connective tissue, Berlin, 1986, *Am J Med Genet* 29:581-594, 1988.

7. Bittles AH, Carson NAJ: Homocystinuria: studies on cystathionine β-synthase, S-adenosylmethionine synthase and cystathionase activities in skin fibroblasts, *J Inherit Metab Dis* 4:3-6, 1981.

8. Boers GHJ et al: Improved identification of heterozygotes for homocystinuria due to cystathionine synthase deficiency by the combination of methionine loading and enzyme determination in cultured fibroblasts, *Hum Genet* 69:164-149, 1985.

9. Boers GHJ et al: Heterozygosity for homocystinuria in premature peripheral and cerebral occlusive arterial disease, *New Engl J Med* 313:709-715, 1985.

10. Boers G et al: Heterozygosity for homocystinuria in premature arterial disease, *New Engl J Med* 314:850-851, 1986.

11. Brenton DP, Cusworth DC, Gaull CE: Homocystinuria: biochemical studies of tissues, *Pediatrics* 35:50-56, 1965.

12. Burke G et al: Intrauterine growth retardation, perinatal death, and maternal homocysteine levels (letter), *New Engl J Med* 326:69-70, 1992.

13. Carey MC et al: Homocystinuria. I. A clinical and pathological study of nine subjects in six families, *Am J Med* 45:7-25, 1968.

14. Carey MC, Fennelly JJ, Fitzgerald O: Homocystinuria. II. Subnormal serum folate levels, increased folate clearance and effects of folic acid therapy, *Am J Med* 45:26-31, 1968.

15. Carson NAJ, Neill DW: Metabolic abnormalities detected in a survey of mentally backward individuals in Northern Ireland, *Arch Dis Child* 37:505-513, 1962.

16. Carson NAJ et al: Homocystinuria: a new inborn error of metabolism associated with mental deficiency, *Arch Dis Child* 39:425-436, 1963.

17. Carter S, Gold AP: Acute infantile hemiplegia, *Pediatr Clin North Am* 14:851-864, 1967.

18. Chou S-M, Waisman HA: Spongy degeneration of the central nervous system: case of homocystinuria, *Arch Pathol* 79:357-363, 1965.

19. Cline JW et al: Adult homocystinuria with ectopia lentis, *Southern Med J* 64:613-617, 1971.

20. Cochran FB et al: Pyridoxine-unresponsive homocystinuria with an unusual clinical course, *Am J Med Genet* 35:519-522, 1990.

21. Collins JE, Brenton DP: Pancreatitis and homocystinuria, *J Inherit Metab Dis* 13:232-233, 1990.

22. Cross CE et al: Oxygen radicals and human disease, *Ann Int Med* 107:526-545, 1987.

23. Cross HE, Jensen AD: Ocular manifestations in the Marfan syndrome and homocystinuria, *Am J Ophthalmol* 75:405-420, 1973.

24. Dietz HC et al: Defects in the fibrillin gene cause the Marfan syndrome: linkage evidence and identification of a missense mutation, *Nature* 352:337-339, 1991.

25. Dunn HG, Perry TL, Dolman CL: Homocystinuria: a recently discovered cause of mental defect and cerebrovascular thrombosis, *Neurology* 16:407-420, 1966.

26. Esmon NL, Owen WG, Esmon CT: Isolation of a membrane-bound cofactor for thrombin-catalyzed activation of protein C, *J Biol Chem* 257:859, 1982.

27. Fleisher LD et al: Cystathionine β-synthase deficiency: differences in thermostability between normal and abnormal enzyme from cultured human cells, *Pediatr Res* 12:293-296, 1978.

28. Fowler B et al: Homocystinuria: evidence for three distinct classes of cystathionine β-synthase mutants in cultured fibroblasts, *J Clin Invest* 61:645-653, 1978.

29. Gaudier B et al: Étude radiologiques des signes osseux de l'homocystinurie (à propos de six observations), *Arch Franc Pediatr* 26:963-975, 1969.

30. Genest JJ Jr et al: Prevalence of familial hyperhomocyst(e)inemia in men with premature coronary artery disease, *Arteriosclerosis Thromb* 11:1129-1136, 1991.

31. Gerritsen T, Vaughn JG, Waisman HA: The identification of homocystine in the urine, *Biochem Biophys Res Commun* 9:493-496, 1962.

32. Gerritsen T, Waisman HA: Homocystinuria: absence of cystathionine in the brain, *Science* 145:588 only, 1964.

33. Gerritsen T, Waisman HA: Homocystinuria, an error in the metabolism of methionine, *Pediatrics* 33:413-420, 1964.

34. Gibson JB, Carson NAJ, Neill DW: Pathologic findings in homocystinuria, *J Clin Pathol* 17:427-437, 1964.

35. Graeber JE et al: Effect of homocysteine and homocystine on platelet and vascular arachidonic acid metabolism, *Pediatr Res* 16:490, 1982.

36. Gröbe H, Belleisen L, Stahl K: Platelet function and morphology in homocystinuria, *Pediatr Res* 13:72 only, 1979.

37. Gu Z et al: Identification of a molecular genetic defect in homocystinuria due to cystathionine β-synthase deficiency (abstr), *Am J Hum Genet* 49:406 only, 1991.

38. Hall J et al: Pneumothorax in the Marfan syndrome: prevalence and therapy, *Ann Thorac Surg* 37:500-504, 1984.

39. Harkness RD: In vitro and in vivo observations on the effect of penicillamine on collagen, *Postgrad Med J* 44(suppl):31-1968.

40. Harker LA et al: Homocystinuria: vascular injury and arterial thrombosis, *New Engl J Med* 291:537-543, 1974.

41. Harker LA et al: Homocystine-induced arteriosclerosis: the role of endothelial cell injury and platelet response in its genesis, *J Clin Invest* 58:731-741, 1976.

42. Harris ED Jr, Sjoerdsma A: Collagen profile in various clinical conditions, *Lancet* 2:707-711, 1966.

43. Henkind P, Ashton N: Ocular pathology in homocystinuria, *Trans Ophthalmol Soc UK* 85:21-38, 1965.

44. Hill-Zobel RL et al: Kinetics and biodistribution of ^{111}In−labeled platelets in homocystinuria, *New Engl J Med* 307:781-786, 1982.

45. Hofman KJ, Bernhardt BA, Pyeritz RE: Marfan syndrome: neuropsychological aspects, *Am J Med Genet* 31:331-338, 1988.

46. Hollister DW et al: Marfan syndrome: immunohistologic abnormalities of the elastin-associated microfibrillar fiber system, *New Engl J Med* 323:152-259, 1990.

47. Holt JF, Allen RJ: Signes radiologiques des amino-aciduries primitives, *Ann Radiol* 10:317-321, 1967.

48. Jensen AD, Cross HE: Surgical treatment of dislocated lenses in the Marfan syndrome and homocystinuria, *Trans Am Acad Ophthalmol Otolaryngol* 76:1491-1499, 1972.

49. Kainulainen K et al: Marfan syndrome: no evidence for heterogeneity in different populations and more precise mapping of the gene, *Am J Hum Genet* 49:662-667, 1991.

50. Kang S-S, Wong PWK, Norusis M: Homocysteinemia due to folate deficiency, *Metabolism* 36:458-462, 1987.

51. Kang S-S et al: Protein-bound homocyst(e)ine: a possible risk factor for coronary artery disease, *J Clin Invest* 77:1482-1486, 1986.

52. Kang S-S et al: Intermediate hyperhomocysteinemia resulting from compound heterozygosity of methylenetetrahydrofolate reductase mutations, *Am J Hum Genet* 48:546-551, 1991.

53. Kang S-S et al: Thermolabile methylenetetrahydrofolate reductase: an inherited risk factor for coronary artery disease, *Am J Hum Genet* 48:536-545, 1991.

54. Kim YJ, Rosenberg LE: On the mechanism of pyridoxine responsive homocystinuria. II. Properties of normal and mutant cystathionine β-synthase, *Proc Nat Acad Sci USA* 71:4821-4825, 1974.

55. Komrower GM, Sardharwalla IB: The dietary treatment of homocystinuria. In Carson NAJ, Raine DN, editors: *Inherited disorders of sulphur metabolism*, London, 1972, Churchill Livingstone, p 254.

56. Komrower GM et al: Dietary treatment of homocystinuria, *Arch Dis Child* 41:666-671, 1966.

57. Kozich V, Kraus JP: Bacterial expression of human cystathionine β-synthase: a rapid method to screen for mutations in patients with homocystinuria and vascular disease (abstr), *Am J Hum Genet* 49:410 only, 1991.

58. Kraus JP et al: Cloning and screening with nanogram amounts of immunopurified mRNAs: cDNA cloning and chromosomal mapping of cystathionine beta synthase and the beta subunit of propionyl-CoA carboxylase, *Proc Nat Acad Sci USA* 83:2047-2051, 1986.

59. Kurczynski TW et al: Maternal homocystinuria: studies of an untreated mother and fetus, *Arch Dis Child* 55:721-723, 1980.

60. Lee B et al: Linkage of Marfan syndrome and a phenotypically related disorder to two different fibrillin genes, *Nature* 352:330-332, 1991.

61. Longhi RC et al: Cystathionine β-synthase deficiency: a qualitative abnormality of the deficient enzyme modified by vitamin B$_6$ therapy, *Pediatr Res* 11:100-103, 1977.

62. MacCarthy JM, Carey MC: Bone changes in homocystinuria, *Clin Radiol* 19:128-134, 1968.

63. Maddox BK et al: Connective tissue microfibrils, *J Biol Chem* 274:21381-21385, 1989.

64. Maslen CL et al: Partial sequence of a candidate gene for the Marfan syndrome, *Nature* 352:334-337, 1991.

65. Maumenee IH: The eye in the Marfan syndrome, *Trans Am Ophthalmol Soc* 79:684-733.

66. McCully KS: Vascular pathology of homocysteinemia: implications for the pathogenesis of arteriosclerosis, *Am J Pathol* 56:111-128, 1969.

67. McCully KS, Ragsdale BD: Production of arteriosclerosis by homocysteinemia, *Am J Pathol* 61:1-8, 1970.

68. McCully KS, Wilson RB: Homocysteine theory of arteriosclerosis, *Atherosclerosis* 22:215-227, 1975.

69. McDonald L et al: Homocystinuria, thrombosis and the blood platelets, *Lancet* 1:745-746, 1964.

70. Moreels CL Jr et al: The roentgenographic features of homocystinuria, *Radiology* 90:1150-1158, 1968.

71. Morrow G III, Barness LA: Combined vitamin responsiveness in homocystinuria, *J Pediatr* 81:945-954, 1972.

71a. Mudd SH: Personal communication, Feb 1992.

72. Mudd SH, Levy HL, Skovby F: Disorders of transulfuration. In Scriver CR et al, editors: *The metabolic basis of inherited disease*, ed 6, New York, 1989, McGraw-Hill, pp 693-734.

73. Mudd SH, Levy HL, Skovby F: Disorders of transulfuration. In Scriver CR et al, editors: *The metabolic basis of inherited disease*, ed 7, New York, 1993, McGraw-Hill. In press.

74. Mudd SH et al: Homocystinuria: an enzymatic defect, *Science* 143:1443-1445, 1964.

75. Mudd SH et al: Homocystinuria due to cystathionine synthase deficiency: the effect of pyridoxine, *J Clin Invest* 49:1762-1773, 1970.

76. Mudd SH et al: A study of cardiovascular risk in heterozygotes for homocystinuria, *Am J Hum Genet* 33:883-893, 1981.

77. Mudd SH et al: The natural history of homocystinuria due to cystathionine beta-synthase deficiency, *Am J Hum Genet* 36:1-31, 1985.

78. Munke M et al: The gene for cystathionine beta-synthase (CBS) maps to the subtelomeric region on human chromosome 21q and to proximal mouse chromosome 17, *Am J Hum Genet* 42:550-559, 1988.

79. Murphy-Chutorian DR et al: Methionine intolerance: a possible risk factor for coronary artery disease, *J Am Coll Cardiol* 6:725-730, 1985.

80. Nimni ME, Bavetta LA: Collagen defect induced by penicillamine, *Science* 150:905-906, 1965.

81. Palareti G et al: Blood coagulation changes in homocystinuria: effects of pyridoxine and other specific therapy, *J Pediatr* 109:1001-1006, 1986.

82. Parvy P et al: A new pitfall in plasma amino acid analysis, *Clin Chem* 35:178 only, 1989.

83. Perry TL et al: Treatment of homocystinuria with a low-methionine diet, supplemental cystine, and a methyl donor, *Lancet* 2:474-478, 1968.

84. Price J, Vickers CF, Brooker FK: A case of homocystinuria with noteworthy dermatological features, *J Ment Defic Res* 12:111-118, 1968.

85. Pyeritz RE: Cardiovascular manifestations of heritable disorders of connective tissue. In Motulsky AG et al, editors: *Progress in medical genetics*, vol 5, Philadelphia, 1983, WB Saunders, pp 191-302.

86. Ratnoff OD: Activation of Hageman factor by L-homocystine, *Science* 162:1007-1009, 1968.

87. Refsum M, Helland S, Ueland PM: Radioenzymic determination of homocysteine in plasma and urine, *Clin Chem* 31:624-628, 1985.

88. Robinson RG: The temporal lobe agenesis syndrome, *Brain* 87:87-106, 1964.

89. Rodgers GM, Kane WH: Activation of endogenous factor V by a homocysteine-induced vascular endothelial cell activator, *J Clin Invest* 77:1909-1916, 1986.

90. Ross R, Bernstein P: The elastic fiber: the separation and partial characterization of its macromolecular components, *J Cell Biol* 40:366-381, 1969.

91. Sakai LY, Keene DR, Engvall E: Fibrillin, a new 350-kD glycoprotein, is a component of extracellular microfibrils, *J Cell Biol* 103:2499-2509, 1986.

92. Sakai LY et al: Purification and partial characterization of fibrillin, a cysteine-rich structural component of connective tissue microfibrils, *J Biol Chem* 266:14763-14770, 1991.

93. Savage CR Jr, Inagami T, Cohen S: The primary structure of epidermal growth factor, *J Biol Chem* 247:7612-7621, 1972.

94. Schimke RN, McKusick VA, Pollack AD: Homocystinuria simulating Marfan's syndrome, *Trans Assoc Am Phys* 78:60-72, 1965.

95. Schimke RN, McKusick VA, Pollack AD: Homocystinuria, a study of 38 cases in 20 families, *JAMA* 193:711-719, 1965.

96. Seashore MR, Durant JL, Rosenberg LE: Studies of the mechanism of pyridoxine-responsive homocystinuria, *Pediatr Res* 6:187-196, 1972.

96a. Seidman CR, Personal communication, March 1992.

97. Shapira E et al: *Biochemical genetics: a laboratory manual*, New York, 1989, Oxford University.

98. Shih VE, Efron ML: Pyridoxine-unresponsive homocystinuria: final diagnosis of M.G.H. Case 19471, 1933, *New Engl J Med* 283:1206-1208, 1970.

99. Skovby F, Krassikoff N, Francke U: Assignment of the gene for cystathionine beta-synthase to human chromosome 21 in somatic cell hybrids, *Hum Genet* 65:291-294, 1984.

100. Skovby F, Kraus J, Rosenberg LE: Homocystinuria: biogenesis of cystathionine β-synthase subunits in cultured fibroblasts and in an in vitro translation system programmed with fibroblast messenger RNA, *Am J Hum Genet* 36:452-459, 1984.

101. Skovby F et al: Immunochemical studies on cultured fibroblasts from patients with homocystinuria due to cystathionine β-synthase deficiency, *Am J Hum Genet* 34:73-83, 1982.

102. Slocum RH, Cummings JG: Amino acid analysis of physiological samples. In Hommes FA, editor: *Techniques in diagnostic human biochemical genetics*, New York, 1991, Wiley-Liss, pp 87-126.

103. Smith SW: Roentgen findings in homocystinuria, *Am J Roentgenol* 100:147-154, 1967.

104. Smolin LA, Benevenga NJ, Berlow S: The use of betaine for the treatment of homocystinuria, *J Pediatr* 99:467-472, 1981.

105. Spaeth GL, Barber GW: Prevalence of homocystinuria among the mentally retarded: evaluation of a specific screening test, *Pediatrics* 40:586-589, 1967.

106. Spiro HR, Schimke RN, Welch JP: Schizophrenia in a patient with a defect in methionine metabolism, *J Nerv Ment Dis* 141:285-290, 1965.

107. Starkebaum G, Harlan JM: Endothelial cell injury due to copper-catalyzed hydrogen peroxide generation from homocysteine, *J Clin Invest* 77:1370-1376, 1986.

108. Steegers-Theunissen RPM et al: Neural-tube effects and derangement of homocysteine metabolism, *New Engl J Med* 324:199-200, 1991.

109. Uhlemann ER et al: Platelet survival and morphology in homocystinuria due to cystathionine synthase deficiency, *New Engl J Med* 295:1283-1286, 1976.

110. Uhlendorf BW, Conerly EB, Mudd SH: Homocystinuria: studies in tissue culture, *Pediatr Res* 7:645-658, 1973.

111. Uhlendorf VW, Mudd SH: Cystathionine synthetase in tissue culture derived from human skin: enzyme defect in homocystinuria, *Science* 160:1007-1009, 1968.

112. Valle D et al: Homocystinuria due to cystathionine beta-synthase deficiency: clinical manifestations and therapy, *Johns Hopkins Med J* 146:110-117, 1980.

113. Wall RT et al: Homocysteine induced endothelial cell injury in vitro: a model for the study of vascular injury, *Thromb Res* 18:113-121, 1980.

114. Wilcken DEL, Dudman NPB, Tyrrell PA: Homocystinuria due to cystathionine beta-synthase deficiency—the effects of betaine treatment in pyridoxine-responsive patients, *Metabolism* 34:1115-1121, 1985.

115. Wilcken DEL, Gupta VJ: Cysteine-homocysteine mixed disulphide: differing plasma concentrations in normal men and women, *Clin Sci* 47:211-215, 1979.

116. Wilcken DEL, Reddy SG, Gupta VJ: Homocysteinemia, ischemic heart disease, and the carrier state for homocystinuria, *Metabolism* 32:363-370, 1983.

117. Wilcken B, Turner B: Homocystinuria: reduced folate levels during pyridoxine treatment, *Arch Dis Child* 48:58-62, 1973.

118. Wilcken DE, Wilcken B: The pathogenesis of coronary artery disease: a possible role for methionine metabolism, *J Clin Invest* 57:1079-1082, 1976.

119. Wilcken DEL et al: Homocystinuria—the effects of betaine in the treatment of patients not responsive to pyridoxine, *New Engl J Med* 309:448-453, 1983.

120. Wiley VC, Dudman NPB, Wilcken DEL: Interrelations between plasma free and protein-bound homocysteine and cysteine in homocystinuria, *Metabolism* 37:191-195, 1988.

121. Wilson RS, Ruiz RS: Bilateral central retinal artery occlusion in homocystinuria: a case report, *Arch Ophthalmol* 82:267-268, 1969.

CHAPTER 5

The Weill-Marchesani Syndrome

Irene H. Maumenee

The Weill-Marchesani syndrome is one of the last remaining connective tissue disorders for which the basic defect and pathogenesis have not been identified. In this generalized hereditary disorder of connective tissue the skeletal features as stressed by Marchesani[19,20] are the antithesis of those seen in the Marfan syndrome: the patients have short stature and stubby hands and feet, and many have stiff joints, especially in the hands. The majority of patients have been described by ophthalmologists, since the most significant morbidity results from the ocular manifestations. Secondary complications are caused by dislocation of the microspherophakic lens, which induces acute or chronic glaucoma, or both, that may lead to blindness. Patients with the Weill-Marchesani syndrome are homozygous for the faulty gene; their heterozygote parents often have short stature.

HISTORICAL NOTE

In 1932 Weill[38] of Strasbourg reported, among eight cases of supposed Marfan syndrome, a 42-year-old woman with ectopia lentis, a height of 142 cm, and "short, swollen fingers permitting only imperfect opening and closing" of the hands. In 1939 Oswald Marchesani,[19,20] then in Munster and later, professor of ophthalmology in Hamburg, gave the first definitive description based on two families. He presented comparative photographs of patients with brachydactyly and arachnodactyly and described an 8-year-old boy whose parents were short and had short hands. In the second family two brothers and a sister were affected; both parents had short stature. Consanguinity was present in one of the families. Autosomal recessive inheritance of spherophakia with brachymorphia and the phenotypic manifestation of the gene in heterozygotes as brachymorphia were discussed. This type of inheritance was further established by Kloepfer and Rosenthal[18] and Rosenthal and Kloepfer[31] on the basis of a family in Louisiana (Fig. 5-1); the family members were reexamined by McKusick in 1971. Marchesani termed the syndrome "brachydactyly and congenital spherophakia." Others have called this disorder the spherophakia-brachymorphia syndrome.[18] The condition is now known as the Weill-Marchesani syndrome, and the abbreviated designation *W-M* is sometimes used.

CLINICAL MANIFESTATIONS
Skeletal Features

Proportionate short stature is present: Weill's original patient [37] was only 142 cm in height. The head is brachycephalic and the face is round. Many affected persons show limitation of joint mobility, especially in the hands,[1,25,38] where neither full extension nor full flexion of the fingers is possible (Figs. 5-2 and 5-3). Seeleman[35] described the fingers and toes in a 3-year-old boy as being capable of only slight flexion. Reduced joint mobility, like short stature, is a feature opposite from the finding in the Marfan syndrome.[31] Rennert[30] described "difficulty in extending his arms over

179

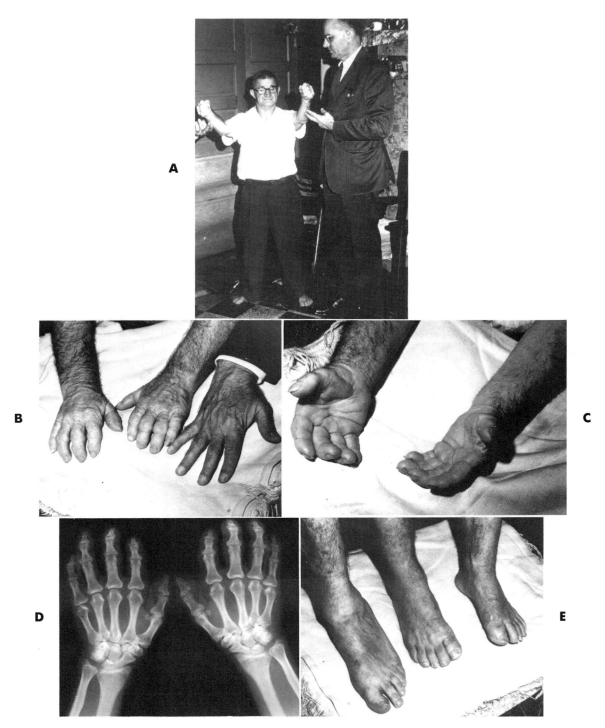

Fig. 5-1. **A** to **E,** Weill-Marchesani syndrome in the proband of the family reported by Kloepfer and Rosenthal.[18] **A,** Short stature and limitation in closure of the fists are demonstrated. Motion is limited at the wrists and elbows. **B,** The short fingers with "knobby" joints are well demonstrated in comparison with the hand of a normal male. **C,** The fingers are held at almost maximal extension. Atrophy of the abductor pollicis brevis muscle, consistent with compression of the median nerve in the carpal tunnel (carpal tunnel syndrome), is present bilaterally. The palmar fascia is irregularly thickened, with puckering of overlying skin. **D,** Radiograph of the hands shows shortening of the tubular bones and hypertrophic osteoarthropathy. **E,** The short feet are compared with the foot of a normal male. (Courtesy Dr. H.W. Kloepfer and Dr. T.F. Thurmon, New Orleans.)

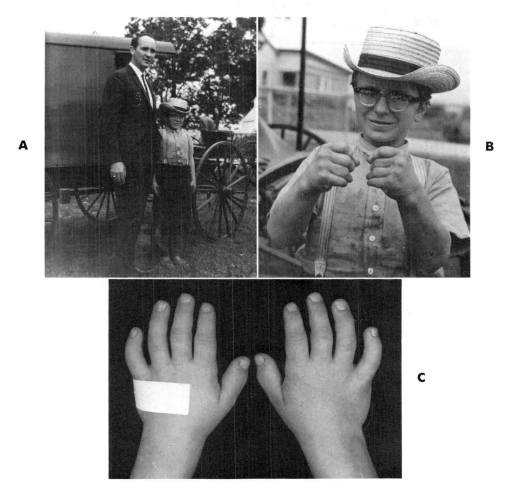

Fig. 5-2. A to **C,** Weill-Marchesani syndrome in an Amish boy. **A** and **B,** The patient, standing with Dr. Charles Scott, is depicted at 15½ years of age. He had worn spectacles for myopia from the age of 10 years. He had always been of short stature. Limitation of joint mobility was striking, especially in the hands, **B.** In addition to having spherophakia and iridodonesis, he intermittently had elevated intraocular pressures, with serious decline in vision. In addition to short fingers, the fifth fingers showed clinodactyly. **C,** The hands of the patient's younger sister, aged 4 years, showed similarly short fingers, limitation in joint mobility, and clinodactyly, as in the hands of brother. The parents were related as first cousins once removed. An affected second cousin had catheterization-confirmed pulmonic stenosis.

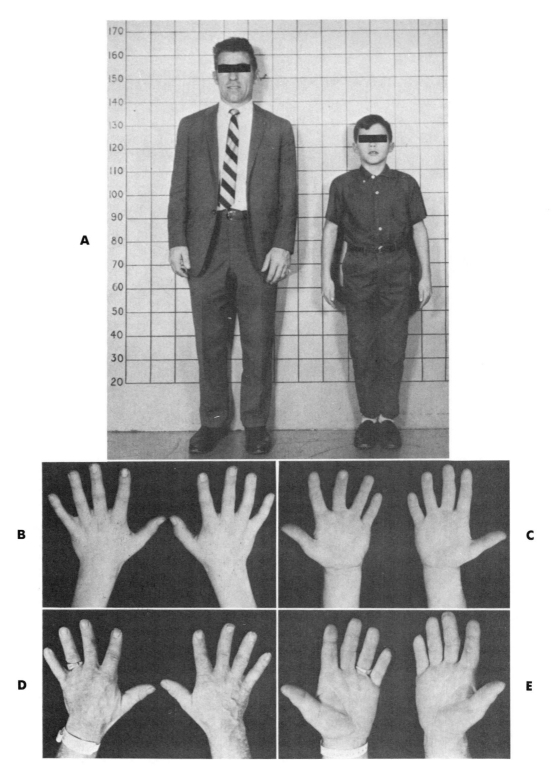

Fig. 5-3. This affected boy, aged 13 years, was 54 cm in length at birth and weighed almost 4 kg. He was found to be myopic when he started school. At the age of 12 years, aspiration of the anteriorly displaced lens and iridectomy were performed in the left eye. His father and mother were unrelated and were 28 and 31 years of age, respectively, at his birth. They were 156 and 152 cm in height, respectively, with stubby fingers. Of five sibs, a sister also had the Weill-Marchesani syndrome. In 1969, at the age of 13 years, the boy was 140 cm in height (below the third percentile for age). **B** and **C,** His hands and feet were stubby. Extension of joints was only slightly limited. In the right eye the lens was microspheric and the anterior chamber was shallow. The left eye showed the signs of extracapsular cataract extraction and superior-sector iridectomy. **A,** Father and son; **B** and **C,** hands of son; **D** and **E,** hands of father.

his head" in a 9-year-old boy. The patients are often strikingly muscular[1,24] (Figs. 5-4 and 5-5). McKusick found evidence of carpal tunnel compression in the then-61-year-old proband of the family described by Kloepfer and Rosenthal.[18]

Ocular Features

Both the horizontal and sagittal diameters of the lens are reduced, and the spheric lens dislocates frequently. The anterior chambers are shallow. Displacement of the lens tends to be forward or downward, or both, inducing further shallowing of the chamber. Microspherophakia appears to

be congenital, but lens dislocation occurs during the first decade of life. Cataracts are frequently a feature. Myopia is present in all affected persons and commonly measures between 10 and 20 diopters,[13,23] but the author has observed myopia with a measurement as high as 42 diopters. This defect has a lenticular and an axial component. Glaucoma seems to be an inexorable complication and usually affects children in late childhood in an acute or a chronic fashion. The rounded-off lens obstructs aqueous flow through the pupil.[4,5,16,39] Intraocular pressure rises and the angle closes. This process may be acute and total or may occur

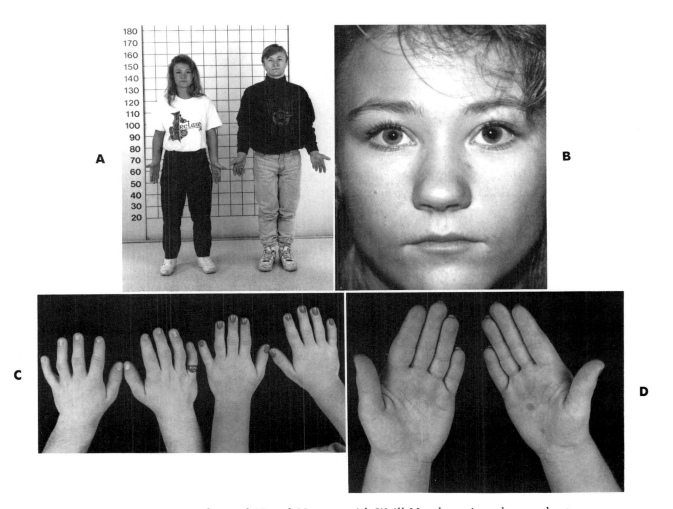

Fig. 5-4. A to **H,** Sibs aged 17 and 19 years with Weill-Marchesani syndrome, short stature, muscular body build, and round facies. Both parents have short stature. **B,** Round facies of sister shown in **A** after right lens extraction. Bilateral laser iridotomy had been performed at the age of 9 years. **C,** Short, broad hands of the same brother and sister. Clinodactyly in the brother and incomplete digital extension in both sibs are evident. **D,** The sister had undergone bilateral carpal tunnel release surgery. *Continued.*

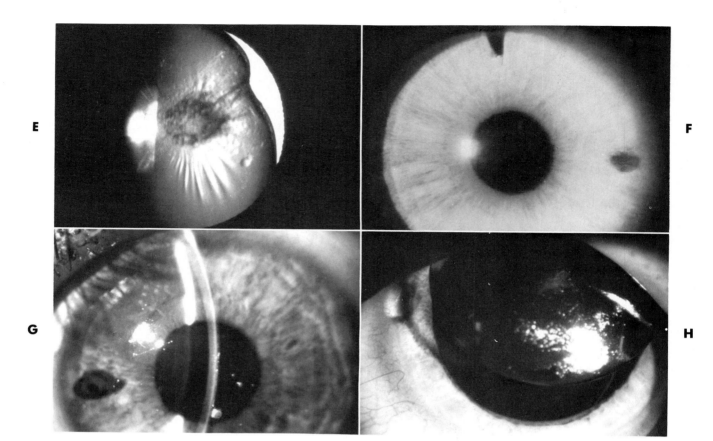

Fig. 5-4, cont'd. E, A right anterior subcapsular cataract developed in the sister's dislocated lens at the age of 11 years. She ascribed this complication to an episode of trauma. **F,** After lens extraction and laser and surgical iridectomies. **G,** The left anterior chamber remains shallow in spite of the presence of a patent nasal laser iridotomy. The lens is microspherophakic. The visual acuities are 20/25 in each eye. There is no evidence of glaucoma to date. **H,** The brother successfully wears contact lenses. The edge of the microspherophakic lens is easily seen. The chambers remain shallow, despite the presence of patent laser iridotomies. The visual acuity is 20/20 in each eye and there is no evidence of glaucoma.

as repeated, self-limited attacks; these ultimately lead to extensive synechiae and chronic angle-closure glaucoma.[3] Chamber-angle anomalies[2] such as those seen in other heritable disorders of connective tissue have been described—bridging pectinate strands, numerous iris processes, fraying of the iris root, and anomalous angle vessels—all of which, however, may be secondary to glaucoma. Since miotics lead to shallowing of the chamber, they are contraindicated in patients with the Weill-Marchesani syndrome, especially during acute attacks of glaucoma.[3] By means of gonioscopy the angle can be observed to "close" on miosis and "open again" on pupillary dilation. An acute attack of angle-closure glaucoma may be in-

terrupted by the administration of mydriatics and by manually repositioning the lens if it has entered the anterior chamber.

Iridotomy is considered the treatment of choice for the prevention of glaucoma in persons with the Weill-Marchesani syndrome.[3,14] Any patient suspected of having the Weill-Marchesani syndrome should be referred for an ophthalmologic evaluation and laser surgery. Glaucoma has been prevented by means of laser surgery in two sibs now in their late teens who have been followed by the author for more than 11 and 12 years, respectively.

Measurement of the cataractous lens removed from a patient with bilateral lens dislocation as

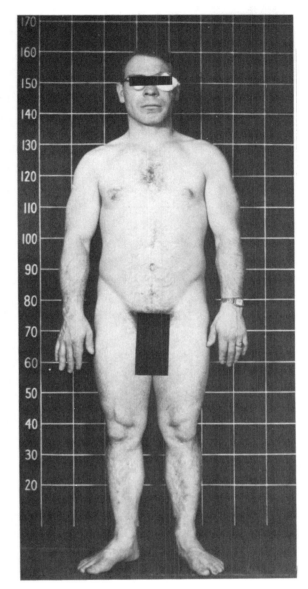

Fig. 5-5. The patient, born in 1925, and his brother have the Weill-Marchesani syndrome. His sister, who has not been examined, also is bilaterally blind, but this abnormality, which dates from childhood, has been attributed to a febrile illness. Because of secondary glaucoma, subluxated spherophakic lenses were removed from both eyes of the patient. He had a retinal detachment in the left eye.

part of the Weill-Marchesani syndrome showed a roughly spheric 7-mm lens. The surface was roughened, with zonules still adherent. In this 11-year-old patient alpha-chymotryposin had been used, followed by removal of the lens with the cryoprobe; although equatorial globule

formation was observed, neither unusual fibers nor abnormalities of the zonules were evident on light microscopy. In a Japanese patient the lens, which was removed during emergency surgery because of a ruptured globe, measured 7 mm in diameter. The anterior capsule was normal. Some cortical fibers remained nucleated. The anterior and posterior cortical fibers were totally liquefied.

Other Features

Anomalies of extraocular motility and ptosis have been described in individual patients. One Amish patient with the Weill-Marchesani syndrome has congenital pulmonic stenosis, which was diagnosed by means of cardiac catheterization. All patients known to the author have normal intelligence. Chromosomes have been normal except for mosaic aneuploidy of the X chromosome in one patient.[6,13,17]

PREVALENCE AND INHERITANCE

Kloepfer and Rosenthal[18] further elaborated Marchesani's conclusions that only homozygotes show the full-blown disorder and that the height of heterozygotes is roughly intermediate between that of unaffected persons and that of homozygotes. The findings of Kloepfer and Rosenthal suggest that about 92% of heterozygotes have abnormally short stature. Probert[28] described a family in which four sibs (three females and one male) had the full syndrome and one of their parents and many relatives had brachymorphism in a dominant pedigree pattern. Meyer and Holstein[25] described four affected sibs whose parents were first cousins; Diethelm[7] described two affected children with first-cousin parents. The high rate of consanguinity among the Amish and in other reported cases[18,36,37,41] is also in keeping with autosomal recessive inheritance.

Families have been reported in which persons in successive generations had presumed Weill-Marchesani syndrome.[32,40] McKusick reinvestigated the family of Italian extraction reported by McGavic and concluded that the family represents an instance of "simple" autosomal dominant ectopia lentis in a generally short-statured family.[21,24] No difference in stature was observed between persons with and without the ocular feature. McKusick suspected that the family of Rousseau and Hermann[24] may have been similarly affected.[24]

The Weill-Marchesani syndrome is one of three

forms of recessively inherited dwarfism frequently found among the Amish people who constitute several American religious isolates.[34] The other two types of dwarfism in the Amish are the Ellis-van Creveld syndrome[22] and cartilage-hair hypoplasia.[23] Because heterozygotes are much more frequent than homozygotes, numerous persons in the Lancaster County (Pennsylvania) Amish community have short stature, possibly as a result of heterozygosity for the Weill-Marchesani syndrome gene.[21]

Fewer than a hundred families with the Weill-Marchesani syndrome have been described, and additional pedigrees are now rarely published, since publication appears to be unwarranted in the absence of significant new information. The Weill-Marchesani syndrome has been documented in several populations. The large kindred studied by Kloepfer and Rosenthal[18] is of French extraction, and other cases have been described in the French literature.[1,4,10,37] Cases have been reported from Pakistan,[29] in a Bengali Muslim boy from India,[33] and from Israel[8] (ethnicity not stated). Two Japanese cases are on record.[15] In addition, there are anecdotal accounts of a large number of persons with the Weill-Marchesani syndrome on the Maldive islands in the Indian Ocean.

SUMMARY

Weill-Marchesani syndrome is a generalized disorder of connective tissues characterized by microspherophakia, ectopia lentis, brachymorphism, and joint stiffness. The full syndrome is inherited as an autosomal recessive trait, whereas heterozygotes show brachymorphism. Ocular complications are conspicuously absent in the heterozygotes. The molecular defect and pathogenesis remain unknown.

REFERENCES

1. Bebe M: Le syndrome de Weill-Marchesani: a propos d'une observation, *Ann Pediatr* 30:673-677, 1983.
2. Burian HM, von Noorden GK, Ponseti IV: Chamber angle anomalies in systemic connective tissue disorders *Arch Ophthalmol* 64:671-680, 1960.
3. Chandler PA: Choice of treatment in dislocation of the lens, *Arch Ophthalmol* 71:765-786, 1964.
4. Combe P et al: Le syndrome de Weill et Marchesani, *Société Francaise de Pédiatrie* 25:433-440, 1971.
5. Cross HE: Ectopia lentis in systemic heritable disorders, *Birth Defects: Original Article Series* 10(10):113-119, 1974.
6. Cummins H, Midlo C: *Finger prints, palms and soles: an introduction to dermatoglyphics*, New York, 1961, Dover.
7. Diethelm W: Über Ectopia lentis ohne Arachnodaktylie und ihre Beziehungen zur Ectopia lentis et pupillae, *Ophthalmologica* 114:16-32, 1947.
8. Feiler-Ofry V, Stein R, Godel V: Marchesani's syndrome and chamber-angle anomalies, *Am J Ophthalmol* 65:862-866, 1968.
9. Feinberg SB: Congenital mesodermal dysmorphodystrophy (brachymorphic type), *Radiology* 74:218-224, 1960.
10. Ferrier S et al: Le syndrome de Marchesani (spherophakie, brachymorphie), *Helv Paediatr Acta* 35:185-198, 1980.
11. Fujiwara H et al: Histology of the lens in the Weill-Marchesani syndrome, *Br J Ophthalmol* 74(10):631-634, 1990.
12. Reference deleted in proofs.
13. Gotz M, Schenk E: Weill-Marchesani syndrome: growth hormone, thyroid and chromosome studies, *Z Kinderheilk* 116:43-49, 1973.
14. Haik GM, Terrell WL: The Weill-Marchesani syndrome: report of two cases and a review, *J Louisiana State Med Soc* 142(12):25-32, 1990.
15. Hazato N et al: Two cases of Marchesani syndrome (in Japanese), *Jpn J Intern Med* 60:431-437, 1971.
16. Jensen AD, Cross HE, Paton D: Ocular complications in the Weill-Marchesani syndrome, *Am J Ophthalmol* 77:261-269, 1974.
17. Jouhaud F, Augustin P, Malbrel C: Syndrome de Weill Marchesani: étude d'un cas, *Bull Soc Ophtalmol Fr* 10:1107-1111, 1984.
18. Kloepfer HW, Rosenthal JW: Possible genetic carriers in the spherophakia-brachymorphia syndrome, *Am J Hum Genet* 7:398-425, 1955.
19. Marchesani O: Brachydaktylie und angeborene Kugellinse als Systemerkrankung, *Klin Mbl Augenheilk* 103:392-406, 1939.
20. Marchesani O: *Jubilee volume for Professor Vogt, part II*, Basel, 1939, Benno Schwage, p 32.
21. McGavic JS: Weill-Marchesani syndrome: brachymorphism and ectopia lentis, *Am J Ophthalmol* 62:820-823, 1966.
22. McKusick VA, Egeland JA, Eldridge R: Dwarfism in the Amish. I. The Ellis-van Creveld syndrome, *Bull Hopkins Hosp* 115:306-336, 1964.
23. McKusick VA et al: Dwarfism in the Amish. II. Cartilage-hair hypoplasia, *Bull Hopkins Hosp* 116:285-326, 1965.
24. McKusick VA: *Heritable disorders of connective tissue*, ed 4, St Louis, 1972, Mosby–Year Book.
25. Meyer SJ, Holstein T: Spherophakia with glaucoma and brachydactyly, *Am J Ophthalmol* 24:247-257, 1941.
26. Obituary, Oswald Marchesani (1900-1952), *Klin Mbl Augenheilk* 120:653-655, 1952.
27. Obituary, Oswald Marchesani, *Graefe Arch Ophthalmol* 152:551-552, 1951-52.
28. Probert LA: Spherophakia with brachydactyly: comparison with Marfan's syndrome, *Am J Ophthalmol* 36:1571-1574, 1953.
29. Rahman M, Rahman S: Marchesani's syndrome, *Br J Ophthalmol* 47:182-183, 1963.
30. Rennert OM: The Marchesani syndrome: a brief review, *Am J Dis Child* 117:703-705, 1969.
31. Rosenthal JW, Kloepfer HW: The spherophakia-brachymorphia syndrome, *Arch Ophthalmol* 55:28-35, 1956.

32. Rousseau, Hermann: Ectopie congenitale du cristallin avec brachymorphie (syndrome de Marchesani), *Bull Mem Soc Fr Ophtalmol* 62:369-373, 1949.

33. Saxena KM et al: Dwarfism with brachydactyly, spherophakia and glaucoma: Marchesani syndrome in an Indian girl, *Indian Pediatr* 3:231, 1966.

34. Scott CI: Weill-Marchesani syndrome. In Bergsma D, editor: *Clinical delineation of birth defects. II. Malformation syndromes*, New York, 1969, National Foundation, March of Dimes, pp 238-240.

35. Seeleman K: Brachydaktylie und angeborene Kugellinse, *Z Kinderheilk* 67:1-6, 1949.

36. Sellem C et al: Syndrome de Weill-Marchesani, *Pediatrie* 25(7):771-775, 1970.

37. Stadlin W, Klein D: Ectopie congénitale du cristallin avec spherophaquie et brachymorphie accompagnée de parésies du regard (syndrome de Marchesani), *Ann Ocul* 181:692-701, 1948.

38. Weill G: Ectopie du cristallins et malformations generales, *Ann Ocul* 169:21-44, 1932.

39. Willi M, Kut L, Cotlier E: Pupillary-block glaucoma in the Marchesani syndrome, *Arch Ophthalmol* 90:504-508, 1973.

40. Young ID, Fielder AR, Casey TA: Weill-Marchesani syndrome in mother and son, *Clin Genet* 30:475-480, 1986.

41. Zabriskie J, Reisman M: Marchesani syndrome, *J Pediatr* 52:159-169, 1958.

The Ehlers-Danlos Syndromes

Peter Beighton

The Ehlers-Danlos syndromes (EDS) are a group of heritable connective tissue disorders that share the common features of skin hyperextensibility, articular hypermobility, and tissue fragility. Considerable clinical and genetic heterogeneity exists, and more than nine separate forms have been recognized. The fundamental biomolecular defect has been elucidated in some types of the disorder, and it is becoming apparent that even greater heterogeneity exists at this level. The abbreviation EDS, which is conventionally employed for both the singular and the plural form of the eponymous designation, is used throughout this chapter.

✦ HISTORICAL NOTE

None of the hereditary disorders of connective tissue, except possibly osteogenesis imperfecta (OI), has a history as ancient as that of EDS. McKusick speculated that a description by Hippocrates of the Scythians of the fourth century B.C. was suggestive that EDS was present in this population.* The first definitive case of this syndrome

seems to have been described in 1682 by Job van Meekeren,[510] a surgeon in Amsterdam. Fig. 6-1 presents van Meekeren's illustration of the "extraordinary dilatability of the skin" in a 23-year-old Spaniard who could pull the right pectoral skin to the left ear, the skin under the chin up over the head like a beard, and the skin of the knee area out about half a yard. On being released, the skin retracted promptly to fit snugly over the underlying structures. This phenomenon was limited to the skin of the right side of the body.

In retrospect, Smith and Worthington[459] suggested that Nicolo Paganini (1782-1840), the violinist "virtuoso in excelsis," had EDS. His slender physique, thoracic deformity, and joint laxity, which in the hypermobility of the fingers is thought to have contributed to his virtuosity, are well documented.

Late in the last century various dermatologists published scattered references to this condition, which was usually observed as a curiosity in fairground side shows. Gould and Pyle[188] published a photograph made in Budapest in 1888 of the "In-

---

*In *Airs, Waters and Places* Hippocrates,[309] in the fourth century B.C., described the Scythians as having markedly lax joints. "I will give you a strong proof of the humidity (laxity?) of their constitutions. You will find the greater part of the Scythians, and all the Nomades, with marks of the cautery on their shoulders, arms, wrists, breasts, hip-joints, and loins, and that for no other reason but the humidity and flabbiness of their constitution, for they can neither strain with their bows, nor launch the javelin from their shoulder owing to their humidity and atony: but when they are burnt, much of the hu-

midity in their joints is dried up, and they become braced, better fed, and their joints get into a more suitable condition." Is it possible that the cigarette-paper scars of EDS were misinterpreted? Against this suggestion is the fact that burning the skin around joints became an established treatment for dislocation of joints in the ancient world. Another statement is of much interest: ". . . they afterwards became lame and stiff at the hipjoint, such of them, at least, as are severely attacked with it." (From Adams F: *The genuine works of Hippocrates*, New York, 1891, William Wood.)

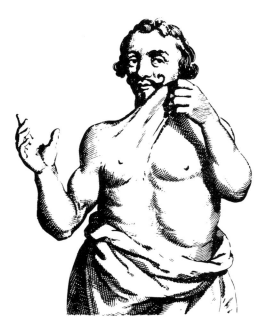

Fig. 6-1. Job van Meekeren's case of "extraordinary dilatability of the skin," described as follows:

In the year 1657, in the presence of the very distinguished John van Horne and Francis Sylvius, professors of medicine in the famous academy of Leyden, as well as of William Piso and Francis vander Schagen, practitioners of Amsterdam, we saw in our hospital a certain young Spaniard, 23 years of age, by the name of George Albes, who with his left hand grasped the skin over his humerus and right breast and stretched it till it was quite close to his mouth. With each hand he first pulled the skin of his chin downward like a beard to his chest, hence he lifted it upwards to the vertex of his head so as to cover each eye with it. As soon as he removed his hand the skin contracted to reassume its proper smoothness. In the same way he pulled the skin of his right knee upwards or downwards, to the length of half an ell; then it easily returned to its natural position. It was worthwhile noting that the skin which covered the forementioned parts on the left side could not be extended since it firmly adhered to them. It has, thus far, not been possible to learn the cause [of this anomaly?]." [Translated from original Latin by Dr. Owsei Temkin.]

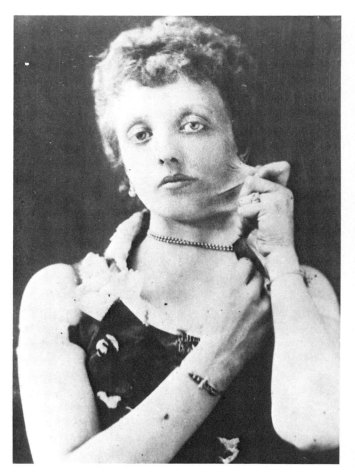

Fig. 6-2. Etta Lake, "Elastic Lady." Miss Lake was a professional exhibitionist in early 1900s. This photograph was found by the author in a fairground peepshow on Hampstead Heath, London, in 1966. The owner of the show and grandson of Miss Lake's former manager, Mr. Tim Bowan, gave his kind permission for the illustration to be published. (From Beighton P: *The Ehlers-Danlos syndrome,* London, 1970, William Heinemann Medical Books.)

dia Rubber Man," an exhibitionist named Felix Wehrle "who besides having the power to stretch his skin could readily bend his fingers backward and forward." Another skin stretching artiste, Etta Lake, was known as the "Elastic Lady" (Fig. 6-2). Kopp,[269] who is widely quoted as first drawing attention to familial incidence by describing an affected father and son, was probably describing cutis laxa, not EDS.

With considerable justification Jansen[244] argues

that Tschernogobow[501,502] is most deserving of credit for the first detailed clinical description of EDS. In 1891 he presented two affected persons at a meeting of the Moscow Dermatologic and Venereologic Society. He described the fragility and hyperelasticity of the skin, the failure of the skin to hold sutures, the hypermobility and luxation of joints, and the molluscoid pseudotumors of the knees, elbows, and other areas. Most important, he tied all these features together as manifesta-

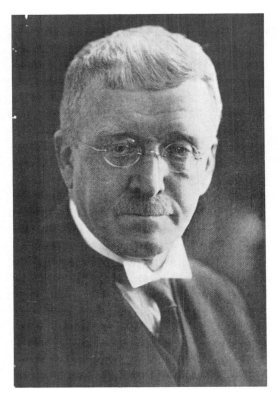

Fig. 6-3. Edvard Ehlers (1863-1937). Edvard Ehlers, born in Copenhagen, Denmark, in 1863 and qualified in medicine in that city in 1891,[123] had a distinguished career as chief of the Dermatological Polyclinic at Fredericks Hospital and as director of the special service for venereal diseases at Commune Hospital. Tall, with fair hair, blue eyes, and a distinguished bearing, Ehlers traveled widely and organized programs of disease control in island communities, including the West Indies, Iceland, and Jutland. Ehlers, a francophile, often participated in clinical meetings of the French Dermatological Society in Paris. In 1899 he presented and subsequently published case details of a law student with recurrent hematomas, lax digits, and extensible skin. This young man came from the island of Bornholm in the Baltic Sea, and it would be of interest to determine whether affected members of this prototype EDS family are still living in that locality. Ehlers died in Copenhagen in 1937 at 74 years of age. (Photograph from Shelley WB, Crissey JT: *Classics in clinical dermatology*, Springfield, Ill, 1953, Charles C. Thomas.)

tions of a fundamental and generalized inadequacy of connective tissue: "Erschlaffung des Bindegewebes" were his words. Denko[129] provided a full translation of Tschernogobow's case report, using the alternative spelling, "Chernogubov." This eponym in the singular or conjoined form is still used in the contemporary Russian literature.[240,513]

One of Tschernogobow's patients[501] was a 17-year-old boy with epilepsy who, in falling frequently, had sustained numerous linear scars on his face. The skin of the knees, elbows, and wrists was unusually spongy and loose. Joint changes were especially pronounced on the left side, where dislocations of the elbow and hip, dating from childhood, were present. In the second patient,[502] a 50-year-old woman, "tumors" were present not only on the elbows and knees but also on the buttocks, presumably near the ischial tuberosities. When one of these "tumors" was removed, it was discovered that sutures did not hold well and dehiscence of the wound occurred within two days. Du Mesnil[147] in 1890, Williams[536] in 1892, working in Unna's laboratory in Hamburg, and Unna himself[509] in 1894 reported on histologic

studies. These authors were puzzled by the absence of specific changes and encountered difficulties in the interpretation of their findings. The contribution in 1901 by Ehlers[154] (Fig. 6-3) consisted of pointing out the associated loose-jointedness and the subcutaneous hemorrhages that are prone to occur. Danlos[122] (Fig. 6-4) in 1908 rounded out the clinical description with inclusion of the posttraumatic tumors that may develop over bony prominences.

Sir Malcolm Morris[343] demonstrated the first British case at a meeting of the Dermatological Society of London in 1900 and subsequently depicted the affected boy in the 1909 edition of his *Diseases of the Skin* (Fig. 6-5, *A*). Beighton[40] provided a picture of the same patient in his eighty-second year (Fig. 6-5, *B*).

In 1934 Tobias[497] reported the first case in the United States, and in 1936 Ronchese[420] of Rhode Island found 24 cases in the literature and added three of his own. At the time of publication of the first edition of this book (1956) the world literature contained less than 100 well-documented reports, but by the time the third edition was published (1966), the estimate had risen to over 300.

Fig. 6-4. Henri-Alexandre Danlos (1844-1912). Henri-Alexandre Danlos was born in Paris in 1844 and qualified in medicine, with distinction, in 1869. After postgraduate experience in chemistry, Danlos trained as a specialist physician and obtained a consultant post at Hôpital Tenon. He subsequently spent an unhappy 5 years in Public Health Services, and in 1885, at 51 years of age, he achieved his life's ambition by gaining a specialist appointment at Hôpital St. Louis, where he spent the remainder of his career. Danlos had special interest in the treatment of skin disease and used his chemical and scientific expertise in developing techniques involving the use of mercurials, arsenicals, and radiation. In 1908, during a meeting of the French Dermatological Society, Danlos discussed the nature of heaped-up lesions on the elbows and knees of a boy in whom a diagnosis of juvenile pseudodiabetic xanthomata had previously been made by his colleagues, Hallopeau and Macé de Lépiny. Danlos recognized that the skin of this patient was fragile and extensible, and he pointed out the similarity of these features to those of the patient presented by Ehlers to the same Society in 1899. Danlos had poor health during most of his adulthood and died in 1912 at 68 years of age. (Courtesy Dr. Pierre Maroteaux, Paris, CMT Assistance Publique, Paris. From Beighton P, Beighton G: *The man behind the syndrome,* Heidelberg, 1986, Springer-Verlag.)

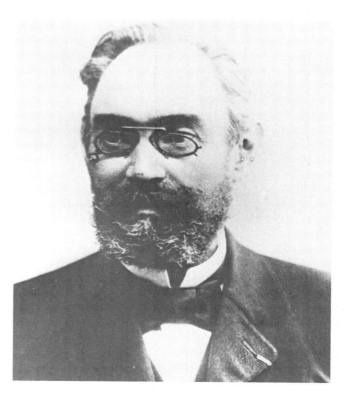

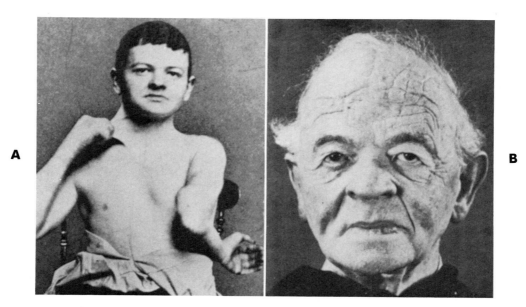

Fig. 6-5. "Lad with elastic skin and multiple cutaneous nodules," a case presented to the Old Dermatological Society of London in 1900 by Sir Malcolm Morris.[342] Beighton[40] suggests that this is the earliest recognizable case of EDS in British medical literature. The picture of the boy, **A,** appeared in the 1909 edition of Morris' *Diseases of the Skin,*[343] where the disorder was described as "fibroma with elastic skin and congenital dislocations." The photograph, **B,** is of same "lad" in his eighty-second year. His activity was limited by degenerative arthritis of the spine, knees, elbows, and hands. (From Beighton P: *The Ehlers-Danlos syndrome,* London, 1970, William Heinemann Medical Books.)

Autosomal dominant inheritance was demonstrated in 1949 by Johnson and Falls[250] on the basis of an extensive kindred containing 32 affected persons. In 1954 Jansen[244] suggested that the basic defect concerns the collagen wickerwork, or basketry, which is excessively loose in this disorder.

Genetic heterogeneity of EDS was proposed in 1960 by McKusick in the second edition of this book. In 1967 Barabas[25] suggested the existence of three types of the disorder, and Beighton et al.[54] subsequently recognized five clinically distinct forms, one an X-linked recessive.[36] A sixth form, an autosomal recessive ocular-scoliotic type, was added to the classification[41]; in this variety of EDS a defect of collagen was identified by Krane, Pinnell, and Erbe[276] and Pinnell et al.[389] and confirmed by Lichtenstein et al.[303,304] This was the first heritable disorder of collagen (other than alkaptonuria) to be elucidated at the biochemical level. Additional forms of EDS were subsequently delineated,[329] and nine major categories of the condition are now recognized.

A book on EDS by Beighton,[40] based on a review of the world literature and personal experience with 130 cases, was published in 1970. This book was dedicated to Victor McKusick and to the "'India Rubber Men' for bending over backwards to help in my investigations, and to the 'Elastic Ladies,' who were always prepared to stretch a point to assist my work." Increasing interest in the syndrome and evolving concepts concerning heterogeneity have prompted numerous articles; in the fourth edition of McKusick's book (1972)[328] accumulated references to the EDS totalled almost 300. Advances in collagen chemistry and the elucidation of the biomolecular pathology in some forms of EDS have given further impetus, and by 1991 more than 500 articles had appeared in the world literature.

Many terms have been used for this syndrome or, more often, for its individual features. In 1936 F. Parkes Weber[524] attempted to bring nosologic order out of the group of conditions with the features of lax skin and loose joints, together or alone, and defended the use of the eponym "Ehlers-Danlos syndrome" as useful for the specific disorder discussed in this chapter. (Tschernogobow's reports were not known to Weber.) As in the case of Marfan syndrome, the eponymic designation seems preferable, since it does not convey any connotations of the invariable occurrence of an individual manifestation or any ill-founded no-

tion of the nature of the basic defect. The conjoined eponym, *EDS* in its abbreviated form, is now in general use.

CLINICAL MANIFESTATIONS[273,327,488]

The diagnostic triad of EDS comprises hyperextensibility of the skin, hypermobility of the joints, and connective tissue fragility (Fig. 6-6). Skin splitting may lead to extensive scarring, and a host of complications can occur in other systems. The various forms of EDS all share the cardinal syndromic features to a greater or lesser extent, but considerable differences exist in severity of involvement. Indeed, some types of the condition are innocuous, whereas others are potentially lethal. It must be emphasized, however, that considerable phenotypic overlap exists and that precise diagnostic subcategorization, especially of a sporadic case, is not always possible.

In addition to the complications of EDS, a number of abnormalities are congenital malformations in the conventional sense and occur often enough to be considered genuine syndromic components. McKusick proposed that these are secondary manifestations and that the underlying hereditary disturbance of connective tissue creates an ontogenetic setting in which certain predictable congenital anomalies occur with increased frequency. In EDS, ureteropelvic anomaly, tetralogy of Fallot, and interatrial defect may fall into this category. Nevertheless, since these malformations have been documented in few affected persons, it is equally reasonable to suspect that the malformations may have occurred by coincidence.

The general manifestations and complications of EDS are reviewed in the first section of this chapter. Thereafter, the various specific types of the disorder are dealt with in greater detail in the section, Heterogeneity.

Cutaneous Features*

The skin in persons with EDS is often velvety in appearance and texture.[106] It has been likened to wet chamois and described by an enthusiast as "the skin you love to feel." In an infant the skin may be impressively white. It is hyperextensible yet not lax; if stretched, it springs back on release to resume its former position.

The term "cutis laxa" has been used in connection with EDS to describe the localized lax or pendulous regions of the skin that sometimes develop

---

*References 58, 83, 264, 385, 411, 420, and 423.

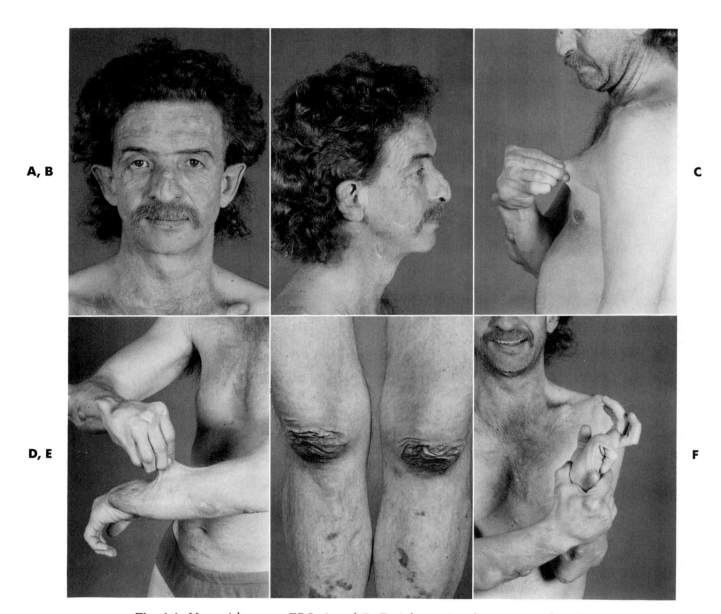

A, B

C

D, E

F

Fig. 6-6. Man with severe EDS. **A** and **B,** Facial scarring due to tissue fragility. **C** and **D,** Skin hyperextensibility. On release, the skin springs back to its former position. **E,** Papyraceous, darkly pigmented scars over the knees and shins. **F,** Joint hypermobility in the left fifth finger.

in adulthood. To avoid any possible confusion, it must be emphasized that cutis laxa[416] per se is a rare genetic entity entirely distinct from EDS. In cutis laxa, which is described in detail in Chapter 7, the skin hangs in pendulous folds, the tissues are not fragile, and the joints are not hypermobile.

In addition to hyperextensibility, the skin in EDS is fragile, leading to the phenomenon termed dermatorrhexis.[420] The skin overlying the bony prominences of the elbows, knees, and shins is particularly vulnerable, and minor trauma may produce gaping, "fish-mouth" wounds. Scars on the forehead and chin often have a linear configuration (Fig. 6-7). In a patient reported by Brown

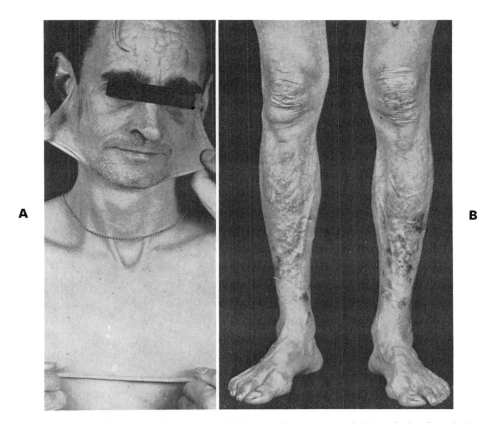

Fig. 6-7. Man, 35 years of age, with EDS. **A,** Hyperextensibility of the facial skin. Linear scars evident on the forehead are a legacy of the man's earlier career as professional boxer. **B,** Knees and shins are covered with thin, pigmented scars.

and Stock,[80] 282 stitches had been taken before count was stopped. Often stitches hold poorly in the skin,[250,421] and the patients and their physicians may resort to the use of adhesive tape or "butterfly" sutures. Thomas, Cordier, and Algan[492] described slow healing of a skin biopsy site and dehiscence of an ocular incision made during removal of an ectopic lens. Packer and Blades[372] observed disruption of an appendectomy scar four times in 30 months. Surgeons have described the tissues during laparotomy as having the consistency of wet blotting paper and have compared attempts at wound closure with "sewing porridge." The tissues at autopsy are also likely to be abnormally friable.

"Cigarette paper" or "papyraceous" scars develop over the knees, shins, and elbows, and the skin in these regions becomes shiny, parchment-thin, and hyperpigmented (Figs. 6-6, *E* and 6-7, *B*). Telangiectases sometimes form in these atrophic scars, and the appearances may resemble those produced by exposure to radiation. Despite this scarring tendency, striae gravidarum do not usually develop in affected women.[250]

The organization and calcification of superficial hematomas sometimes result in pseudotumor formation. These molluscoid pseudotumors,[379,400] which develop at pressure points, notably heels, knees, and elbows (Fig. 6-8), were the basis for the misconceived term, "juvenile pseudodiabetic xanthomatosis," which was used in the early literature by Hallopeau and Macé de Lépinay.[122,204]

Subcutaneous spherules or spheroids are fat-containing cysts, pea-sized or smaller, that slip about under the skin an inch or more without causing the patient any discomfort. The spherules or spheroids may become calcareous[525] or ossified.[261] They are ovoid and occur principally in the subcutaneous tissue of the legs and, to a lesser extent, the arms. On radiographic examination they

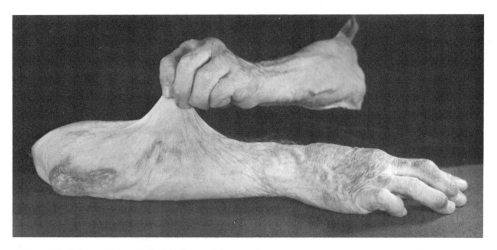

Fig. 6-8. Man with EDS. Molluscoid pseudotumours are present over the elbows.

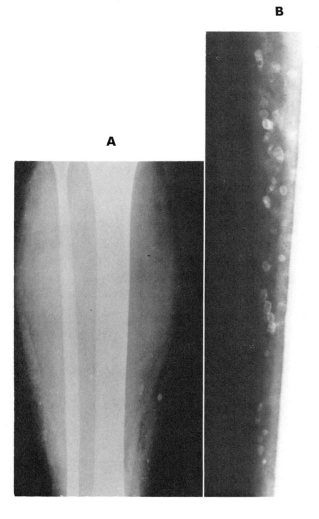

Fig. 6-9. A, Subcutaneous spheroids are evident in this radiograph of the skin of an adult with EDS. **B,** Enlargement showing finer detail of the ring structure of spheroids.

display a diffuse inner calcification with a more dense surrounding shell[69,229] (Fig. 6-9). They are not laminated like phleboliths. These characteristics, together with the facts that they are not present in muscle (as are calcified parasitic cysts) and are too widely distributed to be phleboliths, should permit the radiologist to make a confident diagnosis of EDS.[53,285]

The limitation of the cutaneous changes, particularly hyperelasticity, to one side of the body, as recounted by van Meekeren[510] in 1682, is incredible but possible. In Beighton's investigation[37] in England he observed a young man with striking cutaneous hyperextensibility on the right side of the body and only mild changes on the left side. This unusual situation could be explained by somatic mosaicism. Localized cutaneous hyperextensibility in the left shoulder region of a young woman, which developed in adulthood, has also been documented[117]; this abnormality was probably the result of some acquired process rather than EDS.

Limitation of integumental hyperelasticity to the mucous membranes, specifically those of the mouth and tongue, has been described,[144] and many patients show evidence of hyperelasticity or fragility at these sites.* Gorlin and Pindborg[187] pointed out that many EDS patients display unusual ease in touching the tip of the nose with the tip of the tongue (Fig. 6-10). Duperrat[149] described a patient who was able to hold six golf balls in his mouth, a further demonstration of hyperextensibility of mucous membranes.

The skin of the hands and of the soles of the feet tends to be redundant (unlike most of the skin elsewhere, which fits snugly); with pressure it flattens out like a loose glove or moccasin. A comparable change may develop in later years at the elbows, where the skin may hang lax like a dewlap (Fig. 6-11). Many patients with EDS have markedly wrinkled palms, that is, they have a large number of adventitious palmar creases (Fig. 6-12). Goodman, Katznelson, and Frydman[181] referred to these as secondary skin creases and showed that they may develop in early childhood and that they are well demonstrated by the standard dermatoglyphic techniques. In the wrinkly skin syndrome,[235] which is sometimes confused with EDS, the skin of the dorsal surfaces of the hands and feet is affected, rather than the palms and soles.[181]

---

*References 116, 144. 170, 305, 495, and 532.

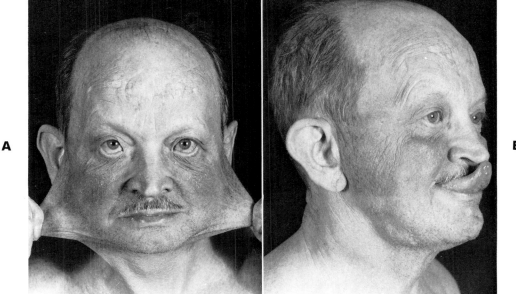

Fig. 6-10. Sixty-year-old man has all the typical features of EDS. No other member of his family is known to be affected. **A,** Excessively stretchable skin and scars of the forehead are demonstrated. **B,** Gorlin's sign: unusual facility in touching the tip of nose with the tip of the tongue.

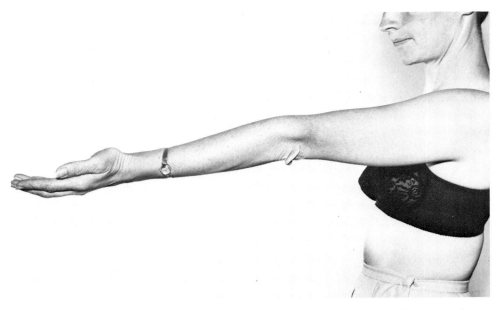

Fig. 6-11. Skin at the elbow may ultimately become redundant and hang in a loose fold.

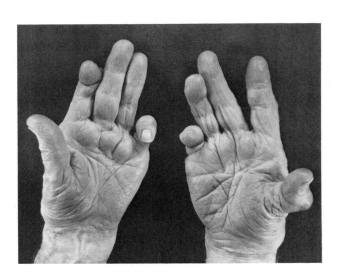

Fig. 6-12. Palms of hands are sometimes excessively wrinkled.

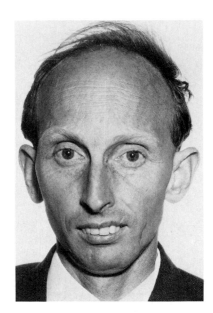

Fig. 6-13. Lack of subcutaneous fat in the face, producing a hollow-eyed appearance.

The skin and other manifestations show qualitative and quantitative differences in the various forms of EDS, although these are by no means absolute. For instance, in many patients with the classical form of EDS IV, fragility and bruisability are striking and the skin is generally thin and translucent, with a clearly evident subcutaneous venous pattern. The skin is not excessively stretchable in these individuals; indeed it is usually tight over the fingers and face, with associated absence of subcutaneous fat (Fig. 6-13).

The altered physical properties of connective tissue that render the skin hyperextensible and fragile also have other ramifications. For instance, "lop ears," ears that project farther than normal from the head and tend to face downward to some extent, are encountered in persons with EDS; "lop ears" also occur as an isolated heritable anomaly.[312] Normally the ear makes a 30-degree angle with the head.[323] The ears in persons with EDS are often unusually stretchable (Fig. 6-14) and can be folded into a ball-like mass.

Acrocyanosis with or without chilblains has been described as a seemingly integral component of EDS, particularly by French authors[166,176,311,345,405] but by others as well,[80,98,423,483,506] and it may be the initial complaint in persons with EDS. For example, Gilbert, Villaret, and Bosviel[176] described a 22-year-old man who had cyanosis of the hands, feet, and ears from birth and displayed the other characteristic features of EDS. In the patient's family several other cases of "cyanosed limbs and ulcerated chilblains" occurred in association with EDS. McKusick recorded the cases of two female patients in whom acrocyanosis was a striking feature. They suffered severely from cold and displayed the Raynaud phenomenon. A woman with EDS reported by Newton and Carpenter[353] had severe symptoms of Raynaud phenomenon and marked acroosteolysis of the terminal phalanges. It is conceivable that abnormal hyperelasticity, either of the supporting tissues about the arterioles or of the connective tissue in the vessel wall itself, interferes with blood flow.[84] McKusick's observations of difficulties in obtaining blood specimens by finger puncture or venipuncture in affected persons may be significant in this connection.

Miescher elastoma, also known as *elastosis perforans serpiginosa*, is an occasional finding in Marfan syndrome, pseudoxanthoma elasticum (PXE), and OI, and it has also been observed in

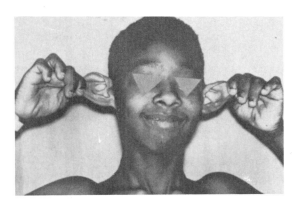

Fig. 6-14. Boy with EDS, 12 years of age, demonstrating stretchability of his ears. (Courtesy Dr. Glenn R. Stoutt, Louisville, Ky.)

EDS.[272,332,333,546] McKusick encountered elastosis perforans serpiginosa in a 13-year-old boy with particularly extensive involvement of the arms and nape of neck (see Fig. 6-33). This patient had EDS IV, in which the elastoma may be especially likely to occur. McKusick also knew of another boy with elastosis perforans who had frequent ecchymoses and died at 18 years of age of a hemorrhage from the thyrocervical trunk.[174]

The combination of neurofibromatosis and EDS in the same person has been reported in at least three instances.[115,179,506] Since the former condition is comparatively common, the association is probably coincidental. Chance could also explain the occurrence of dermatomyositis,[11] epidermolysis bullosa,[274] and systemic lupus erythematosus combined with myasthenia gravis[74] in patients with EDS.

The skin and joint changes in persons with EDS are almost always evident from an early age. However, Jacobs[242] described a patient in whom the manifestations seemed quite clearly to appear first at the age of 29 years. Although the patient had been a pugilist, no friability of the skin had been noted earlier. Golden and Garret[177] reported a similar case, a patient with onset of easy bruising, cutaneous fragility, and poor wound healing after the age of 26 years. It is difficult to conceive of a pathogenetic mechanism for late onset in EDS, and it seems possible that one or both of these reports relate to a condition other than EDS.

Physiologic studies of skin elasticity and tensile strength have been undertaken in individuals with normal skin and persons with EDS, using a variety of techniques.* Skin elasticity† can be measured with the "pinchmeter" of Olmsted, Page, and Corcoran,[364] with the elastometer of Schade, or by the simple, although subjective, method of Ellis and Bundick.[155] In this last technique the skin of the dorsum of the wrist is elevated between the forefinger and thumb and relative elasticity estimated. With aging, normal skin becomes progressively less extensible. This observation may partially explain the tendency for the cutaneous fragility and extensibility in EDS to become less striking as the affected individual ages.

Rollhäuser[419] studied the skin tensile strength of a 35-year-old man with EDS and found it to be quite low (0.34 kg/mm²). This researcher found parallel changes in the tensile strength and extensibility of tendons, suggesting that the properties measured in the skin may be constitutional and generalized. Wenzel[534] found lesser tensile strength in the skin of females and made important observations indicating reduction in the strength of the skin in normal pregnancy and in Cushing syndrome. The fragility of the skin and easy bruisability are similar in EDS and in Cushing syndrome.[282] However, in all likelihood the similarity is only superficial.

Musculoskeletal Features

Hypermobility of the joints is a cardinal feature of EDS. In the past this characteristic, together

---

*References 134, 135, 140, 190, 247, 265, 419, and 534.

†There is so much confusion in the biologic literature with reference to the term *elasticity* that some care must be exercised. Burton[84] writes as follows:

Elasticity is properly defined as the property of materials which enables them to resist deformation by the development of a resisting force or "tension." All coefficients of elasticity are defined as the ratio of this resisting force (which at equilibrium is equal to the applied deforming force, or "load") to the measure of deformation produced. Thus, by the physical definition, material of "high elasticity" resists deformation, e.g., stretching, by a large force; so that it takes a large force to produce a given deformation. A material of "low elasticity" cannot resist deformation so well, and it takes only a small force to produce the same degree of deformation. Thus glass or steel has a much higher elasticity than does rubber.

Most unfortunately, popular usage of the adjective "elastic" connotes the opposite. If a material like rubber is easily stretched, it is popularly said to be "elastic" and glass is "not so elastic" as rubber.

As used in this discussion of EDS, *elasticity* refers to physical properties like those of rubber, specifically, stretchability and restoration after deformation.

with hyperextensibility of the skin, made it possible for some persons to earn a living in fairground sideshows as "india rubber men," "elastic ladies," and "human pretzels." The range of joint movements tends to diminish as the patient becomes older, and the incidence of complications consequent on articular instability also lessens. Carter and Wilkinson[96] developed a scoring system for the semiquantitation of joint laxity in persons with recurrent dislocations. This technique was modified by Wynne-Davies[542] and, later, by Beighton and Horan.[49] In the latter system (Fig. 6-15) patients were given a score of 0 to 5, subsequently modified to 0 to 9 because of bilaterality, one point being assigned for achieving each of the following:
1. Passive dorsiflexion of the fifth finger beyond 90 degrees with the forearm flat on a table, as suggested by Ellis and Bundick[155]
2. Passive apposition of the thumb to the flexor aspect of the forearm
3. Hyperextension of the elbow beyond 10 degrees
4. Hyperextension of the knee beyond 10 degrees
5. Forward flexion of the trunk so that the palms of the hands rest easily on the floor

Population studies of the range of joint movements in individuals with normal joints have been undertaken by Ellis and Bundick,[155] who used measurements of extensibility of the fifth finger, (Fig. 6-16) and by Beighton, Solomon, and Soskolne,[52] who used the 0 to 9 scale (Fig. 6-17). These investigations have confirmed the impression that the normal range of articular movements is age related and that at any age the joints of females tend to be looser than those of males.

Methods for the objective quantitation of joint mobility and the investigation of plasticity, viscosity, and other components of joint stiffness were developed in the early 1970s.[247,248,249,463,541] Since that time further insights have been gained concerning the biomechanics of joint lubrication, which is proving to be a complex matter.[143] Computerized arthrography is now widely used for the assessment of joint stiffness and laxity.[220] The main application of these techniques is in the field of rheumatology, but they have obvious relevance to EDS.

The rheumatologic and orthopedic implications of EDS have been the subject of several reviews.[39,42,49] Joint effusions, especially in the

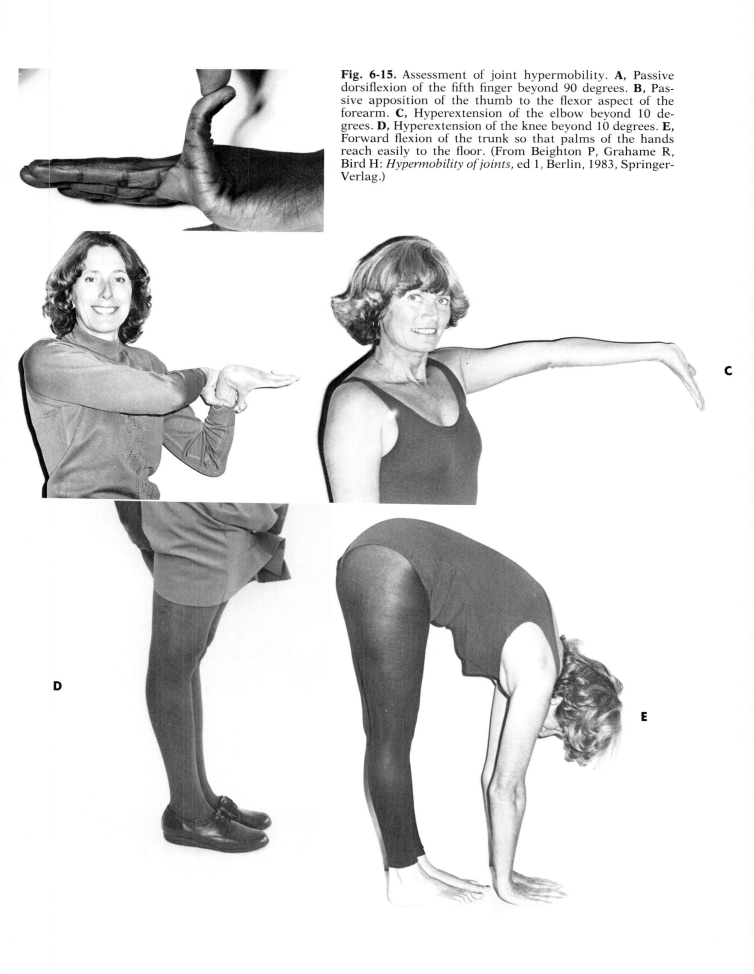

Fig. 6-15. Assessment of joint hypermobility. **A,** Passive dorsiflexion of the fifth finger beyond 90 degrees. **B,** Passive apposition of the thumb to the flexor aspect of the forearm. **C,** Hyperextension of the elbow beyond 10 degrees. **D,** Hyperextension of the knee beyond 10 degrees. **E,** Forward flexion of the trunk so that palms of the hands reach easily to the floor. (From Beighton P, Grahame R, Bird H: *Hypermobility of joints,* ed 1, Berlin, 1983, Springer-Verlag.)

Fig. 6-16. A, Ellis-Bundick method for quantifying joint mobility. **B** and **C,** Joint mobility by sex and age, as determined by the Ellis-Bundick method in 500 subjects. **B,** Women and girls show higher grades of mobility. **C,** Most young children under 5 years of age show at least 90-degree mobility. In the groups of intermediate age, incidence is appreciably greater in women. (**B** and **C** from Ellis FA, Bundick WR: *Arch Dermatol* 74:22, 1956.)

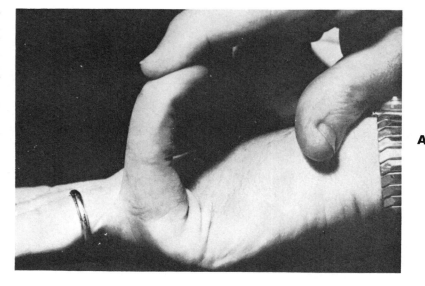

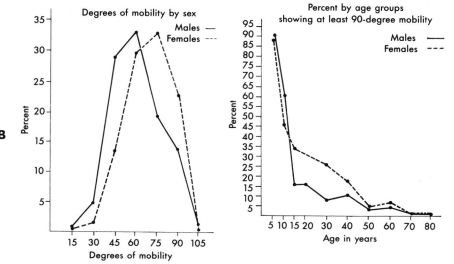

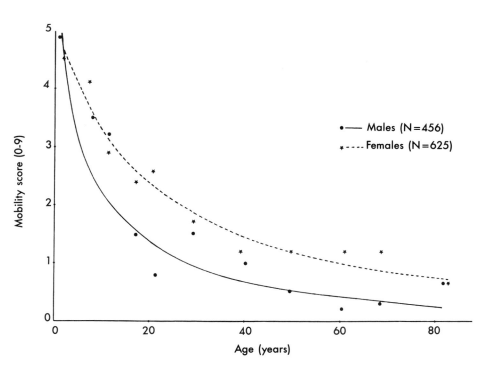

Fig. 6-17. Joint mobility in 1081 normal persons of Tswana stock, measured on the 0 to 9 scale during an epidemiologic survey in a rural community in Western Transvaal and shown as fitted curves. The range of joint movements decreases with age, falling sharply through childhood to early adulthood and more slowly thereafter. At any age females tend to be more loose-jointed than males. (From Beighton PH, Solomon L, Soskolne CL: *Ann Rheum Dis* 32:413-418, 1973.)

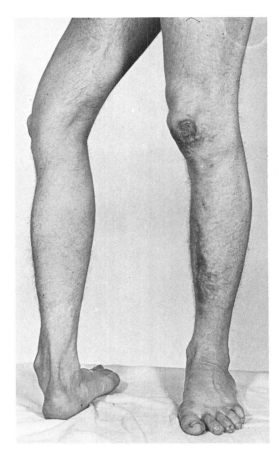

Fig. 6-18. Gross joint laxity in a patient with EDS. This young man could place his feet "back to front" and tuck his big toes into his ears. His knees were unstable, and he had recurrent sprains and effusions.

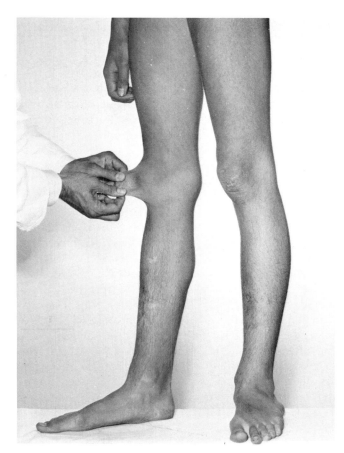

Fig. 6-19. Many persons with EDS have pes planus when weight bearing, due to altered physical properties of the connective tissues, which are responsible for maintaining the integrity of the arches of the feet.

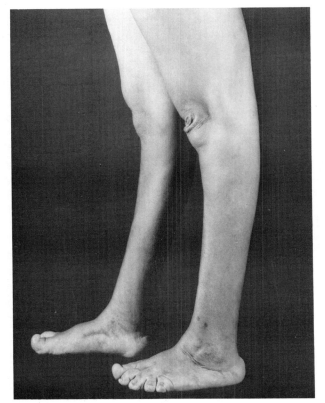

Fig. 6-20. Deformed foot in a 30-year-old schoolteacher. Several operations for clubfoot were performed in childhood. Other cardinal features of EDS were present. Dislocation of the shoulder and of the patella occurred on several occasions. Intracranial hemorrhage, presumably from berry aneurysm, occurred. The patient died at 36 years of age after an operation for a perforated sigmoid colon.

knees, are frequent because of traumatization as a result of joint instability (Fig. 6-18). Hemarthroses also occur.[347,388] Pes planus or flatfoot during weight bearing is common (Fig. 6-19), and clubfoot has been described[70,388] (Fig. 6-20). The loose-jointedness, particularly in the knees, may result in a gait and stance suggesting tabes dorsalis. Recurrent dislocation of the hip,[96,122,360,378,530] patellae,[94,95,146,360,442] shoulder,[95,246a,381] clavicle,[188] and other joints is a frequent feature. Chronic temporomandibular joint subluxation has been described,[179] as has painful subluxation of the carpometacarpal joint of the thumb.[339] Congenital dislocation of the hip is present in about 5% of affected neonates.[6,20,297,483] The recurrent dislocations of the patellae[442] are spontaneously reducible and usually represent no particular incapacitation to the patient. As in Marfan syndrome, the sternal ends of the clavicle may be loose and genu recurvatum[530] may occur. Posterior dislocation of the radial heads is occasionally a complication of joint laxity,[105] but this problem is infrequent in persons with EDS.

Persons with EDS are often able to pull their fingers out longitudinally for an appreciable distance, even to almost twice their length,[378] and allow them to snap back into place on release (Fig. 6-21). The loose-jointed hand is evident in the handshake, and the limp feel has been compared to that of a fine foam-rubber sponge[294] or a "bag of bones."

Joint instability in patients with EDS leads to a variety of mechanical problems in the digits, hands, and wrists.[173,271] In the feet piezogenic papules may cause pain during weight bearing.[255,256] These lesions are the result of herniation of the fat lobules and may share a common pathogenesis with subcutaneous spheroids.

Some patients may show restricted motion in joints such as the elbows and hips,[325] but this feature is probably a consequence of articular damage that results from instability. Radioulnar synostosis[298] has been reported,[432] although bony union is not otherwise a feature of EDS. Likewise, ectopic bone formation with formation of osseous bridges between the acetabula and the femoral trochanters has been described[261]; the pathogenesis may have involved hemorrhage resulting from increased joint mobility.

Spinal malalignment is relatively frequent*

---

*References 126, 360, 419, 445, 482, 483, 506, and 534.

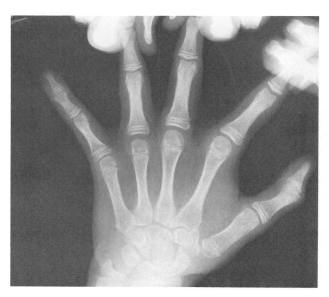

Fig. 6-21. Radiograph of the hand of a young man with EDS, demonstrating how the fingers can often be pulled out longitudinally for an appreciable distance.

(Fig. 6-22, *A*), but cord compression is rare. Coventry[114] observed thoracolumbar kyphoscoliosis with anterior wedging of several vertebrae; long, giraffelike neck; downward curvature of the upper ribs; and a tendency to reversal of the normal spinal curves. It seems plausible that laxity in the joints of the shoulder girdle and downward dragging with gravity may result in sloping shoulders and a long neck. Spina bifida occulta is described,[265] as well as wedge-shaped deformity of vertebral bodies (Fig. 6-22, *B*)[325]; the former is almost certainly a chance concomitant, whereas the latter is probably a result of spinal malalignment.

Spondylolisthesis was a painful problem to two of McKusick's patients during their teens. The patient shown in Fig. 6-23 had spinal fusion at the age of 18 years and has been well since that time. The second patient had spontaneous relief of symptoms. Although atlanto axial dislocation has been encountered in a Japanese patient,[349] it is rare in patients with EDS.

Muscular hypotonicity may be an initial feature in early childhood; thus EDS enters into the differential diagnosis of the "floppy infant" (Fig. 6-24). An initial misdiagnosis of amyotonia congenita was known to McKusick; Smith[458] described a similar experience. The initial manifes-

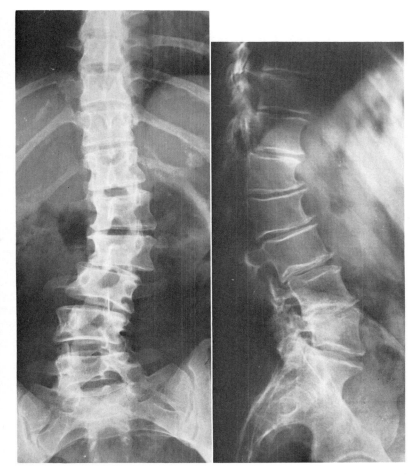

A

B

Fig. 6-22. A, Radiograph of the spine in a young woman with EDS I. She had intermittent backache due to spinal malalignment but did not have any evidence of spinal cord compression. **B,** Mild asymmetric vertebral wedging was probably secondary to the spinal malalignment. (From Beighton P, Grahame R, Bird H: *Hypermobility of joints,* ed 1, Berlin, 1983, Springer-Verlag.)

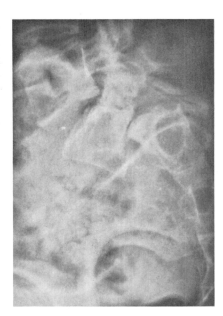

Fig. 6-23. Severe spondylolisthesis in a 17-year-old girl with all the cardinal features of EDS. Fifth lumbar vertebra has almost slipped off the first sacral vertebra.

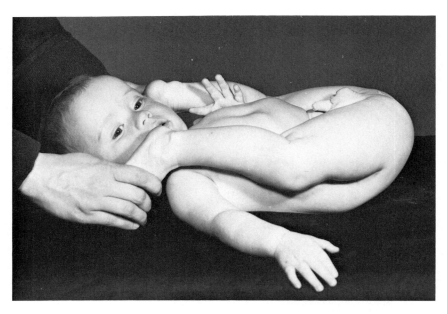

Fig. 6-24. Child with EDS who came to medical attention with hypotonia and was initially misdiagnosed as having a neuromyopathy. EDS enters into the differential diagnosis of any "floppy" infant.

tations of EDS may simulate a primary muscle disease.[22]

Stature and habitus are usually normal in persons with EDS, although affected individuals sometimes have orthopedic problems. Mild thoracic asymmetry is fairly common, either in isolation or as a consequence of kyphoscoliosis[49,544] (Fig. 6-25, *A*).

Severe leg cramps and muscle pains that occur at night and while sitting at rest can be problems in patients with EDS. Beighton[40] observed this feature in 43 of 100 patients; the cramps may result indirectly from the loose-jointedness, although the pathogenetic mechanism is obscure. Kirk, Ansell, and Bywaters[266] had previously noted that cramps and muscle pains were commonly associated with simple joint hypermobility. In the same context, easy fatigability of uncertain origin is a frequent complaint of EDS patients. The limb pains in patients with EDS are occasionally of sufficient severity to mimic rheumatic disease.[368]

Hematologic Features

Many individuals with EDS have bruising after minor trauma,[9a] but in the majority abnormal bleeding usually is not a problem. Persons with

EDS IV are an exception, since vascular phenomena predominate in this form of EDS. It is probable that hemorrhagic complications are the consequence of abnormalities in the walls of large and small blood vessels rather than a reflection of any fundamental defect of the clotting mechanism.

Although little bleeding occurs from the skin wounds, easy bruisability is the rule. Scarring and recurrent unexplained bruising in children with EDS can lead to a misdiagnosis of child abuse,[370,414] and in view of the medical and legal implications, EDS should feature prominently in the differential diagnosis of any "battered child" (Fig. 6-25, *B*).

Bleeding from the gums may occur during brushing of the teeth, from tooth sockets after dental extractions, from the pharynx after tonsillectomy, and at the site of operations performed on the joints.[516] Petechiae in late pregnancy and prolonged postpartum hemorrhage have been described.[433] Gastrointestinal bleeding occurs in some patients.[102,103,242,433,514] Recurrent hemoptysis has been described.[417] In a patient known to McKusick a strain of the tendons of the hamstring muscles at the knee resulted in a subcutaneous hematoma that extended down to the ankle. Despite this apparent tendency to bleed, in some patients

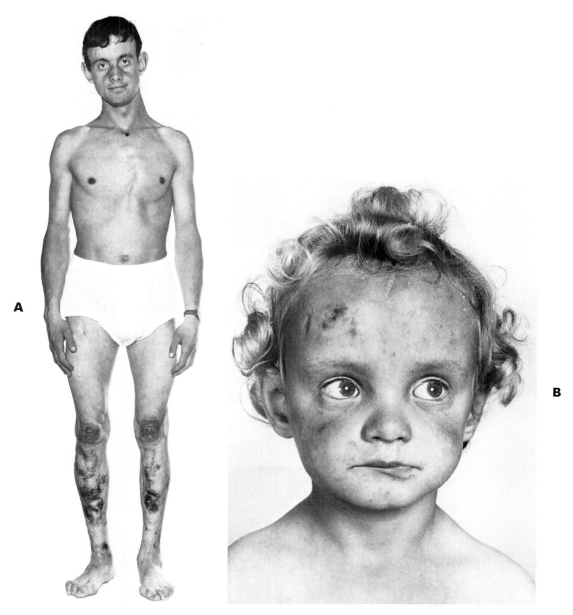

Fig. 6-25. A, Thoracic asymmetry in young man with EDS I. Characteristic darkly pigmented papyraceous scars are evident on shins. **B,** Same patient in infancy. Facial bruising and scarring could easily have led to misdiagnosis of the battered child syndrome. (From Beighton P, Grahame R, Bird H: *Hypermobility of joints*, ed 1, Berlin, 1983, Springer-Verlag.)

it is difficult to obtain blood specimens by finger puncture, and venipunctures also can be difficult, seemingly because of small, collapsed superficial veins.

EDS must be included in the differential diagnosis of familial hemophilia-like states. All results of coagulation tests are usually normal,[81,242,477,504] except that results of the Rumpel-Leede test may be positive.* In a family with EDS that was transmitted through four generations a mother and

---

*References 168, 213, 372, 378, 425, 433, and 506.

daughter showed deficiency of plasma thromboplastin component[308] (Christmas factor, factor IX). A deficiency of Hageman factor in a boy with EDS was described by Fantl, Morris, and Sawers,[158] but a brother without EDS also had the clotting defect. Kashiwagi, Riddle, and Abraham[260] and Green, Schuman, and Barron[193] reported on studies of a patient with EDS, probable deficiency of platelet factor III, and morphologic alteration of platelet structure demonstrable by electron microscopy; the platelets tended to clump and showed osmiophilic blunting of processes with few or no dendrites. Estes[156] observed abnormally large platelets, some of which also showed a functional abnormality, in patients with EDS and in persons with other heritable disorders of connective tissue. Goodman, Levitsky, and Friedman[182] found defective platelet thromboplastic function and clot retraction, as well as a vascular defect. On the other hand, Day and Zarafonetis[125] and Wigzell and Ogston[535] demonstrated normal coagulation in patients with EDS and concluded that the bleeding is the result of defects other than those of platelets or plasma clotting factors. Nevertheless, several other authors have documented abnormalities of platelet morphology or function in patients with EDS[14,100,259,366]; these accumulated observations cannot all be fortuitous, and it is possible that, as with other reported pathologic changes, platelet defects may be present in some forms of EDS and not in others.

Arterial Complications

Complications related to fragility of the aorta and other large arteries are a major cause of death in patients with EDS IV.[*] This situation is presumably a reflection of an underlying abnormality of type III collagen, which is an essential condition of this form of EDS. Since type III collagen is a major constituent of arterial walls, it is not surprising that vascular complications predominate in EDS IV. Indeed, it is likely that the vast majority of reports of serious vascular incidents in patients with EDS concern this type of the disorder.

Spontaneous rupture of large arteries has emerged as a major complication of EDS IV.[25,219,428] In an early report McFarland and Fuller[324] documented a 12-year-old boy who suffered rupture of the right popliteal artery, which apparently occurred spontaneously during sleep. Trauma at play during the previous day could not be ex-

cluded. These authors also reported a 17-year-old boy who died of rupture of the right subclavian artery, which occurred during the course of strenuous cheering at a basketball tournament. Lynch, Larsen, and Wilson[310] described a boy who died after a tear of the lower thoracic aorta. Autopsy showed fistulae between the abdominal aorta and inferior vena cava and the left common iliac artery and vein. After the delineation of EDS IV in the mid-1960s numerous reports were made of arterial catastrophes in this specific form of the condition[*]; in other articles the type of EDS is not specified,[†] but it is likely that some if not all of the affected persons had EDS IV.

Multiple intracranial aneurysms were present in a 47-year-old woman with typical EDS who was studied by Rubinstein and Cohen.[425] (A brother also had EDS. One of her children died at 1 month of age of massive ectasia of the gastrointestinal tract through the abdominal wall. Another child, who had hyperelastic skin, died at 2 years of age of a congenital cardiac defect). François et al.[166] observed a patient with an intracranial arteriovenous aneurysm in whom spontaneous cure occurred as a result of thrombosis in this blood vessel. Intracranial arteriovenous fistulae also were described by Schoolman and Kepes[441] and Graf.[189] In the last instance multiple intracranial aneurysms were found at autopsy.[23] A brother had a spontaneously developing arteriovenous fistula. Bannerman, Ingall, and Graf[23a] reported the cases of a brother and sister with EDS IV who spontaneously developed carotid-cavernous fistulae; a mother and daughter in a collateral branch of their family had died of subarachnoid hemorrhage. Other authors have also reported the occurrence of carotid-cavernous fistulae.[160,164,200,283] McKusick observed a 30-year-old woman with EDS who had a subarachnoid hemorrhage, presumably as a result of an intracranial aneurysm. Cerebrovascular accidents that may have the same basis were described in normotensive middle-aged women by several authors.[192,432,441] Type III collagen has been shown to be faulty in kindreds with congenital intracranial aneurysms,[392] and this substance seems to represent a pathogenetic link between familial aneurysms and EDS IV.

Dissecting aneurysm of the aorta is an uncom-

---

*References 57, 61, 175, 283, 284, and 511.

*References 60, 100, 278, 447, 508, and 538.

†References 27, 35, 101, 148, 232, and 234.

mon but well-established complication.[40,383] In the fourth edition of this book, McKusick gave detailed accounts of the features evident on clinical examination and during autopsy in several persons who died after dissection of the aorta or major arteries. He drew attention to other similar cases in the literature[185,186,340,341]; hindsight permits the assumption that these affected individuals probably had EDS type IV. In addition to dissecting aortic aneurysms in EDS, instances of dilation of the ascending aorta with aortic regurgitation have occurred, which simulate the changes seen in Marfan syndrome.[99,302,504] Excision of an aneurysm of the abdominal aorta was undertaken in an affected 17-year-old boy by Burnett et al.,[82] and rupture and dissection of the abdominal aorta was successfully repaired by Serry, Agomouh, and Goldin.[443]

Aneurysms of the vertebral arteries may occur[26]; Brodribb[77] successfully cured an aneurysm of the left vertebral artery by means of proximal and distal ligation. The aneurysm was probably a false aneurysm, although the distinction from "true" aneurysm can be difficult to make. The same patient was described by Edwards and Taylor.[153] Dales and O'Neill[121] documented a comparable false aneurysm that developed in the left axilla of a 15-year-old boy while he was lifting a mattress. Ballooning of the aneurysm occurred 12 days later. Because of arterial friability, suture of the torn artery was not possible; therefore proximal ligation of the axillary artery was performed. Aneurysm of the internal carotid artery in patients with EDS IV has been documented,[426] as has resection of an aneurysmal dilation of a patent ductus arteriosus in a 3-year-old Chinese girl.[99] Operative occlusion of a hepatic arterial aneurysm also was successful.[359]

The 18-year-old patient of Garrick[174] who had elastosis perforans and frequent ecchymoses and died at 18 years of age of rupture of the thyrocervical arterial trunk, probably had EDS type IV. Anning[9] gave a dermatologic report of another patient who was found to have elastosis perforans at 18 years of age and died of "dissecting aneurysm of the aorta" at 20 years of age. This individual had "multiple tears of the aorta, which was thin walled, and histological examination of the aorta revealed degenerative elastic tissue." Again, EDS IV seems to be a likely diagnostic possibility.

Because of friability of tissues, including those of arterial walls, arteriograms and other procedures requiring arterial puncture[310,428,455] can be hazardous in patients with EDS. An affected woman died of a tear in the ascending aorta that was sustained during investigation of her intracranial arteriovenous fistula,[441] and perforation of the superior vena cava occurred during digital angiography in another person with the disorder.[145] Complications of this type are not inevitable, as demonstrated by uneventful angiography in a patient with EDS and multiple aneurysms.[337] Ultrasound may be useful in demonstrating intraabdominal aneurysms in EDS.[113]

Traumatic vascular accidents in EDS are occasionally followed by neurologic complications. In an 11-year-old girl, Bell's palsy followed a large subgaleal hematoma that was produced by a fall and a blow to the occiput.[477] High median nerve palsy after rupture of the branchial artery has been documented,[73] as has traumatic disruption of the subclavian artery and brachial plexus[119] after simple reduction of a dislocated shoulder. In the latter patient, a Mexican girl, amputation of the arm was ultimately required.

Gastrointestinal Features

One group of gastrointestinal manifestations in patients with EDS can be related to tissue extensibility, and the occurrence of these manifestations generally parallels the severity of the other stigmata of the disorder. These problems include an eventration of the diaphragm[51,386] (Fig. 6-12), hiatus hernia,[547] and rectal prolapse.[142] Diverticula of the stomach, duodenum, and colon may occur together[78] or separately (Fig. 6-26). Megaesophagus, megatrachea, and megacolon have been encountered in the same patient.[345] Ptosis viscerum,[4,369] torsion of the stomach,[307,386] and gastric atony[423] have been reported, as have small bowel dilation[208] and megaduodenum with malabsorption resulting from bacterial overgrowth.[224]

Abnormalities of the viscera sometimes cluster in the same patient. For instance, Schippers and Dittler[440] described the concurrence of diverticula of the colon, bile duct, and urinary bladder; the patient also had multiple arterial aneurysms and spontaneous perforation of the bowel. In a similar report Toyohara et al.[498] documented a case of a Japanese boy with a giant epiphrenic diverticulum of the esophagus and diverticula of the stomach, colon, and urinary bladder. Ectasia of the colon, which produced intractable constipation in an adolescent boy and necessitated colectomy to forestall imminent perforation, was recorded by Shi, Bohane, and Bowring.[448] Iwama et al.[241] re-

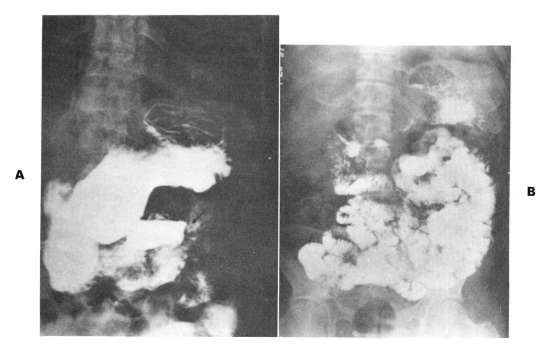

Fig. 6-26. Gastrointestinal radiograph of a 64-year-old man with EDS who had dissection of the ascending aorta and other serious complications. **A,** A large duodenal diverticulum arises in the region of the ligament of Treitz and extends up behind the stomach. **B,** A diverticulum in the second part of the duodenum was also demonstrated.

ported the case of a woman with eventration of the diaphragm and volvulus of the stomach, in whom three episodes of colonic and jejunal perforation had occurred.

Spontaneous perforation of the bowel and severe gastrointestinal hemorrhage are uncommon but potentially lethal complications that occur predominantly in EDS IV.[32,452] In most instances these problems are probably the result of a combination of friability of the bowel wall and fragility of blood vessels. Perforation is often accompanied by hemorrhage and may result from bleeding into the wall of the gut.[34] Perforation occurs most frequently in the colon,* but the small intestine is sometimes involved.[7] The surgical management of perforation can be difficult, since tissue fragility may pose practical problems during operation. The long-term prognosis is poor, since repeated perforations of the bowel may occur.[6] Spontaneous rupture of the esophagus has been documented[198]; splenic rupture is another rare but potentially lethal complication.[209] Hematemesis and melena caused by gastroesophageal reflux[32] represent other hazards in EDS IV. Acute appendicitis[233] and acute pancreatitis[435] are probably chance concomitants, although the latter occurred in two out of eight affected sibs in a large Chilean family with EDS type II, which suggests some common pathogenetic mechanism.

The following experience of McKusick and his colleagues at The Johns Hopkins Hospital in Baltimore provides a valuable perspective of the serious gastrointestinal complications:

A female patient had rupture of the sigmoid colon at the age of 24 years and again at 26 years. Each episode was preceded by rectal bleeding, suggesting that intramural bleeding may be a factor in rupture, along with friability of the bowel wall. The patient died at the age of 36 years after an operation for perforated sigmoid colon. At autopsy multiple intestinal hematomas were found, as well as a large hepatic hematoma. A second patient, who had the phenotype of EDS IV (Fig. 6-27), had an attack of severe abdominal pain at the age of 17 years, three weeks after a mild bout of gastroenteritis.

*References 51, 207, 241, 451, 461a, 462, and 484.

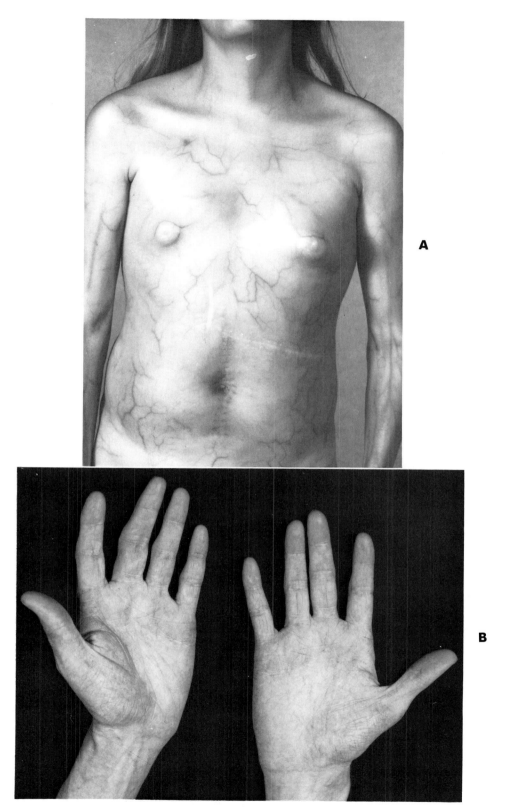

Fig. 6-27. Young woman with EDS IV. **A,** She had thin, translucent skin with an easily visible venous pattern. Surgery had been performed for pyloric stenosis in infancy, traumatic rupture of the spleen at 12 years of age, and spontaneous intestinal rupture at 19 years of age. **B,** Her palms had many creases and a blotchy appearance.

Surgery was not performed, but a subsequent barium enema showed narrowing of the distal colon. When she was 19 years old, a second attack of severe abdominal pain developed while she was sitting quietly at home. Laparotomy revealed a massive intramural hematoma of the jejunum, necessitating resection of an 18-inch-long segment of bowel. At this operation the narrowed area in the colon was found to show mural fibrosis consistent with intramural hematoma at that site two years previously. The patient continues to have episodes of partial intestinal obstruction, apparently due to intramural bowel hemorrhage. She learned to recognize the event when it developed, and conservative measures usually sufficed to "tide her over." This patient had had pyloric stenosis of apparently conventional type which was operated on at the age of 7 weeks. Also, when she was 12 years old, splenic rupture occurred after a fall from a bicycle.

Genitourinary Features

Diverticula of the bladder are probably frequent in patients with EDS.[76,476,545] Diverticula are sometimes found incidentally by contrast studies, but they can also produce micturition difficulties and cause predisposition to urinary infection. Bladder diverticula have been described in a 47-year-old man[151] and in a young infant in whom the diverticulum extended into both a sliding left inguinal and an umbilical hernia.[139] Levard et al.[296] reported an affected 5-year-old boy with two large bladder diverticula, which caused severe micturition disturbance, and identified nine similar cases in the literature. They commented that recurrence after surgical correction was usual and speculated that the diverticula were the result of abnormalities of the vesical wall rather than vesicourethral obstruction. Nevertheless, mechanical impediment to urinary flow can certainly occur, since bladder neck obstruction in a patient with EDS was recorded by Eadie and Wilkins.[151] At a different anatomic level McKusick has encountered bilateral congenital anomalies of the ureteropelvic junction in patients with EDS, and Levine and Michael[297] have described a similar anomaly.

Bannerman, Graf, and Upson[23] reported finding polycystic kidneys in patients with EDS in two of 20 cases of medullary sponge kidney. They considered that this must be more than coincidence and suspected that the condition of medullary sponge kidney[344] can have different causes, among them the connective tissue defect of EDS. A child with polycystic kidneys and EDS was documented by Mauseth, Lieberman, and Heuser.[319] Imahori et al.[239] noted multiple cysts of the kidney and multiple arterial aneurysms in a patient with EDS IV. It may be relevant that in a broader context congenital cystic kidneys and intracranial aneurysms represent a well-known[63] but poorly understood association.

Cardiac Features

Structural cardiac abnormalities occur in low frequency in patients with EDS, without any obvious predilection for any particular type of the disorder.[38,295,449] There have been reports of interatrial septal defect,[167,439] tetralogy of Fallot,[521] partial persistent atrioventricular canal,[158] aneurysm of the sinus of Valsalva,[118,504] coronary artery aneurysms,[138] bicuspid right atrioventricular valve,[324] aortic incompetence,[454] and atrial septal defect.[66,444] McKusick studied a patient with longstanding electrocardiographic evidence of incomplete right bundle-branch block without subjective or other objective cardiovascular manifestations, and Sestak[444] also observed incomplete right bundle-branch block in two patients; in one of these, atrial septal defect was present. Cardiac conduction defects together with mitral valve prolapse have been observed by Cabeen, Jr. et al.[91]

Madison, Bradley, and Castillo[313] described a 17-year-old patient with features of EDS and intractable heart failure that resulted from mitral and tricuspid regurgitation. Autopsy findings seemed to exclude rheumatic heart disease and showed redundant chordae tendineae and valve cusp changes compatible with the same defect as in other connective tissue structures. Papillary muscle dysfunction has also been documented in EDS,[10] and mitral valve prolapse has been recognized in some patients,[75] particularly in those with EDS types III and IV.[243] The chordae tendineae of the atrioventricular valves are tendons, and the cusps themselves and the fibrous skeleton of the heart are largely collagenous. On this basis it is perhaps surprising that serious cardiac difficulties occur so relatively uncommonly in patients with EDS.

Pulmonary Features

Pulmonary complications are uncommon in patients with EDS, although instances of mediastinal and subcutaneous emphysema[372] and spontaneous pneumothorax have been reported.[189,365,457] McKusick drew attention to the autopsy findings in a case of dissecting aneurysm in a patient with

EDS, in which subpleural blebs in the lungs and subcutaneous emphysema were revealed. In another case Clarke, Kuhn, and Vitto[102] described the ultrastructure and biochemistry of collagen in pulmonary tissues.

Hemoptysis is a rare manifestation of the bleeding diathesis in EDS.[117,192,242] André et al.[7] observed a young woman who had many episodes of bleeding from various sites, in whom bilateral hemothorax developed without any obvious precipitating factors. Dilation of the trachea and bronchi has been described[1,345] in patients with presumed EDS. This tracheobronchiomegaly is sometimes termed the Mounier-Kuhn syndrome.[1] Multiple severe pulmonary artery stenoses of uncertain significance have been recorded in an affected child.[293]

In a review of the features of 24 patients with EDS, Ayres et al.[18] documented hemoptysis in five and bullous lung disease in two. One of these latter individuals, who had EDS IV, had experienced three episodes of spontaneous pneumothorax, and he also had tracheobronchomegaly. No consistent spirometric abnormalities were detected, but eight persons had elevated gas-transfer coefficients. The authors speculated that this factor might have been the consequence of an increased intrapulmonary vascular volume.

Neurologic Features

The nervous system is not primarily involved in cases of EDS, but major neurologic dysfunction may result from vascular accidents (see the section, Arterial Complications). In addition, articular dislocations and subluxations can lead to nerve damage and spinal malalignment can cause cord compression, although neither of these problems is common. Attention was drawn to neurologic involvement in EDS by Reed,[407] and these problems were subsequently reviewed by Pretorius and Butler.[402] More recently Hagino et al.[199] outlined the role of computed tomography in the evaluation of central nervous system complications in patients with EDS.

Mental retardation is not a feature of EDS, and in the small number of persons affected in this way the association is probably coincidental[290,305]; in a few, however, mental retardation may be the result of complications associated with prematurity.[133] The infrequent occurrence of epilepsy in patients with EDS may have the same basis. Neuropsychiatric symptoms occasionally oc-

cur in affected persons,[162] although the majority of patients with EDS are apparently well adjusted to their disabilities.

In some persons with EDS, neurologic problems of uncertain pathogenesis have developed. For instance, acute brachial neuropathy without obvious arterial damage has been observed.[262,373,376] In a 19-year-old woman with EDS VII, left-sided hemiplegia developed 3 weeks after a head injury. Dodge and Shillito[139] described the gradual development of an encephalocele (essentially, a cerebral hernia) in an infant with EDS who died in the third year of life.

A few specific neurologic disorders have been encountered in patients with EDS. In one 61-year-old patient EDS coexisted with amyotrophic lateral sclerosis.[354] McKusick found it impossible to agree with the authors' contention[353] that an etiologic connection between the two conditions existed. Familial spastic paraplegia with platelet dysfunction in conjunction with EDS II has been documented[100] in a father and his four offspring. These associations are probably fortuitous. EDS can easily be mistaken for a neuromyopathy if hypotonicity is prominent during infancy. The correct diagnosis usually becomes apparent after specialized investigations or after the characteristic skin scarring develops in early childhood. Misdiagnosis at a later stage is unusual, but in a case known to McKusick, Oppenheim disease (amyotonia congenita)[195] was the initial diagnosis when the patient was first seen at 4 years of age.

Ocular Features

Changes in the ocular adnexa, the cornea, the sclera, the suspensory mechanism of the lens, and the fundus of patients with EDS have been described. These abnormalities occur in all forms of the condition, but additional severe complications, notably, scleral perforation and retinal detachment, are prominent features of EDS VI (ocular-scoliotic type).

Minor ocular manifestations are present in a significant proportion of affected persons with all types of the disorder. For instance, the skin about the eyes often lies in redundant folds (Fig. 6-28) and can be pulled out to a considerable distance, as can the skin elsewhere. Epicanthal folds are frequent*; epicanthus may disappear as the patient grows older, when it is replaced by an appearance

---

*References 8, 58, 250, 356, 401, 438, and 446.

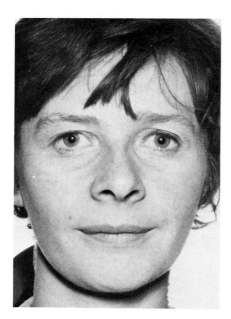

Fig. 6-28. Young woman with EDS I. The redundant skin on her upper eyelids interferred with the application of cosmetics. (From Beighton P: *The Ehlers-Danlos syndrome*, London, 1970, William Heinemann Medical Books.)

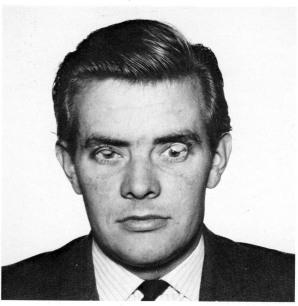

Fig. 6-29. Méténier sign; ease of eversion of the upper eyelids. This young man could fix his upper eyelids in this position by means of a winking maneuver.

of widely spaced eyes. This feature appears to represent not true hypertelorism but a change in the soft tissues at each side of the nose, resulting in telecanthus. In this situation the eyes may have a parrotlike or owllike appearance, as demonstrated in Fig. 6-14. Méténier[334] has lent his name to a frequent phenomenon, namely, unusual ease in everting the upper lid (Fig. 6-29). Internal strabismus is frequent.[30,111,244,446]

In EDS VI, the ocular-scoliotic type, eye manifestations include microcornea, glaucoma, retinal detachment, and rupture of the globe from minor trauma. May and Beauchamp[320] studied a girl with microcornea, cornea plana, keratoconus posticus, stromal haze at the level of Bowman layer, and a peripheral ring opacity suggestive of anterior embryotoxon. Several other ocular abnormalities have been mentioned in isolated case reports published in the early literature; hindsight permits the assumption that many if not all of the affected persons probably had EDS VI. These manifestations include blue sclerae,* microcornea,[438] and megalocornea.[71] Microcornea with associated glaucoma was described in one patient[150] in

whom the small size of the cornea was thought to be responsible, at least indirectly, for an impediment to ocular drainage. The cornea was abnormally large and thin in one reported case.[71] Keratoconus has been encountered,[281,415,493] as has corneal dystrophy.[399] Ectopia lentis occurred in at least one twice-reported patient[492,493] in whom operative repair was complicated by wound dehiscence.

Retinal changes have been reported in a few persons with uncategorized forms of EDS. Bonnet[70] described and illustrated changes in the fundus consisting of retinitis proliferans, pigment spots that were interpreted as residua of microhemorrhages, and detachment of the retina of the secondary type (no retinal tear was detected). Retinal detachment occurred bilaterally in the patient shown in Fig. 6-35, and it has been reported after trauma to the eye[110] and in a family in which several members had associated myopia.[383] Situs inversus of the disc, which has been seen in EDS III,[163] is probably a chance concomitant.

Green, Friedman-Kien, and Banfield[194] found typical angioid streaks in two of six affected members of a kindred with EDS. To the best of their knowledge this was the first description of angioid

---

*References 33, 72, 150, 318, 424, and 493.

streaks in patients with EDS and without skin manifestations of PXE. The relationship of PXE and EDS is discussed on p. 642.

Oral and Dental Features

Periodontosis is a major feature of EDS VIII, although not exclusive to this type of the disorder. Affected persons have progressive breakdown of the gums and destruction of the alveolar bone, with loss of the teeth by early adulthood. Slootweg and Beemer[456] recognized fibrinoid deposits during histologic studies of the gums of a girl with EDS VIII and suggested that this abnormality might be a useful diagnostic aid.

In addition to the preponderance of dental problems in patients with EDS VIII, involvement of oral structures is also a minor nonspecific feature of most forms of EDS.[28,225] The teeth may be maldeveloped,[291] irregularly positioned,[176,273,438] abnormally small,[290,315,400] or even absent. Crenation of the incisors has been noted in the EDS,[305,315] but this feature is also a frequent finding in persons with normal teeth. Easy fracturing of the teeth was thought by Barabas and Barabas[29] to be an expression of the generalized connective tissue defect. Multiple odontogenic keratocysts have been documented in a patient with EDS II[93]; however, dental anomalies are not a specific feature of this form of the condition. Hyperextensibility of the tongue (see Fig. 6-10, *B*) and stretchability of the buccal mucosa have already been mentioned. Cleft lip and palate have been encountered in patients with EDS,[362] although it seems likely that this association was fortuitous.

Gingival fragility, with bleeding after use of a toothbrush[250] and excessive bleeding after dental extractions, sometimes requiring transfusion,[40,184,497] is well known in patients with EDS. A soft toothbrush is recommended for these patients, and the dentist is urged to use special precautions such as avoidance of nerve blocks and extra care during scaling, lest the fragile gums be split. Grant and Aldor[192] described tearing of the buccal mucosa accompanied by severe hemorrhage during dental extraction.

Chronic or recurrent temporomandibular joint dislocation[179,430] may occur. Thexton[490] performed bilateral condylectomy in a young woman who had recurrent dislocations of the jaw; she was found to be a notorious "Munchausen," or peripatetic medical confabulator, who had visited many London hospitals and displayed a variety of dislocated joints. The implications of temporomandibular problems for anesthesia in patients with EDS have been discussed by Myers,[348] and the dental and orthodontic management of EDS has been the subject of several reviews.[112,251,358,431]

Miscellaneous Features

Parathyroid tumor with osteitis fibrosa cystica has been documented in patients with EDS.[384] After surgical correction of the hyperparathyroidism the joint laxity, particularly the scoliosis, and the fragility of the skin apparently decreased. In another patient with possible endocrinologic problems, gigantism, craniostenosis, and melanoderma were associated with EDS.[471] Other abnormalities that have been encountered in patients with EDS include hypophyseal dysfunction,[299] monostotic fibrous dysplasia of bone,[404] and urethra bifida with polydactyly.[314] These anomalies are not recognized components of EDS, and the significance, if any, of these unusual combinations is uncertain.

PREGNANCY

Pregnancy carries risks for both the mother and the baby with EDS; these are maximal in patients with EDS IV, in whom pregnancy is potentially lethal.[380] In a review of a heterogeneous group of EDS patients Beighton[35] recorded experience with pregnancy in 29 affected women who gave birth to 27 affected and 34 unaffected children. Complications included distraction of the pubic symphysis during delivery, postpartum uterine prolapse, and slow healing of perineal wounds. Several authors subsequently discussed various aspects of pregnancy in EDS.* Reports of pregnancy in specific forms of the condition include EDS II,[263] EDS III,[15,335] EDS IV,[130] and EDS X.[205]

The mother with EDS may display an increase in bruisability during pregnancy.[433] Abdominal hernia and varicosities of the leg veins and the vulva may also develop.[40] Rupture of great vessels and of the uterus are special hazards of pregnancy in patients with EDS IV, and maternal death has been recorded in this form of the condition.[380] On the positive side, women with all forms of EDS enjoy remarkable freedom from striae gravidarum.

Excessive bleeding resulting from episiotomy, spontaneous extension of episiotomy, perineal hematoma, and postpartum hemorrhage have been observed as expressions of the mother's friable tis-

---

*References 2, 39, 346, 412, 460, 461, and 487.

sues and bleeding diathesis. After cesarean section, sutures have failed to hold in the uterus and hysterectomy has been necessary.[441] Stoddard and Myers[470] performed an elective cesarean section at 39 weeks of gestation in a woman in whom a similar procedure had been carried out as an emergency procedure during her previous pregnancy. The scar in the uterine wall had completely disrupted, leaving the baby's head covered only by peritoneum and the fetal membranes. Forceps should be used with caution; there is an alarming report of an instance in which the baby was extracted by forceps along with the uterus, the posterior wall of the bladder, and part of a ureter.[40] Tyson[507] informed McKusick of other unpublished examples of uterine rupture, vaginal rupture, or avulsion of the bladder in patients with EDS.

Precocious and precipitous labor can be a complication[380,427,531,543] in pregnant women with EDS. In the presence of lax tissues the increasing weight of the fetus and the contents of the uterus acts to force cervical effacement and dilation, leading to early delivery. Some of the prematurity noted by several observers and attributed to precocious rupture of fetal membranes may be due to these maternal factors in those cases in which the mother is affected. The high incidence of premature labor in patients with EDS was first recorded by Kanof[258] and Mories.[340] Barabas[24] confirmed this observation and advanced the reasonable hypothesis that EDS defect in the connective tissue of the placental membranes (which are of fetal origin) causes predisposition to early rupture of the membranes and precocious delivery. Young et al.[543a] reported amniotic bands in two children with EDS IV and suggested that abnormal collagen in the membranes might be an important factor in band formation. In the same way, the umbilical cord may be friable and lead to difficulty in ligation.

Joint laxity in the fetus causes predisposition to congenital dislocation of the hips[6,96] and clubfoot.[70,388] Thomas, Cordier, and Algan[493] described dislocation of the shoulder in a baby delivered in breech presentation. Macfarlane[325] reported Erb palsy, which may be more likely to occur because of the excessive joint mobility. The infant with EDS is often "floppy," leading to the misdiagnosis of amyotonia congenita[195] or other infantile neuromyopathy. Bleeding in infant boys with EDS has led to the misdiagnosis of hemophilia.

McKusick, quoting the experience of his colleague Tyson,[507] commented as follows:

In the management of pregnancy in severe EDS, elective cesarean section has much to recommend it. The procedure is best performed through a lower midline abdominal incision avoiding, insofar as possible, the use of forceful tissue retraction. The uterus is entered through an incision of the lower uterine segment, with the usual repair following delivery of the infant and placenta. Closure of the abdominal wall should include the use of large retention sutures secured over plastic retention bridges, which remove tension from the suture line. After retention sutures are placed, subcuticular stitching can be performed with a non-absorbable suture. The retention sutures should be left in for 6 weeks or longer.

HETEROGENEITY

The cardinal features of EDS are hyperextensible skin, hypermobile joints, and fragile tissues. Variability in the individual features and differences in inheritance patterns permit delineation of separate forms of the disorder.[54]

With the continuing recognition of new forms of EDS and other heritable connective tissue disorders, problems have arisen concerning syndromic boundaries, classification, and nomenclature. These difficulties were addressed at a workshop held during the Seventh International Congress of Human Genetics in Berlin in 1986, and in committee meetings that followed a consensus was reached concerning syndromic definition and standardization of the nomenclature. The results of these deliberations were published in 1988 as the *International Nosology of Heritable Connective Tissue Disorders,*[56] now generally known as the *Berlin nosology.* The subcategorization of EDS, together with mode of inheritance, basic defect (when known), and the number of the entry in the catalogue, *Mendelian Inheritance in Man,*[330] (MIM number) are listed in the box on p. 217, top.

In the Berlin nosology the categories *EDS IX* and *XI* have been left vacant, since the disorders that previously occupied these slots have been reclassified. New forms of EDS that are delineated in the future will be numbered sequentially in accordance with this format.

Diagnostic features of the various types of EDS are summarized in the box on p. 217, bottom.

It is important to be aware that considerable overlap exists among the different forms of EDS and that accurate subcategorization of EDS in an

Subcategorization of Ehlers-Danlos Syndrome

Type	Basic defect	Mode of inheritance	MIM number
EDS I	Gravis type	AD	(130000)
EDS II	Mitis type	AD	(130010)
EDS III	Hypermobile type	AD	(130020)
EDS IV	Vascular	Heterogeneous	
	IV-A Acrogeric type	AD	(130050)
	IV-B Acrogeric type	AR	(225350)
	IV-C Ecchymotic type	AD	(130050)
	IV-D Others		
	(All forms have defect of type III collagen)		
EDS V	X-linked type	XL	(305200)
EDS VI	Ocular-scoliotic type	AR	(225400)
	VI-A Decreased lysyl hydroxylase activity		
	(VI-B Normal lysyl hydroxylase activity ?)*		
EDS VII	Arthrochalasis multiplex congenita	Heterogeneous	
	VII-A Structural defect of pro alpha 1(1) collagen	AD	(130060)
	VII-B Structural defect of pro alpha 2(1) collagen	AD	(130060)
	(VII-C Procollagen N-Proteinase deficiency ?)*	AR	(225410)
EDS VIII	Periodontitis type	AD	(130080)
EDS IX	Vacant (formerly occipital horn syndrome, or X-linked cutis laxa, now recategorized as a disorder of copper transport)		(304150)
EDS X	Fibronectin abnormality	AR	(225310)
EDS XI	Vacant (formerly familial joint instability, now recategorized with the familial articular hypermobility syndromes)		(147900)

From Beighton P et al: *Am J Med Genet* 29:581-594, 1988.
*The existence of these subtypes is unproven.
AD, autosomal dominant; *AR*, autosomal recessive; *MIM, Mendelian Inheritance in Man* number; *XL*, X-linked.

Diagnostic Features of Ehlers-Danlos Syndrome

Cardinal manifestations
Skin: hyperextensible with soft, velvety, doughy texture
Dystrophic scarring
Easy bruising
Joint hypermobility
Connective tissue fragility

EDS I — Cardinal manifestations in severe degree

EDS II — Cardinal manifestations in mild degree

EDS III — Marked articular hypermobility
Moderate dermal hyperextensibility
Minimal scarring

EDS IV — Variable stigmata
Severe bruising, hyperpigmentation and/or scarring
Thin skin with prominent venous plexus
Vascular rupture
Colonic perforation
Characteristic facial appearance

EDS V — Cardinal manifestations in moderate degree
X-linked inheritance

EDS VI — Cardinal manifestations in severe degree
Eye involvement (microcornea, scleral perforation, retinal detachment)
Scoliosis

EDS VII — Cardinal manifestations with marked articular hypermobility
Short stature
Micrognathia

EDS VIII — Cardinal manifestations in moderate degree
Aggressive periodontitis, gingival recession, early tooth loss

EDS X — Cardinal manifestations but skin texture normal
Petechiae
Striae distensae
Platelet aggregation defect corrected by fibronectin

From Beighton P et al: *Am J Med Genet* 29: 581-594, 1988.

individual patient may be difficult or even impossible. It is also of practical significance that EDS types I, II, and III collectively make up more than 80% of all cases and that the other types are individually rare.

EDS I (Gravis Type)

Skin hyperextensibility, joint hypermobility, and tissue fragility are present in moderate to severe degree in patients with EDS I. The bony prominences bear the characteristic scars; orthopedic complications of articular laxity are commonplace; and manifestations in other systems are not infrequent (Fig. 6-30). Autosomal dominant inheritance of EDS I is well documented; about 40% of all affected persons have this form of the disorder. There is no firm phenotypic evidence for heterogeneity within EDS I, but in the light of precedents for other heritable disorders it is possible that the condition is heterogeneous at the molecular level.

The basic defect in EDS I is unknown. Inconsistent abnormalities of the size, configuration, and organization of skin collagen fibrils have been demonstrated,[65,387,519] but these changes are found in other forms of EDS and they are not of

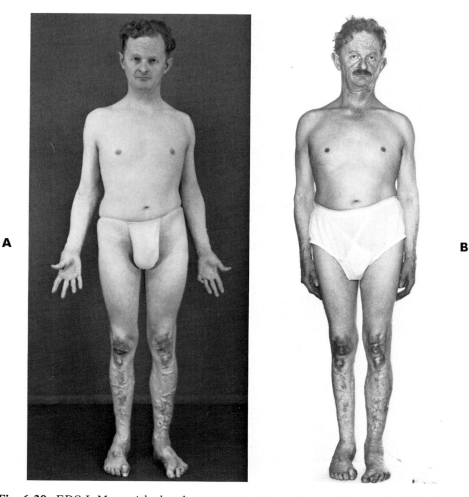

Fig. 6-30. EDS I. Man with the characteristic stigmata, notably, marked skin hyperextensibility and gross joint laxity. Tissue fragility has led to the formation of thin, darkly pigmented scars over his bony prominences. Varicose veins and clubfoot are additional features. This individual is the son of the first affected person to be depicted in the British literature, who is shown in childhood and in old age in Fig. 6-5. **A,** At 20 years of age. **B,** At 50 years of age.

diagnostic value. Defective proliferative activity of cultured skin fibroblasts has been noted,[363] but the significance of this observation is uncertain. It is equally uncertain whether collagen itself is primarily involved or whether the basic defect lies in other components of connective tissue matrix, with which collagen interacts.

Reduced amounts of type III collagen have been demonstrated in an affected father and daughter by De Paepe et al.,[131] but in view of the consistent involvement of this form of collagen in EDS IV and the wide range of phenotypic manifestations in this latter disorder, it is questionable, and perhaps a matter of semantics, whether this family should be regarded as having EDS I.

Linkage studies with the genes for type I collagen, the pro alpha 1 collagen genes (COL1A1 and COL1A2), have yielded negative results, and at present the chromosomal locus of the mutant gene is unknown. Since families with EDS are available for study, it is probably only a matter of time before linkage analyses reveal the site location of the EDS I gene.

EDS II (Mitis Type)

EDS II is a mild version of EDS I, and the skin and joint manifestations are present to a much lesser degree. Scarring is not a serious problem, and significant orthopedic complications are unusual. At the mild end of the clinical spectrum, the phenotype blends into normality, whereas at the severe end the clinical features overlap with those of EDS I.

EDS II is inherited as an autosomal dominant trait, and several large pedigrees have been published (Fig. 6-31). As with EDS I, about 40% of all patients with EDS have this form of the disorder. The condition may be heterogeneous; in this context Holzberg, Hewan-Lowe, and Olansky[230] claimed that they could identify a milder variant of EDS II, which was present in no less than 9% of a population of dermatology patients.

The nature of the basic defect in EDS II is unknown. Abnormal fibrillogenesis of dermal collagen has been recorded, but the significance of this observation is uncertain.[413] By means of linkage investigations Wordsworth et al.[539] excluded the structural gene for type II collagen (COL2A1) as a mutant locus in a large British family with EDS II. In a further series of studies in the same family the structural genes for type I collagen (COL1A1 and COL1A2) and for type III collagen (COL3A1) were also excluded.[539] Scarborough et al.[437] noted an unbalanced translocation between the long arms of chromosomes 6 and 13 in a boy with EDS II. Skin hyperextensibility has also been observed in two other persons with abnormalities of the long arm of chromosome 6[331]; therefore it is possible that the mutant gene is situated in this region of the genome.

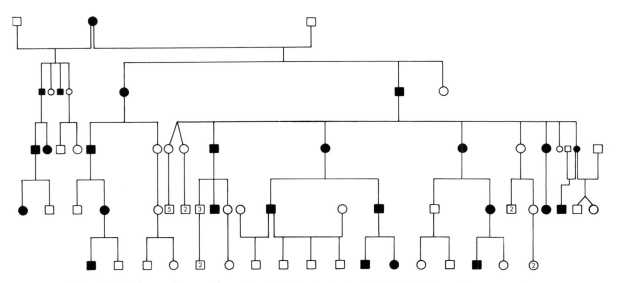

Fig. 6-31. The pedigree of an English kindred with EDS II. Affected persons have mild manifestations, and the condition is little more than a minor nuisance.

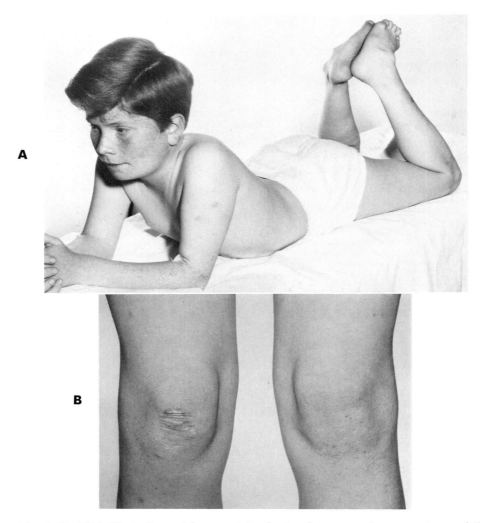

Fig. 6-32. EDS III. **A,** Boy with gross joint laxity demonstrating excessive mobility in the ankle joints. Bruising, which is minor feature of EDS III, is evident on the left upper arm. **B,** Small scars on knees, which have resulted from the mild tissue fragility that characterizes EDS III. (From Beighton P: *The Ehlers-Danlos syndrome,* London, 1970, William Heinemann Medical Books.)

EDS III (Hypermobile Type)

Gross joint laxity is the major feature of this form of EDS, and skin extensibility and splitting are present only to a minor degree (Fig. 6-32). Orthopedic complications are frequent, but the condition is otherwise innocuous.[13] The articular hypermobility decreases with aging, and the liability to sprains, subluxations, and dislocations lessens with the passage of time. About 10% of all affected persons have EDS III. Inheritance is autosomal dominant, with reasonably consistent phenotypic expression.

The basic defect in EDS III is unknown. Morphologic and organizational abnormalities of collagen fibrils have been recorded,[65] but, as in other forms of EDS, these changes are nonspecific.

Differentiation from EDS VII can be difficult; the normality of stature and mandibular configuration and the absence of the specific molecular defects found in EDS VII distinguish EDS III. Equally, there is considerable similarity between EDS III and the familial articular hypermobility syndrome (FAHS). The skin may have a soft, doughy quality in both disorders, but the presence of minor scarring and skin extensibility are suggestive of EDS III.

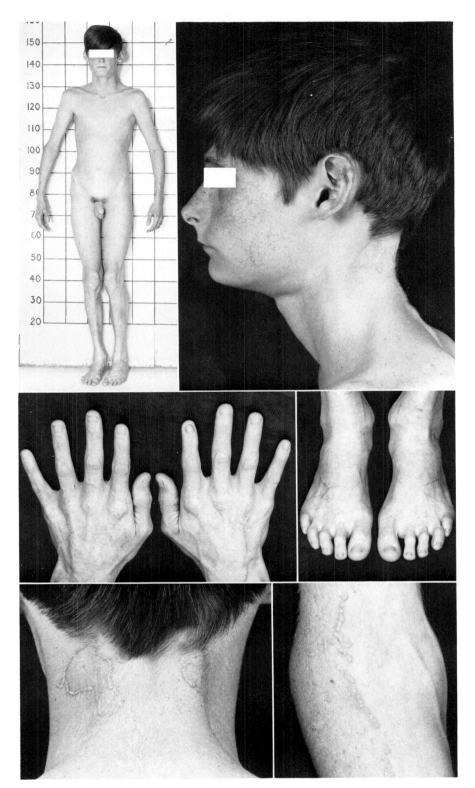

Fig. 6-33. EDS IV in a 13 year-old boy. This boy was the patient in whom Pope et al.[394] first demonstrated the defect in type III collagen. The patient died of acute rupture of the innominate artery, which was sustained at 16 years of age, while lifting a heavy bag of sugar.

EDS IV (Vascular Type)

Although rare, EDS IV is heterogeneous.[89,393,395,491] The classical clinical stigmata consist of joint hypermobility limited to the digits, minimal or absent skin hyperextensibility, and thin, pale skin with a prominent venous network and deeply pigmented scars (Fig. 6-33). The phenotype is variable, however, and some patients have features that resemble those of patients with EDS I and EDS VIII; unifying characteristics are a severe bruising tendency and a liability to the potentially lethal complications of rupture of the aorta and large arteries and spontaneous perforation of the bowel. A number of authors have recorded unusual clinical manifestations in patients with EDS IV[67]; these include organ malformation,[257] myocardial infarction,[267] and acroosteolysis with joint contractures.[300] The following case report of a patient referred to McKusick by Dr. S. Miles Bouton of Lynchburg, Virginia, exemplifies the manifestations and natural history of EDS IV:

The boy died at the age of 14 years, of dissecting aneurysm of the aorta. At the age of 7 years spontaneous rupture of the outer two coats of the sigmoid colon, with intraabdominal bleeding, produced severe pain in the left lower abdomen and required surgical exploration. Two weeks after operation symptoms of partial obstruction of the large bowel appeared but were resolved with conservative measures. Six months later partial bowel obstruction necessitated surgical release of adhesions. Less than 4 weeks later, the child was sitting in school when he was seized with left upper quadrant pain radiating to the shoulder, which doubled him over. Operation revealed peritonitis secondary to perforation of the splenic flexure of the colon. About 3 years later, at the age of 10 years, the boy had perforation of the sigmoid colon and pelvic abscess, which again required operation.

It was noted repeatedly that lacerations of the knees, legs, and scalp occurred unusually readily. However, healing of the skin occurred normally. The boy tended toward constipation.

Later, at the age of 11 years, the boy again suffered a perforation of the colon; the transverse and descending portions of the colon were removed. Four months later the monotonous accident was repeated: the ascending colon ruptured spontaneously; the remainder of the colon was resected, and the ileum was anastomosed to the rectum. In the postoperative period there was intraabdominal hemorrhage with shock, and drainage of a subdiaphragmatic hematoma was necessary.

Three years after the last surgical episode, at the age of 14 years, this apparently healthy boy, who did, however, receive skin lacerations at slight provocation, went to summer camp. One night, while in bed, he suffered the onset of severe pain in the back and abdomen. He died on the way to his home.

Autopsy revealed two transverse intimal tears, one in the descending portion of the arch and the other just proximal to the renal arteries. A large volume of blood occupied the left pleural cavity. The entire aorta and its branches appeared to be unusually delicate. Dissection extended from the reflection of the pericardial sac to the bifurcation of the aorta and into the right iliac artery.

On histologic study the bowel removed at surgery revealed disarrangement, irregular development, and, in places, marked hypoplasia of the smooth muscle elements.

All persons with EDS IV have abnormalities of type III collagen,[16,17,393,397] and a wide variety of mutations have been demonstrated at the molecular level.[403] A major subgroup of EDS IV patients have reduced serum levels of the type III procollagen aminopropeptide. Determination of the serum concentration of this peptide is not difficult and represents a useful diagnostic indicator.[467]

In the Berlin nosology, EDS IV is subcategorized into acrogeric and ecchymotic types, with further subdivision in terms of the mode of genetic transmission. The ecchymotic form is probably the same as the "arterial" type of Barabas[25] and the "status vascularis" documented many years previously by Sack.[429] Pope[391] made the point that there appears to be a continuous clinical spectrum from patients with severe skin changes to patients with almost no skin changes, so distinction between ecchymotic and acrogeric subtypes may be unnecessary. It is clear that the limits of syndromic definition on a basis of the clinical phenotype have been reached in EDS IV. An alternative approach would be to define the disorder in terms of the biomolecular defect, since all affected persons have abnormalities of type III collagen. Even this arrangement is unsatisfactory, however, because some individuals with abnormal type III collagen have familial cerebral aneurysms in the absence of the EDS IV phenotype,[392] whereas in other kindreds the stigmata of EDS IV and cerebral aneurysms coexist.[397] Furthermore, familial aneurysms of the abdominal aorta in the absence of any stigmata of EDS may also result from abnormalities of type III collagen.[270,270a] Pope[391] provided the following information concerning the basic defect in EDS IV:

1. *Genetics.* Despite early reports suggesting recessive inheritance, all cases studied at the biochemical and molecular level have shown evidence of heterozygosity for dominant mutations. In particular, the presumptive autosomal recessive form described by Sulh et al.[474] ("EDS IV D") in the case of two sibs born to consanguineous parents is apparently not associated with defects in type III procollagen synthesis.

2. *Biochemical defects.* Structural defects in pro alpha 1 (III) collagen chains result in reduced or abnormal type III collagen, or both, in tissues. Biochemical phenotypes that can be distinguished in fibroblast cultures follow:

    Synthesis and early intracellular degradation of defective pro alpha 1 (III) chains without significant intracellular storage[478]
    Synthesis of unstable type III procollagen that accumulates within the cell because of impaired secretion[88,479]
    Synthesis of defective type III procollagen that can be secreted, although more slowly than normal, and is rapidly degraded in the extracellular matrix[489]
    Combination of the above

3. *Linkage data.* The findings of structural defects in type III procollagen and the direct demonstration of mutations in the gene imply that the disease is caused by mutations at the COL3A1 gene, which codes for the alpha 1 chain of type III collagen. This gene, which is 38 kilobases (kb) in length, is situated on the long arm of chromosome 2 in the region of bands 31 to 32,3 (2q31 to q32,3). Cosegregation of the disease with COL3A1 restriction fragment length polymorphisms has been demonstrated in several families.[355,496]

4. *Molecular defects.* Numerous single base mutations in COL3A1 that lead to substitution of glycine by other amino acids have been identified.[397,480,499,500] Protein data indicate that amino acid substitutions which lower the stability of the protein are a common cause of EDS IV.[499,500] In-frame genomic deletions[292,326,351,480,518] and splicing errors[109,279,280] within the triple helical coding domain lead to the synthesis of shortened pro alpha 1 (III) chains.[280,480]

With the upsurge of interest in type III collagen and the availability of new laboratory techniques, defects of the COL3A1 gene continue to be recognized. Many other mutations within the COL3A1 gene await elucidation.

EDS V (X-Linked Type)

In patients with EDS V the skin is soft and extensible and has a doughy consistency. Joint hypermobility is limited; tissue fragility, scarring, and bruising are moderate. The phenotype does not differ significantly from other major forms of EDS, and the diagnosis is based on recognition of the X-linked pattern of inheritance (Fig. 6-34).

Beighton[36] initially documented the condition in 1968 in a London family in which three affected brothers had a maternal uncle and male cousin with the disorder. When the family was followed up almost two decades later the clinically normal sister of the affected brothers had produced a son with EDS, whereas the brothers' own offspring were all unaffected. These new pedigree data give further support to the concept of X-linked inheritance.[46] In a second family with presumptive X-linked EDS that was described in the original report,[36] two affected brothers both subsequently produced offspring with "partial" stigmata; the syndromic status of this kindred is uncertain.

Di Ferrante et al.[136,137] reported that lysyl oxidase activity in cultured fibroblasts from a North American family with X-linked EDS was decreased. The phenotype in this kindred differed from that of the English family, and it is uncertain whether these disorders were the same entity. Siegal, Black, and Bailey[450] subsequently investigated the London family and demonstrated the presence of normal lysyl oxidase activity and collagen cross-link formation. The locus of the mutant gene on the X chromosome has not yet been elucidated.

EDS VI (Ocular-Scoliotic Type)

The manifestations of EDS VI are similar to those of EDS I, namely, moderately severe articular hypermobility, skin extensibility, and connective tissue fragility. In addition, there are propensities to spinal malalignment and serious ocular complications.[33,276,303,389,532] Vascular and gastrointestinal catastrophes have also been documented in a few persons with EDS VI.[481] An autosomal recessive mode of inheritance and defi-

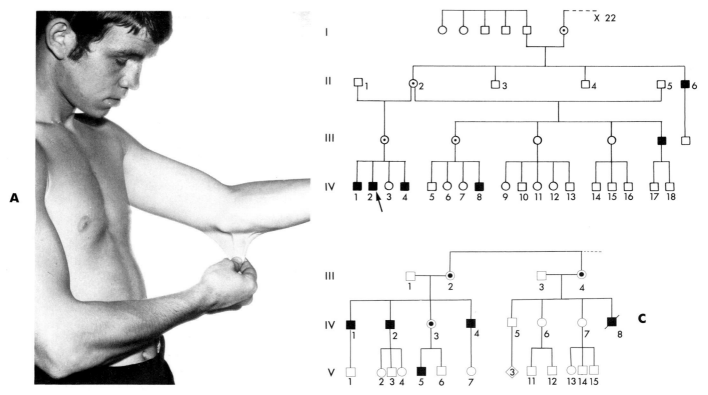

Fig. 6-34. EDS V. **A,** The proband of an English family with EDS V. The skin is markedly hyperextensible, whereas tissue fragility and joint hypermobility are of mild to moderate degree. **B,** The pedigree of the affected kindred. The pattern of transmission in the family is consistent with X-linked inheritance. **C,** The family was reassessed almost two decades after the initial investigation. By this time, the proband and the siblings had procreated. The affected brothers had produced offspring who were normal on clinical examination, whereas their unaffected sister had borne a son with the disorder. These new pedigree data are in accordance with X-linked inheritance. (**B** from Beighton P: *Br Med J* 3:409-411, 1968. **C** from Beighton P, Curtis D: *Clin Genet* 27[5]:472-478, 1985.)

ciency of lysyl hydroxylase,[238,276,389,533] which leads to a paucity of hydroxylysyl residues in collagen, are further distinguishing features.

The existence of this distinct form of EDS was first proposed in 1970 when an adult brother and sister with blindness and cardinal manifestations of EDS were reported by Beighton.[41] Their parents and offspring were unaffected; thus the possibility of autosomal recessive inheritance arose. A review of the literature revealed further instances of severe ocular problems in patients with a similar phenotype in genealogic settings that were compatible with autosomal recessive transmission.[72,104,110,494] Following the lead of Krane, Pinnell, and Erbe[276] and Pinnell,[389] who found the

first molecular defect in a heritable disorder of connective tissue, and acting on McKusick's observation that the phenotype was similar in both families, Lichtenstein[301] and Lichtenstein et al.[303] demonstrated that collagen was deficient in hydroxylysine in this family. Thus syndromic identity was firmly established.

McKusick, who had known the original patients for many years, gave the following graphic description:

In that family a brother and sister (latter shown in Fig. 6-35) had typical cutaneous and articular features of EDS and both had lost their sight after ocular catastrophes. The brother, born in 1915, sustained rupture of the right globe from a minor blow from a car-tire patch

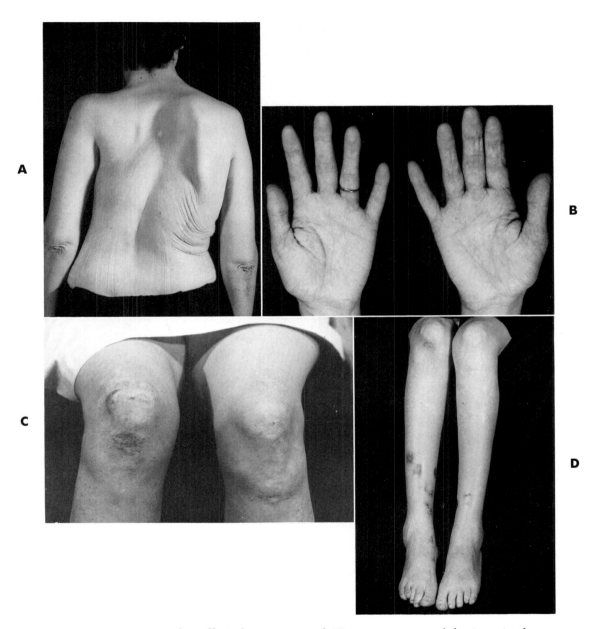

Fig. 6-35. EDS VI. This affected woman, aged 37 years, was an adult sister in the sibling pair on the basis of whom autonomous syndromic identity of EDS VI was first suggested.[41] These sisters were the subject of early reports of biochemical abnormalities in patients with EDS.[276,389] The woman had marked joint laxity, stretchable skin, a propensity to scarring, and acrocyanosis of the digits. **A,** Severe scoliosis. **B,** Acrocyanosis of the fingers. **C,** Distracted papyraceous scars on the knees. **D,** Pigmented scars on the shins.

at 22 years of age. Enucleation was necessary. At the age of 51 years the patient tripped and hit the left side of the head; the left globe ruptured, and although the scleral rent was sutured, he remained blind. The sister, born in 1924, had, like her brother, severe myopia from an early age. She had orthopaedic treatment for club-foot at the age of 12 years and for scoliosis when she was 15 years of age. Her glaucoma, microcornea, and blue sclerae were documented by Durham in 1953.[150] At the age of 36 years she sustained detachment of the left retina, followed a year later by detachment of the right retina. Attempts at repair, during which the surgeons commented on the fragility of the sclera and excessive bleeding, were unsuccessful, and the woman has remained totally blind. She subsequently died in middle age from an acute episode which probably represented a dissecting aneurysm of the aorta. These sibs are 2 among 8 children, the others being unaffected, as are also their parents and the 4 children of the brother. Although the parents were not consanguineous, recessive inheritance is likely.

In 1972 Pinnell et al[389] found hydroxylysine-deficient skin collagen in two sisters, 9 and 12 years of age, with severe scoliosis, a marfanoid habitus, recurrent joint dislocation, and hyperextensible skin and joints. The elder child had small corneas with scattered infiltrates in the anterior part of the stroma and slightly blue sclerae. Her 9-year-old sister had required removal of the left eye after trauma sustained in an automobile accident. The right cornea was small and deeply curved, and the sclerae were slightly blue. She also had a late systolic click and a late systolic murmur consistent with a floppy mitral valve.

In 1974 Sussman et al[481] established that lysyl hydroxylase was deficient in the patient shown in Fig. 6-35. This was the second demonstration of this enzyme defect, but it seems that the condition is heterogeneous, since normal lysyl hydroxylase activity has also been documented.[252] This latter form of the condition is designated EDS VIB to distinguish it from the classical form, EDS VIA, in which the enzyme is abnormal. Biochemical subcategorization has been attempted,[237] and collagen type specificity of defective lysyl hydroxylation in various tissues has been investigated.[46,464,485] The role of ascorbate in the regulation of collagen biosynthesis in this form of the disorder has been explored by Dembure et al.,[128] and the same investigators have pointed out that antenatal diagnosis by assay of lysyl hydroxylase activity in cultured amniotic fluid cells is technically possible.[127]

EDS VII (Arthrochalasis Multiplex Congenita)

Marked joint laxity with multiple dislocations is the major feature of EDS VII, whereas the other cardinal manifestations are mild. Stunted stature and mandibular micrognathia are additional components (Fig. 6-36).

There is semantic confusion concerning the name of this form of EDS, since the term *arthrochalasis multiplex congenita* has also been used loosely for other nonspecific hypermobility syndromes. The solution is further complicated by biochemical heterogeneity and by the possible existence of an autosomal recessive form of EDS VII, in addition to the established autosomal dominant types. EDS VII is rare, and although the diagnosis can be suspected from the phenotype, confirmation and subcategorization depends on demonstration of the characteristic biochemical abnormality.

Persons with EDS VII in whom molecular investigations have been undertaken have all been

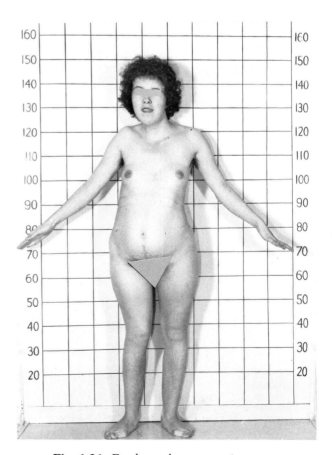

A

Fig. 6-36. For legend see opposite page.

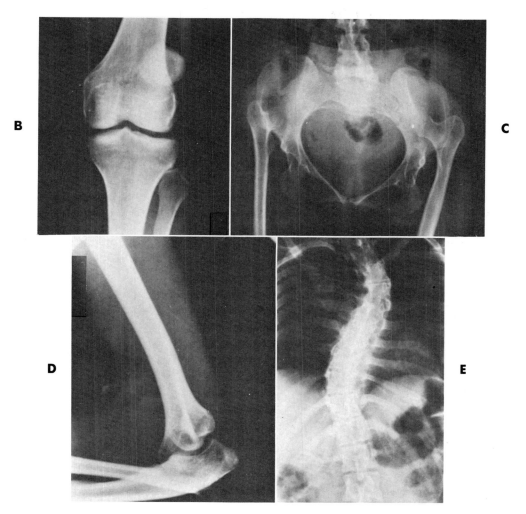

Fig. 6-36 cont'd. EDS VII. The proband in the original family in which defective conversion of procollagen to mature collagen was identified and ascribed to an abnormality of procollagen peptidase by Lichtenstein et al.[304] Steinmann et al.[466] subsequently showed that the abnormality lay in the structure of the procollagen itself rather than in enzymatic control of processing. This woman was 25 years of age at the time of the first investigations and had marked hyperextensibility of many joints, especially those of the hands, feet, shoulders, and spine. Dislocations at both hips and both elbows have resulted in limitation of motion in these joints. The bridge of the nose is broad, and the patient has myopia, microphthalmia, and intermittent exotropia. She is 58 inches tall. The fingers are somewhat webbed. The skin is not excessively stretchable or fragile, but some increased bruisability is present. No "cigarette-paper" scars are present; no striae resulted from pregnancy. No chromosomal abnormality could be identified. A sister had dislocation of the knees about 25 times, beginning at 6 years of age. This woman also has scoliosis and bilateral dislocation of the patellae. A young sister also had habitual dislocation of patellae. Neither parent showed any abnormality resembling those in the children, and the two offspring of the affected sibs show no abnormality. **A,** Patient had stunted stature and dislocations of hips and elbows. **B,** Radiograph of the knee showing lateral dislocation of the patella. **C,** Bilateral dislocation of the hips. **D,** Dislocation of the radial heads. **E,** Scoliosis.

found to be heterozygous for an abnormality of exon 6 of either the COL1A1 (EDS VIIA) gene[107,108,465,466] or the COL1A2 (EDS VIIB) gene.[157,212,527,529,538] The deletion of this exon in general results from point mutations altering the consensus donor or acceptor splice sites in the flanking introns. In one instance a point mutation in the last amino acid of exon 6 in the COL1A2 gene led to both normally and abnormally spliced products from the same allele.[528] The 18 amino acids encoded by exon 6 contain the type I collagen amino-proteinase cleavage site. Deletion of this exon results in incomplete processing of type II procollagen to collagen.[201,304]

EDS VIII (Periodontitis Type)

In the periodontitis form of EDS the gums are boggy and friable, and the teeth are lost by early adulthood because of alveolar bone resorption. Skin fragility leads to pigmented scars over the bony prominences, notably the shins (Fig. 6-37). Cutaneous extensibility and joint hypermobility are variable but usually minor, and except for the early periodontitis the phenotype resembles classical EDS IV.

In the fourth edition of this book McKusick wrote as follows of the condition that is now known as EDS VIII:

A condition unique in my experience, and apparently in the literature as well, is demonstrated by the wife of a colleague of mine and several of her relatives. Lesions on the shins suggest those of EDS, and slow-healing breaks in the skin at that site have occurred after blunt trauma. The skin is not generally fragile, and no unusual bruisability or stretchability of the skin has been noted. The joints are not hyperextensible. A second feature, apparently syndromally related to the lesions on the shins, is absorptive periodontosis, with early loss of the teeth. The dental and skin changes are present also in the proband's father, several sibs of her father, and in a cousin. The lesions on the shins suggested necrobiosis diabeticorum on histologic study, but there is no diabetes in the family, and no abnormality of carbohydrate metabolism is demonstrable in the proband. The small scars on the knees are somewhat like those of EDS, and the skin of the lateral aspect of the soles is wrinkled in the manner demonstrated by EDS patients.

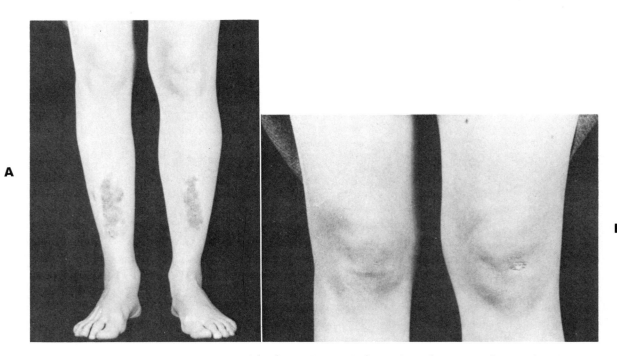

Fig. 6-37. EDS VIII. Patient with absorptive periodontosis and scarring due to skin fragility. Several relatives have the same combination of features. **A,** Skin lesions over the shins. **B,** Scars on the knees.

The condition was further delineated by Stewart, Hollister, and Rimoin[468] in 1977 as a "new variant" of EDS. Other reports followed, and about 20 cases have now been reported.* Although EDS VIII is rare, autosomal dominant inheritance is well established on a basis of two multigeneration pedigrees.[306,468]

Abnormalities of type III collagen have been identified in some persons with EDS VIII[287] but not in others.[210] It is conventional wisdom that type III collagen abnormalities are pathognomonic of EDS IV; in this light and in view of phenotypic similarities between the disorders it might be reasonable to regard EDS VIII as a form of EDS IV. It is equally possible that some patients with early periodontitis and apparent EDS IV might actually have EDS VIII. In the last analysis, collagen studies may be necessary for firm diagnostic categorization.[208]

EDS IX (Vacant)

The nosologic slot for EDS IX was formerly occupied by the occipital horn syndrome, which is also known as X-linked Cutis laxa (see Chapters 7 and 13). The phenotype resembles classical EDS, with the addition of minor changes in the long bones and the development of bony prominences on the occiput in adulthood.[436] Chronic diarrhea and orthostatic hypotension are additional manifestations. The designation *cutis laxa* initially generated some semantic confusion in the EDS context, but this difficulty was resolved when the condition was recategorized after identification of defective copper transport as the basic defect.[382] To avoid confusion in the future, the category EDS IX will remain vacant in the Berlin nosology.

EDS X (Fibronectin Abnormality)

EDS X is a rare autosomal recessive disorder characterized by articular hypermobility, skin extensibility, and fragility with scarring and a bruising tendency. The skin is thin, and in distinction from other forms of EDS, striae distensae may appear during pregnancy. The phenotype otherwise resembles EDS I, with the addition of a propensity to the development of petechiae during upper res-

---

*References 210, 227, 228, 287, 306, 320, 352, and 468.

piratory tract infections or after trauma to the skin.

Fibronectin abnormality was described in 1980 by Arneson et al.[14] in four affected sibs. The authors demonstrated that platelet aggregation was faulty and that this defect could be corrected by fibronectin. In a further report the same group of investigators documented an uneventful pregnancy in one of the affected sibs.[205] A decrease in fibronectin binding sites on polymorphonuclear leucocytes has been identified by Miura et al.[338] in persons with EDS II and VI. Thus it seems possible that the fibronectin mechanism may play a fundamental role in the pathogenesis of various forms of EDS.

EDS XI (Vacant)

EDS XI was formerly the designation for the condition now termed *familial joint instability*. Gross generalized articular hypermobility is the main feature of this disorder, but other stigmata of EDS are lacking. For the sake of nosologic purity, this condition has been reclassified with the familial hypermobility syndromes *(vide infra)*, and the category EDS XI remains vacant.

Other Forms

Several additional forms of EDS have been proposed on a basis of distinctive phenotypic features.[31,169,232,503] Most of these reports have pertained to isolated cases or single families, and the asterisk of confirmed syndromic status has not yet been accorded in the definitive catalogue, *Mendelian Inheritance in Man*.[330]

Progeroid form. In a series of articles Hernàndez et al.[221-223] described a progeroid form of EDS. These authors documented several sporadic individuals who had mild stigmata of EDS along with additional features, including mental retardation, short stature, wrinkled facies, scanty head and facial hair, periodontitis, and cryptorchidism.

Advanced paternal age was suggestive of new dominant mutation. Electron microscopy of the skin revealed fragmentation of the elastic fibers.[223] Fibroblasts have been shown to secrete glycosaminoglycan-free small proteoglycan core protein, and the basic defect is thought to be in proteodermatan sulfate biosynthesis.[277]

Oculoscoliotic phenotype with polyneuropathy. Farag and Schimke[159] observed two Bedouin sibs with EDS VI oculoscoliotic phenotype with polyneuropathy that was confirmed by objective neuromuscular investigations. The parents were consanguineous, and it is possible that this disorder is an autosomal recessive entity.

Overlap Phenotypes

EDS-osteogenesis imperfecta combined form. Blue sclerae are occasionally encountered in patients with EDS. Equally, joint laxity and skin scarring are sometimes found in OI. The combination of EDS and OI in the same person has been observed by Biering and Iverson[62]; these two conditions were not segregating separately in the family, and it seems likely that the affected individual had an autonomous "overlap" syndrome in which pleiotropic manifestations of the mutant gene produced the clinical features of both disorders. More recently Kuivaniemi et al.[279] reported the case of a mother and child with the combined EDS-OI phenotype. These individuals had a 19 base-pair deletion in the region of exon 11 in the pro alpha 2(I) collagen (COL1A2) gene.

The combination of gross articular hypermobility with resultant dislocations, moderate skin extensibility, and mild tissue fragility, together with wormian bones in the cranial sutures, was observed in a Xhosa woman living in Natal and in her four children.[515] These persons were subsequently shown to have a molecular defect that resulted in the loss of exon 6 of the COL1A2 gene.[522] This molecular abnormality has previously been demonstrated in persons with EDS VIIB,[529] and if it is accepted that the Xhosa family had this disorder, the potential range of phenotypic manifestations in EDS VIIB must be wider than previously supposed.

Fragilitas oculi. The ocular form of EDS shares many features with the disorder referred to as *fragilitas oculi*. Both have fragility of the sclera and cornea, with blue sclerae, rupture from minor trauma, and deformation of the cornea, either keratoconus or keratoglobus, and, often, megalocornea. Both have joint hyperextensibility, and both seem to be autosomal recessive disorders.

Zlotogora et al.[547] identified 17 patients with fragilitas oculi in 11 published cases of families and added four additional affected individuals from three kindreds whom they had studied. They

commented that five families were of Tunisian Jewish stock and that these persons had red hair, which is unusual in this population. This association could be explained by chance, pleiotropism of a single mutant gene, or tight linkage of two different genes. There is a parallel with EDS, since there seems to be a high frequency of red hair in some forms of this condition.[46]

EDS and Marfan syndrome. Several individuals with manifestations suggestive of both EDS and Marfan syndrome have been documented.* In this context persons with EDS occasionally have a marfanoid habitus, while loose joints are a variable component of Marfan syndrome. Equally, a nonspecific "marfanoid habitus" is not infrequent in persons with otherwise normal health. Thus potential exists for apparent phenotypic overlap, and the syndromic significance of this apparent concurrence is questionable. It is possible that some of these individuals with stigmata of both EDS and Marfan syndrome had currently undelineated connective tissue disorders. In addition, some of these cases were probably instances of the marfanoid hypermobility syndrome,[520] if this disorder does indeed have separate syndromic identity.

EDS and pseudoxanthoma elasticum. Instances of coincident EDS and PXE have been described.[111,360,381] In Cottini's patient[111] there were angioid streaks together with lesions of the skin of the neck characteristic of PXE (see Chapter 10). In addition, this individual had "cigarette-paper" scars of the elbows and knees and hyperextensible skin and joints characteristic of EDS. The PXE phenotype was not transmitted to a daughter who had acrocyanosis or to a son who had hyperextensible skin and joints, hernia, and varices of the leg veins.

A 22-year-old woman described by Pelbois and Rollier[381] consulted them because of the cosmetically undesirable lesions of PXE involving the skin of the neck and other areas of flexure. As well as having angioid streaks of the fundus (characteristic of PXE), the patient had multiple cicatrices indicative of cutaneous fragility, striking cutaneous hyperelasticity, and articular hypermobility. Her parents were first cousins, a fact significant in the appearance of the autosomal recessive form of

---

*References 64, 117, 161, 180, 183, 245, and 418.

PXE. The parents themselves were unaffected by PXE, although a maternal aunt of the patient had the condition. As for EDS, the patient's mother displayed features of this syndrome and probably had transmitted it as a dominant trait to her daughter.

These cases seem to be examples of accidental coincidence of the two syndromes, one behaving as a dominant and one as a recessive trait.

PATHOLOGY

In none of the disorders of connective tissue discussed in this book is the microscopic anatomy so disputed as in EDS.[273,475] There have been many reports of histologic abnormalities of elastin and even more in which collagen is incriminated. The evidence from recent biomolecular investigations heavily favors a collagen defect, but the pathogenetic mechanisms have not been fully elucidated.

An increase in elastic tissue of the corium has been described by many writers.* Morphologic abnormalities of the elastic fibers have been documented[458,536]; Pautrier[379] found the elastic fibers normal, and Brown and Stock[80] believed them to be *decreased*. To some extent at least, the apparent excess of elastic fibers may be relative. In EDS IV, for instance, the marked deficiency in collagen inevitably leaves the elastic fibers as a predominant fibrous element of the corium.

In 1955 Jansen[246] pointed out with excellent illustrations that "in normal skin, a system of robust, well-directed, crossing and tightly interlacing collagen fibre bundles is present. The whorled disorderly structure in hyperelastic (EDS) skin is remarkable; the collagen bundles seem to have been insufficiently united." Electron microscopy showed the morphologic features of collagen and elastin to be normal. This finding corroborated the earlier finding of Tunbridge et al.,[505] but Jansen[246] was unable to agree that there was an absolute increase in the number of elastic fibers.

In the years that followed Jansen's work, diminution and morphologic abnormalities of collagen fibers have been described by many authors[254,367,458,497,526] (Fig. 6-38, *A*). In 1980 Black et al.,[65] using transmission electron microscopy, demonstrated normal ultrastructure of collagen fibrils in the skin of persons with EDS I, II, and V. At a higher level of morphologic organization, scanning electron microscopy revealed progres-

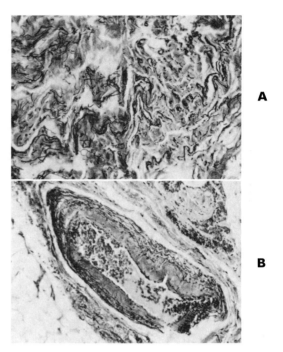

Fig. 6-38. Histologic features of the skin in a 10-year-old boy with typical EDS I. **A,** Loose collagen meshwork and unusually abundant elastic fibers (stained black) in the subcutaneous area overlying pectoral muscle (Verhoeff–van Giesen stain; magnified × 200 and reduced 3/7). **B,** Increased elastic fibers in small artery in pectoral muscle (Verhoeff–van Giesen stain; magnified × 200 and reduced 3/7).

sive increase in fiber bundle disorder from EDS V to II to I. In 1984 Kobayasi, Ogucchi, and Asboe-Hansen,[268] in electron microscopic studies of skin from 13 persons with different forms of EDS, observed collagen fibrils that were bent, curled, or twisted in a distorted arrangement. These changes were present in all subjects and did not permit diagnostic differentiation. After undertaking light and electron microscopic studies of the skin in two adults with EDS IV, in which the researchers demonstrated an increase in the diameter of collagen fibrils and a decrease in the diameter of collagen fiber bundles, Gertsch et al.[175] reached the reasonable conclusion that classification of the different types of EDS by means of electron microscopy is not possible.

The subcutaneous nodules or spherules are apparently fat-containing cysts.[525] They frequently become calcified. It seems likely that they are related to minor traumata and to the general fragil-

---

*References 30, 72, 226, 250, 334, 335, 401, 405, 421, 469, 493, 497, and 526.

ity of the connective tissue in which the fat deposits normally exist. Molluscoid pseudotumors that develop at pressure points are characterized by cyst formation.[244]

Histologic studies do not clarify how much of the bleeding is due to a defect in the supporting tissues and how much is a result of weakness of the vessel walls themselves. Abnormal, dilated, weak-appearing vessels have been described.[305,497] An abnormality (Fig. 6-38, *B*) of the connective tissue of the wall of small arteries was demonstrated in one of McKusick's cases, and similar changes are depicted in Jansen's report.[244] Taking a different approach, François et al.[165] recorded pulse wave velocities in a family with EDS IV in an attempt to elucidate the pathophysiologic features of arterial rupture in this form of the disorder.

Autopsies in affected persons were undertaken more than two decades ago by Lienhart,[305] Nicod,[356] and McFarland and Fuller.[324] The results were unremarkable and threw little light on the pathologic features of EDS. In particular, Lienhart described the autopsy findings in a 22-year-old woman who died of pulmonary tuberculosis; no internal abnormality referable to the connective tissue defect was discovered. Nicod[356] studied bone and cartilage and could detect no abnormality.

Fibronectin, a connective tissue protein, has been shown to have an altered distribution in fibroblasts from persons with unspecified forms of EDS.[120] Fibronectin is involved with collagen fibril formation. In EDS X, defective platelet aggregation can be corrected by fibronectin,[14] and this substance might eventually turn out to be a significant factor in the pathogenesis of other forms of EDS.

Emphasis has shifted from the gross anatomic and the histopathologic features of EDS to the underlying biomolecular abnormality.[85,390a] Type III collagen is consistently abnormal in EDS IV, the enzyme lysyl hydroxylase is defective in EDS VI, and processing of type I procollagen to collagen is incomplete in EDS VII. In the occipital horn syndrome, formally EDS IX, a defect in copper transport has been detected, and in EDS X, fibronectin seems to be faulty. At the molecular level numerous different intragenic mutations have been recognized, especially in EDS IV, and it can be anticipated that many more will be elucidated in the near future. Details of the biomolecular abnormal-

ities in specific forms of EDS are given in this chapter, in the section, Heterogeneity.

THE BASIC DEFECT(S)

In the fourth edition of this book[328] McKusick stated, "I am inclined to favor the view that EDS is another heritable disorder of collagen, biochemically, morphologically, clinically, and, of course, genetically distinct from the others which are under discussion in this book." He commented thus:

> *Superficial consideration of the clinical manifestations of EDS might suggest an abnormality of elastic tissue as the fundamental defect. A super-abundance of elastic fibers in the skin and joint capsules would explain the unusual characteristics, but the histological studies by no means afford unequivocal substantiation of this theory. Brown and Stock[80] suggested, and others,[172] including Jansen,[246] maintained that the defect may reside in the collagen fibers; because of lack of normal tensile strength, this would permit the skin, joint capsules and ligaments to be stretched beyond the normal limits (Fig. 6-39). The elastic fibers may function in connection with the process of restoration of these tissues to a normal configuration. According to the collagen theory, the histologic changes, both quantitative and qualitative, are interpretable as secondary effects of the abnormality of collagen.*

Genetically determined defects of collagen and related substances have now been demonstrated in

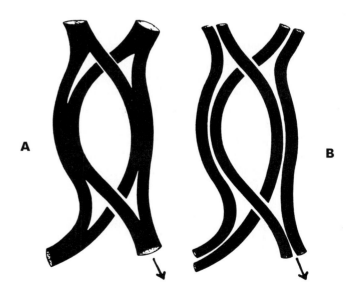

Fig. 6-39. Jansen's schematic representation of the postulated defect in collagen fasciculation in EDS. **A**, Normal. **B**, EDS. (From Jansen LH: *Dermatologica* 110:108-120, 1955.)

EDS IV, VI and VII; thus McKusick's contention has proved to be correct.

In discussing the nature of the basic defect, McKusick continued thus:

The comparative inextensibility of normal collagen may depend on some specific molecular or intermolecular structure which is altered in EDS, with resulting increase in extensibility. This alteration is assumed in the theory of Brown and Stock[80] and has been explicitly stated by Froelich[171] and by others. Jansen[246] advanced a related theory, incriminating collagen but placing the defect at a higher level of organization of collagen. He suggested that EDS is a disorder of the organization of collagen fibrils into bundles and of the bundles into a strong network and referred to the disorder as one of a defective wickerwork of collagen.

McKusick took the view that the evidence Jansen assembled and the clinical aspects of EDS make this version of the "collagen theory" highly probable. The electron microscopic and thermographic normality of collagen[318,357] may support the view of Wechsler and Fisher[526] that, at least in some forms of the condition, there is no qualitative abnormality of collagen but, rather, inadequate collagen production.

It is possible that in some patients and at some subcutaneous and articular locations, production of an excessive number of elastic fibers is stimulated by repeated and excessive stretching. After tissue culture studies Maximow[321] and Bloom[68] thought that the tugging of contractile myocardial cells was a factor in the formation of elastic fibers. Varadi and Hall[512] compared elastin isolated from the skin of four patients with EDS and elastin isolated from normal controls. No abnormality of quantity, amino acid composition, or desmosine cross-linking could be demonstrated, and there were no differences in elastin content between skin of thigh and of knee. This latter observation militates against the possibility of stimulation of elastin synthesis at sites of flexion.

The changes that occur in the skin of the feet and hands and at the elbows of older patients fit in well with the view that the primary defect resides in the collagen fibers: the normal elastic tissue may, with the passage of time, "wear out" from excessive stress imposed on it. In this way the skin becomes somewhat lax in later life.

In Hungary, Banga and Baló,[21] who discovered the elastolytic enzyme in pancreas, also demonstrated that normal serum contains an elastase inhibitor. Hall et al.[203] found in two patients with

EDS a concentration of elastase inhibitor in the blood that was "between 50 and 100 times as great as that in pooled normal serum." Goltz and Hult[178] also found elevated levels of serum elastase inhibitor. In contrast, Carter and Walford[97] could not demonstrate an increase in levels of elastase inhibitor in seven patients whom they studied. It is now generally accepted that the serum elastase inhibitor does not have any significant role in the pathogenesis of most forms of EDS.

The weakness of vessel walls seems an adequate basis for the hemorrhagic diathesis in EDS, and the lack of any consistent abnormality of clotting factors suggests that the defect does not lie in that domain. Owren[371] advanced the plausible suggestion that because of an abnormal structure or a quantitative deficiency, collagen in EDS is ineffective in attracting platelets and triggering liberation of adenosine diphosphate from them. Caen, Legrand, and Sultan[92] reported a case of bleeding diathesis and abnormal wound healing in which the patient's collagen had an abnormal electron microscopic appearance and failed to induce aggregation of normal platelets; the patient's platelets adhered to normal skin collagen.

In view of the defect in collagen type III in EDS IV it cannot be surprising that the bowel is friable in this form of the disorder. In this context it is significant that "surgical gut," which is used as suture material, is made from the submucosa and serosa of sheep and pigs and is almost pure collagen. Obviously collagen is important to the integrity of the bowel.

Abnormalities of the bones themselves are notable in their absence in EDS. Therefore it is difficult to interpret the findings of Julkunen, Rokkanen, and Jounela,[253] that in EDS the collagen of the bone is abnormally irregular, that tetracycline uptake is less than in controls, and that on microradiographic examination decreased mineralization of trabeculae is evident.

The existence of an analogous hereditary disorder in an animal that can be studied experimentally offers promise of providing important new information on the nature of the basic defect. For this reason descriptions of EDS in springer spaniels[523] and in mink[373] are of great interest. In these animals Hegreberg et al.[215,217,218] and Hegreberg, Padgett, and Henson[216] found the same fragility of skin and peripheral arteries and the same hyperextensibility and laxity of skin and joints. In both species inheritance was autosomal dominant, as is true in most forms of EDS in humans.[215] The skin in affected dogs had only one twenty-seventh of the normal tensile strength; in affected mink the tensile strength of skin was one thirteenth of normal.[216,217] The histologic appearances were similar to those in the human disease.[216,217]

A disorder in cattle characterized by extremely fragile skin and called dermatosparaxis has been described.[206,361] Lapière, Lenaers, and Kohn[286] demonstrated the basic defect to be a deficiency of the protease that cleaves procollagen; this condition may be analogous to EDS VII.

In the last analysis it seems probable that collagen or substances functionally related to collagen will prove to be abnormal in all forms of EDS. The abnormalities that have already been recognized in EDS III, VI, VIII, and X, together with their pathologic implications, have been reviewed in detail by Byers[85,86] and Byers and Holbrook,[87] and it seems clear that the physical properties and histopathologic appearances of connective tissue in EDS are explicable in terms of these fundamental defects. It is perhaps surprising that basic defects in EDS I, II, and III have not yet been elucidated, since these are by far the most common forms of the disorder. At least 12 different forms of collagen are known, and further linkage studies might be revealing. It is equally possible that the genetically determined fault in these entities will turn out to be in the regulation of collagen processing rather than in its biosynthesis.

PREVALENCE AND INHERITANCE

EDS has been described principally in Europeans and persons of European extraction. There have also been a number of reports of affected blacks in the United States,[81,122,313] in addition to those mentioned in this chapter, and EDS has been studied in an African (Xhosa) male[375] (Fig. 6-40) and in families of mixed ancestry in South Africa.[537] The condition is well recognized in Japan; the first report was published in 1941.[369] After the publication of a few descriptive articles,[12,434] there have been several recent accounts of serious gastrointestinal or vascular complications in patients from that country.[214,241,267,498] Patients with EDS have also been encountered in India,[98,124,197,346,453] Israel,[299] Scandinavia,[253,483] Iceland,[432] Korea,[336] Russia,[66,240,275,513] Cuba,[5] Egypt,[19] Libya,[22] and Taiwan.[99]

Schaper[438] stated in 1952 that only 93 cases of EDS had been reported. The number had risen to 300 in 1966 and to 500 in 1972; it is now probably well in excess of 1000. A minimum frequency of 1 per 150,000 of the population of southern England was estimated after a large-scale survey was conducted.[40] In 1972 McKusick commented that it is possible that fewer cases of EDS have been re-

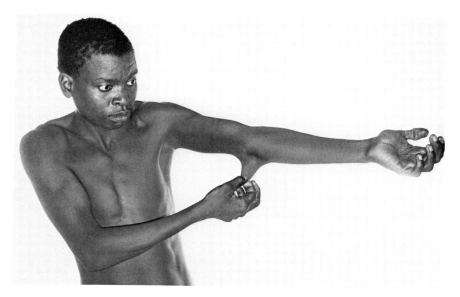

Fig. 6-40. Xhosa boy with EDS I demonstrating marked skin hyperextensibility. (From Pamphlett R, Nelson MM: *S Afr Med J* 48[17]:741-742, 1974.)

ported than of some of the other syndromes discussed in this book. In part this may be the result of greater difficulties in recognizing the condition, since cutaneous and articular hyperelasticity is a graded trait. McKusick stated, "I hazard to say, however, that in actuality this is one of the most frequent of the heritable disorders of connective tissue." As in other instances quoted in this chapter, McKusick's assumption has proved to be correct.

Autosomal dominant inheritance in EDS was suggested by early pedigree data.* In 1949 Johnson and Falls[250] reviewed 16 families reported in the literature[265] as having more than one affected member and concluded that the disorder was inherited as an autosomal dominant trait. In these families a total of 80 affected individuals had been identified, of whom exactly half were male. Two sisters with an unusually severe form of the disease were children of cousins, each with a mild form of the disease; this suggested to the authors that the trait might have occurred in a homozygous state in these affected girls. Similarly a presumed homozygote for EDS I was encountered in a highly inbred kindred by Kaslova et al.[275] Jansen[245] reviewed accumulated pedigree data in 1955; since then several extensive affected kindreds with an autosomal dominant pedigree pattern have been reported.[40,377] EDS has occurred in one member of a pair of twins who were probably fraternal[141] and in monozygous twins.[317]

Autosomal dominant inheritance was firmly established in EDS I, II, and III at the time of their delineation in the mid-1960s. On a basis of intrafamilial phenotypic similarities and interfamilial differences heterogeneity is likely in these forms of EDS. There is some variation in phenotypic expression in most kindreds, but complete nonpenetrance is unusual. All persons with EDS IV have a defect of type III collagen, but the condition has proved to be heterogeneous at the molecular level to the extent that virtually every affected family has a different intragenic defect. The X-linked transmission of EDS V is well established, as is the autosomal recessive nature of EDS VI, in which a deficiency of the enzyme lysyl hydroxylase has been demonstrated. Type VII EDS is an autosomal dominant trait with proven biochemical heterogeneity, whereas EDS VIII and X are respectively autosomal dominant and recessive

traits. It must be emphasized that EDS types V to X are individually rare to the extent that some of them are virtually private syndromes.

The karyotype is normal in EDS.[390] An exception was the child, reported by Vissian et al.,[517] with EDS and the cri-du-chat syndrome (deletion of part of the short arm of chromosome 5). It is uncertain, however, whether the occurrence of EDS in this particular infant was more than coincidence.

A translocation between the long arms of chromosomes 6 and 13 has been documented in a boy with EDS II,[437] and skin hyperextensibility was present in two other patients with deletions involving the long arms of chromosome 6.[331] These cytogenetic observations might provide a hint about the chromosomal locus of a "candidate gene," which might be implicated in the pathogenesis of some forms of EDS.

Somatic mutation is a possible explanation for unilateral involvement, as in the Spanish sailor presented to the Academy of Leiden by van Meekeren[510] and in the young Londoner studied by Beighton.[40] A similar example mentioned by Du Bois[146] is too sketchily reported to permit analysis.

HYPERMOBILITY SYNDROMES

Although articular hypermobility is a cardinal feature of EDS, it may also occur in isolation and as a component of other syndromes and disorders.

"Undifferentiated" hypermobility, in which the range of joint movements is excessive in the absence of other syndromic stigmata, is currently the focus of much attention, particularly in the speciality of rheumatology.[191] Indeed, interest in this topic has prompted the publication of *Hypermobility of Joints*,[47] in which the field is extensively reviewed.

There has been considerable semantic confusion between EDS and the familial undifferentiated hypermobility syndromes. This problem was one of the reasons for the promulgation of the Berlin nosology,[56] in which an attempt was made to separate these groups of disorders. In this document the term *arthrochalasis multiplex congenita*, which has been employed by Hass and Hass[211] for loose jointedness with or without skin changes, was formally accepted as a descriptive title for EDS VII. Furthermore, familial joint instability,[232] which previously had been labelled EDS XI, was reclassified with the familial articular hypermobility

---

*References 79, 147, 236, 341, 345, and 472.

syndrome (FAHS, *vide infra*), and the EDS XI slot was relegated to permanent vacancy.

In addition to the hypermobility syndromes that are briefly reviewed in this section, joint laxity of variable distribution and severity is sometimes a feature of Down syndrome and of connective tissue disorders such as Marfan syndrome and OI. Articular hypermobility is also a component of a number of rare conditions in which it is overshadowed by other syndromic manifestations. The most important of these disorders are Hajdu-Cheney syndrome, FG syndrome, C syndrome,

cutis laxa with joint hypermobility and developmental delay, Aarskog syndrome, Cohen syndrome, multiple endocrine neoplasia, and Coffin-Siris syndrome. Impressive laxity of the digits is encountered in dwarfing dysplasias, including pseudoachondroplasia, Morquio syndrome, cartilage-hair hypoplasia, and acromesomelic dysplasia.

Familial Articular Hypermobility Syndrome

The FAHS comprises generalized joint laxity, with or without subluxations and dislocations, in

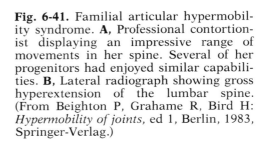

Fig. 6-41. Familial articular hypermobility syndrome. **A,** Professional contortionist displaying an impressive range of movements in her spine. Several of her progenitors had enjoyed similar capabilities. **B,** Lateral radiograph showing gross hyperextension of the lumbar spine. (From Beighton P, Grahame R, Bird H: *Hypermobility of joints,* ed 1, Berlin, 1983, Springer-Verlag.)

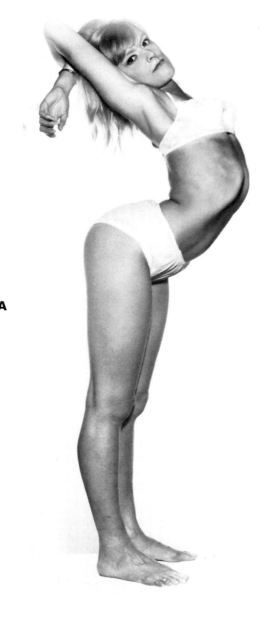

A

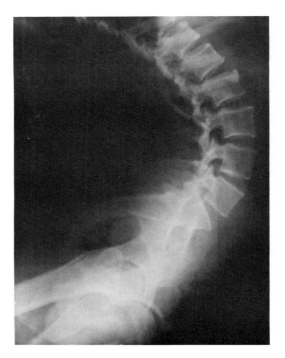

B

the absence of involvement of the skin or other tissues (Fig. 6-41). The EDS group of disorders, notably EDS III (hypermobile type) and EDS VII (arthrochalasis multiplex congenita), are specifically excluded, as are those skeletal dysplasias in which joint laxity is a component.

The FAHS may be innocuous and merely represent a source of innocent amusement to affected persons and onlookers alike by virtue of the opportunities afforded by "double jointedness." Conversely, frequent sprains, subluxations, and dislocations may cause serious physical handicap. The overall presence or absence of these complications is fairly consistent from family to family; on this basis the FAHS has been subdivided into "uncomplicated" and "dislocating" types. Nonspecific limb pains occur in all forms and are often the predominant feature, especially in the rheumatologic context. McKusick has suggested that these pains, which can be severe, may result from excessive stretching of the soft tissues consequent on joint hypermobility. The same mechanism may be responsible for the limb pains that can be troublesome in persons with EDS.

Inheritance of the FAHS is usually autosomal dominant, and several extensive pedigrees have been published.[50,473] An autosomal recessive form of the uncomplicated type has also been documented,[231] but this entity seems to be much less common than the conventional autosomal dominant forms.

Skeletal Dysplasias with Predominant Joint Laxity

Articular hypermobility is a major feature of a number of skeletal dysplasias.[43,45,316] Stunted stature, additional syndromic manifestations, and widespread radiologic changes in the skeleton in these disorders readily permit accurate diagnosis and differentiation from EDS. Nevertheless, these conditions have been misdiagnosed as EDS, so they are accorded brief mention in this chapter.

Larsen syndrome. The Larsen syndrome[288,289] exists in a severe autosomal recessive form and in a mild autosomal dominant variety. The condition comprises multiple congenital dislocations, with osseous anomalies and unusual facies. The elbows, hips, and knees show dislocation, usually bilaterally. Anterior dislocation of the tibia on the femur is especially characteristic. The fingers are cylindric, with short nails; the thumbs are spatulate and the metacarpals short. The facies is characterized by prominent or bossed forehead, flat or depressed nasal bridge, and wide-set eyes. Cleft palate, congenital heart malformation, and hydrocephalus occur in some patients. Decreased rigidity of cartilage in the rib cage, epiglottis, and arytenoid and perhaps in the trachea cause respiratory difficulties in the young child. A juxtacalcaneal accessory ossification center and abnormality of vertebral segmentation, especially in the upper thoracic and cervical spine, are demonstrable on radiographic examination.

Desbuquois syndrome. The Desbuquois syndrome is a rare autosomal recessive disorder in which generalized joint laxity is associated with stunted stature, prominent eyes, broad terminal phalanges, and polydactyly.[132] On radiographic examination supernumerary ossification centers are evident in the carpus (an interesting parallel with Larsen syndrome), and a characteristic prominence of the lesser trochanters of the femurs is present.

Spondyloepimetaphyseal dysplasia with joint laxity. The main manifestations of spondyloepimetaphyseal dysplasia with joint laxity (SEMDJL) are gross joint laxity with progressive spinal malalignment, multiple dislocations, and severe dwarfism.[55] The facies is characteristic, and cardiac defects and palatal clefts may occur. Diagnostic radiographic changes are present in the vertebrae, epiphyses, and metaphyses.

The condition causes serious disability in childhood, as progressive kyphoscoliosis leads to spinal cord compression and cardiorespiratory embarrassment. For these reasons the majority of affected persons fail to reach adulthood.

SEMDJL has been investigated in more than 20 children in the Afrikaans-speaking community of South Africa. Common ancestors have been traced, and an autosomal recessive mode of inheritance is well established.

MANAGEMENT

No specific therapy exists for EDS, but general measures involve minimizing trauma by appropriate regulation of life-style. In view of the great disparity in clinical severity in the different forms of EDS the care of each affected person should be managed on her or his own merits; avoidance of contact sports is a self-evident precaution, and in extreme cases the wearing of protective clothing may be helpful.

The closure of skin wounds can be difficult in some patients because sutures tend to tear out as a result of tissue friability. The scars often distract after healing and produce an unsightly appearance. Careful apposition of wound edges with multiple small stitches or the use of butterfly sutures together with prolonged support produces an optimal result. Cosmetic surgery for scar improvement is not usually worthwhile,[44,196] although occasional favorable outcomes have been documented.[409]

Surgical operations in patients with EDS may be entirely uneventful or fraught with difficulties[48]; the care of each patient must be managed in the light of her or his own past experience. If in doubt, it would probably be wise to err on the side of caution. Surgery in patients with EDS has often been accompanied by wound dehiscence.[242,372] The tissues may be strikingly friable and hold sutures poorly. Hemostasis may be a problem, presumably because of abnormal properties of the walls of small blood vessels rather than because of any inherent coagulation defect (see the section, Hematologic Features). Angiography is especially hazardous.[145,310,428] Obstetric complications and management are discussed in the section, Pregnancy.

Operations that have been successfully performed include thoracoplasty,[422] suture of lacerated tendons,[59,374] aortic valve replacement,[152] appendectomy,[233] homograft of preserved sclera,[350] correction of eventration of the diaphragm and torsion of the stomach,[386] coronary artery vein grafting,[406] repair of cleft lip and palate,[362] and colectomy for colonic ectasia.[448] Sykes[484] made recommendations concerning the optimal surgical approach to acute colonic perforation in patients with EDS. He suggested that since recurrent perforation is frequent, permanent colostomy is preferable to establishment of bowel continuity.

The surgical management of aortic and arterial complications in patients with EDS has been discussed by several authors.[82,278,426,443,540] The management of surgical complications in childhood has been reviewed by McEntyre and Raffensperger.[322]

The genetic management of EDS is largely based on counseling concerning recurrence risks. If there is a clear-cut pattern of inheritance in the family in question, counseling is a straightforward

procedure. Conversely, in a sporadic case the accurate prediction of recurrence risks may be impossible. In the context, assignment of an isolated individual to any particular diagnostic category of the EDS in terms of phenotypic features can be a difficult matter. In the forms of EDS in which a biomolecular defect has been identified, notably EDS IV, VI and VII, antenatal diagnosis by investigation of cultured chorionic or of amniotic fluid cells from at-risk pregnancies or by DNA linkage techniques in suitable families should be possible.[90,127,130,398] Because the relevant laboratory studies require a high level of technical skill, the expertise of a special center is necessary in these circumstances.

The establishment of EDS lay organizations, notably the Ehlers-Danlos National Foundation in the United States* and the Ehlers-Danlos Support Group in Great Britain,† has been of great benefit to affected individuals and their families. These bodies work on the premise that "problems shared are problems halved" and represent a valuable source of information for persons involved with EDS. They also provide an important channel of communication between patients, physicians, researchers, and other professionals through their regular newsletters, which are respectively named "Loose Connections" and "Fragile Links."

SUMMARY

The cardinal features of EDS are loose-jointedness, hyperextensibility, fragility and bruisability of the skin with "cigarette-paper" scarring, and generalized friability of tissues. The major internal manifestations include rupture of great vessels, diaphragmatic and other hernias, gastrointestinal diverticula, and friability of the bowel, which leads to spontaneous perforation.

EDS is heterogeneous, and 10 distinct forms have been identified by clinical and genetic means. Further heterogeneity is evident at a biomolecular level.

The basic defect is thought to concern the organization of collagen bundles into an intermeshing network. Genetically determined abnormalities in collagen structure or processing have been recognized in some forms of EDS.

---

*Ehlers-Danlos National Foundation, P. O. Box 1212, Southgate, Michigan 48195; (313) 282-0180.

†Ehlers-Danlos Support Group, 2 High Garth, Richmond, North Yorks DL10 4DG, England.

REFERENCES

1. Aaby GV, Blake HA: Tracheobronchiomegaly, *Ann Thorac Surg* 2:64-70, 1966.
2. Abouleish E: Obstetric anaesthesia and Ehlers-Danlos syndrome, *Br J Anaesth* 52(12):1283-1286, 1980.
3. Adams F: *The genuine works of Hippocrates. Airs, waters, and places*, paragraphs 20 and 22, vol 1, pp 176-178, New York, 1891, William Wood.
4. Agostini A: Cited by Jansen.[244]
5. Aleman E et al: Sindrome de Ehlers-Danlos, *Rev Cuba Pediatr* 37:35-39, 1965.
6. Aldridge RT: Ehlers-Danlos syndrome causing intestinal perforation, *Br J Surg* 54:22-25, 1967.
7. André R et al: Incidences hémorragiques et viscérales de la maladie d'Ehlers-Danlos, *Bull Soc Méd Hôp Paris* 116:971-976, 1965.
8. Angst H: *Das Ehlers-Danlos syndrome*, doctoral dissertation, Zürich, 1951. Cited by Jansen.[244]
9. Anning ST: Elastoma intrapapillare perforans verruciforme (Miescher), *Proc Roy Soc Med (Sect Derm)* 51:932 only, 1958.
9a. Anstey A, Wilkinson JD, Pope FM: Ehlers-Danlos syndrome with recurrent bruising, *J Roy Soc Med* 83(12):800-801, 1990.
10. Antani JA, Srinivas HV, Shivashanker A: Clinical manifestations of papillary muscle dysfunction in Ehlers-Danlos syndrome, *Jpn Heart J* 16(3):235-242, 1975.
11. Aptekar RG, Reynolds GG: Association of Ehlers-Danlos syndrome with dermatomyositis, *JAMA* 219(6):750, 1972.
12. Araki T: Ehlers-Danlos syndrome occurring in a family, *Orthop Surg* (Tokyo) 17:822-826, 1966.
13. Arendt-Nielsen L et al: Insufficient effect of local analgesics in Ehlers-Danlos type III patients (connective tissue disorder), *Acta Anaesthesiol Scand* 34(5):358-361, 1990
14. Arneson MA et al: A new form of Ehlers-Danlos syndrome. Fibronectin corrects defective platelet function, *JAMA* 224(2):144-147, 1980.
15. Atalla A, Page I: Ehlers-Danlos syndrome type III in pregnancy, *Obstet Gynecol* 71(3;2):508-509, 1988.
16. Aumailley M et al: Biochemical and immunological studies of fibroblasts derived from a patient with Ehlers-Danlos syndrome type IV demonstrate reduced type III collagen synthesis, *Arch Dermatol Res* 269(2):169-177, 1980.
17. Aumailley M et al: Low production of procollagen III by skin fibroblasts from patients with Ehlers-Danlos syndrome type IV is not caused by decreased levels of procollagen III mRNA, *Eur J Clin Invest* 18(2):207-212, 1988.
18. Ayres JG et al: Abnormalities of the lungs and thoracic cage in the Ehlers-Danlos syndrome, *Thorax* 40(4):300-305, 1985.
19. Aziz el AM, el Khashab MM, el Ashmawi S: The Ehlers-Danlos syndrome, *J Egypt Med Assoc* 54(8):579-609, 1971.
20. Badelon O et al: Congenital dislocation of the hip in Ehlers-Danlos syndrome, *Clin Orthop* 255:138-143, 1990.
21. Banga I, Baló J: Elastin and elastase, *Nature* 171:44 only, 1953.
22. Banerjee G et al: Ehlers-Danlos syndrome—masquerading as primary muscle disease, *Postgrad Med J* 64(748):126-127, 1988.
23. Bannerman RM, Graf CJ, Upson JF: Ehlers-Danlos syndrome, *Br Med J* 3:558-559, 1967.
23a. Bannerman RM, Ingall GB, Graf CJ: The familial occurrence of intracranial aneurysms, *Neurology* 20:283-292, 1970.
24. Barabas AP: Ehlers-Danlos syndrome associated with prematurity and premature rupture of foetal membranes: possible increase in incidence, *Br Med J* 2:682-684, 1966.
25. Barabas AP: Heterogeneity of the Ehlers-Danlos syndrome: description of three clinical types and a hypothesis to explain the basic defect(s), *Br Med J* 2:612-613, 1967.
26. Barabas AP: Ehlers-Danlos syndrome with vertebral artery aneurysm, *Proc Roy Soc Med* 62:735 only, 1969.
27. Barabas AP: Vascular complications in the Ehlers-Danlos syndrome, with special reference to the "arterial type" or Sack's syndrome, *J Cardiovasc Surg (Torino)* 13(2):160-167, 1972.Barabas GM:
28. Barabas GM: The Ehlers-Danlos syndrome. Abnormalities of the enamel, the dentine, cementum, and the dental pulp: an histological examination of 13 teeth from 6 patients, *Br Dent J* 126(11):509-515, 1969.
29. Barabas GM, Barabas AP: The Ehlers-Danlos syndrome. A report of the oral and haematological findings in nine cases, *Br Dent J* 123(10):473-479, 1967.
30. Barber HS, Fiddes J, Benians THC: The syndrome of Ehlers-Danlos, *Br J Dermatol* 53:97-112, 1941.
31. Beasley RP, Cohen MM Jr: A new presumably autosomal recessive form of the Ehlers-Danlos syndrome, *Clin Genet* 16(1):19-24, 1979.
32. Bechi P et al: A variety of Ehlers-Danlos syndrome type IV presenting with haematemesis and gastro-esophageal reflux, *Ital J Surg Sci* 17(1):63-66, 1987.
33. Behrens-Baumann W, Gebauer HJ, Langenbeck U: Syndrome of blue sclerae and keratoglobus (ocular type of Ehlers-Danlos syndrome), *Arch Klin Exp Ophthalmol* 204(4):235-246, 1977.
34. Beighton PH: Gastrointestinal bleeding in the Ehlers-Danlos syndrome, *Br Med J* 1:315 only, 1968.
35. Beighton P: Lethal complications of the Ehlers-Danlos syndrome, *Br Med J* 3:656-660, 1968.
36. Beighton P: X-linked recessive inheritance in the Ehlers-Danlos syndrome, *Br Med J* 2:409-414, 1968.
37. Beighton P: Obstetric aspects of the Ehlers-Danlos syndrome, *J Obstet Gynaecol Br Cwlth* 76:97-101, 1969.
38. Beighton P: Cardiac abnormalities in the Ehlers-Danlos syndrome. *Br Heart J* 31(2):227-232, 1969.
39. Beighton P: Ehlers-Danlos syndrome, *Ann Rheum Dis* 29(3):332-333, 1970.
40. Beighton P: *The Ehlers-Danlos syndrome*, London, 1970, William Heinemann Medical Books.
41. Beighton P: Serious ophthalmological complications in the Ehlers-Danlos syndrome, *Br J Ophthalmol* 54(4):263-268, 1970.
42. Beighton P: Articular manifestations of the Ehlers-Danlos syndrome, *Semin Arthritis Rheum* 1(3):246-261, 1972.
43. Beighton P: *Inherited disorders of the skeleton*, ed 2, Edinburgh, 1988, Churchill Livingstone, pp 409-418.
44. Beighton P, Bull JC: Plastic surgery in the Ehlers-Danlos syndrome. Case report, *Plast Reconstr Surg* 45(6):606-609, 1970.
45. Beighton P, Craig J: Atlanto-axial subluxation in the Morquio syndrome, *J Bone Joint Surg* (BR) 55B(3):478-481, 1973.
46. Beighton P, Curtis D: X-linked Ehlers-Danlos syndrome type V: the next generation, *Clin Genet* 27(5):472-478, 1985.
47. Beighton P, Grahame R, Bird H: *Hypermobility of joints*, ed 2, London, 1989, Springer-Verlag, pp 149-170.

48. Beighton P, Horan FT: Surgical aspects of the Ehlers-Danlos syndrome. A survey of 100 cases, *Br J Surg* 56:255-259, 1960.

49. Beighton P, Horan F: Orthopaedic aspects of the Ehlers-Danlos syndrome, *J Bone Joint Surg* 51B(3):444-453, 1969.

50. Beighton P, Horan FT: Dominant inheritance in familial generalised articular hypermobility, *J Bone Joint Surg Br* 52B(1):145-147, 1970.

51. Beighton PH, Murdoch JL, Votteler T: Gastrointestinal complications of the Ehlers-Danlos syndrome, *Gut* 10:1004-1008, 1969.

52. Beighton P, Solomon L, Soskolne CL: Articular mobility in an African population, *Ann Rheum Dis* 32:413-418, 1973.

53. Beighton P, Thomas ML: The radiology of the Ehlers-Danlos syndrome, *Clin Radiol* 20(4):354-361, 1969.

54. Beighton P et al: Variants of the Ehlers-Danlos syndrome. Clinical, biochemical, haematological, and chromosomal features of 100 patients, *Ann Rheum Dis* 28(3):228-245, 1969.

55. Beighton P et al: Spondylo-epimetaphyseal dysplasia with joint laxity and severe, progressive kyphoscoliosis, *S Afr Med J* 64:772-775, 1983.

56. Beighton P et al: International nosology of heritable disorders of connective tissue, Berlin, 1986, *Am J Med Genet* 29:581-594, 1988.

57. Bellenot F et al: Type IV Ehlers-Danlos syndrome with isolated arterial involvement, *Ann Vasc Surg* 4(1):15-19, 1990.

58. Benjamin B, Weiner H: Syndrome of cutaneous fragility and hyperelasticity and articular hyperlaxity, *Am J Dis Child* 65:247-275, 1943.

59. Bennett JB: Flexor tendon laceration in Ehlers-Danlos Syndrome. A case report, *J Bone Joint Surg* (Am) 59(2):259-260, 1977.

60. Beylot C, Bioulac P, Doutre MS: Les manifestations arterielles du syndrome d'Ehlers-Danlos (Arterial manifestations of the Ehlers-Danlos syndrome), *Ann Med Interne (Paris)* 134(5):451-457, 1983.

61. Bhatia SJ et al: Sporadic Ehlers-Danlos syndrome with neurologic, cardiac and dental involvement, *J Assoc Physicians India* 38(5):361-363, 1990.

62. Biering A, Iverson T: Osteogenesis imperfecta associated with Ehlers-Danlos syndrome, *Acta Paediatr* 44:279-286, 1955.

63. Bigelow NH: The association of polycystic kidneys with intracranial aneurysms and other related disorders, *Am J Med Sci* 225:485-494, 1953.

64. Birkenstock WE et al: Combined Ehlers-Danlos and Marfan's syndromes, with a case report, *S Afr Med J* 47(44):2097-2102, 1973.

65. Black CM et al: The Ehlers-Danlos syndrome: an analysis of the structure of the collagen fibres of the skin, *Br J Dermatol* 102(1):85-96, 1980.

66. Bochkova DN, Ternova TI, Petrosian KI: Interatrial septal defect in a child with the Ehlers-Danlos syndrome, *Kardiologiia* 18(7):127-129, 1978.

67. Boullie MC et al: Syndrome d'Ehlers-Danlos type IV a type d'Acrogeria, *Ann Dermatol Venereol* 113(11):1077-1085, 1986.

68. Bloom W: Studies on fibers in tissue culture. II. The development of elastic fibers in cultures of embryonic heart and aorta, *Arch Exp Zellforsch* 9:6-13, 1929.

69. Bolam RM: A case of Ehlers-Danlos syndrome, *Br J Dermatol* 50:174-181, 1938.

70. Bonnet P: Les manifestations oculaires de la maladie d'Ehlers-Danlos, *Bull Soc Ophtalmol Fr* 1:623-626, 1953.

71. Bopp P, Hatam K, Busset P: Cardiovascular aspects of the Ehlers-Danlos syndrome; report of a case with pulmonary artery bifidity and aortic arch anomaly, *Circulation* 32:602-607, 1965.

72. Bossu A, Lambrechts: Manifestations oculaires du syndrome d'Ehlers-Danlos, *Ann Ocul* 187:227-236, 1954.

73. Bowers WH, Spencer JB, McDevitt NB: Brachial-artery rupture in Ehlers-Danlos syndrome: an unusual cause of high median-nerve palsy. A case report, *J Bone Joint Surg* 58(7)1025-1026, 1976.

74. Branch CE Jr, Swift TR: Systemic lupus erythematosus, myasthenia gravis, and Ehlers-Danlos syndrome, *Ann Neurol* 4(4):374-375, 1978.

75. Brandt KD et al: Herniation of mitral leaflets in the Ehlers-Danlos syndrome, *Am J Cardiol* 36(4):524-528, 1975.

76. Breivik N et al: Ehlers-Danlos syndrome and diverticula of the bladder, *Z Kinderchir* 40(4):243-246, 1985.

77. Brodribb AJ: Vertebral aneurysm in a case of Ehlers-Danlos syndrome, *Br J Surg* 57:148-151, 1970.

78. Brombart M, Coupatez G, Laurent Y: Contribution à l'etude de l'étiologie de la hernie hiatale et de la diverticulose du tube digestif; un cas de maladie d'Ehlers-Danlos associée à une hernie hiatale, un diverticule de l'estomac, un diverticule duodénal, une diverticulose colique et une anémie sidéropénique, *Arch Mal Appar Dig* 41:413-420, 1952.

79. Brown A: Ehlers-Danlos syndrome: description of 3 cases, *Glasgow Med J* 27:7-12, 1946.

80. Brown A, Stock VF: Dermatorrhexis: report of a case, *Am J Dis Child* 54:956-957, 1937.

81. Bruno MS, Narashimhan P: The Ehlers-Danlos syndrome: a report of four cases in two generations of a Negro family, *New Engl J Med* 264:274-277, 1961.

82. Burnett HF et al: Abdominal aortic aneurysmectomy in a 17-year-old patient with Ehlers-Danlos syndrome: case report and review of the literature, *Surgery* 74(4):617-620, 1973.

83. Burrows A, Turnbull HM: Cutis hyperelastica (Ehlers-Danlos syndrome), *Br J Dermatol* 50:648-652, 1938.

84. Burton AC: Relation of structure to function of the tissues of the wall of blood vessels, *Physiol Rev* 34:619-642, 1954.

85. Byers PH: Inherited disorders of collagen gene structure and expression, *Am J Med Genet* 34(1):72-80, 1989.

86. Byers PH: Disorders of collagen biosynthesis and structure. In Scriver CR et al, editors: *The metabolic basis of inherited disease*, ed 2, New York, 1989, McGraw-Hill, pp 2802-2845.

87. Byers PH, Holbrook KA: Molecular basis of clinical heterogeneity in the Ehlers-Danlos syndrome. *Ann New York Acad Sci* 460:298-310, 1985.

88. Byers PH et al: Altered secretion of type III procollagen in a form of type IV Ehlers-Danlos syndrome. Biochemical studies in cultured fibroblasts, *Lab Invest* 44(4):336-341, 1981.

89. Byers PH et al: Clinical and ultrastructural heterogeneity of type IV Ehlers-Danlos syndrome, *Hum Genet* 47(2):141-150, 1979.

90. Byers PH et al: Molecular basis of inherited disorders of collagen biosynthesis: implication for diagnosis, *Current Prob Dermatol* 16:158-174, 1987.

91. Cabeen WR Jr et al: Mitral valve prolapse and conduction defects in Ehlers-Danlos syndrome, *Arch Intern Med* 137(9):1227-1231, 1977.

92. Caen JP, Legrand Y, Sultan Y: Platelet collagen interactions, *Thromb Haemost* (suppl)40:181-197, 1970.

93. Carr RJ, Green DM: Multiple odontogenic keratocysts in a patient with type II (mitis) Ehlers-Danlos syndrome, *Br J Oral Maxillofac Surg* 26(3):205-214, 1988.

94. Carter CO, Sweetnam R: Familial joint laxity and recurrent dislocation of the patella, *J Bone Joint Surg* 40B:664-667, 1958.

95. Carter CO, Sweetnam R: Recurrent dislocation of the patella and of the shoulder, *J Bone Joint Surg* 42B:721-727, 1960.

96. Carter CO, Wilkinson J: Persistant joint laxity and congenital dislocation of the hip, *J Bone Joint Surg* 46B:40-45, 1964.

97. Carter PK, Walford RL: Serum elastase inhibitor levels in Ehlers-Danlos syndrome, *Ann Rheum Dis* 22:198-199, 1963.

98. Chakraborty AN, Banerjee AK, Ghosh S: Ehlers-Danlos syndrome (cutis hyperelastica), *J Indian Med Ass* 23:344-345, 1954.

99. Chang JP, Chang CH, Sheih MJ: Aneurysmal dilatation of patent ductus arteriosus in a case of Ehlers-Danlos syndrome, *Ann Thorac Surg* 44(6):656-657, 1987.

100. Chouza C et al: Familial spastic ataxia associated with Ehlers-Danlos syndrome with platelet dysfunction, *Can J Neurol Sci* 11(suppl 4):541-549, 1984.

101. Cikrit DF, Miles JH, Silver D: Spontaneous arterial perforation: the Ehlers-Danlos specter, *J Vasc Surg* 5(2):248-255, 1987.

102. Clark JG, Kuhn C 3rd, Uitto J: Lung collagen in type IV Ehlers-Danlos syndrome: ultrastructural and biochemical studies, *Am Rev Respir Dis* 122(6):971-978, 1980.

103. Clough V et al: Acquired von Willebrand's syndrome and Ehlers-Danlos syndrome presenting with gastro-intestinal bleeding, *Scand J Haematol* 22(4):305-310, 1979.

104. Clunie GJA, Mason HM: Visceral diverticulosis and the Marfan syndrome, *Br J Surg* 50:51-52, 1962.

105. Cockshott WP, Omololu A: Familial congenital posterior dislocation of both radial heads, *J Bone Joint Surg* 40B:483-486, 1958.

106. Coe M, Silver SH: Ehlers-Danlos syndrome (cutis hyperelastica), *Am J Dis Child* 59:129-135, 1940.

107. Cole WG, Evans R, Sillence DO: The clinical features of Ehlers-Danlos syndrome type VII due to a deletion of 24 amino acids from the pro alpha 1(I) chain of type I procollagen, *J Med Genet* 24(11):698-701, 1987.

108. Cole WG et al: Deletion of 24 amino acids from the pro-alpha 1(I) chain of type I procollagen in a patient with Ehlers-Danlos syndrome type VII, *J Biol Chem* 261(12):5496-5503, 1986.

109. Cole WG et al: A base substitution at a splice site in the COL3A1 gene causes exon skipping and generates abnormal type III procollagen in a patient with Ehlers-Danlos syndrome type IV, *J Biol Chem* 265(28):17,070-17,077, 1990.

110. Cordella M, Vinciguerra E: Le manifestazioni oculari nella sindrome d'Ehlers-Danlos, *Minerva Oftal* 8:103-107, 1966.

111. Cottini GB: Association des syndromes de Groenblad-Strandberg et d'Ehlers-Danlos dans le même sujet, *Acta Dermatol (Stockholm)* 29:544-549, 1949.

112. Courtois J, Couchie C: Implications orthodontiques et stomatologiques chez un enfant presentant un syndrome d'Ehlers-Danlos, *Acta Stomatol Belg* 85(4):245-248, 1988.

113. Cremers PTJ, Busscher DLT, Macfarlane JD: Case report. Ultrasound demonstration of a superior mesenteric artery aneurysm in a patient with Ehlers-Danlos syndrome, *Br J Rheumatol* 29:482-484, 1990.

114. Coventry MB: Some skeletal changes in the Ehlers-Danlos syndrome, *J Bone Joint Surg* 43A:855-860, 1961.

115. Crowe JF, Neel JV, Schull WJ: *A clinical and genetic study of multiple neurofibromatosis*, Springfield, Ill, 1956, Charles C Thomas, p 112.

116. Cullen SI: Localized Ehlers-Danlos syndrome, *Arch Dermatol* 115(3):332-333, 1979.

117. Cunliffe WJ, Ead RD: A case of Ehlers-Danlos syndrome occurring with Marfan's syndrome, *Clin Exp Dermatol* 2(2):117-120, 1977.

118. Cupo LN et al: Ehlers-Danlos syndrome with abnormal collagen fibrils, sinus of Valsalva aneurysms, myocardial infarction, panacinar emphysema and cerebral heterotopias, *Am J Med* 71(6):1051-1058, 1981.

119. Curley SA, Osler T, Demarest GB: Traumatic disruption of the subclavian artery and brachial plexus in a patient with Ehlers-Danlos syndrome, *Ann Emerg Med* 17(8):850-852, 1988.

120. Cutolo M et al: Altered fibronectin distribution in cultured fibro-blasts from patients with Ehlers-Danlos syndrome, *Clin Exp Rheumatol* 4(2):125-128, 1986.

121. Dales HC, O'Neill JJ: Management of arterial complications in a case of the arterial type of Ehlers-Danlos syndrome, *Br J Surg* 57(6):476-477, 1970.

122. Danlos M: Un cas de cutis laxa avec tumeurs par contusion chronique des coudes et des genoux (xanthome juvenile pseudo-diabetique de MM Hallopeau et Mace de Lépinay), *Bull Soc Franc Derm Syph* 19:70-72, 1908.

123. Darier MJ: Notice nécrologiques sur M Ehlers (1868-1937), *Bull Acad Med* 117:626-628, 1937.

124. Das M, Saha PK, Mishra Y: Ehlers-Danlos syndrome, *J Indian Med Assoc* 57(11):428-430, 1971.

125. Day HJ, Zarafonetis CJD: Coagulation studies in four patients with Ehlers-Danlos syndrome, *Am J Med Sci* 242:565-573, 1961.

126. Debré R, Semelaigne G: A propos de la maladie d'Ehlers chez le nourrisson, *Bull Soc Méd Hôp Paris* 57:849, 1936.

127. Dembure PP et al: Genotyping and prenatal assessment of collagen lysyl hydroxylase deficiency in a family with Ehlers-Danlos syndrome type VI, *Am J Hum Genet* 36(4):783-790, 1984.

128. Dembure PP et al: Ascorbate regulation of collagen biosynthesis in Ehlers-Danlos syndrome, type VI, *Metabolism* 36(7):687-691, 1987.

129. Denko CW: Chernogubov's syndrome: a translation of the first modern case report of the Ehlers-Danlos syndrome, *J Rheumatol* 5(3):347-352, 1978.

130. De Paepe A et al: Obstetrical problems in patients with Ehlers-Danlos syndrome type IV: a case report, *Eur J Obstet Gynecol Reprod Biol* 33(2):189-193, 1989.

131. De Paepe A et al: Ehlers-Danlos syndrome type I: a clinical and ultra-structural study of a family with reduced amounts of collagen type III, *Br J Dermatol* 117(1):89-97, 1987.

132. Desbuquois G et al: Nanisme chondrodystrophique avec ossification anarchique et polymalformations chez duex soeurs, *Arch Franc Pediatr* 23:573-587, 1966.

133. Dewart P: Maladie d'Ehlers-Danlos, *Arch Derm Syph* 21:397, 1965.

134. Dick JC: Observations of the elastic tissue of the skin with a note on the reticular layer at the junction of the dermis and epidermis, *J Anat* 81:201-211, 1947.

135. Dick JC: The tension and resistance to stretching of human skin and other membranes, with results from a series of normal and edematous cases, *J Physiol* 112:102-113, 1951.

136. Di Ferrante N et al: Lysyl oxidase deficiency in Ehlers-Danlos syndrome type V, *Connect Tissue Res* 3(1):49-53, 1975.

137. Di Ferrante N et al: Ehlers-Danlos type V (X-linked form): a lysyl oxidase deficiency, *Birth Defects* 11(6):31-37, 1975.

138. Di Mario C, Zanchetta M, Maiolino P: Coronary aneurysms in a case of Ehlers-Danlos syndrome, *Jpn Heart J* 29(4):491-496, 1988.

139. Dodge JA, Shillito J Jr: Ehlers-Danlos syndrome associated with acquired encephalocele, *J Pediatr* 66:1061-1067, 1965.

140. Doerks G: Zur klinischen Prüfung der Hautdehnug, *Arch Kinderheilk* 136:1-11, 1949.

141. Dorsch HH: Ueber das Ehlers-Danlos-Syndrom, Veröffentlichung eines Falles bei einem Zwillingskind, *Kinderaerztl Prax* 21:49-55, 1953.

142. Douglas BS, Douglas HM: Rectal prolapse in the Ehlers-Danlos syndrome, *Aust Paediatr J* 9(2):109-110, 1973.

143. Dowson D et al: Lubrication of joints. In Dowson D, Wright V, editors: *Introduction to the biomechanics of joints and joint replacement*, London, 1981, Mechanical Engineering Publications, pp 120-133.

144. Dreyfus G et al: Un cas de maladie d'Ehlers-Danlos, *Bull Soc Méd Hôp Paris* 52:1463, 1936.

145. Driscoll SH, Gomes AS, Machleder HI: Perforation of the superior vena cava: a complication of digital angiography in Ehlers-Danlos syndrome, *Am J Roentgenol* 142(5):1021-1022, 1984.

146. Du Bois: Cutis laxa (abstract), *Zbl Haut-u Geschlkr* 35:52 only, 1931.

147. Du Mesnil: Beitrag zur anatomie und aetiologie bestimmter hautkrankheiten, dissertation, Würzburg, 1890. Cited by Unna.[274]

148. Dunmore PJ, Roach MR: The effects of age, vessel size, and Ehlers-Danlos type IV syndrome on the waviness index of arteries, *Clin Invest Med* 13(2):67-70, 1990.

149. Duperrat B: Le syndrome d'Ehlers-Danlos, *Gaz Med France* 72:4037-4040, 1965.

150. Durham DG: Cutis hyperelastica (Ehlers-Danlos syndrome) with blue scleras, micro-cornea, and glaucoma, *Arch Ophthalmol* 49:220-221, 1953.

151. Eadie DG, Wilkins JL: Bladder-neck obstruction and the Ehlers-Danlos syndrome, *Br J Urol* 39:353-358, 1967.

152. Edmondson P, Nellen M, Ross DN: Aortic valve replacement in a case of Ehlers-Danlos syndrome, *Br Heart J* 42(1):103-5, 1979.

153. Edwards A, Taylor GW: Ehlers-Danlos syndrome with vertebral artery aneurysm, *Proc Roy Soc Med* 62:734-735, 1969.

154. Ehlers E: Cutis laxa, neigung zu haemorrhagien in der haut, lockerung mehrerer artikulationen, *Derm Zschr* 8:173-175, 1901.

155. Ellis FE, Bundick WR: Cutaneous elasticity and hyperelasticity, *Arch Dermatol* 75:32, 1957.

156. Estes JW: Platelet size and function in the heritable disorders of connective tissue, *Ann Intern Med* 68:1237-1249, 1968.

157. Eyre DR, Shapiro FD, Aldridge JF: A heterozygous collagen defect in a variant of the Ehlers-Danlos syndrome type VII: evidence for a deleted amino telopeptide domain in the pro-alpha2(I) chain, *J Biol Chem* 260(20) 11,332-11,339, 1985.

158. Fantl P, Morris KN, Sawers RJ: Repair of cardiac defect in patient with Ehlers-Danlos syndrome and deficiency of Hageman factor, *Br Med J* 1:1202-1204, 1961.

159. Farag TI, Schimke RN: Ehlers-Danlos Syndrome: a new oculoscoliotic type with associated polyneuropathy? *Clin Genet* 35(2):121-124, 1989.

160. Farley MK et al: Spontaneous carotid-cavernous fistula and the Ehlers-Danlos syndromes, *Ophthalmology* 90(11): 1337-1342, 1983.

161. Fazekas A: Simultaneous occurrence of Ehlers-Danlos syndrome and Marfan's syndrome, *Orv Hetil* 117(3):154-158, 1976.

162. Fehlow P, Tennstedt A: Neuropsychiatrische Begleitsymptome bei einem Fall von Ehlers-Danlos-Syndrom. (Concomitant neuropsychiatric symptoms in a case of Ehlers-Danlos syndrome), *Psychiatr Neurol Med Psychol* 37(4): 215-220, 1985.

163. Forman AR: Situs inversus of the disc in the Ehlers-Danlos syndrome, type III, *Ophthalmology* 86(5):844-846, 1979.

164. Fox R et al: Spontaneous carotid cavernous fistula in Ehlers-Danlos syndrome, *J Neurol Neurosurg Psychiatry* 51(7):984-986, 1988.

165. François B et al: Pulse wave velocity recordings in a family with ecchymotic Ehlers-Danlos syndrome, *Int Angiol* 5(1):1-5, 1986.

166. François P et al: Maladie d'Ehlers-Danlos avec anéurysme artérioveineux intra-crànien, *Bull Soc Ophthalmol Fr* 5:392, 1955.

167. Freeman JT: Ehlers-Danlos syndrome, *Am J Dis Child* 79:1049-1056, 1950.

168. Frick PG, Krafchuk JD: Studies of hemostasis in the Ehlers-Danlos syndrome, *J Invest Dermatol* 26:453-457, 1956.

169. Friedman JM, Harrod MJ: An unusual connective tissue disease in mother and son: a "new" type of Ehlers-Danlos syndrome? *Clin Genet* 21(3):168-173, 1982.

170. Fritchey JA, Greenbaum SS: Two cases of Ehlers-Danlos syndrome, *Arch Dermatol Syph* 42:742-743, 1940.

171. Froelich H: Fibrodysplasia elastica generalisata (cutis laxa) und nervensystem, *Nervenarzt* 20:366-371, 1949.

172. Gadrat J, Bazex A: Sur le syndrome d'Ehlers-Danlos, *Ann Dermatol Syph* 78:430, 1951.

173. Gamble JG, Mochizuki C, Rinsky LA: Trapeziometacarpal abnormalities in Ehlers-Danlos syndrome, *J Hand Surg* 14(1):89-94, 1989.

174. Garrick JL: Personal communication, 1972.

175. Gertsch P et al: Changing patterns in the vascular form of Ehlers-Danlos syndrome, *Arch Surg* 121(9):1061-1064, 1986.

176. Gilbert A, Villaret M, Bosviel G: Sur un cas d'hyperélasticité congénitale des ligaments articulaires et de la peau, *Bull Soc Méd Hôp Paris* 59:303-307, 1925.

177. Golden RL, Garret R: Forme fruste of Ehlers-Danlos syndrome, *New York J Med* 64:3017-3020, 1964.

178. Goltz RW, Hult AM: Generalized elastolysis (cutis laxa) and Ehlers-Danlos syndrome (cutis hyperelastica): a comparative clinical and laboratory study, *Southern Med J* 58:848-854, 1965.

179. Goodman RM, Allison ML: Chronic temporomandibular joint subluxation in Ehlers-Danlos syndrome: report of case, *J Oral Surg* 27:659-661, 1969.

180. Goodman RM, Baba N, Wooley CF: Observations on the heart in a case of combined Ehlers-Danlos and Marfan syndromes, *Am J Cardiol* 24:734-742, 1969.

181. Goodman RM, Katznelson MBM, Frydman M: Evolution of palmar skin creases in the Ehlers-Danlos syndrome, *Clin Genet* 3(1):67-72, 1972.

182. Goodman RM, Levitsky JM, Friedman IA: The Ehlers-Danlos syndrome and neurofibromatosis in a kindred of mixed derivation, with special emphasis on hemostasis in the Ehlers-Danlos syndrome, *Am J Med* 32:976-983, 1962.

183. Goodman RM, Wooley CF, Frazier RL: Ehlers-Danlos syndrome occurring together with the Marfan syndrome: report of a case with other family members affected, *New Engl J Med* 273:514-519, 1965.

184. Gordon H: Ehlers-Danlos syndrome, *Proc Roy Soc Med* 35:263-264, 1942.

185. Gore I: Dissecting aneurysm of the aorta in persons under forty years of age, *Arch Pathol* 55:1-13, 1953.

186. Gore I, Seiwert VS: Dissecting aneurysm of the aorta, pathologic aspects: an analysis of 85 fatal cases, *Arch Pathol* 53:121-141, 1952.

187. Gorlin RJ, Pindborg JJ: *Syndromes of the head and neck*, New York, 1964, McGraw-Hill, pp 96-97.

188. Gould GM, Pyle WL: *Anomalies and curiosities of medicine*, Philadelphia, 1897, WB Saunders, p 217.

189. Graf CJ: Spontaneous carotid-cavernous fistula; Ehlers-Danlos syndrome and related conditions, *Arch Neurol* 13:662-672, 1965.

190. Grahame R, Beighton P: Physical properties of the skin in the Ehlers-Danlos syndrome, *Ann Rheum Dis* 28(3):246-251, 1969.

191. Grahame R et al: A clinical and echocardiographic study of patients with the hypermobility syndrome, *Ann Rheum Dis* 40:541-546, 1981.

192. Grant AK, Aldor TA: Haemorrhage into the upper part of the gastrointestinal tract in three patients with heritable disorders of connective tissue, *Aust Ann Med* 16:75-79, 1967.

193. Green GJ, Schuman BM, Barron J: Ehlers-Danlos syndrome complicated by acute hemorrhagic sigmoid diverticulitis, with an unusual mitral valve abnormality, *Am J Med* 41:622-625, 1966.

194. Green WR, Friedman-Kien A, Banfield WH: Angioid streaks in Ehlers-Danlos syndrome, *Arch Ophthalmol* 76:197-204, 1966.

195. Greenfield JG, Cornman T, Shy GM: The prognostic value of the muscle biopsy in the "floppy child," *Brain* 81:461-484, 1958.

196. Guerrerosantos J, Dicksheet S: Cervicofacial rhytidoplasty in Ehlers-Danlos syndrome: hazards on healing, *Plast Reconstr Surg* 75(1):100-103, 1985.

197. Gupta KK, Lal R: Two cases of Ehlers-Danlos syndrome with cardiac abnormalities, *Indian Heart J* 23:296-301, 1971.

198. Habein HC: Ehlers-Danlos syndrome with spontaneous rupture of the esophagus: report of first case, *Rocky Mt Med J* 74(2):78-80, 1977.

199. Hagino H et al: Computed tomography in patients with Ehlers-Danlos syndrome, *Neuroradiology* 27(5):443-445, 1985.

200. Halbach VV et al: Treatment of carotid cavernous fistulas associated with Ehlers-Danlos syndrome, *Neurosurgery* 26(6):1021-1027, 1990.

201. Halila R, Steinmann B, Peltonen L: Processing of types I and III procollagen in Ehlers-Danlos syndrome type VII, *Am J Hum Genet* 39(2):222-231, 1986.

202. Reference deleted in proofs.

203. Hall DA et al: Collagen and elastin in connective tissue, *J Gerontol* 10:388-400, 1955.

204. Hallopeau, de Lépinay M: Sur un cas de xanthoma tubéreaux et de tumeurs juvéniles offrant les charactères du xanthome diabétique, *Bull Soc Dermatol Syph Fr* 17:283-287, 1906.

205. Hammerschmidt DE et al: Maternal Ehlers-Danlos syndrome type X. Successful management of pregnancy and parturition, *JAMA* 248(19):2487-2488, 1982.

206. Hanset R, Ansay M: Dermatosparaxie (peau déchirée) chez le veau; un defaut général du tissu conjonctif, de nature héréditaire, *Ann Méd Vet* 110:451, 1967.

207. Harland D: Ehlers-Danlos syndrome, *Proc Roy Soc Med* 63:286-287, 1970.

208. Harris RD: Small bowel dilatation in Ehlers-Danlos syndrome—an unreported gastrointestinal manifestation, *Br J Radiol* 47(561):623-627, 1974.

209. Harris SC, Slater DN, Austin CA: Fatal splenic rupture in Ehlers-Danlos syndrome, *Postgrad Med J* 61(713):259-260, 1985.

210. Hartsfield JK, Kousseff BG: Phenotypic overlap of Ehlers-Danlos syndrome types IV and VIII, *Am J Med Genet* 37:465-470, 1990.

211. Hass J, Hass R: Arthrochalasis multiplex congenita, *J Bone Joint Surg* 40(A):663-674, 1958.

212. Hata R, Kurata S, Shinkai H: Existence of malfunctioning pro alpha2(I) collagen genes in a patient with a pro alpha2(I)-chain–defective variant of Ehlers-Danlos syndrome, *Eur J Biochem* 174(2):231-237, 1988.

213. Hathaway WE: Bleeding disorders due to platelet dysfunction, *Am J Dis Child* 121:127-134, 1971.

214. Hayakawa A, Fujimoto K, Ibayashi H: Two cases of Ehlers-Danlos syndrome with gastrointestinal complications, *Gastroenterol Jpn* 17(1):61-67, 1982.

215. Hegreberg GA et al: A connective tissue disease of dogs and mink resembling the Ehlers-Danlos syndrome of man. II. Mode of inheritance, *J Hered* 60:249-254, 1969.

216. Hegreberg GA, Padgett GA, Henson JB: Connective tissue disease of dogs and mink resembling Ehlers-Danlos syndrome of man. III. Histopathologic changes of the skin, *Arch Pathol* 90:159-166, 1970

217. Hegreberg GA et al: A heritable connective tissue disease of dogs and mink resembling Ehlers-Danlos syndrome of man. I. Skin tensile strength properties, *J Invest Dermatol* 54(5):377-380, 1970.

218. Hegreberg GA: Animal model of human disease: Ehlers-Danlos syndrome, *Am J Pathol* 79(2):383-386, 1975.

219. Heilmann K, Kolig G: Nierenarterienruptur bei Ehlers-Danlos syndrome, *Z Kreislaufforsch* 60:519-533, 1971.

220. Helliwell PS, Howe A, Wright V: Lack of objective evidence of stiffness—rheumatoid arthritis, *Ann Rheum Dis* 47:754-758, 1988.

221. Hernàndez A et al: A distinct variant of the Ehlers-Danlos syndrome, *Clin Genet* 16(5):335-339, 1979.

222. Hernàndez A et al: Third case of a distinct variant of the Ehlers-Danlos syndrome, *Clin Genet* 20:222-224, 1981.

223. Hernàndez A et al: Ehlers-Danlos features with progeroid facies and mild mental retardation. Further delineation of the syndrome, *Clin Genet* 30(6):456-461, 1986.

224. Hines C Jr, Davis WD Jr: Ehlers-Danlos syndrome with megaduodenum and malabsorption syndrome secondary to bacterial overgrowth: a report of the first case, *Am J Med* 54(4):539-543, 1973.

225. Hoff M: Dental manifestations in Ehlers-Danlos syndrome: report of a case, *Oral Surg Oral Med Pathol* 44(6):864-871, 1977.

226. Hollister DW: Heritable disorders of connective tissue: Ehlers-Danlos syndrome, *Pediatr Clin North Am* 25(3):575-591, 1978.

227. Hollister DW: Clinical features of Ehlers-Danlos syndrome type VIII and IX. In Akeson WH, editor: *Symposium on heritable disorders of connective tissue*, St Louis, 1982, Mosby—Year Book, pp 102-113.

228. Hollister DW et al: Ehlers-Danlos syndrome type VIII, abstract, *Clin Res* 28(1):99A, 1980

229. Holt JF: The Ehlers-Danlos syndrome, *Am J Roentgenol* 55:420-426, 1946.

230. Holzberg M, Hewan-Lowe KO, Olansky AJ: The Ehlers-Danlos syndrome: recognition, characterization, and importance of a milder variant of the classic form. A preliminary study, *J Am Acad Dermatol* 19(4):656-666, 1988.

231. Horan FT, Beighton P: Recessive inheritance of generalized joint hypermobility, *Rheumatol Rehabil* 12:47-49, 1973.

232. Horton WA et al: Familial joint instability syndrome, *Am J Med Genet* 6:221-228, 1980.

233. Hulme JR, Wilmshurst CC: Acute appendicitis in the Ehlers-Danlos syndrome, *Am J Surg* 132(1):103-104, 1976.

234. Hunter GC et al: Vascular manifestations in patients with Ehlers-Danlos syndrome, *Arch Surg* 117(4):495-498, 1982.

235. Hurvitz SA, Baumgarten A, Goodman RM: The wrinkly skin syndrome: a report of a case and review of the literature, *Clin Genet* 38:307-313, 1990.

236. Husebye KO: Tre familiäere tilfelle av Ehlers-Danlos syndrom, *T Norsk Laegeforen* 72:185-188, 1952.

237. Ihme A et al: Biochemical characterization of variants of the Ehlers-Danlos syndrome type VI, *Eur J Clin Invest* 13(4):357-362, 1983.

238. Ihme A et al: Ehlers-Danlos syndrome type VI: collagen type specificity of defective lysyl hydroxylation in various tissues, *J Invest Dermatol* 83(3):161-165, 1984.

239. Imahori S et al: Ehlers-Danlos syndrome with multiple arterial lesions, *Am J Med* 47:967-977, 1969.

240. Iurlov VM: Pathogenesis of bleeding in Chernogubov—Ehlers-Danlos syndrome, *Klin Med (Mosk)* 53(11):93-97, 1975.

241. Iwama T et al: Ehlers-Danlos syndrome complicated by eventration of the diaphragm, colonic perforation and jejunal perforation: a case report, *Jpn J Surg* 19(3):376-380, 1989.

242. Jacobs PH: Ehlers-Danlos syndrome; report of a case with onset at age 29, *Arch Dermatol* 76:460, 1957.

243. Jaffe AS et al: Mitral valve prolapse: a consistent manifestation of type IV Ehlers-Danlos syndrome. The pathogenetic role of the abnormal production of type III collagen, *Circulation* 64(1):121-125, 1981.

244. Jansen LH: *De Ziekte van Ehlers en Danlos*, Gravenhage, 1954, Uitgeverij Excelsor.

245. Jansen LH: Le mode de transmission de la maladie d'Ehlers-Danlos, *J Genet Hum* 4:204-218, 1955.

246. Jansen LH: The structure of the connective tissue, an explanation of the symptoms of the Ehlers-Danlos syndrome, *Dermatologica* 110:108-120, 1955.

246a. Jerosch J, Castro WH: Shoulder instability in Ehlers-Danlos syndrome. An indication for surgical treatment, *Acta Orthop Belg* 56(2):451-453, 1990.

247. Jochims J: Elastometrie an Kindern bei wechselnder Hautdehnung, *Arch Kinderheilk* 135:228-237, 1948.

248. Johns RJ, Wright V: Relative importance of various tissues in joint stiffness, *J Appl Physiol* 17:824-828, 1962.

249. Johns RJ, Wright V: An analytical description of joint stiffness, *Biorheology* 2:87-95, 1964.

250. Johnson SAM, Falls HF: Ehlers-Danlos syndrome: a clinical and genetic study, *Arch Dermatol Syph* 60:82-105, 1949.

251. Jones ML: Orthodontic treatment in Ehlers-Danlos syndrome, *Br J Orthod* 11(3):158-162, 1984.

252. Judisch GF, Waziri M, Krachmer JH: Ocular Ehlers-Danlos syndrome with normal lysyl hydroxylase activity, *Arch Ophthalmol* 94(9):1489-1491, 1976.

253. Julkunen H, Rokkanen P, Jounela A: Bone changes in Ehlers-Danlos syndrome, *Ann Med Intern Fenn* 56:55-59, 1967.

254. Junqueira LC, Roscoe JT: Reduced collagen content and fibre bundle disorganization in skin biopsies of patients with Ehlers-Danlos syndrome, *Histochem J* 17(11):1197-1202, 1985.

255. Kahana M et al: Painful piezogenic pedal papules in a child with Ehlers-Danlos syndrome, *Pediatr Dermatol* 3(1):45-47, 1985.

256. Kahana M et al: Painful piezogenic pedal papules in patients with Ehlers-Danlos Syndrome, *J Am Acad Dermatol* 17(2,1):205-209, 1987.

257. Kahn T et al: The Ehlers-Danlos syndrome, type IV, with an unusual combination of organ malformations, *Cardiovasc Intervent Radiol* 11(5):288-291, 1988.

258. Kanof A: Ehlers-Danlos syndrome: report of a case with suggestion of a possible causal mechanism, *J Dis Child* 83:197-202, 1952.

259. Karaca M, Cronberg L, Nilsson IM: Abnormal platelet-collagen reaction in Ehlers-Danlos syndrome, *Scand J Haematol* 9(5):465-469, 1972.

260. Kashiwagi H, Riddle JM, Abraham JP: Functional and ultrastructural abnormalities of platelets in Ehlers-Danlos syndrome, *Ann Intern Med* 63:249-254, 1965.

261. Katz I, Steiner K: Ehlers-Danlos syndrome with ectopic bone formation, *Radiology* 65:352-360, 1955.

262. Kayed K, Kåss B: Acute multiple brachial neuropathy and Ehlers-Danlos syndrome, *Neurology* 29(12):1620-1621, 1979.

263. Kiilholma P et al: Pregnancy and delivery in Ehlers-Danlos syndrome. Role of copper and zinc, *Acta Obstet Gynecol Scand* 63(5):437-439, 1984.

264. King-Lewis FL: Two cases of Ehlers-Danlos syndrome, *Proc Roy Soc Med* 39:135 only, 1946.

265. Kirk E, Kvorning SA: Quantitative measurements of the elastic properties of the skin and subcutaneous tissue in young adults and old individuals, *J Gerontol* 4:273-284, 1949.

266. Kirk JA, Ansell BM, Bywaters EG: The hypermobility syndrome; musculoskeletal complaints associated with generalized joint hypermobility, *Ann Rheum Dis* 26:419-425, 1967.

267. Kitazono T et al: Two cases of myocardial infarction in type 4 Ehlers-Danlos Syndrome, *Chest* 95(6):1274-1277, 1989.

268. Kobayasi T, Ogucchi M, Asboe-Hansen G: Dermal changes in Ehlers-Danlos syndrome, *Clin Genet* 25(6):477-484, 1984.

269. Kopp: Demonstration zweier Fälle von "Cutis laxa," *München Med Wschr* 35:259, 1888.

270. Kontusaari S et al: Inheritance of an RNA splicing mutation (G+ 1 IVS20) in the type III procollagen gene (COL3A1) in a family having aortic aneurysms and easy bruisability: phenotypic overlap between familial arterial aneurysms and Ehlers-Danlos syndrome type IV, *Am J Hum Genet* 47(1):112-120, 1990.

270a. Kontusaari S et al: A mutation in the gene for type III procollagen (COL3A1) in a family with aortic aneurysms, *J Clin Invest* 86:1465-1473, 1990.

271. Kornberg M, Aulicino PL: Hand and wrist joint problems in patients with Ehlers-Danlos syndrome, *J Hand Surg (Am)* 10(2):193-196, 1985.

272. Korting GW: Elastosis perforans serpiginosa als ektodermales rand Symptom bei Cutis laxa, *Arch Klin Exp Dermatol* 224:437-446, 1966.

273. Korting GW, Gottron E: Cutis laxa, *Arch Dermatol Syph* 193:14, 1951.

274. Kousseff BG: Ehlers-Danlos syndrome and epidermolysis bullosa in the same family, *Cutis* 27(5):519-521, 1981.

275. Kozlova SI et al: Presumed homozygous Ehlers-Danlos syndrome type I in a highly inbred kindred, *Am J Med Genet* 18(4):763-767, 1984.

276. Krane SM, Pinnell SR, Erbe RW: Decreased lysyl-protocollagen hydroxylase activity in fibroblasts from a family with a newly recognized disorder: hydroxylysine-deficient collagen, *J Clin Invest* 51:52a, 1972.

277. Kresse H et al: Glycosaminoglucan-free small proteoglycan core protein is secreted by fibroblasts from a patient with a syndrome resembling progeroid, *Am J Hum Genet* 41:436-453, 1987.

278. Krog M et al: Vascular complications in the Ehlers-Danlos syndrome, *Acta Chir Scand* 149(3):279-82, 1983.

279. Kuivaniemi H et al: A 19-base pair deletion in the pro alpha 1(1) gene of Type I Procollagen that causes in-frame RNA splicing from exon 10 to exon 12 in a proband with atypical osteogenesis imperfecta and in his asymptomatic mother, *J Biol Chem* 263:11,407-11,413, 1988.

280. Kuivaniemi H et al: Identical G^{+1} to A mutations in three different introns of the type III procollagen gene (COL3A1) produce different patterns of RNA splicing in three variants of Ehlers-Danlos syndrome IV. An explanation for exon skipping with some mutations and not others, *J Biol Chem* 265(20):12,067-12,074, 1990.

281. Kuming BS, Joffe L: Ehlers-Danlos syndrome associated with keratoconus: a case report, *S Afr Med J* 21(10):403-405, 1977.

282. Laane CL: Cushing's syndrome associated with obliterative arterial disease and multiple subcutaneous nodules (Ehlers-Danlos syndrome?), *Acta Med Scand* 148:323-325, 1954.

283. Lach B et al: Spontaneous carotid-cavernous fistula and multiple arterial dissections in type IV Ehlers-Danlos syndrome: case report, *J Neurosurg* 66(3):462-467, 1987.

284. Langeron P, Coisne T: Iliac arteriopathy and Ehlers-Danlos disease, *Sem Hôp Paris* 55(5-6):292-295, 1979.

285. Lapayowker MS: Cutis hyperelastica: the Ehlers-Danlos syndrome, *Am J Roentgenol* 84:232-234, 1960.

286. Lapière CM, Lenaers A, Kohn LD: Procollagen peptidase: an enzyme excising the co-ordination peptides of procollagen, *Proc Natl Acad Sci* 68:3054-3058, 1971.

287. Lapière CM, Nusgens BV: Ehlers-Danlos type VIII skin has a reduced proportion of collagen type III, abstract, *J Invest Dermatol* 76:422-429, 1981.

288. Larsen LJ, Schottstaedt ER, Bost FC: Multiple congenital dislocations associated with characteristic facial abnormality, *J Pediatr* 37:574-581, 1950.

289. Latta RJ et al: Larsen's syndrome: a skeletal dysplasia with multiple joint dislocations and unusual facies, *J Pediatr* 78:291-298, 1971.

290. Launay C: Syndrome d'Ehlers-Danlos chez un garçon de onze ans, associé à une arriération mentale, *Bull Soc Méd Hôp Paris* 56:709-711, 1941.

291. Le Coulant P: Hyperélasticité cutanée et articulaire avec fragilité anormale de la peau et tumeurs molluscoides, chez un enfant de treize ans (syndrome d'Ehlers-Danlos), *Gaz Sci Méd Bordeaux* vol 29, 1934.

292. Lee B et al: Characterization of a large genomic deletion associated with a polymorph block of repeated dinucleotides in the type III procollagen gene (COL3A1) of a patient with Ehlers-Danlos syndrome type IV, *Am J Hum Genet* 48:511-517, 1991.

293. Lees MH et al: Ehlers-Danlos syndrome associated with multiple pulmonary artery stenoses and tortuous systemic arteries, *J Pediatr* 75:1031-1036, 1969.

294. Leider M: Forme fruste of Ehlers-Danlos syndrome, *Urol Cut Rev* 53:222, 1949.

295. Leier CV et al: The spectrum of cardiac defects in the Ehlers-Danlos syndrome, types I and III, *Ann Intern Med* 92(2 Pt 1):171-178, 1980.

296. Levard G et al: Urinary bladder diverticula and the Ehlers-Danlos syndrome in children, *J Pediatr Surg* 24(11):1184-1186, 1989.

297. Levine AS, Michael AF: Ehlers-Danlos syndrome with renal tubular acidosis and medullary sponge kidneys: a report of a case and studies of renal acidification in other patients with the Ehlers-Danlos syndrome, *J Pediatr* 71(1):107-113, 1967.

298. Levy-Coblentz G: Radio-ulnar synostosis, *Bull Soc Dermatol Syph Fr* 39:1252, 1932.

299. Lewitus Z: Ehlers-Danlos syndrome: report of two cases with hypophyseal dysfunction, *Arch Dermatol* 73:158-161, 1956.

300. Lewkonia RM, Pope FM: Joint contractures and acroosteolysis in Ehlers-Danlos syndrome type IV, *J Rheumatol* 12(1):140-144, 1985.

301. Lichtenstein JR: Ehlers-Danlos syndrome with probable recessive inheritance and hydroxylysine-deficient collagen, *Birth Defects* 11(2):339, 1975.

302. Lichtenstein JR, McKusick VA: Ehlers-Danlos syndrome with aortic aneurysm, *Birth Defects* 11(2):341-343, 1975.
303. Lichtenstein J et al: Molecular defect in a form of the Ehlers-Danlos syndrome: hydroxylysine deficient collagen (abstract), *Am J Hum Genet* 24:27 only, 1972.
304. Lichtenstein JR et al: Defect in conversion of procollagen to collagen in a form of Ehlers-Danlos syndrome, *Science* 182(109):298-300, 1973.
305. Lienhart O: *La maladie d'Ehlers-Danlos: étude clinique, anatomopathologique et génetique*, thesis de NANCY (No 30), 1945.
306. Linch DC, Acton CH: Ehlers-Danlos syndrome presenting with juvenile destructive periodontitis, *Br Dent J* 147(4):95-96, 1979.
307. Linnemann MP, Johnson VW: Ehlers-Danlos syndrome presenting with torsion of stomach, *Proc Roy Soc Med* 68(5):330-332, 1975.
308. Lisker R, Noguerón A, Sánchez-Medal L: Plasma thromboplastin component deficiency in the Ehlers-Danlos syndrome, *Ann Intern Med* 53:388-395, 1960.
309. Littré E: *Oeuvres complète d'Hippocrate*, vol 2, Paris, 1840, JB Bailliére.
310. Lynch HT, Larsen AL, Wilson R: Ehlers-Danlos syndrome, and "congenital" arteriovenous fistulae, a clinicopathologic study of a family, *JAMA* 194:1011-1104, 1965.
311. Mabille JP et al: Un case de syndrome d'Ehlers-Danlos, avec acro-osteolyse, *Ann Radiol (Paris)* 15(9):781-786, 1972.
312. MacCollum DW: The lop ear, *JAMA* 110:1427-1430, 1938.
313. Madison WJ Jr, Bradley EJ, Castillo AJ: Ehlers-Danlos syndrome with cardiac involvement, *Am J Cardiol* 11:689-693, 1963.
314. Manna R et al: Ehlers-Danlos syndrome (type V) with urethra bifida and polydactyly: an unusual combination, *Minerva Med* 72(26):1725-1730, 1981.
315. Margarot J, Deneze P, Coll de Carrera: Hyperlaxité cutanée et articulaire (syndrome de Danlos) existant chez trois membres d'une même famille, *Bull Soc Dermatol Syph Fr* 40:277-286, 1933.
316. Maroteaux P, Frezal J, Cohen-Solal L: The differential symptomatology of errors of collagen metabolism: a tentative classification, *Am J Med Genet* 24(2):219-230, 1986.
317. Martin GI: The Ehlers-Danlos syndrome: report of two cases in monozygous Philippino-American twins, *J Chronic Dis* 23(3):197-200, 1970.
318. Mason P, Rigby BJ: Ehlers-Danlos syndrome, physical and biochemical aspects, *Arch Pathol* 80:363-364, 1965.
319. Mauseth R, Lieberman E, Heuser ET: Infantile polycystic disease of the kidneys and Ehlers-Danlos syndrome in an 11-year-old patient, *J Pediatr* 90(1):81-83, 1977.
320. May MA, Beauchamp GR: Collagen maturation defects in Ehlers-Danlos keratopathy, *J Pediatr Ophthalmol Strabismus* 24(2):78-82, 1987.
321. Maximow A: Development of argyrophile and collagenous fibers in tissue culture, *Proc Soc Exp Biol Med* 25:439-442, 1928.
322. McEntyre RL, Raffensperger JG: Surgical complications of Ehlers-Danlos syndrome in children, *J Pediatr Surg* 12(4):531-535, 1977.
323. McEvitt WG: The problem of the protruding ear, *Plast Reconstr Surg* 2:481-496, 1947.
324. McFarland W, Fuller DE: Mortality in Ehlers-Danlos syndrome due to spontaneous rupture of large arteries, *New Engl J Med* 271:1309-1310, 1964.
325. Macfarlane IL: Ehlers-Danlos syndrome presenting certain unusual features, *J Bone Joint Surg* 41B:541-545, 1959.
326. McGookey DJ et al: Mosaicism for a deletion in one of the type III collagen alleles indicates that the deletion occurred after identification of cells for recruitment in different cell lineages early in human development, Abstract 0809, *Am J Hum Genet* 45(suppl 4):A206, 1989.
327. McKusick VA: Hereditary disorders of connective tissue, *Bull New York Acad Med* 35:143-156, 1959.
328. McKusick VA: *Heritable disorders of connective tissue*, ed 4, St Louis, 1972, Mosby–Year Book.
329. McKusick VA: Multiple forms of the Ehlers-Danlos syndrome, *Arch Surg* 109(4):475-476, 1974.
330. McKusick VA: *Mendelian inheritance in man*, ed 9, Baltimore, 1990, Johns Hopkins University.
331. McLeod DR et al: Chromosome 6q deletions: a report of two additional cases and a review of the literature, *Am J Med Genet* 35(1):79-84, 1990.
332. Meara RH: Ehlers-Danlos syndrome and elastoma verruciforme perforans (Miescher), *Trans St John Hosp Dermatol Soc* 40:72, 1958.
333. Mehregan AH: Elastosis perforans serpiginosa: a review of the literature and report of 11 cases, *Arch Dermatol* 97:381-393, 1968.
334. Méténier P: *A propos d'un cas familial de maladie d'Ehlers-Danlos*, Thése d'Alger (No 55), 1939.
335. Miguet A: *Le syndrome d'Ehlers-Danlos*, Thése, Louis Arnette, Paris, 1933.
336. Min HK, Lee LDB: Ehlers-Danlos syndrome in a Korean kindred, *Korean J Intern Med* 6:545-550, 1963.
337. Mirza FH et al: Multiple aneurysms in a patient with Ehlers-Danlos syndrome: angiography without sequelae, *Am J Roentgenol* 132(6):993-995, 1979.
338. Miura S et al: Fibronectin receptor on polymorphonuclear leukocytes in families of Ehlers-Danlos syndrome and other hereditary connective tissue diseases, *J Lab Clin Med* 116(3):363-368, 1990.
339. Moore JR, Tolo VT, Weiland AJ: Painful subluxation of the carpometacarpal joint of the thumb in Ehlers-Danlos syndrome, *J Hand Surg (Am)* 10(5):661-663, 1985.
340. Mories A: *An investigation into the Ehlers-Danlos syndrome*, Edinburgh thesis, 1954.
341. Mories A: Ehlers-Danlos syndrome, with a report of a fatal case, *Scot Med J* 5:269-272, 1960.
342. Morris : Case report: elastic skin and numerous cutaneous nodules, *Br J Dermatol* 12:208-209, 1900.
343. Morris M: *Diseases of the skin*, ed 4, Plate XI, New York, 1909, William Woods.
344. Morris RC et al: Medullary sponge kidney, *Am J Med* 38:883-892, 1965.
345. Mounier-Kuhn P, Meyer L: Méga-organes (oesophage, trachée, colon), syndromes de Mickulicz et d'Ehlers-Danlos chez une hérédosyphilitique, *Bull Soc Méd Hôp Lyon*, Nov 9, 1943.
346. Mukerji S: Ehlers-Danlos syndrome with pregnancy, *J Indian Med Assoc* 64(6):149-151, 1975.
347. Murray JE, Tyars ME: A case of Ehlers-Danlos syndrome, *Br Med J* 1:974 only, 1940.
348. Myers DE: Ehlers-Danlos syndrome as a cause of temporomandibular joint disorders, *Anesth Prog* 32(1):23-24, 1985.
349. Nagashima C et al: Atlanto-axial, atlanto-occipital dislocations, developmental cervical canal stenosis in the

Ehlers-Danlos syndrome, *No Shinkei Geka* 9(5):601-608, 1981.

350. Nakazawa M et al: Homograft of preserved sclera for posttraumatic scleral staphyloma in Ehlers-Danlos syndrome, *Arch Clin Exp Ophthalmol* 224(3):247-250, 1986.

351. Narcisi P et al: An alpha 1(1III) CB5 mutation in Ehlers-Danlos syndrome type IV, *Abstract J Med Genet* 26(3):211, 1989.

352. Nelson DL, King RA: Ehlers-Danlos syndrome type VIII, *J Am Acad Dermatol* 5(3):297-303, 1981.

353. Newton JE, Carpenter ME: Ehlers-Danlos syndrome with acro-osteolysis, *Br J Radiol* 32:739-743, 1959.

354. Nicaud P, Lafitte A, Buhot S: Syndrome d'Ehlers-Danlos fruste associé à une atrophic musculaire du type Aran-Duchenne, *Bull Soc Méd Hôp Paris* March 10, 1944.

355. Nicholls AC et al: Linkage of a polymorphic marker for the type III collagen gene (COL3A1) to atypical autosomal dominant Ehlers-Danlos syndrome type IV in a large Belgian pedigree, *Hum Genet* 78(3):276-281, 1988.

356. Nicod M: Un cas de syndrome d'Ehlers-Danlos, *Ann Paediatr* 167:358, 1946.

357. Nordschow CD, Marsolais EB: Ehlers-Danlos syndrome: some recent biophysical observations, *Arch Pathol* 88:65-68, 1969.

358. Norton LA: Orthodontic tooth movement response in Ehlers-Danlos syndrome: report of a case, *J Am Dent Assoc* 109(2):259-262, 1984.

359. Nosher JL, Trooskin SZ, Amorosa JK: Occlusion of a hepatic arterial aneurysm with Gianturco coils in a patient with the Ehlers-Danlos syndrome, *Am J Surg* 152(3):326-328, 1986.

360. Noto P: Cited by Pelbois and Rollier.[205]

361. O'Hara PJ, Read WK, Romane WM, Bridges CH: A collagenous tissue dysplasia of calves, *Lab Invest* 23:307-314, 1970.

362. Okamura H, Matsumoto Y: A case of Ehlers-Danlos syndrome associated with cleft lip and palate, *J Laryngol Otol* 98(3):311-315, 1984.

363. Oku T et al: Growth kinetics of fibroblasts from a patient with Ehlers-Danlos syndrome, *Acta Derm Venereol (Stockholm)* 70(1):56-57, 1990.

364. Olmsted F, Page IH, Corcoran AC: A device for objective clinical measurement of cutaneous elasticity, a "pinchmeter," *Am J Med Sci* 222:73-75, 1951.

365. O'Neill S et al: Pneumothorax in the Ehlers-Danlos syndrome, *Irish J Med Sci* 150(2):43-44, 1981.

366. Onel D, Ulutin SB, Ulutin ON: Platelet defect in a case of Ehlers-Danlos syndrome, *Acta Haematol* 50(4):238-244, 1973.

367. Ormsby OS, Tobin WW: Cutis hyperelastica: case report, *Arch Dermatol Syph* 38:828-829, 1938.

368. Osborn TG et al: Ehlers-Danlos syndrome presenting as rheumatic manifestations in the child, *J Rheumatol* 8(1):79-85, 1981.

369. Ota M, Yasuda T: Erster Fall von "Syndrome d'Ehlers-Danlos" in Japan, *Zbl Haut Geschlechtskr* 66:120, 1941.

370. Owen SM, Durst RD: Ehlers-Danlos syndrome simulating child abuse, *Arch Dermatol* 120(1):97-101, 1984.

371. Owren PA: The nature of the defects in hemorrhagic disorders, *Acta Haematol* 36:141-156, 1966.

372. Packer BD, Blades JF: Dermatorrhexis: a case report, the so-called Ehlers-Danlos syndrome, *Virginia Med Monthly* 81:27-30, 1954.

373. Padgett GA, Gorham JR, Henson JB: Mink as a biomedical model, *Lab Anim Care* 18:258-266, 1968.

374. Palvölgyi R, Bálint BJ, Józsa L: The Ehlers-Danlos syndrome causing lacerations in tendons and muscles, *Arch Orthop Trauma Surg* 95(3):173-176, 1979.

375. Pamphlett R, Nelson MM: The Ehlers-Danlos syndrome in a Xhosa male, *S Afr Med J* 48(17):741-742, 1974.

376. Papapetropoulos T, Tsankanikas C, Spengos M: Brachial neuropathy and Ehlers-Danlos syndrome (letter), *Neurology* 31(5):642-643, 1981.

377. Papp JP, Paley RG: Ehlers-Danlos syndrome: incidence in three generations of a kindred, *Postgrad Med* 40:586-592, 1966.

378. Pascher F: Ehlers-Danlos syndrome, *Arch Dermatol Syph* 67:214, 1953.

379. Pautrier M: Note histologique sur un cas de cutis elastica, avec pseudotumeurs aux genoux et aux coudes, présenté par M Danlos, *Bull Soc Franc Dermatol Syph* 19:72-74, 1908.

380. Peaceman AM, Cruikshank DP: Ehlers-Danlos syndrome and pregnancy: association of type IV disease with maternal death, *Obstet Gynecol* 69(3:2):428-431, 1987.

381. Pelbois F, Rollier F: Association d'un syndrome d'Ehlers-Danlos et d'un syndrome de Groenblad-Strandberg, *Bull Soc Dermatol Syph Fr* 59:141, 1952.

382. Peltonen L et al: Alterations in copper and collagen metabolism in the Menkes syndrome and a new subtype of the Ehlers-Danlos syndrome, *Biochemistry* 22(26):6156-6163, 1983.

383. Pemberton JW, Freeman HM, Schepens CL: Familial retinal detachment and the Ehlers-Danlos syndrome, *Arch Ophthalmol* 76:817-824, 1966.

384. Perreau P, Bangas J, Lecuit P: Osteitis fibro-kystique atypique et syndrome d'Ehlers-Danlos: lesion parathyroidienne, *Bull Soc Méd Hôp Paris* 57:135, 1941.

385. Péyri: Un cas de syndrome d'Ehlers-Danlos, probablement d'origine syphilitique, *Bull Soc Dermatol Syph Fr* 44:1744, 1937.

386. Phadke JG, Johnson VW, Young HB: Ehlers-Danlos syndrome with surgical repair of eventration of diaphragm and torsion of stomach, *J Roy Soc Med* 72(10):781-783, 1979.

387. Pierard GE, Pierard-Franchimont C, Lapière CM: Histopathological aid at the diagnosis of the Ehlers-Danlos syndrome, gravis and mitis types, *Int J Dermatol* 22(5):300-304, 1983.

388. Pierce LE, Tyrrell ME, Day CE: Gastrectomy in Ehlers-Danlos syndrome, *Arch Surg* 96:95-99, 1968.

389. Pinnell SR et al: A new heritable disorder of connective tissue with hydroxylysine-deficient collagen, *New Engl J Med* 286:1013-1020, 1972.

390. Pommerening RA, Antonius JI: Normal chromosomes in a family with Ehlers-Danlos syndrome, *Arch Dermatol* 94:425-431, 1966.

390a. Pope FM: Molecular analysis of Ehlers-Danlos syndrome Type II, *Br J Rheumatol* 30(3):163-166, 1991.

391. Pope FM: Personal communication, 1991.

392. Pope FM, Limburg M, Schievink WI: Familial cerebral aneurysms and type III collagen deficiency, *J Neurosurg* 72:156-157, 1990.

393. Pope FM, Martin GR, McKusick VA: Inheritance of Ehlers-Danlos type IV syndrome, *J Med Genet* 14(3):200-204, 1977.

394. Pope FM et al: Patients with Ehlers-Danlos syndrome type IV lack type III collagen, *Proc Natl Acad Sci USA* 72(4):1314-1316, 1975.

395. Pope FM et al: EDS IV (acrogeria): new autosomal dominant and recessive types, *J Roy Soc Med* 73:180-186, 1980.

396. Pope FM et al: Clinical presentations of Ehlers-Danlos syndrome type IV, *Arch Dis Child* 63(9):1016-1025, 1988.

397. Pope FM et al: Type III collagen mutations in Ehlers-Danlos syndrome type IV and other related disorders, *Clin Exp Dermatol* 13(5):285-302, 1988.

398. Pope FM et al: Prenatal diagnosis and prevention of inherited abnormalities of collagen, *J Inherited Metab Dis* 12(suppl 1):135-173, 1989.

399. Pouliquen Y, Petroutsos G, Papaioannou D: Corneal dystrophy and Ehlers-Danlos syndrome, *J Fr Ophtalmol* 6(4):387-389, 1983.

400. Poumeau-Delille G, Soulié P: Un cas d'hyperlaxité cutanée et articulaire avec cicatrices atrophiques et pseudotumeurs molluscoides (syndrome d'Ehlers-Danlos), *Bull Soc Méd Hôp Paris* 50:593-595, 1934.

401. Pray LG: Cutis elastica (dermatorrhexis, Ehlers-Danlos syndrome), *Am J Dis Child* 75:702-711, 1948.

402. Pretorius ME, Butler IJ: Neurologic manifestations of Ehlers-Danlos syndrome, *Neurology* 33(8):1087-1089, 1983.

403. Pyeritz RE et al: Ehlers-Danlos syndrome IV due to a novel defect in type III procollagen, *Am J Med Genet* 19(3):607-622, 1984.

404. Rao AA: Ehlers-Danlos syndrome with monostotic fibrous dysplasia, *J Postgrad Med* 25(3):186-188, 1979.

405. Raybaud A, Guidoni P: Hyperlaxité ligamentaire et cutanée; trouble du métabolisme calcique; maladie d'Ehlers-Danlos, *Bull Soc Méd Hôp Paris* 54:738-740, 1938.

406. Redington A, McCue J, Lennox S: Coronary artery vein grafting in a case of Ehlers-Danlos syndrome, *Br Heart J* 52(2):237-239, 1984.

407. Reed WB: Ehlers-Danlos syndrome with neurological complications, *Arch Dermatol* 106(3):410-411, 1972.

408. Rees TD, Wood-Smith D, Converse JM: The Ehlers-Danlos syndrome, *Plast Reconstr Surg* 32:39-44, 1963.

409. Ricketson G: The behavior of skin grafts and donor sites in a case of Ehlers-Danlos syndrome, *Plast Reconstr Surg* 20:32-37, 1957.

410. Riedle M et al: A case of prepuberty periodontitis—a classification based on laboratory results, *Dtsch Zahnarztl Z* 44(4):289-292, 1989.

411. Ringrose EJ, Nowlan FB, Perry H: Ehlers-Danlos syndrome: report of a case, *Arch Dermatol Syph* 62:443-448, 1950.

412. Rivera-Alsina ME et al: Complications of the Ehlers-Danlos syndrome in pregnancy: a case report, *J Reprod Med* 20(10):797-799, 1984.

413. Rizzo R et al: Familial Ehlers-Danlos syndrome type II: abnormal fibrillogenesis of dermal collagen, *Pediatr Dermatol* 4(3):197-204, 1987.

414. Roberts DL et al: Ehlers-Danlos syndrome type IV mimicking nonaccidental injury in a child, *Br J Dermatol* 111(3):341-345, 1984.

415. Robertson I: Keratoconus and the Ehlers-Danlos syndrome: a new aspect of keratoconus, *Med J Aust* 1(18):571-573, 1975.

416. Robinson HM Jr, Ellis FA: Cutis laxa, *Arch Dermatol* 77:656, 1958.

417. Robitaille GA: Ehlers-Danlos syndrome and recurrent hemoptysis, *Ann Intern Med* 61:716-721, 1964.

418. Roederer C: Syndrome d'Ehlers-Danlos atypique coincidant avec une dolichosténomélie, *Arch Franc Pédiatr* 8:192-195, 1951.

419. Rollhäuser H: Die Zugfestigkeit der menschlichen Haut, *Gegenbaurs Morphol Jahrb* 90:249, 1950.

420. Ronchese F: Dermatorrhexis, with dermatochalasis and arthrochalasis (the so-called Ehlers-Danlos syndrome), *Am J Dis Child* 51:1403-1414, 1936.

421. Ronchese F: Dermatorrhexis, with dermatochalasis and arthrochalasis (the so-called Ehlers-Danlos syndrome): additional data on a case reported 12 years previously, *Rhode Island Med J* 32:80-83, 1949.

422. Ross M, Dooneief AS: Chest surgery in the presence of cutis hyperelastica (Ehlers-Danlos syndrome), *New York J Med* 57:2256-2259, 1957.

423. Rossi E, Angst H: Das Danlos-Ehlers syndrome, *Helv Paediatr Acta* 6:245-254, 1951.

424. Royce PM et al: Brittle cornea syndrome: an heritable connective tissue disorder distinct from Ehlers-Danlos syndrome type VI and fragilitas oculi, with spontaneous perforations of the eye, blue sclerae, red hair, and normal collagen lysyl hydroxylation, *Eur J Pediatr* 149(7):465-469, 1990.

425. Rubinstein MK, Cohen NH:. Ehlers-Danlos syndrome associated with multiple intracranial aneurysms, *Neurology* 14:125-132, 1964.

426. Ruby ST et al: Internal carotid artery aneurysm: a vascular manifestation of type IV Ehlers-Danlos syndrome, *Conn Med* 53(3):142-144, 1989.

427. Rudd NL et al: Pregnancy complications in type IV Ehlers-Danlos syndrome, *Lancet* 1(8314-5):50-53, 1983.

428. Rybka FJ, O'Hara ET: Surgical significance of the Ehlers-Danlos syndrome, *Am J Surg* 113:431-434, 1967.

429. Sack G: Status dysvascularis: ein Fall von besonderer Zerreisslichkeit der Blutgefässe, *Deutsch Arch Klin Med* 178:663-669, 1936.

430. Sacks H, Zelig D, Schabes G: Recurrent temporomandibular joint subluxation and facial ecchymosis leading to diagnosis of Ehlers-Danlos syndrome: report of surgical management and review of the literature, *J Oral Maxillofac Surg* 48(6):641-647, 1990.

431. Sadeghi EM, Ostertag PR, Eslami A: Oral manifestations of Ehlers-Danlos syndrome: report of a case, *J Am Dent Assoc* 118(2):187-191, 1989.

432. Saemundsson J: Ehlers-Danlos syndrome; a congenital mesenchymal disorder, *Acta Med Scand* 154(suppl 312):399-408, 1956.

433. Samuel MA, Schwartz ML, Meister MM: The Ehlers-Danlos syndrome, *US Armed Forces Med J* 4:737, 1953.

434. Sato J: Case of Ehlers-Danlos syndrome with visceral abnormalities, *Clin Endocri (Tokyo)* 14:565-569, 1966.

435. Sarra-Carbonnell S, Jimenez SA: Ehlers-Danlos syndrome associated with acute pancreatitis, *J Rheumatol* 16(10):1390-1394, 1989.

436. Sartoris DJ et al: Type IX Ehlers-Danlos syndrome: a new variant with pathognomonic radiographic features, *Radiology* 152(3):665-670, 1984.

437. Scarborough PR et al: An unbalanced (6q,13q) translocation in a male with clinical features of Ehlers-Danlos type II syndrome, *J Med Genet* 21(3):226-228, 1984.

438. Schaper G: Familiäres Vorkommen von Ehlers-Danlos Syndrome; ein Beitrag zur Klinik und Pathogenese, *Zschr Kinderheilk* 70:504-526, 1952.

439. Scheinin TM, Dahl M: Repair of atrial septal defect in a patient with the Ehlers-Danlos syndrome, *Scand J Thorac Cardiovasc Surg* 1:114-117, 1967.

440. Schippers E, Dittler HJ: Multiple hollow organ dysplasia in Ehlers-Danlos syndrome, *J Pediatr Surg* 24(11):1181-1183, 1989.

441. Schoolman A, Kepes JJ: Bilateral spontaneous carotid-cavernous fistulae in Ehlers-Danlos syndrome: case report, *J Neurosurg* 26:82-86, 1967.

442. Seaton DG: Bilateral recurrent dislocation of the patellas in the Ehlers-Danlos syndrome, *Med J Aust* 1:737-739, 1969.

443. Serry C, Agomuoh OS, Goldin MD: Review of Ehlers-Danlos syndrome. Successful repair of rupture and dissection of abdominal aorta, *J Cardiovasc Surg* 29(5):530-534, 1988.

444. Sestak Z: Ehlers-Danlos syndrome and cutis laxa: an account of families in the Oxford area, *Ann Hum Genet* 25:313-321, 1962.

445. Shapiro SK: A case of Meekrin-Ehlers-Danlos syndrome with neurologic manifestations, *J Nerv Ment Dis* 115:64-71, 1952.

446. Shaw HB, Hopkins P: A case of a boy, aged seven, showing (a) double-jointedness, (b) dermatolysis ("elastic skin") with great friability of the skin and excessive tendency to bruising, and (c) multiple subcutaneous tumours on the limbs (fibromata, neuronomata), *Proc Roy Soc Med (Clin Sect)* 6:20-22, 1913.

447. Sheiner NM, Miller N, Lachance C: Arterial complications of Ehlers-Danlos syndrome, *J Cardiovasc Surg* 26(3):291-296, 1985.

448. Shi EC, Bohane TD, Bowring AC: Prophylactic colectomy in Ehlers-Danlos syndrome with colonic ectasia, *J Pediatr Surg* 24(11):1187-1188, 1989.

449. Shohet I et al: Cardiovascular complications in the Ehlers-Danlos syndrome with minimal external findings, *Clin Genet* 31:148-152, 1987.

450. Siegel RC, Black CM, Bailey AJ: Cross-linking of collagen in the X-linked Ehlers-Danlos Type V Syndrome, *Biochem Biophys Res Commun* 88(1):281-287, 1979.

451. Sigurdson E et al: The Ehlers-Danlos syndrome and colonic perforation. Report of a case and physiologic assessment of underlying motility disorder, *Dis Colon Rectum* 28(12):962-966, 1985.

452. Silva R et al: Intestinal perforation and vascular rupture in Ehlers-Danlos syndrome, *Int Surg* 71(1):48-50, 1986.

453. Singh SD, Munjal N, Mansharamani RK: Ehlers-Danlos syndrome: Brief review with a case report, *Indian J Pediat* 31:1-5, 1964.

454. Simon AP, Stein PD: Aortic insufficiency in Ehlers-Danlos syndrome, *Angiology* 25(4):290-296, 1974.

455. Slingenberg EJ: Complications during intravascular diagnostic manipulations in the Ehlers-Danlos syndrome, *Neth J Surg* 32(2):56-58, 1980.

456. Slootweg PJ, Beemer FA: Gingival fibrinoid deposits in Ehlers-Danlos syndrome, *J Oral Pathol* 16(3):150-152, 1987.

457. Smit J, Alberts C, Balk AG: Pneumothorax in the Ehlers-Danlos syndrome: consequence or coincidence, *Scand J Respir Dis* 59(5):239-42, 1978.

458. Smith CH: Dermatorrhexis (Ehlers-Danlos syndrome), *J Pediatr* 14:632-641, 1939.

459. Smith RD, Worthington JW: Paganini: the riddle and connective tissue, *JAMA* 199:820-824, 1967.

460. Smith SA, Powell LC, Essin EM: Ehlers-Danlos syndrome and pregnancy, report of a case, *Obstet Gynecol* 32:331-335, 1968.

461. Snyder RR, Gilstrap LC, Hauth JC: Ehlers-Danlos syndrome and pregnancy, *Obstet Gynecol* 61(5):649-650, 1983.

461a. Soucy P, Eidus L, Keeley F: Perforation of the colon in a 15 year old girl with Ehlers-Danlos Syndrome type IV, *J Pediatr Surg* 25(11):1180-1182, 1990.

462. Spiro MJ, Janiak BD: Spontaneous rupture of the sigmoid colon in a patient with Ehlers-Danlos syndrome, *Ann Emerg Med* 13(10):960-962, 1984.

463. Steer G et al: Joint capsule collagen: analysis by the study of intraarticular pressure during joint distension, *Ann Rheum Dis* 30(5):481-486, 1971.

464. Steinmann B et al: Ehlers-Danlos syndrome in two siblings with deficient lysyl hydroxylase activity in cultured skin fibroblasts but only mild hydroxylysine deficit in skin, *Helv Paediatr Acta* 30(3):255-274, 1975.

465. Steinmann B et al: Evidence for a structural mutation of procollagen in a patient with Ehlers-Danlos syndrome type VII, *Eur J Pediatr* 130:203-205, 1979.

466. Steinmann B et al: Evidence for a structural mutation of procollagen type I in a patient with Ehlers-Danlos syndrome type VII, *J Biol Chem* 255(18):8887-8893, 1980.

467. Steinmann B et al: Ehlers-Danlos syndrome type IV: a subset of patients distinguished by low serum levels of the amino-terminal propeptide of type III procollagen, *Am J Med Genet* 34(1):68-71, 1989.

468. Stewart RE, Hollister DW, Rimoin DL: A new variant of Ehlers-Danlos syndrome: an autosomal dominant disorder of fragile skin, abnormal scarring, and generalized periodontitis, *Birth Defects* 13(3B):85-93, 1977.

469. Stillians AW, Zakon SJ: Cutis laxa (cutis hyperplastica), *Arch Dermatol Syph* 35:342-343, 1937.

470. Stoddard FJ, Myers RE: Connective tissue disorders in obstetrics and gynaecology, *Am J Obstet Gynecol* 102:240-243, 1968.

471. Stoll C et al: Ehlers-Danlos syndrome associated with gigantism, craniosynostosis and melanoderma, *Pediatrie* 29(1):81-89, 1974.

472. Stuart AM: Three cases exhibiting the Ehlers-Danlos syndrome, *Proc Roy Soc Med* 30:984-986, 1937.

473. Sturkie PD: Hypermobile joints in all descendants for two generations, *J Hered* 32:232-234, 1941.

474. Sulh HM et al: Ehlers-Danlos syndrome type IV D: an autosomal recessive disorder, *Clin Genet* 25(3):278-287, 1984.

475. Sulica VI et al: Cutaneous histologic features in Ehlers-Danlos syndrome: a study of 21 patients, *Arch Dermatol* 115(1):40-42, 1979.

476. Sullivan JD: The Ehlers-Danlos syndrome; report of case with transient paralysis of vocal cord, *Arch Neur Psychiat* 47:316-318, 1942.

477. Summer GK: The Ehlers-Danlos syndrome; a review of the literature and report of a case with a subgaleal hematoma and Bell's palsy, *J Dis Child* 91:419-428, 1956.

478. Superti-Furga A et al: Ehlers-Danlos syndrome type IV: a multi-exon deletion in one of the two COL3A1 alleles affecting structure, stability, and processing of type III procollagen, *J Biol Chem* 263(13):6226-6232, 1988.

479. Superti-Furga A, Steinmann B: Impaired secretion of type III procollagen in Ehlers-Danlos syndrome type IV fibroblasts: correction of the defect by incubation at reduced temperature and demonstration of subtle alterations in the triple-helical region of the molecule, *Biochem Biophys Res Commun* 150(1):140-147, 1988.

480. Superti-Furga A et al: Molecular defects of type III procollagen in Ehlers-Danlos syndrome type IV, *Hum Genet* 82(2):104-108, 1989.

481. Sussman M et al: Hydroxylysine-deficient skin collagen in a patient with a form of the Ehlers-Danlos syndrome, *J Bone Joint Surg (AM)* 56(6):1228-1234, 1974.

482. Sutro CJ: Hypermobility of bones due to "overlengthened" capsular and ligamentous tissues: cause for recurrent intra-articular effusions, *Surgery* 21:67-76, 1947.

483. Svane S: Ehlers-Danlos syndrome; a case with some skeletal changes, *Acta Orthop Scand* 37:49-57, 1966.

484. Sykes EM Jr: Colon perforation in Ehlers-Danlos syndrome: report of two cases and review of the literature, *Am J Surg* 147(3):410-413 1984.

485. Tajima S, Murad S, Pinnell SR: A comparison of lysyl hydroxylation in various types of collagen from type VI Ehlers-Danlos syndrome fibroblasts, *Coll Relat Res* 3(6):511-515, 1983.

486. Reference deleted in proofs.

487. Taylor DJ, Wilcox I, Russell JK: Ehlers-Danlos syndrome during pregnancy: a case report and review of the literature, *Obstet Gynecol Surv* 36(6):277-281, 1981.

488. Taylor FR: The Meekrin-Ehlers-Danlos syndrome, *Urol Cut Rev* 47:378-379, 1943.

489. Thakker-Varia S et al: An exon deletion in type III procollagen mRNA is associated with intracellular degradation of the abnormal protein in a patient with Ehlers-Danlos syndrome IV, Abstract III-11, Third International Conference on the Molecular Biology and Pathology of Matrix, Philadelphia, June 13-16, *Matrix* 10:249-250, 1990.

490. Thexton A: A case of Ehlers-Danlos syndrome presenting with recurrent dislocation of the temporomandibular joint, *Br J Oral Surg* 2:190-193, 1965.

491. Thivolet J et al: Dysplasie mésenchymateuse complexe: type artériel de l'Ehlers-Danlos syndrome de Sack-Barabas? *Bull Soc Dermatol Syph Fr* 76:817-821, 1969.

492. Thomas C, Cordier J, Algan B: Une étiologie nouvelle du syndrome de luxation spontanée des cristallins: la maladie d'Ehlers-Danlos, *Bull Soc Belg Ophtalmol* 100:375-381, 1952.

493. Thomas C, Cordier J, Algan B: Les altérations oculaires de la maladie d'Ehlers-Danlos, *Arch Ophtalmol (Paris)* 14:691-697, 1954.

494. Thomas C et al: Les manifestations oculaires de la maladie d'Ehlers-Danlos, *Bull Soc Ophtalmol Fr* p.211-217, 1953.

495. Thurmon FM: Ehlers-Danlos syndrome, *Arch Dermatol Syph* 40:120-121, 1939.

496. Tsipouras P et al: Ehlers-Danlos syndrome type IV: cosegregation of the phenotype to a COL3A1 allele of type III procollagen, *Hum Genet* 74(1):41-46, 1986.

497. Tobias N: Danlos syndrome associated with congenital lipomatosis, *Arch Dermatol Syph* 30:540-551, 1934; 40:135-137, 1939.

498. Toyohara T et al: Giant epiphrenic diverticulum in a boy with Ehlers-Danlos syndrome, *Pediatr Radiol* 19(6-7):437, 1989.

499. Tromp G et al: Single base mutation in the type III procollagen gene that converts the codon for glycine 883 to aspartate in a mild variant of Ehlers-Danlos syndrome IV, *J Biol Chem* 264(32):19,313-19,317, 1989.

500. Tromp G et al: A single base mutation that substitutes serine for glycine 790 of the alpha 1 (III) chain of type III procollagen exposes an arginine and causes Ehlers-Danlos syndrome IV, *J Biol Chem* 264(3):1349-1352, 1989.

501. Tschernogobow A: Cutis laxa (presentation at first meeting of Moscow Dermatologic and Venereologic Society, Nov 13, 1891) *Mhft Prakt Derm* 14:76, 1892.

502. Tschernogobow A: Ein Fall von Cutis laxa. Protokoly Moskowskawo wenerologitscheskawo i dermatologitscheskawo Obtschestwa, vol 1, quoted in *Jahresb Ges Med* 27:562, 1892.

503. Tsukahara M et al: A disease with features of cutis laxa and Ehlers-Danlos syndrome: Report of a mother and daughter, *Hum Genet* 78(1):9-12, 1988.

504. Tucker DH, Miller DE, Jacoby WJ Jr: Ehlers-Danlos syndrome with sinus of Valsalva aneurysm and aortic insufficiency simulating rheumatic heart disease, *Am J Med* 35:715-720, 1963.

505. Tunbridge RE et al: The fibrous structure of normal and abnormal human skin, *Clin Sci* 11:315-331, 1952.

506. Turkington RW, Grude HE: Ehlers-Danlos syndrome and multiple neurofibromatosis, *Ann Intern Med* 61:549-555, 1964.

507. Tyson JEA: Personal communication to McKusick, 1972.

508. Umlas J: Spontaneous rupture of the subclavian artery in the Ehlers-Danlos syndrome, *Hum Pathol* 3(1):121-126, 1972.

509. Unna PG: *The histopathology of the diseases of the skin.* Translated from the German by N Walker with the assistance of the author, New York, 1896, Macmillan, pp 984-988.

510. van Meekeren JA: De dilatabilitate extraordinaria cutis. *Observations medicochirugicae*, Chapter 32, Amsterdam, 1682.

511. van Selms WG, Yo TI, Kuiken H: Spontaneous rupture of the external iliac artery in a patient with Ehlers Danlos syndrome type IV, *Eur J Vasc Surg* 4(4):419-421, 1990.

512. Varadi DP, Hall DA: Cutaneous elastin in Ehlers-Danlos syndrome, *Nature* 208:1224-1225, 1965.

513. Vasileva ON, Vasileva NV: Dva nabliudeniia sindroma Chernogubova-Elersa-Danlos, *Vestn Khir* 131(9):110-112, 1983.

514. Verger P et al: Syndrome d'Ehlers-Danlos compliqué d'hémorragies digestives chez l'enfant, *Pediatrie* 25:215-216, 1970.

515. Viljoen D et al: Ehlers-Danlos syndrome: yet another type? *Clin Genet* 32(3):196-201, 1987.

516. Vissian L, Rovinski J: Syndrome d'Ehlers-Danlos chez quatre membres d'une même famille, *Bull Soc Franc Dermatol Syph* 62:62-63, 1955.

517. Vissian L et al: Un nouvel état morbide lié à une anomalie chromosomique: syndrome d'Ehlers-Danlos associé à une maladie du cri du chat chez un nouveau-né, *Presse Méd* 73:2991-2994, 1965.

518. Vissing H et al: Multi-exon deletion in the Procollagen III Gene is associated with mild Ehlers-Danlos syndrome type IV, *J Biol Chem* 266:5244-5248, 1991.

519. Vogel A et al: Abnormal collagen fibril structure in the gravis form (type I) of Ehlers-Danlos syndrome, *Lab Invest* 40(2):201-206, 1979.

520. Walker VA, Beighton PH, Murdoch JL: The Marfanoid hypermobility syndrome, *Ann Intern Med* 71:349-352, 1969.

521. Wallach EA, Burkhart EF: Ehlers-Danlos syndrome associated with tetralogy of Fallot, *Arch Dermatol Syph* 61:750-752, 1950.

522. Wallis G: Personal communication, 1991.

523. Ward GW: Cutaneous asthenia (cutis hyperelastica) of dogs, *Aust Vet J* 46:115 only, 1970.

524. Weber FP: The Ehlers-Danlos syndrome, *Br J Dermatol Syph* 48:609-617, 1936.

525. Weber FP, Aitken JK: Nature of the subcutaneous spherules in some cases of Ehlers-Danlos syndrome, *Lancet* 1:198-199, 1938.

526. Wechsler HL, Fisher ER: Ehlers-Danlos syndrome: pathologic, histochemical, and electron microscopic observations, *Arch Pathol* 77:613-619, 1964.

527. Weil D et al: Identification of a mutation that causes exon skipping during collagen pre-mRNA splicing in an Ehlers-Danlos syndrome variant, *J Biol Chem* 263(18):8561-8564, 1988.

528. Weil D et al: A base substitution in the exon of a collagen gene causes alternative splicing and generates a structurally abnormal polypeptide in a patient with Ehlers-Danlos syndrome type VII, *EMBO J* 8(6):1705-1710, 1989.

529. Weil D et al: Structural and functional characterization of a splicing mutation in the pro-alpha 2(I) collagen gene of an Ehlers-Danlos type VII patient, *J Biol Chem* 265(26):16,007-16,011, 1990.

530. Weill J, Martineau J: A propos d'un cas de maladie d'Ehlers-Danlos; étude anatomoclinique et biologique, *Bull Soc Dermatol Syph Fr* 44:99, 1937.

531. Weinbaum PJ et al: Pregnancy management and successful outcome of Ehlers-Danlos syndrome type IV, *Am J Perinatol* 4(2):134-137, 1987.

532. Weiss RS: Danlos' syndrome, *Arch Dermatol* 40:137-138, 1939.

533. Wenstrup RJ, Murad S, Pinnell SR: Ehlers-Danlos syndrome type VI: clinical manifestations of collagen lysyl hydroxylase deficiency, *J Pediatr* 115(3):405-409, 1989.

534. Wenzel HG: Untersuchungen über die Dehnbarkeit und Zerreissbarkeit der Haut, *Zbl Allg Path* 85:117, 1949.

535. Wigzell FW, Ogston D: The bleeding tendency in Ehlers-Danlos syndrome, *Ann Phys Med* 7:55-58, 1963.

536. Williams AW: Cutis laxa, *Monatsschr Prakt Derm* 14:490, 1892.

537. Winship IM: Ehlers-Danlos syndrome in the Western Cape, *S Afr Med J* 67(13):509-511, 1985.

538. Wirtz MK et al: Ehlers-Danlos syndrome type VIIB. Deletion of 18 amino acids comprising the N-telopeptide region of a pro-alpha 2(I) chain, *J Biol Chem* 262(34):16,376-16,385, 1987.

539. Wordsworth BP et al: Exclusion of the alpha 1(II) collagen structural gene as a mutant locus in type II Ehlers-Danlos syndrome, *Ann Rheum Dis* 44(7):431-433, 1985.

539a. Wordsworth BP et al: Limited heterogeneity of the HLA classII contribution to susceptibility to rheumatoid arthritis is suggested by positive associations with HLA-DR4, DR1 and DRw10, *Br J Rheumatol* 30:178-180, 1991.

540. Wright CB et al: Successful management of popliteal arterial disruption in Ehlers-Danlos syndrome, *Surgery* 85(6):708-712, 1979.

541. Wright V, Johns RJ: The quantitative measurement of joint stiffness (abstract), *J Clin Invest* 38:1056 only, 1959.

542. Wynne-Davies R: Acetabular dysplasia and familial joint laxity: two etiological factors in congenital dislocation of the hip. A review of 589 patients and their families, *J Bone Joint Surg* 52B:704-716, 1970.

543. Yamashita M et al: Uterine rupture in a case with Ehlers-Danlos syndrome type IV—anesthetic considerations, *Middle East J Anesthesiol* 9(3):277-281, 1987.

543a. Young ID et al: Amniotic bands in connective tissue disorders, *Arch Dis Child* 60(11):1061-1063, 1985.

544. Zaida AH: Ehlers-Danlos syndrome with congenital herniae and pigeon breast, *Br Med J* 2:175-176, 1959.

545. Zalis EG, Roberts DC: Ehlers-Danlos syndrome with a hypoplastic kidney, bladder diverticulum, and diaphragmatic hernia, *Arch Dermatol* 96:540-544, 1967.

546. Zambal Z: Sind Hyperkeratosis follicularis in cutem penetrans und Elastoma intrapapillare perforans verruciforme identisch? *Hautarzt* 9:304, 1958.

547. Zlotogora J et al: Syndrome of brittle cornea, blue sclera and joint hyper-extensibility, *Am J Med Genet* 36:269-272, 1990.

CHAPTER 7

Cutis Laxa

F. Michael Pope

In the syndromic context the term "Cutis laxa (CL)" refers to a heterogeneous group of disorders that are characterized by inappropriate symmetric laxity of skin, which hangs in loose folds. The changes are especially evident over the face and trunk and are frequently associated with systemic abnormalities, particularly of the lungs, arteries, and urinary tract. The underlying pathologic process involves primary or secondary changes in elastin.

The classical forms of heritable CL are conventionally subclassified into autosomal dominant and autosomal recessive categories, but other genetic forms of CL have been delineated. In addition, skin laxity is a feature of several rare entities not of genetic origin, and it may also be a minor manifestation of a variety of connective tissue disorders and other conditions.

In addition to the use of "Cutis laxa" as a name for several rare entities of genetic and nongenetic origin, the term is also employed to describe skin laxity resulting from whatever cause, without implying any particular etiology. In this chapter the designation "Cutis laxa" or its abbreviation, "CL," pertains to specific disorders, whereas "cutis laxa" or "cutis laxa (loose skin)" simply implies loose skin.

HISTORICAL NOTE

The terminology of CL is closely entwined with that of the Ehlers-Danlos syndrome (EDS), with which it has often been confused; the reasons have been both semantic and nosologic. Thus semantic failure to distinguish between lax[42,164] and elastic[168] skin led Ehlers,[43] Danlos,[35] and Sequeira[141] to describe their patients as having cutis laxa. Similarly, in the fourth edition of this book McKusick pointed out that Kopp,[82] who clearly documented autosomal dominant transmission of generalized cutis laxa as early as 1888, has often been cited as describing EDS. Part of the confusion also stemmed from the fundamental conceptual failure to recognize that the skin changes in EDS and CL were the result of different pathologic processes. In practice, ironically, some overlap exists between the two disorders in syndromes such as CL with joint laxity and wormian bones and in those unusual cases of individuals with particular forms of EDS who have loose and redundant skin either as infants or as aging adults.

The history of CL is complicated and confusing, but it provides precedents for the accepted subcategories of the modern classification. Indeed, the condition has been recorded under a number of different names in numerous publications dating from 1800 and thereafter (see the box on p. 254). The authors of these articles all documented the redundant nature of the skin but failed to distinguish between generalized and patchy changes. Indeed, it is apparent that several of them (notably, Alibert[2,3]) were describing conditions that are now recognized as plexiform neurofibromas, hypertrophic keloid scarring, nevoid changes, and tumors.[103,146] Lymphatic obstruction, lymphoedema, and, occasionally, fibrosarcomas probably were also included in this group. Later, a distinction emerged between localized cutis laxa (then called *chalazoderma,*[161] *cutis pendula,* or *dermatolysis*) and more generalized inherited forms of the disorder. These familial conditions were clearly described by Graf[61] in 1836 and Tilbury-Fox in

Terminology of Cutis Laxa

Term	Source
Cutis pendula	
Cutis pensilis	
Cutis lapsus	Alibert, 1832,[2] 1855[3]
Cutis rugositas	
Chalazodermie	
Pachydermatocele	Mott, 1854[101]
Atrophie idiopathique de la peau	Pospelow, 1886[121]
Dermatolysis	Dubreuilh[42]
Cutis Laxa	Kopp, 1888[82]
Geromorphisme cutane	Souques and Charcot, 1891[145]
Chalodermie	von Ketley, 1901[161]
Schlaffhaut	von Ketley, 1901[161]
Progeria (premature senility)	Rand, 1914[122]
Peau ridée sénile congenitale	Variot and Cailliau, 1920[159]
Loose skin	Petges and Lecoulant, 1936[117]
Gerodermie infantile	Petges and Lecoulant, 1936[117]

1876[151] and shortly afterward by Rossbach[131] (who reported the same family that Kopp[82] and Dubreuilh[42] reported in 1887). Dubreuilh's patient was a strikingly abnormal 13-year-old girl with an appearance of premature aging caused by lax, soft skin, especially over the face, neck, upper thighs, and abdomen. Four years later, in 1891, she was depicted in much more detail by Souques and Charcot[145] (Fig. 7-1, A). Whereas Dubreuilh[42] named the disorder "generalized dermatolysis," the others called it "geromorphisme cutane." In 1886 Pospelow[121] described both localized and generalized forms of cutaneous atrophy with laxity (in some cases affecting single limbs and in others, the whole body). He called these changes "atrophie idiopathique de la peau" and mentioned a German child with generalized skin laxity and onychogryphosis. At this time other patients whose disorders were labeled "cutis laxa" but who actually had EDS were being reported. Examples included those described by Seifert[139] in 1890, Ehlers[43] in 1901, Cohn[30] in 1907, and Danlos[35] in 1908. Other terms applied to genuine CL included

"peau ridée sénile," which was used by Variot and Cailliau[156] to describe the condition of a 15-month-old girl born with lax skin, which was described by her father as being too large for the child (Fig. 7-1, B). She also had heavy jowls, generalized wrinkling of the abdominal and axillary skin, and a large inguinal hernia. Some authors confused CL with progeria, which itself is probably heterogeneous (as described by Gilford in 1904[54]). Rand[122] in 1914 reported a girl with dwarfism suspected of having progeria. She had obviously lax skin, normal hair, thin skin, joint hypermobility with bilateral congenital dislocation of the hips, pes planus, and wormian bones. Although some of the child's external features (Fig. 7-1, C) have a superficial resemblance to those in progeria, her other manifestations, such as normal hair and boney changes, strongly suggest geroderma osteodysplastica.* Similar cases were also described under such titles as "premature senility."[148]

Weber[164] in 1923 separated generalized CL from EDS but unfortunately failed to clarify the differences among the localized conditions that cause lax skin. In particular, he did not differentiate among scleroderma, calcinosis, and various forms of hypertrophic proliferation and scarring. An excellent analysis of these disorders, written by Petges and Lecoulant,[117] appeared in *Nouvelle Practique Dermatologique, Volume VI*, in 1936. These authors divided the localized forms into hypertrophic and nonhypertrophic categories. The former, which included plexiform neurofibromas, was termed "dermatolyse faciale" by Alibert[2,3] in 1832 and 1855 and "pachydermatocele" by Mott[101] in 1854. Both of these processes and that previously described by Stokes[143] were obvious examples of hypertrophic proliferation. Entities in the nonhypertrophic group included the "dermatolyses" reported by Wise and Snyder[169] in 1914, in which widespread but patchy lichenoid infiltrate was quite different from conventional CL as it is now understood.

Infantile generalized CL was first recorded in 1880 by Houel,[71] but it was not until 1938 that the

---

*The majority of reports concerning this condition have appeared under the title "geroderma osteodysplastica." In 1978 Wiedemann[167] pointed out that "derma" is neuter and that the correct designation should be "geroderma osteodysplasticum" or "gerodermia osteodysplastica." Because the incorrect form has been hallowed by conventional usage, it has been retained in this chapter.

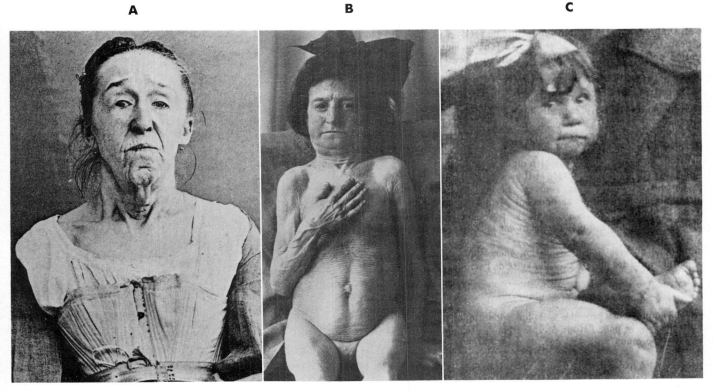

Fig. 7-1. A, A young woman described by Dubreuilh[42] in 1887 and by Souques and Charcot[145] in 1891. In this photograph she is 21 years of age and had a 10-year history of skin laxity. **B,** A girl described by Variot and Cailliau[159] in 1920. She was born with generalized lax skin described by her father as being too large for her. Skin biopsy specimen showed depletion of elastin. **C,** A girl reported in 1914 by Rand[122] as possibly having progeria. She was eleventh of 12 children in a family. She had obvious skin laxity, dwarfism, a pigeon breast, dorsal kyphosis, pes planus, and congenital hip dislocations. Wormian bones were present in the cranial sutures. With hindsight it seems probable that she had geroderma osteodysplastica. (**A** from Souques A, Charcot J-B: *Nouv Iconogr Salpet* 4:169-178, 1891. **B** from Variot, Cailliau: *Arch Med Enfantes* 23:106-111, 1920. **C** from Rand CW: *Boston Med Surg J* 171:107-111, 1914.)

first convincing example of a causative association between skin laxity and pulmonary emphysema in two affected sibs was documented by Siegmund.[144] Since that time there have been many similar examples.* The article of Christiaens, Marchant-Alphant, and Fovet,[28] which depicted the features of generalized CL together with radiographic and gross anatomic and histologic illustrations of generalized emphysema and elastin depletion, was of special importance in this context.

Generation-to-generation transmission of CL was documented as early as 1836 by Graf[61] and

*References 6, 15, 25, 28, 49, 57, 58, and 156.

only a little later by Rossbach[131] and Kopp[82] (who described the other affected member of Rossbach's family). In 1972 Beighton[10] suggested that there were autosomal dominant and autosomal recessive forms of CL. He described several British families with pedigrees that were indicative of these different modes of inheritance and tabulated details of others published between 1836 and 1968. Beighton pointed out that the autosomal dominant and autosomal recessive disorders differed in clinical severity, the former being benign and the latter more likely to be complicated by emphysema. He also speculated that the dominant form might be caused by a structural mutation in the elastin gene, whereas the recessive was likely to be enzymatic in origin.

Byers et al.[22,23] in 1976 and 1980 reported lysyl oxidase deficiency in an X-linked recessive disorder characterized by congenital cutis laxa and bladder diverticula. This condition was subsequently designated "EDS IX" and, later, the "occipital horn syndrome." It is now classified with disorders of copper metabolism,[11] but it is noteworthy that the clinical feature of lax skin is unmistakable and is an important part of this syndrome.

Cutis Laxa with joint laxity and developmental delay has now achieved syndromic status. It was initially termed "cutis laxa with growth retardation" by Sakati et al.[134] and has been designated "cutis laxa recessive type II" by McKusick.[94] Another condition initially described by Rand[122] in 1914 is now known as geroderma osteodysplastica.[8,73,74] Finally, a syndrome of cutis laxa, mental retardation, and corneal clouding was documented by De Barsy, Moens, and Dierckx.[38] This condition is now generally designated by the eponym *De Barsy syndrome*.

Acquired generalized CL was recognized more than a century ago. The first recorded patient, described separately by Dubreuilh[42] in 1887 and Souques and Charcot[145] in 1891, began her progressive illness in childhood with transient, non-itching generalized urticarial rash. Other persons in whom onset of the disorder occurred in adolescence, early adulthood, and even old age[117] were subsequently documented. A good example of adolescent onset is in Rossbach's patient,[131] in whom the disorder began at the age of 18 years. This individual, who had previously been described by Kopp,[82] was employed in hot conditions as a baker's apprentice, and the heat was implicated as a causative factor. Bettman[13] recorded the case of a 62-year-old man in whom relentless progression of late-onset generalized CL had begun 13 years earlier. This patient had eight separate excisions of overhanging eyebrow skin that interfered with his vision and had operations for repair of a ruptured diaphragm and various abdominal hernias. In addition, he had esophageal and colonic diverticula. His skin biopsy specimen showed depleted, distorted, and fragmented elastic fibers. He collapsed and died suddenly of a linear tear in his aorta 6 months after his last series of consultations. Bettman[13] mistakenly considered this patient to have EDS and also suspected chronic adrenal insuffi-

ciency. Goltz and Hult[57] and Goltz et al.[58] subsequently emphasized that generalized systemic elastic degeneration in the lungs, in blood vessels, and in skin is characteristic of this form of late-onset CL.

Generalized elastolysis may be preceded by various cutaneous rashes such as urticaria,[91] eczema,[96] and Sweet syndrome[105] (acute febrile neutrophilic dermatosis). A form of this condition characterized by a skin eruption followed by the development of localized patches of atrophic skin was described in South Africa by Marshall, Heyl, and Weber[97] and in Kenya by Verhagen and Woederman.[160] The association of lax skin with acquired amyloidosis was documented by Hashimoto and Kanzaki[65] in 1975 and by Scott et al.[138] in

---

Classification of Cutis Laxa

Heritable Cutis Laxa	MIM number
Autosomal dominant (AD) Cutis Laxa	AD 123700
Autosomal recessive (AR) Cutis Laxa (AR CL type I)	AR 219100
Cutis Laxa with joint laxity and developmental delay (AR CL type II)	AR 219200
Geroderma osteodysplastica (CL with joint laxity, wormian bones, and osteoporosis)	AR 231070
De Barsy syndrome (CL with mental retardation and corneal clouding)	AR 219151
Occipital horn syndrome (X-linked (XL) recessive Cutis Laxa, formerly EDS IX)	XL 304150
Blepharochalasis	AD 110000

Acquired Cutis Laxa

Primary generalized elastolysis
Generalized elastolysis as a result of cutaneous rashes
Generalized elastolysis as a result of amyloidosis

Cutis Laxa accompanying inherited connective tissue disorders and other conditions

Resulting from connective tissue disorders, notably, pseudoxanthoma elasticum and Ehlers-Danlos syndrome.

MIM, *Mendelian Inheritance in Man.*

1976. Since then, a number of other similar cases have been described. Cutis Laxa occurring mainly around the face in conjunction with hereditary amyloidosis of the Finnish type or lattice dystrophy pattern was reported by Meretojoa[100,101] and commented on in detail by Boysen et al.[17]

Once generalized CL had been differentiated from other disorders such as localized tumors, nevi, and neurofibromatosis, attention was gradually focused on the systemic complications and the genetics of the condition. It then became clear that whereas in some instances the disorder was recognizable at birth and was usually rapidly progressive, in others the onset was delayed until childhood, puberty, or even adulthood. It also became evident that the more severe childhood forms were often associated with pulmonary involvement that progressed to pulmonary hypertension and cardiorespiratory failure. As with other heritable connective tissue disorders, research efforts are currently aimed at the elucidation of the underlying biomolecular defects.

The current classification of CL, with modes of inheritance and the *Mendelian Inheritance in Man (MIM)* numbers, is shown in the box on p. 256.

HERITABLE CUTIS LAXA SYNDROMES
Autosomal Dominant Cutis Laxa

The skin hangs in loose folds, particularly over the face, eyes, and jowls, and is associated with a curved nose, a shortened columella, and a long upper lip.[9,10,128] The person with autosomal dominant CL has a prematurely aged appearance, with "mournful," "bloodhound," or "Churchillian" facies (Fig. 7-2, *A* to *C*). This feature is all the more dramatic in young children because of the impression of aging it conveys; several authors have commented on the social difficulties that such children encounter in such matters as peer taunting and disputes about adult fares on public transport. The range of joint movements is normal. Although systemic complications are uncommon, angiographic abnormalities of the aorta and great vessels have been described in an affected father and his child,[7] and cases of other persons with multiple pulmonary stenoses[81] and generalized carotid ectasia have been documented.[66,147] The natural history of the condition has not been fully established, but accumulating evidence suggests that there may be a propensity to the development of pulmonary and arterial complications in middle age.

In 1972 Beighton[10] distinguished a mild autosomal dominant phenotype from a much more severe recessive form in which pulmonary emphysema was a major complication. He was able to list from the literature seven families with autosomal dominant CL.* To these he added two British families (Fig. 7-2, *D*). About 30 cases have now been reported; the phenotype is reasonably consistent, and syndromic identity is firmly established.

Autosomal Recessive Cutis Laxa Type I

The facies and cutaneous manifestations of autosomal recessive CL type I closely resemble those of the autosomal dominant form, and in a sporadic case it is not possible to deduce the mode of inheritance from the patient's external appearance with any certainty. In general, however, the changes are more severe in autosomal recessive CL, and sagging skin may be a striking feature (Fig. 7-3). The skin changes are usually obvious in infancy and early childhood, but in a few instances the onset has been delayed until adolescence. Occasionally the skin becomes less lax with time.[6,40]

Pulmonary complications include recurrent chest infections, dyspnea, pneumothorax, emphysema,[7,9,63,99] and stenosis of the pulmonary vasculature.[165] Cor pulmonale, arrhythmias, and premature death resulting from cardiorespiratory failure may occur in patients as young as 18 months of age.[57,58,152] In the fourth edition of this book McKusick speculated that respiratory tract obstruction caused by the lax tissues lining the airways might precipitate cardiorespiratory failure, and he suggested that tracheostomy might be valuable in these circumstances. Cosmetic surgery can produce a dramatic improvement in facial appearance (Fig. 7-4).

Van Maldergem et al.[157] described a family with three affected sibs and quoted a thesis for the degree of Doctor of Medicine by Courouge-Dorcier[32] in which the death rate from pulmonary emphysema in 32 published cases was 40%; in addition, 16% of these persons had severe bladder or urinary tract diverticula. Other complications include umbilical, inguinal, and obturator hernias, gastrointestinal diverticula, and prolapse of the rectum and uterus.[21,76] A single report has been made of a patient with abnormalities of bleeding time and platelet aggregation,[76] but hematologic dysfunction is not an accepted feature of CL.

---

*References 7, 61, 66, 82, 88, 124, 131, 142, and 148.

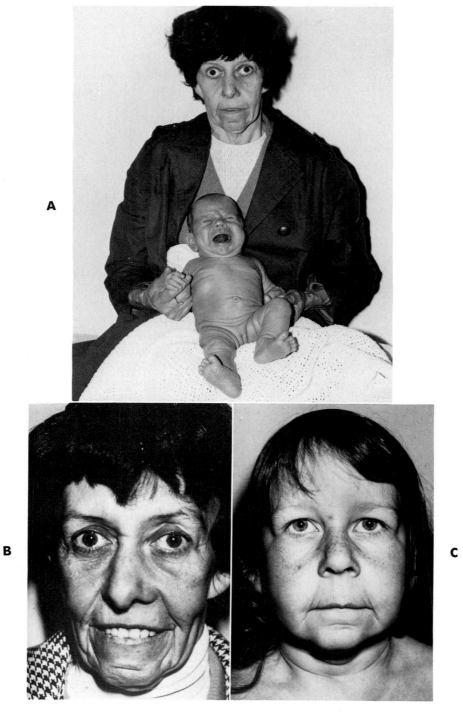

Fig. 7-2. A, Autosomal dominant CL. An infant girl born in 1940 was noted to have loose skin at birth. The cutaneous laxity increased throughout childhood and produced an appearance of premature aging. Her case history was described to the Royal Society of Medicine when she was 8 years of age.[88] In this illustration, which was obtained in 1967, the mother is 27 years of age and the infant is 9 months of age. Clinical appearance of, **B,** proposita and, **C,** daughter in 1990. By 50 years of age the mother had severe generalized emphysema and respiratory failure; her skin biopsy specimen showed fragmented, shortened elastic fibers.

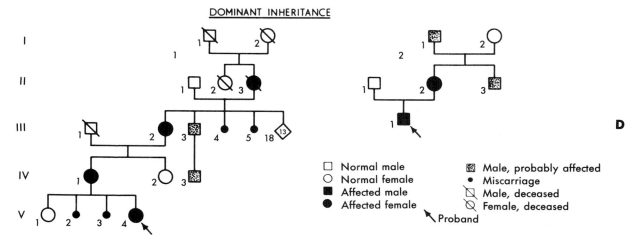

DOMINANT INHERITANCE

□ Normal male   ▨ Male, probably affected
○ Normal female   • Miscarriage
■ Affected male   ⊠ Male, deceased
● Affected female   ⊘ Female, deceased
                      ↖ Proband

D

Fig. 7-2 cont'd. D, Pedigrees published by Beighton[9] of British families with autosomal dominant CL. The mother is *IV-1*, and the affected baby is *V-4* in the pedigree, *left.* (**A** and **D** from Beighton P: *J Med Genet* 9:216-221, 1972.)

Fig. 7-3. Cutis laxa corrected surgically. **A** and **B,** The 16-year-old patient, *left,* appears older than her mother, *right.*

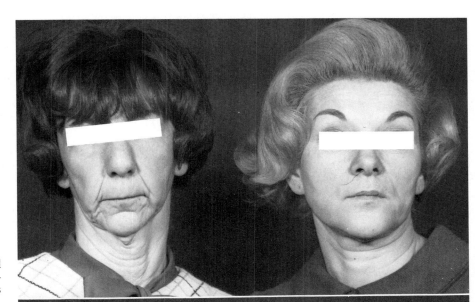

A

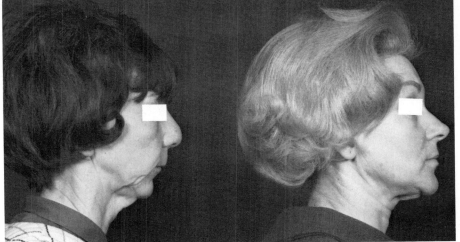

B

Continued.

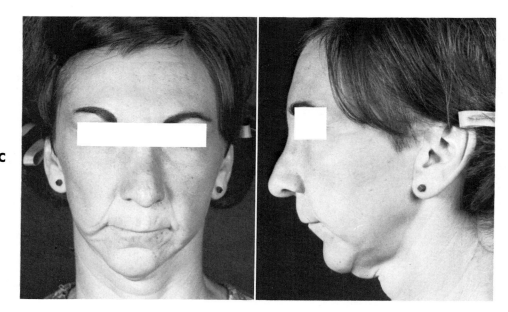

C

D

Fig. 7-3 cont'd. C and **D,** Improvement of appearance after plastic surgery of the face and nose is demonstrated. She was born in 1952 and was reported by Robinson and Ellis,[127] who made the diagnosis of CL when they saw her at the age of 3½ years, and kindly arranged for her to be seen during adolescence for investigations and treatment. The results of plastic surgery were reported by Beighton et al.[9] Somewhat increased wrinkling of skin had been noted at birth. By 6 months of age laxity was marked; several years later, however, the laxity had not seemed to increase. The skin was not unusually fragile or bruisable, and scarring was normal. Her general health was good, and she had no serious illnesses. At no time has she had cardiac or pulmonary symptoms or complications suggesting diverticula of the bladder or gastrointestinal tract. Her intelligence was normal and she performed well in school, although she was limited in social activities by embarrassment about her appearance. Two older sibs and their children were normal. The parents, also normal, were both Italian but presumably not related. The father and mother were 36 and 34 years of age, respectively, when the patient was born. At the age of 16 she had lax, redundant skin of the face and neck, which made her look about three times older than she was. Indeed, she looked older than her mother. The skin was unremarkable except for the laxity and wrinkles. Her peculiar appearance was exaggerated by the conformation of her nose, which was hooked, with prominent bridge and short columnella, and of her upper lip, which was unusually long. Her voice was deep. No other abnormality was detected. Chest radiographic examinations, an electrocardiogram, pulmonary function tests, the karyotype, and dermatoglyphics were all normal. In 1989 McKusick[93] gave a long-term follow-up of the affected girl in his autobiographic article, "Forty Years of Medical Genetics." By 36 years of age she had mild emphysema and had had hypertension for more than 10 years as a result of fibromuscular dysplasia of both renal arteries. The carotid arteries were similarly affected. In view of these complications, it was noteworthy that she was a nonsmoker.

A B C

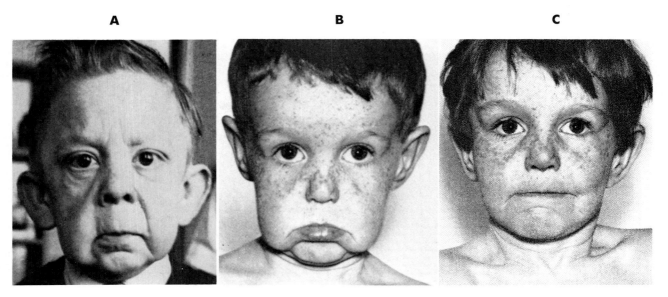

Fig. 7-4. CL autosomal recessive type I. **A,** A boy, shown at 7½ years of age, was born with severe generalized CL. His history[26,27] included congenital pyloric stenosis (corrected at 6 weeks of age), bilateral inguinal hernias (corrected at 9 months of age), and an episode of congestive cardiac failure, possibly associated with redundant aryepiglottic folds and upper respiratory tract obstruction. The boy had emphysema at 3 years of age, and skin biopsy performed at the time showed sparse elastic fibers that were abnormally shortened and clumped. Thereafter, he led a relatively normal life, and no further respiratory problems developed by early adulthood. However, intermittent esophageal obstruction developed as a result of redundancy of esophageal mucosa. Early onset of emphysema is suggestive but not conclusive of autosomal recessive form of CL. Similar child, **B,** before surgery and, **C,** after surgery. Improvement in facial appearance after plastic surgery. (**A** from Chadfield HW: *Br J Dermatol* 81:387-388, 1969. **B** and **C** from Chadfield HW, North JF: *Trans St Johns Hosp Dermatol Soc* 57:181-187, 1971.)

Beighton[10] summarized the evidence for autosomal recessive inheritance, which included several reports of affected sibs with consanguineous heterozygous but clinically normal parents.* He added two examples from his own experience: the first was an infant boy whose parents were first cousins and who had neonatal emphysema and died before 2 years of age of respiratory failure; the second was the offspring of a father and daughter who had an incestuous relationship.

Autosomal Recessive Cutis Laxa Type II (Cutis Laxa with Joint Laxity and Developmental Delay)

The major features of CL type II are lax skin, articular hypermobility, and congenital dislocation of the hips, without pulmonary or urinary tract in-

volvement (Fig. 7-5). The disorder was first described by Debré, Marie, and Seringe[39] in the case of a child with lax skin, loose joints, and a dislocated hip. In 1971 Reisner, Seelenfreund, and Ben-Bassat[125] reported the case of female sibs with intrauterine growth retardation and congenital hip dislocations and suggested that the mode of inheritance might be autosomal recessive with male lethality. Other similar cases can be recognized in the literature.[14,44,53,87,166] Electron microscopic studies of a skin specimen carried out in a single patient revealed subtle morphologic changes in elastic fibril, which suggested absence of amorphous elastin components.[134]

In 1978 Agha et al.[1] proposed that inheritance in CL type II might be X-linked dominant with male lethality. Allanson, Austin, and Hecht[4] described a patient with consanguineous parents and reiterated that very few cases of affected males

*References 25, 27, 49, 58, 142, 144, and 150.

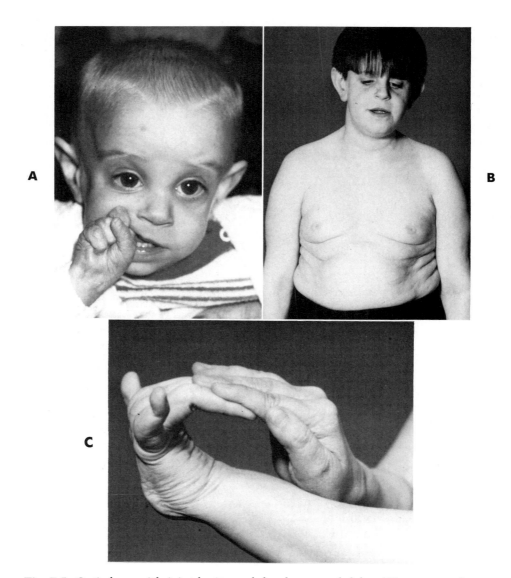

Fig. 7-5. Cutis laxa with joint laxity and developmental delay (CL autosomal recessive type II). This boy born in 1981 was "floppy" at birth and had an inguinal hernia, dislocated hips, and skin that was thin, lax, and translucent. These features were still present when he was examined at 2 years of age. His subsequent progress was good; he never had bladder or urinary problems. Collagen profiles excluded EDS types IV and VII. Lysyl oxidase estimation in his mother showed half normal control levels and less than one tenth activity in his own case. His only current problems are limited to progression of skin laxity, especially over the abdomen, bilateral undescended testes, generalized joint laxity, and a tendency to have knee dislocations. His radiographs showed wormian bones and mild generalized osteoporosis. **A,** Sagging of the jowls and laxity of the skin of the hands was evident during early childhood. **B,** His skin was still lax at puberty, especially over the abdomen. His large ear lobes were an obvious feature. **C,** Joint laxity persisted.

had been recorded. Thereafter Goldblatt et al.[56] documented the case of an affected boy and recognized two other cases in the literature.[50,118] Autosomal recessive inheritance now seems likely, although genetic heterogeneity of this phenotype is still a possibility.[115]

The patients reported by Sakati et al.[134] had lax skin during infancy, but there has been no indication that their skin involvement persisted into later childhood and adulthood. At least some of them may have had unusual forms of EDS with associated dermal laxity. Other atypical cases were recorded by Fitzsimmons et al.,[50] who observed three affected brothers and a sister with variable manifestations, including fatal pulmonary failure in one boy but milder disease and osteoporosis in the others. Reports of other individuals with CL and additional features include the case of a child with unusual facies and massive inguinal hernias;[158] downward slanting lateral palpebral fissures and severe dental caries;[115] kyphoscoliosis, polysyndactyly, ambiguous genitalia, and undercalcification of the calvaria;[77] and multiple skin webs.[108] The family described by Welch et al.,[166] in which cutis laxa and arterial aneurysms coexisted, might have been an example of a homozygous connective tissue collagen mutation. It is evident that atypical CL type II is quite heterogeneous.

Geroderma Osteodysplastica (Cutis Laxa with Joint Hypermobility, Wormian Bones, and Osteoporosis)

In 1950 Bamatter[8] described a Swiss family of children with stunted growth, prematurely aged lax skin, articular hypermobility, and generalized osteoporosis. They were fancifully likened to Walt Disney's animated cartoon dwarfs. Hunter[73] and Hunter et al.[74] subsequently drew attention to mandibular prognathism and a fracturing tendency as components of the disorder (Fig. 7-6, A). Hunter's first report concerned families of Dutch-Russian-Mennonite extraction who had normal skin on histologic study. Thereafter, he and his coworkers documented the case of a French-Canadian girl with similar clinical features and wormian bones in the cranial sutures, severe osteoporosis, and loss of vertebral height.[74] Because of early bruising, her condition had originally been misdiagnosed as an unspecified form of EDS. Skin biopsy revealed elastic fiber fragmentation (but not depletion). Collagen alpha 1 (I) and alpha

2 (I) chains were normal, thus excluding a major abnormality of type I collagen. Her features closely resembled those of the Saudi Arabian children described by Sakati and Nyhan.[133] These sibs also had lax skin, large ears, osteoporosis, and diminished but fragmented dermal elastic fibers. In the opinion of Hunter et al.[73] two of the seven patients listed by Patton et al.[115] as having CL type II with developmental delay also resembled these children.

A lucid report of geroderma osteodysplastica published by Lisker et al.[90] described three young affected Mexican brothers with dysmorphic facies, lax skin, hypertelorism, squints, fleshy noses with protruding eyes, marked joint laxity, kyphosis, severe generalized osteoporosis, brachycephaly, and wormian bones (Fig. 7-6, B and C). Boreux[16] considered the disorder an X-linked recessive condition with inconsistent minor manifestations in the female gene carriers. Accumulated evidence now favors autosomal recessive inheritance. Geroderma osteodysplastica is probably heterogeneous and the clinical manifestations are strongly suggestive of an inherited collagen defect, although the latter remains to be elucidated.

De Barsy Syndrome (Cutis Laxa with Corneal Clouding and Mental Retardation)

De Barsy, Moens, and Dierckx[38] described a 22-month-old infant girl with typical CL together with mental retardation and hypotonia. The skin was elastin depleted. In addition, she had corneal clouding as a result of degeneration of Bowman membrane (subcorneal epithelial basement membrane). Further cases were published by Burck,[19] Hoefnagel et al.,[69] Kunze et al.,[85] Pontz, Zepp, and Stoss,[117] and Riebel.[126] Several of these accounts included features such as athetosis, severe mental retardation, and a progeroid appearance. Histologic studies showed frayed elastic fibers that were deficient in density and number.[119] This condition resembles autosomal dominant and autosomal recessive CL type I, but it may be distinguished by the absence of manifestations of generalized connective tissue involvement and the presence of severe mental retardation and corneal changes.

Occipital Horn Syndrome (Formerly, X-Linked Recessive Cutis Laxa and EDS Type IX)

The occipital horn syndrome, formerly known as X-linked CL and EDS type IX, is characterized

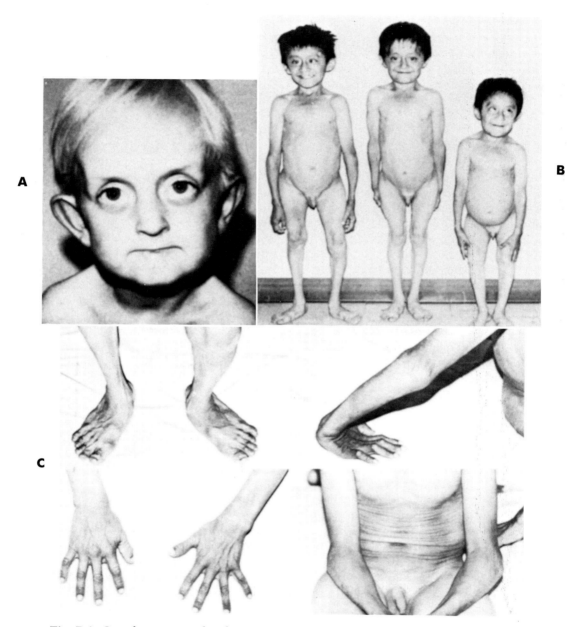

Fig. 7-6. Geroderma osteodysplastica. **A,** Typical facial features. **B,** General characteristics of a family described by Lisker et al.[90]; three affected brothers with normal parents. **C,** Closer views showing pes planus, joint hypermobility, and lax skin in the affected children. (**A** from Hunter AGW: *Hum Genet* 40:311-320, 1978. **B** and **C** from Lisker R et al: *Am J Med Genet* 3:389-395, 1979.)

by mild skin laxity and a hooked nose with a long philtrum. Other variable features include joint hypermobility, thoracic malformations, and carpal synostoses.[86,92] Downward occipital projections that become evident on radiologic examination at puberty are pathognomonic.[22,23] Affected persons may have bladder neck obstruction, chronic diarrhea, and personality disorders. Details of this X-linked condition, which is now classified as a disorder of copper metabolism, are given in Chapter 13.

Blepharochalasis

The term "blepharochalasis" refers to wrinkling and redundancy of the skin of the upper eyelid. When severe, blepharochalasis produces an appearance of premature world-weariness and aging. The British politician Harold McMillan provided a typical example. Although quite common after middle age, blepharochalasis is more distressing in young adults, especially when accompanied by ptosis.

Laxity of the eyelid skin is a feature of the CL syndromes, but isolated blepharochalasis is a separate entity. The several subgroups include a juvenile form, which is characterized by recurrent attacks of unexplained eyelid edema followed by dermal atrophy; a senile variety, which is an almost obligatory concomitant of aging; and a more unusual hereditary form. An impressive case in a three-generation French-Canadian family was described in 1936 by Panneton.[112] The proband was a 21-year-old woman with localized blepharochalasis and bilateral ptosis. The disorder was transmitted through her mother, who although mildly affected, had 50 relatives with the disorder. Histologic study revealed elastic fragmentation and depletion resembling some forms of CL. In 1965 Schulze[137] documented the cases of 14 affected persons in six generations of a German family. The Ascher syndrome[47,51] is a variant of blepharochalasis in which redundancy of the mucosa of the upper lip is associated with eyelid wrinkling.

Surgical treatment of blepharochalasis includes the excision of excess skin, elevation of the ptosed eyelid, and plastic reconstruction of the lid fold. The operative results are usually entirely satisfactory.

ACQUIRED CUTIS LAXA

Acquired skin laxity can develop at any time from infancy to old age. The disorder progresses over months or years and may produce a striking clinical picture. This process occurs in the following circumstances: (1) spontaneously with no obvious cause, (2) in association with a severe but nonspecific urticaria or papular erythema, or (3) in association with generalized primary amyloidosis or as a secondary complication of multiple myeloma. There is a certain amount of overlap in the natural history of these forms of acquired CL, and their autonomous identity is uncertain. Indeed, it is evident that a variety of mechanisms can produce significant skin laxity, and subcategorization is necessarily arbitrary. About 50 cases that fall into one or another of these groups have been described.

None of these acquired forms of CL have a known genetic basis, but they are discussed in this chapter for the purpose of comparison with the genetic types and in view of their importance in differential diagnosis.

Primary Generalized Elastolysis

Primary generalized elastolysis is a rare disorder that develops insidiously in the absence of any major predisposing factors. Minor skin eruptions have preceded the skin laxity in a few instances, but it is uncertain whether these have any pathogenetic significance.

The onset of this disorder can occur at any time between the second and sixth decade. A comprehensive account was given by Reed, Horowitz, and Beighton[123] in their description of two patients: the onset in one occurred in the fifth decade, whereas the other had a teenage onset. In the former the illness commenced with a hypersensitivity to penicillin and rash of brief duration followed over the next 10 years by progressive redundancy of the skin and subcutaneous tissue of the neck (Fig. 7-7, *A*). Other complications included an esophageal diverticulum with dysphagia, an hiatus hernia, and bilateral inguinal hernias. Progressive dyspnea during exertion developed, and chest radiographs revealed severe emphysema, cardiac enlargement, and aortic dilation (Fig. 7-7, *B*). The patient died suddenly, and post mortem examination revealed elastin depletion of the skin and aortic media, and pulmonary alveoli, as well as marked emphysema and evidence of mild pulmonary hypertension. Colonic diverticula and a previous myocardial infarction were also present. A similar example was provided by Bettman's spectacular patient[13] in whom progressive skin laxity

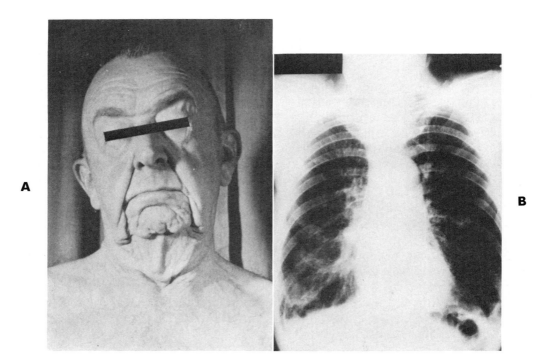

Fig. 7-7. Generalized systemic elastolysis. An engineer at 59 years of age had a 19-year history of CL that began 1 month after a penicillin reaction. A laryngeal diverticulum was removed after he had progressive dysphagia, repair of a hiatus hernia, and cosmetic surgery to remove loose skin from the face and neck. At 56 years of age he had orthopnea, and chest radiographs revealed moderate emphysema and basal fibrosis. When he was 59 years of age, after surgical repair of bilateral inguinal hernias, progressive congestive heart failure developed and he died suddenly 5 months later. On examination after death the heart showed moderate right ventricular hypertrophy, a previous left ventricular infarction, and slight dilation of the aorta. The lungs showed multiple pleural microbullae 1 to 2 mm in diameter, as well as pleural fibrosis and extensive pulmonary emphysema. The gall bladder was distorted, and multiple diverticulae of the descending colon were present. Histologic studies revealed elastin depletion in the upper dermis and elastin fragmentation in the lower dermis. Elastin was also depleted in the aorta and lungs. **A,** Appearance at 50 years of age, before plastic surgery. **B,** Chest radiograph taken 1 month before death, showing generalized emphysema, pulmonary hypertension, and a dilated aorta. (From Reed WB et al: *Arch Dermatol* 103:661-669, 1971.)

developed at the age of 39 years and who died of a ruptured aorta 20 years later. Harris, Heaphy, and Perry[64] described three patients with late-onset disease. The first was a 44-year-old woman in whom a transient erythema was followed by progressive skin laxity and pulmonary emphysema over the next 6 years. Electron microscopy showed aggregation of electron-dense amorphous and microfibrillar material around the elastic fibers. The second was a 56-year-old man with progressive generalized skin laxity, pulmonary fibrosis, a large diaphragmatic hernia, and multiple diverticula in the alimentary tract. In the third patient progressive generalized looseness of the skin developed after the age of 48 years. He received several face-lift procedures and repairs of various hernias and eventually died of a ruptured aorta.

Generalized Elastolysis Secondary to Cutaneous Rashes

Cutis laxa associated with erythematous, eczematous, or vasculitic rashes that precede the onset of cutaneous degeneration can be broadly subcategorized into generalized and localized forms.

These subgroups of secondary generalized elastolysis are sometimes respectively designated acquired CL type I and type II.[48]

Generalized secondary elastolysis is identical in appearance and clinical course to primary generalized elastolysis; the only difference is the prominent occurrence of preceding cutaneous manifestations in the former. The following examples are notable. Marshall, Vogelpol, and Weber[96] described a man whose illness had commenced with the onset of chronic eczema when he was 44 years of age. At the age of 56 years his skin had begun to wrinkle; thereafter, progressive skin laxity and pulmonary emphysema developed. He also had a coincidental gastric ulcer. The patient of McCarthy, Warin, and Read[91] had a history of persistent urticaria over a 13-year-period, and in addition to recurrent pneumothoraces, inguinal and abdominal hernias also developed. Uterine prolapse is another complication that might be attributable to elastin damage in acquired CL.[24] The patient documented by Wanderer et al.,[163] who had a childhood onset, had chronic urticaria associated with tracheobronchiomegaly (also know as the Mounier-Khun syndrome[104]). In the case reported by Kerl et al.[78] the patient had penicillin-induced dermatitis herpetiformis, which appeared at the age of 11 years and was accompanied by progressive skin laxity and emphysema. Similarly, in the 41-year-old patient of Nanko et al.[106] erythema perstans developed coincident with sigmoid colonic diverticula, redundancy of the vocal cords, and disturbed lung function, whereas the patient documented by Heilman and Haustein[67] had isolated cold urticaria and uncomplicated dermal laxity. Lewis et al.[89] documented the case of an American patient in whom postoperative urticaria or erythema resolved over a 2-month period, leaving extensive bloodhoundlike wrinkling of the face, trunk, and buttocks. The atrophic areas were elastin depleted and showed a minor abnormality of elastin organization with abundant microfibrils but sparse elastin matrix. In the patient described by Muster et al.[105] skin laxity developed, and the patient died during childhood of aneurysmal aortitis with aortic regurgitation. This course was similar to that documented by Heye et al.[68] in a British patient who had lax skin and aortitis that followed Sweet disease. Onset in a 3-year-old boy was recorded by Jablonska[75]; in this boy skin laxity was preceded by an erythematous, infiltrative nodular eruption.

Localized secondary elastolysis is typified by the unusual syndrome documented by Marshall, Heyl, and Weber[97] in the cases of five South African girls. In these patients urticarial papules and plaques similar to erythema chronicum migrans evolved into either a series of concentric circles or persistent urticarial plaques. The disease process resulted in either localized areas of cutaneous wrinkling analagous to anetoderma or widespread cutaneous atrophy. Verhagen and Woerdeman[160] described seven affected Kenyan girls and termed the condition "inflammatory elastolysis." Histologic study in the acute phase shows an infiltration with lymphocytes, eosinophils, and polymorphonuclear leucocytes, as well as elastin depletion in the affected areas. It is possible that the skin reaction is a response to initiating antigens from unidentified arthropods, but it is likely that both genetic and environmental influences are operative. Verhagen and Woerdeman[160] suggested that a similar, less fierce immune reaction might explain sporadic anetoderma that is encountered in temperate regions. Fisher, Page, and Wedad[48] described a form of CL that followed recurrent papular urticaria and was localized to the hands and feet. Elastic fibers were depleted, fragmented, and degenerated. This condition seems to be a distinctive entity.

Generalized Elastolysis Secondary to Amyloidosis

Cutis laxa can occur as a complication of both idiopathic primary amyloidosis and amyloidosis secondary to multiple myeloma.[153] In the former circumstance the lax skin is usually generalized, whereas in the latter it is often confined to the face.

Lax facial skin may be a feature of the syndrome of familial amyloidosis with cranial neuropathy and corneal lattice dystrophy.[17,132] This form of hereditary amyloidosis is particularly common in the Finnish population.[100,101] McKusick[94] suggested that three Czech sisters with bulbar palsy, reticular lattice dystrophy, and CL had this disorder. The cranial neuropathy may contribute to the facial appearance in this disorder. The basic defect is deposition of an abnormal protein, gelsolin.[98] Cutis laxa with lattice dystrophy, bulbar palsy, and amyotrophic lateral sclerosis has also been described.[80]

Newton et al.[107] documented systemic amyloidosis with chronic angioedema and chronic renal failure in association with skin laxity of the face, groins, and axillae. Histologic investigations revealed elastin depletion and amyloid deposits surrounding the elastic fibers. The serum showed a transient monoclonal immunoglobulin (IgG) gammopathy, and the bone marrow contained 12% plasma cells, some of which were atypical.

Gonnering and Sonneland[59] described a 65-year-old man with late-onset blepharochalasis. Histologic study of the skin removed at blepharoplasty showed striking amyloid infiltration, and evidence of underlying myeloma was adduced from serologic and bone marrow investigations. An interesting patient with late-onset CL and myeloma but without amyloid was documented by Hashimoto and Kanzaki.[65]

Comment

It is important to be aware that some overlap exists among the various categories of acquired CL. For instance, the patient of Newton et al.,[105] who had CL, generalized cutaneous amyloidosis, and chronic renal failure, had erythematous rashes for 28 years, and the patient described by Tsuji et al.,[154] who had CL and nephrotic syndrome, had occasional episodes of facial edema long before there was any suspicion of involvement of her kidneys.

The pathogenesis of acquired CL remains obscure, but in addition to the preceding cutaneous eruptions, other precursors have included polyarthritis,[60] typhoid fever,[143] and diabetes mellitus.[135] Identical twins, one of whom had localized CL with onset at the age of 13 years, have been reported.[62] This observation is further evidence for the role of environmental rather than genetic determinants in the etiology of this disorder.

CUTIS LAXA ACCOMPANYING OR FOLLOWING INHERITED CONNECTIVE TISSUE DISORDERS AND OTHER CONDITIONS

Lax redundant skin may occur in uncommon forms of certain connective tissue disorders. In these circumstances skin laxity may develop early in life as a temporary phenomenon before disappearing in childhood.[15] Skin laxity also can appear later in life as a complication of long-standing connective tissue disease[149] and as an exaggeration of the normal aging process.

Transient skin laxity in infancy is a rare feature of EDS III, IV, and VII (Fig. 7-8). Objective criteria

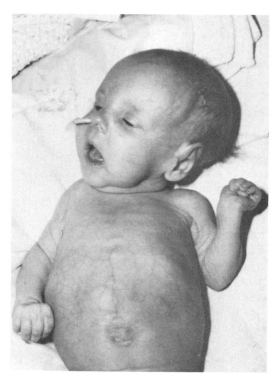

Fig. 7-8. EDS type IV. A baby with generally thin and mildly lax skin over the upper arms and lower abdomen.

that permit differentiation from conventional forms of CL include increased elastin and collagen depletion in EDS IV, variable collagen fibril diameters in EDS IV, irregular collagen fibrils in EDS VII, specific biochemical abnormalities in EDS IV and VII.

Tsukahara et al.[155] recorded an affected mother and daughter with combined CL and EDS. The daughter had "tissue-paper" scars typical of EDS, as well as classical CL, whereas the mother showed no clinical abnormality on clinical examination but had histologic and biochemic changes identical to those of the daughter. Associations between EDS and CL have been recorded previously[125,142] but are of uncertain significance.

Generalized atrophy and wrinkling of the skin is a rare, late complication in some forms of EDS. These patients have exaggerated facial drooping and atrophic loose skin over the trunk and limbs (Fig. 7-9). In families with poorly defined connective tissue disorders, lax skin is associated with

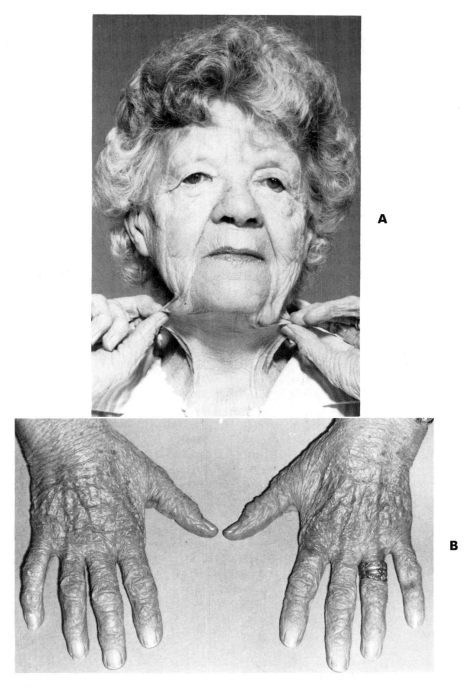

Fig. 7-9. EDS types II and III. **A,** Facial features of a 70-year-old woman with EDS types II/III; skin is lax and hyperextensible. **B,** Generalized skin atrophy and laxity in the dorsum of the hands in the same patient.

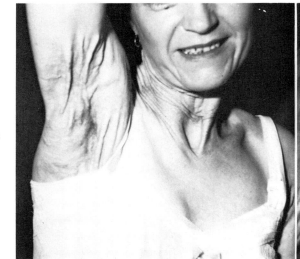

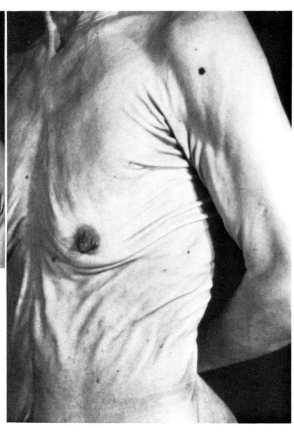

Fig. 7-10. Pseudoxanthoma elasticum. **A,** Lax elastic skin of the neck and axilla. **B,** Severe PXE with marked generalized skin laxity.

cutaneous striae, joint laxity, and ruptured colonic diverticula. The histologic study of skin shows no elastin depletion but does reveal slight dermal thinning and senile purpura.

In adulthood there is clinical overlap between pseudoxanthoma elasticum (PXE) and acquired CL of the elastolytic type. In patients with PXE, skin laxity (Fig. 7-10, A) is usually confined to the axillae and other flexures, although occasionally it may be generalized. (Figure 7-10, B) Histologic investigation settles the diagnostic issue, since the skin in patients with PXE is characterized by calcification and elastin fragmentation. Retinal changes further distinguish PXE, although in rare instances, the generalized cutaneous changes can occur without obvious ophthalmologic signs.

In a few rare syndromes localized cutis laxa is a component. In leprechaunism[34,41] mild cutis laxa is associated with multiple endocrine abnormalities such as hirsuitism, clitoral hypertrophy, Langerhans-cell hyperplasia, ductal hyperplasia of the breasts, and ovarian cysts. Other lepre-

chaunlike disorders include the Patterson syndrome[112-114] and a variant of this condition described by David[36] and David, Webb, and Gordon,[37] in which obvious but minor skin laxity is associated with gross skeletal abnormalities, hyperpigmentation, hirsuitism, and adrenal hyperplasia. Lax skin of the scalp is the major manifestation of isolated cutis verticis gyrata[129] and of a similar condition in which acromegaly and corneal leukoma are additional features.[130]

Laxity of the abdominal skin is a secondary feature of the prune-belly syndrome, a disorder first delineated in 1939 by Frohlich,[52] although an earlier example was described in 1901 by Osler.[110] This nonspecific symptom complex results from the abdominal distention that has occurred *in utero.* Progression leaves both wrinkled abdominal skin and atrophic abdominal muscles.[20,111]

PATHOLOGY AND PATHOGENESIS

In many forms of CL the skin and internal organs, notably, lungs and arteries, show sparsity,

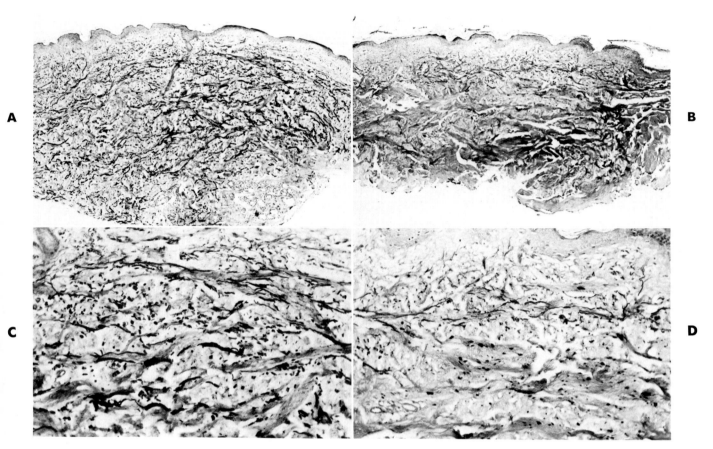

Fig. 7-11. Acquired CL. Sections from normal and abnormal regions of skin stained with hematoxylin and eosin. **A,** Normal region magnified × 50. **B,** Abnormal region magnified × 50. **C,** Normal region magnified × 160. **D,** Abnormal region magnified × 160. The elastin depletion in **B** and **D** is obvious when compared with elastin in **A** and **C.** (Courtesy Dr. George Beveridge, Department of Dermatology, University of Edinburgh.)

fragmentation, and disruption of elastic fibers on light microscopy[57,58,72,75] (Fig. 7-11). The changes in cutaneous elastic fibers were first noted by Variot and Cailliau[159] more than 30 years after Dubreuilh[42] first recognized the disorder in 1887. These histologic abnormalities are present in almost all types of CL, including the autosomal dominant and autosomal recessive forms, de Barsy syndrome, late onset inflammatory and noninflammatory types, and in postinflammatory anetoderma. Furthermore, the elastin is involved in inherited and acquired amyloidosis and in PXE. In amyloidosis the ubiquitous amyloid P protein, which is normally associated with elastin microfibrils,[18] probably acts as a focus for other amyloid deposits, which induce elastolysis[107] (perhaps the result of complement-mediated inflammation and degradation). In PXE, elastic fibers are fragmented and hypercalcified. Elastin abnormalities do not occur consistently in autosomal recessive CL type II (joint laxity and growth retardation form), and are absent in the occipital horn syndrome (X-linked recessive CL) in which collagen fibril diameter is increased.[23] There are also other exceptional families with CL type I or type II in which elastic fibers have a normal histologic appearance.

The elastic fiber abnormalities in many forms of CL are in keeping with the redundant, loose skin and destruction of pulmonary alveolar structure,

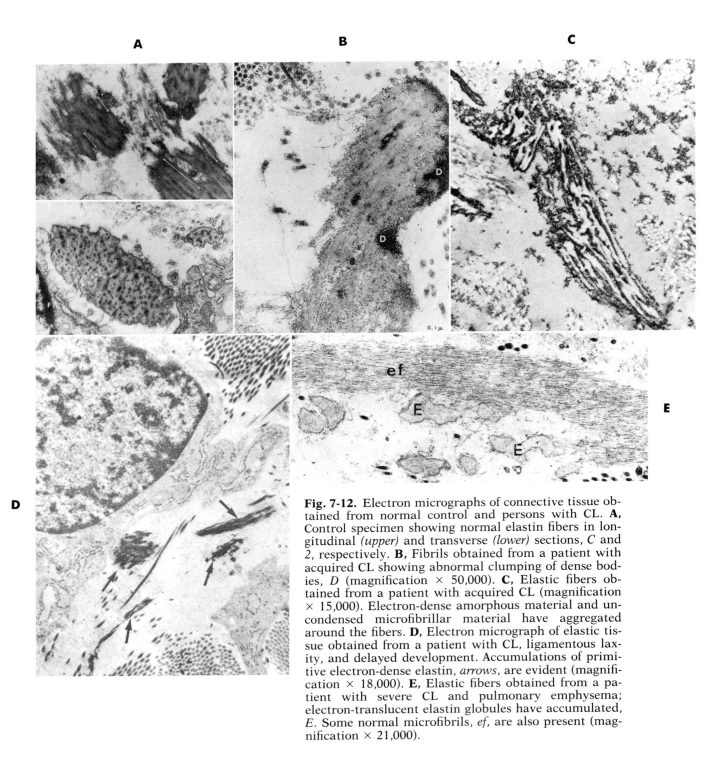

A   **B**   **C**

D   **E**

Fig. 7-12. Electron micrographs of connective tissue obtained from normal control and persons with CL. **A,** Control specimen showing normal elastin fibers in longitudinal *(upper)* and transverse *(lower)* sections, *C* and *2,* respectively. **B,** Fibrils obtained from a patient with acquired CL showing abnormal clumping of dense bodies, *D* (magnification × 50,000). **C,** Elastic fibers obtained from a patient with acquired CL (magnification × 15,000). Electron-dense amorphous material and uncondensed microfibrillar material have aggregated around the fibers. **D,** Electron micrograph of elastic tissue obtained from a patient with CL, ligamentous laxity, and delayed development. Accumulations of primitive electron-dense elastin, *arrows,* are evident (magnification × 18,000). **E,** Elastic fibers obtained from a patient with severe CL and pulmonary emphysema; electron-translucent elastin globules have accumulated, *E.* Some normal microfibrils, *ef,* are also present (magnification × 21,000).

F   G   H

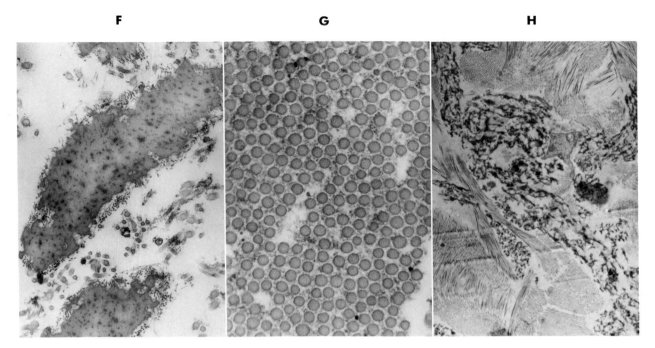

Fig. 7-12 cont'd. F, Normal elastic fibers obtained from a patient with lethal autosomal recessive CL and emphysema. Both microfibrilar and amorphous components are completely normal (magnification × 30,000). **G,** Collagen fibril patterns in transverse section obtained from the patient in **F.** Irregularity in fibril size is present, and generally fibril diameter is larger than normal (magnification × 50,000). **H,** Distorted and prolific elastic fibers obtained from a patient with late-onset blepharochalasia. Both microfibrilar and amorphous components are hypertrophic (magnification × 24,000). (**B** from Hashimoto K, Kanzaki T: *Arch Dermatol* 11:861-862, 1975. **C** from Harris RB et al: *Am J Med* 65:815-822, 1978. **D** from Sakati NO et al: *Pediatrics* 72:850-856, 1983. **E** from Van Maldergem L et al: *Am J Med Genet* 31:455-464, 1988.)

which is often accompanied by pulmonary fibrosis and pleural blebs.* With the use of electron microscopy a variety of subtle structural abnormalities of elastin fibers have been observed (Fig. 7-12, *B* to *G*). These include proliferation of microfibrils,[65] immature elastin fibrils with matrix deficiency,[79,136,158] elastin matrix lacking microfibrils,[70,95] and accumulation of elastin-dense amorphous material.[64] Poorly stained elastin globules without abnormal microfibrils may also be evident.[157] Sakati and Nyhan[133] reported proliferation of elastin microfibrils with absence of amorphous components in the autosomal recessive, delayed development, loose jointed form of CL (Fig. 7-12, *D*). Pope[120] has observed deficient elastic fibrils with sparse microfibrillar and amorphous components in autosomal recessive CL, as well as gross proliferation of microfibrilar components in

*References 10, 26, 28, 57, 58, and 63.

late-onset blepharochalasis (Fig. 7-12, *H*). He has also noted completely normal elastic fibers at the light and electron microscopic levels in a patient with lethal autosomal recessive CL and emphysema (Fig. 7-12, *F* and *G*).

Fibrillin is an extracellular matrix glycoprotein[132] that can be shown by immunofluorescent staining techniques to be deficient in patients with Marfan syndrome[55] (see Chapter 3). Similar changes have been observed in skin biopsy specimens obtained from a few patients with CL; therefore it is possible that abnormalities of fibrillin are implicated in this disorder.[120]

Sephal and Davidson[140] and Olsen et al.[109] demonstrated that elastin messenger RNA levels were consistently reduced in fibroblasts derived from persons with autosomal dominant and autosomal recessive CL (Fig. 7-13). The genes for tropoelastin, which are located on chromosome 2, have been cloned and sequenced. Elastin gene se-

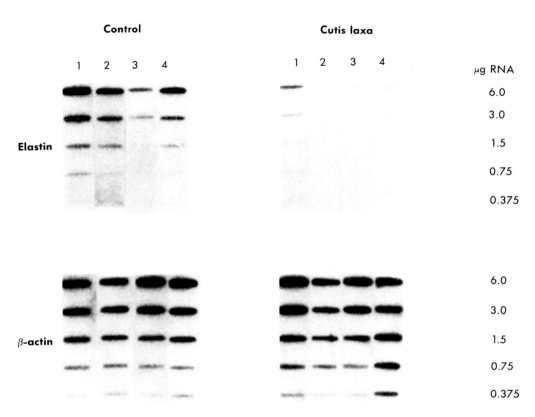

Fig. 7-13. Elastin mRNA levels from normal controls and persons with CL. (From Olsen DR et al: *J Biol Chem* 263:6465-6467, 1988.)

quences have also been identified on the long arm of chromosome 7 within the 7q11 to 21.1 region; it is thus possible that there is more than one elastin gene.[45] It seems likely that an elastin gene might be faulty in the genetic forms of CL, but there is no firm evidence to support this contention.

In the occipital horn syndrome (X-linked CL), lysyl oxidase deficiency was demonstrated by Byers et al.[22,23] by means of radioimmunoassay. Subsequently, several workers have detected accompanying abnormalities of copper metabolism; these include increased copper concentrations secreted into the medium by cultured fibroblasts, low hair and tissue levels,[84] and increased 64Cu incorporation similar to the abnormalities in Menkes syndrome.[116] McKusick[94] has suggested that the occipital horn syndrome might be allelic to Menkes syndrome. Disordered copper metabolism has also been implicated in other forms of CL.[102] For instance, elevated levels of copper in the serum and skin in a 35-year-old woman with acquired CL have been documented by Ferreira and Spina.[46] In contrast, in a 10-month-old infant with

postinflammatory CL, copper metabolism was apparently normal.[89] It seems unlikely that abnormalities of copper play a primary role in the pathogenesis of CL.

Type VI collagen, which has three distinct protein components (alpha 1, alpha 2, and alpha 3) is derived from genes localized on chromosomes 2 and 21. In a study of a family with apparent autosomal recessive CL characterized by mild pectus excavatum and joint laxity and described by Fitzsimmons et al.,[50] Pope and his colleagues noted lower molecular weight forms of alpha 1(VI) or alpha 2(VI) collagen with immunoblots from cultured skin fibroblasts. The alpha 1 and alpha 2(VI) proteins comigrated and could not be distinguished at the protein level. It is uncertain whether this is due to clonal selection, since only some (not all) fibroblast lines obtained from the affected family showed this change.[120] Interestingly, Crawford et al.[33] detected a possible abnormality of type VI collagen in cultured fibroblasts obtained from a patient with autosomal recessive type I CL. Fourteen collagen genes and over 20 proteins have been recognized,[12,83,152,162] and it is possible that other collagen genes and proteins may also be disturbed in CL. Indeed, a shortened alpha 2(I) collagen was detected in an affected mother and daughter with combined CL and EDS.[147] With the availability of modern techniques such as DNA amplification by polymerase chain reaction (PCR),[132] chemical cleavage, mismatch analysis,[31] and denaturing gradient gel electrophoresis, it is probably only a matter of time before specific collagen and elastin abnormalities will be detected in at least some forms of CL.

The acquired late-onset types of CL have some clinical resemblance to the classic autosomal dominant and autosomal recessive forms. On histologic study, too, they resemble these genetic entities, and it is probable that they have similar pathogenic mechanisms. The situation is analagous to that whereby mutations of types III and I collagen can cause both common diseases, such as late-onset aneurysms or osteoporosis, and rare single-gene disorders such as EDS VI and osteogenesis imperfecta.[11,12,84] It is also possible that mutations which cause familial emphysema and familial jejunal and intestinal diverticulosis[5,29] may in the end be found to resemble those causing conventional elastolytic CL. Finally, it is probable that the environmental triggering mechanism of late-onset elastolytic CL associated with eczema, urticaria, Sweet syndrome, nephrotic syndrome, and other disorders operates against a background of abnormal connective tissue.

MANAGEMENT

Cosmetic surgery[9,26,40,88] can lead to a substantial improvement in the appearance of patients with the genetic forms of CL. In addition to face lifting and blepharoplasty, removal of extensive skin from neck, arms, breasts, and abdomen can also be performed. Nose reconstruction is also possible.[9] Tissue fragility, excessive bleeding, and widened scars, which are problems in patients with some forms of EDS, do not occur in patients with CL, so surgery is technically straightforward and carries no special hazards.[125] The results of cosmetic operations are not necessarily permanent, but face lifts can be repeated if laxity returns too quickly.[57,58,88] Hernias and diverticula of the bowel and urinary tract respond to conventional surgery if this should be required. The presence of emphysema in some persons with CL poses risks during anesthesia, and this factor must be taken into account when operative procedures are planned. In patients with CL, progressive pulmonary emphysema, and respiratory or right ventricular heart failure, heart or single-lung transplantation warrants consideration.

SUMMARY

Cutis laxa is a generalized disorder of connective tissue characterized mainly by striking laxity of the skin but also by abnormalities of the lungs and arteries. It is likely that the fundamental defect resides in the elastic fibers. At least two genetic forms exist, one autosomal dominant and the other autosomal recessive; in addition, lax skin is a syndromic component of several other genetic conditions. Acquired types of systemic elastolysis have many features that resemble those of the genetically determined forms; it is probable, however, that these are distinct nongenetic entities.

REFERENCES

1. Agha A et al: Two forms of cutis laxa presenting in the newborn period, *Acta Paediatr Scand* 67:775-780, 1978.
2. Alibert J-L: Quoted by Petges and Lecoulant. In *Nouvelle Practique Dermatologique*, vol 6, Paris, 1936, Masson et Cie.
3. Alibert J-L: Histoire d'un berger des environs de Gisors (dermatose hypermorphe), *Monogr Derm* 2:719, 1855.
4. Allanson J, Austin W, Hecht F: Congenital Cutis laxa with retardation of growth and motor development: a recessive disorder of connective tissue with male lethality, *Clin Genet* 29:133-136, 1986.
5. Anderson LP, Schjoldager B, Halver B: Jejunal diverticulosis in a family, *Scand J Gastroent* 23:672-674, 1988.
6. Bakker BJ: Cutis laxa universalis und Lungenemphysem, *Hautarzt* 10:371, 1959.
7. Balboni FA: Cutis laxa and multiple vascular anomalies, *Bull St Francis Hospital* 19:26-34, 1963.
8. Bamatter F et al: Gerodermie osteodysplastique hereditaire, *Ann Pediatr* 174:126-127, 1950.
9. Beighton P, Bull JC, Edgerton MT: Plastic surgery in cutis laxa, *Br J Plast Surg* 23:285-290, 1970.
10. Beighton P: The dominant and recessive forms of cutis laxa, *J Med Genet* 9:216-221, 1972.
11. Beighton P et al: International nosology of heritable disorders of connective tissue, Berlin, 1986, *Am J Med Genet* 29:581-594, 1988.
12. Beighton P et al: Molecular nosology of heritable disorders of connective tissue, *Am J Med Genet* 42:431-448, 1992.
13. Bettman AG: Excessively relaxed skin and the pituitary gland, *Plast Reconstr Surg* 15:489-501, 1955.
14. Beuren AJ et al: Dysplasia of the systemic and pulmonary arterial system with tortuosity and lengthening of the arteries: a new entity, diagnosed during life, and leading to coronary death in early childhood, *Circulation* 39:109-115, 1969.

15. Bondi R, Gori F, Treves G: Concomitanza e significatao della cutis laxa e dell'enfisema polmonare alveolare infantile in una rara osservazione anatomopatologica, *Arch De Vecchi Anat Pat* 51:801-820, 1968.

16. Boreux G: Osteodysplastic geroderma of sex-linked heredity: a new clinical and genetic entity, *J Genet Hum* 17:137-178, 1969.

17. Boysen G et al: Familial amyloidosis with cranial neuropathy and corneal lattice dystrophy, *J Neurol Neurosurg Psychiat* 42:1020-1030, 1979.

18. Breathnach SM et al: Amyloid P component is located on elastic fibre microfibrils in normal human tissue, *Nature* 293:652-654, 1981.

19. Burck U: De Barsy-Syndrome: eine Weitere Beobachtung, *Klin Paediat* 186:441-444, 1974.

20. Burton BK, Dillard RG: Brief clinical report: Prune Belly syndrome: observations supporting the hypothesis of abdominal overdistension, *Am J Med Genet* 17:669-672, 1984.

21. Butterworth T, Strean P: *Clinical gerodermatology*, Baltimore, 1962, Williams & Wilkins.

22. Byers PH et al: An X-linked form of Cutis laxa due to deficiency of lysyloxidase, *Birth Defects Original Article Series* 12(5):293-298, 1976.

23. Byers PH et al: An X-linked form of Cutis laxa: defective collagen crosslink formation due to decreased lysyloxidase activity, *New Engl J Med* 303:61-65, 1980.

24. Carney RG, Nomland R: Acquired loose skin (chalazoderma): report of a case, *Arch Dermatol Syph* 56:794-800, 1947.

25. Cashman ME: Cutis laxa, *Proc Roy Soc Med* 50:719-720, 1957.

26. Chadfield HW: Cutis laxa, *Br J Dermatol* 81:387-388, 1969.

27. Chadfield HW, North JF: Cutis laxa: a report of three cases, *Trans St John's Hospital Dermatol Soc* 57:181-187, 1971.

28. Christiaens L, Marchant-Alphant A, Fovet A: Emphysème congénital et cutis laxa, *Presse Méd* 62:1799-1801, 1954.

29. Clunie GJA, Mason JM: Visceral diverticula and the Marfan syndrome, *Br J Surg* 50:51-52, 1962.

30. Cohn: Presentation d'une malade avec peaux en caoutochouc (Cutix lax) avec des modifications singulieres circumscribes de la peau, sans forme d'elements brun-rouge depressibles, IXe Congress des Societe Allemandes de dermatologie, 1907, p 415.

31. Cotton RGH et al: Reactivity of cytosine and thymine in single base-pair mismatches with hydroxylamine and osmium tetroxide and its application to the study of mutations, *Proc Nat Acad Sci* 85:4397-4401, 1988.

32. Courouge-Dorcier AM: *Cutis laxa généralisée congénitale à propos d'un cas*, Thèse no 103, vol 1, p 1-160, University Bordeaux. II. Quoted by Van Maldergem et al.[158]

33. Crawford SW et al: Characterisation of type VI collagen related Mr 140,000 protein from cutis laxa fibroblasts in culture, *Biochem J* 227:491-501, 1985.

34. Dallaire L: Discussion (of leprechaunism). In Bergsma D, editor: *Clinical delineation of birth defects. IV. Skeletal dysplasia*, New York, 1969, National March of Dimes Foundation, p 121.

35. Danlos M: Un cas de cutis laxa avec tumeurs par contusion chronique des coudes et des genoux (xanthome juvenile pseudo-diabetique de MM Hallopeau et Macé de Lépinay), *Bull Soc Franc Derm Syph* 19:70-72, 1908.

36. David TJ: Skeletal dysplasia, hyper-pigmentation, endocrine abnormality and mental retardation—the Patterson syndrome, *Prog Clin Biol Res* 104:331-337, 1982.

37. David T, Webb BW, Gordon IRS: The Patterson syndrome, leprechaunism, pseudoleprechaunism, *J Med Genet* 18:294-298, 1981.

38. De Barsy AM, Moens E, Dierckx L: Dwarfism, oligophrenia and degeneration of the elastic tissue in skin and cornea. A new syndrome? *Helv Paediat Acta* 23:305-313, 1968.

39. Debré R, Marie J, Seringe P: "Cutis laxa" avec dystrophies osseuses, *Bull Soc Méd Hôp Paris* 61:1038, 1937.

40. Dingman RO, Grabb WC, O'Neal RM: Cutis laxa congenita: generalized elastosis, *Plast Reconstr Surg* 44:431-435, 1969.

41. Donohue WL, Uchida I: Leprechaunism: a euphemism for a rare familial disorder, *J Pediatr* 45:505-519, 1954.

42. Dubreuilh W: Un cas de dermatolysie generalisée, *Ann Dermatol Syph* 7:529-531, 1887.

43. Ehlers E: Cutis laxa, Neigung zu Hämorrhagien in der Haut, Lockerung mehrerer Artikulationen, *Derm Wschr* 8:173, 1901.

44. Ertugrul A: Diffuse tortuosity and lengthening of the arteries, *Circulation* 36:400-407, 1967.

45. Fazio MJ et al: Human elastin gene: new evidence for localization to the long arm of chromosome 7, *Am J Hum Genet* 48:696-703, 1991.

46. Ferreira ML, Spina V: A case of cutis laxa with abnormal copper metabolism, *Br J Plast Surg* 26:283-286, 1973.

47. Findlay GH: Idiopathic enlargement of the lips: cheilosis granulomatosa, Ascher's syndrome and double lip, *Br J Dermatol* 66:129-138, 1954.

48. Fisher BK, Page E, Wedad H: Acral localized acquired cutis laxa, *J Am Acad Dermatol* 21:33-40, 1989.

49. Fittke H: Über eine ungewöhnliche Form multipler Erbabartung: (Chalodermie und Dysostose), *Z Kinderheilk* 63:510-523, 1942.

50. Fitzsimmons JS et al: Variable clinical presentations of cutis laxa, *Clin Genet* 28:284-295, 1985.

51. Franceschetti A: Manifestation de blepharochasis chez le père, associé à des doubles lèvres apparaissant également chez sa filette agée d'un mois, *J Genet Hum* 4:181-184, 1955.

52. Frohlich F: Der Mangel der Muskeln, innsbesondere der Seitenbauchmuskien, Wurzburg, Dissertation 1839. In McKusick VA: *Mendelian inheritance in man, catalogs of autosomal dominant, autosomal recessive and X-linked phenotypes*, ed 9, Baltimore, 1990, Johns Hopkins University.

53. Gardner LI, Sanders FK, Bifano EM: Congenital cutis laxa syndrome: relation of joint dislocations to oligohydramnios, *Arch Dermatol* 122:1241-1243, 1986.

54. Gilford H: Progeria: a form of senilism, *Practitioner* 71:188-217, 1904.

55. Godfrey M et al: Cosegregation of elastin associated microfibrillar abnormalities with the Marfan phenotype in families, *Am J Hum Genet* 46:652-660, 1990.

56. Goldblatt et al: Cutis laxa, retarded development and joint hypermobility syndrome, *Dysmorph Clin Genet* 1:142-144, 1988.

57. Goltz RW, Hult AM: Generalized elastolysis (cutis laxa) and Ehlers-Danlos syndrome (cutis hyperelactica); a comparative clinical and laboratory study, *Southern Med J* 58:848-854, 1965.

58. Goltz RW et al: Cutis laxa: a manifestation of generalized elastolysis, *Arch Dermatol* 92:373-387, 1965.

59. Gonnering R, Sonneland PR: Ptosis and dermatochalasis as presenting signs in a case of occult primary systemic amyloidosis, *Ophthal Surg* 18:495-497, 1987.

60. Goth A: Über chalodermie (Kerly), *Dermatol Monat* 104:426-435, 1937.

61. Graf (NI): *Örtliche erbliche Erschlaffung der Haut*, Berlin, 1836, Heilk Wschr Ges p 225.

62. Greenbaum SS et al: Localized acquired Cutis laxa in one of identical twins, *Int J Dermat* 28:402-406, 1989.

63. Hajjer BA, Joyner EN III: Congenital cutis laxa with advanced cardiopulmonary disease, *J Pediatr* 73:116-119, 1968.

64. Harris RB, Heaphy MR, Perry HO: Generalized elastolysis (cutis laxa), *Am J Med* 65:815-822, 1978.

65. Hashimoto K, Kanzaki T: Cutis laxa: ultrastructural and biochemical studies, *Arch Dermatol* 11:861-862, 1975.

66. Hayden JG, Talner NS, Klaus SN: Cutis laxa associated with pulmonary artery stenosis, *J Pediatr* 72:506-509, 1968.

67. Heilman VS, Haustein VF: Erworbene post inflammatorische Dermatochalasis nach Kalte-Urtikaria, *Dermatol Monattsch* 169:28-34, 1983.

68. Heye T et al: Post inflammatory cutis laxa and aortitis/acquired systemic elastolysis, *Br J Dermatol* 81(suppl 7):37, 1971.

69. Hoefnagel D et al: Congenital athetosis, mental deficiency, dwarfism and laxity of skin and ligaments, *Helv Paediat Acta* 26:397-402, 1971.

70. Holbrook KA, Byers PH: Structural alterations in the dermal collagen and elastic matrix from the skin of patients with inherited connective tissue disorders, *J Invest Dermatol* 70(suppl 1):75-168, 1982.

71. Houel: *Bulletin de la Societe Anatomique Paris*, Paris, 1880, p 140.

72. Hult AM, Goltz RA, Midtgaard K: The dermal elastic fibers in cutis hyperelastica (EDS) and cutis laxa (generalized elastosis), *Acta Dermatovener* 44:415-420, 1964.

73. Hunter AGW: Is geroderma osteodysplastic underdiagnosed? *J Med Genet* 25:854-857, 1988.

74. Hunter AGW et al: Geroderma osteodysplastica: a report of two affected families, *Hum Genet* 40:311-324, 1978.

75. Jablonska S: Inflammatorische Hautveränderungen, die eine erworhenen Cutis laxa vorausgehen, *Hautarzt* 17:341-346, 1966.

76. Janik J: Cutis laxa and hollow viscus diverticula, *J Pediatr Surg* 17(3):318-320, 1982.

77. Kaye CI, Fisher DE, Esterly NB: Cutis laxa. Skeletal abnormalities and ambiguous genitalia, *Am J Dis Child* 127:115-117, 1974.

78. Kerl H et al: Fatal penicillin-induced generalized post inflammatory elastolysis (cutis laxa), *Am J Dermatopathol* 5:267-276, 1983.

79. Kitano Y et al: Cutis laxa with ultrastructural abnormalities of elastic fiber, *J Am Acad Dermatol* 21:378-380, 1989.

80. Klaus E et al: Familial occurrence of a bulbar paralytic form of amyotrophic lateral sclerosis with reticular corneal dystrophy and cutis hyperelastica in three sisters, *Psychiatr Neurol* 138:79-97, 1959.

81. Koblenzer PJ, LoPresti PJ: Dermatochalasia (dermatomegaly) and congenital pulmonic stenosis, *Arch Dermatol* 97:602-603, 1968.

82. Kopp W: Demonstration zweier Fälle von "Cutis laxa," München, *Med Wschr* 35:259, 1888.

83. Kuivaniemi H, Peltonen L, Kivirikko KI: Type IX Ehlers-Danlos syndrome and Menkes syndrome: the decrease in lysyl oxidase activity is associated with a corresponding deficiency in the enzyme protein, *Am J Hum Genet* 37:798-808, 1985.

84. Kuivaniemi H, Tromp G, Prockop DJ: Mutations in collagen genes. Causes of rare and some common diseases in man, *FASEB J* 5:2052-2060, 1991.

85. Kunze J et al: De Barsy syndrome: an autosomal recessive progeroid syndrome, *Europ J Pediatr* 144:348-354, 1985.

86. Lazoff SG et al: Skeletal dysplasia, occipital horns, intestinal malabsorption, and obstructive neuropathy: a new hereditary syndrome, *Birth Defects Original Article Series* 11(5):71-74, 1975.

87. Lees MH et al: Ehlers-Danlos syndrome associated with multiple pulmonary artery stenosis and tortuous systemic arteries, *J Pediatr* 75:1031-1036, 1969.

88. Lewis E: Cutis laxa, *Proc Roy Soc Med* 41:864-865, 1948.

89. Lewis PG et al: Postinflammatory elastolysis and Cutis laxa, *J Am Acad Dermatol* 22:40-48, 1989.

90. Lisker R et al: Geroderma osteodysplastica hereditaria. Three affected brothers: literature review, *Am J Med Genet* 3:389-395, 1979.

91. McCarthy CF, Warin RP, Read AEA: Loose skin (cutis laxa) associated with systemic abnormalities, *Arch Intern Med* 115:62-67, 1965.

92. MacFarlane JD et al: A new Ehlers-Danlos syndrome with skeletal dysplasia, *Am J Hum Genet* 32 (abstr):118A only, 1980.

93. McKusick VA: Forty years of medical genetics, *JAMA* 261(21):3155-3158, 1989.

94. McKusick VA: *Mendelian inheritance in man, catalogs of autosomal dominant, autosomal recessive and X-linked phenotypes*, ed 9, Baltimore and London, 1990, Johns Hopkins University Press.

95. Marchese P, Holbrook K, Pinnell SR: A familial cutis laxa syndrome with ultrastructural abnormalities of collagen and elastin, *J Invest Derm* 75:399-403, 1980.

96. Marshall J, Vogelpol L, Weber HU: Primary elastolysis, *S Afr Med J* 34:721-727, 1960.

97. Marshall J, Heyl T, Weber HW: Postinflammatory elastolysis and cutis laxa, *S Afr Med J* 40:1016-1022, 1966.

98. Maury CP, Alli K, Baumann M: Finnish hereditary amyloidosis: amino acid sequence homology between the amyloid fibril protein and human plasma gelsoline, *FEBS Letters* 260:85-87, 1990.

99. Maxwell E, Esterly NB: Cutis laxa, *Am J Dis Child* 117:479-482, 1969.

100. Meretojoa J: Familial systemic para-amyloidosis with lattice dystrophie of the cornea, progressive cranial neuropathy, skin changes and various internal symptoms, *Ann Clin Res* 1:314-324, 1969.

101. Meretojoa J: Genetic aspects of familial amyloidosis with corneal lattice dystrophy and cranial neuropathy, *Clin Genet* 4:173-185, 1973.

102. Miller EJ et al: The biosynthesis of elastin cross-links: the effect of copper deficiency and a lathyrogen, *J Biol Chem* 240:3623-3627, 1965.

103. Mott V: Remarks on a peculiar form of tumour of the skin denominated pachydermatocele, *Lond Med Chirurg Trans* 37:155, 1854.

104. Mounier-Kuhn P: Dilatation de la trachie constations radiographiques et bronchoscopiques, *Lyon Med* 150:106, 1932.

105. Muster AJ et al: Fatal cardiovascular disease and cutis laxa following acute febrile neutrophilic dermatosis, *J Pediatr* 102:243-248, 1983.

106. Nanko H et al: Acquired cutis laxa (generalized elastolysis). Light and electron microscopic studies, *Acta Dermato-Venereologica* 59:315-324, 1979.

107. Newton JA et al: Cutis laxa associated with amyloidosis, *Clin Exp Derm* 11:87-91, 1986.

108. O'Brien BM et al: Multiple congenital skin webbing with cutis laxa, *Br J Plast Surg* 23:329-336, 1970.

109. Olsen DR et al: Cutis laxa: reduced elastin gene expression in skin fibroblast cultures as determined by hybridization with homologous cDNA and an exon 1 specific oligonucleotide, *J Biol Chem* 263:6465-6467, 1988.

110. Osler W: Congenital absence of the abdominal muscles and hypertrophied urinary bladder, *Bull Johns Hopkins Hosp* 12:371-333, 1901.

111. Pagon RA, Smith DW, Shepherd TH: Urethral obstruction malformation complex: a cause of abdominal muscle deficiency and the "prune belly," *J Pediatr* 94:900-906, 1979.

112. Panneton P: La blepharochalasis; à propos de 51 cas dans une même famille, *Arch Optalmol Paris* 53:729-755, 1936.

113. Patterson JH: Presentation of a patient with leprechaunism. In Bergsma D, editor: *Clinical delineation of birth defects. IV. Skeletal dysplasias*, New York, 1969, National March of Dimes Foundation, pp 117-121.

114. Patterson JH, Watkins WL: Leprechaunism in a male infant, *J Pediatr* 60:730-739, 1962.

115. Patton MA et al: Congenital cutis laxa with retardation of growth and development, *J Med Genet* 24:556-561, 1987.

116. Peltonen L et al: Alterations in copper and collagen metabolism in the Menkes syndrome and a new subtype of the Ehlers-Danlos syndrome, *Biochem* 22:6156-6163, 1983.

117. Petges G, Lecoulant P: Dystrophies de la peau par relachement et hyper elasticitie. In *Nouvelle Pratique Dermatologique*, Tome VI, Paris, 1936, Masson et Cie, Libraires de l'Academie de Medicine, pp 240-254.

118. Philip AGS: Cutis laxa with intrauterine growth retardation and hip dislocation in a male, *J Pediatr* 93:150-151, 1978.

119. Pontz BF, Zepp F, Stoss H: Biochemical, morphological and immunological findings in a patient with cutis laxa-associated inborn disorder (De Barsy syndrome), *Europ J Pediatr* 145:428-434, 1986.

120. Pope FM: Unpublished observation, April 1992.

121. Pospelow A: Cas d'une atrophie idiopathique de la peau, *Ann Dermatologie* 7 (series 2):505-510, 1886.

122. Rand CW: A case of supposed progeria (premature senility) in a girl of 8 years with remarks, *Boston Med Surg J* 171:107-111, 1914.

123. Reed WB, Horowitz RE, Beighton P: Acquired cutis laxa: primary generalized elastolysis, *Arch Dermatol* 103:661-669, 1971.

124. Reidy JP: Cutis hyperelastica (Ehlers-Danlos) and cutis laxa, *Br J Plast Surg* 16:84, 1963.

125. Reisner SH, Seelenfreund M, Ben-Bassat M: Cutis laxa associated with severe intrauterine growth retardation and congenital dislocation of the hip, *Acta Paediat Scand* 60:357-360, 1981.

126. Riebel T: De Barsy-Moens-Dierckx-syndrome, *Beobachtung bei Gesch Monats Kinderheil* 124:96-98, 1976.

127. Robinson HM, Ellis FA: Cutis laxa, *Arch Dermatol* 77:656-665, 1958.

128. Ronchese F: Dermatomegaly, *Arch Dermatol* 77:666-668, 1958.

129. Rosenthal JW, Kloepfer HW: An acromegaloid, cutis verticis gyrata, corneal leukoma syndrome, *Arch Ophthal* 68:722-726, 1962.

130. Rossbach MJ: Ein merkwurdiger Fall von griesen hafter Veranderung der allgemeinen Korpdecke bei einem achtsehnjahrigen Jungling, *Deutsch Arch Klin Med* 36:197-203, 1884.

131. Sack GA et al: Three forms of dominant amyloid neuropathy, *Johns Hopkins Med J* 149:239-247, 1981.

132. Saiki LY, Keen BR, Engvall E: Fibrillin: a new 350kd glycoprotein is a component of extracellular microfibres, *J Cell Biol* 103:2499-2509, 1986.

133. Sakati NO, Nyhan WL: Congenital cutis laxa and osteoporosis, *Am J Dis Child* 137:452-454, 1983.

134. Sakati NO et al: Syndrome of cutis laxa, ligamentous laxity, and delayed development, *Pediatr* 72:850-856, 1983.

135. Samantray SK: Cutis laxa, *Postgrad Med* 69:65-68, 1981.

136. Sayers CP, Goltz RW, Motte T: Pulmonary elastic tissue in generalized elastic tissue abnormalities (Cutis laxa and Marfan syndrome): a light and electron microscopic study, *J Invest Derm* 65:451-452, 1975.

137. Schultz F: Beitrag zur hereditaren Blepharochalasis, *Klin Mbl Augenheilk* 147:863-877, 1965.

138. Scott MA et al: Acquired Cutis laxa associated with multiple myeloma, *Arch Dermatol* 112:853-855, 1976.

139. Seifert: Ueber cutis laxa, *Zentrablatt fur Klinsche Medicine*, 1890, vol 3, p 49.

140. Sephal G, Davidson JM: Elastin production in human skin fibroblast cultures and its decline with age, *J Invest Derm* 86:279-285, 1986.

141. Sequeira JH: A case of dermatolysis and molluscum fibrosum with congenital morbus cordis and kyphosis, *Br J Dermatol* 28:68-70, 1916.

142. Sestak Z: Ehlers-Danlos syndrome and cutis laxa: an account of families in the Oxford area, *Ann Hum Genet* 25:313-321, 1962.

143. Shah BH, Sindhur CP, James MJ: Cutis laxa, *Indian J Dermatol* 34:152-157, 1968.

144. Siegmund H: Uber das Sog oedema lymphangiectaticum Zentralblatt fur Allegmaine, *Pathologie Pathologische Anatomie* 70:243-247, 1938.

145. Souques A, Charcot J-B: Géromorphisme cutané, *Nouv Iconogr Salpet* 4:169-178, 1891.

146. Stokes W: On excision of a pachydermatocele from the scalp, *Dublin J Med Sci* 61(series 3, no 49):1-6, 1876.

147. Taieb A et al: Collagen studies in congenital cutis laxa, *Arch Dermatol Res* 279:279-308, 1987.

148. Talbot FB: Metabolism study of a case simulating premature senility, *Monats Kinderheil* 25:643-646, 1923.

149. Thaning O, Beighton P: Alimentary bleeding in cutis laxa of late onset, *S Afr Med J* 46:928-930, 1972.

150. Theopold W, Wildhack R: Dermatochalasis im Rahmen multipler Abortungen, *Monats Kinderheil* 99:213-298, 1951.

151. Tilbury-Fox: Quoted by Dubreuilh, 1887, p 529 (see reference 42).

152. Timpl R, Engel J: In Mayne R, Burgeson RE, editors: *Structure and function of collagen types*, New York, 1987, Academic Press, pp 105-143.
153. Ting HC, Foo MH, Wang F: Acquired Cutis laxa and multiple myeloma, *Br J Dermatol* 110:363-367, 1984.
154. Tsuji et al: Acquired Cutis laxa concomitant with nephrotic syndrome, *Arch Dermatol* 123:1211-1216, 1987.
155. Tsukahara M et al: A disease with features of cutis laxa and Ehlers-Danlos syndrome, *Hum Genet* 78:9-12, 1988.
156. Turner-Stokes L et al: Emphysema and cutis laxa, *Thorax* 38:790-792, 1983.
157. Van Maldergem L et al: Severe congenital cutis laxa with pulmonary emphysema: a family with three affected sibs, *Am J Med Genet* 31:455-464, 1988.
158. Van Maldergem L, Ogar G, Yuksel M: Facial anomalies in congenital cutis laxa with retarded growth and skeletal development, *Am J Med Genet* 32:265 only, 1989.
159. Variot, Cailliau: Peau ridée senile chez une enfant deux ans: agenesie des reseaux elastiques due derme, *Arch Med Enfantes* 23:106-111, 1920.
160. Verhagen AR, Woerdeman MJ: Post inflammatory elastolysis and cutis laxa, *Br J Dermatol* 92:183-190, 1975.
161. Von Ketley L: Ein Fall con eigenartiger Hautverand-erung: "chalodermie" (Schlaffhaut), *Arch Dermatol Syph* 56:107, 1901.
162. Vuorio E, de Crombrugghe B: The family of collagen genes, *Ann Rev Biochem* 59:837-872, 1990.
163. Wanderer AA et al: Tracheobronchiomegaly and acquired cutis laxa in a child. Physiologic and immunologic studies, *Pediatrics* 44:709-715, 1969.
164. Weber FP: Chalasodermia, or "loose skin," and its relationship to subcutaneous fibroids or calcareous nodules, *Urol Cutan Rev* 27:407, 1923.
165. Weir EK et al: Cardiovascular abnormalities in cutis laxa, *Eur J Cardiol* 5(3):255-261, 1977.
166. Welch JP et al: Familiar aggregation of a "new" connective tissue disorder, a nosologic problem. In Bergsma D, editor: *Clinical delineation of birth defects. XII. Skin, hair and nails*, Baltimore, 1971, Williams & Wilkins, pp 504-513.
167. Wiedemann H-R: Geroderma osteodysplastica: what would Virchow have thought about it? (letter), *Hum Genet* 43:245 only, 1978.
168. Wile H: The elastic skin man, *Med News* 43:705, 1883.
169. Wise F, Snyder EJ: Diffuse and disseminate dermatolysis: report of a case, *J Cutan Dis* 32:139-144, 1914.

CHAPTER 8

Osteogenesis Imperfecta

Petros Tsipouras

Osteogenesis imperfecta (OI) is a generalized disorder of connective tissue involving bone, skin, ligaments, tendons, fascia, sclera, and the ear. Although the most frequent functionally important manifestation is bone fragility, blueness of the sclera is often a dramatic feature. Thin skin, loose-jointedness, and hernia are other variable manifestations.

The condition is phenotypically and genetically heterogeneous and a variety of subtypes have been defined. Considerable progress has been made in the elucidation of the fundamental defect, and it has been shown that the alpha 1 and alpha 2 chains of type I collagen are implicated in the major forms of the disorder.

HISTORICAL NOTE

It has been suggested[168] that an early case of OI was that of Ivar the Boneless, the mastermind behind the Scandinavian invasion of England in the last quarter of the ninth century. He is said to have had cartilage where bones should have been. He could not walk and was carried into battle on shields. Complete verification of the diagnosis is impossible because so much poetic glorification enshrouds any remaining records, and Ivar's skel-eton is no longer available for study, having been dug up and burned by William the Conqueror. A study of Ivar's descendants turned up no instances of OI or other bone disorder.

A left femur thought to be that of a person with OI was found in an Anglo-Saxon burial ground in England dating from the seventh century A.D.[222] The evidence is at best tenuous. Better evidence was provided in the case of an Egyptian mummy dating from about 1000 B.C. and residing in the British Museum for more than 60 years.[94] The skull showed a mosaic of innumerable wormian bones and "tam-o'shanter" deformity on reconstruction. The teeth were amber-colored, with the roots disproportionately smaller than the crowns. The legs were bowed, and radiographic studies showed the "thick bone" type of change.[94] The recorded history of the development of knowledge about this disorder is given in the box on p. 282.

The terms that have been applied to this syndrome are numerous and include, to mention a few, osteogenesis imperfecta,[217] mollities ossium,[139] fragilitas ossium,[97] and osteopsathyrosis idiopathica.[124] To complicate matters further, the disease is called *la maladie de Lobstein* in the French-speaking portion of the medical world. It is also known as Eddowes[76] syndrome (brittle bones and blue sclerae), van der Hoeve[210] syndrome (brittle bones, blue sclerae, and deafness), and Vrolik[217] disease (osteogenesis imperfecta congenita). Looser[126] suggested the terms "osteogenesis imperfecta congenita" and "osteogenesis imperfecta tarda." The condition called by French authors "periosteal dysplasia of Porak and Durante" is probably the same as osteogenesis imperfecta congenita.

Special thanks are due to Dr. Andrew Poole for assistance with the section on dentinogenesis imperfecta, to Dr. Francis Glorieux for allowing me to use unpublished information generated in his laboratory, and to Dr. Cheryl Greenberg for contributing material on the otologic aspects of osteogenesis imperfecta. Drs. Victor McKusick and Richard Wenstrup reviewed the text and made many useful suggestions. Dr. Peter Byers allowed me to use unpublished material, shared unpublished information with me, and endured repeated questions regarding several aspects of collagen biosynthesis.

Landmarks in the History of Osteogenesis Imperfecta

1788 O.J. Ekman.[77] In medical doctorate thesis at Uppsala, described "osteomalacia congenita" in three generations. (See Seedorff[168] for an extensive translation of Ekman's Latin thesis.)

1831 Edmund Axmann,[7] Wertheim, Germany. Described the disease in himself and his brothers, Paul and Anton. Made reference to the occurrence of articular dislocations and blue sclerae. One of the brothers had been reported by Strach in 1807.[193]

1833 J.C. Lobstein (1777-1838), gynecologist and pathologist, Strasbourg. Wrote about adult form of the disease in his textbook of morbid anatomy.[124]

1849 Willem Vrolik (1801-1863). Dutch anatomist. Described disease in newborn infant[217] (Fig. 8-1).

1859 Edward Latham Ormerod,[139] Brighton, England. Early description of case of 68-year-old woman only 39½ inches tall. Disease was passed to a son and a daughter. The skeleton, in the Royal College of Surgeons, London, is reproduced in Bell's monograph.[28] Use of term "mollities ossium."

1862-1865 Ernest Julius Gurlt[97] (1825-1899), Professor of Surgery, Berlin. Use of term "fragilitas ossium."

1889 H. Stilling,[191] Strasbourg. Histologic studies.

1896 John Spurway,[184] Tring, England. Described blue sclerae with fragility of bones.

1897 M.B. Schmidt,[161] Strasbourg. Proposed fundamental identity of the disease in adults and newborn infants.

1900 Alfred Eddowes,[76] London. Described blue sclerae. Suggested that OI is generalized hypoplasia of mesenchyme.

1903 Leslie Buchanan,[40] Glasgow. Demonstrated that blue sclerae are due to thinness of sclera. Fractures, deafness, or familial incidence not mentioned in his report of "A. M'C—, a girl aet. 9 years."

1906 E. Looser,[126] Heidelberg. Defended identity of disease in adult and newborn infant. Proposed terms "osteogenesis imperfecta congenita" and "osteogenesis imperfecta tarda".

1912 Charles A. Adair-Dighton,[2] Liverpool. Described deafness in OI.

1918 J. van der Hoeve, Groningen, and A. de Kleyn,[210] Utrecht. Emphasized brittle bones, blue sclerae, and deafness as a syndrome.

1920 K.H. Bauer,[21,22] Breslau. Provided histologic support for view that OI is a "hypoplasia mesenchymialis." Described dental histology.

1919, 1922 E. Ruttin,[159] Vienna. Described otosclerotic nature of the deafness in OI.

1928 Julia Bell,[28] of the Galton Laboratory, London. Described dominant pattern of inheritance, especially of blue sclerae, on the basis of a large number of pedigrees.

During the past few years much attention has been focused on the elucidation of the underlying biomolecular defects. Abnormalities of the alpha 1 or alpha 2 chains of type I collagen have been implicated in many affected persons, and a wide variety of mutations have been identified.

CLINICAL MANIFESTATIONS

The clinical variability of OI had been noted in the past by a number of investigators who attempted to define specific phenotypic groups. For many years there was broad subdivision into a severe "congenita" form, which was present at birth, and a milder "tarda" form, which became evident at a later stage. With the accumulation of large series of cases, together with increasing diagnostic sophistication, various attempts at further subcategorization were made. Sillence, Senn, and Danks,[174] using clinical, historical, radiologic and genetic criteria, proposed a classification that is now in general use. In this system OI is subdivided into four types. Although the clinical variability of OI defies any precise categorization,[24] the Sillence classification is widely used in clinical practice because it provides a practical description of diverse phenotypes (see the box on p. 284).

The clinical manifestations of the different types of osteogenesis imperfecta are discussed in the following section.

Musculoskeletal System

A propensity to fracturing on minor trauma is the hallmark of OI. This complication is extremely variable; some affected individuals have hundreds

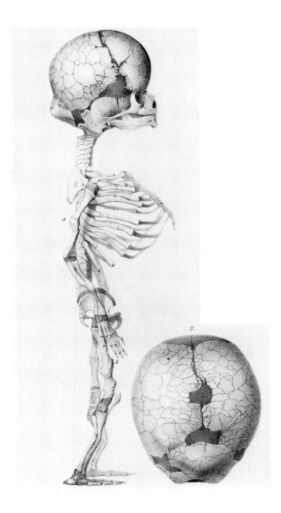

Fig. 8-1. Skeleton in osteogenesis imperfecta. The multiple wormian bones of the caput membranaceum are evident. (From Vrolik W: *Tabulae ad illustrandam embryogenesim hominis et mammalium, tam naturalem quam abnormem,* Amstelodami, 1849.)

of fractures, whereas others have very few.[25] There is no sex difference in the severity of bone fragility. A decrease in the incidence of fractures is observed after puberty in both sexes, with, possibly, an increase in incidence in women after the menopause[144] and in men over 60 years of age. Modification of life-style by the patient may be responsible in part for the improvement after puberty, in addition to possible hormonal influence.

The triviality of the trauma that may cause fracture is well known. Examples include fracture of the forearm during whittling or throwing a ball, of the phalanges in writing, and of the femora when another person sits on the patient's lap or when the patient stretches out in bed. Apert[5] called affected persons "les hommes de verre." In one family several children with the condition were appropriately referred to as "china dolls."

Sudden muscle pulls may fracture bones: the olecranon, for instance, has been pulled off by the triceps muscle during swimming or even less strenuous exercise. Relatively little pain tends to accompany the fracture,[38,121] probably because soft tissue trauma[5,39] is minimal and because the patients become accustomed to the frequent fractures. Persons with the disorder sometimes learn to set their own fractures. The fractures appear to heal at a normal rate, but occasionally the callus is so large as to suggest osteosarcoma.[10,131,164,194] Malignant degeneration is not recognized as a definite complication of OI, although bone neoplasms have been described[107,119] and a few patients have had surgery for suspected osteosarcoma. At times, overgrowth of bone occurs without evident fracture, and exostosis-like abnormalities may develop.

On radiologic examination the sutures of the

	Nosology of Osteogenesis Imperfecta	
Type	**Basic defect**	**Mode of inheritance**
OI type I	Osseous fragility (variable from minimal through moderately severe), distinctly blue sclerae (at all ages), presenile hearing loss	AD (heterogeneous)
OI type II	Lethal perinatal OI. Extremely severe osseous fragility, stillbirth or neonatal death	
	Subgroup A. Radiographs show broad, crumpled long bones and broad ribs with continuous beading	AD New mutation
	Subgroup B. Radiographs show broad, crumpled long bones, ribs show discontinuous beading or are not beaded	AR?
	Subgroup C. Radiographs show thin, fractured long bones and thin, beaded ribs	AR?
OI type III	Moderately severe to severe osseous fragility, normal sclerae (sometimes blue in infancy), variable but severe deformity of long bones and spine, stunted stature; generally nonlethal in the newborn infant	AR, AD?
OI type IV	Osseous fragility with normal sclerae (blue in infancy), variable deformity of long bones and spine	AD

AD, Autosomal dominant; *AR*, autosomal recessive.

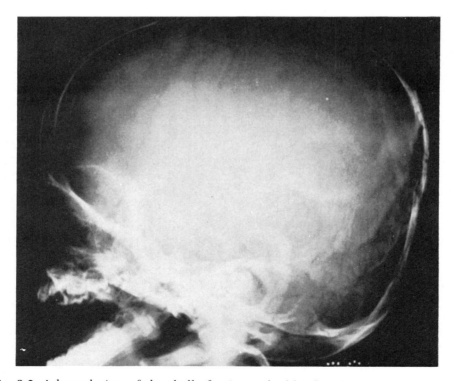

Fig. 8-2. A lateral view of the skull of a 2-month-old infant boy with osteogenesis imperfecta, showing a mosaic of wormian bones and a thin calvarium (caput membranaceum).

skull in all types of OI show numerous wormian bones[64] (Fig. 8-2). This mosaic phenomenon was striking in the case described and illustrated by Volik (Fig. 8-1) in 1849.[217] (This was the first time the name "osteogenesis imperfecta" was used.)

Gross skeletal abnormalities such as kyphoscoliosis, pectus excavatum, and "pigeon chest" are not uncommon in some forms of nonlethal OI.[29] Scoliosis may develop as a result of laxity of ligaments, as well as of vertebral osteoporo-

sis. The spinal malalignment is often extreme in patients with OI type III.[98]

The joints are sometimes excessively mobile, although to a much lesser extent than in the various hypermobility syndromes. The joint laxity is due in part to the presence of weak, stretched tendons and joint capsules and also to deformity and maladaptation of the bony surfaces of the joints. Rupture of the inferior patellar tendon, recurrent dislocation of joints, pes planus, and clubfoot occur in a minority of affected persons. Muscular hypo-

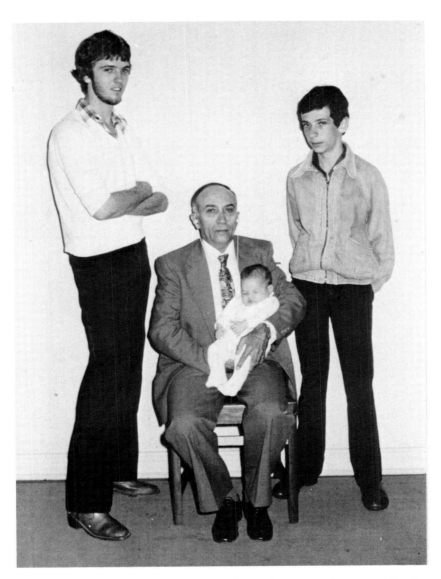

Fig. 8-3. OI type I in a father, his two affected sons, and a grandchild aged 4 months. The fracturing tendency was relatively mild in these individuals, and their stature was not reduced. The father wore hearing aids for bilateral deafness, which developed in early childhood.

tonia and underdevelopment are secondary to the anomalies of the tendons and joints and to general debility associated with reduced muscular activity occasioned by frequent fractures. A few individuals with a phenotype suggestive of both OI and EDS have been described.[63,177] Tardiness in walking of a child with OI is frequent, even in the absence of preceding fractures. This problem could be attributed to the underlying joint laxity. In a minority of affected persons the joints are rigid.[213] This rare form of OI, which may be an autonomous entity, has the eponymous designation, "Bruck syndrome."

In OI type I blue sclerae and bone fragility are the typical presenting features (Fig. 8-3).[174] The first fracture usually occurs in the preschool period, the rate decreases significantly in adolescence, and fractures are unusual in adults. Anterior or lateral bowing of the femora and anterior bowing of the tibiae are present in a minority of affected individuals. Kyphoscoliosis, which is usually comparatively mild, develops in adolescence in about one fifth of patients. Although only a few affected persons are below the tenth percentile in length at birth, by adult life almost 50% have some stunting of stature. Given the absence of significant skeletal deformity in most patients, the shortness of stature appears to be constitutional.[142,174,180] Apart from the presence of wormian bones in the cranial sutures there are no radiologic signs that are characteristic of this type of OI. Indeed, if radiographs are obtained at intervals between fractures, the appearance of the skeleton may be virtually normal.

OI type II is evident at birth, and affected neonates may have significant limb malalignment as a result of multiple intrauterine fractures. Caput membranaceum and micromelia are typical of OI type II (Fig. 8-4).[174,175,183] The chest is small, the limbs are bowed, and the thighs may rest in a characteristic frog-leg position because of abduction and external rotation. On radiologic examination, beading of the ribs that results from calluses is almost always present and the calvarium is severely undermineralized. In many cases the femora have a characteristic "concertina-like" radiologic appearance. The radiologic findings in OI type II are not uniform, but they represent a continuum as seen in Fig. 8-5.[47,130,175] Infants with OI type II are frequently premature, and many are stillborn. In survivors the condition is invariably

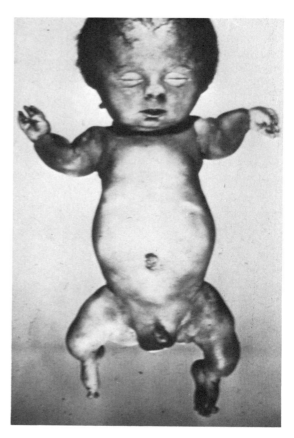

Fig. 8-4. A newborn with OI type II who died within hours of birth. The short, deformed limbs, the broad, abducted thighs, and the angulation of the legs are evident. (From Sillence DO et al: *J Med Genet* 17:407-423, 1984.)

lethal; death results from intracranial hemorrhage, inability to ventilate, or brainstem and cervical cord compression.[145]

OI type III presents at birth with bowing of the limbs (Fig. 8-6).[174,176] In older individuals shortness of stature in OI type III is often severe. Characteristically the adults have short legs in relation to the upper part of the body (Fig. 8-7). The shortness of the lower extremities is due to a combination of the sequelae of fractures in the shafts of the long bones, bowing that results from mechanical forces acting on malleable skeleton, and defective growth. The spine is usually malaligned, and the thorax has a characteristic conical or beehive shape.[176] Because of the softness of the bones of the thoracic cage, "flail chest" may lead to severe,

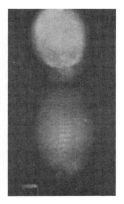
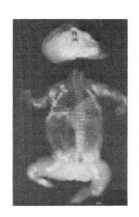
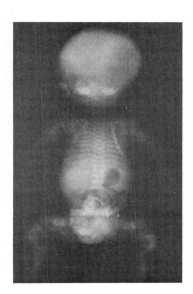
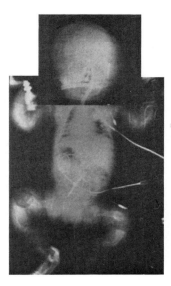

Fig. 8-5. Radiographs of infants with OI type II. (From Byers PH et al: *Am J Hum Genet* 42:237-248, 1988.)

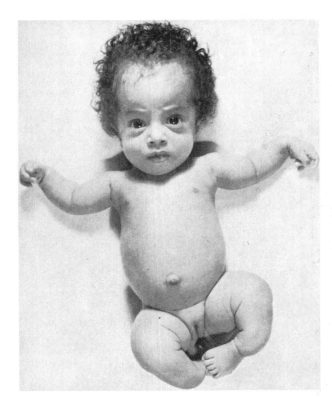

Fig. 8-6. A 3-month-old infant with OI type III. The head is large, and the lower extremities are short and bowed.

Fig. 8-7. A 14-year-old boy with OI type III. Severe angulation deformity of both upper and lower extremities is evident.

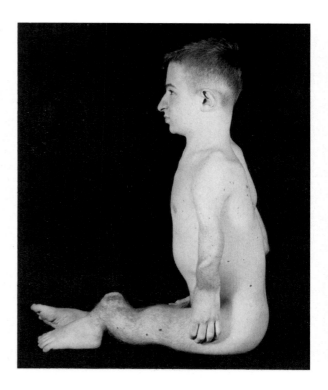

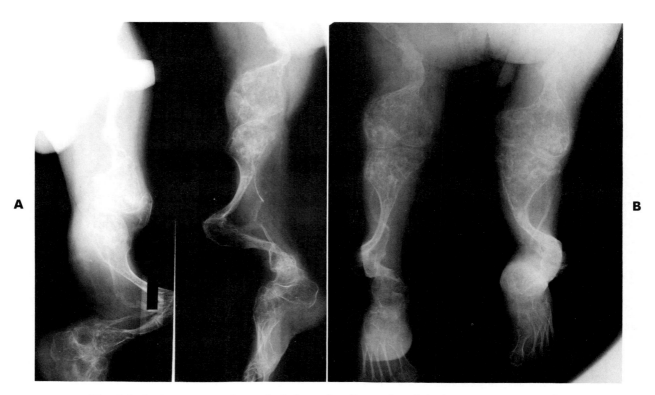

Fig. 8-8. **A,** Anteroposterior and, **B,** lateral radiographs of the lower extremities of a patient with OI type III. The bones are demineralized, with thin cortices and cystic changes in the metaphyses.

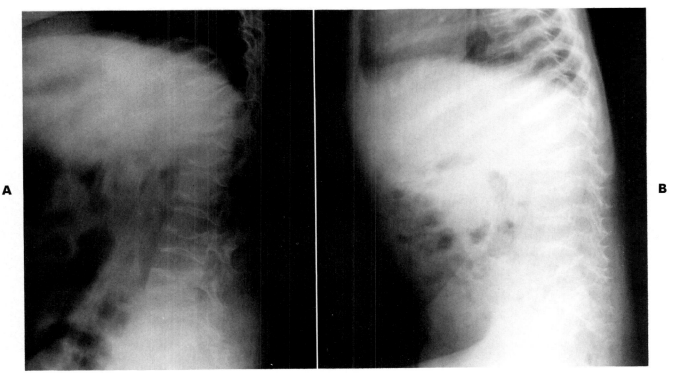

Fig. 8-9. Lateral view of the spine showing the characteristic "codfish" vertebrae. **A,** Patient aged 13 years. **B,** Patient aged 2 years.

often lethal, respiratory embarrassment in the neonate. It is not unusual for individuals with this form of OI to sustain up to 200 fractures in their lifetime, and in the absence of specialized orthopedic care functionally awkward pseudoarthroses may develop.

On radiologic examination all bones in OI type III have thin cortices, and the long bones usually have slender shafts with rather abrupt widening as the epiphysis is approached. In some instances the shafts of the long bones are thick, and in others there is a cystic appearance[79] (Fig. 8-8). During prepubertal years the changes may evolve from thin cortices to the cystic type or to thick cortices.[92] In addition to these changes, the limb bones are often asymmetrically malaligned as a result of fractures and in response to mechanical forces. The pressure of the normally elastic nucleus pulposus on the abnormally soft bone of the vertebral bodies produces a "codfish" or "hourglass" biconcave configuration (Fig. 8-9). In some instances actual herniations of the nucleus pulposus into the substance of the vertebral body may occur. Pro-

trusio acetabulum, which is often severe, imparts a characteristic "wine glass" configuration to the pelvis.

In OI type IV the face is usually triangular, largely as a result of the bulging calvarium and craniofacial disproportion.[174] The forehead is broad and domed, and the temporal areas are overhanging. The presence of an occipital overhang and platybasia result in a characteristic cranial appearance (Fig. 8-10). The onset of fractures is frequently prenatal, and malalignment of the long bones of the extremities is usual. Stature is significantly decreased; in a recent study the birth length in 40% of affected infants was found to be below the tenth percentile, whereas the height in 95% of affected adults was below the third percentile.[143,174]

Ocular Features

Blue sclerae constitute the ocular hallmark of OI. The color of the sclera has been described as "robin's egg," "slate," or "Wedgwood" blue. The color changes with age, and in adults the sclerae

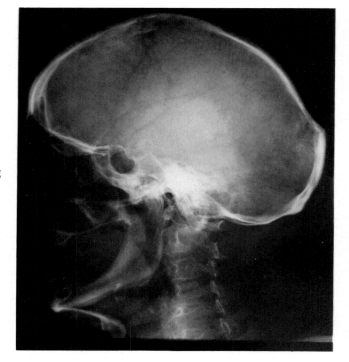

Fig. 8-10. Skull radiograph showing an "overhanging occiput" in a 51-year-old woman with severe OI.

may have a grayish hue. An increase in the blueness of the sclerae during episodes of stress such as fractures has been noted, but the significance of this observation is uncertain.[180] Scleral color is variable, and there is considerable overlap with the curve of normal distribution. Indeed, impressively blue sclerae are occasionally encountered in persons free from all other stigmata of OI. Conversely, the sclerae are usually white in OI types III and IV.[174,176]

The pericorneal region of the sclera is often white and opaque, resulting in the so-called "Saturn's ring." Embryotoxon, a congenital opacity in the periphery of the cornea, also known as arcus juvenilis, is also frequent. Hypermetropia is common in OI. By means of slit-lamp examination the cornea can be demonstrated to be measurably thinner than normal.[180] There is probably some increased risk of traumatic perforation of the sclera, although this is an unusual event. Other ocular abnormalities that have been observed in OI are keratoconus and megalocornea. Infrequently ectopia lentis and glaucoma have been reported in association with OI.

Cutaneous Features

The skin is affected in both the mild and the severe forms of osteogenesis imperfecta.[118] The skin

has been described as soft, smooth, and thin, and it may resemble the atrophic skin of elderly persons. Healing of skin wounds and surgical incisions sometimes results in scars that are wider than usual. Subcutaneous hemorrhages may occur after minor injuries, and results of tests of capillary fragility may be positive. Macular atrophy of the skin and elastosis perforans have been documented in a few affected persons.

Otologic Features

Significant hearing loss, conductive, sensorineural, or mixed, is present in about 50% of affected adults.[146,147,154,155] The clinical pattern of deafness differs in no respect from that of otosclerosis, although the histologic picture may be distinct. In a large Danish study by Pedersen[146,147] it was shown that 40% of patients with OI have a conductive or mixed loss and 10% had a sensorineural loss. An American study by Shapiro et al.[170] suggested that sensorineural hearing loss occurred more commonly than conductive or mixed deafness. These latter authors suggested that there is a loss in the high frequency range which was highly specific for OI. Deafness may have its onset in the teens but is most often a problem in early adult life. Deafness often begins or accelerates during pregnancy. In many individuals the hearing loss is mild, but in

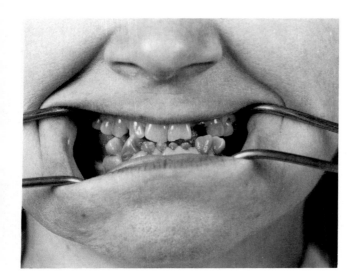

Fig. 8-11. Discoloration and stunting of the incisor teeth in OI type I.

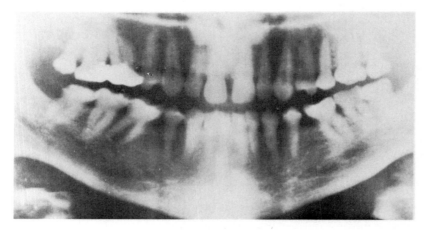

Fig. 8-12. Panoramic radiograph of the permanent teeth from an individual with dominantly inherited OI. The pulp chambers are obliterated in all teeth. Most root canals are obliterated. The coronal-radicular junctions are more constricted than normal. (From Levin LS: *Clin Orthop Related Res* 159:64-74, 1981.)

others it can be moderate, severe, or even profound. Recurrent middle ear infections aggravate the hearing loss. The hue of the tympanic membrane may be blue in a way that is analogous to the scleral color.[110,189]

Persons with OI may have long periods of tinnitus, possibly as an early symptom of stapedial fixation. Attacks of vertigo may indicate labyrinthine involvement,[235] which is sometimes uncomplicated by deafness.[83] A reduced response to vestibule-stimulating maneuvers in the absence of any clinical symptoms has been documented.[120]

Dental Features

The most common dental finding in OI is dentinogenesis imperfecta (DI). Affected teeth are translucent and brown or purple. The enamel is worn away or chipped, and the teeth are often carious (Fig. 8-11). On radiographic examination the crowns are bulbous with increased cervical constriction; obliteration of the pulp chambers is common[165] (Fig. 8-12). On histologic study the dentinal tubules are irregular and odontoblasts are absent, particularly where the pulp is obliterated. Lukinmaa et al.[127] noted a high frequency of thistle-shaped pulp chambers with or without pulp stones, dens invaginatus, and hypodontia of the permanent teeth in individuals with OI.

About 30% of individuals with all forms of OI have DI.[127] It has been suggested that the presence or absence of DI defines a phenotypic subclassification in both OI type I and OI type IV.[23,122,123,127] This situation is not clear-cut, however, since DI is extremely mild in some families. Furthermore, clinical assessment of DI can be difficult, even to the experienced eye. In some affected individuals DI is present in the primary but not the permanent dentition or vice versa, and in some teeth but not in others.[165] In other instances histologic evidence of DI can be adduced, although the teeth are normal on clinical examination.

Dentinogenesis imperfecta can exist in isolation as an autosomal dominant trait.[172,233] In the northern part of the United States the condition can be traced mainly to a passenger on the Mayflower, who was born in 1607. In the Middle Atlantic states affected families are derived from an early Pennsylvania settler from southern Germany. Other families, including those in a biracial isolate in southern Maryland, are traced back to a sea captain from Liverpool who settled in southern Maryland in 1732. He was said to be descended from, or at least related to, a butler of Henry II of England; Butler was the surname of the southern Maryland progenitor.[132]

Cardiovascular Features

Nonprogressive aortic root dilation has been observed in a few patients with different types of OI[65,153]; this abnormality bred true in some families.[106] Mitral valve prolapse also occurs in significant but low frequency.[106] In severely affected persons spinal malalignment may precipitate cor pulmonale.

Easy bruisability of mild degree is found in many affected individuals. Siegel, Friedman, and Schwartz[173] described a 25-year-old man with OI and a hemorrhagic diathesis that was manifested by epistaxes, hemoptyses, easy bruisability, and prolonged bleeding time. Excessive perspiration is a poorly understood but genuine manifestation of OI.[180]

Neurologic Features

Basilar impression, which occurs predominantly in OI types III and IV, can be suspected on clinical examination from the shape of the cra-

nium and confirmed on radiologic examination (Fig. 8-10). Neurologic complications associated with basilar impression, or platybasia, include bilateral, progressive cerebellar disturbance, interference with the function of the lower cranial nerves, and compression of the spinal cord at the level of the foramen magnum.[81,100,116] Backache and leg pains, which may have an element of nerve root compression in their causation, are frequent, but neurologic deficits directly attributable to nerve root compression are less common.[150] Computerized axial tomography (computed tomography [CT]) and nuclear magnetic resonance imaging (MRI) are helpful in delineating the extent of involvement of the central nervous system structures.[100,116]

Low-pressure hydrocephalus may develop in individuals with severe OI type III. In most instances the anterior fontanelle remains open, and CT of the brain reveals a generalized dilation of the ventricular system and cortical atrophy (Fig. 8-13).[205] Macrocephaly is sometimes evident in persons with nonlethal types of OI.[205] These individuals do not have any untoward symptoms or signs, and CT scans are normal. Intelligence is not usually affected in OI.

Pregnancy

Pregnancy is usually uncomplicated in women with mild forms of OI, although fracture of the rami of the pubis and of the coccyx during delivery has been described.[132] If the fetus has the condition, intrauterine fracture of the limbs may lead to malpresentation and delay in labor. In these circumstances cesarean section may be warranted.

In women with severe forms of OI types III or IV, stunted stature and gross pelvic deformity may make pregnancy a difficult undertaking.[111] Delivery by cesarean section is often necessary. In the severe African form of OI type III, no affected woman is known to have reproduced; the marked constriction of the pelvis that characterizes this form of OI[26] would probably preclude normal delivery.

DIFFERENTIAL DIAGNOSIS

Wormian bones are an important diagnostic indicator in OI, but they are far from pathognomonic for this disorder. Wormian bones also occur in pyknodysostosis, cleidocranial dysplasia, Cheney syndrome, progeria, and Menkes syndrome.[133] The

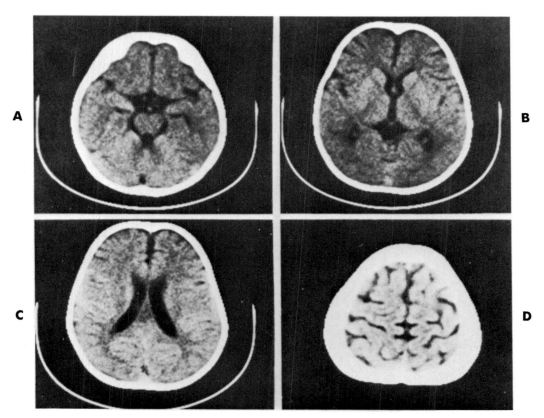

Fig. 8-13. Serial sections of CT scan of the skull in a 6-year-old boy with OI type III. **A,** Prominent basal cisternae. **B,** Dilated third ventricle with prominent cortical markings. **C,** Dilated occipital horns. **D,** Marked prominence of sulci and gyri. (From Tsipouras P et al: *Arch Neurol* 43:150-152, 1986.)

manifestations of pyknodysostosis, an autosomal recessive trait, include bone sclerosis, persistently wide cranial fontanelles, micrognathism with an obtuse angle of the ramus of the mandible, hypoplasia of the clavicles, and osteolysis in the terminal phalanges of the fingers. Cleidocranial dysplasia differs in that it is dominantly inherited and lacks bone sclerosis. The Cheney syndrome resembles OI in the occurrence of multiple wormian bones, osteoporosis with tendency to fracture, basilar impression, and dominant inheritance. Distinctive features include acroosteolysis and hypoplasia of the ramus of the mandible. Progeria is easily recognizable by virtue of premature aging, whereas Menkes syndrome, in which fracturing is not a significant problem, is lethal in infancy.

Idiopathic juvenile osteoporosis is an unusual disorder that begins at about puberty and remits spontaneously 3 to 5 years after onset.[73,179] On ra-diologic examination gross generalized rarefaction of the skeleton is evident, and in severe cases characteristic changes are present in the metaphyses. The age of onset, negative family history, and the normal sclerae and teeth distinguish this disorder from OI. It must be emphasized that idiopathic juvenile osteoporosis is extremely rare and there is some doubt concerning its existence as an autonomous entity.

The osteoporosis-pseudoglioma syndrome is an autosomal recessive disorder in which skeletal fragility is associated with severe ocular abnormalities that can cause blindness and mimic glioma.[84,160] The bone changes closely resemble those of OI, and the conditions can easily be confused with each other.

Hypophosphatasia closely resembles OI in infancy; in particular, blue sclerae and bowing of the legs are common to both disorders. Autosomal recessive inheritance and a low level of serum alkaline phosphatase activity in the former are distinguishing features.[229]

Homocystinuria may be confused with OI by virtue of the presence of osteoporosis, vertebral biconcavity, and susceptibility to fracture. A marfanoid habitus, ectopia lentis, central nervous system involvement, and abnormal urinary metabolites distinguish this disorder (see Chapter 4).

Hereditary opalescent dentin (OD), or DI, is a genetic disorder in which the teeth resemble those in OI; systemic manifestations, however, are lacking. The disorder is inherited as an autosomal dominant trait, and the OD gene locus has been mapped on the long arm of chromosome 4.[12] The opalescent character of the teeth is particularly evident in transmitted light, and the teeth are uniformly affected. In OI, on the other hand, there is wide variability in the extent of dental involvement, even within the same family.

A number of unusual but isolated cases with features that resemble those of OI have been documented. For instance, Cole and Carpenter[58] reported two unrelated children who came to medical attention with multiple fractures, craniosynostosis, hydrocephalus, ocular proptosis, and distinctive facial features. Biochemical studies showed no abnormality in the collagen type I synthesized by means of cultured skin fibroblasts obtained from the two patients.[57]

Nonaccidental Injury

In recent years considerable attention has been focused on the presence of fractures in infants and children suspected to be victims of child abuse.[1,105,112,141] Child abuse warrants consideration when the cause and extent of the injury are not compatible with the given history and when there is lack of or delay in seeking medical attention. Retinal hemorrhages, bruises in unusual places, and evidence of human bites and cigarette burns are other features.[1] The absence of systemic manifestations of OI such as wormian bones, blue sclerae, and DI are other diagnostic indicators. In addition to OI, copper deficiency has been implicated in osseous fragility in infants and therefore enters into the differential diagnosis of nonaccidental injury.[141]

PREVALENCE

With a few exceptions the ethnogeographic distribution of OI is ubiquitous. The frequency of OI type I has been estimated at 2.35 per 100,000 individuals in Japan[113] and 4.7 per 100,000 in Germany.[167] In Victoria, Australia, the frequency was estimated to be 3.4 per 100,000 individuals.[174] The new mutation rate for OI has been calculated to be between 0.7×10^{-5} and 4×10^{-5}.[113,167,178,216] The mean paternal age in the Victoria study was not significantly different from average.[174] OI type I is by far the most common form of the disorder.

The incidence of OI type II has been estimated at about 1 in 40,000 births by Freda, Vosburgh, and Di Liberti,[82] and approximately 1 per 56,000 births by Connor et al.[60] In Victoria, Australia, the incidence of OI type III has been estimated at 1.45 per 100,000 live births.[174]

In the black population of southern Africa, autosomal recessive OI type III is far more common than is the conventional OI type I. The disorder is found in all tribal groups and it is evident that the gene frequency is comparatively high.[26,27] It is uncertain whether this situation reflects a founder effect or represents some form of biologic advantage in the clinically normal heterozygous carrier of the mutant gene.[212]

The frequency of OI type IV is unknown, largely because of uncertainty concerning the phenotypic definition of this disorder. Sporadic atypical cases are relatively frequent, and it is debatable whether these are best regarded as unclassifiable or whether they warrant categorization as OI type IV.

GENETICS
OI Type I

In 1928 Bell[28] reported dominant transmission of blue sclerae and bone fragility in 73 kinships with a total of 463 affected individuals. Since then, scores of well-documented pedigrees leave no doubt that OI type I is inherited as an autosomal dominant trait.[142,174,201,207] The range of phenotypic expression is exceedingly wide, and in some individuals manifestations are at times too mild to be recognized on clinical examination.[154] Indeed, skipping of generations has been described in well-studied families.[59,103] The autosomal dominant pattern of inheritance has been further substantiated by the demonstration of transmission of specific heterozygous mutations in individual families.[43] The OI phenotype usually breeds true within a family. There are, however, certain notable exceptions, which have been explained on the basis of somatic mosaicism in one of the parents, affected with a mild form of OI, who subsequently had children with OI type II.[55,62,90]

OI Type II

In most instances OI type II is an autosomal dominant trait. The proband is usually the only affected child of unaffected parents and represents a new mutation for the faulty gene.[47,203,234] Indeed, a number of individuals affected with OI type II have been found to have heterozygous mutations in either the COL1A1 or the COL1A2 genes, whereas none of their parents were found to carry the same mutation. On the basis of biochemical and genetic findings it is reasonable to conclude that most cases of OI type II are new mutations.

In some families multiple affected offspring with clinical and radiologic pictures typical of OI type II have been documented.[47,55] These multiplex families with OI type II can be explained on the basis of germinal mosaicism, which renders one of the parents heterozygous for a collagen gene mutation in a proportion of gonadal cells.[55] Multiple affected siblings with normal parents can also be explained on a basis of autosomal recessive inheritance. The rare autosomal recessive types of OI type II, which are designated as OI type IIB and OI type IIC, can be distinguished on radiologic examination, although syndromic boundaries are not clear-cut.[36,49,175] An apparent instance of compound heterozygosity in typical OI type II was reported by de Wet et al.[68] The proband inherited a "null" COL1A2 allele from one parent and a de novo mutation in the other COL1A2 allele. The activity of these mechanisms make it difficult to estimate recurrence risks based on mendelian principles, but an empirical risk of about 7% is generally accepted.[47,203]

OI Type III

OI type III has been identified in more than 100 black individuals in southern Africa.[26] Many sets of affected sibs have been encountered, and in every instance the parents were normal. Inheritance is clearly autosomal recessive in this population.[212] In addition, a few OI type III pedigrees in other groups demonstrate a pattern indicative of autosomal recessive inheritance.[3,104,109] Genetic linkage analysis in families with OI type III has shown discordant segregation to both COL1A1 and COL1A2 gene markers.[3] Biochemical studies

in cultured dermal fibroblasts have failed to demonstrate a defect in type I collagen.

Autosomal dominant inheritance has been infrequently documented in OI type III.[195] In a few sporadic patients, biochemical studies have shown a de novo mutation in either the COL1A1 or the COL1A2 gene.[140,152,186,225,228] Homozygosity for a COL1A2 gene mutation in a child with OI type III, who was the offspring of a consanguineous union, has also been demonstrated.[74]

OI Type IV

OI type IV is inherited as an autosomal dominant trait.[174] It differs from the common OI type I by virtue of white sclera and greater severity of skeletal abnormalities.[143,174] These are, however, a matter of degree, and some authorities consider that OI type IV should be categorized with OI type I.

BIOMOLECULAR DEFECT

In 1975 Penttinen et al.[148] reported a decrease in the ratio of collagen I to collagen III synthesized by cultured dermal fibroblasts obtained from an infant with OI type II. The study results suggested for the first time that there might be a causal relationship between OI and collagen I. Since then, a variety of mutations in both the COL1A1 and COL1A2 genes have been found in association with the different types of OI.[43,44,151]

OI Type I

One of the earliest observations in biochemical studies of skin and subsequently of cultured dermal fibroblasts of patients who, in retrospect, would be considered to have OI type I, was the decreased amount of synthesized procollagen I as compared to that in controls. A low ratio of collagen I to collagen III was also observed.[199] It soon became clear that the synthesis of collagen I by cells cultured from individuals with OI type I was about half the normal level, whereas that of collagen III was normal.[14] The structure of the procollagen I was normal, and the decrease in procollagen I production resulted from synthesis of only half the usual amount of the pro alpha 1 (I) chains of procollagen I.

The mechanism by which the synthesis of pro alpha 1 (I) chains is decreased remains elusive. It has been suggested that in at least one family there is a defect in splicing of the nuclear RNA of COL1A1 that prohibits transport of the product of

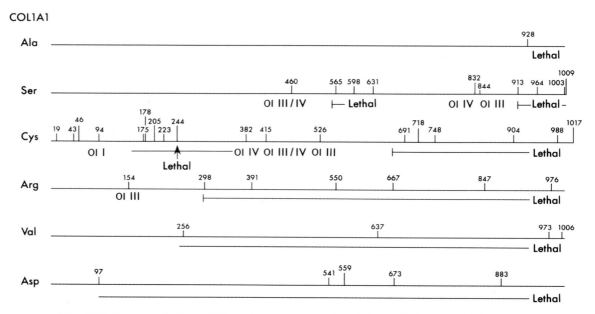

Fig. 8-14. Reported sites of Gly substitutions in the alpha 1 (I) chain in all four types of OI. (Courtesy Dr. Peter H. Byers.)

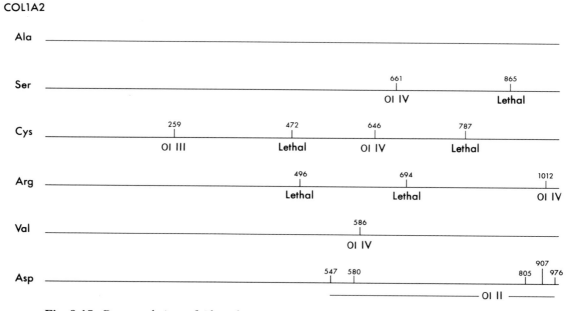

Fig. 8-15. Reported sites of Gly substitutions in the alpha 2 (I) chain in OI. (Courtesy Dr. Peter H. Byers.)

the mutant allele to the cytoplasm, although the precise molecular defect has not yet been characterized.[87] Linkage studies in 38 families demonstrated no evidence of deletion of those regions of the COL1A1 gene used for linkage analysis and confirmed that most individuals with the OI type I phenotype have mutations linked to the COL1A1 gene.[95,200,201] In some families a similar phenotype is thought to result from mutations in the COL1A2 gene.[201,207,218]

A 5-bp deletion near the 3' end of one COL1A1 allele results in a reading frame shift of 12 amino-acid residues from the normal terminus of the chain and predicts an extension of 84 amino acids beyond the normal termination site.[231] Although the abnormal mRNA can be translated in vitro, the protein product is unstable, since no abnormal chains have been identified in cells. This mutation provides a model of how many different mutations in the COL1A1 gene could produce the OI type I phenotype by resulting in the synthesis of half the normal amount of a functional pro alpha 1 (I) chain. In each instance the synthesis of pro alpha 2 (I) chains would be expected to be normal, but about half of them could not be incorporated into intact molecules (because the excess pro alpha 2 (I) chains cannot associate into trimeric molecules) and thus would be degraded.

Structural mutations in COL1A1 and COL1A2. Although structural mutations are less common than "null" allele mutations, there are several examples in which synthesis of abnormal procollagen I molecules can produce the OI type I phenotype. Substitutions of cysteine or another amino acid for glycine within the triple helix of the alpha 1 (I) chain at residues 178, 94, 46, 43, and 19 also produce mild forms of OI, most likely OI type I[44,71,138,186, 209] (Fig. 8-14). Deletion of exon 12 in a COL1A2 gene was found in a patient with blue sclerae, short stature, and hearing loss[46] (Fig. 8-15).

These findings indicate that other point mutations in the COL1A1 gene, and perhaps in the COL1A2 gene (as also suggested by linkage studies) could produce similar phenotypes.

OI Type II

OI type II is the most extensively investigated variety of OI and the best characterized at both

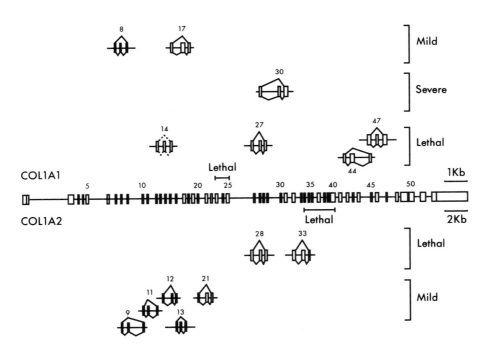

Fig. 8-16. Exon-skipping mutations involving both the COL1A1 and COL1A2 genes in different types of OI. The bold horizontal lines above and below the COL1A1 and COL1A2 gene schematic indicate two multiexon deletions detected with the COL1A1 and COL1A2 genes. (Courtesy Dr. Peter H. Byers.)

the biochemical and the molecular level. A wide array of mutations produces the OI type II phenotype: point mutations in the triple helical domain that result in substitutions for glycine (largely in the COL1A1 gene), multiexon rearrangements, small deletions (usually the result of splicing defects) in the triple-helical domain of either chain, and mutations in the carboxyterminal propeptide that interfere with molecular assembly. In almost all instances the affected individual is heterozygous for the lethal mutations.

Rearrangements. Three multiexon rearrangements involving the COL1A1 and COL1A2 genes have been identified in OI type II (Fig. 8-16). Among the cells initially studied by Penttinen et al.[148] was one from an infant with the lethal form of OI.[101] Although it was recognized that the cells did not produce procollagen I efficiently, the nature of the defect was unclear. Other studies of the same cell strain indicated that decreased production was a consequence of inefficient secretion of molecules that contained one or more pro alpha 1 (I) chains from which the 84 amino acids from 327 to 411 of the triple-helical domain (encoded by exons 23 to 25) had been deleted.[13,230] An intron-to-intron deletion of approximately 650 bp in one COL1A1 allele removed three exons and resulted in a shortened chain.[51] The deletion may have been mediated through a short inverted repeat at the ends of the deleted fragment.[15,53] Because the deletion end points were within introns, the resulting pro alpha 1 (I) chain was predicted to have an intact Gly-X-Y triplet structure that was 84 residues shorter than the product of the normal allele. Cells from this infant synthesized three populations of procollagen I molecules: normal molecules and those that contained either one or two of the short chains. Molecules that contained this shortened chain had a decreased thermal stability (about 32° C, compared with the normal value of 42° C), and virtually none of these molecules was secreted.[13,230] The deletion from the COL1A1 allele probably is sufficient to produce the lethal phenotype, but this cell strain secretes procollagen III, the chains of which have been excessively modified after translation.[230]

Another example of a multiexon rearrangement was the identification of a 4.5-kb, seven-exon deletion from one COL1A2 allele, which resulted in the synthesis of a pro alpha 2 (I) chain lacking 180 amino acids of the triple helix, residues 586 to 765 (Fig. 8-16).[232] Molecules that contained the shortened chain were not secreted but remained in the lumen of the rough endoplasmic reticulum.

Point mutations. The majority of cells from infants with OI type II are heterozygous for point mutations that result in the substitution for single glycine residues within the triple helix of either the pro alpha 1 (I) or the pro alpha 2 (I) chains. These mutations, in general, decrease triple helical stability, interfere with secretion, and affect the formation of fibrils in the extracellular matrix.[117]

The first demonstration that point mutations in the triple helix of the pro alpha 1 (I) chain might be significant came with the recognition that cells from an infant with OI type II contained a cysteine residue within the triple helical domain of the alpha 1 (I) chain[188] (Fig. 8-16). The presence of cysteine within the triple helix could not be recognized by the formation of an alpha 1 (I) chain dimer that resulted from interchain-intramolecular disulfide bonds. A single nucleotide substitution that changed the glycine codon at position 988 in the triple helix to that for a cysteine was found in one of the COL1A1 alleles.[54] All molecules that contained either one or two copies of the chain were less efficiently secreted than the normal molecules, had undergone increased posttranslational modification along the entire length of the molecule, and were less stable to thermal denaturation. A similar pattern of behavior of abnormal molecules was noted in other cell strains from infants with OI type II in which the mutation has not been characterized.[16,31,33]

It is now clear that although most substitutions for glycine within the triple-helical domain of either pro alpha 1 (I) chain or pro alpha 2 (I) chain do result in the clinical picture of OI, the severity of the phenotype is a reflection of the chain in which the mutation appears, the location of the mutation in that chain, and the nature of the substituting residue.* More than 20 point mutations have now been characterized from infants with the lethal OI phenotype[43] (Figs. 8-14 and 8-15).

Exon-skipping mutations and small deletions. Heterozygosity for exon-skipping defects currently comprises the second largest group of mutations

---

*References 11, 17, 18, 61, 62, 214, 219, and 220.

that produce the OI type II phenotype.[85] In general, exon skipping occurs as a result of point mutations in the splice donor or splice acceptor sequences.[43] Some of the reported exon-skipping mutations are presented in Fig. 8-16.

Mutations outside the triple-helical domain. Although far less common than any of the other mutations, alterations in the sequence of the carboxyl-terminal propeptide of the pro alpha 1 (I) chain are now being recognized as causes of the OI type II phenotype. In one instance the insertion of a single nucleotide results in a shift in reading frame and premature termination, alters the ability of the molecules to be secreted, and, in effect, acts as a sink for normal chains. Thus the secretion of procollagen I is reduced to about 25% of the usual amount, apparently insufficient to sustain normal bone formation.[19] This and other investigated mutations all appear to alter the ability of the abnormal chains to form stable trimers and be secreted.

Homozygosity or compound heterozygosity. Although the vast majority of infants with OI type II appear to be heterozygous for mutations in one of the genes that encode the chains of procollagen I, emerging biochemical and molecular genetic information suggests that in some situations two mutant alleles may be necessary to produce the phenotype. In one instance, biochemical and molecular data suggested that the OI type II phenotype resulted from compound heterozygosity for different mutations in the two COL1A2 alleles.[68,69,204]

A more recent example of homozygosity for a mutation provides additional insight into the mechanisms by which OI type II may be produced.[32] The infant described bore two copies of a COL1A1 allele in which there was a point mutation at position +6 in intron 14, just beyond the requisite GT dinucleotide that identifies the beginning of an intron. In cells, because of alternative splicing (deleting exon 14 from the mRNA), both the normal and the abnormally spliced mRNAs appeared in equal proportion. Thus, although the cells were, in effect, heterozygous for a mutation that resulted in abnormal splicing, they were, from a genetic point of view, homozygous for the allele that resulted in inefficient splicing. In this instance, the asymptomatic father was mosaic for the mutation and the mother lacked it altogether.

Further studies indicated that the infant represented an instance of uniparental disomy for all or a portion of chromosome 17. In such an instance, the recurrence risk for OI type II should be negligible but there would still be concern about the effect of heterozygosity (not mosaicism) for the mutant allele (see the preceding discussion of OI type I) in an offspring.

OI Type III

Until recently the molecular nature of OI type III has been elusive because in most individuals cultured cells appear to synthesize only normal procollagen I molecules. The best explanations for these findings are that mutations in collagen I genes are difficult to detect by means of the screening studies normally used and that the primary mutations occur in genes other than those that encode the chains of procollagen I. It is likely that both suppositions are correct. As more individuals are studied, however, it is becoming clear that some do have mutations in the genes that encode the chains of procollagen I.

Autosomal recessive OI type III. In one family the molecular basis of recessively inherited OI type III has been shown to be due to a mutation in a type I collagen gene. The proband was born to phenotypically normal first-cousin parents and recognized to have OI at birth. He had bone fragility, short stature, decreased calvarial mineralization, and moderate bone deformity that increased during childhood.[137] Type I collagen isolated from the proband's skin contained only alpha 1 (I) chains.[52,70,136] Dermal fibroblasts cultured from the child secreted procollagen I molecules that contained only pro alpha 1 (I) chains, and pro alpha 2 (I) chains synthesized by the cells were not incorporated into procollagen molecules. Both COL1A2 alleles contained, near the end of the exon that encodes the carboxyl-terminal end of the pro alpha 2 (I) chain, the same 4-bp deletion that changed the sequence of the final 33 residues of the chain.[74,149] The frame shift deleted the cysteine in carboxyl-terminal propeptide position 245 that normally bonds with a cysteine at position 80 to stabilize the structure of the peptide. Presumably, this resulted in a change in the tertiary structure of the carboxyl-terminal propeptide extension of the pro alpha 2 (I) chains to be incorporated into type I procollagen molecules. In the presence of normal pro alpha 2 (I) chains only, there is little formation of pro alpha 1 (I) homotrimers. In this instance, however, in the absence of normal pro alpha 2 (I) chains, pro alpha 1 (I) homotrimers formed. The chains in these molecules were overmodified along the length of the triple helix (although the thermal stability was unimpaired), and they were secreted more slowly than the normal. It is not clear whether the relatively severe phenotype resulted from the presence in the matrix of only homotrimeric molecules that were overmodified or from the absence of the alpha 2 (I) chain. This mutation demonstrated, to the surprise of many, that the absence of alpha 2 (I) chains in type I collagen can be tolerated.

Autosomal dominant OI type III. The OI phenotype usually results from mutations in the COL1A1 or the COL1A2 gene. Like most infants with OI type II, persons with OI type III have mutations that result in the substitution of individual glycine residues within the triple-helical domain of either the pro alpha 1 (I) or the pro alpha 2 (I) chains of type I procollagen. In all reported instances, molecules that contained one or two abnormal pro alpha chains were assembled and secreted (albeit less efficiently than normal molecules) but were less stable than the normal molecules synthesized and were overmodified aminoterminal to the site of the mutation[140,152,186,211,225] (Figs. 8-14 and 8-15).

OI Type IV

In early studies linkage heterogeneity was recognized among families segregating dominantly inherited OI.[200,201,207,218] In these kindred OI type IV was most often linked to polymorphic markers at the COL1A2 locus, but in some families linkage to the COL1A1 locus was identified. The clinical criteria by which many of these families were classified were often not clearly defined. For these reasons there is some uncertainty concerning the categorization of certain families. The significant point in these studies, however, is that mutations at both COL1A1 and COL1A2 loci can lead to the OI type IV phenotype.

As in other forms of OI, point mutations that result in substitutions for glycine residues in the triple-helical domains of the pro alpha 1 (I) and pro alpha 2 (I) chains of procollagen I, exon-skipping mutations, and a variety of mutations that disrupt the normal sequence of the pro alpha chains can all result in the OI type IV phenotype.

Point mutations in collagen I genes. The first point mutation that was characterized in the COL1A2 gene from a family with OI type IV resulted in the substitution of arginine for glycine at position 1012 of the triple helix of the alpha 2 (I) chain.[224] Additional point mutations in the COL1A2 gene that underlie OI type IV are indicated in Fig. 8-15.[20,182,225] It is of interest that the cysteine-for-glycine substitution in residue 646 has been identified in two unrelated families.

Another example of cysteine-for-glycine substitution in the triple-helical domain of the alpha 2 (I) chain has been recognized. In this instance the affected individual, who has mild OI, is mosaic for a mutation at position 472 that is lethal in his offspring. He was identified by virtue of having fathered two children with lethal forms of OI by different wives. This observation raises the important issue of the role of mosaicism for lethal mutations in producing mild OI phenotypes while, at the same time, putting the mosaic individual at significant risk of having severely affected children.

Identification of mutations in the COL1A1 gene verifies the linkage heterogeneity identified in OI type IV. Several substitutions for glycine that produce the OI type IV phenotype have been reported[48,67,129] (Figs. 8-14 and 8-15).

Exon-skipping mutations. In the first family in which linkage to the COL1A2 gene could be demonstrated,[206] cells from affected individuals synthesized and secreted normal procollagen I and also synthesized a population of molecules with a low thermal stability that was retained within cells.[223] The retained molecules contained a pro alpha 2 (I) chain that carried a small deletion (10 to 20 amino acids) within the triple-helical domain, which appears to be the result of deleting the sequences contained in exon 26 from the mRNA.[227] Several exon-skipping mutations that affect sequences toward the amino terminal end of the pro alpha 2 (I) chain have been reported. The clinical effects of exon-skipping events may vary, and it may be difficult to decide, on clinical grounds, whether the family in question has OI type I or OI type IV[46,115,158,177,197] (Fig. 8-16).

Other mutations. In one family a point mutation that results in the insertion of 6 additional amino acids in the triple helix, between residues 585 and 586 of the alpha 2 (I) chain, produces the

OI type IV phenotype.[197,226] A point mutation changes the T of the obligate GT splice donor sequence and forces the use of a second GT sequence 18 bp 3' to the usual site, resulting in the insertion of 6 residues that interrupt the normal Gly-X-Y triplet at that site.

PATHOGENETIC MECHANISMS
Mechanisms of Mutation in Collagen Genes

For several reasons collagen genes appear to be good reporters of mutations. First, there is a high density of invariant and required glycine residues in the triple-helical domain and substitution of either of the first two nucleotides of the glycine codon changes the encoded amino acid to one with a side chain that does not fit in the central core of the triple helix. Thus an alteration of any two of nine of the nucleotides encoding the triple-helical domain will probably give rise to a phenotypic change in the heterozygote. Second, the large exon number, as well as sensitivity to exon loss regardless of position in the protein, provides more than 200 additional mutation-sensitive sites in each gene. Finally, because type I collagen forms fibrils from identical subunits, the presence of any abnormal molecules in the matrix presumably interferes with the production of a normal fibrillar structure.

Most characterized mutations that produce recognizable forms of OI are single nucleotide substitutions that change a glycine codon to the codon for another amino acid. Few of the catalogued mutations have occurred independently in unrelated individuals.

It is surprising, given the repetitive structure of the type I collagen genes and the higher proportion of multiexon rearrangement in other fibrillar collagen genes (e.g., the COL3A1 gene that encodes the chains of procollagen III gene),[196] that large deletions within type I collagen genes are uncommon. The multiexon deletions that have been identified in collagen I genes occurred as results of intron-exon events.*

Exon-skipping mutations most often occur as the result of point mutations in the consensus splice donor and acceptor domains, but small deletions within the intron and exon may produce similar results. The mechanism by which small deletions occur is unclear, and it is uncertain

*References 15, 42, 45, 53, 56, and 232.

whether they result in exon-skipping events or simply in shorter amino-acid deletions.

Translation of Mutation to Phenotype

The phenotypic consequences of mutations in type I collagen genes reflect the gene in which the mutation occurred, the nature and location of the mutation, and its effect on the behavior of the abnormal chain and molecules in which it is contained. Sykes[198] proposed that mutations could be considered in two major categories: those that resulted in exclusion of the product of the mutant allele from the mature molecule, that is, "excluded mutations," and those that permitted the incorporation of a structurally abnormal chain, or "included mutations."

Effect of Excluded Allelic Products

Excluded mutations can be regarded in two ways: as failure of synthesis of the product of an allele and as failure of the synthesized chain to be incorporated into the protein. Both processes appear to result in mild phenotypes in the heterozygote and are generally found in individuals with OI type I. In the homozygote such mutations appear to be lethal in the case of COL1A1[162] but only moderately severe in the case of COL1A2.[70] Few "excluded" mutations have yet been identified and characterized at the molecular level.[14,87,157] Because the expression of the abnormal (or "null") allele may be low, the mutations must be identified at the genomic level; this is a formidable task with genes that encompass 18 kb and 38 kb and have more than 50 exons apiece. Nonetheless, the phenotypic effects of having too little collagen in bone are apparently far milder than those resulting from the presence of molecules that contain abnormal chains.

The effects on tissue strength of decreased production of procollagen I are not well understood. Bonadio et al.[34] demonstrated that in the mouse a marked decrease in the bone strength is compatible with the tissue that has decreased amounts of collagen I. It is not clear, however, that the decreased mass of collagen is the only effect. The striking morphologic appearance of collagen fibrils in skin of individuals with OI type I suggests that altered ratios of the major components of the matrix may contribute to abnormal tensile strength. Thus even the simplest of mutations is likely to have complex effects on the extracellular matrix.

Effects of Included Abnormal Products

On the whole, the phenotypic effects of mutations that result in the generation of abnormal procollagen I molecules are more deleterious than those of "null" mutations. There is, however, an enormous range in the spectrum of the clinical presentation of these mutations; this situation appears to reflect the gene (chain) in which the mutation occurs, the nature of the mutation, the location of the abnormal sequence in the protein, and the effects of the mutation on the behavior of the chain and of the mature molecule into which it is incorporated.

If an abnormal chain leads to rapid intracellular degradation of molecules that incorporate the chain, the clinical consequences should differ depending on the gene in which the mutations occur. Mutations in the COL1A1 gene may be highly deleterious, even lethal, because they make up three quarters of all the type I procollagen molecules synthesized (half of all molecules will contain one abnormal pro alpha 1 (I) chain and a quarter, two abnormal pro alpha 1 (I) chains). In contrast, a similar mutation in the COL1A2 gene would result in the loss of only half the molecules that are produced and so might be similar in effect to a "null" COL1A1 allele.

The effects of mutations reflect the domain of the procollagen molecule in which they occur and, within that domain, the way in which the specific mutation alters function. For point mutations in the COL1A1 gene that result in the substitution of glycine residues within the triple-helical domain of the chain, there is a broad "phenotypic gradient" such that defects near the carboxyl-terminal end of the chain are generally more severe than those near the amino-terminal end. Because this gradient is modified by the nature of the substituting amino acid, some defects may be lethal along the entire domain (e.g., aspartic acid[11]), whereas others may have a lethal-to-nonlethal transition in the carboxyl-terminal half of the chain (e.g., cysteine[187]).

Point mutations that substitute for glycine residues have several effects on the protein. First, almost all molecules that contain a chain with mutations in the triple-helical domains are less stable than their normal counterparts (i.e., they display a reduced thermal stability[228]. Second, the molecules that result are asymmetric in that they fold normally to the site of the mutant sequence and then appear either to fold slowly or to form a subtly different triple-helical structure amino-terminal to the sequence.[9] Third, as a result of the change in structure or in the rate of propagation of triple helix, the chains in the molecules remain accessible to the post translationally modifying enzymes. They undergo additional hydroxylation of lysyl residues in the triple helix and additional hydroxylysyl glycosylation, further accentuating the asymmetric character of the molecules. Finally, the relative tissue specificity of the effects of these mutations in type I collagen genes may reflect more stringent requirements of bone (rather than skin and other soft tissues) for aspects of molecular structure that can be changed by helix-altering mutations. It is likely that different mutations have different effects on molecular assembly[71]; these will be identified only by means of more detailed experimental study.

PATHOLOGY
Bone

The gross pathology and histological changes of the bone in OI have been reviewed.[41,108] The microscopic appearances of the skeleton vary in the different types of the disorder. Iliac crest bone biopsy specimens obtained from 14 affected children (2 to 14 years of age) were studied by morphometry after dual tetracycline labeling and compared to labeled biopsy specimens from age-matched controls.[91] The authors found the cancellous bone volume and trabecular thickness to be decreased in all types of OI. A mild but definite mineralization defect that was present was probably related to the quantitative or qualitative defect, or both, in collagen synthesis characteristic of OI (Fig. 8-17, A). There was no evidence of increased resorption. In OI type I, cancellous bone contained numerous osteocytes embedded in a lamellar matrix in which tetracycline labeling was included linearly (Fig. 8-17, B); cortical bone was decreased in thickness with a few haversian systems. In OI type III, cancellous bone was made of a mixture of woven and lamellar structures that took up tetracycline in an irregular fashion (Fig. 8-17, C), whereas cortical bone contained no haversian systems. In the marrow fibrosis was evident. The overall appearance of the most severe OI type III biopsy specimens was similar to the disorganization seen in fibrous dysplasia. Thus it appears that the molecular defects described in OI directly in-

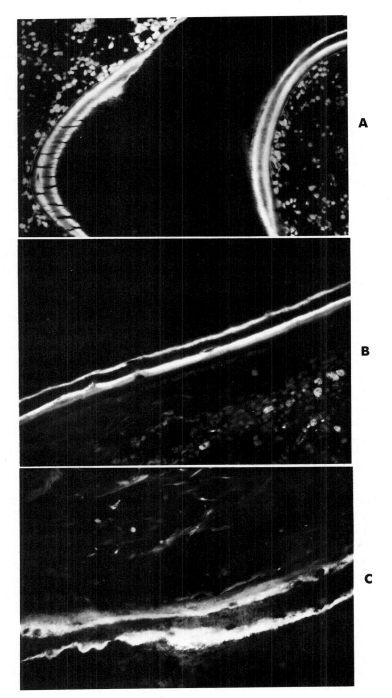

Fig. 8-17. Dual tetracycline labeling on mineralizing surfaces of a trabeculum. **A,** Normal control. The sharp delineation of the two markers can be seen (magnification × 150). **B,** Bone tissue from an individual with OI type I. The labeling shows well-delineated marker lines just under the shadow of osteoblasts (magnification × 250). **C,** Bone tissue from a person with OI type III. The tetracycline uptake is diffuse and irregular and most probably reflects the absence of organization of the matrix on which the mineral is deposited (magnification × 500). (Courtesy Dr. Francis H. Glorieux.)

fluence not only the synthesis of the matrix but also its organization in bone tissue.

PRENATAL DIAGNOSIS

Prenatal detection of fractures in a fetus with the lethal perinatal form of OI was first accomplished with a fetogram in 1933.[135] Since then, a number of cases of OI have been diagnosed in utero by conventional radiology or ultrasonography, usually at an advanced stage of pregnancy.

Several methods are presently available for prenatal diagnosis in OI. These include sonographic imaging of the fetus, collagen biomolecular studies of cultured chorionic villus cells, and genetic linkage studies using COL1A1 and COL1A2 markers. The prenatal detection of OI early in pregnancy gives the parents time to make decisions concerning termination and also facilitates optimal obstetric management should the parents decide to continue with the pregnancy.

Ultrasonography

Transabdominal sonographic imaging is a sensitive technique used extensively in the recognition of OI type II and other lethal or nonlethal chondrodysplasias before 20 weeks of gestation. Criteria used in the diagnosis of OI type II include the length of the femora adjusted for a particular gestational age, the extent of mineralization of the long bones and the calvarium, and evidence of fractures. This approach is effective in the monitoring of pregnancies that are possibly at risk for OI type II because of the previous birth of an affected child.* Sonography can detect intrauterine fractures and bone deformity with considerable precision and can also be used for the midtrimester prenatal diagnosis of OI type III.[8,15,156] In OI type I, in which the fetus is often mildly affected, the absence of fractures and resultant limb deformity may preclude accurate ultrasonographic diagnosis. As a result of the use of routine sonographic screening of all pregnancies, fetuses with previously unsuspected OI type II are being increasingly recognized before 20 weeks of gestation.

Chorionic Villus Biopsy

If a biochemical defect of collagen, or even a specific mutation, has been identified in an affected parent or sibling, prenatal detection can be

---

*References 37, 50, 75, 78, 89, 135, 169, and 190.

accomplished by screening fetal tissue for the presence or absence of that particular defect. Cultured cells grown from chorionic villi provide a source of tissue for collagen studies of this type. Substantial experience has accumulated regarding the electrophoretic characteristics of type I collagen synthesized by cultured chorionic cells, and it has been apparent that there are several limitations to the use of these investigations. First, the collagens synthesized by these cells are normally slightly more modified than those synthesized by skin fibroblasts. This factor necessitates the use of chorionic villus cells rather than dermal fibroblasts as controls (matched according to gestational age and time of biopsy). Second, the slight shift in electrophoretic mobilities makes it difficult to detect abnormal molecules in which the mutation results in only a small change in mobility. For these reasons, in many instances it may be difficult to identify a fetus with OI type III.

Amniotic fluid cells are not useful in establishing the diagnosis of OI because the major population of cells synthesizes a variant of type I procollagen, which contains pro alpha 1 (I) trimers that are dramatically overmodified.[66] Therefore, the effect of mutations in the COL1A1 gene on electrophoretic mobility is lost and mutations in the COL1A2 gene cannot be detected because no pro alpha 2 (I) chains are incorporated into molecules.

Linkage Studies

Genetic linkage studies are currently the diagnostic investigation of choice in families with autosomal dominant OI. A large collaborative study showed that in more than 90% of families with OI type I and OI type IV the condition is genetically linked to either the COL1A1 or the COL1A2 genes.[201] The identification of numerous DNA markers in both type I collagen genes has increased significantly the number of informative families. When genetic linkage studies are used for antenatal assessment, the observation of cosegregation of a COL1A1 or COL1A2 gene-specific marker with the phenotype is sufficient for diagnostic confirmation.[128,208] In this approach fetal chorionic villus tissue obtained between the ninth and eleventh week of gestation can be used for genotyping the fetus.

Comment

It is evident that prenatal diagnosis of the different types of OI is often feasible. Couples at risk for having a child born with the lethal or severe form of OI are likely to avail themselves of the opportunity for pregnancy monitoring. Biomolecular studies performed on chorionic cells facilitate diagnosis during the first trimester and provide ample time for an early termination of the pregnancy. The disadvantage of this approach is the necessity of an invasive procedure to obtain fetal tissue. On the other hand, sonographic imaging is a sensitive, noninvasive technique that is useful for the prenatal diagnosis of severe types of OI. A drawback of sonography is that this technique is unlikely to give definite results before the second trimester. In the future the development of transvaginal sonography might provide the means for first-trimester appraisal.

MANAGEMENT

As might be expected, many kinds of medication have been employed in the treatment of this distressing and long-standing disorder, but all therapeutic approaches have proved to be of doubtful benefit. The situation has been obfuscated by difficulties in evaluating results, the variable course of the disease, and wishful thinking on the part of physicians and patients. For these reasons overly enthusiastic reports have at times been forthcoming.

In the past, medicinal agents used in the treatment of OI included anabolic steroids, calcium,[4] vitamin C, fluoride, magnesium oxide, biphosphonates,[192,221] and flavinoids.[30] These agents have enjoyed a transient vogue, but none has proved to be efficacious and they have all faded from use.

The management of OI presents a challenge to the health professionals who care for individuals with this condition. A prompt diagnosis and a systematic follow-up during the early years of life establish the natural history of the disorder and provide a guide for the design of a plan best suited to the needs of the individual. The needs of infants, children, and adults with OI depend primarily on the severity of their condition, and optimal management of OI requires the participation of specialists in different branches of medicine together with other health professionals.

Lay organizations have an important role to play in the overall care of affected persons and their families. The Osteogenesis Imperfecta Foundation of the United States was incorporated in 1970, and "Brittle Bone" societies have subsequently been established in many countries. These groups represent a valuable source of information and collective wisdom, and their newsletters enable regular contact to be maintained.

Orthopedic Complications

In mild OI type I competent management of fractures minimizes skeletal deformity, and the great majority of affected individuals are able to walk unaided. Scoliosis is treated conservatively with the use of bracing, and if this approach proves to be ineffective, surgical measures remain a further option.

In OI types III and IV, in which ambulation is frequently compromised either permanently or for extended periods, orthopedic management is more complex. The objective in these circumstances is to render the individual functional and not necessarily to correct all existing skeletal deformity. In these conditions various types of osteotomy and subsequent stabilization of the bone with intramedullary metal rods or bone plates may be necessary.[134,181] Orthopedic management coupled with physical therapy aimed at improving muscle strength, as well as the provision of appropriate orthotic devices (bracing),[88] has allowed many individuals with severe OI to live full and productive lives. Many persons with OI type III and some with OI type IV are never able to walk (Fig. 8-18), and they need early instruction in the efficient use of a wheelchair. Scoliosis in individuals with OI types III and IV is frequently intractable and eventually leads to cor pulmonale. Surgical stabilization of the spine has a variable rate of success.[98]

The management of infants with severe OI begins in the nursery with instruction of the parents in the safe handling and lifting of their child. Head control, particularly if the head is enlarged, sometimes poses a problem. Infants with severe OI require multidisciplinary rehabilitation, which ideally is coordinated by a knowledgeable physician.

Neurologic Complications

The head may enlarge rapidly as a result of a communicating hydrocephalus[205]; in most instances this complication is self-limiting and shunting is not required unless nerve impingement or focal neurologic signs develop.

Basilar impression, although an uncommon feature of OI, can produce significant neurologic disability associated mainly with anterior compres-

Fig. 8-18. Osteogenesis imperfecta in a woman 35 years of age. Innumerable fractures have occurred, the first having been recognized at the age of 9 months. The sclerae are blue; hearing is intact. The patient is scarcely taller than a 4-year-old child. She has never walked and is carried about by a husky woman friend. There are pseudoarthroses of the left humerus and left tibia. Of two pregnancies, one was terminated for therapeutic reasons and the other ended in spontaneous abortion. (From McKusick VA: *Bull N Y Acad Med* 35:143, 1959.)

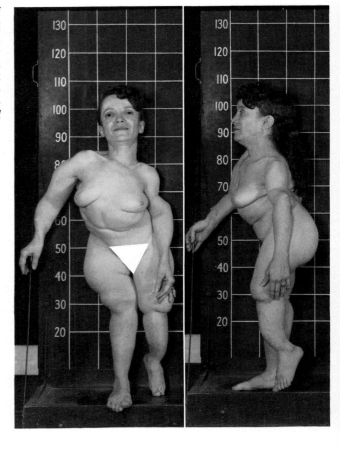

sion of the neuraxis.[100,116] In this process progressive infolding of the foramen magnum results in increasing impingement of the upper vertebral column upon the posterior fossa. The neurologic structures that are compressed include the upper spinal cord, the hindbrain and midbrain, and medial parts of the cerebellum. The clinical manifestations range from those of acute brain-stem compression to variable degrees of facial nerve palsy or spasm. Skull radiographs, CT scans, and MRI are needed to accurately define the extent of involvement of the underlying structures. Operations for cranial decompression and subsequent reconstruction have been undertaken for the relief of neurologic complications, but recurrence is not uncommon and full recovery is not always achieved.[100,116]

Dental Complications

Treatment of DI is aimed at maintaining normal growth and function of the teeth and improving their esthetic appearance. Excessive occlusal wear of the dentition is common in DI; this leads to reduction of the vertical dimension of the face and eventually to decreased arch length resulting from loss of interproximal contact.[102] In turn, the latter causes crowding of the permanent dentition. Occlusal wear occasionally precipitates pulpal involvement and abscess formation, particularly if pulpal obliteration has not occurred.

Stainless-steel crowning of the primary teeth is advocated for the prevention of occlusal wear. These procedures are often difficult to perform because of the bulbous crowns in DI and the necessity of general anesthesia in young children. Extraction of the teeth is not a satisfactory approach because this leads eventually to loss of alveolar bone and lack of ridges for the application of dentures. Space maintenance where primary teeth are lost is essential. Overdentures have also been advocated, but these must be adjusted and refashioned as the child grows. In the adult permanent esthetic crowns may be necessary, particularly in the anterior teeth, but in general, occlusal wear seems to diminish in the secondary dentition.[122] Intraosseous implants after loss of teeth, particularly in the affected adult, are of considerable value.

Hearing Impairment

Hearing impairment is a manifestation of OI that is frequently overlooked. Although the pathogenetic process leading to deafness starts in childhood, its presence usually becomes apparent during or after the third decade of life. Several studies have shown that up to 50% of individuals with OI have a conductive, mixed, or sensorineural hearing loss. The severity of deafness ranges from mild to profound, and the management of this problem begins with its timely diagnosis. Although the age of onset of hearing loss is usually young adulthood, any child with OI who comes to medical attention with speech delay, frequent ear infections, or articulation problems warrants a formal audiologic evaluation. Equally, an affected adult with a subjective complaint of hearing loss or tinnitus (an early symptom of stapedial fixation) requires audiologic examination. The provision of an appropriate hearing aid is often the only step that is necessary. Nevertheless, some adults with OI eventually require surgery to manage the increasing severity of their hearing loss. The objective of the surgical correction is the replacement of the fixed stapedial footplate with a Teflon prosthesis fitted on the oval window. The operation is performed with use of a dissecting operating microscope, and the stapedectomy is undertaken by excision either with scalpel or with argon laser. When appropriate, stapedectomy is the approach of choice for lasting restoration of normal hearing.[6,86,146,171]

ANIMAL MODELS

Two naturally occurring and one recombinant animal model of OI have been described. In 1983 Denholm and Cole[72] reported a lethal condition in cattle characterized by bone fragility, joint laxity, and translucent teeth. The sire was phenotypically normal. Outbreeding suggested that the mutation arose in the germline of the bull, which was therefore mosaic for the mutation. These experiments suggested an autosomal dominant type of inheritance. Analysis of bone collagen from one of the calves[80] was compatible with heterozygosity for a mutation in a collagen gene.

Guenet et al.[96] described a phenotype in the mouse, which resembled OI type III. The disorder in the mouse is inherited as an autosomal recessive trait, but the molecular basis is unknown.

A recombinant strain of mice has been created in which a retrovirus was fortuitously inserted into the first intron of a COL1A1 allele.[99,162] Mice heterozygous for the insertion event, known as the Mov13 mutation, have early-onset hearing loss and increased fragility of their bones compared to controls[34]; most tissues contain about half the normal amount of COL1A1 mRNA. The heterozygous Mov13 mouse could be considered an animal model of OI type I. Mouse embryos homozygous for the Mov13 mutation die at approximately 12 days of gestation of rupture of the heart and arteries.[125] Tissues in those embryos contain no type I collagen, and death appears to result from mechanical failure of the organs. In contrast, teeth synthesize procollagen I in a normal fashion, indicating that the promoter in dentin differs from that in bone and other tissues.[114,166] The pro alpha 2 (I) chains synthesized by means of cultured fibroblasts derived from a Mov13 homozygote can be rescued after transfection with a normal COL1A1 gene.[163] The inverse type of experiment, that is, introduction of a COL1A1 gene bearing a point mutation into normal fertilized mouse eggs, resulted in a phenotype similar to OI type II.[185] Thus a point mutation in a collagen allele is sufficient and necessary to produce the lethal phenotype.

SUMMARY

Osteogenesis imperfecta is a generalized disorder of connective tissue involving, in addition to bone, the skin, ligaments, tendons, fascia, sclera, and middle and inner ear. Although the most frequent functionally important manifestations are brittle bones and deafness, blue sclerae are a dramatic feature and thin skin, loose-jointedness, and hernia occur as manifestations of a single basic defect.

The wide range of phenotypic expression has resulted in division into a number of subtypes. Although this approach has some value in clinical practice, the boundaries of these different conditions are not clear-cut and precise diagnostic categorization is not always possible. It is significant, however, that more than 70% of all affected persons have the classic autosomal dominant form of OI in which a mild to moderate fracturing tendency and blue sclerae are the major features.

Osteogenesis imperfecta has been the subject of intensive molecular investigations in recent years. It has been shown that the majority of families with OI types I and IV have defects in the COL1A1 or COL1A2 gene. Similarly the majority of stillborn neonates with OI type II represent new mutations for the type I collagen gene. In the severe autosomal recessive form of OI type III, which occurs in comparatively high frequency in the black population of southern Africa, the basic defect has thus far defied elucidation.

REFERENCES

1. Ablin DS et al: Differentiation of child abuse from osteogenesis imperfecta, *Am J Roentgenol* 154:1035-1046, 1990.
2. Adair-Dighton CA: Four generations of blue sclerotics, *Ophthalmoscope* 10:188-189, 1912.
3. Aitchison K et al: Homozygous osteogenesis imperfecta unlinked to collagen I genes, *Hum Genet* 78:233-236, 1988.
4. Albright JA: Systemic treatment of osteogenesis imperfecta, *Clin Orthop* 159:88-96, 1981.
5. Apert E: Les hommes de verre, *Presse Méd* 36:805-808, 1928.
6. Armstrong BW: Stapes surgery in patients with osteogenesis imperfecta, *Ann Otol Rhinol Laryngol* 93:634-636, 1984.
7. Axmann E: Merkurdige Fragilitat der Knochen ohne dyskraische Ursache als krankhafte Eigenthumlichkeit dreir Geschwister, *Ann Ges Heilk (Karlrsruhe)* 4:58, 1831.
8. Aylsworth AS et al: Prenatal diagnosis of a severe deforming type of osteogenesis imperfecta, *Am J Med Genet* 19:707-714, 1984.
9. Baker AT et al: Changes in collagen stability and folding in lethal perinatal osteogenesis imperfecta, *Biochem J* 261:253-257, 1989.
10. Baker SL: Hyperplastic callus simulating sarcoma in two cases of fragilitas ossium, *J Pathol Bact* 58:609-623, 1946.
11. Baldwin CT et al: A single base mutation that converts glycine 907 of the alpha 2 (I) chain of type I procollagen to aspartate in a lethal variant osteogenesis imperfecta, *J Biol Chem* 264:3002-3006, 1989.
12. Ball SP et al: Linkage between dentinogenesis imperfecta and Gc, *Ann Hum Genet* 46:35-40, 1982.
13. Barsh GS, Byers PH: Reduced secretion of structurally abnormal type I procollagen in a form of osteogenesis imperfecta, *Proc Natl Acad Sci USA* 78:5142-5146, 1981.
14. Barsh GS, David KE, Byers PH: Type I osteogenesis imperfecta: a nonfunctional allele for pro alpha 1 (I) chains of type I procollagen, *Proc Natl Acad Sci USA* 79:3838-3842, 1982.
15. Barsh GS, et al: Intron-mediated recombination may cause a deletion in an alpha 1 (I) collagen chain in a lethal form of osteogenesis imperfecta, *Proc Natl Acad Sci USA* 82:2870-2874, 1985.
16. Bateman JF et al: Collagen defects in lethal perinatal osteogenesis imperfecta, *Biochem J* 240:699-708, 1986.
17. Bateman JF et al: Lethal perinatal osteogenesis imperfecta due to the substitution of arginine for glycine at residue 391 of the alpha 1 (I) chains of type I collagen, *J Biol Chem* 262:7021-7027, 1987.
18. Bateman JF et al: Substitution of arginine for glycine 664 in the collagen alpha 1 (I) chain in lethal perinatal osteogenesis imperfecta, *J Biol Chem* 263:11627-11630, 1988.
19. Bateman JF et al: A frameshift mutation results in a truncated nonfunctional carboxyl-terminal pro alpha 1 (I) propeptide of type I collagen in osteogenesis imperfecta, *J Biol Chem* 264:10960-10964, 1989.
20. Bateman JF et al: Characterization of a type I collagen alpha 2 (I) glycine-586 to valine substitution in osteogenesis imperfecta type IV: detection of the mutation and prenatal diagnosis by a chemical cleavage method, *Biochem J* 276:765-770, 1991.
21. Bauer KH: Ueber Identitat und Wesen der sogenannten Osteopsathyrosis idiopathica und Osteogenesis imperfecta, *Deutsch Zschr Chir* 160:289, 1920.
22. Bauer KH et al: Uber Osteogenesis imperfecta, *Deutsch Zschr Chir* 154:166, 1920.
23. Beighton P: Familial dentinogenesis imperfecta, blue sclera and Wormian bones without fractures: another type of osteogenesis imperfecta, *J Med Genet* 18:124-128, 1981.
24. Beighton P: Osteogenesis imperfecta: diagnostic considerations. In Noble J, Galasko CSB, editors: *Recent developments in orthopaedic surgery*, Manchester, 1987, Manchester University Press, pp 110-115.
25. Beighton P, Spranger J Versveld G: Skeletal complications in osteogenesis imperfecta: a review of 153 South African patients, *S Afr Med J* 64:565-568, 1983.
26. Beighton P, Versfeld GA: On the paradoxically high relative prevalence of osteogenesis imperfecta type III in the black population of South Africa, *Clin Genet* 27:398-401, 1985.
27. Beighton P et al: Osteogenesis imperfecta in Southern Africa, *Ann N Y Acad Sci* 543:40-46, 1988.
28. Bell J: Blue sclerotics and fragility of bone. In *Treasury of human inheritance*, vol 2. III. Cambridge, 1928, Cambridge University Press.
29. Benson DR, Donaldson DH Millar EA: The spine in osteogenesis imperfecta, *J Bone Joint Surg* 6OA:925-929, 1978.
30. Blumenkrantz N, Asboe-Hansen G: Effect of (+) Catechin on connective tissue, *Scand J Rheum* 7:55-60, 1978.
31. Bonadio J, Byers PH: Subtle structural alterations in the chains of type I procollagen produce osteogenesis imperfecta type II, *Nature* 316:363-366, 1985.
32. Bonadio J Ramirez F, Barr M: An intron mutation in the human alpha 1 (I) collagen gene alters the efficiency of pre-mRNA splicing and is associated with osteogenesis imperfecta type II, *J Biol Chem* 265:2262-2268, 1990.
33. Bonadio J et al: Altered triple helical structure of type I procollagen in lethal perinatal osteogenesis imperfecta, *J Biol Chem* 260:1734-1742, 1985.
34. Bonadio J et al: Transgenic mouse model of the mild dominant form of osteogenesis imperfecta, *Proc Natl Acad Sci USA* 87:7145-7149, 1990.
35. Reference deleted in proofs.

36. Braga S, Passarge E: Congenital osteogenesis imperfecta in three sibs, *Hum Genet* 58:441-443, 1981.

37. Brons JTJ et al: Prenatal ultrasonographic diagnosis of osteogenesis imperfecta, *Am J Obstet Gynecol* 159:176-181, 1988.

38. Bronson E: On fragilitas ossium and its association with blue sclerotics and otosclerosis, *Edinburgh Med J* (new series) 18:240-281, 1917.

39. Bryan RS, Cain JC, Lipscomb PR: Hereditary osteogenesis imperfecta: a mother and son with their family tree, *Mayo Clin Proc* 31:475-477, 1956.

40. Buchanan L: Case of congenital maldevelopment of the cornea and sclerotic, *Trans Ophthal Soc UK* 23:267, 1903.

41. Bullough PG, Davidson DD, Lorenzo JC: The morbid anatomy of the skeleton in osteogenesis imperfecta, *Clin Orthop Related Res* 159:42-57, 1981.

42. Byers PH: A novel mutation causes a perinatal lethal form of osteogenesis imperfecta: an insertion in one alpha 1 (I) collagen allele (COL1A1), *J Biol Chem* 263:7855-7861, 1988

43. Byers PH: Brittle bones-fragile molecules: disorders of collagen gene structure and expression, *Trends in Genetics*, 6:293-300, 1990.

44. Byers PH: Personal communication, 1992.

45. Byers PH, Wallis GA, Willing MC: Osteogenesis imperfecta: translation of mutation to phenotype, *J Med Genet* 28:433-442, 1991.

46. Byers PH et al: Abnormal alpha 2 chain in type I collagen from a patient with a form of osteogenesis imperfecta, *J Clin Invest* 71:689-697, 1983.

47. Byers PH et al: Perinatal lethal osteogenesis imperfecta (OI type II): a biochemically heterogeneous disorder usually due to new mutations in the gene for type I collagen, *Am J Hum Genet* 42:237-248, 1988.

48. Cetta G et al: The substitution of cys for gly in alpha 1 (I) triple helical domain: mutual influence of the mutation with neighboring amino acids, *Fourth International Conference on Osteogenesis Imperfecta (abstracts)*, Pavia, Ital, 1990, p 8.

49. Chawla S: Intrauterine osteogenesis imperfecta in four siblings, *Br Med J* 1:99-101, 1964.

50. Cherveval FA et al: Antenatal sonographic findings of osteogenesis imperfecta, *Am J Obstet Gynecol* 143:228-230, 1982.

51. Chu M-L et al: Internal deletion in a collagen gene in a perinatal lethal form of osteogenesis imperfecta, *Nature* 304:78-80, 1983.

52. Chu M-L et al: Presence of translatable mRNA for pro alpha 2 (I) chains in fibroblasts from a patient with osteogenesis imperfecta whose type I collagen does not contain alpha 1 (I) chains, *Collagen Related Res* 4:389-394, 1984.

53. Chu M-L et al: Multiexon deletion in an osteogenesis imperfecta variant with increased type III collagen mRNA, *J Biol Chem* 260:691-694, 1985.

54. Cohn DH et al: Substitution of cysteine for glycine within the carboxyl-terminal telopeptide of the alpha 1 (I) chain of type I collagen produces mild osteogenesis imperfecta, *J Biol Chem* 263:14605-14607, 1988.

55. Cohn DH et al: Germline and somatic mosaicism in osteogenesis imperfecta. *Fourth International Conference on Osteogenesis Imperfecta (abstracts)*, 1990, p 47.

56. Cohn DH et al: Homology-mediated recombination between type I collagen gene (COL1A1) exons results in an intragenic tandem duplication and lethal osteogenesis imperfecta, *Am J Hum Genet* 47:All0, 1990.

57. Cole DEC: Personal communication, 1991.

58. Cole DEC, Carpenter TO: Bone fragility, craniosynostosis, ocular proptosis, hydrocephalus, and distinctive facial features: A newly recognized type of osteogenesis imperfecta, *J Pediatr* 110:76-80, 1987.

59. Conlon FA: Five generations of blue sclerotics and associated osteoporosis, *Boston Med Surg J* 169:16-18, 1913.

60. Connor JM et al: Lethal neonatal chondrodysplasias in the west of Scotland 1970-1983 with a description of a thanatophoric dysplasialike, autosomal recessive disorder, Glasgow variant, *Am J Med Genet* 22:243-253, 1985.

61. Constantinou CD, Nielsen KB, Prockop DJ: A lethal variant of osteogenesis imperfecta has a single base mutation that substitutes cysteine for glycine 904 of the alpha 1 (I) chain of type I procollagen, *J Clin Invest* 83:574-584, 1989.

62. Constantinou CD et al: Phenotypic heterogeneity in osteogenesis imperfecta: the mildly affected mother of a proband with a lethal variant has the same mutation substituting cysteine for alpha 1 glycine 904 in a type I procollagen gene (COL1A1), *Am J Hum Genet* 47:670-679, 1990.

63. Crawfurd MD'A, Winter RM: A new type of osteogenesis imperfecta, *J Med Genet* 19:158, 1982.

64. Cremin P, Beighton P: Wormian bones in osteogenesis imperfecta and other disorders, *Skeletal Radiol* 8:35-38, 1982.

65. Crisciitiello MG et al: Cardiovascular abnormalities in osteogenesis imperfecta, *Circulation* 31:255-262, 1965.

66. Crouch E, Bornstein P: Collagen synthesis by human amniotic fluid cells in culture: characterization of a procollagen with three identical pro alpha 1 (I) chains, *Biochemistry* 17:5499-5509, 1978.

67. de Vries WN, de Wet WJ: The molecular defect in an autosomal dominant form of osteogenesis imperfecta: synthesis of type I procollagen containing cysteine in the triple-helical domain of pro alpha 1 (I) chains, *J Biol Chem* 261:9056-9064, 1986.

68. de Wet WJ et al: Synthesis of a shortened pro alpha 2 (I) chain and decreased synthesis of pro alpha 2 (I) chains in a proband with osteogenesis imperfecta, *J Biol Chem* 258:7721-7728, 1983.

69. de Wet W et al: Use of R-loop mapping for the assessment of human collagen mutations, *J Biol Chem* 261:3857-3862, 1986.

70. Deak SB et al: The molecular defect in a nonlethal variant of osteogenesis imperfecta: synthesis of pro alpha 2 (I) chains which are not incorporated into trimers of type I procollagen, *J Biol Chem* 258:15192-15197, 1983.

71. Deak SB et al: The substitution of arginine for glycine 85 of the alpha 1 (I) procollagen chain results in mild osteogenesis imperfecta, *J Biol Chem* 266:21827-21832, 1991.

72. Denholm LJ, Cole WG: Heritable bone fragility, joint laxity and dysplastic dentin in Friesian calves: a bovine syndrome of osteogenesis imperfecta, *Aust Vet J* 60:9-17, 1983.

73. Dent CE, Friedman M: Idiopathic juvenile osteoporosis, *Quart J Med* 34:177-210, 1965.

74. Dickson LA et al: Nuclease Sl mapping of a homozygous mutation in the carboxyl-propeptide-coding region of the pro alpha 2 (I) collagen gene in a patient with osteogenesis imperfecta, *Proc Natl Acad Sci USA* 81:4524-4528, 1984.

75. Dinno ND et al: Midtrimester diagnosis of osteogenesis imperfecta type II, *Birth Defects (Original Article Series)* 18(3A):125-132, 1982.

76. Eddowes A: Dark sclerotics and fragilitas ossium, *Br Med J* 2:222, 1900.

77. Ekman OJ: *Dissertatio medica descriptionem et casus aliqot osteomalacia sistens*, Uppsala, Sweden, 1788.

78. Elejalde BR, De Elejalde MM: Prenatal diagnosis of perinatally lethal osteogenesis imperfecta, *Am J Med Genet* 17:407-423, 1983.

79. Fairbank T: *An atlas of general affections of the skeleton*, London, 1951, Churchill Livingston.

80. Fisher LW et al: Mineralized tissue protein profiles in the Australian form of bovine osteogenesis imperfecta, *Calcif Tissue Int* 38:16-20, 1986.

81. Frank E, Berger T, Tew J: Basilar impression and platybasia in osteogenesis imperfecta tarda, *Surg Neurol* 17:116-119, 1981.

82. Freda VJ, Vosburgh GJ, Di Liberti C: Osteogenesis imperfecta congenita: a presentation of 16 cases and review of the literature, *Obstet Gynecol* 18:535-547, 1961.

83. Friedberg CK: Zur Kenntnis des vererbbaren Syndrome: abnorme Knochenbruchigkeit, blaue Skleren und Schwerhorigkeit, *Klin Wochenscrift* 10:830-832, 1931.

84. Frontali M, Stomeo C, Dallapiccola B: Osteoporosis-pseudoglioma syndrome: report of three affected sibs and an overview, *Am J Med Genet* 22:35-47, 1985.

85. Ganguly A et al: Heterozygous mutation in the G+5 position of intron-33 of the pro alpha 2 (I) gene (COL1A2) that causes aberrant RNA splicing and lethal osteogenesis imperfecta, *J Biol Chem* 266:12035-12040, 1991.

86. Garretsen TJTM, Cremers CWRJ: Ear surgery in osteogenesis imperfecta, *Arch Otolaryngol Head Neck Surg* 116:317-323, 1990.

87. Genovese C, Rowe D: Analysis of cytoplasmic and nuclear messenger RNA in fibroblasts from patients with type I osteogenesis imperfecta, *Methods Enzymol* 145:223-235, 1987.

88. Gerber LH et al: Rehabilitation of children and infants with osteogenesis imperfecta, *Clin Orthop* 251:254-262, 1990.

89. Ghosh A et al: Simple ultrasonic diagnosis of osteogenesis imperfecta type II in early second trimester, *Prenat Diagn* 4:235-240, 1984.

90. Gillerot Y, Druart JM, Koulischer L: Lethal perinatal type II osteogenesis imperfecta in a family with dominantly inherited type I, *Eur J Pediatr* 141:119-122, 1983.

91. Glorieux FH, Travers R, Chabot G: Personal communication, 1992.

92. Goldman AB et al: "Popcorn" calcifications: a prognostic sign in osteogenesis imperfecta, *Radiology* 136:351-358, 1980.

93. Gorlin RJ, Cohen MM Jr, Levin LS: Syndromes affecting bone: the osteogenesis imperfectas. In Gorlin RJ, Cohen MM Jr, Levin LS: *Syndromes of the head and neck*, ed 3, Oxford, 1990, Oxford University Press, pp 155-166.

94. Gray PHK: A case of osteogenesis imperfecta associated with dentinogenesis imperfecta, dating from antiquity, *Clin Radiol* 21:106, 1970.

95. Grobler-Rabie AJ et al: Detection of a high frequency Rs alpha I polymorphism in the human pro alpha 2(I) collagen gene which is linked to an autosomal dominant form of osteogenesis imperfecta, *EMBO J* 4(7):1745-1748, 1985.

96. Guenet JL et al: Fragilitas ossium: a new autosomal recessive mutation in the mouse, *J Hered* 72:440-441, 1981.

97. Gurlt E: *Handbuch der Lehre von den Knochenbruchen*, Berlin, 1862, pp 147-154.

98. Hanscom DA, Bloom BA: The spine in osteogenesis imperfecta, *Orthop Clin North Am* 19:449-458, 1988.

99. Harbers K et al: Insertion of retrovirus into the first intron of alpha 1 (I) collagen gene leads to embryonic lethal mutation in mice, *Proc Natl Acad Sci USA* 81:1504-1508, 1984.

100. Harkey HL et al: The operative management of basilar impression in osteogenesis imperfecta, *Neurosurg* 27:782-786, 1990.

101. Heller RH, Winn KJ, Heller RM: The prenatal diagnosis of osteogenesis imperfecta congenita, *Am J Obstet Gynecol* 121:572-573, 1975.

102. Helmers GB, Finn SB: Treatment of dentitions affected by hereditary amelogenesis imperfecta and dentinogenesis imperfecta, *Dent Clin North Am* 43:447, 1966.

103. Holcomb DY: A fragile-boned family: hereditary fragilitas ossium, *J Hered* 22:105-115, 1931.

104. Horan F, Beighton P: Autosomal recessive inheritance of osteogenesis imperfecta, *Clin Genet* 8:107-111, 1975.

105. Horan FT, Beighton P: Infantile metaphyseal dysplasia or "battered babies"? *J Bone Joint Surg* 62B(2):243-247, 1980.

106. Hortop J et al: Cardiovascular involvement in osteogenesis imperfecta, *Circulation* 73:54-61, 1986.

107. Jewell FC, Lofstrom LE: Osteogenic sarcoma occurring in fragilitas ossium, *Radiology* 34:741-743 1940.

108. Jones CJ et al: Collagen defect of bone in osteogenesis imperfecta (OI), *Clin Orthop* 183:208-214, 1984.

109. Kaplan M, Baldino C: Dysplasie periostale paraissant familiale et transmise suivant le mode mendelien reccessif, *Arch Fr Pediatr* 10:943-953, 1953.

110. Kellogg CS: Osteogenesis imperfecta: study of five generations, *Arch Intern Med* 80:358-365, 1947.

111. King JD, Bobechko WP: Osteogenesis imperfecta: An orthopedic description and surgical review, *J Bone Joint Surg* 53(B):72-89, 1971.

112. Knight DJ, Bennett GC: Nonaccidental injury in osteogenesis imperfecta: case report, *J Pediatr Orthop* 10:542-544, 1990.

113. Komai T, Kunai H, Ozaki Y: A note on the genetics of van der Hoeve's syndrome, with special reference to a large Japanese kindred, *Am J Hum Genet* 8:110-119, 1956.

114. Kratochwil K et al: Retrovirus induced insertional mutation in Mov13 mice affects collagen I expression in a tissue-specific manner, *Cell* 57:807-816, 1989.

115. Kuivaniemi H et al: A 19-base pair deletion in the pro alpha 2 (I) gene of type I procollagen that causes in-frame RNA splicing from exon 10 to exon 12 in a proband with atypical osteogenesis imperfecta and in his asymptomatic mother, *J Biol Chem* 263:11407-11413, 1988.

116. Kurimoto M, Ohara S, Takaku A: Basilar impression in osteogenesis imperfecta tarda, *J Neurosurg* 74:136-138, 1991.

117. Lamande SR et al: Characterization of point mutations in the collagen COL1A1 and COL1A2 genes causing lethal perinatal osteogenesis imperfecta, *J Biol Chem* 264:15809-15812, 1989.

118. Lapiere CL: Connective tissue disorders with skin expression, *Ann Dermatol Venereol* 105:905-911, 1978.

119. Lasson U, Harms D, Wiedemann H-R: Osteogenic sarcoma complicating osteogenesis imperfecta tarda, *Eur J Pediatr* 129:215-218, 1978.

120. Leicher H, Haas E: Labyrinthausfall bei Osteopsathyrosis, *Z Laryng* 36:190-194, 1957.

121. Levin EJ: Osteogenesis imperfecta in the adult, *Am J Roentgenol*, 91:973-978, 1964.

122. Levin LS: The dentition in osteogenesis imperfecta syndrome, *Clin Orthop* 159:64-74, 1981.

123. Levin LS, Salinas CF, Jorgenson RJ: Classification of osteogenesis imperfecta by dental characteristics, *Lancet* 1:332-333, 1978.

124. Lobstein *JGCFM: Lehrbuch der pathologischen Anatomie,* Stuttgart, 1835, p 179.

125. Loehler J, Timpl R, Jaenisch R: Embryonic lethal mutation in mouse collagen I gene causes rupture of blood vessels and is associated with erythropoietic and mesenchymal cell death, *Cell* 38:597-607, 1984.

126. Looser E: Zur Kenntnis der Osteogenesis imperfecta congenita et tarda, *Mitt Grenzgeb Med Chir* 15:161, 1906.

127. Lukinmaa PL et al: Dental findings in Osteogenesis imperfecta. I. Occurrence and expression of Type I dentinogenesis imperfecta, *J Craniofac Genet Dev Biol* 7:115-125, 1987.

128. Lynch JR et al: Prenatal diagnosis of osteogenesis imperfecta by identification of the concordant collagen 1 allele, *J Med Genet* 28:145-150, 1991.

129. Marini JC et al: Osteogenesis imperfecta type IV: detection of a point mutation in one alpha-1 (I) collagen allele (COL1A1) by RNA/RNA hybrid mutation, *J Biol Chem* 264:11893-11900, 1989.

130. Maroteaux P, Cohen-Solal L: L'osteogenese imparfaite letale, *Ann Genet* 27:11-15, 1984.

131. McCall R, and Bax JA: Hyperplastic callus formation in osteogenesis imperfecta following intramedullary rodding, *J Pediatr Orthop* 4:361-364, 1984.

132. McKusick VA: *Heritable disorders of connective tissue,* ed 4, St Louis, 1972, Mosby–Year Book, pp 390-454.

133. McKusick VA: *Mendelian inheritance in man,* ed 9, Baltimore, 1990, Johns Hopkins University.

134. Moorefield WG, Miller GR: Aftermath of osteogenesis imperfecta: the disease in adulthood, *J Bone Joint Surg* 62(A)113-119, 1980.

135. Munoz C, Filly RA, Golbus MS: osteogenesis imperfecta type II: prenatal sonographic diagnosis, *Radiology* 174:181-185, 1990.

136. Nicholls AC, Pope FM, Schloon H: Biochemical heterogeneity of osteogenesis imperfecta: a new variant, *Lancet* I:1193, 1979.

137. Nicholls AC et al: The clinical features of homozygous alpha 2 (I) collagen deficient osteogenesis imperfecta, *J Med Genet* 21:257-262, 1984.

138. Nicholls AC et al: Type I collagen mutation in osteogenesis imperfecta and inherited osteoporosis, *Fourth International Conference on Osteogenesis Imperfecta (abstracts)* Pavia, Italy, 1990, p 48.

139. Ormerod EL: An account of a case of Mollities ossium, *Br Med J* 2:735, 1859.

140. Pack M et al: Substitution of serine for alpha 1 (I)-glycine 844 in a severe variant of osteogenesis imperfecta minimally destabilizes the triple helix of type I procollagen, *J Biol Chem* 264:19694-19699, 1989.

141. Paterson CR: Osteogenesis imperfecta and other bone disorders in the differential diagnosis of unexplained fractures, *J Royal Soc Med* 83:72-74, 1990.

142. Paterson CR, McAllion S, Miller R: Heterogeneity of osteogenesis imperfecta type I, *J Med Genet* 20:203-205, 1983.

143. Paterson CR, McAllion S, Miller R: Osteogenesis imperfecta with dominant inheritance and normal sclerae, *J Bone Joint Surg* 65(B):35-39, 1983.

144. Paterson CR, McAllion S, Stellman JL: Osteogenesis imperfecta after the menopause, *New Engl J Med* 310:1694-1696, 1984.

145. Pauli RM, Gilbert EF: Upper cervical cord compression as cause of death in osteogenesis imperfecta type II, *J Pediatr* 108:579-581, 1986.

146. Pedersen U: Hearing loss in patients with osteogenesis imperfecta: a clinical and audiological study of 201 patients, *Scand Audiol* 13:67-74, 1984.

147. Pedersen U: Osteogenesis imperfecta: clinical features, hearing loss and stapedectomy. Biochemical, osteodensitometric, corneometric, and histological aspects in comparison with otosclerosis, *Acta Otolaryngol* (suppl)415:1-36, 1985.

148. Penttinen RP et al: Abnormal collagen metabolism in cultured cells in osteogenesis imperfecta, *Proc Natl Acad Sci USA* 72:586-589, 1975.

149. Pihlajaniemi T et al: Osteogenesis imperfecta: cloning of a pro alpha 2 (I) collagen with a frameshift mutation, *J Biol Chem* 259:12941-12944, 1984.

150. Pozo JL, Crockard HA, Ransford AO: Basilar impression in osteogenesis imperfecta, *J Bone Joint Surg* 66(B):233-238, 1984.

151. Prockop DJ et al: Type I procollagen: the gene-protein system that harbors most of the mutations causing osteogenesis imperfecta and probably more common heritable disorders of connective tissue, *Am J Med Genet* 34:60-67, 1989.

152. Pruchno CJ et al: Osteogenesis imperfecta due to recurrent point mutations at CpG dinucleotides in the COL1A1 gene of type I collagen, *Hum Genet* 87:33-40, 1991.

153. Pyeritz RE, Levin LS: Aortic root dilatation and valvular dysfunction in osteogenesis imperfecta, *Circulation* 64(4):311, 1981.

154. Quisling RW et al: Osteogenesis imperfecta: a study of 160 family members, *Arch Otolaryngol* 105:207-211, 1979.

155. Riedner ED, Levin LS, Holliday MJ: Hearing patterns in dominant osteogenesis imperfecta, *Arch Otolaryngol* 106:737-740, 1980.

156. Robinson LP et al: Prenatal diagnosis of osteogenesis imperfecta type III, *Prenat Diagn* 7:7-155, 1987.

157. Rowe DW et al: Diminished type I collagen synthesis and reduced alpha 1 (I) collagen messenger RNA in cultured fibroblasts from patients with dominantly inherited (type I) osteogenesis imperfecta, *J Clin Invest* 76:604-611, 1985.

158. Rowe DW et al: Molecular mechanisms (real and imagined) for osteopenic bone disease, *Fourth International Conference on Osteogenesis Imperfecta (abstracts)*, Pavia, Italy, 1990, p 57.

159. Ruttin E: Ohrbefund bei Osteopsathyrose, *Mschr Ohrenheilk* 53:305, 1919.

160. Saraux H et al: Pseudo-gliome et fragilite osseuse hereditaire a transmission autosomal recessive, *Ann Oculis* 200:225-226, 1967.

161. Schmidt MB: Die allgemeinen Entwicklungshemmungen der Knochen, *Ergebn Allg Path* 4:612, 1897.

162. Schnieke A, Harbers K, Jaenisch R: Embryonic lethal mutation in mice induced by retrovirus insertion into the alpha 1 (I) collagen gene, *Nature* 304:315-320, 1983.

163. Schnieke A et al: Introduction of the human pro alpha 1 (I) collagen gene into pro alpha 1 (I)-deficient Mov-13 mouse cells leads to formation of functional mouse-human hybrid type I collagen, *Proc Natl Acad Sci USA* 84:764-768, 1987.

164. Schwarz E: Hypercallosis in osteogenesis imperfecta, *Am J Roentgenol* 85:645, 1961.

165. Schwartz S, Tsipouras P: Oral findings in osteogenesis imperfecta, *Oral Surg Oral Med Oral Pathol* 57:161-167, 1984.

166. Schwarz M, Harbers K, Kratochwil K: Transcription of a mutant collagen I gene is a cell-type and stage-specific marker for odontoblast and osteoblast differentiation, *Development* 108:717-726, 1990.

167. Scroder G: Osteogenesis imperfecta, *Z Mensch Vereb Konstitut* 37:632-676, 1964.

168. Seedorff KS: *Osteogenesis imperfecta: a study of clinical features and heredity based on 55 Danish families comprising 180 affected persons*, Copenhagen, 1949, Ejnar Munksgaard.

169. Shapiro JE et al: Prenatal diagnosis of lethal perinatal osteogenesis imperfecta (OI type II), *J Pediatr* 100:127-133, 1982.

170. Shapiro JR et al: Hearing and middle ear function in osteogenesis imperfecta, *JAMA* 247:2120-2126, 1982.

171. Shea JJ, Smyth GDL, Altman F: Surgical treatment of the hearing loss associated with osteogenesis imperfecta, *J Laryngol Otolaryngol* 77:679-690, 1963.

172. Shields ED, Bixler D, El-Kafrawy AM: A proposed classification for heritable human dentine defects with a description of a new entity, *Arch Oral Biol* 18:543-553, 1973.

173. Siegel BM, Friedman IA, Schwartz SO: Hemorrhagic disease in osteogenesis imperfecta: study of platelet functional defect, *Am J Med* 22:315, 1957.

174. Sillence DO, Senn A, Danks DM: Genetic heterogeneity in osteogenesis imperfecta, *J Med Genet* 16:101-116, 1979.

175. Sillence DO, et al: Osteogenesis imperfecta, type II. Delineation of the phenotype with reference to genetic heterogeneity, *Am J Med Genet* 17:407-423, 1984.

176. Sillence DO et al: Osteogenesis imperfecta type III: delineation of the phenotype with reference to genetic heterogeneity, *Am J Med Genet* 23:821-832, 1986.

177. Sippola M, Kaffe S, Prockop DJ: A heterozygous defect for structurally altered pro alpha 2 chain of type I procollagen in a mild variant of osteogenesis imperfecta, *J Biol Chem* 259:14094-14100, 1984.

178. Smars G: *Osteogenesis imperfecta in Sweden: clinical, genetic, epidemiological and sociomedical aspects*, Stockholm, 1961, Scandinavian University Books.

179. Smith R: Idiopathic osteoporosis of the young, *J Bone Joint Surg* 62(B)417-427, 1980.

180. Smith R, Francis MJO, Houghton GR: *The brittle bone syndrome: osteogenesis imperfecta*, London, 1983, Butterworths.

181. Sofield HA, Millar EA: Fragmentation, realignment, and intramedullary rod fixation of deformities of the long bones in children, *J Bone Joint Surg* 41(A):1371-1391, 1959.

182. Spotila LD et al: Mutation in a gene for type I procollagen (COL1A2) in a woman with postmenopausal osteoporosis: evidence for phenotypic and genotypic overlap with mild osteogenesis imperfecta, *Proc Natl Acad Sci USA* 88:5423-5427, 1990.

183. Spranger J, Cremin B, Beighton P: Osteogenesis imperfecta congenita, *Pediatr Radiol* 12:21-27, 1982.

184. Spurway J: Hereditary tendency to fracture, *Br Med J* 2:844, 1896.

185. Stacey A et al: Perinatal lethal osteogenesis imperfecta in transgenic mice bearing an engineered mutant pro alpha 1 (I) collagen gene, *Nature* 332:131-136, 1988.

186. Starman BJ et al: Osteogenesis imperfecta: The position of substitution for glycine by cysteine in the triple helical domain of the pro alpha 1 (I) chains of type I collagen determines the clinical phenotype, *J Clin Invest* 84:1206-1214, 1989.

187. Steinmann B, Nicholls A, Pope FM: Clinical variability of osteogenesis imperfecta reflecting molecular heterogeneity: cysteine substitutions in the alpha 1 (I) collagen chain producing lethal and mild forms, *J Biol Chem* 263:8958-8964, 1986.

188. Steinmann B et al: Cysteine in the triple-helical domain of one allelic product of the alpha 1 (I) gene of type I collagen produces a lethal form of osteogenesis imperfecta, *J Biol Chem* 259:11129-11138, 1984.

189. Stenvers HW: Radiological studies on the patients by J. Van der Hoeve and A. de Kleyn *Archives fur Ophthalm (Leipzig)* 95:94-96, 1918.

190. Stephens JD et al: Prenatal diagnosis of osteogenesis imperfecta type II by real-time ultrasound, *Hum Genet* 64:191-193, 1983.

191. Stilling H: Osteogenesis imperfecta, *Virchows Arch* 115:357, 1889.

192. Storm T et al: Effect of intermittent cyclical etidronate therapy on bone mass and fracture rate in women with postmenopausal osteoporosis, *N Engl J Med* 322:1265-1271, 1990.

193. Strach E: Beobachtung von Fragilitat der Knochen in der Jugend, ein Beitrag zu der Lehre von den Knochenkrankheiten, *J Pract Arzneyk Wundarzneyk*, 1807.

194. Strach EH: Hyperplastic callus formation in osteogenesis imperfecta: report of a case and review of the literature, *J Bone Joint Surg* 35(B):417, 1953.

195. Suen VF, Harris V, Berman JL: Osteogenesis imperfecta congenita, *Clin Genet* 5:307-311, 1974.

196. Superti-Furga A et al: Molecular defects of type III procollagen in Ehlers-Danlos syndrome type IV, *Hum Genet* 82:104-108, 1988.

197. Superti-Furga A et al: Clinical variability of osteogenesis imperfecta linked to COL1A2 and associated with a structural defect in the type I collagen molecule, *J Med Genet* 26:358-362, 1989.

198. Sykes B: The molecular genetics of collagen, *BioEssays* 3:112-117, 1985.

199. Sykes B, Francis MJO, Smith R: Altered relation of two collagen types in osteogenesis imperfecta, *New Engl J Med* 296:1200-1203, 1977.

200. Sykes B et al: Osteogenesis imperfecta is linked to both type I collagen structural genes, *Lancet* 2:69-72, 1986.

201. Sykes B et al: Consistent segregation of dominantly inherited osteogenesis imperfecta to the type I collagen loci: COL1A1 and COL1A2, *Am J Hum Genet* 46:293-307, 1990.

202. Tenni R et al: Anomalous cysteine in type I collagen: localization by chemical cleavage of the protein using 2-nitro-5-thiocyanobenzoic acid by mismatch analysis of cDNA heteroduplex, *Matrix* 10:1026, 1990.

203. Thompson EM et al: Recurrence risk and prognosis in severe sporadic osteogenesis imperfecta, *J Med Genet* 24:390-405, 1987.

204. Tromp G, Prockop DJ: Single base mutation in the pro alpha 2 (I) collagen gene that causes efficient splicing of RNA from exon 27 to exon 29 and synthesis of a shortened but inframe pro alpha 2 (I) chain, *Proc Natl Acad Sci USA* 85:5254-5258, 1988.

205. Tsipouras P, Barabas G, Matthews WS: Neurologic correlates of osteogenesis imperfecta, *Arch Neurol* 43:150-152, 1986.

206. Tsipouras P et al: Restriction fragment length polymorphism associated with the pro alpha 2 (I) gene of human type I procollagen: application to a family with an autosomal dominant form of osteogenesis imperfecta, *J Clin Invest* 72:1262-1267, 1983.

207. Tsipouras P et al: Molecular heterogeneity in the mild autosomal dominant forms of osteogenesis imperfecta, *Am J Hum Genet* 36:1172-1179, 1984.

208. Tsipouras P et al: Prenatal detection of osteogenesis imperfecta (OI type IV): exclusion of inheritance using a collagen gene probe, *J Med Genet* 24:406-409, 1987.

209. Valli M et al: A de novo G to T transversion in a pro alpha 1 (I) collagen gene for a moderate case of osteogenesis imperfecta: substitution of cysteine for glycine 178 in the triple helical domain, *J Biol Chem* 266:1872-1878, 1991.

210. Van der Hoeve J, de Kleyn A: Blaue Sclerae, Knochenbruchigkeit und Schwerhorigkeit, *Arch Ophthalmol* 95:81, 1918.

211. van der Rest M et al: Lethal osteogenesis imperfecta with amniotic band lesions: collagen studies, *Am J Med Genet* 24:433-446, 1986.

212. Viljoen D, Beighton P: Osteogenesis imperfecta type III: an ancient mutation in Africa? *Am J Med Genet* 27:907-912, 1987.

213. Viljoen D, Versfeld G, Beighton P: Osteogenesis imperfecta with congenital joint contractures (Bruck syndrome), *Clin Genet* 36:122-126, 1989.

214. Vogel BE et al: A point mutation in a type I procollagen gene converts glycine 748 of the alpha 1 chain to cysteine and destabilizes the triple helix in a lethal variant of osteogenesis imperfecta, *J Biol Chem* 262:14737-14744, 1987.

215. Reference deleted in proofs.

216. Vrba M: Heredity and incidence of osteogenesis imperfecta tarda in the South Moravian region, *Cesk Pediatr* 21:509-512, 1968.

217. Vrolik W: *Tabulae ad illustrandam embryogenesim hominis et mammalium, tam naturalem quam abnormem,* Amstelodami, 1849.

218. Wallis GA et al: Mutations linked to the pro alpha 2 (I) collagen gene are responsible for several cases of osteogenesis imperfecta type I, *J Med Genet* 23:411-416, 1986.

219. Wallis GA et al: Variable expression of osteogenesis imperfecta in a nuclear family is explained by somatic mosaicism for a lethal point mutation in the alpha 1 (I) gene (COL1A1) of type I collagen in a parent, *Am J Hum Genet* 46:1034-1040, 1990.

220. Wallis GA et al: Substitution of arginine for glycine at position 847 in the triple-helical domain of the alpha 1 (I) chain of type I collagen produces lethal osteogenesis imperfecta, *J Biol Chem* 265:18628-18633, 1990.

221. Watts NB et al: Intermittent cyclical etidronate treatment of postmenopausal osteoporosis, *New Engl J Med* 323:73-79, 1990.

222. Wells C: Osteogenesis imperfecta from an Anglo-Saxon burial ground at Burgh Castle, *Suffolk Med Hist* 9:88, 1965.

223. Wenstrup RJ, Tsipouras P, Byers PH: Osteogenesis imperfecta type IV: Biochemical confirmation of genetic linkage to the pro alpha 2 (I) gene of type I collagen, *J Clin Invest* 78:1449-1455, 1986.

224. Wenstrup RJ et al: Arginine for glycine substitution in the triple helical domain of the products of one alpha 2 (I) collagen allele (COL1A2) produces the osteogenesis imperfecta type IV phenotype, *J Biol Chem* 263:1172-1179, 1988.

225. Wenstrup RJ et al: Distinct biochemical phenotypes predict clinical severity in nonlethal variants of osteogenesis imperfecta, *Am J Hum Genet* 46:975-982, 1990.

226. Wenstrup RJ et al: The effects of different cysteine for glycine substitutions within alpha 2 (I) chains: evidence of distinct structural domains within the type I collagen triple helix, *J Biol Chem* 266:2590-2594, 1990.

227. Wenstrup RJ et al: Osteogenesis imperfecta (OI) type IV: analysis in two families for mutations in alpha 2 chains of type I collagen by alpha 2–specific cDNA synthesis and amplification by polymerase chain reaction (PCR), *Ann N Y Acad Sci* 580:560-561, 1990.

228. Westerhausen A, Kishi J, Prockop DJ: Mutations that substitute serine for glycine alpha 1-598 and glycine alpha 1-631 in type I procollagen: the effects on unfolding of the triple helix are position-specific and demonstrate that the protein unfolds as cooperative blocks, *J Biol Chem* 265:13995-14000, 1990.

229. Whyte MP: Hypophosphatasia. In Scriver CR et al, editors: *The metabolic basis of inherited disease,* ed 6, New York, 1989, McGraw-Hill, pp 2843-2856.

230. Williams CJ, Prockop DJ: Synthesis and processing of a type I procollagen containing shortened pro alpha 1 (I) chains by fibroblasts from a patient with osteogenesis imperfecta, *J Biol Chem* 258:5915-5921, 1983.

231. Willing MC, Cohn DH, Byers PH: Frameshift mutation near the 3' end of the COL1A1 gene of type I collagen predicts an elongated pro alpha 1 (I) chain and results in osteogenesis imperfecta type I, *J Clin Invest* 85:282-290, 1990.

232. Willing MC et al: Heterozygosity for a large deletion in the alpha 2 (I) collagen gene has a dramatic effect on type I collagen secretion and produces perinatal lethal osteogenesis imperfecta, *J Biol Chem* 263:8398-8404, 1988.

233. Witkop CJ: Hereditary defects in enamel and dentin, *Acta Genet* 7:236, 1957.

234. Young ID, Harper PS: Recurrence risk in osteogenesis imperfecta congenita, *Lancet* 1:432, 1980.

235. Zerba L, Stucchi GF: Considerations on the cochleovestibular picture in Lobstein's disease, *Annali Laryngol Otol Rinol Faringol* 65:45-53, 1966.

CHAPTER 9

Alkaptonuria

Peter Beighton
Peter Berman
Štefan Sršen

Alkaptonuria is an autosomal recessive disorder in which defective activity of the enzyme homogentisic acid (HGA) oxidase leads to darkening of the urine and deposition of black pigment in collagenous tissues. Degenerative arthropathy predominates, but complications may also occur in the cardiovascular and renal systems.

Alkaptonuria was the first genetic metabolic disorder to be extensively elucidated, and it formed the basis of Archibald Garrod's one-gene–one-enzyme concept. To a large extent the clinical manifestations are the consequence of involvement of collagen in the ochronotic process; thus alkaptonuria is both a heritable disorder of connective tissue and an inborn error of metabolism.

HISTORICAL NOTE

Garrod[62] gave the following early history of alkaptonuria:

Until the early years of the nineteenth century no distinction was drawn in medical writings between urines which were black when passed and such as darkened on exposure to air, but it is difficult to suggest any other diagnosis than that of alkaptonuria for some cases referred to in works of the sixteenth and seventeenth centuries, such as that mentioned by G.A. Scribonius (in 1584) of a schoolboy who, although he enjoyed good health, continuously excreted black urine, and that cited by Schenck (in 1609) of a monk who exhibited a similar peculiarity and stated that he had done so all his life. The most interesting record of this kind is to be found in the work of Zacutus Lusitanus, published in 1649. The patient was a boy who passed black urine and who, at the age of fourteen years, was submitted to a drastic course of treatment which had for its aim the subduing of the fiery heat of his viscera which was supposed to bring about the condition in question by charring and blackening his bile. Among the measures prescribed were bleedings, purgation, baths, a cold and watery diet, and drugs galore. None of these had any obvious effect, and eventually the patient, who tired of the futile and superfluous therapy, resolved to let things take their natural course. None of the predicted evils ensued, he married, begat a large family, and lived a long and healthy life, always passing urine black as ink.*

In 1859 Boedeker[18] recognized that the reducing properties of the urine from a patient with alkaptonuria differed from those of urine containing glucose. Bismuth hydroxide, for example, was not reduced. Because of the avid uptake of oxygen in alkaline solutions, he gave the name alkaptonuria to the condition: ". . . in alkalischer Lösung bei gewöhnlicher Temperatur den Sauerstoff begierig zu verschlucken und nannte ihn danach Alcapton (freilich recht barbarisch zusammengesetzt aus dem arabischen *al kali* und dem griechischen καπτειν, begierig verschlucken)."† In 1861

---

*Knox called attention to this interesting historical note.

†From Boedeker C: *Z Rat Med* 7:130, 1859. Translation: ". . . in alkaline solution at ordinary temperature avidly to absorb the oxygen and named it accordingly alcapton (admittedly somewhat barbarously compounded from the Arabic *al kali* and the Greek καπτειν, to suck up greedily)."

Boedeker[19] spelled the name *alkaptonurie,* a practice that has been followed in the German literature. The French spell it *alcaptonurie,* and English writers use *c* and *k* interchangeably.

The morbid anatomy of ochronosis was described by Virchow[198] in 1866 on the basis of findings in a 67-year-old man. Although the gross coloration was gray to blue-black, an ochre color was observed on microscopic examination—hence Virchow's designation *ochronosis.* Not until the early part of this century was the connection between ochronosis and alkaptonuria recognized—by Albrecht[3] in 1902 and by Osler[139] in 1904. Boedeker's patient[18,19] had severe pain in the lumbar spine, "so severe that he lay mostly in bed and could take only a few steps." The development of severe arthritis in the course of alkaptonuria with ochronosis was emphasized by Gross and Allard[72] in 1907. The characteristic roentgenographic appearance of the spine in ochronosis was described by Söderbergh[168] in 1913.

The chemical structure of "alkapton" was established in 1891 by Wolkow and Baumann,[207] who identified it as 2, 5-dihydroxyphenylacetic acid and named it *homogentisic acid (HGA)* because of its close structural similarity to gentisic acid (2, 5-dihydroxybenzoic acid).

Alkaptonuria is par excellence Garrod's disease.[32,63,90] Archibald Garrod (Fig. 9-1) greatly extended knowledge of the nature of the disorder

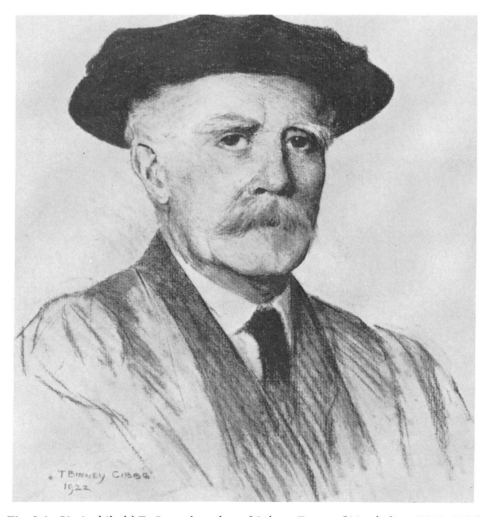

Fig. 9-1. Sir Archibald E. Garrod, author of *Inborn Errors of Metabolism* (1909, 1923) and successor to Osler as Regius Professor of Medicine at Oxford. (From a previously unpublished crayon drawing made in 1922. Reproduced here through the kindness of Sir Archibald's daughter, Miss Dorothy A.E. Garrod.)

and on the basis of these studies conceived the principle underlying most inborn errors of metabolism, the last being his terminology. As Beadle[12] pointed out in his Nobel prize acceptance lecture, the concept of one-gene—one-enzyme was essentially Garrod's. As Garrod[62] stated in 1908: "Of inborn errors of metabolism, alkaptonuria is that of which we know most, and from the study of which most has been learnt." In most research, which followed the lead of Wolkow and Baumann,[207] alkaptonuria had been viewed as a specific form of infection of the alimentary tract—a concept that was undoubtedly influenced by the thinking of the "bacteriology era" in which he worked—but Garrod[61] thought of alkaptonuria as an enzyme defect:

> We may further conceive that the splitting of the benzene ring in normal metabolism is the work of a special enzyme, [and] that in congenital alcaptonuria this enzyme is wanting. . . . The experiments of G. Embden and others upon perfusion of the liver suggest that organ as the most probable seat of the change.[61]

Garrod's contemporaries, such as Osler,[139] considered alkaptonuria to be a "freak" of metabolism comparable to morphologic freaks and to be of no pathologic importance. Indeed it is likely that many of Garrod's contemporaries viewed his work in alkaptonuria as a harmless but practically noncontributory pastime. There is the tone of the *apologia* in Garrod's writings on the value of studying rare diseases. Clearly Garrod was ahead of his time.

The juxtaposition of Garrod and Bateson and the rediscovery of Mendel's work were important factors in the development of the concept of inborn errors of metabolism. Bateson's *Mendel's Principles of Heredity* did much to acquaint the English-speaking world with "genetics," the term he applied to this field.[10] Because of the occurrence of affected sibs with normal parents and the high proportion of parents who are consanguineous, he suggested to Garrod that alkaptonuria is a recessively inherited disorder. In 1932 Hogben, Worrall, and Zieve[79] analyzed statistically the family data on alkaptonuria and supported the recessive hypothesis. There were, however, anomalous pedigrees in which alkaptonuria was transmitted through many successive generations, suggesting dominant inheritance, for example, that of Pieter,[144] reported from Santo Domingo. However, the interpretation that the inheritance was quasidominant because of marriage in successive generations of affected homozygous persons with heterozygous carriers in an inbred population was demonstrated by restudy in the Dominican Republic by Milch.[122]

The question as to whether HGA is a normal metabolite that, in alkaptonuria, accumulates in unusual concentration behind an enzyme block (the view of Garrod) or whether it is an abnormal compound formed by an abnormal series of reactions was resolved by 1928 in favor of the former view by Neubauer[133] and by others.

In 1958 La Du et al.[98] succeeded in demonstrating deficiency of homogentisic oxidase in liver, as predicted by Garrod. The importance of ochronotic connective tissue changes in the production of arthritis and cardiovascular pathology has become generally recognized only in more recent times, although some contemporaries of Garrod[77,196] emphasized this pathogenetic relationship. In 1963 O'Brien, La Du, and Bunim[136] reviewed the clinicopathologic manifestations in 604 reported cases. Thereafter, Gaines[55] presented an update of the pathologic features of alkaptonuric ochronosis based on six cases and 45 others culled from the literature.

Alkaptonuria occurs in high frequency in Slovakia, as evidenced by the large series of cases reported more than three decades ago.[30,164] Since 1968, the condition has been extensively investigated at the Research Laboratory for Clinical Genetics in the Medical Faculty of Komensky University, Martin, Czechoslovakia, and by 1990, 187 persons with alkaptonuria had been studied. Numerous publications about various aspects of alkaptonuria have emanated from this group of researchers,[135,172,174-186] including a comprehensive review[171] and a book in the Slovak language written by Štefan Sršen in 1984.[173] Alkaptonuria has been encountered in many other parts of the world, as well as in Czechoslovakia, and the total number of published cases now exceeds 1000. Current interest centers around identification of the chromosomal locus of the faulty gene and the development of methods for the identification of heterozygotes.

CLINICAL MANIFESTATIONS

The phenotypic features of alkaptonuria are blackness of urine, pigmentation of cartilaginous and collagenous structures (ochronosis), and degenerative joint and vascular changes.

The urine turns dark on sitting. Darkening is

hastened by alkalinization of the urine. Black diapers are sometimes the first clue to the presence of the disease. Washing with soap exaggerates the pigmentation of the diaper rather than removing it. Some patients never note black urine, the conditions for darkening apparently never being present. One patient first noted dark urine at age 93.[58] Garrod[61] observed that in the first hours after birth alkaptonuria may not be demonstrable, although it appears in the second day of life and continues without interruption thereafter. It is probable that immaturity of the enzyme systems involved in tyrosine oxidation accounts for the failure of expression from the very beginning. Acting as a reducing substance, HGA produces a positive reaction in some urinary tests for glycosuria, such as that using Benedict solution, but of course not in enzyme tests specific for glucose. The proper interpretation of an atypical test for reducing substance in the urine is the most frequent means of diagnosing alkaptonuria.

Pigmented prostatic calculi were described by Young[211] and by others and probably occur in all men with alkaptonuria who are more than 50 years of age. These calculi are usually calcified, as well, and evident by radiographic study. Enlargement of the stone-filled prostate may require prostatectomy.[17,81,92] Savastano, Quigley, and Scala[155] described palpable prostatic calculi. Death as a result of prostatic obstruction in patients with uremia has been observed.[11,140] Apparently the alkalinity of the prostatic secretions promotes polymerization of HGA, and this pigment then affords a nidus for stone formation. Urinary calculi are also black in this disorder.[191]

Renal stones are a feature of ochronosis.* Pigment may be deposited in the renal parenchyma, and nephrocalcinosis has been reported.[67] Ochronotic nephropathy with ochronotic pigment casts is thought to occur[29] but cannot be considered fully documented. Patients with alkaptonuria who have renal failure as a result of an unrelated renal abnormality show greatly aggravated ochronosis.[6]

Ochronotic pigmentation of blue-black hue is most evident in the sclera and in ear cartilages, but pigmentation of many cartilaginous and collagenous structures is found during surgical operation or autopsy, for example, costal cartilages and heart valves. As a rule, pigmentation does not become evident until the twenties or thirties. The scleral pig-

*References 48, 76, 78, 92, 104, 114, 117, and 140.

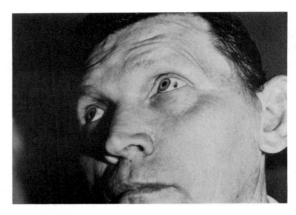

Fig. 9-2. The eye in alkaptonuria. A patch of ochronotic pigmentation is evident in the sclerae. (From Sršen Š: *Alkaptonuria*, Martin, Czechoslovakia, 1984, Osveta.)

mentation is usually concentrated about midway between the corneal limbus and the inner and outer canthi at the sites of insertion of the rectus muscles (Fig. 9-2). Pigmentation of the cornea concentrated peripherally at the three- and nine-o'clock positions has been observed,[167,204] as well as pigmentation of the tarsal plates and eyelids. In one case[165] the pigmentation was mistaken for melanosarcoma and the eye was removed.

Pigmentation of the nasal cartilages is sometimes evident at the tip of the nose. Pigmentation of the pinnae is best demonstrated by transillumination. The ear becomes stiff, also, so that it cannot be folded with the normal ease. Calcification and even ossification are radiographically demonstrable.[131,205] Other conditions accompanied by calcification of the ear cartilages include Addison's disease, diabetes mellitus, cold hypersensitivity,[111] and diastrophic dysplasia.[112] The cerumen is jet black, and the eardrum often shows steel blue pigmentation. Pigmentation of tendons in the hand may be evident through the skin, and a bluish gray discoloration of the fingernails[52] and the teeth has been described.[161]

The pigment is excreted in the sweat. Clothing in contact with the axilla may be stained, and the skin of the axillary and inguinal area, as well as the malar area of the face, may show brownish coloration. Hoke, Maibach, and Epstein[80] showed that apocrine sweat stimulated by intradermal injection of epinephrine is bluish black (Fig. 9-3), whereas eccrine sweat stimulated by intradermal

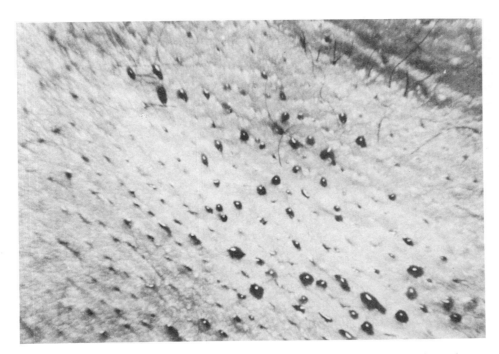

Fig. 9-3. Pigmentation of apocrine sweat in patient with ochronosis. Enlarged view of axilla, photographed 1 minute after stimulation with intradermal injection of epinephrine. Darkly pigmented sweat around hair follicles is evident. Clear eccrine sweat between hair follicles is less clearly demonstrated. Punch biopsy of skin in axillary area showed pigment outlining secretory tubules. (Courtesy Dr. Axel W. Hoke, San Francisco.)

injection of acetylcholine is clear. They also demonstrated, by means of punch biopsy of the axillary area, pigment outlining apocrine coils and ducts.

Ochronotic arthropathy was succinctly and graphically described by O'Brien, La Du, and Bunim[136] in the following manner:

> The anatomic distribution and sequence of spinal and peripheral joint involvement in ochronosis are characteristic. The course is chronic and progressive, beginning early in the fourth decade with back pain and stiffness. During the ensuing ten years the knees become involved and later the shoulders and hips are affected. The patient becomes increasingly crippled and by sixty years of age may be totally disabled.

Two acute manifestations may develop during the chronic course: herniation of the intervertebral disks and synovial effusion after negligible trauma. Acute rupture of a nucleus pulposus may be the first manifestation of ochronotic spondylosis. It occurs principally in men in early adult life. Articular structures in ochronosis seem to be vulnerable; pain and effusion may follow minor injuries. The friable articular cartilages are readily fragmented and embedded in the synovial lining with consequent effusion and pain.

In men joint involvement occurs more frequently, develops at an earlier age, and is of greater severity than in women. Ruptured disks are especially more common in men.

Low-back pain, limitation of motion in the lumbar spine, and symptoms of root pressure that result from an extruded intervertebral disk[44,45,109] are matched by the radiographic finding of narrowing of the intervertebral space and collapse and calcification of the intervertebral disks of the lumbar spine (Fig. 9-4). The calcified disks present a spindle shape on lateral projection. Mueller et al.[131] and others[37,89] described a vacuum phenomenon. Joint spaces can be demonstrated by gas if traction is applied to produce a partial intraarticular vacuum, for example, in the shoulder joints of children when the arms are raised above the head for chest radiographic studies or in the symphysis pubis in pregnant women at term. Intraarticular

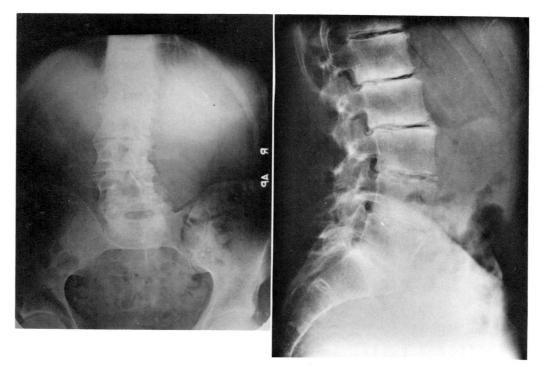

Fig. 9-4. Characteristic spinal changes of ochronotic arthropathy in a 34-year-old man.

vacuum is a consistent finding in the ochronotic spine, being located, on lateral projection, anterior to the calcified disk. Some degree of fusion of the vertebral bodies occurs. Unlike rheumatoid spondylitis, alkaptonuria is accompanied by little calcification of spinal ligaments. The radiographic findings are sufficiently typical that studies of Egyptian mummies[162,202] have led to the conclusion that certain of them are the bodies of persons with alkaptonuria.

Large joints such as the hips and knees usually show degenerative changes on radiographic examination, with calcium deposits around the joint or present as loose bodies in the joint.[27,138,156,192] Frequently ochronotic arthritis is of such severity as to keep the patient bedridden for many years. Severe pain over the symphysis pubis occurs frequently.[76,110,126,192] On radiographic examination, the pubic synchondrosis in such cases may present irregular sclerosis, narrowing, and destructive changes.[145] The shoulder joint sometimes shows degenerative changes of severity rarely seen in non–weight-bearing joints except in syringomyelia and in this disorder. Suppurative arthritis was superimposed on ochronotic arthritis in one case.[29] Rupture of the Achilles tendon has been reported in several instances,[2,41,105] and the cartilagenous menisci of the knee joint may also be involved.[118] It has been suggested that the human lymphocyte antigen (HLA) B27 might be an aggravating factor in the development of ochronotic rheumatism in persons with alkaptonuria.[64,147]

Degenerative arthropathy in the hip joint is not usually troublesome until middle age; however, if warranted by the severity of the symptoms, prosthetic joint replacement gives satisfactory results.[35] In severe ochronotic arthopathy, involvement of the craniovertebral joints may lead to cervicomedullary compression.[158] The joints in persons with alkaptonuric arthropathy have been studied in some detail by conventional radiography.*

A review of case reports of alkaptonuria indicates a high frequency of cardiovascular abnormality.[166] Generalized arteriosclerosis[34,58] and abnormalities of the heart valves, in particular, calcific aortic stenosis,[39,56,199] are frequent. Aortic

*References 86, 99, 140, 145, 162, 187, and 214.

Table 9-1. Cardinal clinical manifestations of alkaptonuria in relation to age

Cardinal features	Age (in years)								
	1	1-5	5-10	10-15	15-20	20-30	30-40	40-50	50
Dark urine	+++	+++	+++	+++	+++	+++	+++	+++	+++
Dark ear cerumen	+++	+++	+++	+++	+++	+++	+++	+++	+++
Skin pigmentation in the axilla	—	—	±	+	++	+++	+++	+++	+++
Auricle changes	—	—	—	±	±	+	++	+++	+++
Scleral pigmentation	—	—	—	±	±	+	++	+++	+++
Ochronotic arthropathy	—	—	—	—	—	±	+	++	+++

From Sršen S, Srsnova K, Lanyi A: *Bratisl Lek Listy* 77(6):662-669, 1982.
The frequency and intensity of the manifestations is expressed by the number of crosses.

valve replacement is an appropriate therapeutic option.[39,56,102,199] Myocardial infarction is said to be a common cause of death,[200] although no firm incidence statistics are available.

The ear ossicles and the tympanic membrane may be affected by the ochronotic process,[143] and hearing may be impaired.[136] Long-standing, severe hoarseness,[69] fixed vocal cords, and pigmentation of the larynx observed by direct laryngoscopy[83] have also been documented.

Alkaptonuria has been encountered in association with the Klinefelter syndrome,[23,169] in successive generations with the tetralogy of Fallot,[73] and in a patient with Parkinson disease[153]; it seems probable that these are chance concurrences. The development of diabetes mellitus[40] in association with alkaptonuria may be the consequence of the pancreatic involvement in the ochronotic process, although this is apparently a rare complication.

The natural history of alkaptonuria is lifelong, slow progression, with the onset of clinically significant complications in adulthood. Alkaptonuria can be diagnosed in the neonatal period by the recognition of the characteristic discoloration of diapers and linen and by means of simple biochemical tests of the urine.[182] Darkening of the urine and ear cerumen[170] is a consistent feature from early childhood onward, and pigmentation in the axillary regions appears at the end of the first decade.[177-179] Orthopedic problems usually appear in early adulthood, with disk rupture and vertebral arthrosis preceding arthopathy of the large joints.[30,136,180] Arteriosclerosis and aortic stenosis have a propensity to develop in middle age, as have prostatic and renal calculi.[48,74,140,211] The age relationship of the major manifestations of alkaptonuria in the series of Czechoslovakian patients is shown in Table 9-1.[181]

In view of the potential complications in cases of alkaptonuria, the question of decreased life expectancy has been the subject of considerable debate. This issue was resolved when Sršen et al.[186] investigated life span in 90 Czechoslovakian families comprising 132 affected persons and their 208 unaffected sibs.[186] There were no significant differences in longevity in these two groups; therefore it seems probable that the significant morbidity in cases of alkaptonuria is not paralleled by increased mortality.

DIAGNOSIS

The demonstration of HGA in urine establishes the diagnosis of alkaptonuria. Adults with alkaptonuria usually excrete 4 to 8 g of HGA daily.[82,96,203] HGA is the only detectable abnormal urinary metabolite.

The reducing properties of HGA form the basis of a number of screening tests, including the reduction of molybdate,[24] silver,[82,201] or cupric[82] ions. Although these tests are relatively nonspecific, the error introduced by other substances with reducing properties similar to HGA is negligible at the high levels of HGA encountered in alkaptonuric urine.[160] HGA produces a false-positive result in the Benedict test for glucose, since HGA reduces the cupric ions to yield a yellow-orange precipitate and is itself darkened by the alkalinity of the reagent. The net result is an orange precipitate in a muddy-brown solution.[82,96] Treatment for diabetes has been administered erroneously to patients.[110] Paradoxically HGA interferes with the specific glucose oxidase test for glucose by reducing the hydrogen peroxide (H_2O_2) formed, thereby preventing its reaction with the peroxidase and dye system. Thus a false-negative result for glucose is obtained.[115] Interference by HGA in the biochemical investigation of urine is reviewed by Koska.[93]

Other commonly employed screening tests for alkaptonuria include the transient blue-green color produced by the addition of ferric chloride[82,201] and the prompt darkening of urine on addition of alkali. A simple screening test was devised by Sršen,[171] in which filter paper strips presoaked in 10% sodium hydroxide are dipped into urine. Immediate darkening of the strip confirms the presence of HGA (Fig. 9-5). Darkening of urine not caused by HGA is seen in patients receiving levodopa, for treatment of Parkinson disease,[22] quinacrine for treatment of rheumatoid arthritis,[96] and carbolic acid dressings for treatment of skin ulcers.[96] Gentisic acid, a minor urinary metabolite of salicylate, can give a false-positive result in the previously mentioned screening tests for HGA.[53] The diagnosis of alkaptonuria should be considered in the case of a patient with arthritis who is receiving salicylate therapy and who has dark urine. Of all the screening tests the most reliable appears to be ammoniacal silver nitrate, which forms an immediate black precipitate with urine containing HGA.[53]

If the results of one or more qualitative tests prove positive, the presence of HGA can be confirmed by paper chromatography,[53] thin layer chromatography,[46,82] gas liquid chromatography[20] or high-pressure liquid chromatography,[22,85] or nuclear magnetic resonance spectroscopy[210] or by specific enzyme assays utilizing HGA oxidase.[160] Detection of heterozygotes by oral tyrosine or HGA loading tests is not possible because large reserves of HGA oxidase activity are present in liver.[82,96] HGA is rapidly cleared by the kidney, which accounts for the invariably low plasma levels of HGA encountered in patients with alkaptonuria, even after phenylalanine loading.[134]

HGA oxidase is a cytosolic enzyme with the highest activity in liver tissue and less in kidney tissue.[97] It is not detectable in any other tissue; hence confirmation of HGA oxidase deficiency requires liver or kidney biopsy. Since the enzyme is not expressed in fibroblasts or amnion cells, prenatal diagnosis is not feasible. Enzyme assays are based on oxygen consumption or production of maleylacetoacetate in tissue homogenates incu-

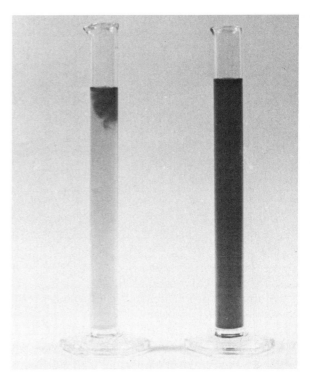

Fig. 9-5. Alkaptonuric urine. A brown ring has formed after the addition of a few drops of 10% solution of sodium hydroxide, *left*. The pigmentation gradually diffuses throughout the specimen, *right*. (From Sršen Š: *Alkaptonuria,* Martin, Czechoslovakia, 1984, Osveta.)

bated with HGA. Maleylacetoacetate can be conveniently monitored spectrophotometrically at 330 nm.[96,160]

PATHOLOGY

Deficient activity of the enzyme HGA oxidase leads to elevation of levels of HGA, and oxidation of this substance causes black pigmentation of urine and sweat. A polymerized form of HGA binds to connective tissues throughout the body, producing the coal black ochronotic pigmentary changes. Ochronotic pigmentation is present in connective tissues, notably, in articular cartilage, tendons, ligaments, joint capsules, sclerae, larynx, bronchial tract, tympanic membranes,[27] and cardiac valves. It is also seen in areas of fibrosis such as healed myocardial and cerebral infarcts.[104] In addition, there is a strong propensity for pigmentary accumulations in atheromatous plaques in the intima of blood vessels. The autopsy findings and histopathologic changes in cases of alkaptonuria were comprehensively reviewed by

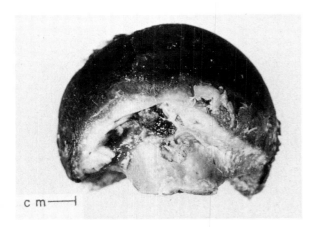

Fig. 9-6. Femoral head from a 62-year-old woman with advanced ochronotic arthropathy. The articular cartilage is darkly pigmented. (From Gaines JJ: *Hum Pathol* 20[1]:40-46, 1989.)

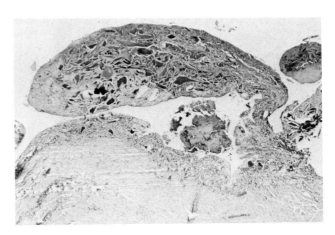

Fig. 9-7. A synovial polyp filled with innumerable shards of ochronotic cartilage (hematoxylin-eosin stain; magnification × 10). (From Gaines JJ: *Hum Pathol* 20[1]:40-46, 1989.)

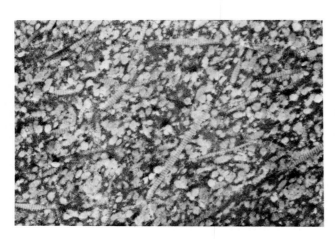

Fig. 9-8. Collagen fibrils in a shard of cartilage surrounded by ochronotic pigment (magnification × 35,100). (From Gaines JJ, Tom GD, Khankhanian N: *Hum Pathol* 18[11]: 1160-1164, 1987.)

O'Brien, La Du, and Bunim[136] in 1963 and by Gaines[55] in 1989.

In the joints the articular cartilage is darkly pigmented,[124] (Fig. 9-6), whereas the tendons,[106] ligaments, and joint capsules[65] are affected to a much lesser extent. The ochronotic articular cartilage is brittle, and there is a tendency to fragmentation and the formation of spicules or shards[54,55,57] (Fig. 9-7). These bodies provoke synovitis and synovial hypertrophy. The ochronotic manifestations in the skeleton are age related and maximal in the large joints. In the late stages the articular cartilage is deeply eroded, and the resultant degenerative arthropathy may cause serious physical handicap. Histologic and electron microscopic investigations reveal ochronotic pigment surrounding collagen fibrils and within chondrocytes[57,94,128] (Fig. 9-8).

In the spine the main effects are in the intervertebral disks, where pigmentation is marked (Fig. 9-9). Degeneration of the disks causes predisposition to spontaneous rupture of the nucleus pulposus, which often occurs in early adulthood. In the later stages the vertebral bodies may ankylose, and extensive osteophytosis frequently develops.

It has long been recognized that ochronosis of the aortic and mitral valves[13,104] (Fig. 9-10) and generalized arteriosclerosis[58] represent the major autopsy findings in the cardiovascular system. Involvement of the aortic valve may lead to calcification and stenosis in late middle age.[56] The endo-

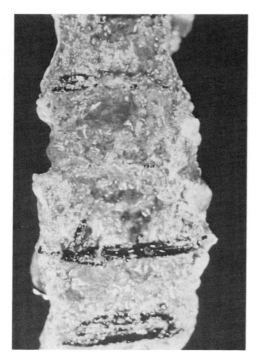

Fig. 9-9. Pathologic changes in the lumbar spine. The intervertebral disks are dystrophic, darkly pigmented, and calcified. (From Sršen Š: *Johns Hop Med J* 145:217-226, 1979.)

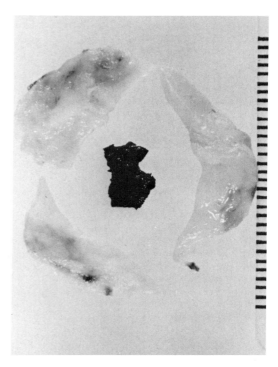

Fig. 9-10. Aortic valve leaflets and a portion of annulus fibrosis, *center*, with deposits of ochronotic pigment. (From Gaines JJ: *Hum Pathol* 20[1]:40-46, 1989.)

cardium is deeply pigmented, and healed myocardial infarcts are also affected.[70,104,148,150] In the arteries pigmentation is maximal in the intima (Fig. 9-11), and atherosclerotic plaques are heavily stained. No obvious affinity for elastin fibers exists, and the mechanical properties of the arterial walls are not compromised.[56] Indeed, although arterial ochronosis may be extensive, it does not seem to predispose to aneurysm formation or cerebrovascular accidents.

In the kidney, pigmentation may be present in the pyramids, Bowman's capsule, and atheromatous arterial plaques. On microscopic examination granules of pigment can be demonstrated in the tubular epithelial cells, whereas ochronotic casts are seen in the tubules. In a high proportion of affected persons, soft black renal calculi develop,[91,193] which may cause urinary tract obstruction and secondary infection. The prostate gland is usually ochronotic, and it is often packed with pigmented calculi. Enlargement of the prostate can lead to obstruction or can mimic carcinoma.[194]

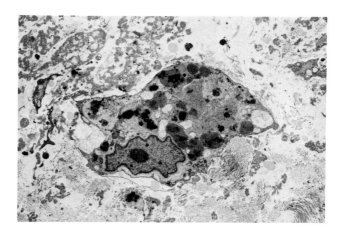

Fig. 9-11. Macrophage from intima of aorta containing membrane-bound ochronotic pigment granules (uranyl acetate-lead citrate, original magnification × 4000). (From Gaines JJ, Pac GM: *Arch Pathol Lab Med* 111:991-994, 1987.)

The eye is frequently involved in the ochronotic process, and patches of dark pigment are present in the sclerae and in the tendons of the extrinsic ocular muscles.[151] Slit lamp examination reveals pigmentation in the cornea and conjunctiva,[59] and at the microscopic level pigmentary granules are evident in association with disorganized collagen bundles[5,8,36] in the affected areas. The retina is spared and, despite the widespread involvement of the other components of the eye, vision is not disturbed.

BASIC DEFECT AND PATHOGENESIS

Patients with alkaptonuria have an absolute deficiency of HGA oxidase.[98] It is not known whether enzyme protein is present but lacks normal activity or whether no protein whatever is produced. Since no alternative pathway of HGA degradation exists, this compound is excreted in the urine. HGA is an intermediate metabolite in phenylalanine and tyrosine catabolism (Fig. 9-12), so excretion of HGA reflects the rate of catabolism of these two amino acids. HGA output in persons with alkaptonuria varies with the phenylalanine and tyrosine content of the diet[206] and decreases markedly during starvation.[96]

The reaction catalyzed by HGA oxidase involves cleavage of the benzene ring of HGA, with the addition of both atoms of molecular oxygen. The enzyme contains essential sulphydryl groups and nonheme iron, which must be maintained in the ferrous state (Fe^{2+}) by intracellular reductants.[96] No known organic cofactor requirement exists. Ascorbate is required only insofar as it keeps the iron atom in the reduced (Fe^{2+}) state. Experimental alkaptonuria is induced in animals by α,α'-dipyridyl, which chelates the essential iron atom, and concomitant administration of tyrosine.[96] In common with the other enzymes of tyrosine catabolism, HGA oxidase is confined to the cytosol. HGA is rapidly excreted by the kidneys, both by glomerular filtration and by tubular secretion, so the HGA clearance of 400 to 500 ml/min approximates total renal plasma flow.[134] The high renal clearance is unusual for an endogenously produced compound. The efficient renal elimination of HGA explains how low plasma levels of HGA (less than 0.04 mmol), are maintained in the face of high urine HGA output (25 to 50 mmol/day) in alkaptonuria[22] and represents an important defense against HGA retention and development of ochronosis.[96,134]

The biochemical mechanism of ochronosis is poorly understood. It is believed that ochronosis is not due to HGA per se but rather to its oxidation product, benzquinone acetic acid (BQAA), which binds either directly or after polymerization to biologic components, including collagen[213] (Fig. 9-13). BQAA forms nonenzymatically in urine exposed to oxygen at an alkaline pH. In the relatively anoxic and neutral pH environment of connective tissue, BQAA formation is believed to proceed enzymatically by the action of HGA polyphenol oxidase, a copper-containing enzyme present in skin and cartilage.[125,213] BQAA can polymerize and can form addition products with sulphydryl[97] and amino[190] residues of connective tissue proteins, particularly collagen, which affects their mechanical properties and metabolic turnover.[43] Polymers formed by oxidation of HGA have been shown to inhibit enzymes present in joint tissue, including hyaluronidase[71] and lysyl hydroxylase.[132] Ascorbic acid inhibits oxidation of HGA to BQAA and has been shown to prevent the urine darkening characteristic of alkaptonuria.[201,206] Although ascorbic acid decreased the binding of isotopically labeled (^{14}C) HGA to connective tissue of rats with experimental alkaptonuria,[108] the therapeutic use of ascorbic acid in established ochronosis has been disappointing.[50]

Recent evidence suggests that oxygen radicals generated by HGA autoxidation may be implicated in the pathogenesis of ochronosis.[66,116] Superoxide radicals ($O_2^-\cdot$) arising from autoxidation may spontaneously or enzymatically dismute to form H_2O_2, which in the presence of ferric ions (Fe^{3+}) generates hydroxyl radicals ($\cdot OH$). These highly reactive oxidizing agents are capable of depolymerizing hyaluronic acid, the major component of synovial fluid. Depolymerization of hyaluronic acid, caused by HGA and ferric ions, can be prevented by catalase and dimethylsulphoxide, which scavenge H_2O_2 and hydroxyl radicals, respectively.[116]

The chromosomal location of the gene that codes for HGA oxidase and the nature of the mutation giving rise to alkaptonuria are unknown. Alkaptonuria has been observed in association with Gilbert syndrome,[26] with sucrase-isomaltase deficiency,[60] and with neonatal severe primary hyperparathyroidism (NSPHP)[188] in offspring of consanguineous marriages. It could be speculated that the genes coding for HGA oxidase, sucrase isomaltase, and the protein deficient in

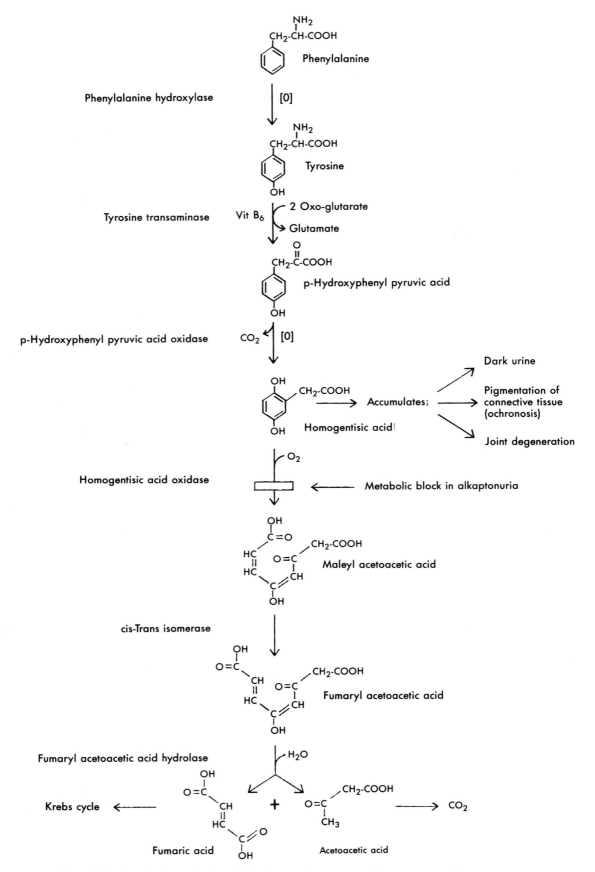

Fig. 9-12. Catabolism of phenylalanine and tyrosine. The position of homogentisic acid on the main catabolic pathway is shown. Enzymes are indicated to the left of the reactions they catalyze; *[0]* indicates oxidation step.

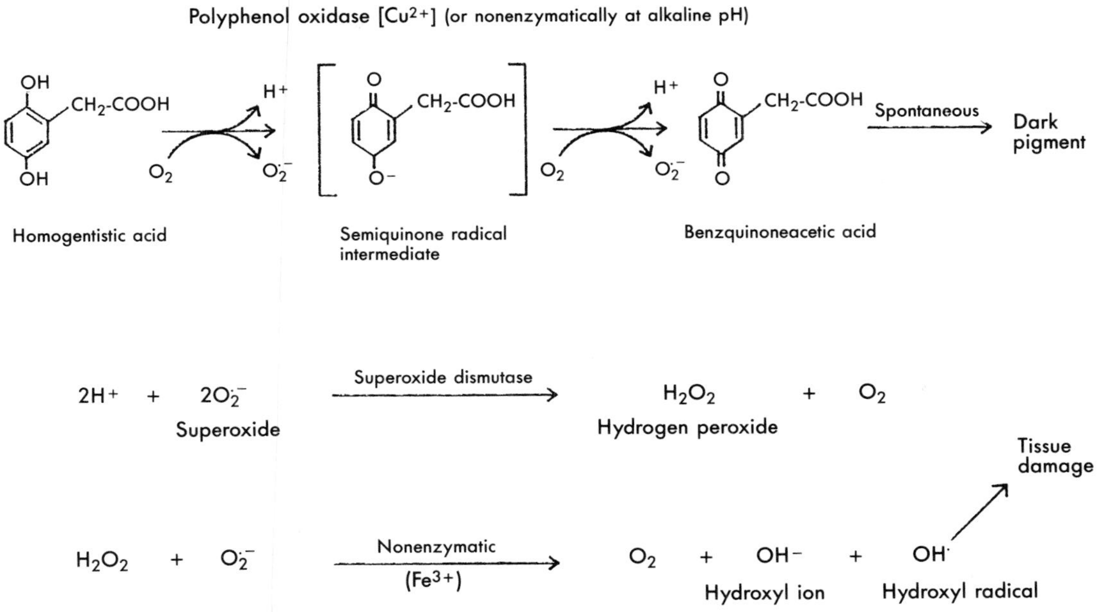

Polyphenol oxidase [Cu^{2+}] (or nonenzymatically at alkaline pH)

Fig. 9-13. Oxidation of homogentisic acid to benzquinone acetic acid, *top*, and generation of reactive oxygen species, *bottom*.

NSPHP are closely linked on the same chromosome.

INHERITANCE AND PREVALENCE

Autosomal recessive inheritance of alkaptonuria was demonstrated by the work of Hogben, Worrall, and Zieve,[79] who used alkaptonuria to test the so-called Lenz-Hogben, or *a priori*, method of segregation analysis. The usual unaffected state of parents of affected sibships likewise supports the hypothesis of recessive inheritance, as does the high frequency of parental consanguinity.[129]

Alkaptonuria is comparatively common in the Dominican Republic[122] and in Slovakia.[30,135,164,172] In areas such as these, where there are high rates of inbreeding and a significant population frequency of the defective gene, transmission of alkaptonuria through several generations can create a pedigree pattern simulating dominance[89,121] (Figs. 9-14 and 9-15). This quasidominance is clearly the result of a high frequency of marriage between homozygous affected persons and heterozygous carriers. No evidence for the existence of a dominant form of alkaptonuria (or more than one basically distinct recessive form) has been discovered.

In a Czechoslovakian program of population screening by urinalysis, 611,000 persons were examined and 187 affected individuals were identified. Routine screening of newborns revealed an incidence of 1 in 19,000 neonates. An incidence figure of 1 in 44,800 was obtained by neonatal screening in Wales[75]; therefore it seems likely that the causative allele is present in significant frequency throughout Europe. In certain areas of Czechoslovakia,[184] such as the Trencin district[183] and the Upper Hron region,[175] there is a tenfold increase in the gene frequency.[175,183,184] This situation is probably the consequence of the founder effect, geographic isolation, and endogamy.[172,176,184,185] As a result of the breakdown of population isolation that has taken place in Czechoslovakia since World War II, it is likely that the incidence of alkaptonuria and other autosomal recessive disorders in this region will fall.

Alkaptonuria has wide ethnic and geographic distribution; in addition to its high frequency in Dominica and Czechoslovakia it has been documented on many occasions in the United States and western Europe. It has also been described in Japanese,[2,119,195] Asian Indians,* and American blacks,[1] and in a gypsy,[29] and it has been encoun-

---

*References 31, 113, 120, 142, 149, 154, 163, and 197.

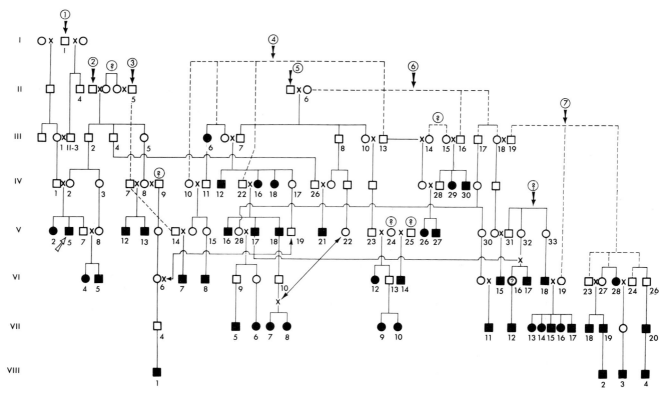

Fig. 9-14. Pedigree of inbred group in Dominican Republic with many cases of alkaptonuria, some in successive generations. The circled numbers indicate separate branches of this extensive family. (From Milch RA: *Am J Hum Genet* 12:76-85, 1960.)

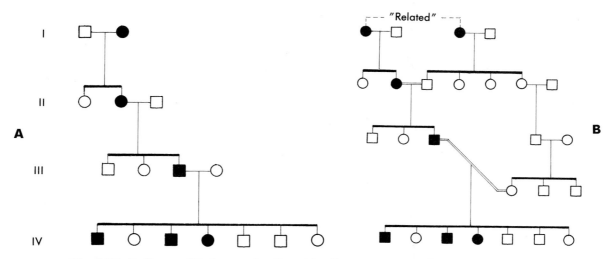

Fig. 9-15. Pedigree of Lebanese family with alkaptonuria. **A,** The pedigree suggests autosomal dominant inheritance. **B,** Consanguinity is indicated by the more complete pedigree. Spouses of the affected persons in the first, second, and third generations are presumably heterozygotes. (Based on data from Khachadurian A, Abu Feisal KA: *J Chronic Dis* 7:455, 1958.)

tered in Filipinos,[137] Lebanese,[89] and Bedouins[127] and in persons in Central Africa,[9] Mexico,[4] Spain,[51,68] Ethiopia,[101] Chile,[150] Taiwan,[201] and Italy.[38] It is evident that the alkaptonuria gene is an ancient mutation, since typical ochronotic spondylosis has been observed in Egyptian mummies.[162,202] (Biochemical confirmation that the ochronotic pigment was indeed HGA was subsequently obtained.[100,189])

In the study of Hogben, Worrall, and Zieve[79] it was noted that the reported cases included 100 males and 46 females. Since the proband was much more often a man, they concluded that the more frequent urine examination of men in connection with insurance, military service, and employment accounted for the distorted sex ratio. The explanation was supported by the finding that among infants, slightly more girls than boys were detected. A higher frequency of arthritis in men with alkaptonuria may contribute to the higher number of ascertained cases in men.

In the review of reported cases by O'Brien, La Du, and Bunim[136] 60% of 520 patients were male.

The recognition of heterozygotes would be important in genetic counseling, but no objective methods are available. Oral loading tests with HGA or tyrosine show no difference between the relatives of persons with alkaptonuria and normal controls.[95,136,152]

The chromosomal locus of the faulty gene is unknown. Investigations of possible linkage between alkaptonuria and the amylase locus[174] and other polymorphic systems[87] have yielded negative results.

OTHER CONSIDERATIONS

Treatment with vitamins, brewer's yeast, tyrosinase, insulin, adrenocortical extract,[58] vitamin B$_{12}$,[49] and cortisone[15,212] has no effect on alkaptonuria. Thiouracil[30,42] was reported to relieve clinical symptoms but had no influence on the amount of HGA excreted in the urine.[207]

As long ago as 1940 it was suggested that therapy with ascorbic acid might be beneficial in patients with alkaptonuria.[157] This viewpoint received support in 1970, when Lustberg, Schulman, and Seegmiller[108] demonstrated that ascorbic acid in high doses decreased the binding of radioisotopically labelled HGA in connective tissues of rats with experimental alkaptonuria. In a clinical trial involving two affected siblings, ascorbic acid in a dose of 500 mg twice daily was administered

for 12 months; alkaptonuria in one of the siblings improved, whereas in the other the condition worsened, and it was concluded that ascorbic acid was not efficacious.[51] In a further study involving two adults and three infants with alkaptonuria,[206] it was shown that the putative toxic metabolite of HGA, BQAA, disappeared from the urine after the administration of large doses of ascorbic acid. It is not known whether these biochemical changes would be followed by clinical improvement, and the role of ascorbic acid in the treatment of alkaptonuria remains controversial.

Dietary manipulation is a possible approach to the management of alkaptonuria, since a diet quite low in phenylalanine and tyrosine results in the increase of urinary HGA.[207] It is uncertain, however, whether any clinical benefit would result, and it is also unlikely that an affected person would accept long-term compliance with a restrictive diet of this type. In the future it might be possible to cure alkaptonuria by replacing the defective enzyme, but this approach is not yet feasible.

Presumed spontaneous alkaptonuria in a rabbit[103] and an orangutan,[88] together with ochronosis in cattle, dogs, and horses[117,146] may be homologous to the disease in man. Conversely, it has been demonstrated that a generalized pigmentation of connective tissues in the silky bantam fowl is not due to alkaptonuria.[98]

Alkaptonuria can be produced in animals such as the rat by giving a diet enriched with phenylalanine[141] or tyrosine,[16,21] and alkaptonuria has also been observed in rats with experimental tryptophan deficiency.[208] Furthermore, clinical arthritis and typical joint changes of ochronosis follow the injection of HGA into the joints of rabbits.[130]

An excellent example of a phenocopy (a nongenetically produced phenotype resembling a gene-determined one) is provided by the ochronosis that develops after the prolonged use of carbolic acid dressings for treatment of chronic cutaneous ulcers.[13,14,25,47,77] After prolonged administration, quinacrine[107] also causes an ochronotic change with pigmentation in many of the same sites as in alkaptonuria and probably with a comparable arthrosis.

In the differential diagnosis of alkaptonuria the several causes of black diapers must be considered.[33] Drummond et al.[42] described the "blue diaper syndrome" in two brothers. Hypercalcemia and nephrocalcinosis were features. A defect in intestinal transport of tryptophan led to excessive indole production by intestinal bacteria. Conversion of indican to indigo blue appeared to account for the staining of the diapers. The urine of patients receiving methyldopa (Aldomet) for treatment of hypertension becomes dark red and almost black when mixed with hypochlorite solution used in a proprietary lavatory cleanser.[28] The urine of patients receiving a mixture of the D and L isomers of dihydroxyphenylalanine (D- and L-dopa) for treatment of parkinsonism turns black, whereas the urine of patients receiving pure L-dopa remains unchanged.[7] The excretion of HGA when D-dopa is administered is probably the result of inefficiency of HGA oxidase in handling the D-isomer. Melanuria sometimes accompanies melanomas.[84]

Also to be considered in the differential diagnosis of alkaptonuria is apocrine chromhidrosis.[159] In this disorder colored sweat is secreted by the apocrine glands. The pigment is a lipofuscin. Axillary chromhidrosis is not seen until after puberty, when apocrine secretory activity is activated; it occurs much more frequently among blacks than among whites. The appearance is the same as that in a patient with alkaptonuria.

SUMMARY

Alkaptonuria is an inborn error of metabolism inherited as an autosomal recessive disorder in which important connective tissue changes occur. The clinical manifestations are dark urine, urinary and prostatic calculi, pigmentation of connective tissues (especially cartilage), progressive arthropathy of characteristic type, and cardiovascular lesions, including valvular sclerosis and accelerated arteriosclerosis. The biochemical defect is a deficiency of HGA oxidase, an enzyme normally present in liver and kidney tissue.

REFERENCES

1. Abbott LD Jr, Mandeville FB, Rein WJ: Complete roentgen and ophthalmologic examination for ochronosis in two alcaptonuric children, *Virginia Med Monthly* 70:615-617, 1943.
2. Abe Y et al: Thirteen cases of alkaptonuria from one family tree with special reference to osteo-arthrosis alkaptonuria, *J Bone Joint Surg* 42(A):817-831, 1960.
3. Albrecht H: Ueber Ochronose, *Z Heilk* 23:366-378, 1902.
4. Alcala O, Alarcon-Corredor OM, Sanchez de Molina D: Alkaptonuria: presentation of a case in a 2-year-old child, *Bol Med Hosp Infant Mex* 43(1):61-65, 1986.
5. Allen RA, O'Malley C, Straatsma BR: Ocular findings in hereditary ochronosis, *Arch Ophthalmol* 65:657-668, 1961.
6. Arcangeli A, Colloridi V, Chiarini M: Una eccezionale associazione morbosa congenita: rene policistico ed alcaptonuria con ochronose, *Arch Ital Pediatr* 20:66-80, 1959.
7. Arras M: Metabolism of D- vs L-DOPA, *New Engl J Med* 282:813 only, 1970.
8. Ashton N, Kirker JG, Lavery FS: Ocular findings in a case of hereditary ochronosis, *Br J Ophthalmol* 48:405-415, 1964.
9. Baldachin BJ, Rothman WT: Alkaptonuric arthritis: report of a case in a Bantu, *Cent Afr J Med* 5:287-290, 1959.
10. Bateson W: *Mendel's principles of heredity*, London, 1902, Cambridge University.
11. Bauer O: Ueber Steinbildungen in den Harnwegen bei Ochronose (Lithiasis ochronotica), *Mitt Grenzgeb Med Chir* 41:451-462, 1929.
12. Beadle GW: Genes and chemical reactions in neurospora, *Science* 129:1715-1719, 1959.
13. Beddard AP: Ochronosis associated with carboluria, *Quart J Med* 3:329-336, 1910.
14. Beddard AP, Plumtre CM: A further note on ochronosis associated with carboluria, *Quart J Med* 5:505-508, 1912.
15. Black RL: Use of cortisone in alkaptonuria, *JAMA* 155:968-970, 1954.
16. Blivaiss BB et al: Experimental ochronosis: induction in rats by long-term feeding with L-tyrosine, *Arch Pathol* 82:45-53, 1966.
17. Bluefarb SM: Alkaptonuria and ochronosis, *Quart Bull Northwest Univ Med Schl* 32:101-105, 1958.
18. Boedeker C: Ueber das Alcapton; ein neuer Beitrag zur Frage: welche Stoffe des Harns Können Kupferreduction bewirken? *Z Rat Med* 7:130-145, 1859.
19. Boedeker C: Das Alkapton; ein Beitrag zur Frage: welche Stoffe des Harns können aus einer alkalischen Kupferoxydlösung Kupferoxydul reduciren? *Ann Chem Pharmacol* 117:98, 1861.
20. Bondurant RE, Greer M, Williams CM: Gas chromatography of urinary homogentisic acid, *Anal Biochem* 15:364-366, 1966.
21. Bondurant RE, Henry JB: Pathogenesis of ochronosis in experimental alkaptonuria of the white rat, *Lab Invest* 14:62-69, 1965.
22. Bory C et al: Homogentisic acid determined in biological fluids by HPLC, *Clin Chem* 35:321-322, 1989.
23. Bosmansky K, Sršen Š, Hermanek S: Klinefelter's syndrome and alkaptonuria, *Cas Lek Cesk* 118(20):628-630, 1979.
24. Briggs AP: A colorimetric method for the determination of homogentisic acid in urine, *J Biol Chem* 51:453-454, 1922.
25. Brogren N: Case of exogenetic ochronosis from carbolic acid compresses, *Acta Dermatovener* 32:258-260, 1952.
26. Brown NK, Smuckler EA: Alkaptonuria and Gilbert's syndrome: report of two affected siblings and hepatic ultrastructure in one sibling, *Am J Med* 48:759-765, 1970.
27. Brunner H: Ueber die Verändergungen des Schläfenbeines bei der Ochronose, *Mchr Ohrenheilk* 63:997-1018, 1929.
28. Cardwell JB: Red urine associated with methyldopa treatment (letter) *Lancet* 2:326 only, 1969.
29. Case records of the Massachusetts General Hospital: Case 9-1966, *New Engl J Med* 274:454-462, 1966.
30. Cervanansky J, Sitaj Š, Urbánek T: Alkaptonuria and ochronosis, *J Bone Joint Surg* 41(A):1169-1182, 1959.

31. Chaudhary HR et al: Alcaptonuria: two cases, *J Assoc Physicians India* 31(10):676-678, 1983.

32. Childs B: Sir Archibald Garrod's conception of chemical individuality: a modern appreciation, *New Engl J Med* 282:71-77, 1970.

33. Cone TE Jr: Diagnosis and treatment: some syndromes, diseases, and conditions associated with abnormal coloration of the urine or diaper, *Pediatrics* 41:654-658, 1968.

34. Coodley EL, Greco AJ: Clinical aspects of ochronosis, with report of a case, *Am J Med* 8:816-822, 1950.

35. Cottini E: Hip prosthesis in alkaptonuric arthropathy of familial type, *Clin Orthop* 25(1):44-59, 1974.

36. Daicker B, Riede UN: Histological and ultrastructural findings in alkaptonuric ocular ochronosis, *Ophthalmologica* 169(5):377-388, 1974.

37. Deeb Z, Frayha RA: Multiple vacuum discs; an early sign of ochronosis: radiologic findings in two brothers, *J Rheumatol* 3(1):82-87, 1976.

38. Del Sasso L, Brambilla S, Pampuri M: Alkaptonuria and ochronosis: presentation of a clinical case, *Chir Ital* 36(3):422-430, 1984.

39. Dereymaeker L et al: Ochronosis and alkaptonuria: report of a new case with calcified aortic valve stenosis, *Acta Cardiol* 45(1):87-92, 1990.

40. Desai HJ et al: Alcaptonuria with diabetes mellitus (a case report with review of literature): *Indian J Med Sci* 32(7-8):77-79, 1978.

41. DiFiore JA: Ochronosis: report of a case, *Arthritis Rheum* 3:359-363, 1960.

42. Drummond KN et al: The blue diaper syndrome; familial hypercalcemia with nephrocalcinosis and indicanuria: a new familial disease, with definition of the metabolic abnormality, *Am J Med* 37:928-948, 1964.

43. Eberle P, Mohr W, Claes L: Biomechanical studies on the pathogenesis of ochronotic arthopathy, *Z Rheumatol* 43(5):249-252, 1984.

44. Eisenberg H: Alkaptonuria, ochronosis, arthritis and ruptured intervertebral disk complicated by homologous serum reaction, *Arch Intern Med* 86:79-86, 1950.

45. Feild JR, Higley GB Sr, DeSaussure RL Jr: Ochronosis with ruptured lumbar disc: case report, *J Neurosurg* 20:348-351, 1963.

46. Feldman JM, Bowman J: Urinary homogentisic acid: determination by thin-layer chromatography, *Clin Chem* 19(5):459-462, 1973.

47. Fishberg EH: Ueber die Carbolochronose, *Virchow Arch Path Anat* 251:376-418, 1924.

48. Fisher RG, Williams J: Ochronosis associated with degeneration of an intervertebral disc, *J Neurosurg* 12:403-406, 1955.

49. Flaschenträger B, Halawani A, and Nabeh I: Alkaptonurie und Vitamin B$_{12}$, *Klin Wschr* 32:131-133, 1954.

50. Forslind K et al: Alkaptonuria and ochronosis in three siblings: ascorbic acid treatment monitored by urinary HGA excretion, *Clin Exp Rheumatol* 6:289-292, 1988.

51. Frasquet Frasquet A, Garcia Carrillo M: Alkaptonuria and ochronosis: apropos of a case, *Rev Esp Reum Enferm Osteoartic* 22(4):259-304, 1979.

52. Friderich H, Nikolowski W: Endogene Ochronose, *Arch Dermatol Syph* 192:273-289, 1951.

53. Frohlich J, Price GE, Campbell DJ: Problems in the laboratory diagnosis of alcaptonuria, *Clin Chem* 19(7):770-773, 1973.

54. Gaines JJ Jr: Ochronotic arthropathy: a comparative scanning electron microscopic and light microscopic study of the synovium in ochronosis, *Am J Clin Pathol* 87:762-765, 1987.

55. Gaines JJ Jr: The pathology of alkaptonuric ochronosis, *Hum Pathol* 20(1):40-46, 1989.

56. Gaines JJ Jr, Pai GM: Cardiovascular ochronosis, *Arch Pathol Lab Med* 111(10):991-994, 1987.

57. Gaines JJ Jr, Tom G, Khankhanian NK: An ultrastructural and light microscopic study of the synovium in ochronotic arthropathy, *Hum Pathol* 18:1160-1164, 1987.

58. Galdston M, Steele JM, Dobriner K: Alcaptonuria and ochronosis with a report of three patients and metabolic studies in two, *Am J Med* 13:432-452, 1952.

59. Garrett E: Ocular ochronosis with alkaptonuria, *Am J Ophthalmol* 55:617-620, 1963.

60. Garnica AD et al: Alkaptonuria and sucrase-isomaltase deficiency in three offspring of a consanguineous marriage, *Acta Vitaminol Enzymol* 3:157-169, 1981.

61. Garrod AE: About alkaptonuria, *Lancet* 2:1484-1486, 1901.

62. Garrod AE: The Croonian lectures on inborn errors of metabolism. Lecture II. Alkaptonuria, *Lancet* 2:73,142,214, 1908.

63. Garrod AE: *Inborn errors of metabolism*, London, 1909, Frowde, Hodder & Stoughton.

64. Gaucher A et al: HLA-B27 antigen and alkaptonuria, *Rev Rhum Mal Osteoartic* 44(4):273-277, 1977.

65. Gaucher A et al: Synovial membrane from ochronotic arthropathy of the hip joint: scanning electron microscopic study, *Z Rheumatol* 39(7-8):231-235, 1980.

66. Gerasimov AM, Zakharov AS: Free radical mechanism of homogentisic acid in alkaptonuria, *Vopr Med Khim* 34(1):112-115, 1988.

67. Goldberg BH et al: Alkaptonuria with nephrocalcinosis, *J Pediatr* 88(3):518-519, 1976.

68. Gomez Mateos JM, Rubio Rubio F: Alkaptonuria-ochronosis: apropos of a case (letter), *Rev Clin Esp* 177(4):197-198, 1985.

69. Gonnermann R: Kasuistischer Beitrag zur Ochronose, *Beitr Path Anat* 100:598-607, 1938.

70. Gould L et al: Cardiac manifestations of ochronosis, *J Thorac Cardiovasc Surg* 72:788-791, 1976.

71. Greiling H: Beitrag zur entstehung der ochronose bei alkaptonurie, *Klin Wochenschr* 35:889 only, 1957.

72. Gross O, Allard E: Untersuchungen über Alkaptonurie, *Z Klin Med* 64:359-369, 1907.

73. Haiya PP et al: Tetralogy of Fallot and alkaptonuria in successive generations, *Indian Pediatr* 17(1):83-85, 1980.

74. Hammond G, Powers HW: Alkaptonuric arthritis: report of a case, *Lahey Clin Bull* 11:18-22, 1958.

75. Harper PS, Bradley DM: Screening for alkaptonuria in the newborn in Wales (letter), *Lancet* 2(8089):576-577, 1978.

76. Harrold AJ: Alkaptonuric arthritis, *J Bone Joint Surg* 38(B):532-538, 1956.

77. Heile: Ueber die Ochronose und die durch Formol verursachte pseudo-ochronotische Färbung der Knorpel, *Virchow Arch* 160:148, 1900.

78. Hendel H, Ben-Assa BJ: Report about a Bedouin family affected by alkaptonuria (comprising two cases of urolithiasis), *Ann Paediatr* 195:77-87, 1960.

79. Hogben L, Worrall RL, Zieve I: The genetic basis of alkaptonuria, *Proc Roy Soc Edinburgh* 52:264-294, 1932.

80. Hoke AW, Maibach HI, Epstein WL: Physiologic and histologic studies of chromidrosis due to ochronosis. Presentation to American Medical Association meeting, June 19, 1971.

81. Hollingsworth RP: Homogentisic acid stone: a rare form of prostatic obstruction, *Br J Urol* 40:546-547, 1968.

82. Ibbott FA: Homogentisic acid. In Henry RJ, Cannon DC, Winkelman JW, editors: *Clinical chemistry: principles and techniques,* ed 2, New York, 1974, Harper & Row, pp 622-626.

83. Janacek M: Ochronotic (alkaptonuric) osteoarthrosis, *Lek Listy* 2:536-540, 1947.

84. Jeghers H: Medical progress: pigmentation of the skin, *New Engl J Med* 231:88 Only, 1944.

85. Jellum E et al: Advances in the use of computerized gas chromatography–mass spectrometry and high-performance liquid chromatography with rapid scanning detection for clinical diagnosis, *J Chromatogr* 468:43-53, 1989.

86. Justesen P, Anderson PE Jr: Radiologic manifestations in alkaptonuria, *Skeletal Radiol* 11(3):204-208, 1984.

87. Kapralik I et al: Association between alkaptonuria and selected polymorphic systems, *Bratisl Lek Listy* 85(2):194-201, 1986.

88. Keeling ME, McClure HM, Kibler RF: Alkaptonuria in an orangutan (Pongo pygmaeus), *Am J Phys Anthropol* 38(2):435-438, 1973.

89. Khachadurian A, Feisal AK: Alkaptonuria: report of a family with seven cases appearing in four successive generations with metabolic studies in one patient, *J Chronic Dis* 7:455-465, 1958.

90. Knox WE: Sir Archibald Garrod's *Inborn errors of metabolism.* II. Alkaptonuria, *Am J Hum Genet* 10:95-124, 1958.

91. Koar J, Krizek VL: Roentgen signs of alkaptonuric ochronosis, *Fortschr Geb Rontgenstr* 109:203, 1968.

92. Koonce DH: Ochronosis: report of three cases in siblings, *J Tenn Med Assoc* 51:85-89, 1958.

93. Koska L: Artifacts produced by homogentisic acid in the examination of urine from alkaptonurics, *Ann Clin Biochem* 23:354 only, 1986.

94. Kutty MK, Iqbal QM, Teh EC: Ochronotic arthropathy: an electron microscopical study with a view on pathogenesis, *Arch Pathol Lab Med* 98:55-57, 1974.

95. La Du BN: Alcaptonuria. In Stanbury JB, Wyngaarden JB, Fredrickson DS, editors: *The metabolic basis of inherited disease,* ed 1, New York, 1960, Blakiston Division, McGraw-Hill, pp 394-427.

96. La Du BN: Alcaptonuria. In Stanbury JB, Wyngaarden JB, Fredrickson DS, editors: *The metabolic basis of inherited disease,* ed 4, New York, 1978, McGraw-Hill, pp 268-282.

97. La Du BN, Zannoni VG: Oxidation of homogentisic acid catalyzed by horseradish peroxidase, *Biochem Biophys Acta* 67:281-287, 1963.

98. La Du BN et al: The nature of the defect in tyrosine metabolism in alkaptonuria, *J Biol Chem* 230:251-260, 1958.

99. Lagier R, Steiger U: The role of ochronotic arthropathies in rheumatology, *Bull Schweiz Akad Med Wiss* 35(4-6):389-402, 1979.

100. Lee SL, Stenn FF: Characterization of mummy bone ochronotic pigment, *JAMA* 240(2):136-138, 1978.

101. Lester FT, Tereschenko OI: Alkaptonuria in an Ethiopian, *East Afr Med J* 55(12):593-595, 1978.

102. Levine HD et al: Aortic valve replacement for ochronosis of the aortic valve, *Chest* 74:466-467, 1978.

103. Lewis JH: Alcaptonuria in rabbit, *J Biol Chem* 70:659-661, 1926.

104. Lichtenstein L, Kaplan L: Hereditary ochronosis: pathological changes observed in two necropsied cases, *Am J Pathol* 30:99-125, 1954.

105. Logroscino CA, Sacchettoni Logroscino G, Caporale M: Subcutaneous Achilles tendon rupture in alkaptonuria; clinical contribution: microscopic and ultrastructural features, *Arch Putti Chir Organi Mov* 32:307-311, 1982.

106. Logroscino CA, Sacchettoni Logroscino G: Alkaptonuria ochronosis: ultrastructural features, *Arch Putti Chir Organi Mov* 32:381-398, 1982.

107. Ludwig GD, Toole JF, Wood JC: Ochronosis from quinacrine (Atabrine), *Ann Intern Med* 59:378-384, 1963.

108. Lustberg TJ, Schulman JD, Seegmiller JE: Decreased binding of ^{14}C-homogentisic acid induced by ascorbic acid in connective tissue of rats with experimental alkaptonuria, *Nature* 228:770-771, 1970.

109. McCollum DE, Odom GL: Alkaptonuria, ochronosis, and low-back pain: a case report, *J Bone Joint Surg* 47(A):1389-1392, 1965.

110. McKenzie AW, Owen JA, Ramsay JHR: Two cases of alkaptonuria, *Br Med J* 2:794-796, 1957.

111. McKusick VA, Goodman RM: Pinnal calcification: observations in systemic diseases not associated with disordered calcium metabolism, *JAMA* 179:230-232, 1962.

112. McKusick VA, Milch RA: The clinical behavior of genetic disease: selected aspects, *Clin Orthop* 33:22-39, 1964.

113. Mam MK, Sethi TS: Alkaptonuria and ochronotic arthropathy, *J Indian Med Assoc* 84(7):218-220, 1986.

114. Manson-Bahr P, Ransford ON: Some pigmentations of the skin occurring in patients from the tropics: carotinaemia, haemochromatosis and alkaptonuria, *Trans Roy Soc Trop Med Hyg* 32:395-404, 1938.

115. Manthorpe R: Failure to detect glucose with paper strips in alkaptonuric urine, *Dan Med Bull* 20(4):126-128, 1973.

116. Martin JP Jr, Batkoff B: Homogentisic acid autoxidation and oxygen radical generation: implications for the etiology of alkaptonuric arthritis, *Free Radic Biol Med* 3(4):241-250, 1987.

117. Martin WJ, Underdahl LO, Mathieson DR: Alkaptonuria: report of three cases, *Proc Mayo Clin* 27:193-200, 1952.

118. Mathias K, Diezemann E: Alkaptonuric ochronosis: rare cause of bilateral meniscopathy, *Z Orthop* 118(2):270-273, 1980.

119. Matsuda H et al: Alkaptonuria, *Nippon Rinsho* 31(8):2404-2412, 1973.

120. Meundi DB, Bhandari SG: Alkaptonuria (a case report), *Indian Pediatr* 15(5):445-446, 1978.

121. Milch RA: Direct inheritance of alkaptonuria, *Metabolism* 4:513-518, 1955.

122. Milch RA: Studies of alcaptonuria: inheritance of 47 cases in eight highly inter-related Dominican kindreds, *Am J Hum Genet* 12:76-85, 1960.

123. Milch RA: Studies of alcaptonuria: infra-red spectra of deuterated homogentisic acid solutions, *Arthritis Rheum* 8:1002-1005, 1965.

124. Milch RA, Robinson RA: Studies of alcaptonuria: content and density of the water and solid phases of ochronotic cartilage, *J Chronic Dis* 12:409-416, 1960.

125. Milch RA, Titus ED: Studies of alkaptonuria: absorption spectra of homogentisic-chondroitin sulphate solutions, *Arthritis Rheum* 1:566-568, 1958.

126. Minno AM, Rogers JA: Ochronosis: report of a case, *Ann Intern Med* 46:179-183, 1957.

127. Modilevsky T, Manor E, Marmor A: Alkaptonuria: prevalence among Bedouins related by consanguinity, *Monogr Hum Genet* 9:123-125, 1978.

128. Mohr W, Wessinghage D, Lenschow E: Ultrastructure of hyaline cartilage and articular capsule tissue in alkaptonuric ochronosis, *Z Rheumatol* 39(3-4):55-73, 1980.

129. Molony J, Kelly DJ: Alkaptonuria, ochronosis, and ochronotic arthritis, *J Irish Med Assoc* 63:22-24, 1970.

130. Moran TJ, Yunis EJ: Studies on ochronosis. II. Effects of injection of homogentisic acid and ochronotic pigment in experimental animals, *Am J Pathol* 40:359-369, 1962.

131. Mueller MN et al: Alkaptonuria and ochronotic arthropathy, *Med Clin North Am* 49:101-115, 1965.

132. Murray JC, Lindberg KA, Pinnell SR: In vitro inhibition of chick embryo lysyl hydroxylase by homogentisic acid: a proposed connective tissue defect in alkaptonuria, *J Clin Invest* 59:1071-1079, 1977.

133. Neubauer O: Intermediärer Eiweisstoffwechsel, *Handb Norm Pathol Physiol* 5:671, 1928.

134. Neuberger A, Rimington C, Wilson JMG: Studies on alkaptonuria. II. Investigations on a case of human alkaptonuria, *Biochem J* 41:438-457, 1947.

135. Neuwirth A et al: Analysis of alkaptonuria incidence in one region of Northwest Slovakia: a preliminary report, *Birth Defects* 10(10):244-249, 1974.

136. O'Brien WM, La Du BN, Bunim JJ: Biochemical, pathologic and clinical aspects of alkaptonuria, ochronosis and ochronotic arthropathy: review of world literature (1584-1962), *Am J Med* 34:813-838, 1963.

137. Oda RE: Alkaptonuria: report of two cases in siblings, *Am J Dis Child* 106:301-303, 1963.

138. Orzincolo C et al: Ochronotic arthropathy in alkaptonuria. Radiological manifestations and physiopathological signs, *Radiol Med (Torino)* 75(5):476-481, 1988.

139. Osler W: Ochronosis: the pigmentation of cartilages, sclerotics and skin in alkaptonuria, *Lancet* 1:10 only, 1904.

140. Pagan-Carlo J, Payzant AR: Roentgenographic manifestations in a severe case of alkaptonuric osteoarthritis, *Am J Roentgenol* 80:635-638, 1958.

141. Papageorge E, Lewis HB: Comparative studies of the metabolism of the amino acids. VII. Experimental alkaptonuria in white rat, *J Biol Chem* 123:211-220, 1938.

142. Parikh A et al: Alkaptonuria: a series of seven cases, *J Assoc Physicians India* 36(9):565-566, 1988.

143. Pau HW: Involvement of the tympanic membrane and ear ossicle system in ochronotic alkaptonuria, *Laryngol Rhinol Otolaryngol* 63(10):541-544, 1984.

144. Pieter H: Une famille d'alcaptonuriques, *Presse Mèd* 33:1310 only, 1925.

145. Pomeranz MM, Friedman LJ, Tunick IS: Roentgen findings in alkaptonuric ochronosis, *Radiology* 37:295-303, 1941.

146. Poulsen V: Ueber Ochronose bei Menschen und Tieren, *Beitr Path Anat* 48:437-498, 1910.

147. Pourel GJ et al: HLA antigens and alkaptonuria, *J Rheumatol* 3(suppl):97-100, 1977.

148. Ptacin M, Sebastian J, Bamrah VS: Ochronotic cardiovascular disease, *Clin Cardiol* 8:441-445, 1985.

149. Reddi YR, Rao MN, Laxman S: Alkaptonuria in siblings, *Indian J Pediatr* 40(308):330-331, 1973.

150. Reginato AJ et al: Alkaptonuria, ochronotic arthropathy and aortic stenosis, *Rev Med Chile* 100:529-533, 1972.

151. Rones B: Ochronosis oculi in alkaptonuria, *Am J Ophthalmol* 49:440-446, 1960.

152. Roth M, Felgenhauer W-R: Recherche de l'excretion d'acide homogentisique urinaire chez des heterozygotes pour l'alcaptonurie, *Enzym Biol Clin* 9:53-58, 1968.

153. Sandler M, Karoum F, Ruthven CRJ: Parkinsonism with alkaptonuria: a new syndrome? (letter), *Lancet* 2:770 only, 1970.

154. Sarin LR, Bhargava RK: Alkaptonuria with ochronosis, *J Indian Med Assoc* 28:481 only, 1987.

155. Savastano AA, Quigley DG, Scala ME: Spontaneous fractures associated with cortisone therapy in a patient with ochronosis, *Am J Orthop Surg* 11:116-120, 1969.

156. Schumacher HR, Holdsworth DE: Ochronotic arthropathy. I. Clinicopathologic studies, *Semin Arthritis Rheum* 6:207-246, 1977.

157. Sealock RR, Galdston M, Steele JM: Administration of ascorbic acid to an alkaptonuric patient, *Proc Soc Exp Biol Med* 44:580-583, 1940.

158. Sharma RR et al: Cervico-medullary compression secondary to ochronotic arthritis affecting cranio-vertebral joints: syndesmodental ochronotic arthritis, *J Postgrad Med* 34(4):253-257, 1988.

159. Shelley WB, Hurley HJ Jr: Localized chromhidrosis: a survey, *Arch Dermatol Syph* 68:449-471, 1954.

160. Seegmiller JE et al: An enzymatic spectrophotometric method for the determination of homogentisic acid in plasma and urine, *J Biol Chem* 236:774-777, 1961.

161. Siekert RG, Gibilisco JA: Discoloration of the teeth in alkaptonuria (ochronosis) and parkinsonism, *Oral Surg* 28:197-199, 1970.

162. Simon G, Zorab PA: The radiographic changes in alkaptonuric arthritis, *Br J Radiol* 34:384-386, 1961.

163. Sinha HK: A case of alkaptonuria, *Indian Med Gaz* 65:153-154, 1930.

164. Sitaj S, Urbànek T: Alkaptonuria, *Rev Czech Med* 2:288-292, 1956.

165. Skinsnes OK: Generalized ochronosis: report of an instance in which it was misdiagnosed as melanosarcoma, with resultant enucleation of eye, *Arch Pathol* 45:552-558, 1948.

166. Smith HP, Smith HP Jr: Ochronosis: report of two cases, *Ann Intern Med* 42:171-178, 1955.

167. Smith JW: Ochronosis of the sclera and cornea complicating alkaptonuria: review of the literature and report of four cases, *JAMA* 120:1282-1288, 1942.

168. Söderbergh G: Ueber Ositis deformans ochronotica, *Neur Zbl* 32:1362-1363, 1913.

169. Sršen Š: Simultaneous occurrence of alkaptonuria and of Klinefelter syndrome in one patient, *Pädiatr u Pädol* 12(2):174-175, 1977.

170. Sršen Š: Dark pigmentation of ear cerumen in alkaptonuria (letter), *Lancet* 2(8089):577 only, 1978.

171. Sršen Š: Alkaptonuria, *Johns Hopkins Med J* 145(6):217-226, 1979.

172. Sršen Š: Analysis of the causes of the relatively frequent incidence of alkaptonuria in Slovakia, *Čas Lék čes* 122(51):1585-1587, 1983.

173. Sršen Š: *Alkaptonuria*, Martin, Czechoslovakia, 1984, Publishing House Osveta.

174. Sršen Š, Kamaryt J, Srsnova K: The study of gene linkage between the locus of the alkaptonuric allele and amylase loci, *Cas Lek Cesk* 125(30):937-939, 1986.

175. Sršen Š, Koska L, Kapralik I: Alkaptonuria in the Upper Hron Region in Slovakia, *Cas Lek Cesk* 117(49):1517-1522, 1978.

176. Sršen Š, Koska L, Kapralik I: Incidence of alkaptonuria in relation to genetic isolation and degree of inbreeding in several selected localities in Slovakia, *Čas Lék čes* 117(12):353-360, 1978.

177. Sršen Š, Neuwirth A: Alkaptonuria in childhood: our hitherto experiences, *Cesk Pediatr* 29(9):475-477, 1974.

178. Sršen Š, Srsnova K: Diagnosis of alkaptonuria in children, *Pädiatr u Pädol* 14(2):163-167, 1979.

179. Sršen Š, Srsnova K: Research on alkaptonuria and the care of the child, *Čs Pediat* 39(5):249-252, 1984.

180. Sršen Š, Srsnova K, Lanyi A: Clinical aspects of alkaptonuria, *Vutr Boles* 21(5):42-48, 1982.

181. Sršen Š, Srsnova K, Lanyi A: Clinical manifestation of alkaptonuria in relation to age, *Bratisl Lek Listy* 77(6):662-669, 1982.

182. Sršen Š, Varga F: Screening for alkaptonuria in the newborn in Slovakia (letter), *Lancet* 2(8089):576 only, 1978.

183. Sršen Š et al: Alkaptonuria in the Trencin District of Czechoslovakia, *Am J Med Genet* 2(2):159-166, 1978.

184. Sršen Š et al: Detection of alkaptonuria and mapping of its occurrence in Slovakia, *Czech Med* 2(4):186-197, 1979.

185. Sršen Š et al: Random and non-random component of inbreeding coefficient in localities with high incidence of alkaptonuria in Slovakia, *Bratisl Lek Listy* 71(2):144-151, 1979.

186. Sršen Š et al: Analysis of the life span of alkaptonuric patients, *Čas Lék čes* 124(41-2):1288-1291, 1985.

187. Steiger U, Lagier R: Combined anatomical and radiological study of the hip-joint in alcaptonuric arthropathy, *Ann Rheum Dis* 31(5):369-373, 1972.

188. Steinmann B et al: Severe neonatal primary hyperparathyroidism and alkaptonuria in a boy born to related parents with familial hypocalciuric hypercalcemia, *Helv Paediatr Acta* 39(2):171-186, 1984.

189. Stenn FF et al: Biochemical identification of homogentisic acid pigment in an ochronotic Egyptian mummy, *Science* 197:566-568, 1977.

190. Stoner R, Blivaiss BB: Homogentisic acid metabolism: A 1,4-addition reaction of benzquinone-2-acetic acid with amino acids and other biological amines, *Fed Proc* 24:656 only, 1965.

191. Sussman T: Alkaptonuria, *Proc Roy Soc Med* 62:485 only, 1969.

192. Sutro CJ, Anderson ME: Alkaptonuric arthritis: cause for free intra-articular bodies, *Surgery* 22:120-124, 1947.

193. Sutor DJ, Wooley SE, Křižek V: The composition of calculi from patients with alkaptonuria, *Br J Urol* 42:386-388, 1970.

194. Suarez GM, Roberts JA: Ochronosis of prostate presenting as advanced carcinoma, *Urology* 22:168-171, 1983.

195. Tsunashima T et al: A case of alkaptonuria with fatal cardiovascular disturbance, *Acta Med Okayama* 30(2):87-94, 1976.

196. Umber G, Burger M: Zur Klinik intermediärer Stoffwechselstörungen (Alkaptonurie mit Ochronose und Osteo-Arthritis deformans: Zystinurie), *Deutsch Med Wschr* 39:2337-2341, 1913.

197. Vaishnava S, Pulimood BM: Alkaptonuria, *Indian J Pediatr* 25:518-523, 1958.

198. Virchow R: Ein Fall von allgemeiner Ochronose der Knorpel und knorpelähnlichen Theile, *Arch Pathol Anat* 37:212-219, 1866.

199. Vlay SC, Hartman AR, Culliford AT: Alkaptonuria and aortic stenosis (letter), *Ann Intern Med* 104(3):446 only, 1986.

200. Wagner LR et al: Clinical and pathological findings in ochronosis, *J Clin Pathol* 13:22-26, 1960.

201. Wang TR, Hwu WL: Alkaptonuria in a Chinese baby, *J Inherited Metab Dis* 12(3):327 only, 1989.

202. Wells C, Maxwell BM: Alkaptonuria in an Egyptian mummy, *Br J Radiol* 35:679-682, 1962.

203. White AG, Parker J, Block F: Studies in human alkaptonuria: effect of thiouracil, para-aminobenzoic acid and diiodotyrosine on excretion of homogentisic acid, *J Clin Invest* 28:140-143, 1949.

204. Wirtschafter JD: The eye in alkaptonuria, *Birth Defects* 12(3):279-293, 1976.

205. Wittenberg J: Gastrointestinal bleeding and arthropathy, *JAMA* 195:1048-1050, 1966.

206. Wolff JA et al: Effects of ascorbic acid in alkaptonuria: alterations in benzoquinone acetic acid and an ontogenic effect in infancy, *Pediatr Res* 26(2):140-144, 1989.

207. Wolkow M, Baumann E: Ueber das Wesen der Alkaptonurie, *Z Physiol Chem* 15:228-285, 1890-1891.

208. Woodford VR, Quan L, Cutts F: Experimental alkaptonuria in the rat induced by tryptophan deficiency, *Can J Biochem* 45:791-796, 1967.

209. Yamaguchi S, Koda N, Ohashi T: Diagnosis of alkaptonuria by NMR urinalysis: rapid qualitative and quantitative analysis of homogentisic acid, *Tohoku J Exp Med* 150(2):227-228, 1986.

210. Yamaguchi S, Koda N, Yamamoto H: Analysis for homogentisic acid by NMR spectrometry to aid diagnosis of alkaptonuria, *Clin Chem* 35:1806-1807, 1989.

211. Young HH: Calculi of prostate associated with ochronosis and alkaptonuria, *J Urol* 51:48-58, 1944.

212. Yules JH: Ochronotic arthritis: report of a case, *Bull New Engl Med Center* 16:168-173, 1954.

213. Zannoni VG, Lomtevas N, Goldfinger S: Oxidation of homogentisic acid to ochronotic pigment in connective tissue, *Biochim Biophys Acta* 177:94-105, 1969.

214. Zocholl G et al: Roentgenologic and nuclear medicine findings in alkaptonuric ochronosis, *Rontgenblatter* 39(4):85-88, 1986.

CHAPTER 10

Pseudoxanthoma Elasticum

Denis Viljoen

Pseudoxanthoma elasticum (PXE) is a heterogeneous disorder involving predominantly the skin, the eye, and the cardiovascular system. The characteristic clinical manifestations are yellow, papular lesions of the skin flexures, loss of visual acuity as a result of recurrent retinal hemorrhage and sclerosis, and premature arteriosclerosis of small and medium-sized blood vessels, which leads to hypertension, stroke, and hemorrhagic episodes.

The designation pseudoxanthoma elasticum *is appropriate for this disorder, since the condition originally had been classified with the xanthomatoses until primary involvement of the* elastic* *fiber was recognized. The eponymic form,* Grönblad-Strandberg syndrome, *is found occasionally in the European literature but is not widely used elsewhere. In this chapter the abbreviation* PXE *replaces the longer title of the disorder.*

HISTORICAL NOTE

The first description of the skin changes that occur in PXE was written by Rigal[138] in 1881, and Balzer[7] provided the first autopsy report in 1884. Because of the yellow, elevated appearance of the skin lesions, the disorder was grouped with the xanthomatoses by Rigal and Balzer and by Chauffard.[26] The disease was identified as a sepa-

rate and nonxanthomatous entity by Darier[36] in 1896.

Ferdinand Jean Darier was born of French parents on April 26, 1856, in Budapest.[20] He was educated in Geneva and then emigrated to Paris at the age of 20 years. After receiving the degree of Doctor of Medicine in 1885, he worked in Louis Antoine Ranvier's laboratory at the College de France. He became one of the "immortal Big Five" who made the Paris School of Dermatology world renowned; the other four members were Ernest Henri Besnier, LAJ Brocq, Raymond Sabouraud, and Alfred Fournier.

Darier described keratosis follicularis and acanthosis nigricans in 1889, and in 1909 his masterpiece, *Précis de dermatologie*, was translated into English, German, Spanish and Japanese. The doyen of international dermatology, he was described as "highly cultured, urbane, modest, full of fun and perenially young. . . ." A man of great energy, Darier began his eight-volume work, *Nouvelle pratique dermatologique* (Paris, 1936), at the age of 80, only 2 years before he died after a protracted illness.

In 1889 Chauffard, at a meeting of the Société Médicale des Hôpitaux in Paris, described a patient destined to occupy a prominent role in the history of PXE.

Anatole Chauffard was born in Avignon on August 22, 1855, to medically distinguished parents. His father, Emile, was professor of general pathology in Paris. Anatole Chauffard had a brilliant career and made several original contributions to medicine, including the first description of hereditary spherocytosis (familial hemolytic jaundice). He pioneered the use of emetine in the treatment of amebic dysentery and was among the first to describe bovine tuberculosis infections in humans. Chauffard also contributed to knowledge of the pathogenesis of jaundice in

---

*Throughout this chapter the term "elastic" is used in preference to "elastin" because the elastic fiber is made up of elastin and other components, including fibrillin (see p. 354, Basic Defect).

carcinoma of the pancreas. He was honored as president of the International Congress of Medicine in 1900 and as president of the French Academy of Medicine in 1923. He died of bronchopneumonia on November 1, 1932, at 77 years of age[19]

The case described by Chauffard was separately reported during the next fifteen years by Besnier and Doyon,[17] by Darier, who established the histopathology and offered the name *pseudoxanthoma elasticum* with the alternative *elastorrhexis*, and by Hallopeau and Laffitte,[71] who described dramatic changes in the fundus oculi. The patient's well-documented case history demonstrates the typical features of the syndrome: changes in the skin, repeated massive gastrointestinal hemorrhages, weak peripheral pulse rates, and failing vision. Chauffard's description follows[26]:

This is a man of 35 years. . . . At 24 years of age, while doing his military service in New Caledonia, he suffered a large hematemesis. This accident repeated itself several times (at ages 26, 31, and 33). This summer he was admitted to the Hotel Dieu for a hematemesis.

In 1880 L. was discharged and returned to France; and it was shortly afterward, he states, when he noted the beginning of his skin affection. . . . The xanthomatous eruption is composed of a series of evolving groups, perfectly symmetrical and confined exclusively to several flexural folds—the base of the neck, the two axillary creases, the folds of the elbows, the anterior abdominal wall, especially just below the umbilicus, the two inguinal triangles, the inferior aspect of the penis, around the anus, the two popliteal fossae. . . . The center of the group is formed by an almost confluent agglomeration of intradermal plaques, soft to the touch, projecting to some extent like papules, separated by small folds of skin. Their coloration is rather pale, resembling that of fresh butter or yellow chamois; the size of the largest plaque is scarcely greater than that of a pea. . . . If one retracts both lips, one sees that the mucosa of the inner aspect is involved. It demonstrates a cluster of small, yellowish intramucosal nodules, resting on a richly vascular background traversed by numerous dilated and tortuous capillaries. . . . In February there developed an unusual phenomenon, of which there is today scarcely any trace remaining. The peripheral zone of the eruptive groups in the skin was traversed by rather large, violaceous rose networks that were not elevated and formed a congestive halo around the yellow plaques. . . . Today traces of this perinodular hyperemia remain only in the pectoral regions, on the anterior extension of the axillary groups. . . .

The pulse is feeble and compressible and gives with the sphygmomanometer of Verdin a tension of 650, rather than of 750, the average normal figure.

In August 1896 at the Third International Dermatologic Congress in London Darier reported histologic studies of the skin of Chauffard's patient. By 1903 amblyopia had developed in this patient; at this time Hallopeau and Laffitte reported that there was "chorioretinitis of the central region, involving the macula, with secondary atrophy of the optic disc."

Although Hallopeau and Laffitte in 1903 speculated that there might be some connection between the changes in the skin and those in the fundus oculi of Chauffard's patient, it was not until 1929 that the relationship between angioid streaks and PXE was established by Ester Grönblad,[65] an ophthalmologist, and James Strandberg,[157] a dermatologist, both of Stockholm.

Ester Elisabeth Grönblad was born in Uppsala, Sweden, in August 1888. She qualified in medicine in Stockholm in 1916 and later specialized in ophthalmology. A Doctor of Philosophy degree was awarded to her for her research on angioid streaks in PXE. Further papers on disorders in which both eye and skin manifestations occurred together followed. These included an investigation in collaboration with Sjögren and the subsequent delineation of the syndrome named after him.

James Victor Strandberg was born in Stockholm on March 9, 1883. He was educated in that city and graduated with the degree of Doctor of Medicine in 1909. As a private practitioner, he was the first to diagnose smallpox in the great epidemic of 1920. He became a dermatology registrar at the Royal Caroline Institute in 1922 and was appointed to the full chair of dermatology and syphilology in 1936. He held this position until his death, which resulted from a cerebral hemorrhage in 1942.

Strandberg was an exceptional diagnostician and teacher, with research interests in occupational eczema, solar elastosis, and tuberculosis of the skin. Although he published widely in dermatologic subjects, he is best remembered for his combined contribution with Ester Grönblad in the description of PXE.

Angioid streaks had been described by Doyne[40] in 1889, and the descriptive term was assigned by Knapp[93] in 1892. Knapp thought angioid streaks had a vascular basis. Their origin as a result of breaks in Bruch membrane was first suggested by Kofler[94] in 1917.

Involvement of the peripheral arteries in this syndrome and the physiologic consequences thereof have been studied by Carlborg,[24] Van Embden Andres,[167] Scheie and Freeman,[145] Urbach and Wolfram,[166] Prick,[130] Guenther,[67] and Wolff, Stokes, and Schlesinger,[177] among others. Gastrointestinal hemorrhage was emphasized by several of these authors, particularly by Revell and Carey[137] in 1948. During the early 1950s the suggestion that the condition is an abnormality of collagen fibers rather than elastic fibers was advanced by Hannay,[73] who used standard histologic techniques, and by Tunbridge et al.,[165] who used electron microscopy. A return to the view that the elastic fiber is primarily involved followed the work of Rodnan, Fisher, and Warren,[139] Fisher, Rodnan, and Lansing,[51] Goodman et al.,[63] and others.

Pseudoxanthoma elasticum is the name usually given this syndrome. With the renewed evidence that the elastic fiber is the main site of abnormality, "elasticum" seems accurate, and the skin and arterial changes certainly justify the designation "pseudoxanthoma." In the present understanding Touraine's term,[163] *élastorrhexie systématisée*, is appropriate, although potential exists for confusion with systemic elastolysis, which is an alternative designation for the acquired form of Cutis Laxa.

Recent History

Several comprehensive studies of various aspects of PXE have been undertaken during the past three decades.* In a large-scale investigation Connor et al.[33] reported data relating to angioid streaks in 106 patients. These authors stressed the progressive nature of the retinal lesions that lead to loss of visual acuity and, in some instances, blindness.

Goodman et al.[63] performed an extensive clinical and histopathologic study of 25 individuals at the Johns Hopkins Hospital in Baltimore. A decade later Pope investigated 180 patients in a national survey that extended throughout England and Wales. He presented the data as a doctoral thesis to the University of Wales in 1972.[126] Pope distinguished four groups of patients, two in which the disorder was inherited as an autosomal dominant trait[127] and two in which autosomal recessive inheritance was likely.[128] In this way he suggested for the first time that PXE might be heterogeneous. Pope also conducted a retrospective

---

*References 2, 33, 63, 119, 126, and 171.

literature survey encompassing all the previously published cases of PXE and identified similar heterogeneity in these individuals.[129]

Important recent studies have included the ultrastructural appearance of the skin by Reeve et al.,[135] mitral valve prolapse in PXE,[97] and the role of calcium in the diet.[136] Neldner[119] comprehensively appraised the clinical, biochemical, and histologic manifestations in 100 persons with PXE.

In an investigation of 86 individuals with PXE in South Africa Viljoen, Pope, and Beighton[174] delineated an apparently autonomous form of PXE in Afrikaners, in whom severe retinal complications posed a serious threat to vision. Gynecologic and obstetric complications[172] and cosmetic surgery[173] were aspects of the condition that were reviewed in detail.

Recombinant deoxyribonucleic acid (DNA) techniques have been used to investigate the structure of the human elastin gene.[9] For a time localization of the elastin gene was disputed; some evidence suggested that it was situated on the long arm of chromosome two, band 31 to long arm terminal (2q31-qter),[44] whereas other data supported localization on the long arm of chromosome 7.[47] Boyd[23] demonstrated linkage between the phenotype and elastin probes on the chromosome-2 site in two families with PXE. There is now firm evidence for localization of the gene to chromosome 7q11.2. It can be anticipated that further studies currently underway will provide evidence to refute or support the concept of heterogeneity in PXE.

CLINICAL MANIFESTATIONS

Pseudoxanthoma elasticum is a heterogeneous disorder with considerable variability in clinical manifestations. The clinical stigmata of PXE are found mainly in three areas: the skin, the eye, and the cardiovascular system. Because of the widespread involvement of the media of the arteries, hemorrhagic and thrombotic complications referable to virtually every organ system may occur. These include bleeding from the gastrointestinal tract, stroke phenomena involving the central nervous system, and minor problems involving the musculoskeletal system, the genital tract in women, and the lungs.

Skin and Mucosa

The changes in the skin often are not recognizable on clinical examination before the second de-

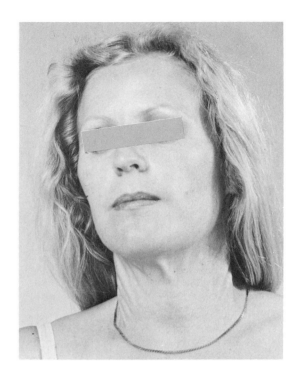

Fig. 10-1. A woman with PXE at 36 years of age. The cervical skin is lax, thickened, and has a yellowish tint.

Fig. 10-2. A to **D**, Accentuated facial folds and creases in four patients with PXE. Patients in **A, B,** and **D** are sibs. (From Goodman RM et al: *Medicine* 42:297-339, 1963.)

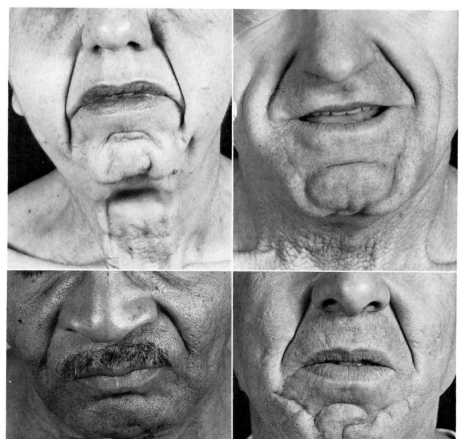

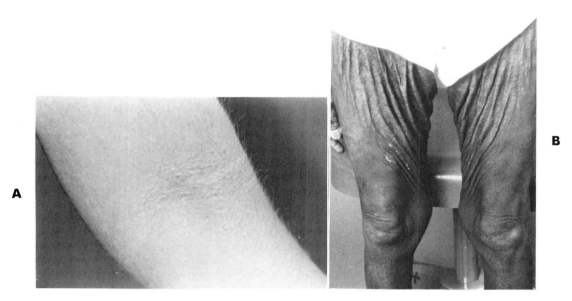

Fig. 10-3. A, Mild peau d'orange changes are evident in the antecubital fossa. **B,** A 52-year-old woman with PXE. The skin of the thighs is lax and discolored.

cade of life or later. The face, neck (Fig. 10-1), axillary folds, cubital regions, inguinal folds, and periumbilical area are particularly prone to involvement. The skin in the perioral area, including the nasolabial creases, another zone of particular wear and tear, is especially likely to show changes (Fig. 10-2).

The cutaneous stigmata of PXE may progress in an erratic manner.[63,119] In most persons the skin in the cervical region is initially affected and the axillary region tends to become involved in early adulthood. In women the next area of predilection is the inguinal region, whereas in men the antecubital fossa is more likely to be affected.[171] (Fig. 10-3).

The skin in the affected areas becomes thickened and grooved like coarse-grained Moroccan leather. The elevated yellowish regions between the grooves may be diamond shaped, rectangular, or polygonal. *Cutis rhomboidalis nuchae* and *peau citreine* are nonspecific descriptive terms that have been used[159]; "crepelike" and "plucked-chicken" skin are other suggested descriptions.[117,120] In the later stages the skin in the involved areas becomes lax, redundant, and relatively inelastic. In women the cosmetically undesirable appearances of the skin, especially that of the neck, are often occasion

for consulting a physician. Exaggeration of nasolabial folds and chin creases is striking and may create a "hound dog" appearance of the face. The skin in the neck, axillary folds, and abdominal wall may be extremely lax. Changes in the skin of the inguinal regions and on the penis occur in some patients with PXE.

The mucous membrane of the palate frequently shows changes, which on gross and histologic examination are identical to those in the skin[59,114]; the inner aspect of the lips and the buccal mucosa are also commonly affected areas[120] (Fig. 10-4). At times the mucosa of the rectum and vagina is affected.[24] On gastroscopic examination most patients with PXE show linear or nodular submucosal lesions that are yellow and are similar to the xanthoma-like skin changes.[29,63]

In some patients the cutaneous manifestations are exceedingly mild, despite advanced ocular and arterial changes. This situation was particularly evident in South African Afrikaners with PXE[174] and in individuals described by Van Embden Andres in Holland.[167] In several instances in these persons no changes in the skin were detectable on clinical examination, yet there were positive findings on biopsy. Goodman et al.[63] described similar experiences. Rubbing or stretching of the skin

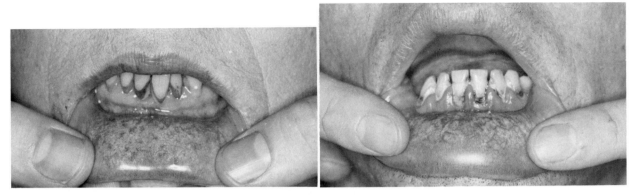

Fig. 10-4. Lesions of the labial mucosa.

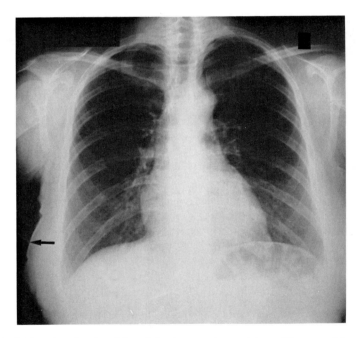

Fig. 10-5. Calcification in the skin of the breast *(arrow)* in a 35-year-old woman with PXE.

may make the lesions more evident.[120] Sometimes patients report expressing "matter" from the nodular lesions of the neck and about the chin. Suppuration and ulceration of PXE lesions have been described.[62,77,84,171]

In addition to the classic features, some patients have localized skin changes of a different type on the neck, axilla, or anterior abdominal wall. These lesions consist of large (3 by 4 cm) circinate plaques of closely grouped, hyperkeratotic papules, 1 to 2 mm in diameter. A hyperkeratotic cap can be dislodged to leave a small, bloody depression. This lesion is termed "reactive perforating elastoma" (elastoma perforans serpiginosa or Miescher elastoma).[152] The lesion occurs not only in PXE but also, occasionally, in other heritable disorders of connective tissue such as Marfan syndrome, Ehlers-Danlos syndrome (EDS), and osteogenesis imperfecta (OI).[109,148]

The skin changes about the neck were noted at

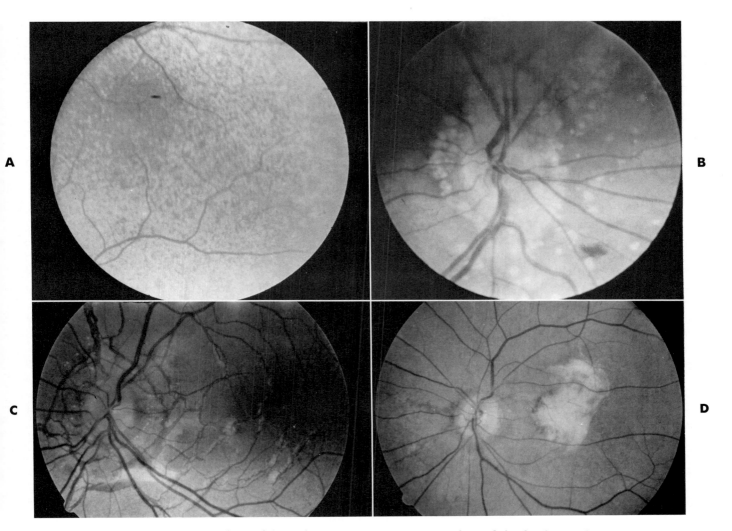

Fig. 10-6. A, Pseudoxanthoma elasticum. Pigmentary mottling of the fundus in the early stages of retinal degeneration. **B,** "Salmon spots" (colloid bodies or drusen) are evident in the fundus. These lesions are precursors of angioid streaks. **C,** Peripapillary angioid streaks are seen encircling the optic disc. **D,** Sclerotic changes and disciform scarring have occurred as a consequence of retinal hemorrhage. (**C** from Viljoen D: *J Med Genet* 25:488-490, 1988. **D** from Viljoen DL, Pope FM, Beighton P: *Clin Genet* 32:100-105, 1987.)

birth by the mother of one patient known to McKusick.[108] In others they have been recognized in early childhood. Some patients are unaware of the involvement of their skin until the changes are pointed out by the physician consulted because of complications such as failing vision or gastrointestinal hemorrhage.

Calcification in the middle and deeper layers of the dermis is identifiable by use of low-dose radiographic techniques[63,171] (Fig. 10-5). There is a ten-

dency toward keloid formation after surgery or trauma.[173] Knuckle pads have been described in cases of PXE, but it is likely that their presence was coincidental.[155]

Ocular Features

The characteristic changes in the eye are demonstrated on funduscopic examination. Some patients show only pigmentary mottling of the fundus,[63,150] which is sometimes described as *peau d'orange* of the retina. This feature is the earliest ophthalmologic manifestation of PXE (Fig. 10-6, *A*) and is thought to represent loss of regularity of the elastic fibers in Bruch membrane. These pigmentary changes were observed in 41 of 54 South African patients of Afrikaner stock during a recent survey.[171]

Progressive degeneration and fragmentation of elastic fibers leads to thickening of Bruch membrane and short interruptions in its integrity. These events give rise to the formation of "salmon spots" (colloid bodies or drusen), circular, light-colored lesions that are initially scattered in the periphery of the fundus but later become more centralized (Fig. 10-6, *B*). Salmon spots are considered the precursors of angioid streaks and are present in up to 13% of adults with PXE.[171]

It has been postulated that disruption of the elastic fibers in Bruch membrane eventually results in the formation of angioid streaks.[68,108,119,168] This term was coined initially by Knapp[93] in 1892 and reflected the view that these retinal abnormalities are "vessel like" in appearance. Angioid streaks vary from dusky red or maroon to nearly black. The absence of pigmentation in the streaks can be demonstrated by applying pressure to the eye to occlude the retinal artery.[63] Pallor of the avascular retina is produced by this maneuver and leads to virtual disappearance of the streaks. That the streaks are cracks in a membrane beneath the retina is substantiated on clinical examination by observation of their tapering and their complementary zigzag borders. They always underlie the retinal vessels and radiate from the optic disc like spokes of a wheel. If they encircle the disc, they are termed "peripapillary streaks" (Fig. 10-6, *C*). Histologic studies have confirmed that breaks in Bruch membrane, which is thickened and calcified, are the basic cause of angioid streaks.[58,92] Angioid streaks may cross the macula and fovea, and more than 50 may be present in each eye.[119] The streaks cause no visual disturbance but fundamentally weaken the retinal structures.

Secondary changes within angioid streaks are common in patients with PXE. Fibrovascular tissue from the underlying choriocapillaris layer may grow into and around the breaks, causing "cuffing," which may become apparent on retinoscopic examination.[41,108] These channels from the choriocapillaris allow the formation of neovascular membranes, which may leak and cause retinal detachment. A tendency toward frank retinal hemorrhage and subsequent disciform scarring also exists (Fig. 10-6, *D*). These sclerotic changes are probably the consequence of both fibrous "cuffing" and resolution of retinal hemorrhages, and they culminate in derangement of the light-sensitive rods and cones, leading to severe impairment of vision.

The angioid streaks are probably not present at birth, but like the skin changes, they usually develop in the second decade or later. Neldner[119] found that only 30% of a large series of individuals under 10 years of age had angioid streaks but that most persons who are more than 50 years of age with PXE have these lesions.[27,33,63,119,171] When chorioretinal scarring and accompanying retinal pigment proliferation are extensive, angioid streaks may be obscured, although distinct remnants of streaks usually persist at the periphery of such scars. Retinal hemorrhage and chorioretinal scarring have ominous implications. Blindness according to the legal definition (visual acuity of 20/200 or less) is common after the fourth decade of life in particular groups such as the Afrikaner community in South Africa.[170,171,175] Although this complication of PXE arises among other populations,[119] it is less frequent; heterogeneity in PXE is a probable explanation for this finding. Nevertheless, between 4% and 40% of all individuals with PXE may be legally blind before 50 years of age as a consequence of the effect of retinal hemorrhage on the foveal or macular areas of the retina.

In many instances retinal hemorrhage may be related to trauma, and the onset of visual symptoms after head injury in PXE has been well documented.[22,66,98] Indeed, more than 100 years ago Doyne[40] ascribed the retinal changes he had visualized to trauma only, not to the underlying disorder of PXE. Fine[48] described 28 patients with PXE and macular hemorrhages, seven of whom sustained trauma to the orbit 24 hours before the onset of visual loss. It may be unusual, however, for retinal hemorrhage after injury to develop in young persons with PXE, since this complication has been reported in only a few young individuals.[98,119,158,171]

In some instances the use of xenon photocoagulation or argon laser therapy for the treatment of neovascular membrane formation appears to have beneficial effects. Conversely, prophylactic photocoagulation of the angioid streaks may make the situation worse.[27]

Although angioid streaks are the ocular hallmark of PXE, not infrequently a less specific central chorioretinitis only is present.[13,167] Indeed, this may have been the case with Chauffard's famous patient. Like the hemorrhages, the central chorioretinitis is a grave threat to vision because of involvement of the macular areas.[4]

Cardiovascular System

On clinical examination the arterial involvement is expressed by pulse volume changes and symptoms of arterial insufficiency in the limbs, by symptoms of coronary insufficiency, by hemorrhage in one or more of many different areas, and by hypertension. On radiographic study evidence of premature medial calcification of peripheral arteries is present (Fig. 10-7).

Weakness or absence of pulses in the extremities is a frequent finding, and fatigability or frank intermittent claudication may occur in the legs. The development of these manifestations by the third decade of life or earlier and the involvement of both the arms and the legs aid in the differentiation of these changes from those of ordinary arteriosclerosis.

The radial or ulnar pulse, or both, are frequently absent in patients with PXE, and arterial pulsation in an anomalous position near the middle of the volar surface of the wrist may substitute for the normal pulse. Although ischemic symptoms are unusual in the upper limbs, especially when considered in relation to the high frequency of drastic angiographic changes, easy fatigability of the arms, for example, in washing clothes, may occur.[32] Ischemic resorption of the terminal phalangeal tufts and the need for surgical amputation of digits[85] have been reported. By means of angiography several authors have demonstrated narrowing or occlusion of radial or ulnar arteries, or both, as well as dilation of the interosseous arteries.[25,63] In cases of occluded radial and ulnar arteries, terminal collaterals from the interosseous arteries provided apparently adequate filling of the arterial system in the hand. These changes are illustrated in Fig. 10-8. Selective diminution of blood supply to a finger was depicted by James, Eaton, and Blazek.[85]

The pulse-wave velocity in the arteries of the

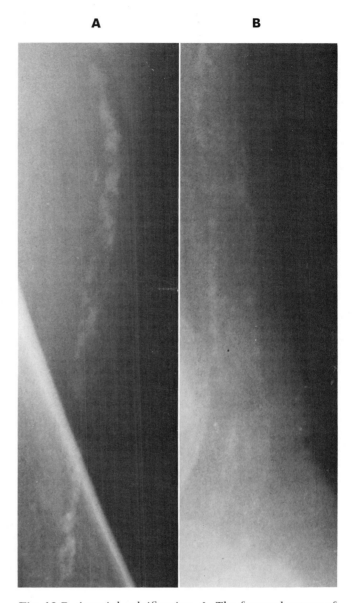

A　　　　　**B**

Fig. 10-7. Arterial calcification. **A,** The femoral artery of a 52-year-old man shows intimal (dense patches) and medial (fine mottling) calcification. **B,** The radial artery of a 58-year-old man shows medial calcification. (From Goodman RM et al: *Medicine* 42:297-339, 1963.)

limbs is diminished in most persons with PXE.[24,167] The pulse wave is, furthermore, of reduced amplitude and has a plateau configuration. The dicrotic notch may be lost, and the peak is attained more slowly than normal.[6] A 9-year-old child studied by Bafverstedt and Lund[6] showed these changes in

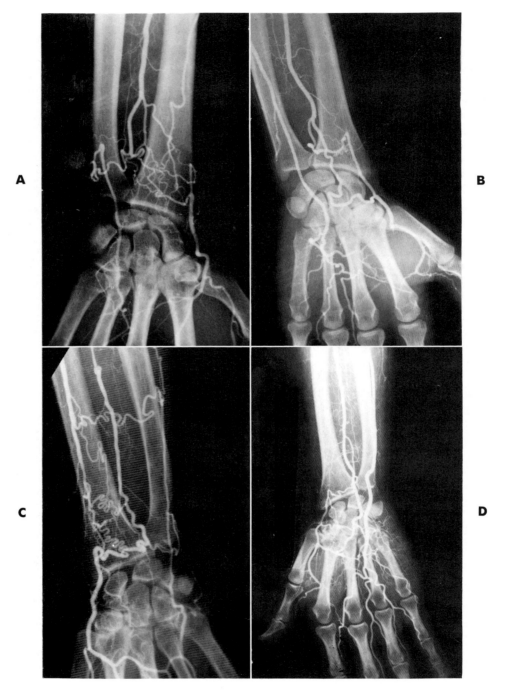

Fig. 10-8. Findings of brachial arteriography in patients with PXE. **A,** Obstruction of both the radial and the ulnar artery, with refilling from a dilated interosseous artery in a 65-year-old man. **B,** Obstruction of the radial artery, with refilling from the interosseous artery in a 33-year-old man. **C,** Occlusion, narrowing, and irregularity of the main forearm arteries, with marked collateral formation in a 54-year-old woman. **D,** Occlusion of the radial artery in a 50-year-old woman.

the pulse curves, despite normal arteriograms, which suggests that occlusive changes are not essential to the alterations in these waves but that changes in the arterial wall compliance are involved.

Angina pectoris,[55] electrocardiographic changes compatible with myocardial ischemia, radiographic evidence of coronary artery calcification,[120] and myocardial infarction have been observed in patients with PXE and leave little doubt that the coronary arteries are involved in this disorder.

Przybojewski et al.[132] described a man with angina and PXE in whom coronary arteriography was performed. Neither atherosclerosis nor calcification could be demonstrated. Endocardial biopsy showed an absence of coronary arterioles, and the authors postulated that much of the mechanical and electric disturbance of cardiac function in patients with PXE can be attributed to "small coronary arteriopathy" without involvement of the larger epicardial coronary arteries. In contrast to these findings, Levine described a girl who had onset of angina pectoris at the age of 11 years.[108] Coronary arteriograms made when the patient was 18 years of age showed disease of three vessels; a triple graft was performed when the patient was 19 years of age, with satisfactory results.

Mitral valve prolapse has been reported in individuals with PXE; prevalence varied between 4%[119] and 71%.[97] Ten patients in a South African series had a diagnosis of mitral valve prolapse, but no adverse sequelae were associated with this diagnosis.[171] In connective tissue disorders such as Marfan syndrome, EDS, OI, and PXE, mitral valve prolapse is common and not always innocuous.[97,124] Several complications that may have severe consequences in persons with PXE may arise in association with mitral valve prolapse, including supraventricular tachycardia, cerebral ischemic events, and mitral valve incompetence.[124]

Hemorrhage constitutes the major medical problem in most cases of PXE that come to the attention of the internist. Gastrointestinal hemorrhage reportedly is common[90] and may be fatal.[68,164] In this context two large series of PXE patients surprisingly failed to reveal one person with gastrointestinal hemorrhage attributable to the disorder.[38,171] Thus the many reports of hemorrhage in patients with PXE may represent an as-

certainment bias of a relatively infrequent, although dramatic, event.

Hemorrhages may occur as a result of a lesion such as peptic ulcer or hiatal hernia, which per se can produce hemorrhage, but in most cases of PXE the source of gastrointestinal bleeding is not evident on clinical or gastroscopic study. Superficial ulceration has occasionally been discovered by gastroscopic study[102] or during gastrectomy,[90] and hemorrhage from the jejunum has been described.[142] McKusick encountered gastrointestinal bleeding in a patient with PXE younger than 7 years of age,[108] and hematemesis in patients 3 years of age[169] and 12 years of age[61] has been described.

Some individuals have repeated abdominal surgery for exploration of unexplained bleeding and repair of some lesion such as hiatal hernia, which may or may not be incidental. The reports of massive gastrointestinal hemorrhage during pregnancy in four women with PXE suggest that pregnancy has an aggravating influence.[107,178] These occurrences may be isolated events, and no instances of excessive bleeding occurred in 64 pregnancies in 22 South African women with PXE.[171]

In addition to gastrointestinal bleeding, hemorrhage may be subarachnoid, retinal, renal, uterine,[167] vesical, or nasal. Subarachnoid hemorrhage is occasionally a cause of death in individuals with PXE.[82,149] Fasshauer et al.[46] described a 59-year-old patient with multiple cerebral infarcts. Spontaneous hemarthroses rarely occur.[167] Excessive bleeding from cutaneous lacerations does not seem to be a problem, although hemorrhages in the skin lesions have been described.[57,103] Foerster's patient[53] sought medical advice because of purpura on the legs and, later, on the left forearm. McKusick studied a patient with PXE who had a severe illness diagnosed as "black (hemorrhagic) measles" at the age of 16 years.[108] It is possible that the connective tissue abnormality was responsible for the hemorrhagic manifestations of the measles in this individual.

Hypertension is frequently found in patients with PXE, and in some instances it has been convincingly shown to be the result of vascular disease of the PXE type in the renal vessels. The occurrence of hypertension is unfortunate because of its aggravating influence on the tendency toward cerebral hemorrhage. Dixon[39] reported a 29-year-old patient with an intracranial "berry" aneurysm in association with skin changes and angioid streaks. Scheie and Hogan[146] documented a similar case. Another patient, who was reported twice, had severe hypertension and pronounced albuminuria and died of cerebral hemorrhage at the age of 43 years.[83,137]

Cerebrovascular accident in a 40-year-old man has been reported.[95] A teenager with severe hypertension and calcification of both renal arteries was known to McKusick.[108] Parker et al.[122] reported two sisters with PXE in whom the initial manifestation was hypertension, which occurred in one at 10 years of age and in the other at 6 years of age. Farreras-Valenti et al.[45] described "unilateral renal hypertension" associated with an angiomatous change in the posterior branch of the right renal artery in a 27-year-old man with severe hypertension. Right nephrectomy resulted in cure. Bardsley and Koehler[8] observed the same type of angiomatous change in the abdominal viscera in two patients with PXE. In

one it involved an intrahepatic artery and the splenic artery above the left kidney.

Second to gastrointestinal hemorrhage, abdominal angina resulting from celiac artery stenosis is probably the most frequent abdominal complication in patients with PXE. The symptoms usually consist of pain that begins within 40 to 45 minutes after eating. Gallbladder disease is often mistakenly suspected.

Calcification in peripheral arteries (both arms and legs) has been recognized on radiographic examination by a number of observers.* Both medial and intimal calcification can be demonstrated (Fig. 10-7). Arterial calcification in childhood may occur; Wolff, Stokes, and Schlesinger[177] documented a 9-year-old child affected by repeated attacks of melena in whom intermittent claudica-

---

*References 24, 63, 131, 143, 145, 151, 177, and 180.

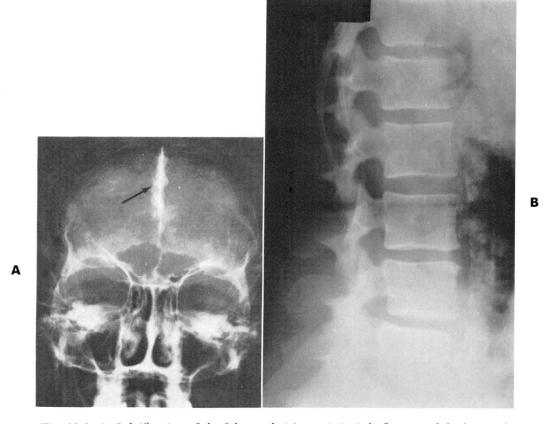

Fig. 10-9. A, Calcification of the falx cerebri *(arrow).* **B,** Calcification of the lower abdominal aorta in a 35-year-old woman.

tion and loss of pulsations in the distal arteries of the limbs were associated with calcification of the arteries; a brother, 25 years of age, had similar manifestations. Arterial changes may be evident in infancy; arterial calcification has been observed in a 2-year-old infant boy with PXE who was admitted to the hospital with septicemia.[171] During the illness swelling and tenderness of both arms developed, and radiographs of the radius and ulna were obtained to exclude osteomyelitis. Calcification of the radial and ulnar arteries was demonstrated; this abnormality disappeared within 4 weeks of resolution of his illness. Subsequently, typical dermatologic and vascular signs of PXE developed. The cause of vascular calcification in this infant was not determined, but it presumably was related to the PXE.

In a 31-year-old woman Nellen and Jacobson[120] demonstrated calcification of the coronary arteries on radiographic examination. Calcification of the choroid plexus, falx cerebri (Fig. 10-9, A), and posterior clinoid processes has been documented. Other sites of blood vessel calcification reported in patients with PXE are carotid artery aneurysms,[146] the aortic arch and its branches,[100] the abdominal aorta (Fig. 10-9, B), and in the bifurcation of this vessel.[108]

Dilation of the aorta has been mentioned in several reports of patients with PXE,[86,104] but it is uncertain whether this finding bears a direct relationship to the fundamental defect of PXE.

Gynecologic and Obstetric Features

A study of the gynecologic manifestations in 27 women with PXE revealed an increased propensity for menorrhagia and pelvic ligament laxity.[171] The latter feature in four persons with PXE led to surgical repair of rectocele or cystocele, or both, and confirms McKusick's contention that abiotrophy of elastic fibers occurs as a result of PXE.[108] Pelvic ligament laxity was particularly evident in women who had had several pregnancies.

Gastrointestinal hemorrhage was recorded in eight of 24 pregnancies in women with PXE whose cases were reviewed by Berde, Willis, and Sandberg.[15] Lao, Walters, and De Swiet[96] briefly outlined the case histories of two pregnant women with PXE, one of whom had mild hypertension, and Elejalde et al.[43] described a pregnancy in detail, with special emphasis on the fetal ultrasonographic findings. Other authors have alluded to

obstetric complications in patients with PXE,[3,70] but the data presented have been insufficient for analysis. In an investigation involving 64 pregnancies in 22 women with PXE, Viljoen[171] documented two adverse factors: a moderately increased risk of first-trimester miscarriage (25%) exists, and most women with PXE claimed a deterioration in the cosmetic appearance of the abdominal skin during pregnancy. Gastrointestinal hemorrhage and complications resulting from hypertension were not encountered. The former finding may reflect a bias in previous reports in which only abnormal confinements may have been described. In the previously mentioned obstetric investigation the level and control of blood pressure improved with the duration of pregnancy in those women with hypertension, suggesting that the increasing low-resistance vascular bed provided by the placenta may have helped in lowering blood pressure levels. An additional important finding in this study was that only one of 48 live-born babies had a congenital malformation (a severe cardiac anomaly), which led to death at 4 days of age. Since the rate of congenital abnormalities in all neonates is considered to be from 1% to 2%, it appears from these data that maternal PXE does not increase the risk of congenital malformation.

A contentious issue in the care of women with PXE is the choice of the method of birth control. Oral contraceptives containing high levels of estrogen are known to increase the risk of deep-vein thromboses. In view of the additional risks of embolic and hemorrhagic complications in persons with PXE, estrogenic compounds administered for the purpose of pregnancy prevention are probably best avoided and methods such as the use of an intrauterine device are advocated for women with PXE.[172]

Other Features

Joint manifestations are conspicuously absent in persons with PXE. Sairanen, Itkonen, and Kangas[141] reported polyarthritis beginning at the age of 65 years in a man with PXE, but the condition may have been coincidental. Immunoglobulin levels (IgG and IgA) were reportedly elevated in eight patients with PXE,[87] but this finding has not been confirmed in subsequent investigations.[119] Psychiatric disorders seem to occur with abnormally high frequency in patients with PXE.[64] It is difficult to know whether these can be explained on the basis of cerebrovascular involvement. Cer-

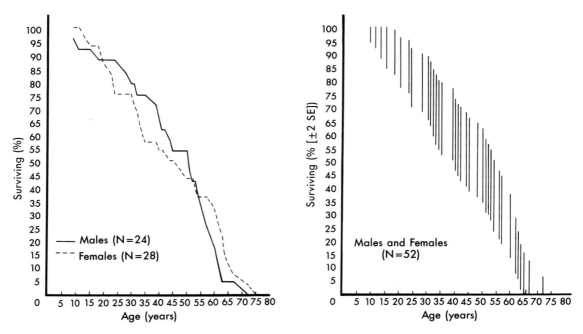

Fig. 10-10. Survivorship analysis in PXE, based on 52 cases.

tainly the high incidence of neurologic abnormalities is attributable to the vascular disease and hypertension. The neurologic abnormalities are highly variable, yet per se they are not unlike those customarily encountered in patients with advanced arteriosclerosis or hypertension, or both. The unusual feature is the relatively early age at which the neurologic accidents and deterioration occur.

Complete dental clearance because of excessive caries was recorded in 30 of 39 individuals with PXE in one study.[171] It was postulated that the small nutrient arteries of the teeth may be compromised by arteriosclerosis in PXE patients, leading to enamel deterioration and decay.

Mortality

In some patients death occurs at an early age as a result of the occlusive or hemorrhagic complications of arterial involvement in PXE. Indeed, McKusick recorded the case of a 13-year-old who died after frequent massive gastrointestinal hemorrhages.[108] McKusick also pointed out that other individuals survive beyond 70 years of age and die of causes probably unrelated to the generalized connective tissue disorder. A life-table type of

analysis of survivorship in 52 cases from the records of the Johns Hopkins Hospital is shown in Fig. 10-10.

DIFFERENTIAL DIAGNOSIS

Angioid streaks are most frequently found in patients with PXE but have also been reported in patients with many other conditions (see the box on p. 349, top). Other than PXE the most commonly associated disorders are Paget disease of bone[116] and the sickle cell hemoglobinopathies. Paget disease of bone, in which progressive bony deformity develops and in which the serum alkaline phosphatase value is elevated, is easily distinguishable from PXE. Angioid streaks usually appear after 60 years of age in about 8% to 15% of patients with Paget disease.[27,147,160] Progression to retinal hemorrhage and retinal sclerosis occurs in a minority of individuals.

Retinopathy in sickle cell disease has been recognized since 1959[99] and is said to occur in 1% to 2% of affected individuals.[27] The frequency of angioid streaks increases with age, and they are seldom apparent before early adulthood. Complications of hemorrhage and retinal detachment seldom occur. The disorders listed in the box

---

Systemic Conditions with Angioid Streaks

Acromegaly
Ehlers-Danlos syndrome
Diabetes mellitus
Hemochromatosis
Acquired hemolytic anemia
Hypercalcemia
Hyperphosphatasia
Lead poisoning
Neurofibromatosis type I
Paget disease
Senile elastosis
Sickle cell hemoglobinopathies
Sturge-Weber syndrome
Tuberous sclerosis

From Clarkson JG, Altman RD: *Surv Ophthalmol* 26:235-246, 1982.

Disorders Mimicking Cutaneous PXE

Solar or actinic elastosis
Aging process
Penicillamine therapy
Tumoral calcinosis
Hypervitaminosis D
Cutis Laxa
Exogenous exposure to calcium salts
Periumbilical perforating PXE
Elastosis perforans serpiginosa
Elastic tissue nevus

---

on this page, top, are usually readily identified by their characteristic clinical manifestations.

The most important disorders in which the dermatologic features are similar to those of PXE are listed in the box on this page, bottom.

Solar or actinic elastosis is an acquired process in which the skin degenerates as a result of excessive and prolonged exposure to sunlight. In this disorder large amounts of amorphous elastic-staining material accumulate in clumps in the upper dermis; this appearance contrasts with the histologic features seen in cases of PXE, in which the changes in elastic fibers occur predominantly in the middle and deep dermal structures. On clinical examination the stigmata of actinic elastosis and mild PXE are similar,[153] especially in sun-exposed flexural regions. However, PXE can usually be differentiated by the presence of peau d'orange changes that occur in nonexposed areas and by the associated characteristic changes in the retina and cardiovascular system.

The normal aging process of skin can closely mimic the changes seen in PXE. The elastic fibers in the former tend to mineralize and swell with age, but frank disruption, calcification, and clumping of these structures is infrequent. Patients with Wilson disease, a hereditary disorder of copper metabolism, frequently receive penicillamine treatment for prolonged periods. The drug is a potent chelator of copper and, through disruption of lysyl-oxidase links in the trophoelastin molecule, produces a generalized, yellowish papular rash and a tendency for the skin to become lax.[14,76,111] Differentiation is usually easily made, since individuals receiving penicillamine lack the ocular manifestations and cardiovascular changes usually seen in patients with PXE. Cutis Laxa may mimic PXE, since skin redundancy can be a prominent feature in both disorders.

Exposure to exogenous calcium salts, especially calcium chloride in road workers and coal miners, has infrequently produced localized PXE-like lesions.[28,179] This condition is easily differentiated by the history of exposure and the localization of the skin abnormalities

An unusual and infrequent disorder occurring predominantly in multiparous, obese black women was described by Hicks, Carpenter, and Reed[78] and designated "periumbilical perforating PXE." Periumbilical lesions resembling PXE, as well as several instances of perforating transepidermal elimination papules, developed in the affected persons. Other than a high incidence of hypertension in these individuals, none of the ocular and cardiovascular stigmata associated with PXE was apparent.

Occasionally elastosis perforans serpiginosa may be confused with PXE.[134] The lesions usually occur in the cervical region and consist of grouped, slightly keratotic, shiny papules that are readily differentiated from PXE lesions on histologic examination. As the name "pseudoxanthoma elasticum" implies, physicians at the end of the nineteenth century had difficulty in distinguishing the condition from the xanthomatoses and other lipid storage disorders. The subsequent discovery of ocular and vascular manifestations in many patients with PXE has reduced the number of conditions with which it may be confused, and most are now easily identified.

PATHOLOGY

Confirmation of a diagnosis of PXE can be made by tissue biopsy, usually of skin, and histologic demonstration of characteristic fragmentation, disruption, and calcification of elastic fibers of the middle and deep zones of the coria (Fig. 10-11). The use of hematoxylin-eosin staining in biopsy specimens permits the demonstration of these changes in PXE lesions that are well established. Less affected elastic fibers with mild calcification can be detected more readily with the von Kossa stain, which is specific for carbonate and phosphate radicals of calcium. The Verhoeff–van Gieson stain is specific for elastic fiber, but this tissue only takes up the stain after fragmentation of the fiber, which occurs late in the pathogenesis of the disorder. By use of these three basic stains, a positive diagnosis of PXE can be made at any stage of the disease process.

After rupture of the elastic fiber has occurred, a granular material is evident on microscopic examination in the lower dermis. Occasionally, rodlike structures are seen, whereas tuberculoid areas with giant cells occur in the area of degeneration. Calcification of the degenerated material may be pronounced,[50,101] and actual bone formation may occur.[10] Goodman et al.[63] have presented evidence that calcium deposition in elastic fibers is the earliest demonstrable histopathologic change in cases of PXE. For example, elastic fibers surrounding sweat glands may show early changes. Later, the

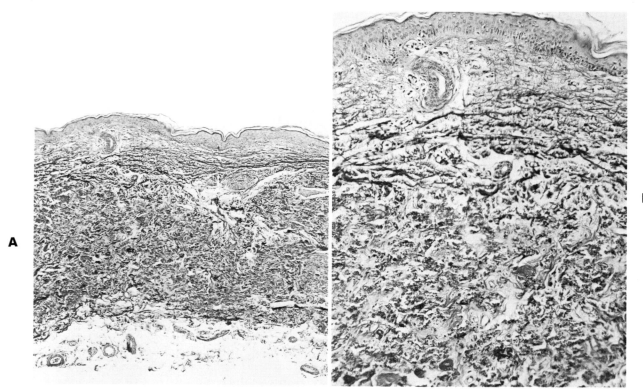

Fig. 10-11. A, Fragmentation and calcification of elastin fibers are evident in the corium by use of an elastic tissue stain (magnification × 50). **B,** Disruption of the elastin fibers is shown (magnification × 125).

elastic fibers become fragmented (Fig. 10-12). Exposure of the tissue section to collagenase does not alter the appearance of the foci of calcified elastic fibers. Elastase, however, removes many of the elastic fiber ends that project from the edge of large concretions. Densely calcified fibers are usually not affected by elastase treatment.

The ultrastructural composition of skin in patients with PXE has been examined repeatedly in numerous investigations by use of transmission and scanning analysis techniques.[37,75,79,140] Electron microscopic studies demonstrate that the site of primary involvement in PXE is the elastic fiber and that a process of degeneration unique to the disorder ensues. The normal elastic fiber is a nonhomogeneous structure with peripheral microfibrils and small, electron-dense deposits throughout the fiber. In PXE a characteristic solid, central core of material appears, which represents mineralization with carbonate and phosphate cal-

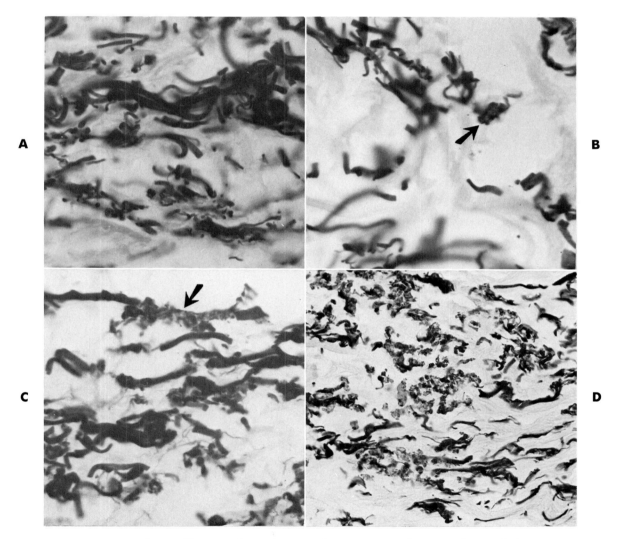

Fig. 10-12. Elastic fibers in skin. **A,** Normal. **B,** Arrow indicates a focus of altered elastic tissue in the skin of a patient with PXE. **C,** More extensive granular degenerative change in PXE. Arrow indicates granular appearance of elastic fiber. **D,** Advanced elastic tissue change in PXE.

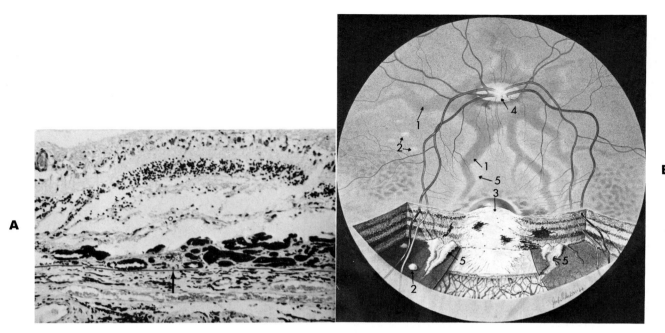

Fig. 10-13. A, Histopathologic appearance of angioid streaks. Bruch membrane is indicated by the arrow. Breaks are shown in the right of the illustration. **B,** Diagram correlating the funduscopic and histologic features of the eye in PXE. *1,* Angioid streaks. *2,* Drusen of Bruch membrane. *3,* Mound of vascularized scar tissue at the macula. *4,* Hyaline body of the optic disc. *5,* Fibrous tissue cuffing an angioid streak. In the lower part of the diagram the retina is shown in cross-section and between two angioid streaks. Bruch membrane and the choriocapillaris have been cut away, showing the pattern of underlying choroidal vessels. (Courtesy David Paton, MD.)

cium salts. The process progresses in the central core, and the outer rim of the fiber thickens. Eventually the elastic fiber becomes enormously enlarged to the point of rupture and fragmentation, discharging its contents into the surrounding dermis.[171]

Most histologic studies of the eye* have shown basophilia and tears in the lamina elastica of Bruch membrane (Fig. 10-13, *A*). No primary abnormality is observed in the inner cuticular layer of Bruch membrane.[113] Advanced sclerotic changes have been found in the choroidal vessels. When tears are present in Bruch membrane, scar tissue tends to occupy the breaks or extend beneath the pigment epithelium[36] (Fig. 10-13, *B*). The breaks correspond to the streaks seen on funduscopic examination. Basophilia of the lam-

---
*References 12, 21, 58, 68, 92, and 168.

ina elastica is not infrequent in the eyes of elderly individuals, although it occurs more regularly and at a younger age in persons with PXE. Descemet membrane of the cornea has chemical, physical, and tinctorial resemblances to the lamina elastica of Bruch membrane. However, clinical or histologic evidence of involvement of the cornea has apparently not been recorded in cases of PXE.

Gross and histologic studies of the cardiovascular system in persons with PXE are few. In the original case of Balzer[7] whitish thickening of the endocardium of the right atrium was described, as well as plaques of the same description on the pericardium and on the ventricular endocardium. On histologic examination degeneration, thought to involve elastic elements, was demonstrated at these sites and in the walls of the pulmonary alveoli. McKusick mentioned identical changes in two

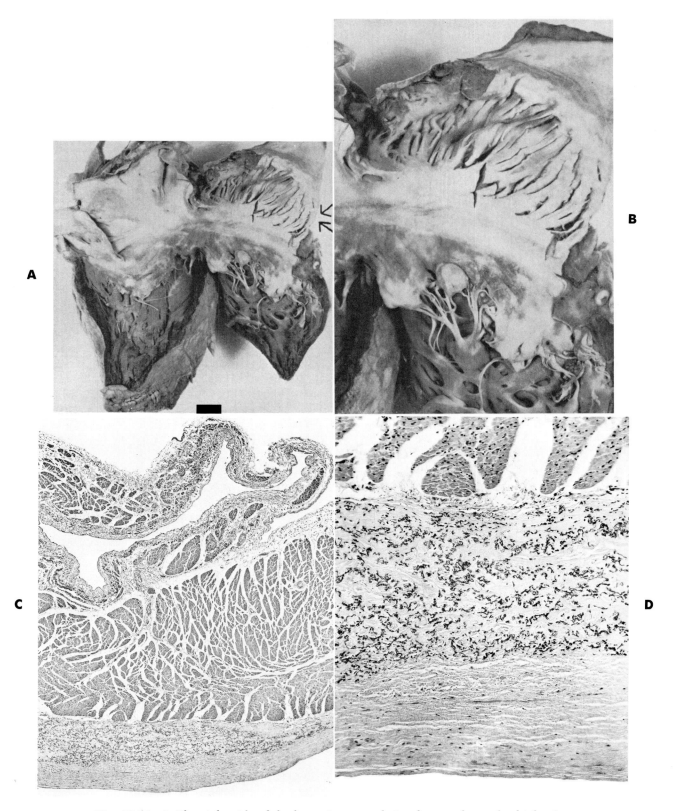

Fig. 10-14. A, The right side of the heart is exposed. An abnormal, pearly thickening of the endocardium with yellowish, irregular nodules is in the area indicated by the arrows. The latter lesions are similar to those in the skin. **B,** Enlarged view of part of the heart shown in **A. C,** Wall of the right atrium. One of the opaque elevated plaques is seen in section, stained with hematoxylin and eosin (magnification × 25). **D,** An enlarged view of part of the field seen in **C** (magnification × 100). Striking similarity to the changes in the skin is evident.

of five cases in which autopsy was performed[108] (Fig. 10-14). Histologic changes interpreted as degeneration of elastic fibers were described in the coronary, renal, pancreatic, uterine, cutaneous, and mesenteric arteries, as well as in the splenic trabeculae, hepatic veins, and Bruch membrane of the eye.

Widening of major blood vessels such as the aorta and the brachial and cerebral arteries has been reported.[86,104] Coffman and Sommers[31] thought specific aortic changes occurred in their patient, and they also attributed valvular disease to PXE; mitral stenosis in one other individual was thought to have this basis.[108]

Mitral valve prolapse occurs in some patients with PXE, as in other connective tissue disorders such as Marfan syndrome and EDS. The first description of "snapping" systolic sounds in cases of PXE was made by Coffman and Sommers[31] in 1959. Lebwohl et al.[97] found echocardiographic evidence in 10 of 14 patients, and Pyeritz[133] reported similar findings. Autopsy findings of fibroelastotic changes involving the mitral valve probably account for prolapse and, in some instances, stenosis.

Early coronary artery disease resulting from fibrous intimal changes has been documented in two adolescents[18,144] and fibrous thickening of the atria, ventricles, and atrioventricular valves in association with congestive heart failure has been reported.[118] Other findings include calcification of the deep endocardial layer,[110] degeneration of the small intramural coronary vessels,[132] and widespread calcification of the coronary vessels in a 6-week-old infant.[72] The infant's mother had PXE, but there was no evidence of the disorder in the baby.

Other blood vessels in which elastic fiber degeneration and calcification have been reported are the thyroid arteries,[91] the ulnar vessels,[145] the vessel of the stomach,[35,52,178] and the vessels in the peritonsillar tissues of one patient.[137]

Degenerative changes involving the elastic fibers in the walls of the pulmonary alveoli have occasionally been documented,[7] as has miliary mottling of the lungs.[177] It is possible that repeated small interstitial hemorrhages with resultant hemosiderosis are responsible for the latter findings. Calcification in small vessels is another possible explanation. No abnormality of residual air volume, maximum breathing capacity, or vital capacity has been attributed to PXE.[167]

In the fourth edition of this book McKusick described autopsy findings in five patients.[108] Other investigators who have reported post mortem details concerning persons with PXE are Prick,[130] Urbach and Wolfram,[166] and Carlborg et al.[25] Navarro-Lopez et al.[118] reviewed the cardiac manifestations of PXE in 15 cases in which autopsy was performed.

Many patients with PXE have advanced and premature arterial changes indistinguishable from ordinary atherosclerosis and arteriosclerosis. By producing changes in the tunica media, PXE probably sets the stage for the development of intimal changes unusually early in life and to an unusually severe degree.

BASIC DEFECT

Whether PXE is a dystrophy of elastic fibers or of collagen fibers has been much debated. Certainly the degenerate material that develops in the skin has certain tinctorial characteristics of elastin. The accumulated evidence now indicates that the defect is indeed one primarily of the elastic fiber, as initially proposed in 1896 by Darier.[36] The degenerated material found in the deep dermal layers has a striking resemblance to elastic tissue. According to Rodnan, Fisher, and Warren[139] and Moran and Lansing,[115] this claim is supported by the presence of brilliant autofluorescence, lack of periodicity in ultrastructure, susceptibility to digestion by elastase, inhibition of affinity for elastic tissue dyes after methylation, and strong proclivity to calcium incrustation. Other electron microscopic studies also support the elastic fiber theory.[75,79]

Elastic fibers are comprised of two distinct components, a more abundant amorphous component (elastin) and the microfibrillar component. Elastin is composed largely of glycine, proline, and other hydrophobic residues and contains multiple lysine-derived cross-links such as desmosines, which link the individual polypeptide chains into a rubberlike network. The hydrophobic regions of the chains between the cross-links are highly mobile. The hydrophobic and cross-linking domains are coded by separate, small (27 to 114 bp) exons that are separated by large introns. The initial translation product is a 72,000-dalton polypeptide, designated "tropoelastin."

An increase in the total amount of elastic fibers in PXE-affected dermis has been much debated but is generally thought to exist.[75,123] The cause of increased elastogenesis is unknown, but it may be due to destruction and loss of calcified elastic fibers.[119] The latter phenomenon is not age related but could reflect abnormalities of the elastic fiber itself.[105]

Calcification of the elastic fibers has been viewed as a secondary phenomenon comparable to the calcification of degenerated tissues that occurs in chronic inflammation, atherosclerosis, and hematomas. Goodman et al.,[63] after finding that calcium accretion on elastic fibers is the earliest demonstrable histologic change, proposed that deposition of calcium may lead to brittleness and subsequent fracture of these fibers. If this view of the pathogenesis is accurate, the issue of the nature of the basic defect resolves itself into the question of what causes the increased affinity of the elastic fibers for calcium. Smith, Davidson, and Taylor[154] concluded that an increase of acid mucopolysaccharides, particularly hyaluronic acid and, to some extent, chondroitin sulfate B (dermatan sulfate), is involved in the calcification process. Johnson and Helwig[88] also concluded that hyaluronic acid coats the elastic fibers and is implicated in calcification.

Findlay[49] reported that the enzyme elastase removes the degenerate material from sections of skin in patients with PXE. An earlier objection was that elastase is not entirely specific; for example, it is said to dissolve mucoproteins and therefore to behave fundamentally as a mucase. Furthermore, other studies indicate that elastase has some effects on normal collagen.[108] Elastase has been purified, and it has been demonstrated that elastase digestion is relatively specific for elastic tissue. Serum elastase levels are known to decrease with age by up to 35%,[69] but this factor has not been studied in patients with PXE over a broad age range. A role for elastase or elastase inhibitor in the pathogenesis of PXE cannot be confirmed or refuted.

The pathogenesis of angioid streaks, although unresolved, is probably related to calcification of elastic fibers within Bruch membrane, which renders them brittle and predisposed to the development of cracks.[27] The initial studies of Böck[21] and Hagedoorn[68] of the eyes in patients with PXE showed evidence of basophilia and calcification of Bruch membrane that corresponded to the clinical location of the angioid streaks. Adelung[1] demonstrated that the lines of force within the eye, which result from the pull of the intrinsic and extrinsic ocular muscles on the relatively fixed side of the optic nerve, have the same configuration as the peripapillary interlacement and radial extensions of angioid streaks. Such forces, acting on a weakened Bruch membrane, may account for the distribution of angioid streaks.

Pseudoxanthoma elasticum is likely to be heterogeneous, and patients with the autosomal recessive form of the disorder may have some sort of enzyme defect. McKusick suggested that some as yet unidentified metabolic defect damages the elastic fibers in such a way that degeneration occurs.[108] A further alternative is that an enzyme important to the integrity of the elastic fiber protein or a substance closely associated with it may be deficient. Neldner[119] proposed that since the fibroblast made all the connective tissue components, including the enzymes required for their ultimate metabolic turnover, this cell most likely was the source of the abnormal structural protein or enzyme in PXE.

A structural defect of elastin may well exist in persons with autosomal dominant PXE. A structural abnormality of the elastic fiber would make it more susceptible to degenerative changes and calcification, which occur in PXE. However, posttranslational events may also have a pathogenetic role in elastic fiber degeneration. Details regarding molecular investigations in patients with PXE are discussed further in the section, Laboratory Investigations.

DISTRIBUTION, PREVALENCE, AND SEX PREDISPOSITION

The disorder is widely distributed and has been described in persons in many European countries[104]; it has also been observed in Japanese.[121] Four autopsies at the Johns Hopkins Hospital recorded by McKusick[108] were in affected blacks, and several other black patients with PXE have been reported.[55,56,112] Some indication of the frequency of PXE is provided by the following facts: 125 instances of associated skin and fundus changes and 68 cases with skin changes alone had been described before 1910[159]; more than 1000 persons with PXE have now been reported.

Berlyne, Bulmer, and Platt[16] estimated the frequency to be between 1 in 160,000 and 1 in 1 million persons. McKusick considered that PXE occurs with greater frequency than 1 in 160,000.[108] Viljoen[171] calculated a minimum prevalence of 1 in 23,000 for PXE within the Afrikaner population of South Africa.[171] Founder effect was proven within this community in a detailed genealogic investigation.[162] Although ascertainment of all persons with PXE was not complete, minimum prevalences of PXE in South Africa were estimated at 1 in 120,000 for whites, 1 in 330,000 for the mixed-ancestry group, and 1 in 650,000 for blacks. These calculations imply that a heterozygous gene frequency as high as 1 in 76 for the Afrikaner population may exist (1 in 289 for the mixed-ancestry group and 1 in 408 for blacks) and that homozygous persons with PXE may number 250 persons in a total population of 30 million individuals.

Tabulations of cases of PXE in the literature show a preponderance of affected women and girls.[30,42,119,164,171] Since women are more prone to seek medical advice, especially regarding the cosmetic problems created by the skin involvement, the apparent female preponderance may be spurious. A review of 106 cases from the Mayo Clinic showed a male-to-female ratio of 1:1.2.[33] Within this group there were 32 with angioid streaks only; the male-to-female ratio in the latter group was 2.2:1. In a literature review of 200 cases, Eddy and Farber[42] found a male-to-female ratio of 1:1.7, whereas Neldner's patients[119] were more disparate, with a ratio of 1:2.33. The male-to-female ratio in a South African series was 1:1.53.[171]

GENETICS

Pseudoxanthoma elasticum has long been considered a heritable disorder of connective tissue, and in most literature contributions before 1970 the condition was thought to be inherited as an autosomal recessive trait. Increased frequency of parental consanguinity,* the occurrence of multiple affected sibs, and the rarity of the disorder in successive generations[31,80,108] supported this supposition.

Discussion regarding possible heterogeneity in PXE followed several reports describing individuals with PXE in two generations of a single kindred.[16,60,176] In the opinion of Wise,[176] who found 20 examples of parent-child transmission, this indicated the existence of a dominant form of PXE. Other investigators also have reported PXE kindreds with autosomal dominant inheritance.[35] In the fourth edition of this book McKusick postulated that these individuals may have represented "quasidominance" or "pseudodominance" or that the cause may have been the mating of a homozygote with a heterozygous carrier of the gene (Fig. 10-15). An alternative explanation was "the occasional expression in the heterozygote."

It remained for Pope's extensive studies[126] in England and Wales to demonstrate that PXE truly is a genetically heterogeneous entity. Pope delin-

---

*References 54, 74, 106, 114, 161, and 167.

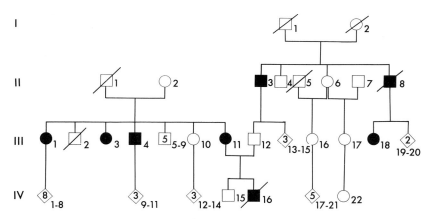

Fig. 10-15. The pedigree of a South African kindred showing "pseudodominant" inheritance between patients II,8 and III,18 and individuals III,11 and IV,16.

eated two autosomal recessive[128] and two autosomal dominant[127] forms of the disorder. The characteristic features of persons with the more common type I autosomal recessive form of PXE were moderate eye, cardiac, and skin manifestations, whereas the rare type II autosomal recessive group had severe cutaneous features only. Individuals with autosomal dominant type II PXE had mild cardiac manifestations associated with a marfanoid habitus. Persons with the less prevalent autosomal dominant type I PXE had severe cardiac complications but lacked the marfanoid features. To substantiate his findings, Pope[129] was able to confirm genetic heterogeneity in previously reported PXE patients by means of a retrospective search of the literature.

As with other connective tissue disorders, problems have arisen concerning syndromic boundaries, classification, and nomenclature. These difficulties were addressed at a workshop held during the Seventh International Congress of Human Genetics in Berlin in 1986.[11] A concensus now known as the Berlin nosology was published; the section relating to PXE is given in the box below.

A further apparently autonomous entity in which serious ophthalmologic complications occurred was subsequently described in the Afri-

kaner population of South Africa by Viljoen, Pope, and Beighton [174] in 1987. On pedigree analysis of 58 affected persons, it was apparent that this latter condition is inherited as an autosomal recessive trait and occurred with a high prevalence in the Afrikaner population. The Afrikaner antecedents were derived from Western European countries and consisted mainly of Dutch, German, and French Huguenot settlers. It is therefore of interest that De Paepe et al.[38] confirmed the occurrence of this form of PXE in patients of Belgian stock. The founder effect in the Afrikaner population is thought to account for the high prevalence of PXE in this subgroup.[162]

Apparently, in light of the foregoing, five autonomous entities are classified as "pseudoxanthoma elasticum." Three of these disorders are inherited as autosomal recessive traits; two are apparently transmitted as autosomal dominant conditions. At present the autonomous status of these entities remains unconfirmed. A summary of the clinical features of these forms of PXE is presented in Table 10-1.

Anomalies of inheritance of PXE have been reported in a few individuals.[16] These discrepant pedigrees could not be explained on the basis of mendelian principles. Berlyne, Bulmer, and

---

Pseudoxanthoma Elasticum

Cardinal changes

Skin: Yellow infiltrated lesions, maximal in the flexures

Eyes: Angioid streaks and retinal hemorrhage

Cardiovascular: Calcification of the media of medium-sized arteries, with progressive occlusion and occasional rupture

Elastic fibers are characteristically fragmented and calcified in skin biopsy specimens, but the basic defect is unknown.

Mode of inheritance	MIM number
PXE, AD form (probably heterogeneous)	177850
PXE, AR form (probably heterogeneous)	264800

MIM, Mendelian Inheritance in Man; AD, autosomal dominant; AR, autosomal recessive.

Table 10-1. Comparison of the clinical features within different types of pseudoxanthoma elasticum

Classification	Clinical features
AD type I	Severe retinal and cardiovascular features; classical flexural changes
AD type II	Mild retinal and cardiovascular changes; marfanoid features: highly arched palate, joint laxity, blue sclerae, arachnodactyly
AR type I	Moderate retinal and vascular lesions; classical peau d'orange skin manifestations
AR type II	Severe generalized cutaneous lesions only
AR "Afrikaner" type	Severe retinal complications; moderately severe cardiovascular lesions; mild cutaneous manifestations

AD, autosomal dominant; AR, autosomal recessive.

Platt[16] claimed to be able to identify persons heterozygous for PXE on the basis of funduscopic changes in choroidal vascular pattern. These claims could not be substantiated on the basis of clinical examination by subsequent investigators.[63] However, elucidation of the genetic defect at the molecular level may eventually allow identification of heterozygous carriers of PXE.

LABORATORY INVESTIGATIONS

No biochemical or histopathologic abnormalities presently permit differentiation among the various forms of PXE. Investigators using recombinant DNA techniques have studied the possibilities that the genetic defects for PXE may reside within either the type I collagen gene or the human elastin gene. Following the investigations of Viljoen[171] in two South African Afrikaner kindreds with PXE, it seems that the type I collagen gene is an unlikely candidate. In particular, no linkage could be established by the use of probes for the pro alpha 1 (type I) and pro alpha 2 (type I) collagen genes.

The structure of the human elastin gene has been elucidated,[9] and it has been shown that the gene is 45 kb in size and contains 34 exons separated by relatively large introns. Despite this knowledge, localization of the elastin gene is disputed on the basis of evidence that it is either on chromosome 2[44] or on the long arm of chromosome 7 (7q).[47] Current evidence favors the latter locus.

Initially Emanuel et al.[44] provisionally assigned the elastin gene to the long arm of chromosome 2, between band 31 and the long arm terminal (2q31-qter). They used messenger RNA (mRNA) obtained from fetal human aorta to synthesize complementary DNA (cDNA), which was cloned into the PstI site of pBR322. The recombinant clones were screened with sheep elastin cDNA, and a human clone that hybridized strongly was isolated.[81] The labeled clone was used for in situ hybridization in normal metaphase chromosomes and in cells with a translocation of the short arm of chromosome 1, band 36, to the long arm of chromosome 2, band 31 (t[1;2][p36;q31]).[44] In later studies Fazio et al.[47] used human elastin cDNAs in both in situ hybridization and Southern blot analysis of hybrid cells of humans and rodents to map the elastin gene to the long arm of chromosome 7, band 11.2 (7q11.2). A problem in the investigation of elastin as a possible candidate gene causing PXE is the remarkable conservation of the human elastin gene within populations throughout the world. Indeed, until 1990, according to Boyd,[23] polymorphisms for elastin had been demonstrated only in the Finnish population. Although there is now firm evidence to indicate that the elastin gene is on chromosome 7, there is still a hint of involvement of a locus on chromosome 2. It can be anticipated that this issue will eventually be resolved by means of further molecular investigations.

MANAGEMENT

Individuals with PXE are prone to cosmetic deterioration of skin, hypertension with vascular stroke phenomena, and subretinal hemorrhages with consequent visual loss. No definitive treatment of the disorder exists, but changes in general life-style and a healthy diet can help modify the severity of these complications.

The major adverse prognostic factors associated with skin deterioration in individuals with PXE are obesity, frequent and rapid changes in body mass, prolonged exposure to ultraviolet light, and multiple pregnancies.[119,171] Women with PXE are advised to limit family size and to use ultraviolet ray screening lotions when exposed to direct sunlight. General measures such as annual medical examination to detect hypertension and other cardiovascular sequelae of the disorder are advocated. Similarly, the dietary restriction of polyunsaturated fatty acid intake, regular exercise, and the avoidance of cigarette smoking are recommended.

It has been suggested that dietary calcium intake during childhood and adolescence correlates positively with severity of clinical manifestations in patients with PXE.[119,136] The authors claimed that dietary restriction of calcium may, in some instances, be associated with regression of the cutaneous stigmata of PXE. However, the problems associated with retrospective dietary studies were emphasized by the authors in both investigations, and the benefits of a calcium-restricted diet in PXE patients, particularly in elderly persons who are at risk for osteomalacia, must remain doubtful.

Persons with PXE are advised not to participate in contact sports such as boxing, rugby, soccer, and the martial arts, in order to limit the risks of retinal hemorrhage and impairment of vision. Annual ophthalmologic appraisal by an experienced ophthalmologist is advised. In the event of neovascularization into angioid streaks and subretinal membrane formation, argon or krypton-red laser therapy can be employed to prevent imminent retinal hemorrhage. Once hemorrhage has occurred, laser therapy is thought to be of little value and may be contraindicated.[119]

Drug therapy for hypertension in most instances is commenced by prescription of thiazide diuretics and propranalol. This choice of diuretic is contentious, since thiazides may induce hypercalcemia in a minority of individuals. Neldner[119] has advocated furosemide as the diuretic of choice in patients with PXE, since this drug promotes calcium excretion in the urine. Because the role of calcium in the pathogenesis of PXE is still unknown, the use of thiazide diuretics, which are less costly and generally have few side effects, is probably warranted. Pentoxyfylline can be employed for improving vascular flow in patients with intermittent claudication associated with PXE. This drug lowers blood viscosity and enhances erythrocyte flexibility.

Tocopherol (vitamin E) was said to effect dramatic improvement in the skin and eyes of some patients.[156] Others have also claimed such improvement.[5,141] Conversely, no beneficial effect

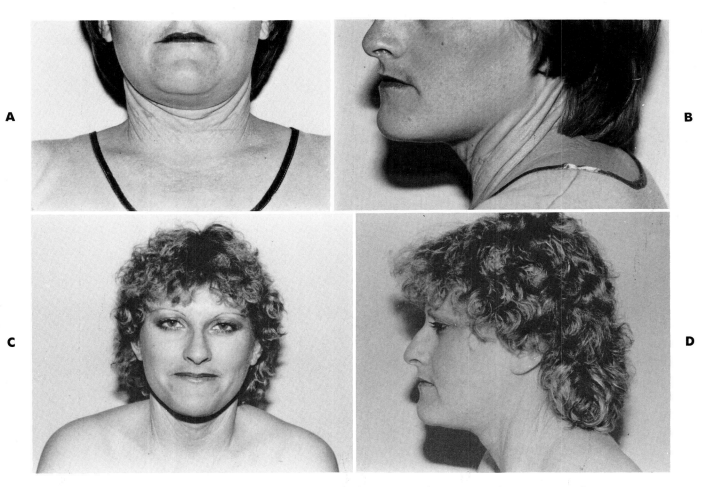

A, Fig. 10-16. **A,** Anteroposterior and, **B,** lateral views of a 25-year-old woman with typical cervical skin laxity resulting from PXE. **C** and **D,** The same patient 5 years later, after plastic surgery. Considerable improvement in her cosmetic appearance is evident.   *Continued.*

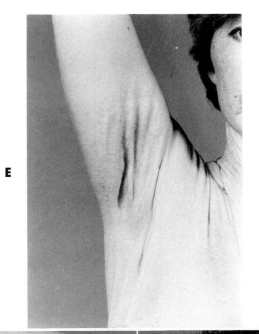

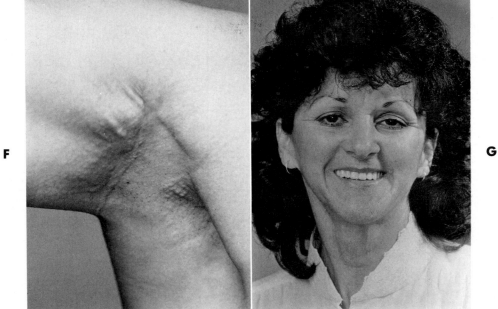

Fig. 10-16, cont'd. E and **F,** The benefit of cosmetic surgery in the axillary area is evident in a 36-year-old woman. **E,** Before surgery and, **F,** after surgery. **G,** Cosmetic surgery had been performed in the cervical region in a 38-year-old woman with PXE. Prominent nasolabial folds remain 8 years after surgery. (**A** to **D, F,** and **G** from Viljoen D, Bloch C, Beighton P: *Plast Reconstr Surg* 85[2]:233-238, 1990. **E** from Viljoen D: *J Med Genet* 25:488-490, 1988.)

was observed in a patient studied by McKusick.[108] Adrenocortical steroids have been used in several patients, but no clear benefit has been noted. Although the reactive process in the skin, eyes, and arteries might be reduced by such treatment, the chronic, indeed, life-long nature of the disease process makes corticosteroid therapy impractical. Cosmetic creams containing agents that block ultraviolet rays and other products containing lanolin, vegetable oils, and perfumes have all been advocated for use in patients with PXE[156]; there is, however, little evidence of their efficacy.

Good cosmetic effects have been reported by plastic surgeons, who have removed the loose, excess skin around the neck, which may be distressingly unsightly, especially in women.[34,89,90,125] Viljoen, Bloch, and Beighton[173] evaluated the effects of cosmetic surgery in nine women who had plastic surgical repair to the skin of the neck, axillae, abdomen, breast, and thighs. The follow-up period ranged from 4 months to 15 years, and there was little regression of the generally excellent operative results. No problems were associated with hemostasis or anesthesia. Fig. 10-16 portrays the good cosmetic outcome achieved. An unusual manifestation in two persons with severe PXE was the extrusion through the surgical scars of spicules of calcium, which caused localized areas of wound dehiscence. Mild keloid formation was also evident in two individuals. Despite these minor complications, cosmetic surgery is useful in women with PXE.

SUMMARY

The clinical manifestations of PXE include (1) characteristic skin changes, especially in areas of wear and tear, (2) angioid streaks of the fundus oculi, and (3) hemorrhage, symptoms of ischemia, and hypertension, all of which result from arterial degeneration. Gastrointestinal hemorrhage is the complication of most importance to the internist, although this occurrence may be rare. The elastic fiber is primarily involved in this condition; PXE behaves as an abiotrophy. The condition is inherited as an autosomal recessive trait in most instances, but at least one autosomal dominant form exists and the disorder is evidently heterogeneous. Current molecular studies have confirmed linkage of the phenotype in two autosomal dominant families to a probe linked to elastin. The elastin gene has been localized to the long arm of chromosome 7, but the possiblity of further nonallelic heterogeneity still remains. Further studies will elucidate the exact nature of anomalies in the elastin gene and its protein product and may eventually permit therapeutic intervention.

REFERENCES

1. Adelung JC: Zur Genese der Angioid Streaks (Knapp), *Klin Mbl Augenheilk* 119:241-250, 1951.
2. Alinder I, Bostrom H: Clinical studies on Swedish material of pseudoxanthoma elasticum, *Acta Med Scand* 191:273-282, 1972.
3. Altman LK et al: Pseudoxanthoma elasticum: an underdiagnosed genetically heterogeneous disorder with protean manifestations, *Arch Intern Med* 134:1048-1054, 1974.
4. Anderson B: Familial central and peripapillary choroidal sclerosis associated with familial pseudoxanthoma elasticum, *Trans Am Ophthal Soc* 46:326, 1948.
5. Ayres S Jr, Mihan R: Pseudoxanthoma elasticum, *Arch Dermatol* 100:119-120, 1969.
6. Bafverstedt B, Lund F: Pseudoxanthoma elasticum and vascular disturbances with special reference to a case in a nine-year-old child, *Acta Dermatovener* 35:438-445, 1955.
7. Balzer F: Récherches sur les charactéres anatomiques du xanthélasma, *Arch Physiol* 4 (series 3):65-80, 1984.
8. Bardsley JL, Koehler PR: Pseudoxanthoma elasticum: angiographic manifestations in abdominal vessels, *Radiology* 93:559-562, 1969.
9. Bashir MM et al: Characterization of the complete human elastin gene, *J Biol Chem* 264:8887-8891, 1989.
10. Beeson BB: Pseudoxanthoma elasticum (Darier) associated with formation of bone, *Arch Dermatol Syph* 34:729-730, 1961.
11. Beighton P et al: International nosology of heritable disorders of connective tissue, Berlin, 1986, *Am J Med Genet* 29:581-594, 1988.
12. Benedict WL: The pathology of angioid streaks in the fundus oculi, *Tr Sect Ophthal AMA*:17-24, 1937.
13. Benedict WL, Montgomery H: Pseudoxanthoma elasticum and angioid streaks, *Am J Ophthalmol* 18:205-212, 1935.
14. Bentley-Phillips B: PXE-like skin changes induced by penicillamine, *J R Soc Med* 78:787 only, 1985.
15. Berde C, Willis DC, Sandberg EC: Pregnancy in women with pseudoxanthoma elasticum, *Obstet Gynecol Surv* 38:339-344, 1983.
16. Berlyne GM, Bulmer HG, Platt R: The genetics of pseudoxanthoma elasticum, *Quart J Med* 30:201-212, 1961.
17. Besnier E, Doyon PAA: Annotations et appendices en traité des maladies de la Peau, de Kaposi (1891). Cited by Darier, reference 36.
18. Bete JM et al: Coronary artery disease in an 18-year-old girl with pseudoxanthoma elasticum, *Am J Cardiol* 36:515-520, 1975.
19. Bett WR: Historical note: Anatole Chauffard (1855-1932), *Med Press* 234:192, 1955.
20. Bett WR: Historical note: Ferdinand Jean Darier (1856-1938) of "Darier's disease," *Med Press* 235:329-330, 1956.

21. Böck J: Zur Klinik und Anatomie der gefässähnlichen Streifen im Augenhintergrund, *Z Augenheilk* 95:1-50, 1938.

22. Britten MJ: Unusual traumatic retinal haemorrhages associated with angioid streaks, *Br J Ophthalmol* 50:540-542, 1966.

23. Boyd C: Personal communication, March 1991.

24. Carlborg U: Study of circulatory disturbances, pulse wave velocity and pressure pulses in larger arteries in cases of pseudoxanthoma elasticum and angioid streaks: a contribution to the knowledge of the function of the elastic tissue and the smooth muscles in larger arteries, *Acta Med Scand* 151(suppl):1-209, 1944.

25. Carlborg U et al: Vascular studies in pseudoxanthoma elasticum and angioid streaks, *Acta Med Scand* 350:1-17, 1959.

26. Chauffard A: Xanthélasma disséminé et symétrique sans insuffisance hèpatique, *Bull Soc Mèd Hôp Paris* 6(series 3):412-419, 1889.

27. Clarkson JG, Altman RD: Angioid streaks, *Surv Ophthalmol* 26:235-246, 1982.

28. Clendenning WE, Auerbach R: Traumatic calcium deposition in skin, *Arch Dermatol* 89:360-363, 1964.

29. Cocco AE et al: The stomach in pseudoxanthoma elasticum, *JAMA* 210:2381-2382, 1969.

30. Cockayne EA: *Inherited abnormalities of the skin and its appendages*, London, 1933, Oxford University and Humphrey Milford, pp 319-332.

31. Coffman JD, Sommers SC: Familial pseudoxanthoma elasticum and valvular heart disease, *Circulation* 19:242-250, 1959.

32. Collomb H, Graveline J, Diop M: Systemix elastorrhexia in a sicklemia patient, *Bull Soc Med Afr Noire Lang Franc* 10:597-602, 1965.

33. Connor PJ et al: Pseudoxanthoma elasticum and angioid streaks: a review of 106 cases, *Am J Med* 30:537-543, 1961.

34. Crikelair GF: Pseudoxanthoma elasticum treated surgically, *Plast Reconstr Surg* 12:152-158, 1953.

35. Cunningham JR et al: Pseudoxanthoma elasticum: treatment of gastrointestinal hemorrhage by arterial embolization and observations on autosomal dominant inheritance, *Johns Hopkins Med J* 147:168-173, 1980.

36. Darier J: Pseudoxanthoma elasticum, *Monatsschr Prakt Derm* 23:609-617, 1896.

37. Dawber R, Shuster S: Scanning electron microscopy of dermal fibrous tissue networks in normal skin, solar elastosis and pseudo-xanthoma elasticum, *Br J Dermatol* 2:130-134, 1971.

38. De Paepe A et al: Pseudoxanthoma elasticum: similar autosomal recessive subtype in Belgian and Afrikaner families, *Am J Med Genet* 38:43-45, 1990.

39. Dixon JM: Angioid streaks and pseudoxanthoma elasticum with aneurysm of the internal carotid artery, *Am J Ophthalmol* 34:1322-1323, 1951.

40. Doyne RW: Choroidal and retinal changes: the result of blows on the eyes, *Trans Ophthalmol Soc UK* 9:129, 1889.

41. Dreyer R, Green WR: The pathology of angioid streaks: a study of twenty-one cases, *Trans PA Acad Ophthalmol Otolaryngol* 31:158-167, 1978.

42. Eddy DD, Farber EM: Pseudoxanthoma elasticum; internal manifestations: a report of cases and a statistical review of the literature, *Arch Dermatol* 86:729-790, 1962.

43. Elejalde BR et al: Manifestations of pseudoxanthoma elasticum during pregnancy: a case report and review of the literature, *Am J Med Genet* 18:755-762, 1984.

44. Emanuel BS et al: Chromosome localization of the human elastin gene, *Am J Hum Genet* 37:873-882, 1985.

45. Farreras-Valenti P et al: Grönblad-Strandberg-Touraine syndrome with systemic hypertension due to unilateral renal angioma: cure of hypertension after nephrectomy, *Am J Med* 39:355-360, 1965.

46. Fasshauer K et al: Neurological complications of Grönblad-Strandberg syndrome, *J Neurol* 231(5):250-252, 1984.

47. Fazio MJ et al: Human elastin gene: new evidence for the localization to the long arm of chromosome 7, *Am J Hum Genet* 48:696-703, 1991.

48. Fine SL: Angioid streaks, *Int Ophthalmol Clin* 17:173-182, 1977.

49. Findlay GH: On elastase and the elastic dystrophies of the skin, *Br J Dermatol Syph* 66:16-24, 1954.

50. Finnerud CW, Nomland R: Pseudoxanthoma elasticum; proof of calcification of elastic tissue: occurrence with and without angioid streaks of the retina, *Arch Dermatol Syph* 35:653-662, 1937.

51. Fisher ER, Rodnan GP, Lansing AI: Identification of the anatomic defect in pseudoxanthoma elasticum, *Am J Pathol* 34:977-991, 1958.

52. Flatley FJ, Atwell ME, McEvoy RK: Pseudoxanthoma elasticum with gastric hemorrhage, *Arch Intern Med* 112:352-356, 1963.

53. Foerster OH: Transactions of the Dermatological Conference of the Mississippi Valley, *Arch Dermatol Syph* 30:280-282, 1934.

54. Fontan P, Merand A, Pfister R: Syndrome de Groenblad-Strandberg, *Bull Soc Franc Syph* 62:101-107, 1955.

55. Fountain RB, Bett D: Pseudoxanthoma elasticum, *Proc R Soc Med* 58:1091 only, 1965.

56. Fountain RB, Bett D: Pseudoxanthoma elasticum, *Proc R Soc Med* 58:1091-1093, 1965.

57. Franceschetti A, Roulet EL: Le syndrome de Groenblad et Strandberg (striés angioides de la rétina et pseudoxanthoma élasticum) et ses rapport avec les affections du mèsenchyme, *Bull Mém Soc Fr Ophtalmol*, 916-922, 1935.

58. Friedenwald JS et al: *Ophthalmic pathology: an atlas and textbook*, Philadelphia, 1952, WB Saunders.

59. Giesen H: *Beitrag zur Kasuistik des Pseudoxanthoma elasticum*. Inaugural dissertation, Erlangen, 1936.

60. Gills JP Jr, Paton D: Mottled fundus oculi in pseudoxanthoma elasticum: a report on two siblings, *Arch Ophthalmol* 73:792-795, 1965.

61. Goedbloed J: Syndrome of Groenblad and Strandberg: angioid streaks in the fundus oculi, associated with pseudoxanthoma elasticum, *Arch Ophthalmol* 19:1-8, 1938.

62. Gold SC: Still's disease with pseudoxanthoma elasticum, *Proc R Soc Med* 50:473-476, 1957.

63. Goodman RM et al: Pseudoxanthoma elasticum: a clinical and histopathological study, *Medicine* 42:297-339, 1963.

64. Goto K: Involvement of the central nervous system in pseudoxanthoma elasticum, *Fol Psychiatr Neurol* 29:263-277, 1975.

65. Grönblad E: Angioid streaks: pseudoxanthoma elasticum; voorläufige Mitteilung, *Acta Ophthalmol* 7:329-336, 1929.

66. Grönblad E: Color photographs of angioid streaks in the late stages, *Acta Ophthalmol* 36:472-474, 1958.

67. Guenther E: Untersuchungen über den Pulsverlauf in den grösseren distalen Arterien der Extremitaten in einigen Fallen von Pseudoxanthoma elasticum cum angioid streaks (Grönblad-Strandbergs Syndrom), *Acta Med Scand* 123:482-509, 1946.

68. Hagedoorn A: Angioid streaks, *Arch Ophthalmol* 21:746, 935 only, 1939.

69. Hall DA, Reed R, Tunbridge RE: Structure of elastic tissue, *Nature* 170:264-266, 1952.

70. Hall JG: Pseudoxanthoma elasticum (PXE): disorders of connective tissue and skeletal dysplasias. In Shulman JD, Simpson JL, editors: *Genetic diseases in pregnancy*, New York, 1981, Academic, pp 63-64.

71. Hallopeau H, Laffitte P: Nouvelle note sur un cas de pseudoxanthome élastique, *Ann Dermatol Syph (Paris)* 4:595, 1904.

72. Hamilton-Gibbs JS: Death from coronary calcinosis in the baby of a mother presenting with pseudoxanthoma elasticum, *Aust J Dermatol* 11:145-147, 1970.

73. Hannay PW: Some clinical and histopathological notes on pseudoxanthoma elasticum, *Br J Dermatol* 63:92-99, 1951.

74. Hartung H: Ueber familiäre angioide Pigmentstreifenbildung des Augenhintergrundes, *Klin Mbl Augenheilk* 88:43-60, 1932.

75. Hashimoto K, Dibella RJ: Electron microscopic studies of normal and abnormal elastic fibers of the skin, *J Invest Dermatol* 48:405-423, 1967.

76. Hashimoto K, McVoy B, Belcher R: Ultrastructure of penicillamine-induced skin lesions, *J Am Acad Dermatol* 4:300-315, 1981.

77. Heyl T: Pseudoxanthoma elasticum with granulomatous skin lesions, *Arch Dermatol* 96:528-531, 1967.

78. Hicks J, Carpenter CL Jr, Reed RJ: Periumbilical perforating pseudoxanthoma elasticum, *Arch Dermatol* 115:300-303, 1979.

79. Huang SN et al: Ultrastructural changes of elastic fibers in pseudoxanthoma elasticum, *Arch Pathol* 83:108-113, 1967.

80. Hubler WR: Two cases of pseudoxanthoma elasticum, *Arch Dermatol Syph* 50:51-54, 1944.

81. Indik Z et al: Alternative splicing of human elastin mRNA indicated by sequence analysis of cloned genomic and complementary DNA, *Proc Natl Acad Sci* 84:5680-5684, 1987.

82. Iqbal A, Alter M, Lee SH: Pseudoxanthoma elasticum: a review of neurological complications, *Ann Neurol* 4:18-20, 1978.

83. Jacoby MW: Pseudoxanthoma elasticum and angioid streaks: report of a case, *Arch Ophthalmol* 11:828-831, 1934.

84. Jacyk WK, Lodder JV, Dreyer L: Pseudoxanthoma elasticum in South African black patients: a report on seven cases, *S Afr Med J* 74(4):184-186, 1988.

85. James AE Jr, Eaton SB, Blazek JV: Roentgen findings in pseudoxanthoma elasticum (PXE), *Am J Roentgenol* 106:642-647, 1969.

86. Joffe E, Joffe M: Classification and etiology of xanthoma, *Urol Cutan Rev* 36:557-559, 1933.

87. Johnson JG, Bloch KJ: Immunoglobulin levels in retinal vascular abnormalities and pseudoxanthoma elasticum, *Arch Ophthalmol* 812:322-324, 1969.

88. Johnson WC, Helwig EB: Histopathology of the acid mucopolysaccharides of skin in normal and in certain pathologic conditions, *Am J Clin Pathol* 40:123-131, 1963.

89. Kaplan EN, Henjyoji EY: Pseudoxanthoma elasticum: a dermal elastosis with surgical implications, *Plast Reconstr Surg* 58(5):595-600, 1976.

90. Kaplan L, Hartman SW: Elastica disease: case of Grönblad-Strandberg syndrome with gastrointestinal hemorrhage, *Arch Intern Med* 94:489-492, 1954.

91. Kat W, Prick JJG: A case of pseudoxanthoma elasticum with anatomico-pathological irregularities of the thyroid arteries, *Psychiatr Neurol (Basel)* 44:417-421, 1940.

92. Klein BA: Angioid streaks: a clinical and histopathologic study, *Am J Ophthalmol* 30:955-968, 1947.

93. Knapp H: On the formation of dark angioid streaks as an unusual metamorphosis of retinal hemorrhage, *Arch Ophthalmol* 21:289-295, 1892.

94. Kofler A: Beitrag zur Kenntnis der Angioid Streakes (Knapp), *Arch Augenheilk* 82:134-137, 1917.

95. Kutty PK, Sadasivan PB: Pseudoxanthoma elasticum, *J Indian Med Assoc* 44:200-201, 1965.

96. Lao TT, Walters BN, De Swiet M: Pseudoxanthoma elasticum and pregnancy, *Br J Obstet Gynaecol* 91(10):1049-1050, 1984.

97. Lebwohl MG et al: Pseudoxanthoma elasticum and mitral-valve prolapse, *New Engl J Med* 307:228-232, 1982.

98. Levin DB, Bell DK: Traumatic retinal hemorrhages with angioid streaks, *Arch Ophthalmol* 95:1072-1073, 1977.

99. Lieb WA, Gerraets WJ, Guerry D III: Sickle-cell retinopathy, ocular and systemic manifestations of sickle-cell disease, *Acta Ophthalmol* 58(suppl), 1959.

100. Lieberman A: The case of the rocky ripples, *J Indiana Med* 62:804-807, 1969.

101. Lobitz W, Osterberg AE: Pseudoxanthoma elasticum: microincineration, *J Invest Dermatol* 15:297-298, 1950.

102. Loria PR et al: Pseudoxanthoma elasticum (Grönblad-Strandberg syndrome): a clinical, light- and electron-microscope study, *Arch Dermatol Syph* 76:609-619, 1957.

103. Marchesani O, Wirz F: Die Pigment-streifenerkrankung der Netzhaut-das Pseudoxanthoma elasticum der Haut-eine Systemerkrankung, *Arch Augenheilk* 104:522-595, 1931.

104. Marchionini A, Turgut K: Ueber Pseudoxanthoma elasticum hereditarium, *Derm Wschr* 114:145-155, 1942.

105. Martinez-Hernandez A et al: Resolution and repair of elastic tissue calcification in Pseudoxanthoma elasticum, *Arch Pathol Lab Med* 102:303-305, 1978.

106. Matras A: Pseudoxanthoma elasticum, *Zbl Haut Geschl Kr* 50:280-287, 1935.

107. McCaughey RS, Alexander LC, Morrish JA: The Grönblad-Strandberg syndrome: a report of three cases presenting with massive gastrointestinal hemorrhage during pregnancy, *Gastroenterology* 31:156-168, 1956.

108. McKusick VA: Pseudoxanthoma elasticum. In McKusick VA: *Heritable Disorders of Connective Tissue*, ed 4, St Louis, 1972, Mosby—Year Book, pp 475-520.

109. Mehregan AH: Elastosis perforans serpiginosa: a review of the literature and report of 11 cases, *Arch Dermatol* 97:381-393, 1968.

110. Mendelsohn G, Bulkley BH, Hutchins GM: Cardiovascular manifestations of pseudoxanthoma elasticum, *Arch Pathol Lab Med* 102:298-302, 1978.

111. Meyrick-Thomas PH, Kirby JD: Elastosis perforans serpiginosa and pseudoxanthoma elasticum-like skin change due to D-penicillamine, *Clin Exper Dermatol* 10(4): 386-391, 1985.

112. Messis CP, Budzilovich GN: Pseudoxanthoma elasticum: report of an autopsied case with cerebral involvement, *Neurology* 20:703-709, 1970.

113. Mitchell A: Angioid streaks, *Boston Med Quart* 15:22-38, 1964.

114. Miyake H et al: A new finding in oral cavity in pseudoxanthoma elasticum, *Nagoya J Med Sci* 29:251-259, 1967.

115. Moran TJ, Lansing AI: Studies on the nature of the abnormal fibers in pseudoxanthoma elasticum, *Arch Pathol* 65:688-696, 1958.

116. Morrison WH: Osteitis deformans with angioid streaks, *Arch Ophthalmol* 26:79-84, 1941.

117. Moschella SL, Greenbaum CH, Fleischmajer R: Pseudoxanthoma elasticum, *Arch Dermatol* 96:97-98, 1967.

118. Navarro-Lopez F et al: Restrictive cardiomyopathy in pseudoxanthoma elasticum, *Chest* 78:113-115, 1980.

119. Neldner KH: Pseudoxanthoma elasticum, *Clin Dermatol* 6:1-157, 1988.

120. Nellen M, Jacobson M: Pseudoxanthoma elasticum (Grönblad-Strandberg disease) with coronary artery calcification, *S Afr Med J* 32(26):649-651, 1958.

121. Ohno T: Ueber Pseudoxanthoma elasticum und dessen Histologie, *Arch Dermatol Syph* 149:420-424, 1925.

122. Parker JC et al: Pseudoxanthoma elasticum and hypertension, *New Engl J Med* 271:1204-1206, 1964.

123. Pasquali-Ronchetti I et al: Pseudoxanthoma elasticum: biochemical and ultrastructural studies, *Dermatologica* 163:302-325, 1981.

124. Perloff JK: Evolving concepts of mitral-valve prolapse, *New Engl J Med* 307(6):369-370, 1982.

125. Pickrell KL, Kelley JW, Marzoni FA: The plastic surgical treatment of pseudoxanthoma elasticum, *Plast Reconstr Surg* 3:700-706, 1948.

126. Pope FM: *Pseudoxanthoma elasticum*, degree of Doctor of Medicine thesis submitted to the University of Wales, 1972.

127. Pope FM: Autosomal dominant pseudoxanthoma elasticum, *J Med Genet* 11:152-157, 1974.

128. Pope FM: Two types of autosomal recessive pseudoxanthoma elasticum, *Arch Dermatol* 110:209-212, 1974.

129. Pope FM: Historical evidence for the genetic heterogeneity of pseudoxanthoma elasticum, *Br J Dermatol* 92:493-509, 1975.

130. Prick JJG: *Pontine pseudobulbar-paralyse bei Pseudoxanthoma elasticum: eine klinische anatomische Studie*, doctoral thesis, Maastricht, 1938.

131. Prick JJG, Thijssen HOM: Radiodiagnostic signs in pseudoxanthoma elasticum generalisatum (dysgenesis elastofibrillaris mineralisans), *Clin Radiol* 28:549-554, 1977.

132. Przybojewski JZ et al: Pseudoxanthoma elasticum with cardiac involvement, *S Afr Med J* 59:268-275, 1981.

133. Pyeritz RE, Weis JL, Renie WA: Pseudoxanthoma elasticum and mitral valve prolapse (letter), *New Engl J Med* 307:1451-1452, 1982.

134. Reed RJ, Clark WH, Mihm MC: The cutaneous elastoses, *Hum Pathol* 4:187-199, 1973.

135. Reeve EB et al: Development and calcification of skin lesions in thirty-nine patients with pseudoxanthoma elasticum, *Clin Exper Dermatol* 4:291-301, 1979.

136. Renie WA et al: Pseudoxanthoma elasticum: high calcium intake in early life correlates with severity, *Am J Med Genet* 19:235-244, 1984.

137. Revell STR Jr, Carey TN: Pseudoxanthoma elasticum as a disseminated disease, *Southern Med J* 41:782-790, 1948.

138. Rigal D: Observation pour servir à l'histoire de la chéloide diffuse xanthélasmique, *Ann Dermatol Syph* 2:491-501, 1881.

139. Rodnan GP, Fisher ER, Warren JE: Pseudoxanthoma elasticum: clinical findings and identification of the anatomic defect, *Clin Res* 6(abstract):236-237, 1958.

140. Ross R, Fialkow PH, Altman LK: Fine structure alterations of elastic fibers in pseudoxanthoma elasticum, *Clin Genet* 13:213-223, 1978.

141. Sairanen E, Itkonen A, Kangas S: Pseudoxanthoma elasticum (PXE) and joint manifestations, *Acta Rheum Scand* 16:130-135, 1970.

142. Sames CP: Pseudoxanthoma elasticum: severe melaena from the jejunum treated by resection, *Proc R Soc Med* 54:519, 1961.

143. Sanbacka-Holstrom I: Das Grönblad-Strandbergische Syndrom: Pseudoxanthoma elasticum-angioid streaks-Gefässveränderungen, *Acta Dermatovener* 20:684-708, 1939.

144. Schachner L, Young D: Pseudoxanthoma elasticum with severe cardiovascular disease in a child, *Am J Dis Child* 127:571-575, 1974.

145. Scheie HG, Freeman NE: Vascular disease associated with angioid streaks of the retina and pseudoxanthoma elasticum, *Arch Ophthalmol* 35:241-250, 1946.

146. Scheie HG, Hogan TF: Angioid streaks and generalized arterial diseases, *Arch Ophthalmol* 57:855-868, 1957.

147. Scholz RO: Angioid streaks, *Arch Ophthalmol* 26:677-695, 1941.

148. Schutt D: Pseudoxanthoma elasticum and elastosis perforans serpiginosa, *Arch Dermatol* 91:151-152, 1965.

149. Sharma NGK et al: Subarachnoid haemorrhage in pseudoxanthoma elasticum, *Postgrad Med J* 50:774-776, 1974.

150. Silvers S: Pseudoxanthoma elasticum with angioid streaks of retina, *Arch Dermatol Syph* 42:155-156, 1940.

151. Silvers SH, Wolfe HE: Pseudoxanthoma elasticum with angioid streaks: the syndrome of Grönblad-Strandberg, *Arch Dermatol Syph* 45:1142-1147, 1942.

152. Smith EW et al: Reactive perforating elastoma: a feature of certain genetic disorders, *Bull Johns Hopkins Hosp* 11:235-251, 1962.

153. Smith JG Jr, Davidson EA, Clark RD: Dermal elastin in actinic elastosis and pseudoxanthoma elasticum, *Nature* 195:716-717, 1962.

154. Smith JG Jr, Davidson EA, Taylor RW: Cutaneous acid mucopolysaccharides in pseudoxanthoma elasticum, *J Invest Dermatol* 43:429-430, 1964.

155. Stankler L: Pseudoxanthoma elasticum with a knuckle pad on the thumb, *Acta Dermatovener* 47:263 only, 1967.

156. Stout OM: Pseudoxanthoma elasticum with retinal angioid streaks, decidedly improved on tocopherol therapy, *Arch Dermatol Syph* 63:510-511, 1951.

157. Strandberg JV: Pseudoxanthoma elasticum, *Z Haut Geschlechtskr* 31:689-693, 1929.

158. Tanenbaum HL, de Margerie J: Sudden bilateral loss of central vision in pseudoxanthoma elasticum: fluorescence photography of the ocular lesions, *Can J Ophthalmol* 1:221-227, 1966.

159. Temine P: *Contribution à l'etude de l'elastorrhexie systematisee,* Paris thesis, Paris, 1940, Jouve & Cie.

160. Terry TL: Angioid streaks and osteitis deformans, *Trans Am Ophthalmol Soc* 32:555-573, 1934.

161. Throne B, Goodman H: Pseudoxanthoma elasticum, *Arch Dermatol Syph* 6:410-447, 1921.

162. Torrington M, Viljoen D: Founder effect in twenty Afrikaner kindreds with pseudoxanthoma elasticum, *S Afr Med J* 71:7-11, 1990.

163. Touraine AL: Elastorrhexie systématiseé, *Presse Med* 49:361 only, 1941.

164. Touraine A, James: Pseudoxanthoma elastique (elastorrhexis), *Bull Soc Franc Dermatol Syph* 47:217-219, 1940.

165. Tunbridge RE et al: The fibrous structure of normal and abnormal skin, *Clin Sci* 11:315-331, 1952.

166. Urbach E, Wolfram S: Ueber Veranderungen des elastischen Gewebes bei einem autoptisch untersuchten Falle von Gröndblad-Strandbergschem Syndrom, *Arch Dermatol Syph* 176:167-175, 1938.

167. Van Embden Andres GH: Afwijkingen, aan die indwendige organen bij Psudoxanthoma elasticum en Angioide Stregpen, Groningen, 1952.

168. Verhoeff FH: Histological findings in a case of angioid streaks, *Br J Ophthalmol* 32:531-599, 1948.

169. Vickers HR: Discussion: pseudoxanthoma elasticum, *Proc R Soc Med* 58:1093 only, 1965.

170. Viljoen D: Pseudoxanthoma elasticum (Grönblad-Strandberg syndrome), *J Med Genet* 25:488-490, 1988.

171. Viljoen DL: *Pseudoxanthoma elasticum in southern Africa,* doctoral thesis, University of Cape Town, South Africa, 1991.

172. Viljoen DL, Beatty S, Beighton P: The obstetric and gynaecological implications of pseudoxanthoma elasticum, *Br J Obstet Gynaecol* 94:884-888, 1987.

173. Viljoen DL, Bloch C, Beighton P: Plastic surgery in pseudoxanthoma elasticum: experience in nine patients, *Plast Reconstr Surg* 85(2):233-238, 1990.

174. Viljoen DL, Pope FM, Beighton P: Heterogeneity of pseudoxanthoma elasticum: delineation of a new form? *Clin Genet* 32:100-105, 1987.

175. Viljoen DL et al: Pseudoxanthoma elasticum in South Africa: genetic and clinical implications, *S Afr Med J* 66:813-816, 1984.

176. Wise D: Hereditary disorders of connective tissue. In Gottron HA, Schnyder UW, editors: *Vererbung von Hautkrankheiten,* Berlin, 1966, Springer Verlag, pp 467-532.

177. Wolff HH, Stokes JF, Schlesinger BE: Vascular abnormalities associated with pseudoxanthoma elasticum, *Arch Dis Child* 27:82-88, 1952.

178. Woo JC Jr, Chandler FW: Pseudoxanthoma elasticum with gastric hemorrhage: report of a case, *Ann Intern Med* 49:215-222, 1958.

179. Zachiem H, Pincus H: Calcium chloride necrosis of the skin, *Arch Dermatol* 76:244-246, 1957.

180. Zentmayer W: Angioid streaks of the fundus oculi observed over a period of 36 years: report of a case, *Arch Ophthalmol* 35:541-595, 1946.

CHAPTER 11

The Mucopolysaccharidoses

Chester B. Whitley

The mucopolysaccharidoses are a heterogeneous group of inborn errors of lysosomal glycosaminoglycan metabolism characterized by the accumulation of excess mucopolysaccharides in various organs and by the excretion of these substances in urine. The combined incidence of the MPS disorders may be as high as 1:10,000 live births.[358]

Although the clinical phenotypes of these disorders are disparate, common features permit provisional diagnosis. Short stature, hepatosplenomegaly, corneal clouding, deafness, cardiac valve dysfunction, coronary artery occlusion, and joint contractures occur in the majority of these conditions. They all share characteristic skeletal abnormalities that fall under the rubric "dysostosis multiplex."

The mucopolysaccharidoses have been designated mucopolysaccharidosis (MPS) types I through VII, with subtypes based on clinical and biochemical findings. Because the evolving nosology has been driven by investigations of the fundamental biochemical and genetic defects, the names applied to the clinical disorders sometimes encompass mild and severe phenotypes. Advances that identify specific mutations promise to improve categorization but may also necessitate revision of the nomenclature.

GENERAL CONSIDERATIONS
Historical Note

The disorders now referred to as mucopolysaccharidoses were said by Henderson[334] to have been recognized in three sibs by John Thompson of Edinburgh in the early years of the twentieth century. The patient documented by Berkhan[73] in 1907 may have been a child with Hurler syndrome. The first definitive description was made by Charles H. Hunter* (Fig. 11-1), whose paper appeared in the Proceedings of the Royal Society of Medicine in 1917,[378] while he was serving in England as a major in the Canadian Army Medical Corps. This beautifully detailed and descriptive report concerned two brothers, 8 and 10 years of age, who were admitted to the Winnipeg General Hospital in 1915. Dwarfism, deafness, widely spaced teeth, short neck, protuberant abdomen with hepatosplenomegaly, inguinal hernias, hands that were short, broad, thick, and stiff, semiflexed knees, and noisy respiration were the major features. "The face [was] very large, of deep burnt-red colour, as after much exposure, with a tinge of cyanosis in cheeks and lips . . . In the younger child, strips of skin 1½ inches wide extended from the angles of both scapulae parallel to the ribs forward to the midaxillary lines; these are pinhead elevations, grouped closely and regularly, smooth of surface, normal in colour . . ." The elder boy had cardiomegaly and "a distinct diastolic murmur audible in the third and fourth left interspaces close to the sternum; at the apex, a systolic murmur was conducted towards the axilla." Twelve illustrations, including many radiographs demonstrating typical changes (such as "shoe-shaped" sella turcica), were presented by Hunter. The boys appeared to be normally intelligent; the cornea was not cloudy; the spine was straight, with loss

---

*Charles Hunter (1873-1955) was professor of medicine at the University of Manitoba, Winnepeg.

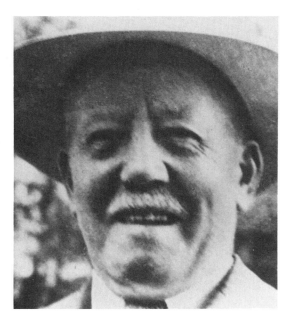

Fig. 11-1. Dr. Charles Hunter (1873-1955). Charles Hunter was born on February 7, 1873, at Auchterlass, Aberdeenshire, Scotland and studied medicine at the University of Aberdeen. After qualification he undertook postgraduate training in London and Berlin before moving to Canada, where he later settled into practice in Winnipeg as a specialist in internal medicine. In 1917, during World War I, while serving in Europe as an army medical officer, Hunter gave a presentation at the Royal Society of Medicine, London, entitled "A Rare Disease in Two Brothers." Hunter subsequently reported the patients in the Society proceedings, giving details of their clinical and radiographic features. McKusick followed up on the family several decades later and confirmed that they had the condition now known as MPS type II, or Hunter syndrome. Hunter was regarded as the leading diagnostician in western Canada for many years. (From Beighton P, Beighton G: *The man behind the syndrome*, New York, 1986. Springer-Verlag, pp 78-79.)

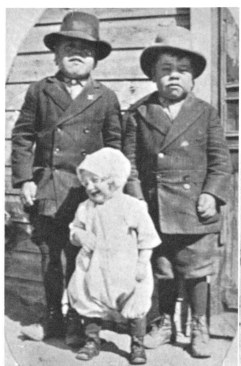

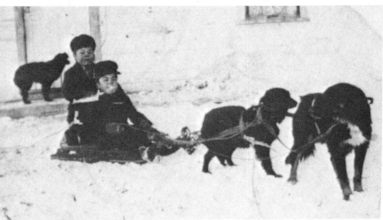

Fig. 11-2. Photographs of the patients Hunter described in 1917.[218] The younger brother (G.B.C., born in 1907) died in 1918 of pneumonia, and the elder one (R.W.C., born in 1904) died in 1920 of "dropsy." The youngest sibling was apparently unaffected. The characteristic facies and hand deformity are evident. These brothers are thought to have had the X-linked recessive form of mucopolysaccharidosis, Hunter syndrome. (Photographs and follow-up information courtesy Dr. Nancy Gemmell and Dr. L.G. Bell, University of Manitoba, Winnipeg.)

Fig. 11-3. Dr. Gertrud Hurler (1889-1965). Gertrud Hurler was born on September 1, 1889, at Taberwiese in the district of Rastenburg, Prussia, where her father was a general practitioner. She was educated in Konigsberg and qualified in medicine at the University of Munich. In 1919, while training in pediatrics, Hurler described a syndrome of corneal clouding, dwarfing skeletal dysplasia, spinal malalignment, and mental retardation. Her report was based on two infants previously presented by her chief, Professor von Pfaundler, at the Munich Pediatric Society. Pfaundler's own case report was published in 1920, but his name never became firmly associated with the condition. Hurler was an exceptional clinician and was greatly liked and respected by her patients. In addition to her clinical activities, she was associated with the local orphanage, served on many medical committees, and was a pioneer in the establishment of a maternal postnatal service. (From Beighton P, Beighton G: *The man behind the syndrome*, New York, 1986, Springer-Verlag, pp 82-83.)

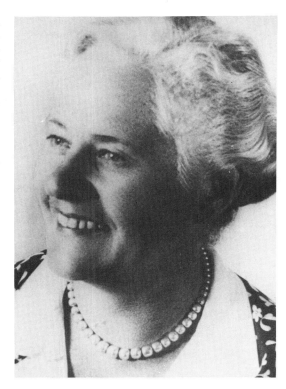

of the normal contour, but there was no gibbus. Follow-up indicates that Hunter's patients clearly had the X-linked MPS which now carries his name and the designation *MPS type II* (Fig. 11-2).

In 1919 Gertrud Hurler* (Fig. 11-3) of Munich published case reports[379] of two patients who had previously been presented to the Munich Society for Pediatrics by Meinhard von Pfaundler,[666] the chief of the University Clinic of Pediatrics. The patients of Hurler and Pfaundler were infants; gibbus was present, as were corneal clouding and retardation of intellect. They probably had the condition once known as Hurler-Pfaundler syndrome but now commonly known as Hurler syndrome.

It is surprising that Hunter's classic article, compared to Hurler's report, received relatively little attention. Subsequently, even in the English-speaking medical world, it was principally Hurler's paper that was cited and the names of Hurler and Pfaundler that became most firmly associated with the syndrome. A similar situation existed in connection with the Morquio syndrome, which

was described in England by Brailsford* of Birmingham slightly earlier than by Morquio† of Montevideo, Uruguay (Fig. 11-4). The first case from the United States was reported by Putnam and Pelkan[678] in 1925 under the title "Scaphocephaly with Malformations of the Skeleton and Other Tissues." The nosography of the Hurler syndrome has now advanced to the point that the limits of the syndrome and its clinical and pathologic features are reasonably well described, although mildly affected persons (i.e., Scheie syndrome) are still difficult to identify with certainty except by means of biochemical investigation. A tabular survey of the cases reported up to 1950 was presented by Jervis.[394] By 1954 Emanuel[231] estimated that over 200 cases had been reported; broader recognition has led to increasingly earlier

---

*James F. Brailsford (1888-1961) was an academic radiologist in Birmingham, England.

†Luis Morquio (1867-1935) was born in Montevideo, Uruguay, and graduated in medicine there in 1892. He studied pediatrics at the Hôpital des Enfants Malades in Paris from 1893 to 1894. In 1899 he was appointed professor of pediatrics at Montevideo and continued in that post until his death. He retained his close links with France, and most of his scientific publications were written in the French language.

---

*Gertrud Hurler (1889-1965) practiced as a pediatrician in Neuhausen, Germany.

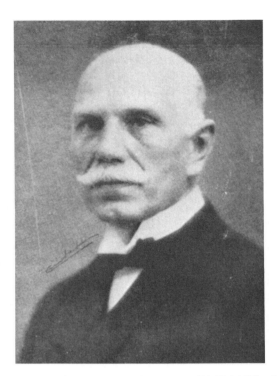

Fig. 11-4. Professor Luis Morquio (1867-1935). Luis Morquio was born in Montevideo, Uruguay, on January 3, 1867, and was graduated in medicine there in 1892. He studied pediatrics at the Hôpital des Enfants Malades in Paris from 1893 to 1894. In 1929 Morquio described a form of "familial skeletal dystrophy" in four of five children of consanguineous Swedish parents. (Concurrently the British radiologist James Brailsford described the clinical and radiologic features of a child with "chondro-osteo-dystrophy," hence the alternate eponym "Morquio-Brailsford syndrome," which has gradually fallen into disuse.) In 1899 Morquio was appointed professor of pediatrics at Montevideo and continued in that post until his death in 1935.[380] Morquio was the author of numerous publications and two pediatrics textbooks, served as president of the International Save the Children Society (Geneva), and became an officer of the French *Légion d'Honneur*.

diagnosis in more recent times.[918]

Probable examples of the Morquio syndrome were reported as cases of achondroplasia by William Osler[637] and by Voisin and Voisin.[867] In 1929, independent reports by Morquio[573] and by Brailsford[102] of England provided definitive descriptions. Thereafter the disorder became known as the Morquio syndrome or, less frequently, as the Morquio-Brailsford syndrome. Patients featured in early reports by Ruggles,[712] White-

side and Cholmeley,[890] and Gasteiger and Liebenam[270] probably also had the condition. Other designations used in the literature of that era included chondro-osteodystrophy and eccentro-osteochondrodysplasia.

The sibs reported by Morquio[573,574] were of Swedish extraction, and their parents were first cousins. Of five offspring, only the first, a male, was unaffected. The second, Maria, born in 1913, was described in the initial report in 1929[573]; she died of pulmonary complications in the 1930s. The third child, Arturo, born in 1915, died of the same cause in 1939. The fourth, Julio, born in 1917, was said to have no sign of cardiac abnormality. The fifth child, Carlos, was born in 1919 and died of pulmonary complications. Maroteaux and Lamy obtained confirmation of the presence of corneal clouding in the affected children.[522]

During a 30-year period after the publication of Morquio's and Brailsford's descriptions, a wide variety of cases found their way into the literature under the Morquio sobriquet.[187,672,689,769] Many of these, in the light of increased knowledge of hereditary skeletal disorders, are no longer considered to have been the same condition as that described by Morquio. Cases initially categorized with the Morquio syndrome but now known to be distinct include X-linked spondyloepiphyseal dysplasia,[388] multiple epiphyseal dysplasia,[775] diastrophic dysplasia,[550] metatropic dysplasia,[524,564] parastremmatic dysplasia,[689] spondyloepiphyseal dysplasia congenita,[179] and other entities.[120,333] The eponym "Morquio-Ullrich syndrome" was subsequently employed[896,938] for patients having corneal changes in addition to the typical skeletal features documented by Morquio and Brailsford. This phenotype then became known as Morquio syndrome, and when the condition was found to be an MPS, it was designated MPS type IV.

Although males with clinical features now recognized as being typical of the Hunter syndrome (MPS type II) were reported by many workers, beginning with the brothers described by Hunter himself, the earliest pedigree clearly indicating X-linked inheritance for that condition was published in 1942 by Wolff,[914] who did not, however, comment on sex linkage. In 1946 Njå[606] in Norway presented an X-linked pedigree, specifically proposed this mode of inheritance, and emphasized lack of corneal clouding as a hallmark of the X-linked cases. Having overlooked Wolff's publication (in "Laryngoscope" during World War II),

Nja observed that "this type of heredity in gargoylism has not been described previously."

Many different names have been suggested for the group of disorders termed mucopolysaccharidoses. Most are now of only historic interest. Hurler[379] suggested the term "dysostosis multiplex," which is now applied to the spectrum of radiographic skeletal changes that characterizes the mucopolysaccharidoses. Ellis et al.,[228,229] Cockayne,[151] and other English authors used the term "gargoylism." This designation has now been discarded because of its unpleasant connotations. Washington[882] suggested "lipochondrodystrophy," believing this disorder to be one of lipid metabolism. The term is a misnomer, however, as indicated by present evidence bearing on the basic defect of the disease.

In 1952 Brante[104] classified the Hurler syndrome as a "mucopolysaccharidosis" after he isolated dermatan sulfate from the liver of two affected children. Brown[115] isolated heparan sulfate from the liver of a similar patient. Discovery of mucopolysacchariduria by Dorfman and Lorincz[217] and by Meyer et al.[561] firmly established the biochemical nature of the disorder. With the identification of urinary glycosaminoglycan excretion as a marker, three new MPS syndromes appeared in the literature shortly thereafter. A case of heparansulfaturia was included in a report by Meyer et al.[561] in 1958 and noted as a possible new genotype by Harris[317] in 1961. This newly recognized condition, which manifested with symptoms of mental retardation, minimal skeletal and somatic changes, and a specific pattern of heparan sulfate excretion, was then more fully described in five patients by Sylvester Sanfilippo et al.[718] in 1963. Radiographic features were delineated by Langer and Carey.[476] As additional cases were reported,[212,525,781,876] the phenotype became known as Sanfilippo syndrome and was designated MPS type III.

In 1962 and 1963 the ophthalmologist Harold "Hank" Scheie* (Fig. 11-5) described an affected sibship with a relatively mild phenotype, which included joint contractures, corneal clouding, and relatively normal intellect.[730] The condition became known as Scheie syndrome and was originally designated MPS type V; subsequent studies, however, showed that this disorder was allelic to

---

*Harold Scheie was Professor of Ophthalmology at the University of Pennsylvania until his retirement in 1975.

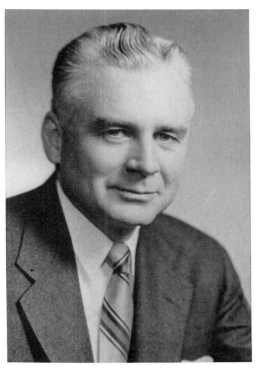

Fig. 11-5. Professor Harold "Hank" Scheie. Harold Scheie, who died in 1990, was born on March 24, 1909, into a homesteading family in North Dakota and spent his early years living in a sod house on the Berthold Indian Reservation. He worked his way through the University of Minnesota, graduating with honors in 1935. He completed his training in ophthalmology at the University of Pennsylvania and then joined the faculty. In 1962 he published observations on adult siblings with a previously unrecognized condition of progressive corneal clouding, near-normal intelligence, and glycosaminoglycanuria. Scheie served as departmental chairman from 1960, was founding director of the Scheie Eye Institute, and published several books and more than 200 articles. He was best known for his innovative surgical techniques and philanthropic endeavors.

Hurler syndrome,[899] and demonstration of the same enzymatic defect[39] led to reclassification of the disorder as MPS type I S.

A later follow-up by Scheie[728] of the original sibs illustrated the course of the condition. The brother was reevaluated in 1970 at the age of 37 years,[156] 12 years after the initial presentation. His facies was still normal, but his vision had failed considerably (to only "hand movements") and he had aortic valve murmurs, cardiomegaly, and enlargement of the liver and spleen. He subse-

Table 11-1. The genetic mucopolysaccharidoses

MPS type	Enzymatic defect	Gene locus	Glycosaminoglycan*	Clinical diagnosis	Distinguishing clinical features
I	α-L-iduronidase	4p16.3	DS, HS	Hurler syndrome	Diagnosis before age 2 yr, early corneal clouding and kyphoscoliosis, mental retardation, death before age 10 yr
				Hurler-Scheie syndrome	Intermediate age of diagnosis, mild to severe skeletal involvement, corneal clouding, early death
				Scheie syndrome	Late corneal clouding, normal intellect, virtually normal longevity
II	Iduronate 2-sulfatase	Xq27. 3	DS,HS	Hunter syndrome, severe	Diagnosis before age 4 yr, absence of corneal clouding and kyphoscoliosis, mental retardation, death before age 15 yr
				Hunter syndrome, mild	Absence of corneal clouding and kyphoscliosis, moderate skeletal and respiratory involvement, survival into adulthood with little or no intellectual impairment
IIIA	Heparan N-sulfatase (Sulfamidase)	—	HS	Sanfilippo syndrome, type A	Diagnosis after age 2 yr, minimal physical abnormalities, progressive dementia
IIIB	α-N-acetylglucosaminidase	—	HS	Sanfilippo syndrome, type B	Same as for type A
IIIC	Acetyl-CoA:α-glucosaminide N-acetyltransferase	—	HS	Sanfilippo syndrome, type C	Same as for type A
IIID	N-acetylglucosamine 6-sulfatase	12q14	HS	Sanfilippo syndrome, type D	Same as for type A
IVA	Galactose 6-sulfatase	—	KS	Morquio syndrome, type A	Variable extreme-to-mild short stature, corneal clouding, thin tooth enamel, progressive spinal cord damage, survival into adulthood
IVB	β-galactosidase	3p21-cen	KS	Morquio syndrome, type B	Variable extreme-to-mild short stature, corneal clouding, progressive cervical spinal cord damage
VI	N-acetylgalactosamine 4-sulfatase	5q11-q13	DS	Maroteaux-Lamy syndrome	Variable extreme-to-mild short stature, frequent kyphoscoliosis, corneal clouding, cardiopulmonary failure, normal intellect, variable survival
VII	β-glucuronidase	7q11.2-q22	DS,HS,CS	Sly syndrome, neonatal	Hydrops fetalis, lethal in newborn
				Sly syndrome, infantile	Mental retardation, moderate skeletal involvement
				Sly syndrome, juvenile	Mild mental retardation

*DS, Dermatan sulphate; HS, heparan sulfate; KS, keratan sulfate; CS, chondroitin.

quently died at 40 years of age. His affected younger sister had a spontaneous esophageal rupture in 1985, followed by aortic valve problems, but she was surviving, at 55 years of age, in 1989.

In 1965, Maroteaux* and Lamy† presented the first description of patients with a phenotype resembling other mucopolysaccharidoses but distinguished by normal intelligence and dermatansultaria.[521,526] The disorder was subsequently termed Maroteaux-Lamy syndrome and designated MPS type VI.[776,782]

By 1965 (as reflected in the third edition of this book[551]) six distinct mucopolysaccharidoses had been differentiated by means of combined clinical, genetic, and biochemical study. These six were designated MPS types I through VI, as shown in Table 11-1. The Hurler syndrome, as the prototype MPS, was termed MPS type I. The X-linked disorder, Hunter syndrome, was labelled MPS type II. MPS type III (Sanfilippo syndrome), MPS type V (Scheie syndrome), and MPS type VI (Maroteaux-Lamy syndrome) had previously been considered "Hurler variants." MPS type IV (Morquio syndrome) was by 1965 known to have both a characteristic mucopolysacchariduria and distinctive skeletal features.

Van Hoof and Hers, in Louvain, Belgium, suggested that the electron microscopic findings[856] and the natural history of the mucopolysaccharidoses are consistent with their being "lysosomal diseases."[339,340] In the first edition of this book[547] McKusick had written the following:

Tissue culture of fibroblasts is possibly one of the more promising, although as yet unexplored, techniques for the study of heritable disorders of connective tissue. (In general, tissue culture has been too little used in physiologic genetics.) . . . In connection with the heritable disorders of connective tissue, the first objective of tissue culture studies should be the in vitro replication of the morphologic abnormalities. In the Hurler syndrome one can with justification anticipate success in demonstrating morphologic abnormality, . . . i.e., the 'gargoyle cell.'. . . If the initial morphologic studies are consonant with the view that a fibroblast strain growing in the test tube represents the original donor's disease 'in pure culture,' then intensive studies should be undertaken of the chemical characteristics.

McKusick's prediction was fulfilled by Danes

and Bearn's demonstration[173, 175] that fibroblasts show cytoplasmic metachromasia, that is, the "gargoyle cell" does exist in culture. Concomitantly the work of Neufeld and her colleagues indicated that cultured fibroblasts from patients with several of the mucopolysaccharidoses had a defect in the degradation of glycosaminoglycans[251] and that a diffusible factor produced by normal cells or by cells from a different mucopolysaccharidosis corrected this metabolic defect in vitro[252] (Fig. 11-6).

The nosology of the mucopolysaccharidoses was greatly influenced after 1968 by the work of Neufeld and her colleagues on specific corrective factors that could, by means of studies of fibroblasts in vitro, be shown to be deficient in various forms of these disorders. Some surprises were forthcoming, for instance, that the Hurler syndrome and the Scheie syndrome, although clinically quite different, are deficient in the same corrective factor.[39,248,899] Equally, two forms of the Sanfilippo syndrome with indistinguishable phenotypes could be differentiated by mutual cross-correction studies of the metabolic defect exhibited in cultured fibroblasts.[457,458,618] In 1972, using the test substrate, phenyl-L-iduronide, prepared by Bernard Weissmann and Santiago,[887] Matalon and Dorfman,[531] and Bach et al.[39] showed that Hurler syndrome was due to deficiency of the enzyme α-L-iduronidase. These and other advances have permitted the revised classification given in Table 11-1. McKusick et al.[557,558] postulated allelism at the loci of MPS types I, II, and VI and presented cases that satisfy the criteria for a genetic compound at the MPS I locus.

Although the Scheie syndrome was initially designated MPS type V, in vitro cross-correction studies[899] necessitated reclassification of Scheie syndrome as a forme fruste of MPS type I. To avoid confusion, the numeric designation "MPS type V" was thereafter excluded from the medical literature.[558] In the same way, the demonstration of different genetic and enzymatic defects in forms of the Sanfilippo and Morquio syndromes have ultimately led to differentiation of four subtypes of MPS type III, (subtypes IIIA, IIIB, IIIC, and IIID) and two subtypes of MPS IV (subtypes IVA and IVB).

In 1973 William Sly* and colleagues described a new MPS characterized by short stature, hepato-

---

*Pierre Maroteaux was born in Versailles in 1926 and had a distinguished career at the Hôpital des Enfants Malades, Paris.

†Maurice Lamy, (1895-1975) was Professor of Medical Genetics at the University of Paris from 1950 to 1967.

---

*William Sly was appointed Chairman of the Department of Biochemistry, St. Louis University School of Medicine in 1984.

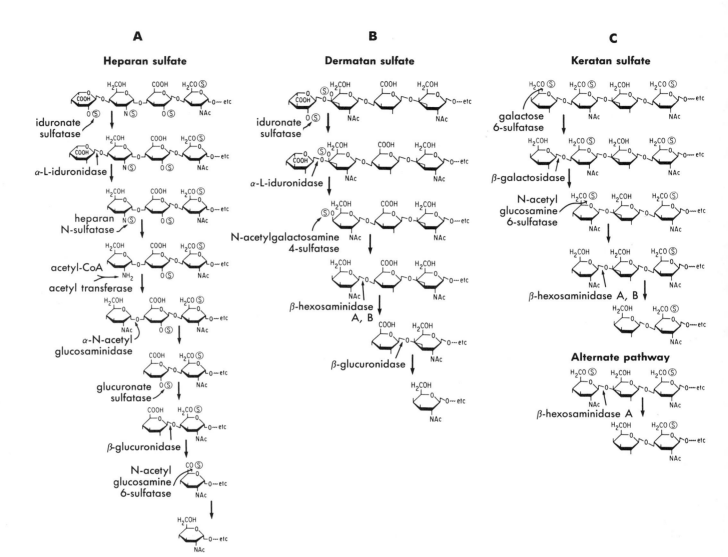

Fig. 11-6. Degradative pathways for the pathologically significant glycosaminogly-cans. **A,** Heparan sulfate; **B,** dermatan sulfate; and, **C,** keratan sulfate. (Modified from Neufeld EF, Muenzer, J: The mucopolysaccharidoses. In Scriver CR et al, editors: *The metabolic basis of inherited disease,* New York, 1989, McGraw-Hill, pp 1565-1587.)

splenomegaly, progressive skeletal deformity, developmental delay, and glycosaminoglycanuria.[774] Cultured skin fibroblasts had been sent to the Neufeld laboratory for cross-correction studies and in the process of establishing normal levels of various lysosomal enzymes in a series of cell lines, Hall and colleagues serendipitously discovered complete deficiency of β-glucuronidase activity in the patient's cells and half the normal levels in first-degree relatives.[311] Thus the basic defect of this disorder, its mode of inheritance, and even an

approach to potential therapy were discovered when only one case was known. (More recently the Sly syndrome was one of the first conditions shown to be completely correctable by gene transfer in a murine model.[773]) Other enzymatic defects in glycosaminoglycan degradation probably exist, although affected persons have not yet been identified.[358]

A number of conditions with clinical or biochemical features, or both, that resemble those of the mucopolysaccharidoses have been delineated.

These include the conditions that combine features of the mucopolysaccharidoses and the sphingolipidoses; these have been termed mucolipidosis types I, II, and III by Spranger and Wiedemann.[780] These three disorders were initially called, respectively, lipomucopolysaccharidosis, I-cell disease, and pseudo-Hurler polydystrophy. Additional Hurler-like conditions are generalized gangliosidosis, fucosidosis, and mannosidosis.

When Neufeld and her colleagues discovered that "corrective factors" could be exchanged between cultured cells,[129,131,177,253,758] an approach to therapy became apparent. It was originally proposed that the uptake mechanism was a means of recapturing enzymes lost to the extracellular environment. More recent teleologic explanations suggest, however, that lysosomal enzyme "maturation" serves to accomplish trafficking and compartmentalization of enzymes through the Golgi–endoplasmic reticulum–lysosome (GERL) system. Nevertheless, the therapeutic applications of enzyme uptake into lysosomes continue to be a fertile field of basic research and clinical investigation.

Initial trials of "enzyme replacement" by means of plasma infusion,* infusion of leukocytes,[411,410,445,576] subcutaneous implantation of fibroblasts[191,192,276] or amniotic membranes,† and liver transplantation sometimes offered tantalizing "trace" effects but failed to demonstrate a response sufficient to motivate continued therapeutic application.

In 1981 Hobbs et al.[343,344] first reported successful engraftment of normal bone marrow into a child with Hurler syndrome. Although highly controversial, continuing clinical trials have substantiated several biochemical and pathophysiologic correlates that have been collectively described as "metabolic correction."[698,893] Subsequent animal studies of bone marrow transplantation were undertaken in a feline model of Maroteaux-Lamy syndrome,[269] a canine model of Hurler-Scheie syndrome,[762,764,766] a murine model of Sly syndrome[86] and a number of other lysosomal storage diseases. The long-term outcome for patients with MPS who receive transplantation, the morbidity, and the limitations of treatment continue to be elucidated as children who have received grafts mature.

---

*References 96, 191, 196, 208, 236, 380, and 923.

†References 6, 7, 11, 582, 838, and 924.

At the threshold of the molecular genetics revolution several genes for MPS diseases have been cloned. In 1987 the full-length complementary DNA (cDNA) sequence for human β-glucuronidase (Sly syndrome) was reported.[635] The gene for β-galactosidase (Morquio syndrome type B) was cloned in three laboratories,[636,921] as was the gene for N-acetylgalactosamine-4-sulfatase (Maroteaux-Lamy syndrome).[499,663,738] The genes for glucosamine-6-sulfatase (Sanfilippo syndrome type D)[705,706] and for iduronate sulfatase[906] have also been cloned. Most recently, cloning of the human α-L-iduronidase gene has been accomplished.[746]

The availability of cloned genes has allowed for more precise localization of chromosomal loci (Table 11-1) and identification of the specific mutations, and has provided the basis for initial attempts to study gene therapy in vitro[913] and in animal models.

The first 75 years of research since the initial clinical description of the mucopolysaccharidoses have witnessed biochemical characterization of this group of disorders, differentiation of distinct forms, and initial attempts at treatment. The challenges of the future will be identification of additional inborn errors of glycosaminoglycan catabolism, recognition of specific molecular defects that can be correlated with the clinical phenotype (e.g., to differentiate patients with relatively "mild" and "severe" forms), development of a practical method for presymptomatic mass newborn screening, and attempts at more satisfactory systemic treatment.

Development of Concepts Concerning the Biochemical Basis of the Mucopolysaccharidoses

That the disorders discussed in this chapter involve a defect in glycosaminoglycan metabolism was suspected in 1952 by Brante[104] on the basis of the nature of the stored material. This supposition was given strong support in the demonstration by Dorfman and Lorincz[217] and by Meyer et al.[561] of excess "mucopolysacchariduria," that is, glycosaminoglycanuria. The glycosaminoglycans excreted in the urine in excess in the mucopolysaccharidoses are of lower molecular weight than are those found in normal urine,[148] indicating partial degradation.

In the early 1960s Hers[339] developed the concept of lysosomal diseases, and in the next few years he and others amassed evidence indicating that the Hurler syndrome satisfied the criteria for inclusion in this category. The archetypic lysosomal disease was glycogenosis type II (acid maltase deficiency); continued investigations have led to characterization of molecular defects, and some three dozen lysosomal storage diseases have now been defined.[598] The characteristics of a lysosomal disorder are as follows:

1. Undegraded enzyme substrates are stored, as demonstrated by the accumulation of glycosaminoglycan in the mucopolysaccharidoses.

2. Storage material may be somewhat heterogeneous, since the degradative enzymes are not strictly specific. For example, heterogeneity of substrate accumulation is evidenced by the urinary excretion of at least two different glycosaminoglycan species in MPS types I, II, and VII. Heterogeneity may also be tissue specific, as illustrated by Hurler syndrome, for which the predominant storage material in brain is ganglioside but in liver is glycosaminoglycan.

3. Deposition of storage material is chiefly intracellular and "vacuolar," that is, membrane bound in secondary lysosomes.

4. The defect is generalized or "systemic;" thus all tissues are enzyme deficient. Some tissues are more significantly affected than others, depending on the amount of substrate normally metabolized by the tissue in question. Because macrophages are active in glycosaminoglycan degradation, these cells (in bone marrow or liver biopsy specimens) are invariably involved in the mucopolysaccharidoses and can be used to provide histochemical or ultrastructural confirmation for diagnosis.

5. As increasing quantities of lysosomal storage material accumulate, the pathophysiologic features of the disease progress and become increasingly apparent at the clinical level. Although infants with an MPS often appear normal at birth, characteristic physical features and clinical problems gradually develop during early childhood.

Replacement therapy by means of the mechanism of endocytosis of enzyme into lysosomes is theoretically possible, as demonstrated in the cross-correction studies of Neufeld and her colleagues. In fact, such "correction factors," which are absent in cultured fibroblasts from affected persons, have now become potential therapeutic agents. This principle found support with early in vitro and short-term clinical studies,[514] which have evolved to actual clinical application in trials of enzyme replacement for Gaucher disease[50,51] and bone marrow transplantation.*

Support for the idea that Hurler syndrome and related disorders are lysosomal diseases was provided by the electron microscopic studies of Van Hoof and Hers,[857] which were published in 1968. These researchers demonstrated that accumulation of material occurred in membranous structures that had the characteristics of lysosomes. To state that a condition is a lysosomal disorder is equivalent to concluding that the defect is in degradation. This concept, however, was not immediately apparent, and in the early stages of the evolution of knowledge many investigators considered excessive synthesis of glycosaminoglycan to be the basic defect.

Danes and Bearn[173] demonstrated cytoplasmic metachromasia in the cultured fibroblasts from patients with mucopolysaccharidoses. Thereafter, in 1968, Fratantoni, Hall, and Neufeld[251] provided definitive proof of a degradative defect: cultured fibroblasts accumulated excessive amounts of $^{35}SO_4$-labeled glycosaminoglycan, and washout of the radioactive label occurred abnormally slowly when the fibroblasts were placed in "cold" medium.

Fratantoni, Hall, and Neufeld[252] initiated the seminal experiments, mixing fibroblasts from patients of different clinical types and demonstrating mutual correction of the metabolic defects. They showed that the medium in which cells of a different MPS type or normal cells had grown would also correct the metabolic defect, as would an extract prepared from the urine of unaffected persons. These observations indicated the existence of diffusible substances that are produced by fibroblasts which are essential to the normal degradation of glycosaminoglycans; one of these substances is deficient in each of the mucopolysaccharidoses. The substance deficient in each clinical syndrome was initially termed the "corrective factor" for that condition, that is, Hurler corrective factor, Hunter corrective factor, and the like. The nature of the "corrective factors" as proteins was delineated, and their specific en-

---

*References 145, 343, 344, 419, 462, 488, 801, and 893.

zymatic properties were subsequently characterized.

Surprises coming from the Neufeld approach included the following discoveries: (1) the Hurler and Scheie syndromes, although clinically quite different, behave the same in cross-correction studies (i.e., have deficiency of the same enzyme),[52,899] (2) the clinical picture of Sanfilippo syndrome can result from any one of four different genetic defects, and (3) Morquio syndrome can result from either of two different mutations.

Biochemical Basis of the Mucopolysaccharidoses

Each type of MPS results from deficiency of an enzyme required in the sequential process of dismantling complex carbohydrate glycosaminoglycan molecules (Fig. 11-6). Deficiency of any one of 10 enzymes in the degradative pathway results in a pathologic phenotype. The clinical features are manifestations of the consequent cell dysfunction, injury, or death in the tissues most involved in accumulation of the specific glycosaminoglycan(s).

Glycosaminoglycans. The important glycosaminoglycans in humans are heparan sulfate, dermatan sulphate, keratan sulfate, and chondroitin sulphate. In affected persons glycosaminoglycans are synthesized normally and are integral constituents of the proteoglycans in many forms of connective tissue. Only when glycosaminoglycans are phagocytosed into the lysosomal compartment do the specific enzymatic defects become manifest. Progressive accumulation of undegradable glycosaminoglycans in the lysosome gradually distend the cell, impair normal cell function, and may result in cell death and tissue damage. In some circumstances it appears that excessive extracellular glycosaminoglycan accumulation may also contribute to the pathophysiologic process. For example, coronary artery occlusion in the mucopolysaccharidoses may in part be the result of an aberrant signal for intimal proliferation.

Several reviews have been written on the clinical, biochemical, and molecular aspects of the mucopolysaccharidoses.[296,358,598,599] A number of principles have been evolved that not only help in the understanding of these conditions, but also have become basic tenets of the pathophysiology of inborn errors of lysosomal metabolism.

Specificity of glycosaminoglycan accumulation. Accumulation of heparan sulfate (Hurler, Hunter, Maroteaux-Lamy, and Sly syndromes) is associated with severe skeletal abnormalities. Accumulation of dermatan sulfate (in Hurler, Hunter, and Sanfilippo syndromes) is associated with central nervous system damage due in part to secondary mechanisms such as meningeal impingement on neural tissues and to a poorly-understood accumulation of gangliosides. Keratan sulfate accumulates in Morquio syndrome and impairs skeletal growth, although other organ systems are also involved.

Severity of disease. In general the rate of glycosaminoglycan accumulation probably determines the severity of the disease process. Although it has not been directly proven on experimental study, it is clear that children in whom significant physical changes develop early in life have a more severe condition, for example, Hurler syndrome (MPS type I H). For such individuals the tempo of progression is likely to continue to be rapid; thus there will be greater morbidity and early mortality. In contrast, affected persons with a slower progression may come to medical attention later in childhood, in adolescence, or even in adulthood, for example, persons with Scheie syndrome (MPS type I S). Such individuals have a slower accumulation of glycosaminoglycans and less severe pathophysiologic changes, thus having a relatively better prognosis.

Determinants of glycosaminoglycan degradation. Although lysosomal enzymes may be present extracellularly (and can even be quantitated in plasma as an indicator of zygosity), these catabolic enzymes do not function except intracellularly, where several other factors, possibly including "substrate channeling" through a lysosomal enzyme complex,[258] determine substrate turnover. If these degradative enzymes were active extracellularly, the body's proteoglycans would be in a constant state of siege and continuous turnover of the basic connective tissue framework would be required. Rather, glycosaminoglycans are important extracellular structural and informational molecules that determine tissue integrity and cell interactions, functions that require a high degree of molecular stability. In the lysosomal compartment actual physiologic enzymatic activity may be regulated by the acidity of the lysosomal pH, by the presence of enzyme or substrate activators, by substrate concentration, by molecular "microenvironments" (with unusual hydrophilicity, ionic strength, or other characteristics), and even by organization of enzymes into complexes.

A second important aspect of glycosaminoglycan metabolism may be the terminal-acting nature of the degradative enzymes. Because most lysosomal enzymes are active only on terminal residues, the bulk of the molecule is immune to the action of an occasional lysosomal hydrolase that escapes the cell into the extracellular compartment. Thus the structure at the terminus of the glycosaminoglycan limits its degradation and stabilizes the molecule as a whole.

MUCOPOLYSACCHARIDOSIS TYPE I H (HURLER SYNDROME)

As the paradigm for the mucopolysaccharidoses, Hurler syndrome (MPS I H) is described in detail. This condition is characterized by coarse facial features, hepatosplenomegaly, a pattern of severe skeletal abnormalities (dysostosis multiplex), progressive neurologic deterioration, and death before the age of 10 years in most instances. The disorder is usually recognizable in infancy. Indeed, clinical diagnosis before the age of 2 years serves as an operational definition of Hurler syndrome for differentiation from the other, milder phenotypes that result from defective activity of the enzyme α-L-iduronidase.

Clinical Manifestations

Natural history. In children with Hurler syndrome the disease is almost always fatal before 10 years of age. In one series of 27 patients the average age at death was 6.25 years, the oldest patient being 10.9 years of age at death.[918] The cause of death is usually cardiac disease (congestive heart failure or myocardial infarction), pneumonia, or respiratory complications related to tracheostomy and anesthesia.

The affected infant is of normal appearance at birth and appears to be developing normally for a few months. Indeed, the patient is characteristically large in the first year of life,[482] giving the impression of robust and healthy physical development.

By 2 years of age (Fig. 11-7) multiple abnormalities become apparent and usually lead to the clinical diagnosis of Hurler syndrome. The most important of these are lumbar kyphoscoliosis and hepatosplenomegaly; walking is often delayed and chronic rhinitis is a common complaint. Although corneal clouding is not obvious in the early stages, affected children often exhibit photophobia.

The clinical diagnosis is corroborated by the identification of excessive glycosaminoglycan in the urine and by the finding of metachromatic granules in cells (Fig. 11-8) such as circulating lymphocytes or bone marrow cells. Methods for these tests are detailed later. The wide availability of synthetic substrates for the assay of α-L-iduronidase renders biochemical confirmation of the diagnosis rapid and reliable.

The line along which development occurs is so characteristic that affected children, although unrelated, tend to resemble each other more than they resemble their unaffected siblings. As the child grows older, dwarfing and articular contractures are accompanied by radiologic changes in the skeleton that are more or less typical of this specific entity (Fig. 11-7, C and E). Progressive clouding of the cornea occurs in all cases and may conceal concurrent retinal degeneration. The liver and spleen become increasingly enlarged as a result of glycosaminoglycan deposition. Mental development, which appears to be normal for the first year or so of life, thereafter becomes delayed in comparison to that in unaffected children of the same age. Hydrocephalus may be obvious but frequently goes unrecognized, since it often develops slowly. After the sutures become fused, increased intracranial pressure may result from meningeal thickening caused by glycosaminoglycan deposits; this rise in pressure becomes manifest in the form of communicating hydrocephalus with cerebral atrophy. Obstructive airway disease is usually apparent and particulary marked during sleep.

In the terminal stages children have severe obstructive airway disease and usually have had palliative tonsilectomy, adenoidectomy, or tracheostomy. Neurologic regression may occur and become evident as loss of language and other skills. The anatomic basis for the cardiac manifestations is the deposition of glycosaminoglycan in the tunica intima of the coronary arteries, in the endocardium, and in the heart valves. Although some affected children have lethal complications during infancy,[788] most die between the ages of 4

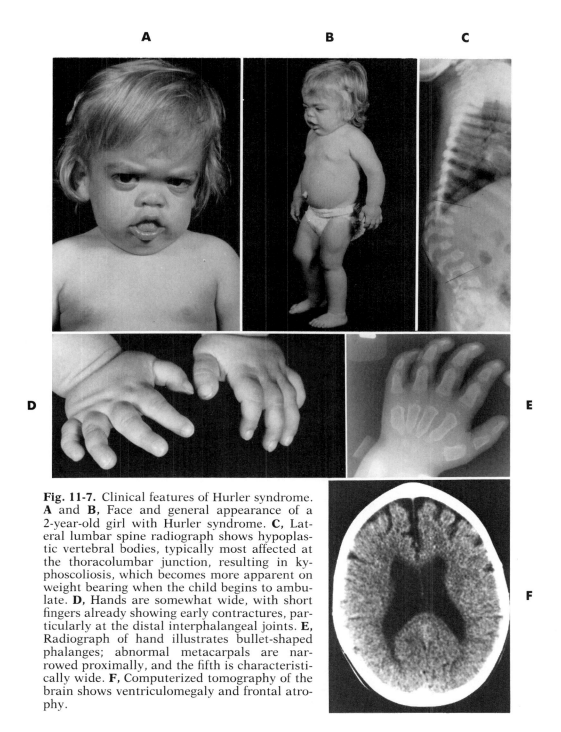

Fig. 11-7. Clinical features of Hurler syndrome. **A** and **B**, Face and general appearance of a 2-year-old girl with Hurler syndrome. **C**, Lateral lumbar spine radiograph shows hypoplastic vertebral bodies, typically most affected at the thoracolumbar junction, resulting in kyphoscoliosis, which becomes more apparent on weight bearing when the child begins to ambulate. **D**, Hands are somewhat wide, with short fingers already showing early contractures, particularly at the distal interphalangeal joints. **E**, Radiograph of hand illustrates bullet-shaped phalanges; abnormal metacarpals are narrowed proximally, and the fifth is characteristically wide. **F**, Computerized tomography of the brain shows ventriculomegaly and frontal atrophy.

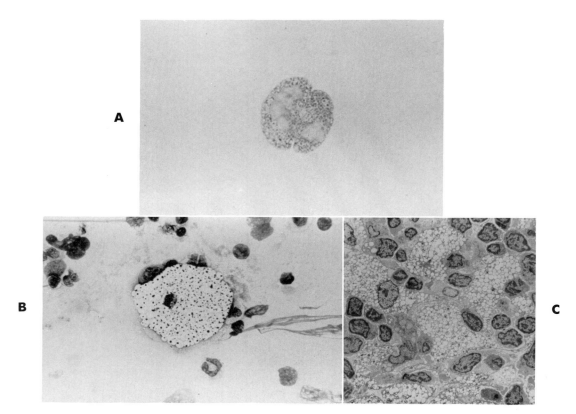

Fig. 11-8. Cytoplasmic inclusions in Hurler syndrome. **A,** This vacuolated polymor-phonuclear leukocyte of the type described in peripheral blood by Reilly[435] (type II polymorph) was identified in cerebrospinal fluid (toluidine blue stain), illustrating the ubiquity of morphologic abnormalities. **B,** In bone marrow a macrophage is grossly distended with lysosomal inclusions (Wright stain). **C,** In a 3-year-old girl with Hurler syndrome, electron microscopy of tissue from an enlarged tonsil reveals densely packed macrophages whose foamy cytoplasm is the ultrastructural corre-late of glycosaminoglycan accumulation.

and 10 years. The usual causes of death are respi-ratory infection and cardiac failure.

Head, neck, and spine. The head is large[612] and the scalp veins are often prominent in small chil-dren. The nose has a flattened bridge, a broad tip, and wide nostrils. Hypertelorism is usual. The skull is often scaphocephalic (i.e., shaped like the keel of a boat) as a result of premature closure of the sagittal suture. This craniosynostosis may be associated with a hyperostosis that creates a ridge along the saggital suture and on the forehead. Al-ternatively some children have a broad face and head as a result of premature fusion of the coronal sutures (Fig. 11-7, *A*). There is usually no difficulty in distinguishing the Hurler syndrome from other conditions associated with "acrocephaly" and "scaphocephaly," although in the earlier days of the nosography of Hurler syndrome such confu-sion did occur.[395]

The facial features have traditionally been de-scribed as "coarse" because of the appearance of thick skin laid upon a facial skeleton of relatively hypertrophic bone and cartilage. The presence of large and patulous lips, an open mouth, and an enlarged, protruding tongue may lead to consider-ation of a diagnosis of congenital hypothyroidism. The teeth are late to erupt and are usually small, short, widely spaced, and somewhat malformed. In many patients there is hypertrophy both of the bony alveolar ridges and of the overlying gums.[166] Dentigerous cysts[124] and a bone cyst of the alveolar ridge have been reported.[122,915] Chronic rhinor-rhea accompanied by noisy mouth breathing, which is virtually universal, results from choanal stenosis and thickened soft tissues of the upper airways.

Radiographs of the skull and face usually show marked abnormalities. The inferior surface of the sphenoid bone approximates to the back of the hard palate, thus narrowing the nasopharyngeal airway. A mass of adenoid tissue often obliterates the remaining air shadow. Changes in the sella turcica, in the form of unusual length and depth and an anterior "pocketing," are often designated as the "J-shaped sella" that characterizes the mucopolysaccharidoses. The sella turcica has also been described as "bowl shaped."[839] Neuhauser et al.[601] documented the features of arachnoid cysts on radiographic study and on autopsy in children with Hurler syndrome. Such cysts have also been observed in the Scheie syndrome (MPS type I S) but not in the Hunter and Sanfilippo syndromes (MPS types II and III). A favored location for cyst development is anterior to the sella turcica; erosion of the body of the sphenoid bone and of the anterior clinoids results. Enormous optic foramina are often demonstrable by means of special radiographic views.

The neck is so short that the head appears to rest directly on the thorax. Functional integrity of the cervical spinal cord is endangered. Vertebral subluxation with cord compression may occur if the odontoid process is hypoplastic.[824] The cord is at special risk for damage during vigorous hyperextension, particularly at anesthetic intubation.[63] The abnormal oropharyngeal anatomy renders intubation increasingly difficult[238] as the child becomes older. Infants can be readily intubated but by 2 years of age the size of the tongue, short pharynx, and limited nasal airway pose problems at oral intubation, and the tube often must be passed blindly through the cords. At this age failed intubation, traumatic intubation with bleeding, and laryngospasm are frequent problems. Such major difficulties and the consequent risks of morbidity and mortality constitute valid reasons for referral of the patient to a medical center experienced in the management of children with the Hurler syndrome.[63] As the child grows older, the airway becomes increasingly precarious and management is progressively more difficult. Quadraparesis and death resulting from subluxation of the cervical spine have occurred during attempts at intuba-

tion. The intervertebral ligaments are generally not excessively lax, however, and the shortness of the neck offers some protection against cervical subluxation (in marked distinction to the neck in Morquio syndrome, for which ligamentous laxity poses the major risk to cord integrity). Chiropractic manipulation of the neck is dangerous and strictly contraindicated. Equally, physical therapists should be advised against the use of any neck traction.

In addition to the problem of cervical spine subluxation, bony stenosis of the cervical canal, together with progressive thickening of the meninges, also places the cord at risk. In a few patients this complication has been associated with quadraparesis, and surgical decompression has been unsuccessful in at least two cases.

A thoracolumbar gibbus is often present, but the spinal cord is unlikely to be compromised at this level. Radiologic examination usually shows a wedge-shaped abnormality of the vertebral body at the apex of the gibbus. This vertebra often has an anterior, hooklike projection, or "beaking." In some instances this beaking appears to be caused by anterior herniation of the nucleus pulposus[62] accompanied by pressure atrophy of the upper anterior margin of the subjacent vertebral body (usually the second lumbar) (Fig. 11-7, *C*). Thoracolumbar kyphoscoliosis may be evident during infancy but is not often recognized until the infant begins to sit. At this stage the child is likely to assume a posture which has been compared to that of a sitting cat. Recognition of the kyphoscoliosis is frequently an important diagnostic pointer that leads the patient into evaluation and initial diagnosis.

Nervous system. Progressive loss of mental capabilities as a result of organic brain disease is the most prominent and devastating nervous system manifestation of Hurler syndrome. The accumulation of glycosaminoglycans and gangliosides in central nervous system tissue is progressive, causing direct injury to the brain. Superimposed on this pathologic condition, other aspects of nervous system disease are significant; some involve the peripheral nervous system, and some are treatable, such as hydrocephalus, hearing impairment, and median nerve compression.

Hydrocephalus. Mental retardation is a conspicuous feature of all cases of MPS I H and may be associated with frank hydrocephalus in severely affected infants.[29,493] Impairment is progressive, especially in the late stages of the disease, and there may be accompanying neurologic signs such as motor paralysis, increase in muscular tone, and a positive Babinski sign. True high-pressure hydrocephalus may be present; in such patients ventricular dilation is often too marked to be accounted for on the basis of cortical atrophy alone (Fig. 11-7, *F*). In the author's personal experience the phenomenon may be partially reversible by means of placement of a ventriculoperitoneal shunt or by means of bone marrow transplantation. In most children with hydrocephalus the usual signs of acute increase in intracranial pressure (ataxia, decreased level of consciousness, and the like) do not become evident; therefore these children do not receive treatment. Some patients may show simple dilation of the ventricles as a result of cortical atrophy, that is, hydrocephalus *ex vacuo*.[9,400,839,884]

Hearing impairment. Deafness of mixed conductive and perceptive type is frequent in the Hurler syndrome. Contributory factors include the predisposition to middle ear infections and, possibly, the accumulation of glycosaminoglycans in the receptive and neurologic components of the hearing mechanism. Furthermore, the ossicles are abnormal, with limitation of motion as in other joints and bones in this condition.[725,914] For these reasons, although neurosensory hearing deficit is often apparent on testing of auditory brain stem response, a conductive element in the deafness of some patients is to be expected.

Carpal tunnel syndrome. In normal anatomic circumstances the median nerve passes freely between the scaphoid and pisiform carpal bones to supply the abductor pollicis brevis muscle, which is crucial for the oppositional action of the thumb in gripping and grasping. This nerve also provides sensory innervation of the dorsal surface of the distal index, middle, and half of the ring finger, together with the volar aspect of the thumb. The abnormal wrist anatomy of children with Hurler syndrome[304,673,677,916] and other mucopolysaccharidoses leads to median nerve compression. In contrast to the carpal tunnel syndrome commonly encountered in normal adults, however, median nerve entrapment in children with Hurler syndrome is typically asymptomatic. Nevertheless, in a large series of young children (ages 1.5 to 7 years) studied by the author and colleagues, several had markedly delayed median nerve conduc-

tion velocity with diminished amplitude, and two had prominent weakness and atrophy of the abductor pollicis brevis muscle. All those with abnormalities detected by means of electrophysiologic testing had visibly narrowed median nerves at surgery; significant recovery followed division of the transverse carpal ligament in every instance.

Ocular features. The main ocular manifestations of Hurler syndrome are early photophobia, progressive corneal clouding, retinal pigmentary dystrophy, swelling of the optic nerve head, optic atrophy, and glaucoma.[154,611] Clouding of the cornea develops in all affected persons. The cornea usually has merely a steamy appearance in the early stages; this feature is most apparent when light is shone on the cornea from the side, and slit-lamp examination confirms the finding. The opacities are located in the medial and deeper layers of the cornea, and the epithelium and endothelium are largely spared. It seems that stromal cells synthesize glycosaminoglcyans, which are secreted into the extracellular space for as long as these cells maintain functional and structural integrity. In the Hurler syndrome, however, glycosaminoglycans accumulate and distend the cell and are eventually released into the surrounding stroma.[709]

Ocular abnormalities such as buphthalmos and megalocornea[74,229,394,563] have been described. A retinal element may be present in visual impairment, since changes in the retina have been documented on histopathologic study[494] and the electroretinogram is diminished or entirely extinguished in many patients.[136,279,801] Glaucoma[145] and blindness caused by central lesions (in the author's personal experience) are infrequent complications.

Respiratory system. Nasal congestion, noisy mouth breathing, and frequent upper respiratory infections occur in all patients with the Hurler syndrome; the malformation of the facial and nasal bones is probably in large part responsible.[229] Progressive glycosaminoglycan accumulation in oropharyngeal structures and tracheal connective tissue (Fig. 11-9) leads to airway obstruction,[4,662] which typically becomes manifest as sleep apnea[512,753,757,893] but also results in hypoxemia during waking hours in severely affected children. Tonsillectomy, adenoidectomy, and radical

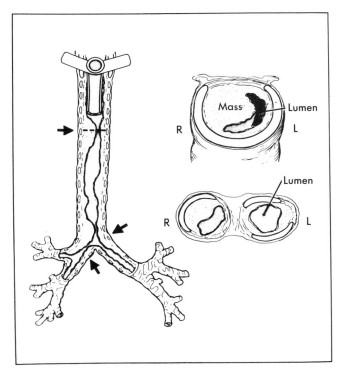

Fig. 11-9. Extensive tracheal and bronchial airway obstruction in a patient with Hurler syndrome, drawn from endoscopic and radiographic observations. Arrows indicate the sites of cross-sectional views. *R,* Right; *L,* left. (From Adachi K, Chole RA: *Arch Otolaryngol Head Neck Surg* 116:1205-1207, 1990.)

pharyngoplasty provide some relief of airway obstruction but are only transiently useful, since airway obstruction recurs. Constant positive airway pressure (CPAP) administered by means of nasal mask (nasal CPAP) and tracheostomy have been used to treat upper airway obstruction. Laser excision of tracheal lesions has also been undertaken to remove tracheal obstruction.[4] All these measures are temporary and generally unsatisfactory. Gingival hypertrophy and severe upper airway obstruction are reversed, however, by allogeneic bone marrow transplantation.[512,893]

Spinal malalignment, thoracic deformity, and abnormalities of the bronchial cartilage contribute to a restriction of chest expansion[231] and diminished vital capacity. Although asthma is not exceptionally common in Hurler syndrome, wheezing is a common auscultatory finding in affected children with intercurrent infections or as a sign of congestive heart failure. In children who do have asthma, the severity of asthmatic crises may be aggravated by accumulation of storage material and mucoid secretions in the lining cells of bronchioles.

Cardiovascular system. The best specific descriptions of the cardiovascular aspects of the Hurler syndrome are those of Lindsay[493] and Emanuel.[231] Cardiac murmurs and the echocar-

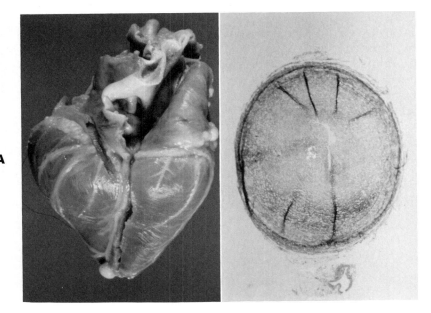

Fig. 11-10. A, External view of the heart of a 2-year-old child with Hurler syndrome who died of coronary insufficiency. Coronary arteries have been largely replaced with bands of fibrous tissue. **B,** Cross-section of a coronary artery showing more than 95% occlusion of the vascular lumen by glycosaminoglycan and collagenous material.

diographic findings in the Hurler syndrome have been described by several authors.[301,399,785,918] In a series of 27 children, the majority had clinical evidence of valvular heart disease and in the five in whom detailed postmortem studies were undertaken, multiple valvular lesions and severe coronary artery occlusion were found.[918] Catheterization and angiocardiographic studies were undertaken by Krovetz, Lorincz, and Schiebler,[463] who demonstrated increased total systemic, total pulmonary, and pulmonary arterial resistance in children with the Hurler syndrome. The significance of pulmonary hypertension is further emphasized by the author's observation that a small number of patients have had sudden, often lethal pulmonary hemorrhage during the stress and thrombocytopenia associated with bone marrow transplantation.

Occlusion of the coronary arteries by a matrix of glycosaminoglycan and collagenous fibers is a common, if not uniform, occurrence (Fig. 11-10). Although most children do not appear to be symptomatic, this problem may be severe and may occur in the first years of life. What was interpreted as angina pectoris occurred[166] at as early as 4¾ years of age in an affected child, who died at the age of 7 years. Extensive occlusion of all the coronary arteries is often discovered at autopsy in affected children and may be the cause of sudden death in many patients with the Hurler syndrome. Brosius and Roberts[114] described occlusion of the major epicardial coronary arteries, which was identified at autopsy in six children ranging from 3 to 16 years of age. Remarkably, none of them had symptoms of cardiac dysfunction or evidence of myocardial ischemia during life. Coronary artery angiography has not been a reliable means of evaluating this occlusion because the narrowing is relatively uniform throughout the extent of each vessel and because there are no standardized methods of measuring vessel caliber in children.[106]

Accumulation of glycosaminoglycan may occur in other vessels; in this way, congenital aortic stenosis has been simulated in an affected child.[107]

Rarely children may come to medical attention in congestive heart failure with cardiomegaly, suggesting an acute viral cardiomyopathy with endocardial fibroelastosis (Fig. 11-11).[213] Some degree of endocardial fibroelastosis has been an incidental finding in various forms of mucopolysaccharidosis in 20% of 68 autopsies that in-

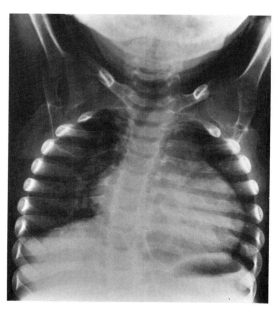

Fig. 11-11. Chest radiograph showing cardiomegaly in a child with Hurler syndrome who subsequently died at 2 years of age of congestive heart failure with endocardial fibroelastosis.

cluded cardiovascular pathologic examination.[464] Stephan et al.[725] described the postmortem diagnosis of Hurler syndrome in two infant girls who died at 8 and 9 months of age; their deaths were attributed to endocardial fibroelastosis. These cases serve to illustrate that cardiac failure may precede recognition of the features of Hurler syndrome on clinical and radiographic examination.

Skeletal system. During the first year of life the hands often appear to be essentially normal, but by 2 years of age, they are broad and the fingers are relatively short and "stubby." The fifth fingers are often bent radially, and there is a partial flexion contracture of each finger. (Fig. 11-7, *D* and *E*). This characteristic appearance of the hand results from stiffening of the phalangeal joints, with incapacity for full extension.

By two years of age, limitation in extensibility of the larger joints is usually striking.[379] This feature may be due in part to abnormalities of the joint surfaces, but it is more likely to be the result of changes in the tendons and ligaments surrounding the joints. Thus patients often find it necessary to walk on their toes, especially when they have been in bed for extended periods. A deformity of the wrist may superficially suggest rickets, but the stiff joints (along with many other features) help distinguish the Hurler syndrome.[374] The limitation of motion of joints seems to extend to the thorax, which often is relatively fixed in position.[231]

The anteroposterior radiograph of the hand provides several helpful diagnostic signs, which are apparent after the second year of life (Fig. 11-7, *E*). These include the bullet-shaped phalanges (so-appearing as a result of undermodeling of the diaphyses), narrowing of the proximal metacarpals, a notably wide fifth metacarpal, and angulation of the distal end of the radius and ulna. The tubular bones show progressive cortical thinning and increase in diameter of their shafts because of expansion of their medullary cavities.[122] These changes tend to be more striking in the bones of the upper rather than the lower limbs. A curious narrowing of the proximal third of the femora to a caliber less than half that of normal has been noted.[21] The ribs are characteristically broad, saber-shaped, or spatulate (Fig. 11-11). The vertebral ends of the ribs are unusually narrow, particularly in comparison with the remainder of the rib.

Genu valgum, coxa valga, pes planus, and other deformities are frequent features. Abnormalities of the sternum are infrequently present, but "funnel chest" was present in one of Hurler's original patients[394,404] and in a child documented by McKusick.

Abdomen and viscera. The abdomen is protuberant (Fig. 11-7, *B*) as a result of a combination of hepatosplenomegaly, abnormalities of the supporting tissues, and kyphosis of the spine. Both liver and spleen may be so large that their lower borders dip into the pelvis. Function of these organs is usually unimpaired, and biochemical markers of liver function are entirely normal. In an isolated instance, however, pancytopenia and epistaxes developed, possibly because of hypersplenism.[781]

Loose stools or frank diarrhea is a common and underreported problem in the Hurler syndrome. This complication appears to result from neurologic dysfunction, and there has been no evidence of malabsorption.

Diastasis recti and umbilical hernia are almost invariably present;[352] inguinal hernia is frequently present. The author has also encountered diaphragmatic hernia in an isolated case. Engel[235] described a patient with scrotal hernias that were the size of a child's head. Bilateral hydrocele may also occur.[332] McCormick[542] reported fatal rupture of the stomach in a 6-year-old boy who had repeated episodes of gastric dilation.

Integument. The skin is generally somewhat thick. Nevertheless, the type of nodular, "pebbled" lesions of the skin described in the section on MPS type II are extremely unusual in MPS type I H. In most affected children the entire surface of the body, including both trunk and limbs, is covered by fine, lanugo-like fuzz. In older patients hairiness remains striking, especially over the back, arms, and hands; hirsutism is a feature of all the mucopolysaccharidoses.

Endocrine system. No consistent endocrine abnormality is evident on clinical examination, in spite of histologic evidence of cellular deposits in most glands of internal secretion. Thyroid enlargement without dysfunction is probably related to the infiltration with glycosaminoglycans. The abnormal configuration of the sella turcica is a reflection of the disordered skeletal development, not a result of enlargement of the pituitary gland. A systematic survey of young patients, in the author's experience, has failed to reveal abnormalities of thyroid function or of serum concentrations of growth hormone, luteinizing hormone, follicle-stimulating hormone, and testosterone.

Pharmacologic response. The dose of premedication required for cardiac catheterization in patients with the Hurler syndrome was found to be two or three times greater than that usually required for comparable unaffected children.[463] Similarly, relative resistance to sedation is a common experience. Indeed, difficulties with sedation and problems with airway obstruction after the child has been successfully sedated are commonplace.

The following narrative by an intelligent and observing father outlines the evolution of the Hurler syndrome in his daughter up to the age of about 4 years:

My impression is that her most difficult period was roughly that of her first to second year. Deafness appeared, so far as we could tell, shortly after her first birthday, becoming complete by about 16 to 18 months of age. Around this time the more pronounced abdominal swelling also began to show, and she was sick much of the time. Nights were very difficult for her and everyone during this time, and until a bit beyond 2 years of age, she would cry for hours, perhaps in pain. On the other hand, she has seemed to be a bit less sensitive to outside pain than the other children. After the crying spells began to diminish, her personality became more buoyant. During the last year or more, angelic would scarcely be too strong a word. She radiates love and affection and thoughtfulness, coupled with a good sense of humor. Her motor skills have kept up remarkably well; she ate with a spoon before 1 year and has kept it up with normal increase in proficiency; she was diaper-trained by about 2½ years and bed-trained by about 3¼ years, with no unusual effort; although the gait is a bit awkward because of underdevelopment of leg muscles and a very large abdomen, she loves to run and dance and slide and swing. Picture books are great favorites; animals are adored, as are dolls and cuddly toys, toward which she is quite maternal. Vision seems still acute, although cloudiness is apparent in the cornea. She dresses and undresses herself as far as her build permits and is almost fastidious about putting away clothes, hanging things up, removing dishes to the sink after eating, etc. Simple cutout jigsaw puzzles she handles well. She understands gestures and expressions perfectly and uses them herself for very efficient communication. During April and May of this year (at the age of 3¾ years) she was a day pupil at a nursery school for the deaf. Since September she has been a Monday-to-Friday boarding pupil at a state institution for deaf children. Here a very capable teacher seems to be making progress with lip reading and vocalization instruction. Other than the direct Hurler's symptoms, her general health has been reasonably good: chickenpox, several periods of respiratory infection each year, and occasional (every 6 weeks or so?) flash fevers to about 103° F, which are over in a few hours, leaving her worn out for a day. Her teeth have never developed fully, even now being little more than widely separated stumps; however, she can handle, and seems to enjoy, practically any kind of food.

My wife and I feel that, at least until quite recently, her intelligence has been essentially normal. She usually learns new patterns of action, or placement of objects, or play, after only one or two repetitions—unless something arouses the stubbornness, of which she has a powerful streak. She watches the other children playing, with close comprehension of their actions and antics, often either joining or copying, nearly always enjoying. She knows all the clothing in the house, often bringing the appropriate items, in proper order, to those of us getting dressed. In driving, she will often back-seat drive, telling me which turns to take, by murmurs and gestures, even when we are several miles from home but headed for it. She sets great store on the proper way of doing things! Her sleep is now peaceful, 11 hours a

night and usually an hour's nap; even when she is tired her personality holds up cheerfully. When hurt in any way she usually cries but little; however, the offended member must be kissed to make the hurt go away.

It is possible that her rate of development is slowing down; she is learning, or at least responding, among the slowest members of her eighteen-pupil nursery class. Also, recently there has been pronounced increase in the abdominal swelling. Our local pediatrician believes that the liver is almost entirely responsible for the more than double normal girth, and that x-ray treatment might offer her a palliative. Should the swelling become much greater, walking will become extremely difficult. Difficulties with respiratory disease might have been too much for her system already, before modern drugs; except for a couple of summer months, there is a constant nasal discharge of varying rate of flow. Her circulation seems to have its troubles, in that lips and fingernails are often very blue.

Pathology

The first autopsy reported in the literature on MPS type I H was undertaken by Tuthill,[837] an American working in Munich, who examined one of Hurler's original patients. At least 40 autopsies, many of which were individual case reports, have now been recorded.*

Abnormalities have been identified in cartilage, fasciae, tendons, periosteum, blood vessels, heart valves, meninges, and cornea, among other sites. All these tissues may contain cells that are thought to be of the fibroblast line and are distended with large amounts of deposited material. The cells were appropriately termed "clear cells" (in a patient with Hunter syndrome) by Millman and Whittick.[566] Similar inclusions are seen in Kupffer and parenchymal cells of the liver, the reticulum cells of the spleen and lymph nodes, and the epithelial cells of several endocrine organs such as the pituitary.

Nervous system. Extensive changes in the meninges have been reported.[189,298,508] Millman and Whittick[566] found thickening of the leptomeninges over the cerebral hemispheres and "clear cells" on histologic study. Hydrocephalus may be the result of interference with cerebrospinal fluid drainage by deposits of glycosaminoglycan. The frequency of hydrocephalus has been underesti-

---

*References 29, 60, 106, 198, 231, 298, 324, 335, 394, 446, 460, 468, 494, 508, 735, 772, 794, 797, 837, 846, and 882.

mated, and it is probably an important factor in the cerebral impairment in affected persons.

Neuhauser et al.[601] described the features of arachnoid cysts on autopsy. Although they are situated predominantly in the area anterior to the sella turcica, they are also found below the cerebellum. The cysts are apparently related to leptomeningeal fibrosis. No ill effects of the cysts per se have been noted, but they may contribute to blockage in cerebrospinal fluid flow and therefore to the hydrocephalus. There has been no evidence of damage to the pituitary, hypothalamus, or visual tracts.

A peculiar feature of Hurler syndrome is the presence of greatly enlarged perivascular spaces in the centrum semiovale and medullary cores of the gyri. (Recent investigations with computed tomography and magnetic resonance imaging have demonstrated similar lesions in the other mucopolysaccharidoses, although correlation on pathologic study is currently lacking.)

Material, presumably identical to that in the fibroblasts, balloons the nerve cells of both the central nervous system and the peripheral ganglia. The nerve cells in the nuclear layer of the retina are similarly involved.[494] Mental retardation is presumably explained by these deposits. Secondary accumulation of specific gangliosides is known to accompany the primary glycosaminoglycan storage, but the role of ganglioside accumulation in specific neuronal geometry (meganeurite formation) and in synaptic connectivity remains an interesting area of speculation.[874,875]

Connective tissue. Collagen fibers in affected areas are swollen, homogeneous, and lacking in the normal fibrillary characteristics.[493] Enlargement and vacuolization of the chondrocytes and osteocytes, as well as of the periosteal cells, has been described[87,494]; these changes are probably intimately related to the skeletal malformation, as well as the gums and dentition and the sensory organs of the ear. In the author's experience bone marrow transplantation may result in the resumption of more normal linear growth of long bones but does not alter preexisting abnormalities of bone shape and ultrastructure.

Cardiovascular system. In the heart the valves and associated structures, the coronary arteries, and the myocardial muscle itself are in-

volved.[106,463,697] Dermatan sulfate normally plays a role in the extracellular organization of collagen, and an excess of dermatan sulfate may induce extensive collagen deposition at inappropriate sites. In persons who have died after a few years of life the aortic and mitral valves almost invariably have shown some degree of nodular thickening,[231,494] together with changes in the chordae tendineae.[87] Functionally both stenosis and regurgitation can result. The histologic picture in the heart valves is dominated by the presence of cells containing storage material. On gross pathologic examination the coronary arteries may "stand out like white cords."[106,231] Cells laden with glycosaminoglycan material may be present in coronary arteries,[106,165,494,508] and almost complete occlusion may result from the extensive intimal deposits.[166,189] The aorta[107,508] and pulmonary artery[231] may also show intimal deposits, presumably of the same material that forms the vacuoles of the cells of various organs. The myocardial cells may show marked ballooning by vacuoles. Patchy thickening of the endocardium and epicardium has been described.[231,494,660,785,797] Changes have been encountered in the peripheral arteries of the brain, spleen, pancreas, and kidney, as well as in the mesenteric, carotid, radial, and anterior tibial arteries.

Respiratory system. Abnormality of the tracheobronchial cartilages and the upper airways may be responsible for the susceptibility to respiratory infection. Bronchopneumonia is a frequent cause of death.[388]

Kidney. Kobayashi[447] demonstrated the presence of granules of acid mucopolysaccharide (i.e., glycosaminoglycan) in the epithelial cells of the glomeruli of three patients. Nephrotic syndrome has been observed rarely.[810]

Eye. The literature on the histopathologic study of the cornea has been reviewed by Scheie et al.[730] The basal layer of the corneal epithelium shows edema, cytoplasmic vacuolization, and the presence of metachromatic cytoplasmic granules.[494] Bowman's membrane is replaced in part by large cells with vacuolated cytoplasm and metachromatic cytoplasmic granules.[74] Corneal corpuscles in the stroma also contain metachromatic granules. The connective tissue of the conjunctiva contains monocytes with toluidine blue–positive granules in their cytoplasm. (These corneal and conjunctival findings are also present in MPS type I S,[680] MPS type IV, and MPS type VI.[430]) Conjunctival biopsy specimens provide useful material for electron microscopic investigation, and at one time biopsy was recommended[730] as a simple diagnostic procedure.

Skin. Hambrick and Scheie[314] gave the following account of the histopathology of the skin: "The characteristic cellular lesion of Hurler syndrome was present within the skin from all sites, clinically normal or abnormal. This consisted of a peculiar, granular vacuolization of the cytoplasm of epithelial cells and fibrocytes of the dermis. The degree of involvement of the epidermis may be quite extensive, particularly in the skin of the involved fingers."

The cytoplasmic granules have metachromatic tinctorial properties and results are positive for stains that are relatively specific for glycosaminoglycans. Cole et al.[153] interpreted a histologic study of a skin section as showing marked fragmentation of collagen fibers and mucinous degeneration.

General considerations. Some reported failures in staining postmortem tissues may have occurred because formalin or alcohol dissolves the vacuolar material.[87,189,494,794] Dioxane-dinitrophenol fixative has been useful in preserving the deposited material.[494] The best method in the study of tissue glycosaminoglycans is to cut frozen sections of unstained tissue, then fix in a 1:1 mixture of tetrahydrofuran and acetone, in the opinion of Haust and Landing.[324] In their view, lead acetate is an inadequate fixative because it preserves glycosaminoglycan poorly and interferes with metachromatic staining. Scheie, Hambrick, and Barness[730] found that absolute alcohol, Carnoy's solution, trichloroacetic acid, acridine, and lead acetate, in descending order, gave the best preservation of glycosaminoglycan in skin biopsy specimens.

A few researchers have reported that the intracellular deposits take conventional fat stains.[84,161,322,400,837] The majority, however, have found either that the vacuoles do not stain as fat or that they stain atypically. Analyses of hepatic and splenic tissue for fat reveal no increase.[335,794] The material that displays striking metachromasia[846] may stain with periodic acid–Schiff reagent

or with Best's carmine. Bishton, Norman, and Tingey[87] suggested that even when precautions are taken to prevent solution of the material deposited in the liver, satisfactory staining of "heparin-type" polysaccharides by means of the periodic acid–Schiff technique cannot be expected. They recommended use of toluidine blue as a stain in these cases.

Histochemical studies led Lindsay et al.[494] to suspect that the storage material was glycoprotein. Brante[104] isolated a polysaccharide material having 0.9% sulfur, 27% hexosamine, and 26% glucuronic acid, containing no fatty acids on hydrolysis, and representing 10% of the dry weight of the liver. Uzman[846] described the following storage materials isolated from the liver and spleen of affected persons: first, a complex polysaccharide containing glucose, galactose, hexosamines, and sulfate, soluble in water and formaldehyde but insoluble in other organic solvents, and staining metachromatically with toluidine blue; second, a glycolipid soluble in water and ethanol but not in other organic solvents and containing fatty acids, sphingosine, neuraminic acid, hexuronic acid, hexosamines, glucose, and galactose. Brown[115] proposed a possible molecular structure of the material isolated in large amounts from the liver of patients with the Hurler syndrome and referred to it as an oligosaccharide. By his evidence the material is composed exclusively of D-glucosamine and D-glucuronic acid units combined in glycosidic linkage. The material in point is heparan sulfate.[560] Meyer et al.[561] found large amounts of heparan sulfate in the liver of one patient.

Dawson[189] thought that the deposits in the brain consisted of phospholipid, although those elsewhere seemed to be glycosaminoglycan. Meyer found that glycosaminoglycan (both dermatan sulfate and heparan sulfate) was deposited in the brain in appreciable amounts.

An extensive literature has accumulated concerning the electron microscopic changes in the liver* and, to a lesser extent, in other tissues.[193,220,854] These findings, together with the general natural history of the Hurler syndrome, led to the characterization of this and related disorders as lysosomal diseases.[340] The same changes are found in noncultured (i.e., in situ) fibroblasts and macrophages of skin[193] and conjunctiva[428]

---

*References 125, 126, 325, 424, 466, 500, and 856.

and in cultured skin fibroblasts.[48] "Membranous cytoplasmic bodies" have also been described in ganglion and satellite cells of intramural plexi of the rectal wall obtained by means of biopsy[230] in a patient with the Hunter syndrome (MPS type II) and probably would be found also in patients with MPS type I. These changes are thought to be causally related to chronic diarrhea which occurs in the mucopolysaccharidoses.

Fundamental Defect

Excessive urinary excretion of dermatan sulfate and heparan sulfate[217,561] in patients with MPS type I H was an early observation which indicated that a defect in glycosaminoglycan metabolism is the basic fault. Glycosaminoglycan levels are elevated in the plasma of affected individuals.[124,717] Although excessive synthesis of glycosaminoglycans and other disturbances[561] were once postulated, it is now well recognized that Hurler syndrome results from a defect in the degradation of glycosaminoglycans. Although theories of abnormality of substances other than glycosaminoglycans have been proposed previously,* it is now presumed that either these concepts are incorrect or the observed changes are secondary to the primary defect (i.e., abnormal α-L-iduronidase enzyme activity).[39,531] The explanation for the appearance of two glycosaminoglycans in the urine in MPS type I is illustrated in Fig. 11-6: both dermatan sulfate and heparan sulfate have iduronide as a component of their polysaccharide side chains. Iduronidase has been well characterized[258,708,739] and has high-uptake and low-uptake forms.[740] It is a lysosomal enzyme with a relatively acidic optimum pH of about 3.5,[887,893] and it is probably catalytically active only within the acidic lysosome. Studies of the kinetics of residual enzyme activity in cultured fibroblasts from patients with various forms of defective α-L-iduronidase have revealed correlations with the severity of disease; investigations of this type have potential application as a prognostic test. Animal models have been identified.[320]

Genomic clones and a full-length cDNA clone encoding human α-L-iduronidase have been isolated. The messenger RNA (mRNA) of 2.3 kb is derived from a gene consisting of 14 exons extending over approximately 20 kb.[747] Such clones have been used to localize the gene to the short arm of chromosome 4, region 16.3 (4p16.3) by means of in situ hybridization.[746] This locus has also been confirmed by Southern blot analysis of human mouse cell hybrids. Molecular genetic investigations are now able to identify specific defects in the α-L-iduronidase gene and to provide even greater diagnostic specificity.

Prevalence and Inheritance

Mucopolysaccharidosis I H is inherited as an autosomal recessive trait.[313] Parental consanguinity[93,313] is frequent, and multiple affected sibs of both sexes, without the occurrence of affected individuals in the preceding generation, have often been observed. There are no well-documented descriptions of abnormalities in close relatives of patients that might suggest partial expression of the trait in the heterozygous state. The occurrence of the condition in identical twin sisters[610] and in a twin brother and sister[195] has been documented.

The Hurler syndrome has been reported in Caucasians, in Africans[224] and Afro-Americans,* in Chinese,[144,235] in Oriental Indians,[299,406,538] and in Egyptians.[33] In British Columbia, Lowry and Renwick[503] estimated the frequency to be about 1 in 100,000, an entirely plausible value.[778] Another survey in Australia indicated a frequency of 1 in 50,000.[358] It is likely that such studies underestimate the actual frequency because of early deaths and other causes of incomplete ascertainment. The Hurler syndrome has an unusually high frequency in the province of L'Aquila in Italy,[21] but no other similar ethnogeographic predeliction has been observed.

Management

Dietary manipulation. Despite numerous attempts, no form of dietary therapy has been shown to be helpful. Hurler,[379] in one of her original cases, observed that dietary supplementation with desiccated thyroid, although having no measurable effect, produced subjective improvement in her patient.

Supplemental vitamin A therapy has been tried in patients with the Hurler and Hunter syndromes because vitamin A cleared metachromasia in fibroblasts cultured from these individuals.[77,176,507] No substantiated benefit could be observed in the affected persons, and possible harm can be caused by aggravation of hydrocephalus.[275,575]

---

*References 153, 229, 494, 794, 797, and 882.

*References 34, 215, 236, 277, 393, 471, 798, and 823.

Vitamin C exaggerates the formation of glycosaminoglycan by fibroblasts in culture.[727] For this reason a scorbutigenic diet has been tried in the management of the Hurler syndrome. Although there was no unequivocal improvement, the patient seemed unusually resistant to the development of scurvy; this observation led to speculation that affected persons might have an unusually low vitamin C requirement.[194]

Large doses of prednisone had no effect on urinary excretion of glycosaminoglycan.[303]

Psychosocial implications. Crocker[167] and Crocker and Cullinane[168] have discussed general problems in the management of patients with mucopolysaccharidoses and the impact of the disorder on the family. A clinic with a multidisciplinary staff for children with developmental disabilities usually provides the most satisfactory long-term management.

Corneal transplantation. In a child with Hurler syndrome a lamellar corneal graft in one eye and a penetrating graft in the other were performed.[434] Whereas the former resulted in improved vision, the latter never healed, with consequent complete loss of sight. The results of eye surgery are influenced not only by severity of the generalized disease but also by progressive retinal degeneration, which is now recognized as a feature of some of the mucopolysaccharidoses.

Carpal tunnel syndrome. Although not widely recognized in the past, compression neuropathy of the median nerve is common if not universal in Hurler syndrome.[304,916] For unknown reasons affected children do not usually complain of pain in their hands. Equally, the examiner cannot elicit the Tinel sign (the production of a tingling sensation by light percussion on the radial side of the palmaris longus tendon). Median nerve conduction progressively deteriorates, however, with eventual loss of apositional function of the thumb. Before clinical trials of bone marrow transplantation therapy (discussed later in this chapter) were performed, affected children did not undergo corrective surgery to divide the transverse carpal ligament. The improved prognosis of children engrafted with normal marrow has led to the practice of annual testing of median nerve conduction. When indicated, surgical decompression of the carpal tunnel consistently yields good results.

Anesthesia. Anesthesia may be required in the management of the Hurler syndrome for a number of procedures, including hernia repair, myringotomy, ventriculoperitoneal shunt placement, relief of airway obstruction, and spine and joint surgery. Against this background it is important to be aware that affected children are at a number of special risks associated with the use of anesthesia. These potential complications are related to preexisting disease in the upper and lower airways, the heart, and the cervical spine,* and the perioperative mortality has been estimated to be as high as 20%. The most common anesthetic complication in the Hurler syndrome is difficult endotracheal intubation, which becomes significant after the age of 2 years and is more problematic as the disease progresses. Thus, failed intubation and failed tracheostomy are common in older children. Other serious problems include occlusion of the endotracheal or tracheostomy tube caused by thick mucoid secretions, postoperative obstructive apnea, stridor, and respiratory arrest. Nasal intubation is almost always unsuccessful because of choanal stenosis, and traumatic failed attempts may lead to airway obstruction caused by an aspirated blood clot. Other life-threatening complications that have occurred during operation include spinal cord damage due to atlantoaxial subluxation and myocardial infarction due to coronary artery disease.

Helpful preoperative measures[63] may include a preoperative examination of the airway by the anesthesiologist, chest radiograph, lateral cervical spine radiographs to assess atlantoaxial stability, electrocardiography, and consultation with a cardiologist and an otorhinolaryngologist. Optimal anesthetic management is achieved by anticipating the potential need for special interventions, including fiberoptic intubation and emergency tracheostomy. Parents should be informed of the high risk of complications, including cervical spine subluxation[109] and mortality inherent in anesthetic management of children with the mucopolysaccharidoses.

Enzyme replacement therapy. DiFerrante et al.[208] concluded that plasma infusions had a positive effect in the Hurler syndrome. The rationale of this approach has been to supply the defective "correction factor"; this is now recognized as "enzyme replacement" with α-L-iduronidase. Correc-

---

*References 40-42, 63, 164, 426, 433, 753, 770, 771, and 900.

tion of metachromasia by addition of normal plasma to cultured fibroblasts from affected persons had been studied.[366] In one patient, administration of normal human plasma containing, presumably, iduronidase was followed by decreased urinary excretion of glycosaminoglycans of relatively large molecular weight and by increased excretion of their products of degradation.[208] Assays of enzyme activity in blood, however, showed a low level of activity. Despite the promising results of this early attempt at enzyme replacement, plasma infusion has not been regarded as an efficacious or a feasible approach to treatment.

Amnionic membrane implant. Subcutaneous transplantation of amniotic membranes was initially thought to offer the benefits of minimal risk and the possibility of providing a long-term supply of a small number of enzyme-producing cells. Despite early claims of success,[6,7,11] however, subsequent studies could not establish any significant biochemical or physiologic response or evidence of long-term survival of donor tissue.[582]

Bone marrow transplantation. Transplantation of bone marrow from a normal or heterozygous donor provides a constant source of enzymatically replete cells to the affected recipient. Hurler syndrome was the first lysosomal disease to be treated by means of bone marrow transplantation,[343,344,793,893] and during the decade that followed, approximately 75 children received transplantation. The risks of the procedure are relatively well established. Children receiving marrow from a human lymphocyte antigen–identical sibling donor have approximately an 80% probability of surviving the transplantation (i.e., 1-year survival rate); this estimate is borne out, in the author's experience, in a series at the University of Minnesota in which 10 of 13 patients have survived. Use of any other donor (closely matched relative, closely matched unrelated donor, or mismatched donor) carries a much greater risk of death, in large part because of graft-versus-host disease and its complications.

Long-term clinical trials have confirmed many encouraging aspects of response but have also demonstrated significant limitations. Bone marrow transplantation reverses hepatosplenomegaly and obstructive airway disease,[512,893] prevents hydrocephalus, and increases longevity. Current means of transplantation, however, fall short of providing a complete "cure," especially when undertaken in older children. An optimal response would be anticipated in infants who receive transplantation immediately after birth. Indeed, the irreversible brain damage and the skeletal malformation that occur early in the course of Hurler syndrome provide strong motivation to identify affected infants by means of newborn screening.[895]

MUCOPOLYSACCHARIDOSIS I S (SCHEIE SYNDROME)

The condition discussed here was described by Scheie, Hambrick, and Barness[730] as a variant of Hurler syndrome, which, indeed, further studies showed it to be. The same enzyme, α-L-iduronidase, is deficient in both the Hurler and the Scheie syndrome, as a result of allelic mutations. These disorders define the ends of a spectrum of clinical severity and share several features in common, including progressive clouding of the cornea, joint contractures, and valvular disease of the heart. Nevertheless, the physical findings in Scheie syndrome are minimal and occur so late in life that affected individuals actually bear no resemblance to those with Hurler syndrome. Whereas children with Hurler syndrome come to medical attention during the first 2 years of life, Scheie syndrome typically remains undiagnosed in affected individuals until adulthood. Normal intelligence and longevity are characteristic of Scheie syndrome.

Clinical Manifestations

General features. The manifestations of the Scheie syndrome are so mild that the condition is never diagnosed during infancy. Only rarely are affected individuals identified during childhood (Fig. 11-12), and in most patients the Scheie syndrome is diagnosed on the basis of symptoms that occur later in life. In retrospect affected adults recall childhood complaints of stiff fingers, difficulties in grasping, and nocturnal pain in the hands. These findings have been incorrectly attributed to an atypical form of arthritis but are actually due to the combination of early joint contractures and carpal tunnel syndrome.[171,778] Umbilical and inguinal hernias may also be present in childhood.

The affected adolescent has a normal facial appearance and growth pattern but may exhibit mild contractures of the hands, mild hepatosplenomegaly, murmurs indicative of aortic and mitral valve disease, and mild corneal clouding.[683,778] Hirsutism is usual at this stage. Radiographic findings may include retarded bone age, palm frond–shaped ribs, vertebral and pelvic

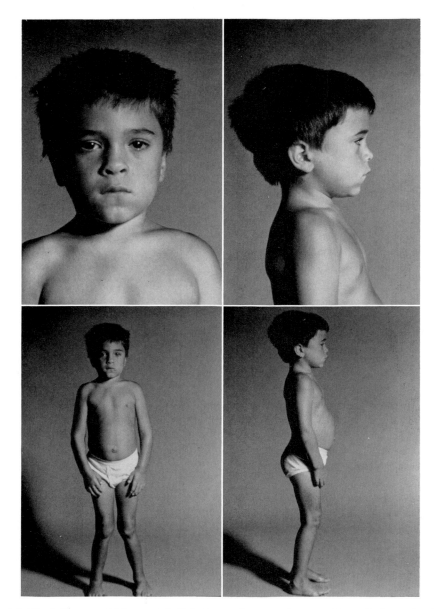

Fig. 11-12. A 5-year-old boy with Scheie syndrome who was identified on the basis of a "metabolic screen" battery of tests undertaken during evaluation for mild hearing loss at 4 years of age. Slightly wide wrists and mild knock-knee stance are the only remarkable clinical features in this child, who has complete deficiency of leukocyte α-L-iduronidase enzyme activity measured with 4-methylumbelliferone substrate.

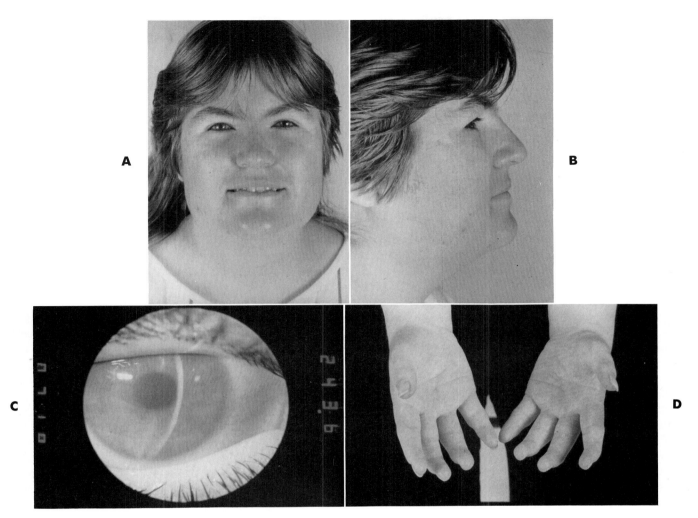

Fig. 11-13. A 24-year-old woman with Scheie syndrome. **A** and **B**, Normal facial features. **C**, Corneal clouding shown by slit-lamp microscopy. **D**, Atrophy of the abducens pollicis brevis muscle caused by compression of the median nerve, that is, carpal tunnel syndrome. Contractures of the distal interphalangeal joints are evident.

anomalies, and short first metacarpals.[423] If tested, the level of urinary glycosaminoglycan excretion is shown to be abnormally elevated.

In early adulthood the subtle features that first become evident during adolescence progress and motivate the patient to seek medical intervention, thus leading to establishment of the diagnosis. Joint contractures, especially of the hands, are a major complaint and may be confused with arthritis. Bilateral carpal tunnel syndrome is often present. Corneal clouding is progressive, and visual limitation sometimes leads to consideration of corneal transplantation. Heart murmurs may

be evident. Stature is typically below average in the low-normal range.

Head and neck. The face is relatively normal (Fig. 11-13), and the coarse appearance generally attributed to other mucopolysaccharidoses is not present. The face is broad and accentuated in the lower part as a result of an increased height of the midface and mandibular prognathism.[778,934] The nasal bridge is often somewhat flat (making it difficult to wear spectacles), the nose tends to be broad, and the nares are wide. Characteristically the cheeks are full. The mouth is wide, with downturned angles, and macroglossia is sometimes present. The skull is slightly enlarged relative to the trunk and limbs, and the neck is short and appears to be placed on a stocky, muscular body. Radiographic studies reveal that the pituitary fossa is shoe shaped or slipper shaped. Magnetic resonance imaging of the brain has failed to detect any significant intracranial abnormalities.[586]

Ocular features. Corneal clouding is a striking feature in adults with Scheie syndrome and may be the presenting complaint that leads to diagnosis (Fig. 11-13, *C*). This clinical finding helps distinguish Scheie syndrome from the mild form of Hunter syndrome, which lacks corneal opacification. Clouding of the cornea has been identified in a 4-year-old child,[421] but it is usually not apparent until adulthood. Corneal clouding is progressive and may cause severe visual impairment or complete blindness.[934] The clouding is most dense peripherally in some patients, although in others, particularly in the earlier stages, involvement is uniform. Glaucoma developed in two reported sibs (see Cases 1 and 2, later in this chapter) at the ages of 51 and 40 years, respectively. Corneal grafts have been helpful[934] but have become opacified in some patients.[470,730]

Corneal clouding often obscures the fundus, but abnormal retinal pigmentation may be present and can be mistaken for other forms of primary retinitis pigmentosa. By adulthood the electroretinogram may be completely extinguished, consistent with neuroepithelial degeneration.

Nervous system. The intellect is impaired slightly or not at all. The original patients described by Dr. Harold Scheie were said to be of "near genius" intelligence, and a patient reported by McKusick was an attorney of more than average intelligence. Psychosis was a feature, however, in two of the four adults studied by McKusick.

Hearing deficit is a variable feature that may result from a cochlear lesion.[553] Median nerve compression in the carpal tunnel ("carpal tunnel syndrome") is frequently present in the Scheie syndrome (Fig. 11-13, *D*).

Cardiorespiratory manifestations. Aortic and mitral valve disease is a feature of the Scheie syndrome,[119,287,553,688] but most patients are without symptoms. The first successful valve replacement in Scheie syndrome was undertaken in a 42-year-old patient who had severe valve stenosis with thickened chordae, calcification, and irregular valve edges that resembled dyplastic nodules.[119] Cardiomyopathy may be present.[390] In distinction to persons with other mucopolysaccharidoses, individuals with Scheie syndrome appear to have relatively normal respiratory function and are not known to have obstructive sleep apnea.

Skeletal system. The skeletal changes of mild dysostosis multiplex are occasionally present (Fig. 11-14) but usually are not severe. Joint movements may be limited, and contractures of the digits and wrists may develop (Fig. 11-13, *D*). Multiple cysts, which caused pathologic fracture in the right femur and necessitated total hip replacement in a patient at the age of 37 years, have been documented.[473] At that time the patient also had generalized joint rigidity, numbness and contractures in the first three digits of both hands, wasting of the thenar eminences, and thick longitudinal nodules in the palms.

Abdomen and viscera. The liver is enlarged in about 50% of affected persons, whereas splenic enlargement is rare. Inguinal or umbilical hernia, or both, are frequent.[423,778] Chronic intestinal pseudoobstruction has been reported.[382]

Natural history. Although no systematic study of longevity has been undertaken, the prolonged survival of several reported patients suggests that a normal or near-normal life expectancy should be anticipated. Aggressive medical intervention may be required (e.g., cardiac valve replacement, corneal transplantation, or carpal tunnel release).

The following clinical histories of two patients, brother and sister, which were documented by McKusick,[553] are instructive (Fig. 11-14).

CASE 1

The proband, a male attorney, was born in 1917. Deformed feet and stiff fingers were noted at 7 years of age. He was considered the most intelligent member of his family and more intelligent than his unaffected brother. He was class valedictorian in high school, for example. Progressive difficulty with night vision began at the age of 27 years, with restriction of the fields of vision in daylight. "Steamy corneas" were first observed

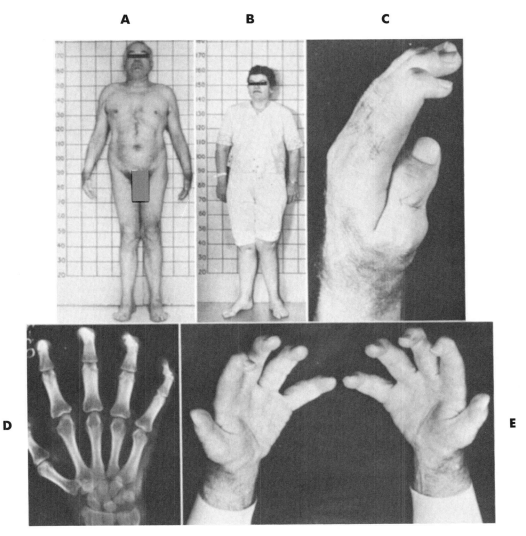

Fig. 11-14. The brother and sister with Scheie syndrome detailed (as Case 1 and Case 2) in the text. **A** and **B,** General appearance includes a relatively broad mouth, hypertrichosis, genu valgum, and a misshapen foot. **C,** The hand of the brother shows generalized contractures of the digits, especially at the distal interphalangeal joints. **D,** Radiograph of hand shown in **C. E,** Atrophy of the abducens pollicis brevis muscle, due to compression of the median nerve in the carpal tunnel (carpal tunnel syndrome), in the brother.

at age 13 years by his ophthalmologist. Right inguinal herniorrhaphy was performed at 42 years of age. Hearing deficit in the right ear was noted at 46 years of age. Intellect may have deteriorated somewhat in later life.

The findings, when the patient was investigated in 1962 and again in 1964, included height of 175 cm; short neck and coarse features, with broad mouth and jaw and fleshy tongue; stiff, contractured hands with carpal tunnel syndrome and stiff wrists; short feet with high arches and overlapping fifth toe; marked clouding

of the cornea, which was more dense peripherally; and extensive bilateral retinitis pigmentosa. The diastolic murmur of aortic regurgitation (blood pressure, 145/65 mm Hg) was present, and the aortic second sound was exceptionally ringing. The distal phalanges were flexed at about 90 degrees with the rest of the fingers but could be straightened passively. The wrists could not be extended beyond the neutral position. He could not supinate the forearms more than about 60 degrees. Except for the foot abnormalities, all other peripheral joints had normal range of motion. The liver was palpable and probably somewhat enlarged.

Radiographs showed spatulate ribs and cystic changes in the bones of the wrists and hands.

The presence of carpal tunnel syndrome was indicated by numbness of the fingers supplied by the median nerve, marked wasting of the abducens pollicis brevis muscle, and characteristic nerve conduction changes: stimulation at the elbow evoked no thumb movement or muscle action potential. Antidromic sensory velocity (stimulating at the wrist and recording at the elbow) was estimated at 26.8 M per second as compared with a velocity of 63.6 M per second in the unaffected ulnar nerve.

The hearing loss was largely limited to the right ear, and audiologic findings suggested a cochlear location of the lesion. The electroretinogram was almost completely extinguished, consistent with neuroepithelial degeneration.

The urine showed 48 to 63 mg per liter of glycosaminoglycan, which was dermatan sulfate and heparan sulfate in the proportion of 3 to 1.[413] Bone marrow and circulating leukocytes showed no definite lysosomal inclusions.

In 1971, at the age of 51 years, the patient developed bilateral narrow-angle or closed-angle glaucoma.

CASE 2

The sister of the patient previously described was born in 1930. Stiff hands and wrists and deformed feet were first noted at the age of 5 years. At as early as 7 years of age an appearance suggesting "mongolism" was noted by her ophthalmologist. Clouding of the cornea was recognized at about 20 years of age. She was regarded by her parents as a slow learner. Nevertheless, she succeeded in completing a 4-year college course, of which the last year was spent in a teachers' college. She attempted to teach school but had a "nervous breakdown," for which she was hospitalized and received electroshock therapy. Other treatments have been necessary since that time. She has noted numbness and anesthesia of the fingers.

At physical examination in 1964 she had a height of 160.5 cm, the same facial characteristics as in her brother (Fig. 11-14, *A*), and hand and foot deformities, which were less severe (Fig. 11-14, *B*). On gross clinical examination the corneal clouding seemed more diffuse than in the brother; however, slit-lamp examination showed possible peripheral concentration. The fundi showed retinal pigmentation, and the electroretinogram was almost completely extinguished. The heart had a harsh systolic murmur with characteristics of aortic stenosis. The abducens pollicis brevis muscle was strikingly atrophied.

In the peripheral blood approximately 1% to 3% of the lymphocytes showed indistinct, poorly formed metachromatic granules in the cytoplasm. Metachro-

matic inclusions were demonstrated in macrophages.

The urine contained 131 mg per liter of glycosaminoglycan, which was dermatan sulfate and heparan sulfate in the proportion of approximately 3 to 1.

In this family one other sib is completely normal; interestingly, he is slightly shorter than the affected brother and in the past has been considered less competent intellectually.

From the age of 23 years the patient had been night blind, presumably as a result of the pigmentary degeneration of the retina that she and her brother demonstrate. In 1971, at the age of 40 years, she developed narrow-angle or closed-angle glaucoma.

CASES 3 AND 4

Through the courtesy of Dr. Scheie it was possible for McKusick to examine the brother and sister in whom the entity was first described. The facial resemblance to the previously described patients was so striking that they could all pass for sibs. Other clinical features were also similar. Both patients, a 33-year-old man and his 31-year-old sister, had aortic regurgitation. The brother had a psychotic episode. Leukocyte studies revealed no obvious metachromatic granules. Urine glycosaminoglycan analyses showed both dermatan sulfate and heparan sulfate in a proportion of about 2 to 1 (see the follow-up by Constantopoulos, Dekaban, and Scheie[156]). The sister gave birth to a healthy son in 1965.

Pathology

In general the skin,[314] cornea, and conjunctiva show on histologic study the same changes as those observed in Hurler syndrome. When the carpal tunnel has been explored for relief of nerve compression, an excess of collagenous tissue has been found.

Histochemical and ultrastructural analyses were undertaken on a penetrating keratoplasty specimen from a patient with Scheie syndrome.[934] Numerous vacuoles containing fibrillogranular material were found in the corneal epithelial cells, keratocytes, and endothelial cells. It is possible that damage to the corneal epithelium may be induced by a microenvironment modified by the presence of abnormal amounts of dermatan sulfate and heparan sulfate or by the inhibition of collagen synthesis by dermatan sulfate. The unique findings of a markedly attenuated Bowman's layer and fibrous long-spacing collagen are abnormalities that may be specific to Scheie syndrome (not observed in the cornea in Hurler or Hurler-Scheie syndrome) and result from the altered glycosaminoglycan composition of the extracellular matrix.

The precise nature of the aortic valve lesion is not known, but presumably the changes are similar to those in other mucopolysaccharidoses. Electron microscopic studies of conjunctiva and skin[20] showed multiple vacuolations in fibroblasts and in conjunctival epithelial cells. Inclusions were single-membrane limited, contained a granulofibrillar material, and were associated with the Golgi bodies. Skin epithelium was normal. Remarkably, no autopsy observations have yet been reported.

Fundamental Defect

Patients with the Scheie syndrome excrete excessive amounts of dermatan sulfate and heparan sulfate in the urine. Although the total amount excreted is not as great in adults as it is in children with the Hurler syndrome (on a per mg creatinine basis), the proportion of the two glycosaminoglycans is usually 70 to 30.[413] The pattern of glycosaminoglycan excretion in the Scheie syndrome resembles that of patients with the Hurler syndrome.

The Hurler and Scheie syndromes, despite the striking clinical differences, show identity by means of the Neufeld cross-correction method in cultured skin fibroblasts.[899] In both conditions cells are corrected by purified Hurler factor (i.e., α-L-iduronidase[52]) and have deficiency of the same enzyme, α-L-iduronidase.[39] These observations led to reclassification of the Hurler and Scheie syndromes as subtypes of MPS type I, which are designated MPS type I H and MPS type I S, respectively.

Results of complementation analysis by use of the method of cell fusion to form heterokaryons have indicated that Hurler, Scheie, and Hurler-Scheie syndromes constitute a single complementation group. No measurable induction of α-L-iduronidase activity was present after fusions between fibroblasts from patients with these different phenotypes. Similar studies of ^{35}S-glycosaminoglycan metabolism in heterokaryons showed persistent glycosaminoglycan accumulation, thus further suggesting allelism of Hurler and Scheie mutations.[248] The Hurler, Scheie, and Hurler-Scheie phenotypes are all presumed to result from allelic mutations of a single gene for α-L-iduronidase.[579] Delineation of such mutations is currently the subject of molecular genetic investigations.

That deficiency of a single enzyme should result in differing clinical pictures is no longer surprising.[159] This phenomenon has been demonstrated in the infantile and adult forms of metachromatic leu-

kodystrophy, the classic and juvenile forms of Tay-Sachs disease, the infantile and visceral forms of the Niemann-Pick disease, three forms of Gaucher disease, and other lysosomal storage diseases. In some of these disorders differences have been identified in the kinetics of the defective enzyme and associated with different mutations at the molecular genetic level. Analogous observations that have been made by comparison of residual α-L-iduronidase in cultured fibroblasts from patients with the Hurler and Scheie syndromes provide an explanation for the clinical differences. Low residual activity of the enzyme in persons with the Scheie syndrome may be sufficient to sustain normal flux rate of substrates in the nervous system but not in cells with a high glycosaminoglycan turnover rate. This phenomenon would account for the lack of mental retardation in the presence of mild or moderate somatic abnormalities.[264] Quantitation of residual α-L-iduronidase by use of oligosaccharide substrates[530a] and evaluation of enzyme kinetics with a monoclonal antibody–based immunoquantification assay[31] provide further evidence for the role of residual enzymatic activity in producing a mild phenotype. This approach may provide tests of prognostic significance.

Prevalence and Inheritance

By 1969 Rampini[683] was able to identify the Scheie syndrome in at least seven previous reports* in addition to the cases studied by Scheie, Hambrick, and Barness[730] and of McKusick et al.[556] (Cases 1 and 2 in this chapter). Since that time, numerous additional cases have been documented and syndromic identity is well established. In British Columbia, Lowry and Renwick[503] estimated the frequency of the Scheie syndrome to be 1 in 500,000 births.

The autosomal recessive mode of inheritance of the Scheie syndrome was suggested by early reports of affected sibs with normal parents.[556,730] This form of transmission is now fully substantiated.

Management

Corneal transplantation. Corneal opacification is progressive and often results in significant visual impairment. In early cases of MPS I S reported by Scheie et al.[730] transplantation grafts became opacified; it is likely, however, that the

*References 233, 427, 454, 609, 674, 732, and 839.

opacification was due to an acute graft rejection because it occurred within a few weeks after surgery. More recently, full-thickness and split-thickness corneal grafting has been successfully performed in patients with Scheie syndrome and the grafts have remained clear.[118,934]

Carpal tunnel syndrome. Carpal tunnel release has been performed to eliminate extrinsic compression of the median nerve and has restored sensation and relieved pain. In patients who are treated relatively late, however, nerve conduction studies show abnormally increased terminal latency,[171] which is indicative of permanent damage. Generalized contractures of the hands have been unsuccessfully treated by means of surgical removal of palmar tendon nodules.[473] A patient with limited mobility and arthralgia of the knees underwent arthroscopic aspiration of viscous joint fluid and had some improvement. The author observed that she later had recurrence of joint movement limitation and discomfort.

Herniorrhaphy. Inguinal herniorrhaphy is often necessary in patients with Scheie syndrome. The operation does not require any special precautions.[473]

Cardiac valve replacement. Severely diseased and calcified aortic and mitral valves have been successfully replaced with a 20-mm Hall valve and a 25-mm St. Jude mitral prosthesis.[119]

MUCOPOLYSACCHARIDOSIS TYPE I HS (HURLER-SCHEIE SYNDROME)

In a previous edition of this book, McKusick described a girl initially labeled as having the Maroteaux-Lamy syndrome. Unlike in other patients with MPS type VI, however, the fibroblasts of this child did not show cross-correction with those of persons with the Hurler and Scheie syndrome. The phenotype, which was less severe than Hurler syndrome yet more severe than Scheie syndrome, led to the conclusion that she might possess both a Hurler allele and a Scheie allele. The compound disorder was designated the Hurler-Scheie syndrome.

McKusick reported six other patients in whom the clinical picture and results of fibroblast studies were consistent with the Hurler-Scheie syndrome. In addition, Neufeld found that cultured fi-

broblasts from a brother and sister reported by Horton and Schimke[368] had the corrective characteristics of the Hurler and Scheie syndromes and showed deficiency of α-L-iduronidase. The intermediate phenotype, in combination with the enzymatic studies, indicates that these patients have Hurler-Scheie syndrome. Several more patients with an intermediate phenotype have been found to lack α-L-iduronidase, thus furthering the hypothesis that such individuals may represent genetic compounds with Hurler and Scheie alleles.[152] However, the same phenotype has been encountered in the offspring of consanguineous parents,[186,248] which suggests that homozygosity for a "Hurler-Scheie allele" is an alternate possibility. It is also significant that other, different phenotypes[710] have been associated with α-L-iduronidase deficiency, including that of normal individuals,[273,892] thus leading to the conclusion that multiple α-L-iduronidase alleles must exist and can be associated with a variety of phenotypes.

The literature contains relatively few reports of patients with Hurler-Scheie syndrome, although the clinical experience of Whitley and colleagues (presented in the following section) provides additional examples of such intermediate phenotypes. It is of considerable interest that the original report of Scheie syndrome and subsequent follow-up[729] indicates that the sibs who represent the prototype of the Scheie syndrome actually fit the Hurler-Scheie category in terms of current diagnostic criteria.

Clinical Manifestations

General features. Differentiation of phenotypes intermediate to the Hurler and Scheie syndromes is challenging insofar as they form a continuum and the most meaningful categorization of affected persons is sometimes retrospective.[239,423] In general, patients with Hurler-Scheie syndrome have significant physical abnormalities that lead to diagnosis during childhood yet have more prolonged survival than those with Hurler syndrome. Pregnancy, which was artificially terminated, has been documented in an affected woman.[553]

Head and neck. The facial features are mild but distinctive, somewhat resembling those of the Hurler syndrome (Fig. 11-15). The bridge of the nose is depressed or wide, the chin may be small, and the mouth is typically broad. On radiographs

A   **B**   **C**

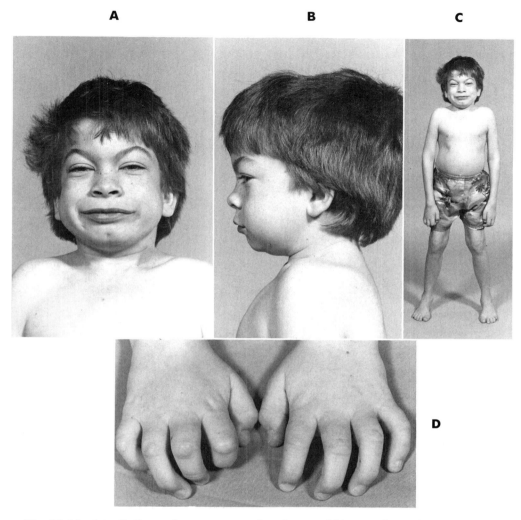

D

Fig. 11-15. A to **C,** General appearance of an 8-year-old boy with Hurler-Scheie syndrome with normal intellect and distinctive but relatively mild physical features. Slight frontal bossing and thick hair are evident. Minimal kyphoscoliosis results in the appearance of a short spine relative to limb length and slight protuberance of the abdomen. The joints are somewhat wide. **D,** Contractures of the fingers are prominent, especially at the distal interphalangeal joints.

patients exhibit a hypoplastic mandible with notched lower borders and bilateral condylar aplasia.

Intraorally, pronounced gingival hypertrophy and macroglossia are present.[559] The teeth appear to be normal in size and configuration, but radiographic studies reveal cystic radiolucencies in the crowns of the teeth. These lesions appear to be accumulations of glycosaminoglycan, probably dermatan sulfate.

Nervous system. Glycosaminoglycan deposits in the meninges may cause hydrocephalus, cervical myelopathy, radiculopathy, and arachnoid cysts. Cortical atrophy may be present (Fig. 11-16) sometimes with cavitary lesions.[692] In one patient with severe obstructive airway disease, electoencephalogram changes suggested cerebral hypoxia.[423] Left hemiplegia later developed, and this patient died at the age of 26 years.

Median nerve compression (carpal tunnel syn-

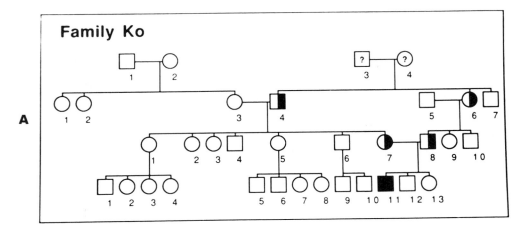

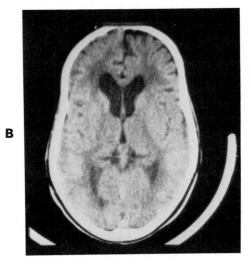

Fig. 11-16. **A,** Family pedigree of an 11-year-old boy with an intermediate phenotype resulting from α-L-iduronidase deficiency. Homozygosity for a single Hurler-Scheie allele is suggested by the close consanguinity of his parents. **B,** Computerized tomography of the head shows the scaphocephalic skull and mild atrophy of the frontal lobes.

drome) is usually asymptomatic but frequently present when evaluated by nerve conduction studies.

Mental functions are usually preserved, but some patients have intellectual decline or exhibit significant behavior problems as they grow older.[221]

Ocular features. Corneal clouding and an abnormal electroretinogram are characteristic ocular findings, but other abnormalities have been reported, including defective dark adaptation, retinal degeneration, optic atrophy, ptosis, strabismus (esotropia), and glaucoma. Limited ocular mobility resulting from mechanical limitation of the superior oblique tendon (Brown syndrome) has been reported in one patient.[101] It was speculated that shortening of this small tendon paralleled shortening of the tendons of the limbs and extremities.

Respiratory system. Frequent chest infections, limited chest expansion, and difficulties with endotracheal intubation are characteristic of the advanced stages of the disorder. The flat configuration of the nose predisposes to snoring, and obstructive sleep apnea has been described in two brothers.[661] In one of these sibs airway obstruction progressed and eventually necessitated tracheostomy.[423] The subsequent response was dramatic and resulted in marked reduction in the frequency and severity of apneic episodes. Tonsillectomy and adenoidectomy provide partial relief of airway obstruction.

Cardiovascular system. Some affected individuals have thickening of the valve leaflets and aortic and mitral regurgitation, which has required valve replacement.[423] Ventricular extrasystoles have been observed after apneic episodes in an affected teenager.

Skeletal system. The radiographic features of Hurler-Scheie syndrome are intermediate in the spectrum of dysostosis multiplex.[733] The hands are characteristically broad and short, with stubby digits and contractures of the interphalangeal joints (see Fig. 11-17, *D*). Supination of the forearms is limited and the feet are short, with high arches.[171] Radiographs reveal retarded bone age, spatulate ribs, and cystic changes in the bones of the wrists and hands.[423]

Integument. Affected individuals are moderately hirsute, particularly over the back and shoulders. The skin is firm, with increased thickness and decreased elasticity, because of storage of glycosaminoglycan. A simple test involving pinching of the skin of the arm has been proposed to evaluate thickness and elasticity.[934]

Prognosis. The life span in the Hurler-Scheie syndrome is variable and not well defined. Most affected persons survive beyond the age of 10 years, and individuals surviving into the third decade are known.

In the fourth edition of this book McKusick described, as follows, an affected woman.

CASE REPORT

A female born in 1950 represents a sporadic example of the Hurler-Scheie syndrome. Her parents were not known to be related, and an older sister was normal.

The patient's infancy was marked by neonatal pneumonia and persistent feeding difficulties. Physical developmental milestones lagged. She attended public school through the sixth grade and received home tutoring thereafter. Her performance deteriorated coincident with progressive physical impairment. Beginning at the age of 10 years, she frequently experienced momentary loss of vision and at the age of 15 years became totally blind. Four weeks before the development of blindness she had facial hemiparalysis and inability to speak or walk. She later regained these functions. Her hearing steadily declined, and severe frontal headaches developed. A clear rhinorrhea began at about the age of 14 years; this was subsequently identified as cerebrospinal fluid. At 19 years of age she was still able to get about, write, and make handicrafts, despite severe physical and sensory handicaps.

The diagnosis of the Hurler syndrome was suggested at 18 months of age because of hypertelorism, mild kyphosis, enlarged wrists, cardiomegaly, hepatosplenomegaly, and umbilical hernia. By 9 years of age she was described as having grotesque facies, mild mental retar-dation, corneal clouding, enlarged tongue, hepatosplenomegaly, generalized limitation of joint mobility, and clawhand deformity.

Examination (1969) showed a short girl (135 cm) weighing 47 kg (Fig. 11-17). The head circumference measured 55 cm. The facies was characterized by prominent forehead, depressed nasal bridge, anteverted nostrils, ocular proptosis with esotropia and corneal clouding, and thick lips. The tongue was enlarged, and the teeth were widely spaced. A systolic murmur was heard at the left lower sternal border. The abdomen was protuberant, with right inguinal and umbilical herniorrhaphy scars. A hernia in the right inguinal area measured 3 cm. The liver extended 12 cm and the spleen 5 cm below their respective costal margins. The breast and vulva showed adult development, but pubic and axillary hair was scant. Decreased mobility was evident in all joints. The hands were broad, with short, clawlike fingers, and mild spinal scoliosis was present.

By means of psychologic testing designed to take account of her visual and auditory handicaps, her maximal mental performance and primary verbal skills were estimated at an intelligence quotient (IQ) equivalent of 63.

Radiographic findings included mild cortical thickening of the skull with multiple small radiolucent areas and a diffusely enlarged sella turcica (Fig. 11-17, *C*). Body section radiographs made with the polytome and a carotid arteriogram showed changes suggesting an anterior encephalocele extending through the cribriform plate into the posterior nasal cavity and protruding into the anterior part of the nasopharynx. (This was thought to be related to the patient's rhinorrhea.) Thoracolumbar scoliosis was present, and the vertebral bodies were variably malformed. The long bones of the upper limbs were short and broad, with metaphyseal and epiphyseal abnormalities. The carpal bones were hypoplastic, and the metacarpals were short and broad, with proximal tapering (Fig. 11-17, *D*). Similar but milder changes were present in the lower limbs.

Further investigations confirmed the theory that the rhinorrhea was cerebrospinal fluid. Electroencephalogram suggested severe cerebral disturbance involving primarily the frontal lobes. Echoencephalogram demonstrated enlargement of the lateral ventricles, as did the carotid arteriogram.

Urinary screening for glycosaminoglycans by means of toluidine blue, cetyltrimethyl-ammonium bromide (CTAB), and acid albumin turbidity methods gave strongly positive results. Urinary excretion of glycosaminoglycans was 215 mg/24 hr; dermatan sulfate accounted for 80%, the remainder being heparan sulfate.

The patient lacked the striking metachromatic inclusions that are seen in the cells of persons with MPS type VI.

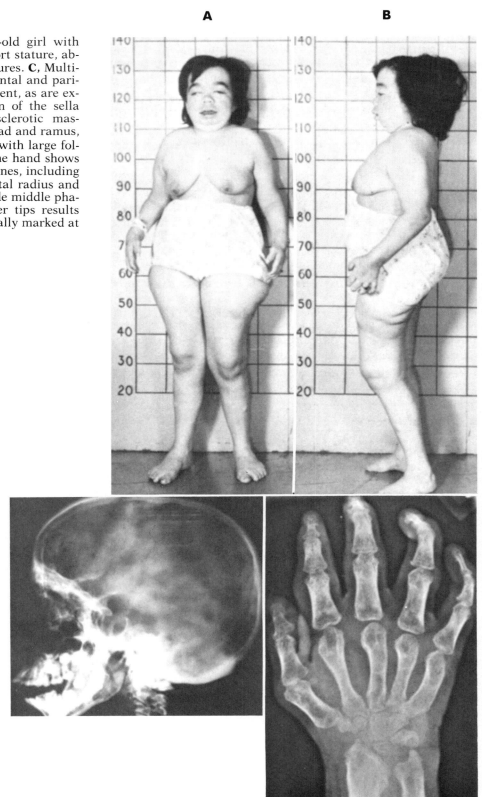

Fig. 11-17. A and **B,** A 19-year-old girl with Hurler-Scheie syndrome with short stature, abnormal facies, and joint contractures. **C,** Multiple oval radiolucencies in the frontal and parietal parts of the calvaria are evident, as are extensive destruction in the region of the sella turcica and cribriform plate, sclerotic mastoids, hypoplastic mandibular head and ramus, and impaction of second molars with large follicular cysts. **D,** Radiograph of the hand shows generalized abnormality of all bones, including angulation of the ends of the distal radius and ulna, small carpal bones, and wide middle phalanges. The position of the finger tips results from contractures that are especially marked at the distal interphalangeal joints.

Fundamental Defect

As stated earlier, mixing fibroblasts from patients with Hurler syndrome with those from patients with Scheie syndrome fails to show mutual correction of the metabolic defect, which can be observed by monitoring metachromasia and handling of ^{35}S-labeled substances; cocultivation and somatic-cell hybridization studies demonstrate this lack of complementation. Both disorders have deficient α-L-iduronidase, yet on clinical examination they are clearly distinct entities. The explanation for the intermediate phenotype and biochemical findings is allelism for different mutations of the same α-L-iduronidase structural gene. As a consequence the enzyme molecule is altered in different ways; the severity of the catalytic defects is different and thus associated with correspondingly mild and severe clinical disorders.

Roubicek, Gehler, and Spranger [710] reported patients with well-documented deficiency of α-L-iduronidase and pathologically high levels of glycosaminoglycan excretion who have atypical clinical features. Such observations suggest the existence of underlying genetic heterogeneity beyond the alleles for Hurler, Hurler-Scheie, and Scheie syndromes.

Whitley, Krivit, and Gorlin[892] reported the mother of a child with Hurler syndrome who, herself, had exceedingly low levels of α-L-iduronidase activity, as measured with the fluorogenic methylumbelliferyl substrate. Further studies suggested that this low level of enzyme was due to a nonpathologic allele for low enzyme activity. Although such an allele resulted in a normal phenotype, it posed special problems for prenatal diagnosis. Concurrently another such family was reported by Gatti et al.[273] in which studies of radiosulfate accumulation of cultured amniocytes provided an accurate means of prenatal diagnosis.

Prevalence and Inheritance

The Hurler-Scheie phenotype has been observed by the author in children from several ethnogeographic backgrounds, mainly European[290,634,777,908] but also Japanese[407-409] and Saudi Arabian. There appears to be no population with an unusually high incidence of this disorder.

As previously mentioned, an explanation for the phenotype intermediate to Hurler syndrome and Scheie syndrome could be that the Hurler-Scheie phenotype represents an individual who is a compound heterozygote for the two allelic disorders. In the absence of consanguinity, and given a frequency of 1:200 for the Hurler syndrome gene (q_H) and 1:700 for the Scheie syndrome gene (q_S), the frequency of the disorders ($q_H{}^2$ and $q_H{}^2$) should be 1:40,000 and 1:490,000, respectively. The compound disorder would be expected to occur in a frequency of 1:70,000 ($2q_H q_S$). Parental consanguinity should not be increased in the case of the compound disorder.

Despite the foregoing, the birth of children with the Hurler-Scheie phenotype to consanguineous parents[186,392,407,408,450] serves to prove the existence of specific Hurler-Scheie alleles. The determination of the actual frequency of these alleles will require a population study. In actual fact it is likely that many alleles are giving rise to a spectrum of phenotypes.[710]

Management

Hearing impairment. Hearing is often improved by the placement of ventilation tubes and the use of hearing aids.

Carpal tunnel syndrome. Median nerve compression is initially asymptomatic but progresses and leads to loss of grasp. Surgical intervention is warranted.

Corneal transplantation. Loss of vision resulting from progressive corneal clouding has been treated by corneal transplantation. The relative merits of operation must be evaluated on an individual basis, weighing the degree of visual impairment, anticipated benefit, and patient compliance with necessary follow-up.

Airway management. Patients with obstructive airway disease may benefit from nasal continuous positive airway pressure (CPAP), sometimes supplemented with oxygen and usually administered only at night. Tonsillectomy, adenoidectomy, and tracheostomy have been performed to reduce respiratory obstruction.[116,423]

Cardiac disease. Cardiac management is symptomatic and may include the use of diuretics, digoxin, and valve replacement.[423]

Bone marrow transplantation. An animal model of Hurler-Scheie syndrome[158,763,765] has been treated with bone marrow transplantation with somewhat encouraging results.[108,157,762,764,766] There has been limited human experience; a girl with Hurler-Scheie syndrome survived bone marrow transplantation at 9 years, 10 months of age.[634] Two months after bone marrow transplantation, α-L-iduronidase activity levels were similar to donor levels and urinary glycosaminglycan excretion decreased, reaching near-normal levels within 18 months. The positive clinical response included some improvement of abnormal facial features and acceleration of growth (10 cm in 24 months). Hepatomegaly was reduced (measured at 10 cm below the inferior costal margin before engraftment, receding to 1 cm by 2 months after transplantation, and lying at the costal margin by 24 months after transplantation). Skeletal abnormalities, cardiac valve thickening, and psychomotor function were not improved, although the girl continued to attend a normal school program and had below-average performance.

MUCOPOLYSACCHARIDOSIS TYPE II (HUNTER SYNDROME)

Historically, and in clinical practice, the Hunter and Hurler syndromes have often been considered together, although the Hunter syndrome is usually less severe than the Hurler syndrome. As in the Hurler syndrome, the predominant features are stiff joints, severe short stature, hepatosplenomegaly, and coarse facial features (which were responsible for the archaic designation "gargoylism"). In the Hunter syndrome, however, mental deterioration progresses at a slower rate than in the Hurler syndrome and lumbar gibbus does not occur.

Hunter syndrome is further differentiated on clinical examination by lack of corneal clouding and longer survival, on genetic study by an X-linked recessive mode of inheritance, and on biochemical study by a different pattern of urinary glycosaminoglycan excretion and deficiency of the enzyme iduronate sulfatase. Recent advances in molecular genetics are unraveling the mutations that cause the spectrum of relatively mild and severe forms of the Hunter syndrome, which differ with respect to length of survival and severity of neurologic involvement.

Clinical Manifestations

General features. Two clinical extremes of the Hunter syndrome are usually recognized, the severe type (Figs. 11-18 and 11-19) and the

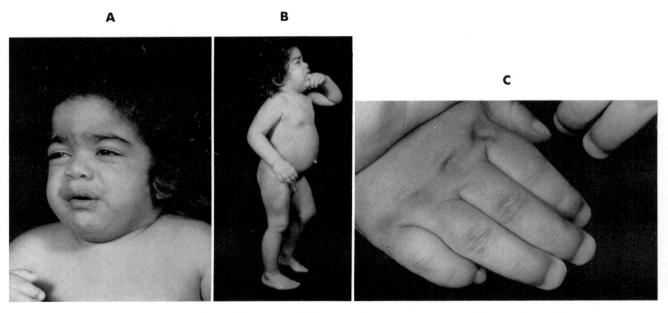

A   **B**   **C**

Fig. 11-18. **A,** The face of a 3-year-old boy with severe Hunter syndrome shows the characteristic appearance. **B,** Minimal curvature of the spine is the usual finding (in contrast to the more severe kyphoscoliosis typical of Hurler syndrome). **C,** Moderate flexion contractures of the fingers are present, especially affecting the distal interphalangeal joints.

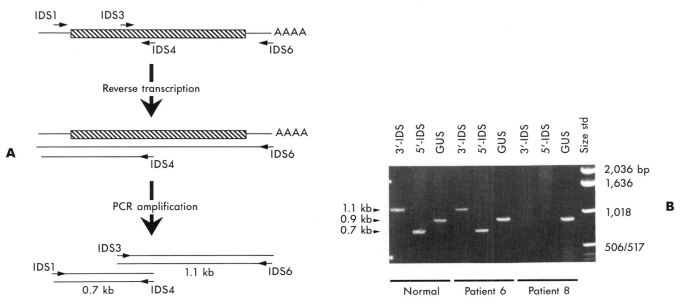

Fig. 11-19. A, Strategy for amplification of iduronate-2-sulfatase mRNA from leuko-cytes to cDNA by means of reverse transcription (RT) linked to polymerase chain reaction (PCR). The arrows indicate the positions of oligonucleotide primers (*IDS1*, *IDS3*, *IDS4*, and *IDS6*) relative to the coding sequence of the iduronate-2-sulfatase transcript with polyadenylation *(AAAA)*. **B,** By means of this RT-PCR method a child with Hunter syndrome (shown in Fig. 11-18) was found to have no detectable mRNA as a result of a partial or complete deletion of the iduronate-2-sulfatase gene. Each lane shows the reaction product amplified for the 3'-end *(3'-IDS)* or 5'-end *(5'-IDS)* of the iduronate sulfatase gene relative to molecular size standards *(Size std); GUS* de-notes a control reaction amplifying a segment of β-glucuronidase mRNA. Study of an unaffected individual (normal) and another child with Hunter syndrome (Patient 6) indicated successful amplification of iduronate sulfatase gene transcript. (From Crotty PL, Whitley CB: *Hum Genet* [in press].)

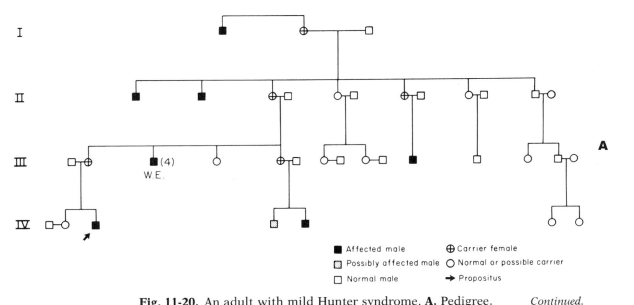

Fig. 11-20. An adult with mild Hunter syndrome. **A,** Pedigree.   *Continued.*

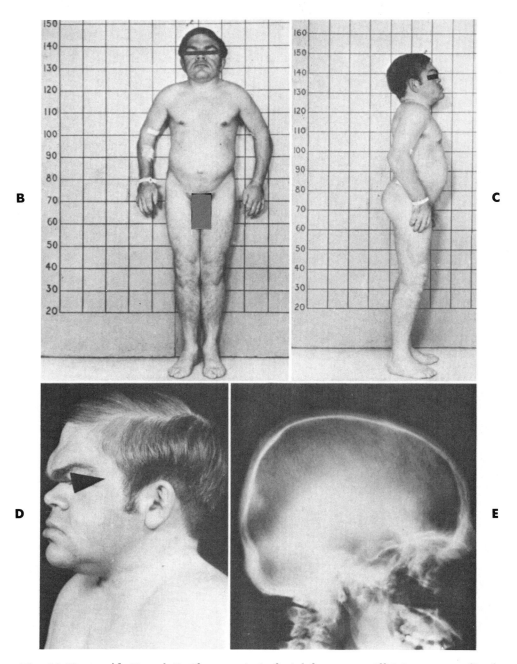

Fig. 11-20, cont'd. B and **C,** Characteristic facial features, stiff joints, generalized contractures of the thumb and fingers, and short stature are evident. **D,** Prominent supercilliary ridges are demonstrated. **E,** Lateral radiographic view of the skull, showing brachycephaly and prominent supercilliary ridge.

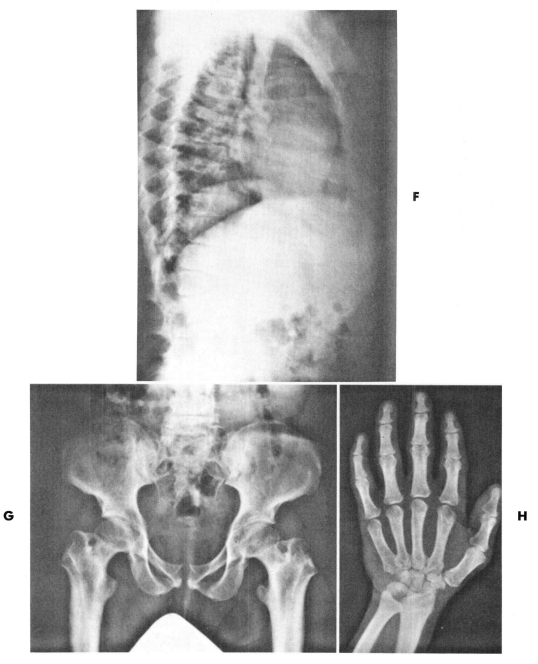

Fig. 11-20, cont'd. F, Lateral radiographic view of the spine, showing hypoplasia and recessing of the second lumbar vertebra. **G,** Radiograph of the pelvis, showing bilateral narrowing in the area above the acetabulum, irregularity of the acetabulum, flattened femoral heads. **H,** Radiograph of the hand and wrist, showing hypoplasia or absence of the proximal row of carpal bones and lipping in the proximal ends of the middle and distal phalanges.

Definite and probable cases

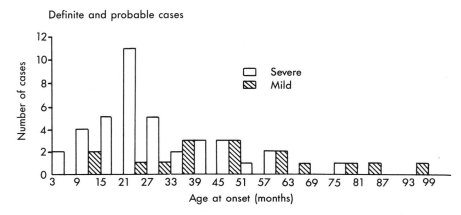

Fig. 11-21. Hunter syndrome, mild and severe forms; age of onset at which either a parent or a health care professional became seriously concerned about the child's health. (From Young ID et al: *J Med Genet* 10:408-411, 1982.)

mild type (Fig. 11-20).[487,834,929,930] These can be differentiated by the presence of mental deterioration in patients with the severe type. The severe form becomes evident early; the diagnosis is usually made between 18 months and 3 years of age (Fig. 11-21). The severe form typically advances to cachexia[5] and death before 15 years of age. The mild form is diagnosed somewhat later, and patients have more prolonged survival, typically living into adulthood.[61] Young and Harper[925]and Young and others[929,930] have attempted to differentiate the characteristics of mild and severe forms of Hunter syndrome. In general the mild type is much more rare. Several different mutations at a unique X-chromosome locus[481,704,843,907] probably account for the variable severity of the disease. Some of these mutations, at least, are known to involve major gene deletions.[169,641,906,907]

Before molecular genetic studies were undertaken, McKusick et al.[556] suggested an alphabetic nomenclature for the severe and mild forms of the Hunter syndrome (types A and B, respectively). This format is now expected to be replaced by designations that reflect the actual mutations which cause the range of phenotypes.

Head and neck. The head is large and hydrocephaly is often present. The facies are coarse, with a large, flattened nose and a depressed nasal bridge, frontal bossing, hypertelorism, and a thickened tongue.[243] The teeth are widely spaced

and drooling is often excessive.[927] Dentigerous cysts are frequent.[506] Condylar abnormalities can be detected radiographically; presumably these are responsible for limited temporomandibular joint movements and contribute to the tendency for patients to have an open mouth. Symmetric otosclerotic foci are located in the bony labyrinthine capsule.[935] Pseudopapilledema (with normal cerebrospinal fluid pressure) is common,[925] but true papilledema reflecting increased cerebrospinal fluid pressure, and even frank hydrocephalus, may develop as the disease progresses.

Nervous system. In severe forms of the Hunter syndrome, mental impairment is usually evident on formal psychometric examination by 4 years of age and progressively becomes a major problem. Young[927] recognized three stages in the mental degeneration; the first consists of the "insidious" onset of mental retardation in conjunction with developmental delay. In the second stage, which lasts from 4 to 8 years, the mental age levels off and behavior problems become more pronounced. The terminal stage is characterized by increasing disability. The progressive neuronal degeneration results from abnormal neuronal storage of dermatan sulfate and heparan sulfate.

Neuroradiologic studies in the mild form of Hunter syndrome are relatively few. Wende and colleagues found age-dependent dilation of the ventricles and low density of white matter. In a 44-year-old man with the mild form, cranial MRI revealed a honeycomb-like appearance in the thalamus and the basal ganglia.[761] The deep white matter showed high signals in the T2 weighted image. Deposition of glycosaminoglycan or glycolipids, or both, were thought to be responsible for these changes.

Compressive myelopathy occasionally results from traumatic cervical spine dislocation (e.g., when attempting intubation) but also occurs atraumatically as a result of the combination of progressive thickening of the dura with glycosaminoglycan deposition (pachymeningitis cervicalis) and stenosis of the spinal canal.[405] Atlantoaxial subluxation resulting from odontoid hypoplasia is not usually a significant problem, but in occasional cases it may place the cord at additional risk.

Hearing loss is a frequent feature in the Hunter syndrome and can be both conductive (relating to chronic eustachian tube obstruction, to recurrent otitis media, and to a mucoid otitis media, possibly caused by glycosaminoglycan infiltration) and sensorineural (as a result of nerve cell changes within the otic ganglion).[757,935]

As in other types of MPS, individuals with the Hunter syndrome may have symptomatic or asymptomatic carpal tunnel syndrome because of median nerve compression[916,930] and other nerve entrapment.[416] Surprisingly the carpal tunnel syndrome is recognized more frequently in patients with mild Hunter syndrome than in those with the more severe type.[930]

Ocular features. Corneal clouding is usually absent in the Hunter syndrome. Isolated instances of corneal opacities, however, have been documented in two patients, one of whom had an extremely severe form of Hunter syndrome; the other had an unusually mild variety of the disorder.[783] In older patients with Hunter syndrome, slight corneal clouding may be evident on the slit-lamp microscopic examination but the involvement is minimal. Nevertheless, glycosaminoglycan deposits in the cornea are demonstrable in affected adults on histologic[292] and ultrastructural[627] study.

Bilateral uveal effusion syndrome characterized by serous detachment of the peripheral choroid and ciliary body, with concurrent detachment of the retina, have been documented in the mild form of the Hunter syndrome.[865] The predominant cause of this uveal effusion syndrome is a scleral thickening resulting from deposition of glycosaminoglycan, which predisposes the eye to vortex vein obstruction and acts as a barrier to the transport of extravascular protein out of the eye. The vortex vein obstruction and increased tissue colloid osmotic pressure result in chronic exudative detachments of the uvea and retina.

Atypical retinitis pigmentosa in which the electroretinogram becomes extinguished sometimes occurs in the Hunter syndrome.[278,351] Delleman and DeJong[199] reported pigmentary changes in the retinal epithelium that blocked background fluorescence at all stages of the fluorescein angiogram. This abnormality has been named pigment epithelial pattern dystrophy. There is a slight diminution in visual acuity in some patients, although a reduced electrooculogram is a consistent finding. Disk edema related to infiltration of glycosaminoglycan has also been reported.[57]

Respiratory system. The upper airways are obstructed by adenoid hypertrophy, nasal congestion, and thick rhinorrhea. Choanal stenosis contributes to the virtually uniform practice of mouth breathing. As children grow older, pharyngeal hypertrophy, tongue enlargement, and supraglottic swelling may result in sonorous breathing, frank obstructive sleep apnea, and death. Infections of the upper respiratory system are common. Rhinitis and chronic rhinorrhea occur in the majority of patients, irrespective of the phenotypic category of disease.[929,930] There is a suggestion that immunologic incompetence may be involved, since selective immunoglobulin A (IgA) deficiency has been found in a child with relatively mild Hunter syndrome.[133] The significance of this observation is uncertain because these researchers excluded IgA deficiency in two other children with relatively severe disease.

Tracheal stenosis and gradual deformation and collapse of the trachea have been documented in several cases (Fig. 11-22).[103,720,757] Sasaki et al.[720] described five patients with mild Hunter syndrome whose demise appeared to be a result of progressive obstruction that sequentially involved the upper, middle, and lower airway. Fig. 11-23 shows the gradual tracheal collapse in a patient at 15 years of age and later, at 22 years of age.

Cardiovascular system. Cardiovascular disease is present in a high proportion of patients with both forms of Hunter syndrome.[927] Cardiac valve

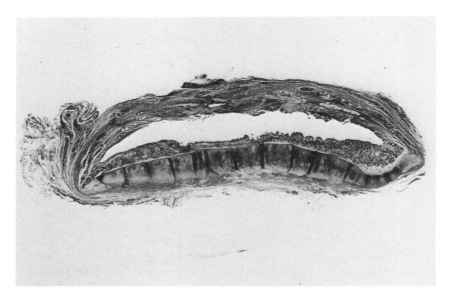

Fig. 11-22. Hunter syndrome. Histopathologic appearance of flattened tracheal cartilage showing loss of the normal curvature and lumen. In the natural course of the disease, progressive anteroposterior narrowing begins proximally below the cricoid and advances toward the carina. Patients are helped somewhat by positive end expiratory pressure ventilation, which maintains distal patency until cartilaginous deformity and mucosal swelling extend into the distal bronchi. (From Sasaki CT et al: *Laryngoscope* 97:280-285, 1987.)

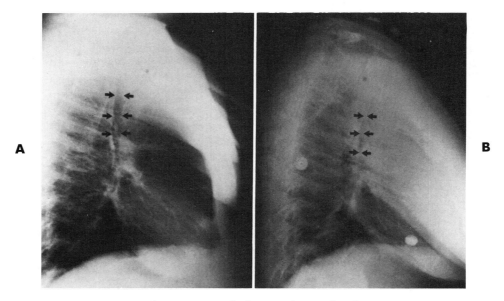

Fig. 11-23. Hunter syndrome. Lateral chest radiographs showing progressive tracheal collapse, **A,** in a patient at 15 years of age *(arrows)* and, later, at age 22 years, **B.** As affected children grow older, pharyngeal hypertrophy, tongue enlargement, and supraglottic swelling produce airway obstruction. Sonorous breathing and sleep apnea may necessitate adenotonsillectomy, which often provides temporary relief. To cope with gradually progressive tracheal deformation and compression, custom-made tracheostomy cannulas have been fashioned to bypass the flattened upper trachea. Eventual involvement below the carina exhausts surgical ingenuity. (From Sasaki CT et al: *Laryngoscope* 97:280-285, 1987.)

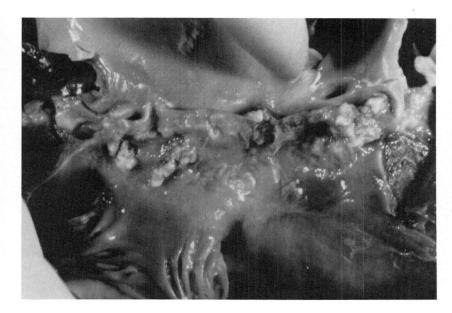

Fig. 11-24. Hunter syndrome. Aortic valve with calcified micronodules ("waxed droppings") disposed along the line of closure and most pronounced in the center third of each leaflet. The nodules extend inferiorly to the myocardium and are ulcerated. (From Zimmermann B III et al: *Clin Cardiol* 11:723-725, 1988.)

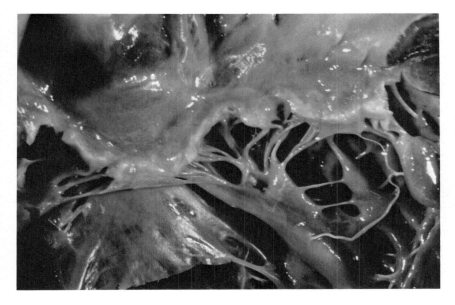

Fig. 11-25. Hunter syndrome. Mitral valve with early changes of micronodular thickening along the line of closure. Chordea tendineae are mildly thickened and shortened, but the commissures are not fused. Early thickening of the leaflets and mitral valve regurgitation can usually be demonstrated by means of echocardiography or heart catheterization during the first few years of life. (From Zimmermann B III et al: *Clin Cardiol* 11:723-725, 1988.)

involvement may cause congestive heart failure; indeed, heart failure appears to be the leading cause of death in affected persons. Zimmerman et al.[940] reported a 30-year-old man with Hunter syndrome and systemic lupus erythematosus who had severe progressive aortic stenosis, which led to his death (Fig. 11-24). At autopsy the heart was found to be enlarged (590 g) with moderate, four-chambered dilation and diffuse biventricular hypertrophy. The mitral valve had diffuse micronodular thickening, especially around the line of closure (Fig. 11-25). Mild thickening and shortening of the chordae tendinae contributed to the regurgitant valve dysfunction. Typical advanced mitral valve involvement, with nodular growths on the valve cusps, is depicted in Fig. 11-26. In a study of echocardiographic abnormalities in the mucopolysaccharidoses, all patients with Hunter syndrome had echographic thickening of mitral valve.[301]

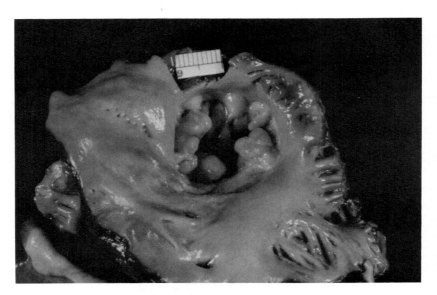

Fig. 11-26. Hunter syndrome. The mitral valve with advanced deforming, calcified granulations is especially involved in progressive glycosaminoglycan accumulation. Surgical valve replacement in older patients is extremely difficult in the face of co-existent coronary artery occlusion, cardiomyopathy, and respiratory disease, thus probably accounting for the paucity of reports of successful procedures. (From Sasaki CT et al: *Laryngoscope* 97:280-285, 1987.)

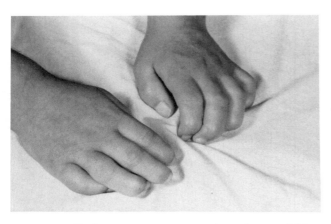

Fig. 11-27. Early joint contractures in a 6-year-old boy with severe Hunter syndrome. These contractures of the fingers occurred despite successful bone marrow transplantation at 3 years of age.

Skeletal system. Digital contractures are a typical feature of Hunter syndrome (Fig. 11-27). The joints of the limbs are held in partial flexion, and their range of motion is limited. Young and Harper[925] described typical changes in a 31-year-old man with ". . . clawed hands with limitation of movement at all joints, particularly wrists, elbows and shoulders. All movements at both hips were severely limited and painful, and were accompanied by clicking. He also showed mild pectus excavatum, but no spine deformity." Changes in the head of the femur, with precocious osteoarthritis, are usually present in older patients. The foot is of the pes cavus type and the fifth toe is often overlapping.

The abnormalities evident on radiographic study in patients with the Hunter syndrome are similar to those in persons with the Hurler syndrome but tend to be less severe. Involvement of the pelvis and spine, in particular, are less striking in the Hunter syndrome. Nevertheless, occasional patients with Hunter syndrome have fairly severe bony abnormalities, which are indistinguishable from those of mild Hurler syndrome. The radiographic skeletal changes in the two conditions thus form a continuum, which is referred to as dysostosis multiplex.

Abdomen and viscera. Clinical and biochemical manifestations of hepatic dysfunction are usually minimal, despite long-standing hepatosplenomegaly.[645]

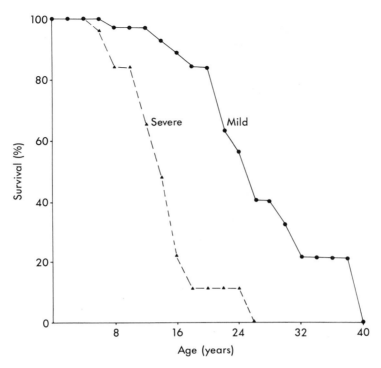

Fig. 11-28. Survival of patients with mild and severe Hunter syndrome (From Young ID et al: *J Med Genet* 10:408-411, 1982.)

Umbilical and inguinal hernias are often present. Diarrhea is frequent; Young and Harper[927] documented persistent diarrhea in 22 of 34 patients, which was "profuse, offensive, and unexplained." These authors proposed that the diarrhea is possibly secondary to neuronal degeneration. The frequency of these episodes seems to increase as the disease progresses.

Endocrine system. The short stature associated with Hunter syndrome was once believed to be secondary to anterior pituitary dysfunction and deficient secretion of growth hormone. Young and Harper,[926] in necropsy studies of a patient with mild Hunter syndrome, found few eosinophilic cells and extensive degenerate cells in the pituitary. By contrast, Nelson and Carson[594] described a 13-year-old patient with mild Hunter syndrome in whom anterior pituitary function and, in particular, growth hormone secretion were normal. In addition, cortisol, thyroid stimulating hormone, prolactin, lutenizing hormone, and follicle stimulating hormone levels were all within the normal range. These findings have been confirmed by the author's observations of three patients ranging in age from 2 to 4 years. A number of surviving men have had offspring,[130,658,922] which suggests a normal reproductive capability.

Integument. Nodules or papules may be present over the scapula, upper arms, thorax and lateral regions of the thighs.[20,153] These lesions usually begin to develop in the second or third year of life and progress slowly.[243] Hypertrichosis is often striking; it is present in the normal distribution of lanugo but to an exaggerated degree and is sometimes expressed as synophrys (confluent dense eyebrows).

Adult patients with Hunter syndrome tend to have a "high coloration" or "rosy cheeks." F. Parkes Weber, in a discussion of Hunter's historic paper,[378] noted that a "remarkable feature" of these individuals "is a 'precociously plethoric' appearance of their facies," like "that of a middle-aged farmer who is fond of malt liquor, and whose work naturally exposes him much to the weather."

Prognosis. The mean age of death (Fig. 11-28) in a combined series of patients with both forms of the Hunter syndrome was 11.77 years for children with the severe form and 21.7 years for those with the mild form.[927]

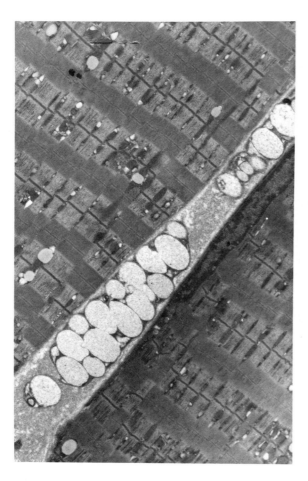

Fig. 11-29. Vacuolated fibroblasts in the endomysium of a patient with severe Hunter syndrome. Accumulation of glycosaminoglycans in muscle tissue may be an additional factor contributing to gradual motor impairment, although the slight dysfunction of muscle is likely to be masked by predominant involvement of the central nervous system. (From Wakai S et al: *Pediatr Neurol* 4:178-180, 1988.)

Pathology

In general the pathologic changes are identical to those in the Hurler syndrome, and virtually every tissue is involved.[627,883] Involvement of the skeletal muscle is an additional feature; Wakai et al.[872] described their investigations of a muscle biopsy specimen from a patient with severe Hunter syndrome. The muscle fibers and interstitial cells contained metachromatic granules which suggest the storage of sulfated glycosaminoglycans. Fig. 11-29 shows a section of skeletal muscle with vacuolated fibroblasts in the endomysium.

On histologic study the cornea may show changes qualitatively similar to those in Hurler syndrome, although clouding is not clinically evident.[543] Deposition of abnormal glycosaminoglycan is minimal in the stroma, but heavy concentrations are present in the corneal endothelium, in the epithelial structures of the iris and ciliary body, and in the markedly thickened sclera.

Hydrocephalus may be associated with thickened, milky leptomeninges.[606] The hydrocephalus[713] may be the result of interference with drainage, which is produced by glycosaminoglycan deposits.

Ferrer et al.[241] observed focal dendritic swellings in secondary dendrites of Purkinje cells in post mortem samples of the cerebellum. The focal dendritic swellings had smooth surfaces, but secondary formation of spinelike appendages was absent; in contrast, terminal, spiny branches were preserved.

Parfrey and Hutchins[645] described hepatic fibrosis in six patients with mucopolysaccharidoses, including two patients with Hunter syndrome. Extensive hepatocyte and Kupffer-cell vacuolization was also present. In the past the fibrosis has been thought to be as a secondary response to the abnormal accumulation of some hepatotoxic metabolite. An alternate possibility is that extracellular glycosaminoglycan contributes to exaggeration of the normal mechanisms that lay down collagen.

By means of electron microscopic study membranous cytoplasmic bodies have been described in ganglion and satellite cells of intramural plexi in a biopsy specimen of the rectal wall.[230] The changes at this site may be causally related to chronic diarrhea, which is a notable feature of the condition.

Fundamental Defect

Patients with Hunter syndrome excrete excessive amounts of dermatan sulfate and heparan sulfate in the urine. Knecht and Dorfman[443,444] showed that two types of heparan sulfate can be identified in tissues from normal individuals and also from patients with Hurler syndrome. Maroteaux[518] found that although the proportion of total heparan sulfate to dermatan sulfate is not clearly different in the Hurler and Hunter syndromes, the proportion of the two types of heparan sulfate does distinguish the two disorders in individual patients. On the other hand, others[295,413,821] could distinguish Hurler syndrome and Hunter syndrome by means of the ratios of dermatan sulfate and heparan sulfate, which were about 70:30 in both the Hurler and the Scheie syndromes and about equal (50:50) in the Hunter syndrome.

The primary biochemical defect is deficient lysosomal iduronate-2-sulfatase,[38,190] the enzyme responsible for cleavage of sulfate from iduronic acid moieties of heparan sulfate and dermatan sulfate (see Fig. 11-6). The same enzyme is deficient in mild and severe forms.[898]

Molecular genetics. Hopwood's group[906] has purified the human iduronate-2-sulfatase enzyme from liver and isolated and sequenced a 2.3-kilobase cDNA clone that includes the entire coding region. Analysis of the deduced 550–amino-acid precursor indicates that the enzyme has a 25–amino-acid amino-terminal signal sequence, followed by eight amino acids, which are removed from the proprotein. An internal proteolytic cleavage occurs to produce the mature iduronate-2-sulfatase that is present in human liver. The sequence has strong homology with other sulfatases from human and animal sources, suggesting that a family of genes may have arisen by gene duplication and divergent evolution. Some patients with the most severe forms of Hunter syn-

drome have been shown to have major structural alterations and gross deletions of the gene.[169,641,906] Patients with mild disease likely have single-base substitutions, which diminish but do not obliterate enzyme activity.[170] Molecular analysis suggests[577,704,802,907] that the following is the orientation of the gene and flanking loci: Xqter-DXS304(5')IDS (3')-DXS296-DXS297-DXS369-Xcen.

Prevalence and Inheritance

An abundance of pedigree data provides ample evidence of X-linked recessive inheritance in the Hunter syndrome.[72,207] Indeed, the gene for iduronidate sulfatase has now been localized by in situ hybridization to Xq27.3,[802,907] near the locus of the gene for the Fragile-X syndrome.

The incidence of the Hunter syndrome in British Columbia has been estimated at 1 in 100,000 births.[503] A study in Great Britain indicated a frequency of 1 in 171,132 male live births (0.584 per 100,000 births) and a prevalence of 1.79 million males (0.115 per 100,000 births).[928]

No particular ethnic concentration of cases of an X-linked recessive trait such as Hunter syndrome would be expected. It has been postulated, however, that there may be a relatively high frequency of the syndrome among Ashkenazi and Moroccan Jews in Israel.[724] Prenatal biologic selection favoring the Hunter allele was proposed as an explanation.[944,945]

Hunter syndrome in females. Females that meet the clinical and biochemical criteria of Hunter syndrome are exceedingly rare.[146,147] Carrier females are always normal on clinical examination. In heterozygotes the lack of physical findings and normal glycosaminoglycanuria suggest that the population of enzyme-deficient cells lyonized to express the mutant allele achieve metabolic correction by uptake of enzyme from neighboring cells that are lyonized to expression of the normal gene.

It is possible that the exceedingly rare females with Hunter syndrome occur by homozygosity for a Hunter allele through one of the following mechanisms: (1) as the offspring of a carrier female born to an affected male or an unaffected male whose sperm carry a new mutation; (2) uniparental disomy of the mutant X-chromosome from a heterozygous female or an affected male; or (3) genetic rearrangement, for example, translocation or deletion resulting in nonrandom lyonization toward expression of a mutant allele.[111]

Early reports of girls and women with the physical stigmata of Hunter syndrome and deficiency of iduronate sulfatase suggested the possibility of an autosomal recessive form of the disease.[600] Subsequent studies demonstrated that one of the affected girls had multiple sulfatase deficiency, a distinct entity resulting from deficiency of several sulfatase enzymes (caused by a postulated defective factor required by several sulfatases). Another girl with clinical features of Hunter syndrome and profound enzyme deficiency was found to have a balanced reciprocal translocation, 46,XX,t(X;5), which presumably disrupted the iduronate sulfatase gene.[577] A further occurrence of Hunter syndrome in a female was attributed to partial deletion of the long arm of one X chromosome, which resulted in nonrandom inactivation and selective expression of a mutant iduronate sulfatase gene on the other X chromosome. A fourth female with Hunter syndrome[146] was found to have a break at the Xq27-Xq28 junction, which caused both disruption of the iduronate sulfatase locus on her paternal X chromosome and an unbalanced inactivation of the nonmutant maternal X chromosome.[147] This observation served to localize the iduronate sulfatase gene to the locus Xq27.3. There is no evidence of another autosomal gene affecting iduronate sulfatase activity. From the foregoing it follows that girls and women with the Hunter syndrome and deficient iduronate sulfatase activity warrant investigation to exclude multiple sulfatase deficiency and X-chromosome rearrangements.

Management

Otologic complications. Management of otologic complications includes tympanostomy,[720] adenoidectomy,[263] and the provision of hearing aids.[655] Placement of ventilation tubes in the tympanic membranes is frequently undertaken for the treatment of recurrent ear infections, with beneficial results.[133] Because long-term drainage may be necessary, the use of flanged "permanant" tubes should be considered so that repeated procedures are avoided.

Sleep apnea. Management of airway problems is symptomatic but based on the characteristic evolution of airway disease.[720] Airway involvement is progressive, beginning with noisy respiration derived from relative choanal stenosis and swelling of nasopharyngeal tissues. This situation is complicated by the increasing dependence of patients on nasal breathing because of enlargement of the tongue, tonsils, and gingiva, together with the small mandibular ramus and temporomandibular ankylosis. Most affected children compensate by holding the mouth open and protruding the tongue to enlarge the airway at the posterior pharynx. Accumulation of storage material in small airways may contribute to respiratory symptoms.[133] In adults with relatively mild Hunter syndrome, diffuse airway obstruction may be manifest as daytime somnolence, snoring, and alveolar hypoventilation. It has been speculated that central apnea and hyponea in the mucopolysaccharidoses results from cervical spinal cord compression caused by glycosaminoglycan deposition in the vertebrae and leptomeninges.[661,753] Cord compression has not been demonstrated, however, and polysomnography invariably shows severe obstructive sleep apnea.[281] As pharyngeal hypertrophy and macroglossia progress, tonsillectomy and adenoidectomy may be transiently helpful. In the experience of Whitley et al.[371] and Steven[789] nasal continuous positive airways pressure has been a successful treatment. Addition of supplemental oxygen has been a successful adjuvant that minimizes desaturation. In many patients significant obstruction occurs exclusively during sleep; thus nasal continuous positive airway pressure may be required only at night. These modalities warrant a trial before uvulopalatopharyngoplasty or tracheostomy is considered. As the large airways become progressively narrowed, tracheostomy may be required.[662] Progressive anteroposterior narrowing begins proximally below the cricoid and advances toward the carina. Gross and histopathologic examination of the trachea demonstrate a peculiar flattening of tracheal cartilages, which results in loss of their normal curvature and in anteroposterior collapse. Custom-designed tracheal cannulas are usually required because of the disproportionate length-to-diameter ratio. An adjustable single-lumen armored tube has been considered useful in allowing for gradual extension, to bypass proximal tracheal narrowing.[720] Distal airway obstruction eventually develops in many patients; this complication necessitates continuous positive airway pressure delivered by tracheostomy.[103,720,753]

Ventriculoperitoneal shunting. Hydrocephalus is a relatively rare complication of Hunter syndrome. Some children have received a shunt, although the indications are unclear, since hydrocephalus may be asymptomatic.

Anesthesia. Difficulties during anesthesia are major and have been the subject of a growing literature.[40-42,433,753,771] In particular, rigidity of the thoracic cage, abdominal distention, macroglossia, temporomandibular ankylosis, and atlantoaxial instability may present significant problems in the management of anesthesia. Furthermore, the neck is short and wide, which renders intubation and management of a tracheostomy particularly difficult.[720]

Autopsy studies indicate that coronary artery disease and cardiomyopathy may be present, although the electrocardiogram, echocardiogram, and results of heart catheterization are relatively normal. Thus appropriate precautions should be taken at the time of general anesthesia to avoid anemia, to ensure euvolemia, and to maintain maximal oxygenation throughout induction, during the procedure, and at extubation.

Cardiac disease. Multiple abnormalities contribute to cardiac disease, and annual chest radiograph, electrocardiogram, and echocardiogram would be a judicious schedule of monitoring. Although cardiac disease may not be evident as auscultatory or echogenic regurgitation, the recognition of early valve lesions on microscopic study suggests that appropriate antibiotic prophylaxis should be used for at-risk procedures as soon as the diagnosis of MPS is suspected.

Hernia. Inguinal and umbilical hernias are common in Hunter syndrome. Repair of an inguinal hernia on one side provides an opportunity for surgical exploration of the contralateral side. In this way a second sack can be identified, thus eliminating the need for a second procedure.

Carpal tunnel syndrome. Although many affected persons do not have the classic symptoms of carpal tunnel syndrome, electrophysiologic evidence of progressive median nerve compression is common. To preserve apposition of the thumb, annual studies are recommended and surgical release is indicated at the earliest sign of an electrophysiologic abnormality, even though the individual may be asymptomatic.

Dental care. Dental care is often difficult because of lack of patient cooperation. Enlargement of the tongue and gums, together with the limited aperture of the mouth (resulting from decreased motion at the temporomandibular joint), compounds the problem. The poor state of the teeth is frequently aggravated by the prolonged use of sucrose-containing medications. Defective oral hygiene and mouth breathing result in hyperplastic gingivitis.

Gastrointestinal complications. Intermittant diarrhea, possibly resulting from autonomic dysregulation and, perhaps, aggravated by frequent use of antibiotics is a common complaint. Including yogurt or other sources of lactobacillus in the diet may be useful in preventing overgrowth of bacteria. For patients who are inactive because of severe debilitation, constipation may necessitate occasional use of enemas.

Musculoskeletal complications. Skeletal abnormalities constitute long-term problems and, because they are generalized and progressive, are exceptionally resistant to conventional orthopedic treatment. Kyphoscoliosis is only mildly progressive and does not usually result in spinal cord compression. For this reason there seems to be little indication for, and virtually no experience with, surgical stabilization of the spine. Although each affected child may be different, many children do not tolerate back bracing for kyphoscoliosis. Use of shoe orthotics and ankle braces are better tolerated and useful in maintaining mobility. Some patients with advanced disease have benefited from Achilles tendon release.

Systemic treatment. A number of attempts at systemic treatment have been undertaken in the Hunter syndrome. Administration of normal human plasma (presumably containing iduronate sulfatase) in two patients was followed by a transient decrease in urinary excretion of glycosaminoglycan of relatively large molecular weight and a concomitant increased excretion of the products of degradation.[208] This approach was not, however, seen as feasible for long-term treatment. Transplantation of normal human fibroblasts has also been undertaken[192] but lacked substantial effect. Knudson, DiFerrante, and Curtis[445] transfused leukocytes into a patient with the Hunter syndrome and reported clinical improvement, as well as a rise in glycosaminoglycan levels, particularly partially degraded ones, in the urine. Infusion of leukocytes (HLA-matched) was shown to reduce airway complications, but progression of cardiac disease and neurologic deterioration seemed unaltered. Despite early reports of success[6,7] with transplantation of amniotic membrane implants under the abdominal skin, this approach to treatment provided neither long-term tissue engraftment nor any biochemical or physiologic response.[582]

Bone marrow transplantation. In a limited number of children bone marrow transplantation has been carried out in an attempt at systemic treatment of Hunter syndrome. Reduction in hepatosplenomegaly, improvement in airway disease, and reduction in urinary glycosaminoglycan excretion have been reported,[880] but the child in question died unexpectedly 3 years after transplantation. The long-term prognosis for longevity, cardiac complications, and neurologic outcome after marrow transplantation remains to be determined.

MUCOPOLYSACCHARIDOSIS TYPE III (SANFILIPPO SYNDROME, HEPARANSULFATURIA)

Sanfilippo syndrome was first delineated as a distinct biochemical and clinical phenotype by Sanfilippo in 1963,[717,718] although cases had been previously observed by Meyer et al.[561] in 1958 and noted as a possible new genotype by Harris in 1961.[317] The condition is an autosomal recessive disorder characterized by the accumulation of excessive amounts of heparan sulfate glycosaminoglycan in lysosomes and by the excretion of large amounts of heparan sulfate in urine. There are few stigmata other than severe and progressive mental retardation.

Failure to degrade heparan sulfate can result from deficiency in any one of four lysosomal enzymes; thus there are four forms of Sanfilippo syndrome that are clinically indistinguishable but are each characterized by the deficiency of a different enzyme. Patients with Sanfilippo syndrome, type A have deficient heparan N-sulfatase activity,[457] those with Sanfilippo syndrome, type B have deficient α-N-acetylglucosaminidase activity,[618,868] those with Sanfilippo syndrome, type C have deficient acetyl-CoA: α-glucosaminide N-acetyltransferase activity,[442] and those with Sanfilippo syndrome, type D have deficient N-acetylglucosamine 6-sulfatase activity.[459]

Clinical Manifestations

General features. The main clinical characteristics are profound, progressive mental retardation and behavioral disturbances; somatic changes are relatively less severe. There is great variability, however, in the clinical expression of this syndrome both between the types and within each type.

Marked variation in clinical expression of the somatic phenotype was documented in a large study of Sanfilippo syndrome, types A, B, and C in the Netherlands[849,850] and is also apparent in the relatively few cases of type D.[162] Intrafamilial variation may be considerable, and mild and severe phenotypes have been observed within the same sibship.[22,850]

Most children with Sanfilippo syndrome appear normal at birth, and their intellectual and social development is usually not recognizably different from that of their peers until the age of 4 to 6 years (Fig. 11-30). A decline in cognitive function becomes apparent thereafter. Mental decline begins with regression in language and memory. The first signs of the disorder often are sleep disturbances[54,755,845] and behavioral disorders such as aggressiveness, hyperactivity, and short attention span.* Behavioral problems intensify coincidentally with mental deterioration.[54]

The disease has been known to become evident in early infancy[755] or to remain unapparent until adulthood. Indeed, in a series of seven adult patients with Sanfilippo syndrome, type B in whom dementia occurred late in the course of the disease, three were employed until adulthood (ages 18, 20, and 24 years) and another worked as a household helper until the age of 32 years.[861] In general the intellect deteriorates progressively: by school age mental retardation is evident, and by the teens it constitutes a major disability.

The rate at which the mental retardation progresses is variable,[850] as shown graphically in several patients (Fig. 11-31). Wraith, Danks, and Rogers[917] described a 4-year-old child with Sanfilippo syndrome, type B who showed no signs of regression and continued to make developmental progress,[917] whereas Sewell, Pontz, and Benischek[755] documented a girl with Sanfilippo syndrome, type C at the age of 1 year who was severely retarded, made no attempt to sit up or roll over, and could not even control her head move-

---

*References 54, 162, 271, 415, 604, 614, 845, and 861.

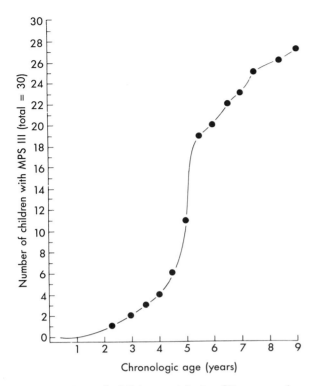

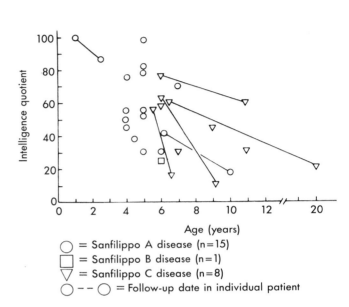

○ = Sanfilippo A disease (n=15)
□ = Sanfilippo B disease (n=1)
▽ = Sanfilippo C disease (n=8)
○ – – ○ = Follow-up date in individual patient

Fig. 11-30. Age of children with Sanfilippo syndrome when parents first noted regression of developmental milestones. Mean = 5.5 years; standard deviation = 1.54 years. In three of 30 children with Sanfilippo syndrome (ages 11 months, 5 years 6 months, and 5 years 7 months) signs of regression had not yet been noted. (From Nidiffer FD, Kelly TE: *J Ment Defic Res* 27:185-203, 1983.)

Fig. 11-31. Intelligence quotient (IQ) scores for 22 patients with Sanfilippo syndrome illustrate the individual difference in intelligence level and the rapid decline in some patients in contrast to the more gradual changes in others. (From Van de Kamp JJP et al: *Clin Genet* 20:152-160, 1981.)

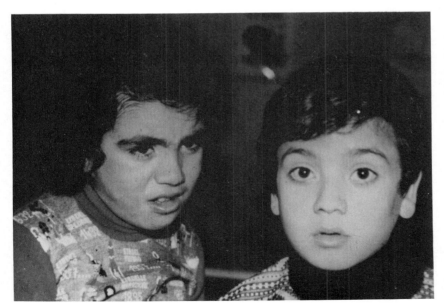

Fig. 11-32. Two siblings with Sanfilippo syndrome, type B illustrate the clinical variability of this disorder. Patient (at 11 years of age, *left*) had coarse facial features, a large tongue, thick lips, generalized hirsutism with synophrys and significant developmental delay. By 26 years of age she had lost contact with the environment as a result of progressive dementia. In contrast, the mildly affected brother (*right,* at 9 years of age) lacked significantly dysmorphic facial features and was only moderately developmentally delayed. At 23 years of age he was working in a shop and had an IQ (Weschler scale) of 44. (From Andria G et al: *Clin Genet* 15:500-504, 1979.)

ments. Coppa[162] observed two boys in whom the diagnoses of Sanfilippo syndrome, type D were made by means of enzyme assay, who showed marked variation in the rate at which their intellect declined. One, a 9-year-old, was functioning fairly normally in third grade, whereas the other was severely retarded, with a profound lack of verbal understanding, by the age of 5 years. Andria et al.[22] noted marked variation in the physical appearance (Fig. 11-32) and the rate and severity of mental degeneration in a brother and sister with Sanfilippo syndrome, type B. When the boy was observed at the age of 11 years, he had mild retardation but was able to read, write, and count and was attending school. His sister, on the other hand, was never able to attend school, and at the

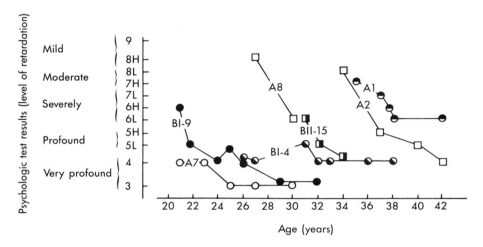

Fig. 11-33. Psychologic test results for seven adult patients with a relatively mild form of Sanfilippo syndrome, type B. Two of the patients, *A1* and *A2*, were living at home and working in a sheltered workshop at 30 years of age. Subsequently dementia and severe mental retardation became evident, thus indicating the progressive nature of neurologic deterioration, even in patients with relatively mild disease. (From Van Schrojenstein-de Valk HMJ, van de Kamp JJP: *Am J Med Genet* 28:125-129, 1987.)

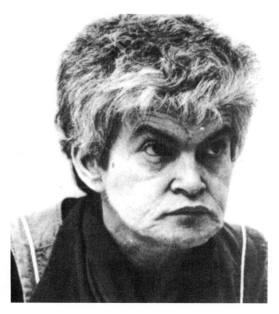

Fig. 11-34. A 43-year-old woman with a relatively mild form of Sanfilippo syndrome, type B. (From Van Schrojenstein-de Valk HMJ, van de Kamp JJP: *Am J Med Genet* 28:125-129, 1987.)

age of 9 years she could communicate only with her parents and used a poor vocabulary.

Although recognition of the disease typically occurs later than for other MPS conditions, Sanfilippo syndrome is no less lethal. Affected children follow a clinical course of progressive dementia and usually die in the second decade of life.[755] Rare individuals with mild disease, however, may survive much longer, possibly to 40 years of age (Figs. 11-33 and 11-34).

Head and neck. Although the facial features are often sufficiently normal to escape early recogni-

tion, some abnormalities may be apparent (Figs. 11-35 to 11-38). The orbital ridges tend to be somewhat prominent, and the eyebrows are generally thick. A broad nose and relatively flat nasal bridge are often present, and a thickened upper lip and a protruding tongue are frequent characteristics. Nearly all patients are described as having thick, abundant scalp hair.* Van de Kamp[845] has reported that 29 of 60 patients had head circumferences that were greater than two standard deviations above the mean. The teeth are normal on

_____
*References 54, 271, 327, 415, 755, and 845.

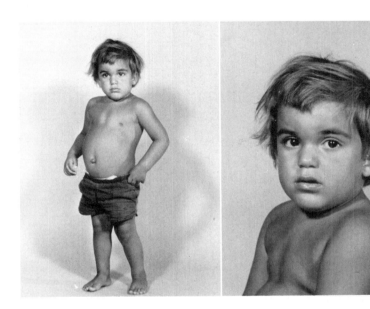

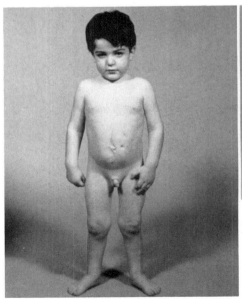

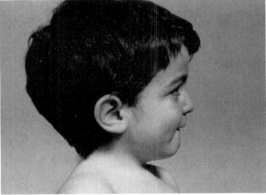

Fig. 11-35. General appearance of a 3-year-old boy with Sanfilippo syndrome, type A.

Fig. 11-36. General appearance of a 2-year-old boy with Sanfilippo syndrome, type B.

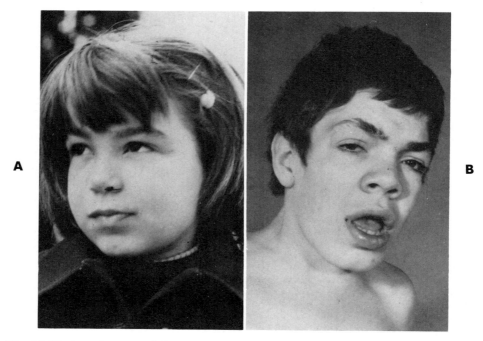

Fig. 11-37. A and **B,** Facial features of a girl and boy with Sanfilippo syndrome, type C. (From Bartsocas CS et al: *Eur J Pediatr* 130:251-258, 1979.)

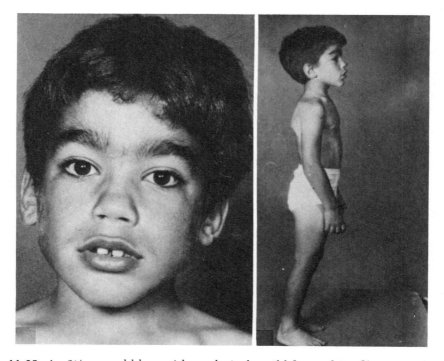

Fig. 11-38. An 8½-year-old boy with a relatively mild form of Sanfilippo syndrome, type D. Macrocephaly, coarse facies, generalized hirsutism with synophrys, and inability to extend the elbows are evident. (From Kaplan P, Wolfe LS: *J Pediatr* 110:267-271, 1987.)

gross examination, but obliteration of pulp cavity has been observed.[885]

Ocular features. Gross clouding of the cornea does not occur. Some problems with vision have been noted in the late stage but are difficult to identify because of the presence of severe mental retardation. A marked loss in photoreceptor cells may take place during the course of the disease and eventually lead to blindness. Pigmentary degeneration similar to that in retinitis pigmentosa has been observed.[200]

Nervous system. It has been suggested that the term "mentally retarded" may be inappropriate in the condition insofar as it connotes a static state of mental deficiency, whereas in Sanfilippo syndrome mental degeneration is progressive. A mother's statement that "she (or he) doesn't recognize me anymore" rather than that "she (or he) never knew me" poignantly illustrates this distinction.[327] The syndrome might be better described as a progressive dementia.

Brain involvement usually starts in the areas of mentation, and motor activities typically remain intact until later in the course of the disease.[200,327,836] Twenty-three of the 73 Dutch patients evaluated by van de Kamp et al.[850] reported difficulties in walking, and most patients are unable to walk in the later stages.[54,664,845] There are exceptions, however; a patient with Sanfilippo syndrome, type A was ambulatory until his death, which resulted from pneumonia, at the age of 36 years.[910] Diarrhea is a common problem,[184,850] and loss of bowel control is often noted about midway through the deterioration process.[54,327] Sometimes toilet and bowel control are never achieved.[162]

Another area influenced by the great clinical variability of the disorder is speech. It may develop normally,[54,271,836] be developmentally delayed, or never be acquired at all.[162] If acquired, speech is usually lost as cognitive function declines.[200,845] Epilepsy has been reported in several instances,[614,807] but this is not a constant feature. Van de Kamp[849] reported that 18 of 46 patients had a history of seizures.

Magnetic resonance imaging of the cranial contents shows altered signal intensity, which suggests that myelination may be deficient and that infiltration or deposition of glycosaminoglycan oc-

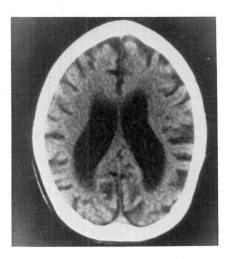

Fig. 11-39. Diffuse cerebral atrophy with hydrocephalus ex vacuo is revealed in CT of the head of an 8-year-old boy with Sanfilippo syndrome, type A. This boy, although ambulatory, had moderately severe mental retardation.

curs in the brain. Small spherical lesions in the brain demonstrated by means of CT or by MRI seem to correspond to areas of tissue rarefaction around blood vessels. Periventricular T2 prolongation is often seen in conjunction with mild ventricular dilation (often also evident on CT as relatively hypodense periventricular areas). These changes are thought to result from low-grade periventricular edema or abnormalities in myelination.[586] Diffuse cerebral atrophy with hydrocephalus *ex vacuo* is the long-term outcome (Fig. 11-39).

Respiratory and cardiovascular systems. Copious nasal discharge and repeated upper respiratory tract infections are early signs of the syndrome.[162,271,327] Respiratory infections and pneumonia were listed as the cause of death in several cases.[910] In general, however, affected persons are not predisposed to obstructive apnea or pneumonia, although the lung radiographs may show increased interstitial markings suggestive of mild fibrosis.

Cardiac signs and symptoms are relatively rare in the Sanfilippo syndrome[337]; nevertheless, the heart is certainly involved in the same pathologic process as in other mucopolysaccharidoses (discussed elsewhere in this chapter) but probably to a much lesser degree.

Skeletal system. Whereas some patients with each of the four types of Sanfilippo syndrome have skeletal abnormalities, others with the same form of the condition may show no such abnormalities. In particular, stature may be stunted, although height is usually normal.[184,664,861]

On radiographic examination the skeleton may show a mild degree of dysostosis multiplex or may be entirely normal.[22,664,861,918] A typical example is illustrated in Fig. 11-40. The severity of skeletal involvement increases with the progression of the disease.[836] Indeed, in patients with severe bone changes the abnormalities may be indistinguishable from those in patients with the mild bone changes of the Hunter syndrome. Sanfilippo syndrome thus represents the mildest example of the dysostosis multiplex continuum, with Hurler syndrome representing the severe end of the spectrum and Hunter syndrome occupying an intermediate position.

Increased thickness and density of the posterior portion of the calvaria is a fairly specific radiographic finding in the Sanfilippo syndrome.[200,226] This thickening in the parietal and interparietal portion of the occipital bone is illustrated in the lateral skull film of a 15-year-old boy (Fig. 11-41).

Another distinctive but nonspecific skeletal characteristic that may be present is a biconvex configuration of the vertebral bodies in the thoracic and lumbar regions[162,271,415] (Fig. 11-42). The ribs may be moderately thickened. Although bone maturation is often delayed,[54,224] bone age is sometimes normal.[273,325]

Stiffness of all joints occurs, as in the Hunter and the Hurler syndromes, but it is usually mild and instances have been reported in which there has been no articular rigidity.[24,162,917] Typically the first or only joint to be affected is the elbow.[54,271,415]

Abdomen and viscera. Hepatomegaly is only slight or moderate, and in many patients no enlargement of the liver is present.[325,910] Andria et al.[22] reported two sibs, one with marked hepatosplenomegaly and one in whom no such feature was present. Splenomegaly may be moderate or absent.[162,415] Umbilical hernias may occur,[271,415] but often no hernias are present.[59]

Endocrine system. Some patients have normal puberty[836,845] and sexual development, but in others secondary sexual characteristics do not devel-

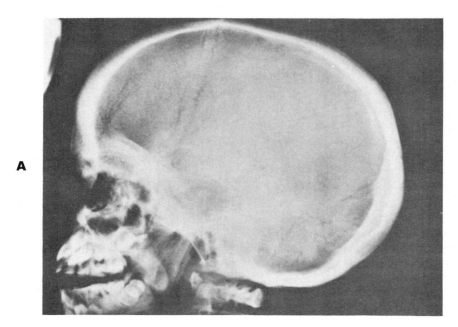

Fig. 11-40. The typically mild radiographic findings in a 9-year-old boy with Sanfilippo syndrome, type A are shown in **A** through **D.** In a lateral view of the skull, **A**, the entire cranial vault appears thickened, as are the orbital plates; the mastoids are underdeveloped and sclerotic.

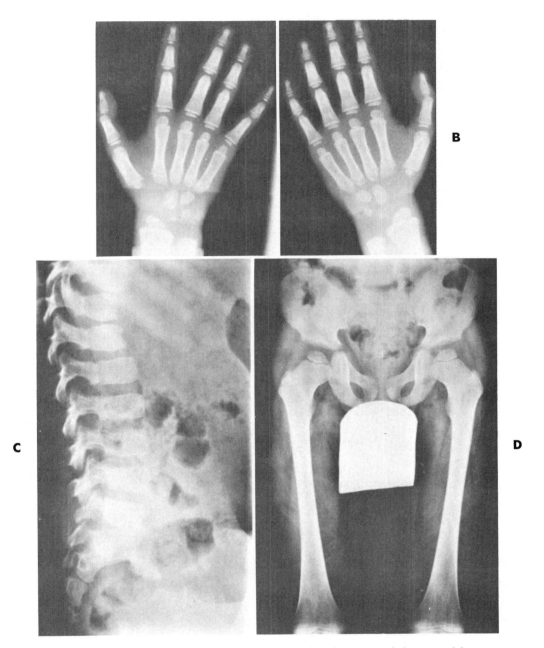

Fig. 11-40, cont'd. The hands, **B,** show delay in development of the carpal bones, a mild notch at the proximal end of the fifth metacarpal, and somewhat coarse trabecular architecture of the tubular bones. The lower spine, **C,** shows hypoplasia of the bodies of vertebrae T12 and L1, and the latter is mildly hooked. The view of the pelvis and femurs, **D,** is notable for its relative normality. Coxa valga is present, and the capital epiphyses are somewhat small.

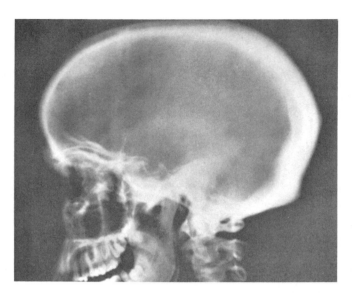

Fig. 11-41. In a lateral view of the skull of a 15-year-old boy with Sanfilippo syndrome, type B, thickening of the calvaria is striking, especially in the posterior parietal and occipital areas. Mastoids are sclerotic but the sella turcica is normal, as is usual in this disorder.

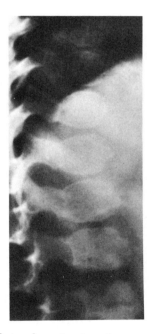

Fig. 11-42. In lateral projection the vertebral bodies of a 6-year-old boy with Sanfilippo syndrome are biconvex in the thoracic and upper lumbar region. Significant kyphosis seldom occurs. The end-plate biconvexity usually disappears in late childhood and adolescence. Irregularity of the end-plates may persist in areas of previous ossification defect. (From Haust MD et al: *Am J Med Genet* 22:1-27, 1985.)

op.[54,807] In addition, problems with menstruation sometimes arise.[861] These complications are likely to have their basis in central nervous system involvement.

Integument. Hypertrichosis is often present, especially on the back.[54,162,271] Variation is evident in this feature; Andria et al.[22] noted marked hirsutism in one sib with Sanfilippo syndrome, type B and the absence of this feature in another.

Pathology

The findings in several autopsies have been reported* and material from aborted fetuses, premature infants, young adults, and older adults has

*References 200, 323, 326, 327, 567, 807, and 910.

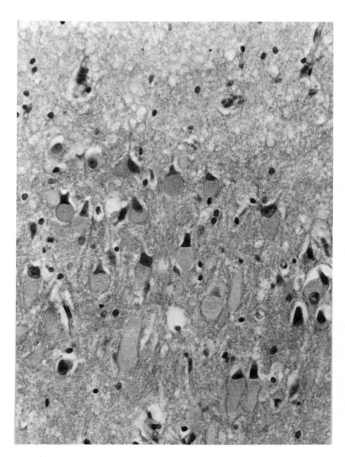

Fig. 11-43. Sanfilippo syndrome. The temporal cortex shows distended neurons, dendrites, and axons containing storage materials (hematoxylin-eosin stain, magnification × 200). (From Tamagawa K et al: *Brain Dev* 7:599-609, 1985.)

been examined at macroscopic, light microscopic, electron microscopic and histochemical levels.

Enlargement of the liver, spleen, kidney, and endocrine glands has been observed. Haust[323] reported the presence of a basically normal heart; conversely, slight or moderate hypertrophy of one or both ventricles has been noted, with thickening and nodularity of the bicuspid and tricuspid valves. Atrophy of skeletal muscle is probably secondary to central nervous system deficits.

In the eye of a female with Sanfilippo syndrome, type A, Del Monte et al.[200] observed extensive intracellular accumulation of glycosaminoglycan in cells of the cornea, iris, lens, sclera, and retina (in ganglia cells and optic nerve cells). Similar findings were noted in a 17-year-old boy with Sanfilippo syndrome, type B. It was concluded that accumulation of glycosaminoglycan resulted in degeneration of photoreceptors.

The brain is usually reduced in size, with cortical atrophy. Dekaban and Patton[197] detailed the changes in the brain of an affected girl who died at the age of 4 years. Layers II and IV of the cerebral cortex were more severely affected than layers III and V, and the authors suggested that a relationship exists between this feature and the early, severe mental deterioration concommitant with relatively good preservation of motor function that characterizes MPS type III.

The presence of lipidlike storage material has been detected in nervous tissue by use of lipid-specific dyes.[323] Tamagawa et al.[807] noted abundant vacuolation and distention of neurons and neural processes throughout the nervous system (Fig. 11-43), and Wisniewski observed a similar distention in the pyramidal cells of the temporal cortex (Fig. 11-44). Lipid inclusions were found not only inside vacuoles of cell bodies but also in the proximal

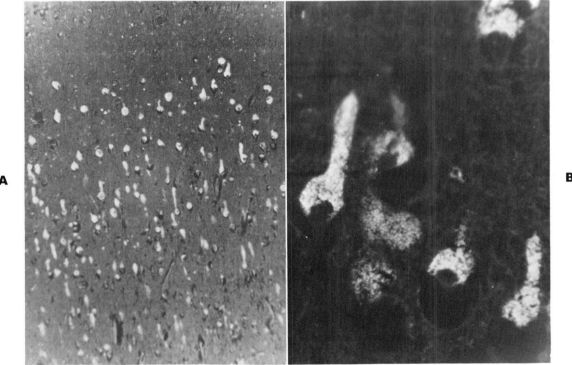

Fig. 11-44. Sanfilippo syndrome. Light microscopic appearance of the cerebral cortex showing a mild to moderate loss of nerve cells with glial cell replacement. **A,** In the temporal isocortex, pyramidal neurons of layers II-IV showed autofluorescent perikaryal granular material (UV 360 nm, magnification × 157). **B,** Pyramidal neurons have distended contours and fusiform enlargement of the initial portions of their axons. Note negative eccentric nuclear contour (ultraviolet 400 nm, magnification × 100). (From Wisniewski KE: *Ann NY Acad Sci* 477:285-311, 1986.)

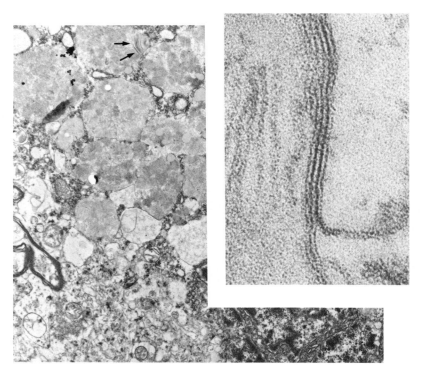

Fig. 11-45. Sanfilippo syndrome. On electron microscopy neurons of the cerebral cortex at necropsy show fused cytoplasmic inclusions whose content appears almost homogeneous. Only on close inspection do some seem to consist of stacks of fine membranes. In a few areas these are reminiscent of the zebra bodies *(arrows)* (magnification × 3000). The inset shows similar areas of membranous arrangements at higher power with the periodicity of 5.9 nm typical of zebra bodies (magnification × 335,000). (From Haust MD et al: *Am J Med Genet* 22:1-27, 1985.)

portions of axons. Loss of nerve cells and a marked decrease in stellate cells were present in the brain of a 36-year-old patient with the Sanfilippo syndrome. Stellate cells may play a part in higher brain function, and their reduction in Sanfilippo syndrome may be related to the marked impairment in brain function that is characteristic of the disease. Tamagawa et al.[807] found brain lesions to be particularly apparent in the thalamus and suggested that they were the result of a primary derangement rather than secondary damage resulting from the storage disorder.

Microscopic examinations conducted during the autopsies of several adults revealed the presence of abundant vacuoles with metachromatically staining inclusions in cells taken from virtually all organs.[327] Greenwood observed metachromatic inclusions in liver tissue at autopsy of a third-trimester fetus with Sanfilippo syndrome, type A, but no inclusions of any kind were found in nervous tissue. Cultured fibroblasts from an aborted fetus were found to stain metachromatically with the use of alcian blue.[567]

Numerous electron-lucent vacuoles have been observed in ultrastructural studies of visceral organ cells taken from patients with Sanfilippo syndrome during biopsy. A finely distributed granu-

loreticular material, presumably remnants of glycosaminoglycan, was present inside the vacuoles. Because glycosaminoglycans are extremely water soluble, special methods must be used for their preservation.[323]

Haust et al.[327] examined the ultrastructure of hepatocytes, white blood cells, precursor cells in bone marrow, and cells in nervous system tissue obtained by means of biopsy from a patient with Sanfilippo syndrome. The same cells were restudied in specimens taken at autopsy 7 years later. Remarkable changes had occurred. The hepatocytes from the biopsy specimen were extremely vacuolated and contained abundant glycosaminoglycan, but hepatocytes from the autopsy were mostly collapsed and showed little glycosaminoglycan accumulation. The leukocytes during the initial study also had numerous vacuoles and a large amount of stored glycosaminoglycan, whereas at autopsy they contained no stored glycosaminoglycan. Tamagawa et al.[807] also observed empty vacuoles in liver, spleen, white blood cells, and endothelial cells at the time of autopsy.

Inclusions found in nervous tissue are different on ultrastructural study from inclusions in visceral organ cells. By electron microscopy, neurons were shown to contain lipid cytosomes similar

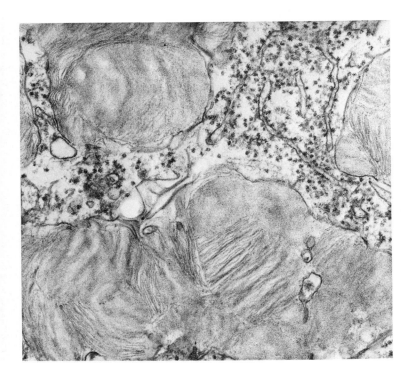

Fig. 11-46. Sanfilippo syndrome. Rectal biopsy specimen reveals a neuron in the myenteric plexus containing inclusions with membranous organization typical of zebra bodies, explaining, perhaps, intermittent soft stool and diarrhea in children with Sanfilippo syndrome.

to those in Tay-Sachs disease; these bodies had alkaline phosphatase activity, which indicated a lysosomal origin. In nerve tissue, vacuoles may contain electron-dense material that has lipidlike characteristics. Also, gangliosides may be stored in the nervous system as membranous material arranged in stacks and termed "zebra bodies" (Fig. 11-45) or as concentric membranous whorls known as membranous cytoplasmic bodies (MCBs) (Fig. 11-46).

Fundamental Defect

The sulfated glycosaminoglycan heparan sulfate is normally degraded from the nonreducing end by the sequential action of several lysosomal enzymes (Fig. 11-47). Defects of four enzymes are associated with Sanfilippo syndrome, and each type (A, B, C, and D) of the syndrome is caused by the deficiency of a different enzyme.

Undegraded heparan sulfate accumulates inside the lysosomes in various tissues and is excreted in urine. This accumulation is presumed to be the primary cause of mental retardation and skeletal deformities, although secondary accumulation of gangliosides has been postulated to be neurotoxic.

Early cross-correction studies in fibroblasts indicated the existence of two clinically indistinguishable forms of heparan-sulfate–excreting MPS that were arbitrarily designated Sanfilippo

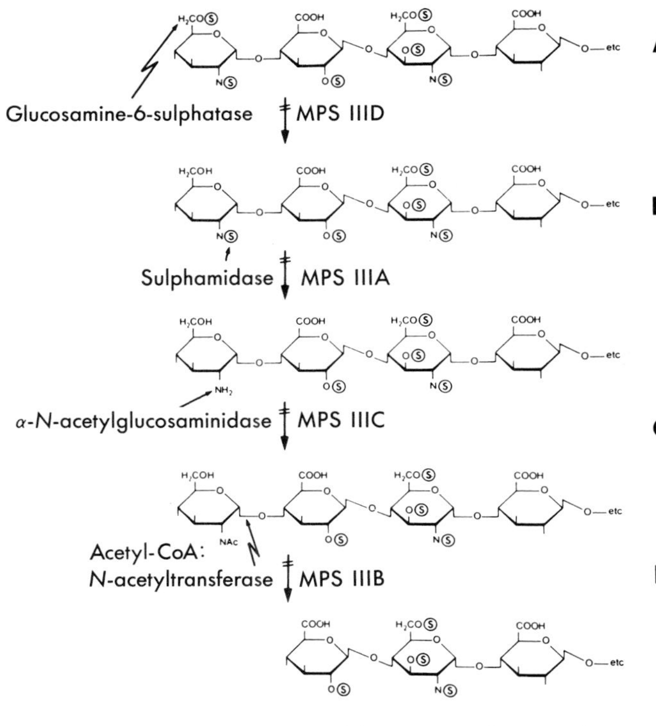

Fig. 11-47. The degradation of heparan sulfate and enzymatic defects responsible for Sanfilippo syndrome are illustrated. **A,** N-acetylglucosamine-6-sulphate sulphatase; **B,** sulfamidase; **C,** α-N-acetylglucosaminidase; **D,** acetyl-CoA:α-glucosaminide N-acetyltransferase.

syndrome, types A and B. The enzyme deficient in Sanfilippo syndrome, type A is heparan sulfate sulfatase (2-deoxyglucoside-2-sulfamate sulfatase).[456-458,532] Because this enzyme removes sulfate groups linked to the amino group of glucosamine, it is also referred to as heparan N-sulfatase or, more commonly, sulfamidase. Deficiency of the enzyme α-N-acetylglucosaminidase results in Sanfilippo syndrome, type B.[618,868,869]

In 1975 and 1976 patients with clinical stigmata of Sanfilippo syndrome but with normal levels of sulfamidase and α-N-acetylglucosaminidase were documented.[54] It was subsequently discovered that this form of the syndrome was caused by deficiency of an enzyme that catalyzed transfer of an acetyl group from acetyl-CoA to the amino group that was desulfated by sulfamidase. This third enzyme is acetyl-CoA:α-glucosaminide N-acetyltransferase, and the third disorder was designated Sanfilippo syndrome, type C.

In 1980 Kresse et al.[459] reported on the biochemical defect in two patients with Sanfilippo syndrome resulting from a new, fourth enzymatic defect. This entity, Sanfilippo syndrome, type D, results from deficiency of the enzyme N-acetylglucosamine 6-sulfate sulfatase, which normally releases inorganic sulfate from heparan sulfate. These patients were found to have normal enzymatic activity against keratan sulfate fragments bearing the same residue, thus arguing against the existence of a new disorder, MPS type VIII, postulated to result from defective 6-sulfatase–sharing of heparan and keratan sulfate substrates. The metabolic blocks in degradation of heparan sulfate are illustrated in Fig. 11-47.

There appears to be no correlation between the measured activity of the enzyme N-acetylglucosamine-6-sulfate sulfatase in cultured skin fibroblasts and the severity of the phenotypic manifestations. For example, five children with equivalent enzyme activity exhibited great variation in the progress and severity of clinical involvement. It was also postulated that the enzyme activity measured in skin fibroblasts may not be a true reflection of the activity in other organs and that significant differences of activity in tissues might explain the variable rate of progression of the disease in different individuals.

Various mechanisms have been proposed to explain the interfamilial variability in the clinical expression of Sanfilippo syndrome. It is possible that there is an allelic mutation of the gene coding for the same lysosomal enzyme or that mutations in the mild and severe cases reside in different genes, each coding for a different subunit of the enzyme. It is also possible that the interfamilial variation could arise from differences in other regions of the genome (epistasis) or in environmental influences. Andria et al.[22] suggested that three mutant alleles might account for the different degrees of severity in children with Sanfilippo syndrome. They also considered the possibility of mosaicism in which the enzyme may be present in some cells and tissues but not in others.

Prevalence and Inheritance

Each of the four types of Sanfilippo syndrome is inherited as an autosomal recessive trait, and males and females are affected with about equal frequency. The parents are invariably normal, and some instances of consanguinity have been documented.[525,781]

Sanfilippo syndrome ranks among the most common of the mucopolysaccharidoses,[295] although current estimates of frequency are even less reliable than in MPS types I and II. Some patients are probably not recognized as having the Sanfilippo syndrome because of the relatively inconspicuous somatic features. The condition may occur appreciably more often than in 1 of 100,000 to 200,000 individuals as suggested by Terry and Linker,[821] and as frequently as 1 in 24,000 to 47,000 as estimated by van de Kamp.[849]

From the existing data it appears that types A and B are more frequent than the others and that type A is more common than type B.[70] In 1981 Vance et al.[848] tested 360 presumed-normal controls for N-acetylglucosamine-6-sulfate sulfatase activity and found that one tested in the heterozygote range, which would mean that the population frequency of Sanfilippo syndrome type B carriers is 1 in 360. Type A is the most common form in Great Britain, Canada, Australia, and Germany,[831] and type B is the most frequent type diagnosed in Greece.[70] Type B is also found in Japan. Type C is more rare than type A or B but has been reported in patients of Dutch, Greek, and German ancestry[54] as well as in patients in Japan,[632] Sweden,[845] Algeria,[755] South Africa,[664] and Turkey.[845] The few reported persons with type D have their origins in Italy or have been of Italian descent.[162,271,415]

Management

Many problems that occur in the other mucopolysaccharoidoses are not an issue in the Sanfilippo syndrome. Specifically, carpal tunnel syndrome, corneal clouding, hydrocephalus, and airway obstruction have not been reported. Recurrent otitis media and respiratory tract infections occur and are managed in a conventional manner. Skeletal changes in Sanfilippo syndrome are minimal and do not require medical intervention.

Central nervous system disease is the major clinical problem to be confronted. Of the central nervous system manifestations, seizures are uncommon and are responsive to conventional medications. Because good bodily strength is combined with severe mental defect, management of affected persons is often difficult.[604] Drug therapy was of little help in managing the aggressive behavior of seven adult patients with Sanfilippo syndrome, type B.[861] In a survey of the attitudes and experiences of 30 parents of children with Sanfilippo syndrome, Nidiffer and Kelly found that slightly over one third claimed that their child's hyperactivity, aggression, and destructive tendencies could be controlled using behavioral techniques.[604] About 20% of the parents reported that the same problems were resolved or partially resolved by use of drug management. Some of the suggestions made with regard to managing the child with Sanfilippo syndrome are the following: (1) obtain the most appropriate special education placement; (2) physically modify the home environment to provide a safe place for the child to play without moment-to-moment supervision; (3) identify and utilize professional and community resources such as the MPS Society for information exchange and emotional support; and (4) of primary importance, secure available respite care opportunities.

In the terminal stages patients who are bedridden may benefit from the use of a wheelchair for transportation, physical therapy to maintain joint mobility, and muscle relaxants for painful spasms. A gastrostomy may be necessary to maintain adequate nutrition. Prospective planning of management of medical emergencies and written orders regarding resuscitation may be useful.

MUCOPOLYSACCHARIDOSIS TYPE IV (MORQUIO SYNDROME, KERATAN SULFATURIA)

The Morquio group of disorders shares significant growth failure with the other mucopolysaccharoidoses but differs in that the joints are lax rather than rigid. The facial features are relatively fine, there is no significant organomegaly, and the intellect remains unimpaired. The Morquio syndromes are also distinguished by a unique glycosaminoglycanuria, namely, the excretion of excessive keratan sulfate. Currently two biochemically distinct forms of the Morquio syndrome are well recognized: Morquio syndrome, type A (galactosamine 6-sulfatase deficiency) and Morquio syndrome, type B (β-galactosidase deficiency). A third condition, Morquio syndrome, type C, has been suggested, although no enzymatic defect has yet been identified.[58]

Clinical Manifestations

General features. Affected children are dwarfed, with a barrel chest, "pigeon breast," and a short neck (Fig. 11-48). Clinical abnormalities are not evident at birth, and psychomotor development is normal in the first year, although changes may be detectable on radiographs at that time.[707] In infancy the lumbar spine may show beaking similar to that in the Hurler syndrome; nevertheless, MPS type IV is difficult to distinguish at this stage by any means except the urinary pattern of glycosaminoglycan excretion. Later, the changes evident on radiographs in MPS type IV differ from those of MPS type I, flat vertebrae being particularly characteristic of the former condition.

In the second or third year of life awkward gait, retarded growth, knock-knees, sternal bulging, flaring of the rib cage, flat feet, prominent joints, dorsal kyphosis, or some combination of these anomalies usually brings the child to medical attention. With advancing age all these abnormalities are exaggerated, and in older children the skeletal changes are quite distinctive. Growth slows remarkably, and patients with MPS type IV are strikingly short in stature, achieving a maximum height of 85 to 100 cm, usually by 7 or 8 years of age.

Although early observations suggested that patients with Morquio syndrome, type A might have more severe disease than do patients with type B, continued observation has indicated that a range of severity exists both within and between these entities. Based on study of the phenotype in 12 patients with type A, Nelson et al.[825] proposed the division of this condition into three groups: the severe "classical" type, an intermediate type, and a mild type, all resulting from deficiency of N-acetylgalactosamine-6-sulfatase activity. According to these investigators, the level of residual activity may be an important prognostic indicator.

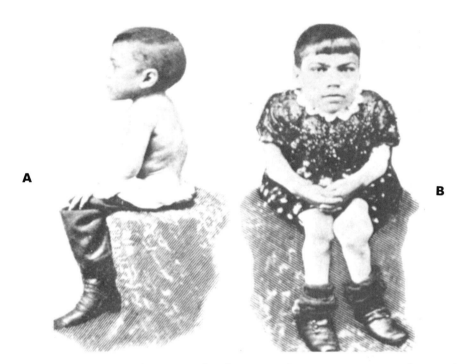

Fig. 11-48. Morquio syndrome in a brother, **A,** and sister, **B,** in a French-Canadian family reported by Osler in 1897. (From Osler W: *Trans Cong Am Phys* 4:169, 1897.)

Head and neck. In contrast to the other mucopolysaccharidoses, the facies in the Morquio syndrome are usually fine; characteristics typically include a broad mouth, prominent maxilla, short nose, and widely spaced teeth (Fig. 11-49). The neck is short, and neurologic complications frequently result from spinal cord and medullary compression.

Dental changes in children with MPS type IVA are distinctive and may serve to distinguish such individuals from persons with the other forms of the Morquio syndrome (Fig. 11-50).[267,268,484,596,751] Garn and Hurme[268] described abnormality of both the deciduous and the permanent teeth in three affected sibs. The changes consisted of thinness of enamel, shown by radiographs, a tendency for the enamel to fracture and flake, and a dull, grayish appearance of the crowns of the teeth. The molars are sharp, with pointed cusps. Because of the thin enamel, the teeth are vulnerable to caries, a feature noted by Brailsford[102] in his 4-year-old patient. Persons with Morquio syndrome, type B have normal enamel, a clinical finding that may be useful in distinguishing type A from type B disease. Although the abnormal morphologic appearance of the tooth is highly specific for type A, it is quite variable and in some instances demonstrable only on radiographs.[596]

Ocular features. The corneas become diffusely opacified,[862,870] but this process progresses slowly and clouding is usually not evident to the unaided eye until after the age of 10 years. Grossly the corneal clouding has the appearance of a filmy haze rather than that of ground glass as seen in MPS types I and VI.

As in the other mucopolysaccharidoses, glaucoma has been observed in Morquio syndrome[123] and is presumed to be related to accumulation of glycosaminoglycan in the trabecular meshwork of the intraocular drainage system.[386] Retinal involvement has also been reported.[183]

Nervous system. Although persons with MPS type IVA usually have normal intelligence,[59] changes may be seen on CT with increasing patient age.[595] These abnormalities have included white matter of low density and gross dilation of the ventricles, the basal cisterns, and the subarachnoid space. Progressive mental regression

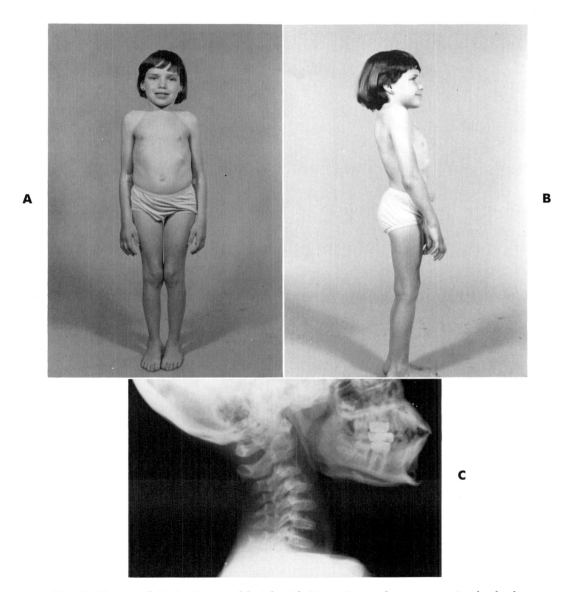

Fig. 11-49. A and **B,** An 8-year-old girl with Morquio syndrome, type A who had a history of progressively diminished exercise tolerance and generalized weakness. At the time of examination she was so weak at the end of the day that she had to crawl on hands and knees to go up stairs. **C,** Lateral view of the cervical spine shows platyspondyly of the cervical vertebrae. Odontoid hypoplasia, in combination with ligamentous laxity, resulted in intermittent trauma to the cord and irreversible damage that accounts for the patient's symptoms.

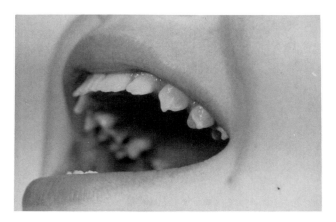

Fig. 11-50. Morquio syndrome. The deciduous and permanent teeth have dull, gray crowns with pitted enamel that tends to flake off, giving the appearance of hypoplastic teeth. The anomaly is characteristic of type A disease but not of type B and has been proposed as a means to distinguish the two disorders.

has been observed in two patients with MPS type IVB.[285]

Neurologic symptoms often result from spinal cord and medullary compression.[597] Spastic paraplegia is frequent, and respiratory paralysis occurs in the late stages.[19] High spinal cord compression related to ligamentous laxity and hypoplasia of the odontoid is a major complication of the Morquio syndrome,[91,226,342,477,497] and five of six affected adults reported by Langer and Carey[477] had long-tract signs referable to an abnormality at the upper cervical area. Ligamentous laxity comparable to that evident at the wrists contributes to the spinal cord compression. A usual history is that by 7 or 8 years of age the child manifests decreasing physical endurance and increasing difficulty in walking up stairs and through snow. He or she may complain that the legs tend to "buckle." Severe genu valgum is often blamed for the disability, but osteotomies for leg straightening fail to relieve the symptoms. As pointed out by Kopits,[553] the level of physical endurance is one of the best indications of the state of the atlantoaxial region. Odontoid aplasia or marked hypoplasia is probably present in all persons with MPS type IV, and the majority sooner or later develop serious spinal cord compression from atlantoaxial subluxation.

Progressive perceptive deafness usually has its onset in the teens and is present in almost all patients who survive to the third decade of life or later. Mixed or sensorineural hearing loss may also occur.[721]

Respiratory and cardiac systems. Cardiac involvement is a well-recognized component of the Morquio syndrome, and aortic valve incompetence is frequent.[556] There is a high prevalence of silent cardiac abnormalities in patients with predominantly left-sided valve involvement. Aortic regurgitation has been reported.[632] Echocardiographic evaluation of 10 persons with type A disease[398] detected abnormalities in six persons, with mitral valve involvement in five and aortic valve changes in four. One patient had severe mitral leaflet thickening to the point of mitral stenosis, and two others had echocardiographic evidence of ventricular hypertrophy. All these lesions were of little hemodynamic significance in these relatively young patients (median age, 12.5 years), but the long-term significance of cardiac abnormalities remains incompletely defined.

Cardiorespiratory embarassment results from a combination of thoracic deformity, spinal malalignment, and aortic incompetence. Respiratory paralysis resulting from cervical cord and medullary compression occurs in the late stages.[19]

Skeletal system. The stance is often semicrouching, and knock-knees are usual. The wrists are enlarged and the hands are misshapen. Some joints, notably, the wrists, may be hyperextensible.

A characteristic radiographic feature of MPS type IV is universal platyspondyly with kyphoscoliosis and thoracic deformity.[59] In the early stages the thoracic vertebrae are ovoid. Growth in height of the vertebrae is slow between the ages of 2 and 6 years, and an anterior projection, or tongue, develops during this stage. In the adult the vertebral bodies are flattened and rectangular, with wide disk spaces, and the odontoid process is hypoplastic or absent. Flaring of the ilia is particularly striking because of narrowing above the acetabula. In the early years the femoral capital epiphyses are normal but progressive flattening and fragmentation, with coxa valga, eventually develop. In the adolescent and adult the femoral heads may disappear, resulting in erosion and widening of the femoral necks. The carpal centers are small and retarded in development. The distal ends of the radius and ulna are inclined toward

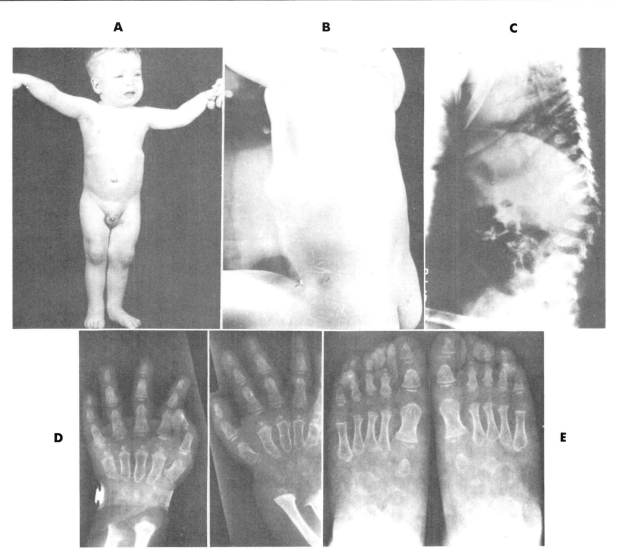

A   B   C

D   E

Fig. 11-51. **A,** The general appearance of a 21-month-old boy with Morquio syndrome (see text, below). **B,** Lumbar gibbus and flared lower ribs are demonstrated. **C,** Lateral view of the spine, showing hypoplastic lumbar vertebrae similar to those seen in Hurler syndrome. **D,** Anteroposterior radiographic views of the hand, showing proximally conical metacarpals. The ulnar and radial growth plates are dysplastic, and that of the ulna is angled toward the radius. **E,** Feet with features analogous to those of the bones of the hands.

each other, and the metaphyses are wide and irregular. The long bones are short and undertubulated, especially in the upper limbs. Spatulate ribs, a bulging sternum, and dorsal kyphosis are also evident on radiographs.

Integument. The skin is loose, thickened, tough, and inelastic, particularly over the limbs, and telangiectasia may be present, especially on the face and limbs.[297]

CASE REPORT

The boy (Fig. 11-51) is the only child of parents who are not known to be related. No similarly affected persons are known in the family of either parent.

The child was first investigated at the age of 21 months because of skeletal abnormalities, which had first been noted at the age of 4 months: flaring of the lower rib cage and a lump on the lumbar spine. Mental and physical development had otherwise been normal. He stood with support at 8 months of age, walked at 17 months, and spoke two-word sentences at 19 months. At the age of 6 weeks he had been hospitalized for two weeks with vomiting, jaundice, and mild enlargement of the liver. Neonatal hepatitis was diagnosed. A right hydrocele was found at that time.

Main features of the examination at the age of 21 months are shown (Fig. 11-51). The flaring of the lower ribs and the lumbar gibbus are striking. The hands are stubby and less extensive than would be expected for a child of this age. The liver was palpated 3 cm below the right costal margin, the tip of the spleen was palpable, and a small umbilical hernia and a hydrocele on the right side were present. The child initially was thought to have the Hurler syndrome.

The following significant investigations were made. Slit-lamp examination revealed fine, gray stippling of the corneal stroma bilaterally, most markedly in the periphery. Radiographs showed a gibbus at the first lumbar vertebral level, a slight reduction in height of the vertebral bodies, and an anteroinferior lipping of the lumbar vertebral bodies. The metacarpals and phalanges showed swelling of the shafts, with distal tapering. Carpal ossification was delayed, and the bones were small and severely misshapen. The metacarpals and phalanges were short and wide, with relatively normal constriction in their diaphyses. Coxa valga was present. No lymphocyte inclusions were found in the peripheral blood; however, the cytoplasm of approximately 50% of the polymorphonuclear leukocytes contained clusters of small, clearly defined metachromatic granules.

On study of the urine, 92.7 mg/L of glycosaminoglycan was recovered, most of it being keratan sulfate. A second study made 2 months after the first yielded similar results. The result of the cetyltrimethylammonium bromide screening test 1 was strongly positive.

CASE REPORT

The patients shown in Fig. 11-52 were 5 and 15 years of age at the time of study. Five sibs were normal. Another sib, an infant boy, died 33 hours after birth. He may have been affected with the Morquio syndrome. The father and mother were of English and English-Irish ancestry, respectively, and were not known to be related.

The elder brother had clubbed feet at birth. The diagnosis of Morquio syndrome was made at the age of 13 months. In the younger brother the diagnosis was made at birth because his facial appearance resembled that of his brother and because motion at the elbows was limited. An inguinal hernia was repaired at the age of 14 months in the younger brother.

A diffuse corneal haze was noted when the elder brother, then 8 years old, was first seen by an ophthalmologist. Examination 4 years later showed little change.

The findings of the physical and radiographic examinations are well shown in Fig. 11-52. Intelligence was normal. The elder brother (15 years old) had lax wrists,

the murmur of aortic regurgitation, and diffuse, grayish clouding of the cornea bilaterally. Slit-lamp examination showed the corneal changes to be primarily in the posterior stroma and to be uniformly distributed.

The 5-year-old brother had slight but definite clouding of the cornea, demonstrable only by slit-lamp examination. A granular appearance of the fundus in the macular area was observed. Urine from the younger brother contained 60 to 70 mg/L of keratan sulfate. Examination of peripheral blood smears from both boys revealed no lymphocytic metachromatic granules, but the majority of the polymorphonuclear leukocytes showed varying numbers of small clusters of clearly defined metachromatic granules within the cytoplasm (i.e., Reilly granulation).

The younger brother died unexpectedly in his sleep at the age of 7 years. The elder brother died at the age of 21 years, after being confined to a wheelchair for several years because of tetraparesis.

CASE REPORT

A 33-year-old woman who was born in 1938, was one of the oldest patients with Morquio syndrome known to McKusick (Fig. 11-53). Because increased glycosaminoglycan excretion is often not identifiable in adults with Morquio syndrome, the diagnosis in this patient was based on clinical grounds.

There was no history of a similar disorder in the family, and the parents were not related. A brother and two sisters were normal. At birth the patient weighed 9 pounds and measured 51 cm in length. Development was considered normal until the age of 2 years, when she fell from a hayloft. Thereafter her growth was limited. At the age of 7 years surgical procedures for leg straightening were performed. By 20 years of age, the corneas were noted to be grossly cloudy. Hearing began to fail when she was in her twenties. At 30 years of age a hearing aid was fitted, with good results. She wore complete dentures from the age of 22 years. Examination revealed markedly short stature (height, 86 cm) with kyphoscoliosis, short neck, protruding sternum, hyperextensible and unstable joints, mild hirsutism, and long-tract signs in both arms and legs, presumed related to the demonstrable aplasia of the odontoid process and cervical (C1-2) vertebral laxity. The poor stability at the wrists made it difficult for her to continue the handiwork that was her main pasttime. Casts applied to the wrists greatly improved hand function, and surgical fusion of the wrists was considered but not performed. Breast development was normal. (Menses occurred at the age of 15 years.) Intelligence was apparently normal.

Tests indicated bilateral neurosensory hearing loss.

Radiographic studies showed severe genu valgum; dislocation of both hips, with no femoral heads; short, broad, eburnated femoral necks; marked, generalized platyspondyly; and characteristic deformity of the ribs, sternum, and hands.

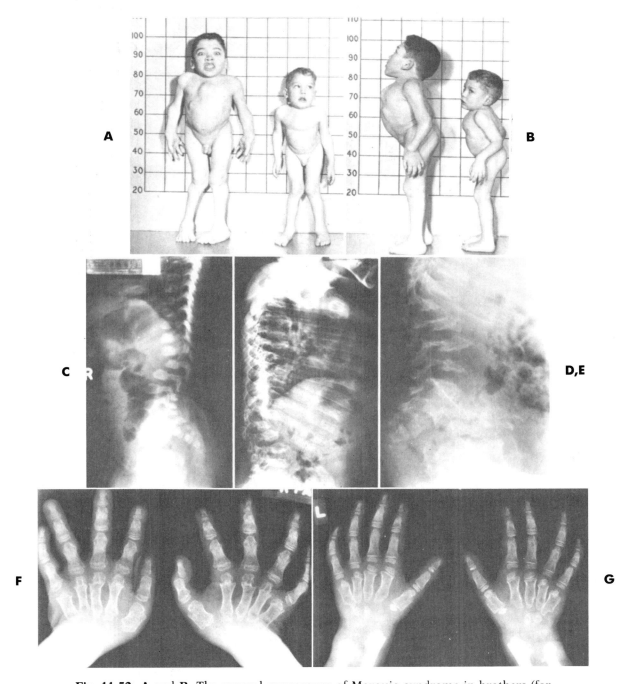

Fig. 11-52. **A** and **B,** The general appearance of Morquio syndrome in brothers (for case reports, see text). **C** to **E,** Spine at the ages of 13 months 8 years and 15 years, respectively. The early changes are indistinguishable from those of Hurler syndrome. Marked osteoporosis and platyspondyly are later developments. **F** and **G,** Hands at 15 years of age, **F,** and at 5 years of age, **G.** Osteoporosis and abnormal shapes of all bones are demonstrated. Carpal bones ossify late and are small and severely misshapen. The shafts of the metacarpals and phalanges are relatively normally constructed. *Continued.*

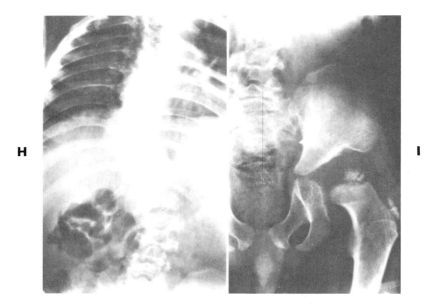

Fig. 11-52, cont'd. H, Spinal curvature at 5 years of age. **I,** Left hip at 5 years of age. (From McKusick VA et al: *Medicine* 44:445, 1965.)

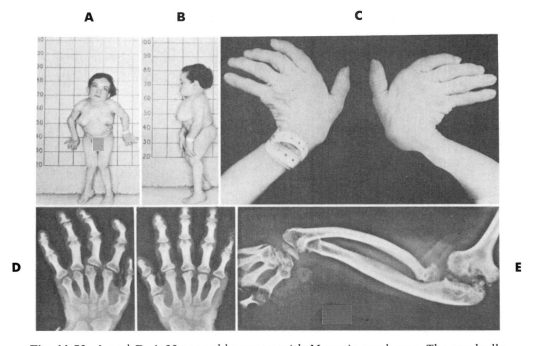

Fig. 11-53. A and **B,** A 33-year-old woman with Morquio syndrome. The markedly short stature and skeletal deformities, which are typical, are evident. **C,** Marked ulnar deviation of the hands related to instability of the wrists. **D,** Radiographic views of the hands and wrists show relatively short ulnas, which contribute to the ulnar deviation; fingers are subluxated at the metacarpophalangeal joints. **E,** Radiographic view of the right forearm, showing marked bowing of the radius and many loose osseous bodies in the region of the elbow.

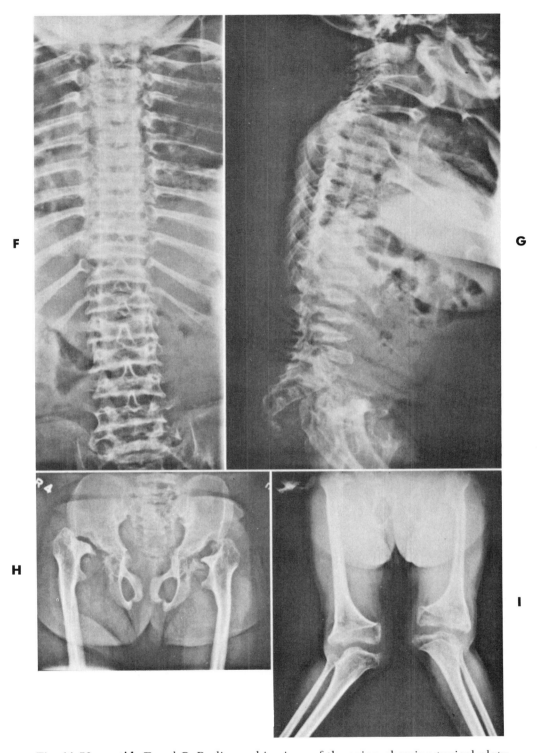

Fig. 11-53, cont'd. F and **G,** Radiographic views of the spine, showing typical platyspondyly in severe form. **H,** No femoral heads can be identified, although the largest of the loose bodies in the region of the left acetabulum may be a remnant. The hips are dislocated. The constriction above the acetabulum is typical of Morquio syndrome. **I,** Marked genu valgum is present.

Prognosis. Before the era of specific management for Morquio syndrome, most patients died before the age of 20 years. In part the deaths were due to cardiorespiratory failure precipitated by respiratory infection. Many died suddenly in their sleep, however, possibly as a result of acute atlantoaxial subluxation. Respiratory arrest during induction of surgical anesthesia may have the same basis, and manipulation of the head for intubation can be dangerous. Surgical fusion of the upper cervical spine (see the section on management) is a life-prolonging measure in this disorder.[597]

Although the prognosis in MPS type IV was generally considered "poor" or "guarded," McKusick drew attention to the potential for prolonged survival by recording seven affected women and an affected man who were 21 years of age or older.[553] One remarkable woman had two children (both of whom, at ages 8 and 7 years, were appreciably taller than their mother). The potential for relatively mild disease with prolonged survival in persons with MPS type IVA and persons with MPS type IVB was subsequently documented.[58]

It has been proposed that affected females fare better than males. It was once speculated that because females may pursue a less active life-style, they were at less risk for the complications of atlantoaxial subluxation.[553] The better prognosis in girls and women was borne out by two affected brother-sister pairs. In each pair the brother was dead, whereas the sister was living at an age well beyond that at which the brother had died. It is notable that the original patient reported by Morquio was a male and was still surviving at age 55 years.[553]

Pathology

Autopsy findings have been reported by Einhorn, Moore, and Rountree,[225] and bone biopsy findings have been documented by several workers.[8,19,540,541,749] Zellweger, Giaccai, and Firzli[937] found Reilly granules in the leukocytes of their patients. These granules, however, may be absent in early stages.[731]

Tondeur and Loeb[830] studied the ultrastructure of the liver in two affected children. The Kupffer cells contained membrane-bound inclusions, whereas fewer, smaller inclusions were found in hepatic cells. Bona, Stanescu, and Ionescu[94] studied the histologic appearance of cartilage, and Schenk and Haggerty[731] demonstrated accumulation of glycosaminoglycan in chondrocytes.

In the eye of a patient with MPS type IVA variable degrees of glycosaminoglycan deposition were present, primarily in the structures of the anterior segment.[386] Transmission electron microscopy demonstrated fibrogranular and multimembranous membrane-bound inclusions in the cornea and trabecular meshwork, to lesser extent in the conjunctiva and sclera, and sparsely in the retinal pigment epithelium.

Tissue from the epiphyseal plate of patients with MPS type IVA, which was studied by means of histochemical and ultrastructural techniques, showed various degrees of vacuolation.[541,749] The normal, orderly proliferating structure of the epiphyseal plate was absent, and calcification was markedly reduced. The morphologic appearance of related bone tissue was normal, although quantity was reduced.

Persons with the Morquio syndrome excrete excessive amounts of keratan sulfate in the urine.[49,520,523,656,787] In normal children keratan sulfate excretion is also relatively high but falls to low levels after 20 years of age. (The excretion of uronic acid containing glycosaminoglycan is also increased somewhat in persons with MPS type IV. This increase may not be unexpected, since keratan sulfate is part of the same protein complex as chondroitin-6-sulfate and may be excreted as such.[413]) Keratan sulfate precipitates with cetyltrimethylammonium bromide (CTAB), thus giving a positive result by this method. Keratan sulfate is more difficult to quantitate than the uronic acid containing glycosaminoglycans, which can be measured specifically by analysis of microsamples for constituent monosaccharide units. For keratan sulfate, isolation on a preparative scale is necessary.[414,495]

The occurrence of abnormally thin dental enamel in MPS type IV[268] may not be surprising in view of the observation, on the basis of staining with toluidine blue and alcian blue, that the enamel matrix is relatively rich in glycosaminoglycans.[419] Islocki and Sognnaes[909] demonstrated toluidine blue metachromasia in the developing enamel. Some of the metachromasia remained after hyaluronidase digestion, suggesting the presence of some highly sulfated glycosaminoglycans.

Metachromatic granules in fibroblasts of patients with the Morquio syndrome were simultaneously and independently discovered by Fraccaro et al.[249] and by Danes and Bearn.[175] Magrini et al.[509] showed a strict parallelism between S^{35} labeling and metachromasia. They further suggested the existence of heterogeneity in the Morquio syndrome on the basis of two affected sisters whose fibroblasts showed negative results by the previously mentioned criteria, despite visceral involvement and excess keratan sulfate in the urine.

Robins, Stevens, and Linker[707] concluded that one group of patients with the Morquio syndrome phenotype excrete, during childhood at least, excessive amounts of chondroitin-4-sulfate in the urine. The clinical characterization of this group will be important in establishing clinical and pathologic correlations in the disorder.

Fundamental Defect

The common biochemical feature that distinguishes Morquio syndrome from other mucopolysaccharidoses and underlies the phenotype is ineffective keratan sulfate catabolism. Pathologic accumulation of keratan sulfate and oligosaccharides[565] thus appears to cause the pathophysiologic features of this condition, which primarily involves the ocular, cardiac, and skeletal tissues.

McKusick's speculation that there were allelic forms of MPS type IV has proved to be correct.[553] MPS type IVA disease results from defective lysosomal galactosamine 6-sulfate sulfatase, that is, galactose 6-sulfatase.[536,768]

The defect in MPS type IVB is deficient β-galactosidase enzymatic activity.[24,300,779,851] Interestingly, a similar abnormality is present in patients with G_{M1}-gangliosidosis. Somatic cell hybridization studies have shown that complementation does not occur between G_{M1}-gangliosidosis and MPS type IVB cell strains; this observation suggested that mutations for these conditions are allelic. Nevertheless, cultured fibroblasts from patients[598] with MPS type IVB exhibited catabolism of G_{M1}-ganglioside comparable with that of controls. Fibroblasts from different types of galactosialidosis (the autosomal recessive disorder associated with a coexistent β-galactosidase and neuraminidase deficiency) all showed degradation of ingested G_{M1}-ganglioside. There are animal models for disorders in this category. In particular, interspecific complementation studies using somatic-cell hybrids constructed from patients with MPS type IVB showed that a disease in sheep results from a mutation of the β-galactosidase gene.[10]

Prevalence and Inheritance

All forms of Morquio syndrome are inherited as autosomal recessive traits. The condition has been recognized in consanguineous families and has occurred in a Hutterite kindred found to have a high inbreeding coefficient.[504] Morquio's original report[573] described four affected sibs of Swedish stock whose normal parents were first cousins. The frequency of the Morquio syndrome is unknown, but in clinical practice it is certainly far less common than the Hurler and Hunter syndromes. No particular geographic or ethnic predeliction has been recorded.[240]

Management

Spinal cord compression. Spinal cord compression as a result of atlantoaxial subluxation at the craniovertebral junction is a major cause of disability and death in the patients. Surgical fusion of the upper cervical spine, as developed by Kopits and Steingass[451] and Kopits et al.,[452] can be lifesaving and is indicated in most patients. Decompression by resection of the spinal lamellae is not beneficial because the compression is anterior; indeed, this procedure may be harmful. A special "halo" brace fixation is used for immobilization before, during, and after surgery. One group has suggested that the conventional posterior approach to occipitocervical fusion is unsafe because of significant anterior compression and has proposed a combined anterior transoral decompression with posterior fusion to deal with this difficult problem.[30]

Genu valgum. Growth ceases at the age of 7 or 8 years. For this reason alignment osteotomies of the lower limbs performed after this age do not need to be repeated. Kopits and Robinson[891] have performed bilateral varus osteotomies of the tibias and posterior fusion of the first and second cervical vertebrae during a single hospitalization. An instance of osteogenic sarcoma of the femur associated with steel staples used in fixation of an osteotomy site has been noted.[749]

Wrists. The instability of the wrists is a serious impediment to use of the hands. Special wrist splints have been used with some success.

Antibiotic prophylaxis. Prophylaxis for bacterial endocarditis has been advised for those persons with structural cardiac abnormalities,[398] but it would be reasonable for this regime to be extended to all patients with MPS type IV, since some have cardiac lesions that remain undiagnosed.

Systemic therapy. Experiments in vitro have shown that cDNA for human β-galactosidase is expressed in COS-1 cells and that a precursor form of the enzyme, excreted into the culture media, is taken up and normally processed by cultured fibroblasts from patients with MPS type IVB.[635] These observations may form a basis for the ultimate development of a method for therapy. Amniotic tissue transplantation has been accomplished but without convincing clinical benefit.[838] A small number of patients with Morquio syndrome have received treatment by means of bone marrow transplantation[419]; it is too early to comment on the clinical response.

MUCOPOLYSACCHARIDOSIS TYPE VI (MAROTEAUX-LAMY SYNDROME, POLYDYSTROPHIC DWARFISM)

Mucopolysaccharidosis type VI was first delineated on clinical and chemical grounds by Maroteaux and Lamy and their colleagues.[521,526] It is characterized by clinical features that resemble those of Hurler syndrome, including extreme short stature, but is distinguished from the other mucopolysaccharidoses, except MPS types I S and IV, by retention of normal intelligence and by a preponderant urinary excretion of dermatan sulfate. The greater severity of the skeletal changes (dysostosis multiplex) and of the other somatic features together with the more limited survivorship in MPS type VI distinguish it from MPS type I S.

Clinical Manifestations

General features. Growth retardation is first noted at the age of 2 or 3 years. Stunting of both the trunk and the limbs is usually present, together with genu valgum, lumbar kyphosis, and anterior sternal protrusion (Fig. 11-54). Although the facial features are not as striking as in Hurler syndrome, they suggest that the patient's condition falls into the general category of the mucopolysaccharidoses. Articular movements are progressively restricted, and the carpal tunnel syndrome contributes to the hand abnormality. In some affected persons[782] the subcutaneous tissues of the volar surface of the fingers are thickened, as in Dupuytren contracture. Some patients have

A   **B**   **C**

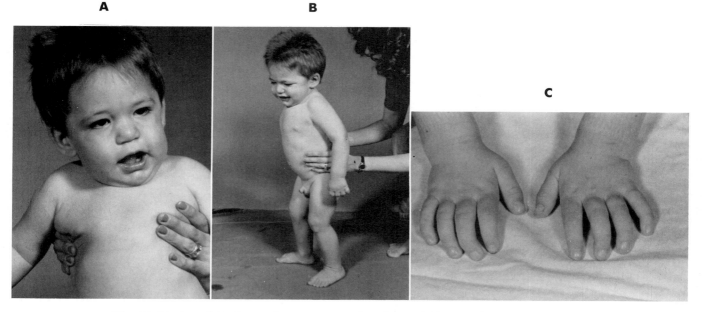

Fig. 11-54. A and **B**, General appearance of a 2-year-old boy with Maroteaux-Lamy syndrome. Early development was normal (Bayley Scales of Infant Development, 113 at 2 years 3 months of age). **C**, Hands show slight shortening of the fingers. Despite normal intellectual development, cranial CT scan showed changes typical of the mucopolysaccharidoses. The possibility of multiple sulfatase deficiency was considered but excluded on the basis of lack of ichthyosis and normal levels of activity of other sulfatase enzymes.

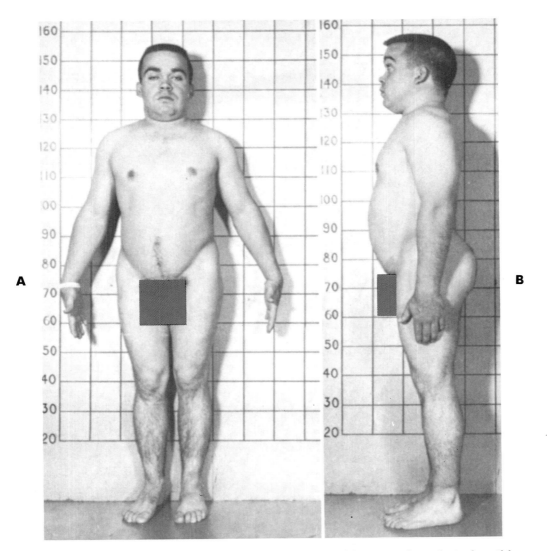

Fig. 11-55. A and **B,** General appearance of a 30-year-old man with a relatively mild form of Maroteaux-Lamy syndrome. The patient was treated for bilateral Legg-Perthes disease when he was between 8 and 12 years of age. Bilateral inguinal hernias were repaired at 20 years of age. Mild stiffness of the hands and corneal clouding were first noted at the age of about 20 years. A grade 3 to 4 systolic ejection murmur was heard at its loudest at the left sternal border. He was of normal intelligence and worked as an automotive mechanic. Leukocytes showed striking metachromatic inclusions. He completed high school. At the age of 30 years he was short (155 cm in height, as compared with heights of more than 180 cm in several of his six sibs) and had mild joint stiffness and carpal tunnel syndrome.   *Continued.*

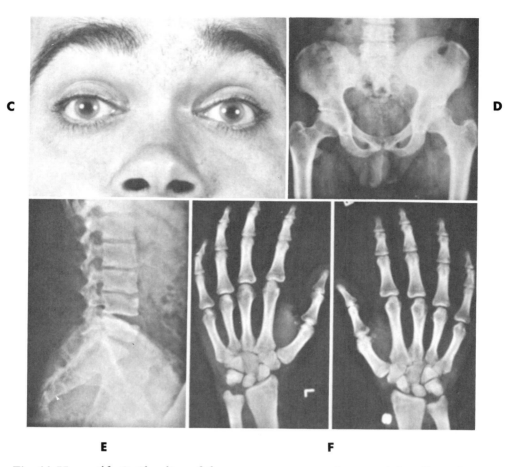

Fig. 11-55, cont'd. C, Clouding of the corneas was most dense peripherally and posteriorly. (Neither pigmentary changes in the retina nor night blindness was present.) **D,** Radiologic changes in the pelvis consisted of shallow acetabulae with femoral heads of about normal size extending beyond the acetabular margins. The left femoral head was flattened, with irregular ossification. **E,** Generalized platyspondyly with decreased width of the vertebral disks, sparing the cervical spine. **F,** Carpal bones, especially the proximal row, were somewhat smaller than average. The metacarpal and phalangeal bones appeared normal. Contractures of the digits appeared to be related to soft tissue changes.

come to medical attention as supposed examples of bilateral Perthes disease.[782] There is a spectrum of mild[209,648] to severe disease.[702] Although patients are occasionally of normal height,[722] most have severe short stature.

Head and neck. The skull is often severely involved and cannot be distinguished from that in MPS type I. In some affected persons, however, the facial appearance and skull involvement are much milder (Fig. 11-55). Dentigerous cysts are seen,[703] analogous to those of the Hurler and Hunter syndromes.

Nervous system. The major neurologic complications are hydrocephalus[293] and spastic paraplegia resulting from compressive myelopathy.[43, 686] Mental retardation is rare.[809,863] Deafness, which is present in some patients, may be due in part to recurrent otitis media. Carpal tunnel syndrome may occur in childhood or later (Fig. 11-56).

Ocular features. Corneal opacities develop fairly early. The cornea is increased in thickness, especially at its periphery, where clouding is most dense (Fig. 11-55, *C*). Glaucoma is a significant

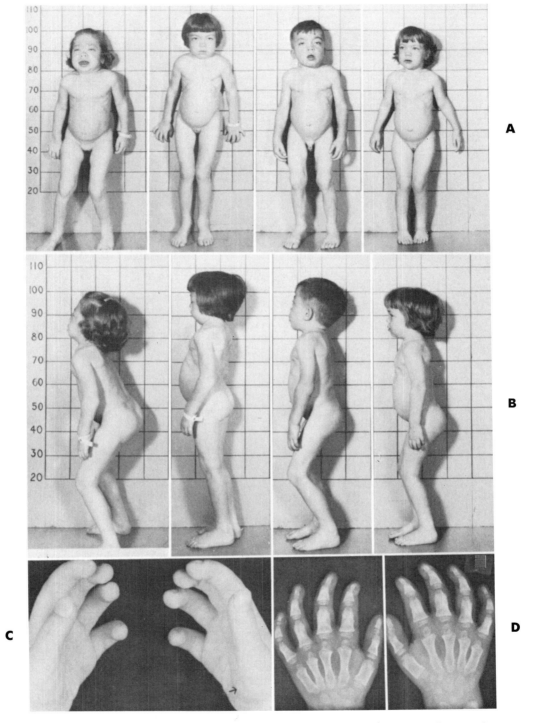

Fig. 11-56. A and **B,** Four siblings with Maroteaux-Lamy syndrome. **C,** Contraction hand deformity in a child with Maroteaux-Lamy syndrome, with atrophy of the abductor pollicis brevis muscle *(arrow)* indicative of compression of the median nerve in the carpal tunnel. **D,** Radiographic views of the hands show skeletal features of dysostosis multiplex: short, bullet-shaped phalanges and wide metacarpals with coarse trabeculation and proximal narrowing.

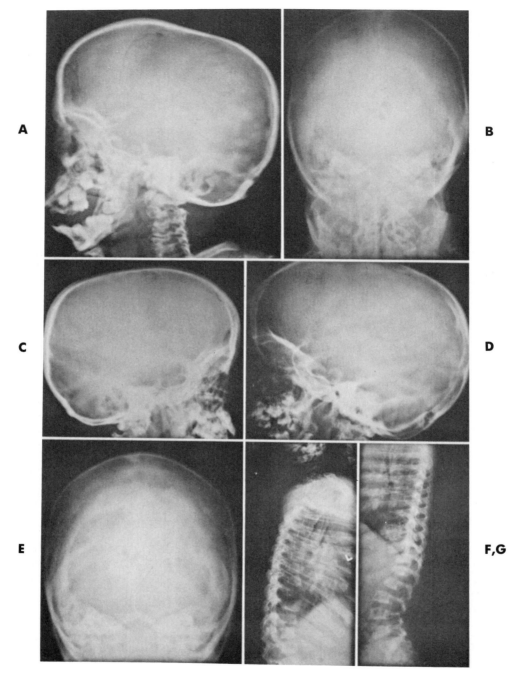

Fig. 11-57. Radiographic features of Maroteaux-Lamy syndrome. **A** to **E**, Representative skull views of children, ages 6 to 8 years (shown in Fig. 11-56), show dolichocephaly, suggesting that the sagittal suture closed first. In all four sibs large, irregular occipital radiolucencies are demonstrated. The radiolucencies may be caused by deposits of glycosaminoglycan within the calvaria or by large emissary vessels. In each child the tuberculum sellae turcicae is eroded and the chiasmatic sulcus greatly enlarged, presumably because of an adjacent dural or arachnoid cyst. **F,** Lateral spine views of a 10-year-old show that the two lowest thoracic vertebrae are shorter than the others and mildly recessed. **G,** Spine in a 9-year-old shows changes that are more severe than those evident in **F.** Vertebral bodies T12 and L1 are short and recessed, with the resulting gibbus. The lumbar pedicles are long.

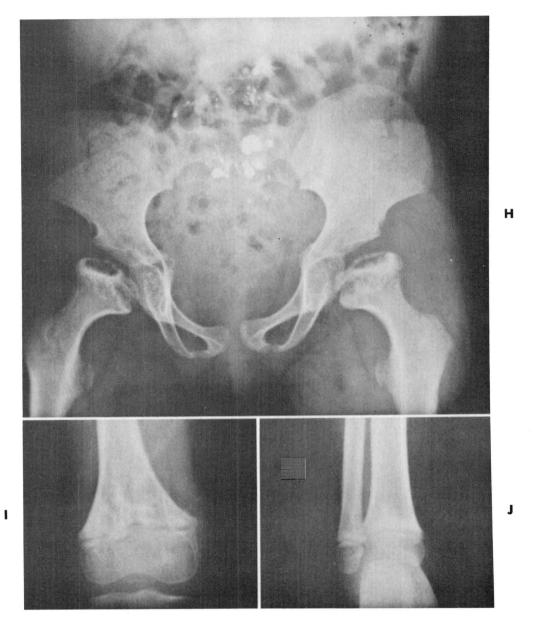

Fig. 11-57, cont'd. H, Pelvis and hip radiograph of a 10-year-old shows flat femoral capital epiphyses with large, cystlike radiolucencies and surrounding sclerosis. The femoral necks are narrow. The acetabulae are shallow, with oblique roofs. **I,** and **J,** The distal femur and tibia show irregular longitudinal radiolucent and radiodense bands with minimal metaphyseal cupping.

clinical problem,[128] and pigmented retinopathy has been described.

Cardiovascular system. Serious cardiac abnormality with murmurs and echocardiographic findings indicative of valvular involvement develop in adolescence and adulthood. The clinical characteristics (except for the later onset of heart failure) and the pathogenetic mechanisms are analogous to those in MPS type I. Endomyocardial fibroelastosis may be an early complication in MPS type VI. In 1987 Fong et al.[245] reported on two sibs, less than a year of age, who each came to medical attention with a dilated cardiomyopathy but without other physical findings of MPS type VI; the diagnosis was subsequently confirmed by means of biochemical studies. Autopsy in one patient revealed endocardial fibroelastosis, and electron microscopy of fibroblasts in the myocardium showed distention with membrane-bound vacuoles consistent with an MPS. Endocardial fibroelastosis developed in these sibs before other clinical manifestations of the Maroteaux-Lamy syndrome. Myocardial biopsy specimens show infiltration by foamy macrophages with lamellar bodies typical of MPS disease.[329]

Skeletal system. Growth is severely retarded and in many patients virtually ceases after the age of 7 or 8 years. The ultimate height ranges from 107 to 138 cm, a point of differentiation from the Scheie syndrome, in which height is usually greater than 144 cm.

The radiographic osseous abnormality in MPS type VI is quite variable in severity (Fig. 11-57), rivaling that in MPS type I in the most severely affected patients. The diaphyses of the long bones, however, are usually less expanded than in MPS type I, and there is also a characteristic localized constriction of metaphyses. This constriction is particularly striking in the neck of the humerus, where it combines with marked varus deformity to give the upper humerus a hatchetlike appearance. At the elbows and wrists the epiphyses and metaphyses may be quite irregular. The proximal one third of the humerus is usually bowed anteriorly. The radius and ulna may also be bowed, and their distal surfaces usually slope toward each other. Although the tibial shaft may be expanded, the femur is usually normally or excessively constricted. As in all the mucopolysaccharidoses, the long bones below the hips are less affected than those in the upper limbs.[302]

The odontoid process is hypoplastic. In some patients the vertebral bodies show little change, but in most the superior and inferior margins are convex, whereas the anterior and posterior margins are concave. Hypoplasia and beaking of the first and second lumbar vertebrae are common. Although these vertebra are usually recessed, little or no gibbus results.

Narrowing of the vertebral ends of the ribs may extend considerably farther laterally than in MPS type I H, so the ribs have the shape more of canoe paddles than of oars. The medial thirds of the clavicles are expanded, and their internal portions are relatively narrow and bowed superiorly, with pointed ends that are directed inferiorly at the shoulders. The scapulae are small and high, with hypoplastic glenoid fossae.

Changes in the pelvis are striking. The iliac wings flare above constricted bodies, and the acetabulae are small, with oblique roofs. Ossification of the femoral head is irregular in most patients, leading to a misdiagnosis of bilateral Perthes disease in some. The femoral necks tend to be long, excessively constricted, and turned outward.

The degree of involvement of the short bones of the hands and feet is variable. These bones may be almost unaffected, but more commonly the ends of the shafts are widened and the metacarpal bases pointed. When the diaphyses are constricted, the appearance is suggestive of MPS type IV. In some affected persons the shafts are more expanded than the ends, and a distinction from MPS type I H may be impossible.

Abdomen and viscera. The liver is consistently enlarged in patients over the age of 6 years, and the spleen is enlarged in about 50% of affected persons. Inguinal hernias often require surgical repair in the first years of life. Frequent episodes of diarrhea have necessitated hospitalization in some instances.

Prognosis. A patient reported by Spranger et al.[782] died at 25 years of age of progressive heart failure, but few other cases have been reported in the literature. In the author's experience death in late childhood or early adult life is usual, often during or after surgical procedures that are complicated by cardiopulmonary disease.

Pathology

Of the six major mucopolysaccharidoses, cytoplasmic inclusions are most striking in MPS type VI[485]; with proper staining and search, coarse and fine granulations can be found in 90% to 100% of granulocytes and in up to 50% of lymphocytes.[177]

Accumulation of glycosaminoglycans occurs in all corneal layers,[681,799] in fibrous tissue, in chondrocytes, and in ganglion cells of the central nervous system.[425] In a case in which compressive cervical myelopathy contributed to the patient's demise, the vertebral canal was reduced to a slit-like space caused by massive thickening of the soft tissues and dislocation of the posterior arch of the atlas.[425]

The atrioventricular valves of the heart are thickened, and the endocardium and bundle of His may be fibrotic.[425] Autopsy in one of two sibs who came to medical attention with dilated cardiomyopathy at less than 1 year of age showed endocardial fibroelastosis.[245] Myocardial fibroblasts were distended with membrane-bound vacuoles.

Fundamental Defect

The increased urinary excretion of glycosaminoglycan is two to fifteen times greater than normal. Dermatan sulfate accounts for 70% to 95% of the excreted glycosaminoglycan, and the remainder has the characteristics of heparan sulfate.

Neufeld found that the fibroblasts from affected children were distinguishable on biochemical study from those in patients with Hurler syndrome, although the abnormality in cells from patients with Maroteaux-Lamy syndrome was only marginally corrected by secretions from other cell lines. Correction did occur in the MPS type VI cells with a factor that is present in urine and is different and separable from all the other correction factors. The enzymatic defect was subsequently determined to be deficiency of N-acetylgalactosamine-4-sulfatase[53] (also known as arylsulfatase B). There is no direct relationship between the level of 4-sulfatase activity in patient samples and the observed severity of clinical phenotype,[113,139,201,365] although patients accumulate dermatan sulfate at levels that approximately correlate to clinical phenotype.[358]

In normal fibroblasts a precursor of 66 kd is rapidly processed intracellularly within 6 hours to a polypeptide of 57 kd composed of disulfphide-linked polypeptides of 43 kd and 8 kd.[811] All fibroblast lines obtained from patients with MPS type VI, who exhibited characteristics ranging from a minor stigmata to the severe classic phenotype, incorporated radioactivity into immune-purified 4-sulfatase at a rate 10% less than that of normal fibroblasts. Maturation of the residual 4-sulfatase variously showed features that may be indicative of delay in intracellular transport, decreased intracellular stability, failure of lysosomal targeting, or resistance to enzyme processing. Development of a sensitive monoclonal antibody-based immunoquantification assay[112] and study of cultured skin fibroblasts from enzyme-deficient subjects[113] have led to speculation that as little as 5% of normal catalytic capacity may be sufficient to prevent accumulation of glycosaminoglycan and manifestation of the Maroteaux-Lamy phenotype. Thus the prospects for enzyme-replacement therapy and gene therapy would seem good, if this amount of enzyme can be achieved in each cell.

Animal models. Genetic deficiency of 4-sulfatase has been studied extensively in cats.* In these animals, this enzymatic defect produces a phenotype which is quite analogous to the human Maroteaux-Lamy syndrome. These cats have been used experimentally to assess metabolic correction and clinical outcome after bone marrow transplantation.[358] (see below).

Prevalence and Inheritance

The Maroteaux-Lamy syndrome is comparatively rare, and there are no good estimates of the frequency of occurrence. It is clear that inheritance is autosomal recessive, since sibships with two or more affected members have been reported several times.[82,90,668,840] The parents have always been normal, and they were consanguineous in several instances.[82,90] The condition has been principally documented in persons of European stock, but it has also been encountered in Vietnamese[316] and German-Acadian "Cajuns."[90] The gene has been localized to the short arm of chromosome 5, bands 11 to 13 (5p11-13).[242]

On clinical grounds Spranger et al.[782] and others[684] raised the question of heterogeneity in the Maroteaux-Lamy syndrome. The major discriminant is the severity of changes evident on radiographs, especially in the bones of the hand. How-

---

*References 17, 318, 319, 397, 545, 795, and 796.

ever, some affected individuals also have central nervous system disease. Undoubtedly the range of phenotypes will be explained by relatively "mild" and relatively "severe" alleles, together with the existence of compound heterozygotes. In this context it is noteworthy that a number of individuals now thought to represent Hurler-Scheie phenotype were initially considered to have MPS type VI.

Management

Corneal dystrophy. Progressive opacification of the cornea as a result of accumulation of heparan sulfate causes significant visual impairment; this problem has been successfully treated by means of keratoplasty.[743,799] Rosen et al.[709] performed penetrating keratoplasty on two patients with an MPS. Since these persons were 13 and 15 years of age at the time of report and one was specifically described as having normal intelligence, the disorder may have been MPS type VI. The transplants remained clear for 3 and 2 years, respectively, after operation, but the older patient remained blind, seemingly because of underlying optic atrophy. Lahdensuu[470] noted opacification of corneal transplants in one of four sibs who were labeled "Pfaundler-Hurlerschen Krankheit" but, as noted earlier, more likely had MPS type I S or MPS type VI. Keratoplasty is accepted as a successful procedure in the management of Maroteaux-Lamy syndrome.[517,591] Recurrence of glycosaminoglycan accumulation in the corneal epithelium and adjacent tissues has been reported. This may indicate that corneal grafts have a limited duration of clarity in some patients and suggests that repeat transplantation may sometimes be required.[743]

Glaucoma. Glaucoma has been increasingly noted as a significant clinical problem in MPS type VI. Standard peripheral iridectomy is inadequate for treatment of this complication because of the considerably increased thickness of the peripheral cornea that occurs in these patients.[128]

Compressive cervical myelopathy. Progressive accumulation of glycosaminoglycan in the dura of the cervical spinal cord is a major cause of morbidity and mortality.* This process may initially be-

---

*References 420, 665, 668, 808, 873, and 931.

come evident on clinical examination with long-tract signs, notably, clonus, but progresses to lower-extremity weakness and then to disabling paraplegia or quadriplegia. To monitor this complication it would be reasonable to initiate regular neurologic examination and imaging studies as soon as the diagnosis is established. Spinal CT with intrathecal metrizamide injection[808] has been used to characterize such lesions, but somatosensory evoked potentials and MRI are now superior methods for evaluating this problem. Early decompression can be beneficial for patients with significant spinal cord compression.

Hydrocephalus. Hydrocephalus is a relatively rare complication of Maroteaux-Lamy syndrome and can be treated with ventriculoperitoneal shunting.[685,686]

Congestive heart failure. Cardiac and respiratory impairment may result in congestive heart failure.[81,686] Conventional medical and surgical treatment, including tracheostomy and valve replacement, are usually helpful but ultimately are limited by progression of the underlying lesions.

Systemic treatment. Bone marrow transplantation has been performed in the treatment of Maroteaux-Lamy syndrome and resulted in decreased inclusions in liver and likely contributed to improved cardiopulmonary function.[462,546] The human N-acetylgalactosamine-4-sulfatase cDNA has been subcloned into a retroviral construct that included an internal thymidine kinase promotor.[663] When packaged through an amphotropic cell line and used to infect fibroblasts from a patient with Maroteaux-Lamy syndrome, cells produced enzyme activity up to 36 times higher than that in fibroblasts from normal individuals.

MUCOPOLYSACCHARIDOSIS TYPE VII (SLY SYNDROME, β-GLUCURONIDASE DEFICIENCY)

Mucopolysaccharidosis type VII, resulting from β-glucuronidase deficiency, was first described by Sly et al.[774] in 1973. Since then, a broad spectrum of clinical variability has been documented. Deficiency of lysosomal β-glucuronidase activity in all tissues results in the inability to degrade the glycosaminoglycans containing β-linked glucuronic acid residues: dermatan sulfate, heparan sulfate, and chondroitin sulfate. The basic defect of this disorder, its mode of inheritance, and the approach to potential therapy were discovered at a time when only one case was known, a record probably matched only by oroticaciduria. Recently β-glucuronidase deficiency became one of the first conditions to be completely corrected by means of gene transfer in an animal model.[465]

Clinical Manifestations

General features. The clinical picture of Sly syndrome spans a broad phenotypic spectrum, but in general the condition is characterized by greater or lesser degrees of short stature, hepatosplenomegaly, progressive dysostosis multiplex, and intellectual impairment. Since the original description was given, approximately two dozen cases have been reported.* These have been categorized into three forms based on clinical criteria[76,182,756] ranging from severely affected (neonatal type) to moderately affected (infantile type) to mildly affected (juvenile type). The clinical variability may be the result of allelic mutations of a single β-glucuronidase gene; this situation is analogous to the range of mild and severe forms of MPS type I disorders, that is, Hurler, Hurler-Scheie, and Scheie syndromes.

Neonatal form. The neonatal type presents as non-immune hydrops fetalis and thus can be diagnosed at birth (Fig. 11-58).* Hepatomegaly, ascites, and hyperbilirubinemia are suggestive of fulminant liver disease and affected infants usually die in the neonatal period.

Infantile form. The infantile type, represented by the original case of Sly et al.,[774] has physical features and a clinical course which are similar to those of the Hurler syndrome (Fig. 11-59). The main manifestations are short stature, hepatosplenomegaly, progressive skeletal abnormalities in the thorax and spine, and mental retardation,

---

*References 56, 132, 178, 250, 274, 283, 286, 307, 311, 371, 480, 503, 511, 516, 572, 592, 667, 756, 774, 822, and 916.

---

*References 56, 132, 178, 383, 592, and 905.

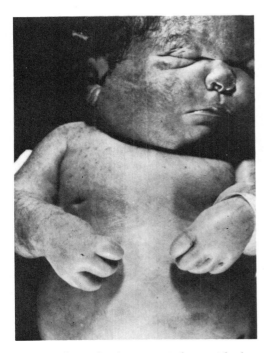

Fig. 11-58. Hydrops fetalis in an infant with the neonatal-lethal form of Sly syndrome. (From Irani D et al: *Ann Neurol* 14:486-490, 1983.)

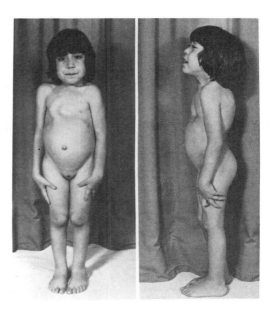

Fig. 11-59. A 6-year-old girl with an intermediate form of Sly syndrome showing mild facial features, a protuberent abdomen, and kyphoscoliosos. (From Sewell AC et al: *Clin Genet* 21:366-373, 1982.)

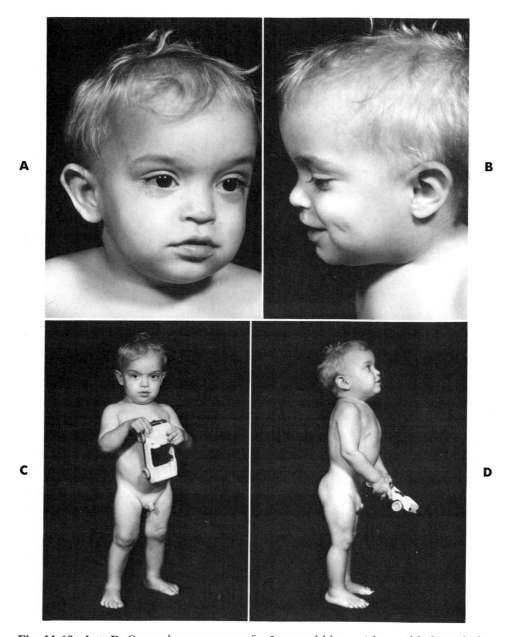

Fig. 11-60. A to **D,** General appearance of a 2-year-old boy with a mild clinical phenotype, which probably represents the juvenile-onset form of Sly syndrome. The patient was diagnosed fortuitously during the newborn period when persistent jaundice led to examination of the bone marrow; toluidine blue stain demonstrated large metachromatic inclusions.

which is marked especially by speech delay.[274,307,774]

Juvenile form. The juvenile form usually presents during adolescence (Fig. 11-60)[56,178,282] with mild kyphosis or scoliosis. However, despite this spinal malalignment, dysostosis multiplex is not radiographically evident.

Head and neck. In the neonatal form, and to some extent in the infantile form, there are moderate Hurler-like facial characteristics with macrocephaly, hypertelorism, depressed nasal bridge, and anteverted nostrils. The corneas appear cloudy in the neonatal form, but are relatively clear in the infantile and juvenile forms.

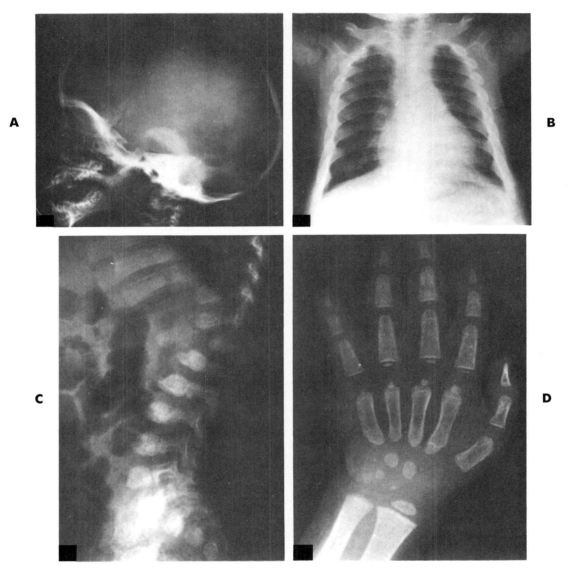

Fig. 11-61. Radiographic features of a boy with Sly syndrome showing mild dysostosis multiplex. **A,** A lateral skull radiograph made of the patient at 1 year of age shows macrocephaly with a J-shaped sella, hypoplastic odontoid, and fused saggital suture. **B,** Chest radiograph shows expansion of the medial portions of the ribs and clavicles. **C,** The thoracolumbar spine is slightly kyphotic as a result of hypoplasia of the T12 and adjacent vertebral bodies. **D,** At age 2 years the bones of the hand are slightly osteopenic, and metacarpals are wide, with proximal narrowing. (From Sly WS et al: *J Pediatr* 82:249-257, 1973.)

Nervous system. Swelling of the optic nerve head, which may precede the development of optic atrophy, has been observed.[154] Hydrocephalus with ventriculomegaly and increased spinal fluid pressure has been documented.[371]

Cardiorespiratory system. The neonatal form is characterized by severe respiratory complications, which are due, to a considerable extent, to the hydropic condition. Recurrent respiratory infections, including pneumonia, are also common in the infantile form,[774] but persons with the juvenile form do not have pulmonary complications.

Skeletal system. In the infantile form, short stature becomes apparent in the second year of life, the height falling below the third percentile. The head is large, with frontal prominence and premature closure of the sagittal and lambdoidal sutures. Pectus excavatum or carinatum and thoracolumbar gibbus, already present in infancy, increase with age. Progressive joint contractures are typical of the infantile form. Metatarsus varus was reported in the original case[774] and is common. Atlantoaxial instability has been reported.[669] Skeletal involvement is minimal in the juvenile form, and spinal malalignment is the only frequent feature.

In the neonatal and infantile forms radiographs reveal moderately severe changes of dysostosis multiplex (Fig. 11-61) with premature closure of cranial sutures. Odontoid hypoplasia and a J-shaped sella are other features. The ribs are wide, especially in their midportions, and there are hooklike protuberances on the lower portions of the ilia. The humeri are shortened and show medullary expansion in their proximal portions. The radii and ulnae are also somewhat expanded, and the capital femoral epiphyses are dysplastic. There is shortening of the tubular bones of the hands and feet, with proximal pointing of the metacarpals.

In contrast to the neonatal and infantile forms, there is little or no dysostosis multiplex in the juvenile form.[140]

Abdomen and viscera. Moderate hepatosplenomegaly is usually present in all forms of MPS type VII. The neonatal form has a clinical course suggesting fulminant liver failure, and prolonged neonatal jaundice has been observed in several pa-tients. Edema and ascites may also be present. The mechanism of their production is not known, but it has been suggested that congestive heart failure and the presence of storage material in the hepatic sinusoidal reticuloendothelial cells, together with hypoproteinemia related to liver disease, may be involved.[383]

Despite progressive enlargement, liver and spleen function are generally normal in the infantile and juvenile forms. Visceral enlargement has the secondary consequence of diminishing the size of the chest cavity and may compromise the respiratory system. Inguinal and umbilical hernias are common.

Prognosis. The neonatal form of Sly syndrome usually becomes evident as nonimmune hydrops fetalis[383] with ascites, hepatosplenomegaly, and dysostosis multiplex. Affected children do not survive more than a few months.

In addition to the neonatal presentation, other patients have a more mild phenotype of developmental delay or degeneration,[877] mild sensorineural hearing deficit, and mild skeletal abnormalities. These individuals survive into adolescence, and ultimate longevity is unknown. The oldest known affected individual has survived to 34 years of age. He has mild mental retardation and epileptic seizures but few other somatic problems.[76] Although the temptation exists to regard "mild" and "severe" forms as distinct entities, experience with other mucopolysaccharidoses indicates that a range of clinical phenotypes in a single disorder should be expected.

Pathology

Patients with Sly syndrome have pathologic findings that are characteristic of the mucopolysaccharidoses,[905] notably, coarse metachromatic inclusions in peripheral granulocytes and granulocyte precursors in the bone marrow.[311] On ultrastructural study clear vacuoles and granular inclusions are evident in nearly all granulocytes and mononuclear cells[516]; this key feature can provide an important clue to the correct diagnosis (Fig. 11-62). Although they are a dramatic and useful laboratory sign, no known functional hematologic problem is associated with these leukocyte granulations. Analogous staining of abnormal inclusions can be observed in cultured skin fibroblasts.[911]

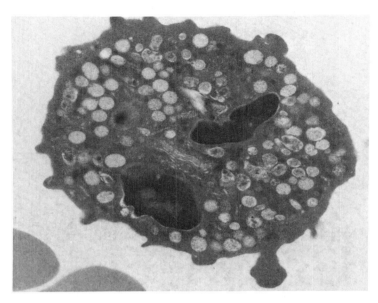

Fig. 11-62. Granulocyte from a patient with Sly syndrome, with vacuoles containing light-floccular material (magnification × 9900). (From Bernsen PLJA et al: *J Neurol Neurosurg Psychiatry* 50:699-703, 1987.)

Fundamental Defect

Molecular defect. Mammalian β-glucuronidase is a tetrameric glycoprotein composed of identical subunits. The human gene has been mapped to 7q21.1-q22.[250,880]

Cloning and characterization of the human β-glucuronidase gene has been reported.[13,635] The workers isolated a cosmid clone containing GUSB, the human gene encoding β-glucuronidase. The 21-kb gene contains 12 exons ranging from 85 to 376 bp in length. Comparison of the human gene organization with that reported for the murine β-glucuronidase gene revealed several similarities. In fact, the substantial similarity of the translated portion of the β-glucuronidase mRNA sequence from humans, rats, mice, and *Escherichia coli* indicates that the genes encoding these products are derived from a common ancestral gene.[310,570,605,741]

Mutations causing β-glucuronidase deficiency have been identified.[828,829] In a 6-year-old girl, sequencing of the full-length mutated cDNA revealed a cytosine-to-thymidine transition, a mutation causing an alanine-to-valine amino acid substitution. (The authors designated this variant βG$_{Gifu}$.) This change is detected by loss of the cleavage site for the enzyme Fnu4HI in the mutant cDNA. On the basis of the loss of Fnu4HI restric-tion site, the patient was shown to be a homozygote with the βG$_{Gifu}$ mutation, whereas her parents and brother were heterozygotes. This mutation disrupts a highly conserved functional domain and obliterates catalytic activity.

Animal models. Relative deficiency of β-glucuronidase is known in mice. In 1950 Morrow and colleagues identified a line of C3H mice with only 5% to 10% as much enzyme in the liver as other mouse lines. In the hands of Paigen[638,639] and others this enzyme system has been useful in elucidating many aspects of mammalian biochemical genetics. These include the genetics of enzyme realization (the set of processes acting to produce the final phenotypic characteristics of the enzyme, such as catalytic properties, intracellular localization, tissue distribution, regulation of synthesis, and breakdown). Deficiency of the enzyme produces few obviously pathologic consequences in the C3H mouse; for this reason interpretation of experimental bone marrow transplantation results was somewhat limited.[348]

Birkenmeier et al.[85] and Volger et al.[866] have evaluated a line of mice found at Bar Harbor, Maine, which represent a close model of the human disease. In particular, the mice have a generalized deficiency of β-glucuronidase enzyme activity and progressive accumulation of glycosaminoglycan, with the phenotypic features of skeletal abnormalities and a shortened lifespan. The availability of this murine model has facilitated important studies, which have revealed that bone marrow transplantation results in significant correction of the phenotype.[86] This positive result is surpassed only by the complete prevention of abnormalities by means of embryonic transfection of the normal human gene by means of microinjection of retrovirus gene constructs.[465]

A model of human MPS type VII in a dog has been studied extensively by Haskins et al.[321] The affected animals have had extensive skeletal disease, generalized hepatomegaly, thickening of the atrioventricular heart valves, and generalized polyarthropathy. The activity of lysosomal β-glucuronidase was reduced to less than 2% of the normal mean value of unaffected controls.

A characterization of the defective β-glucuronidase activity in canine MPS type VII[741] revealed that only 22% of the residual β-glucuronidase activity in canine MPS type VII liver was membrane associated, compared with 65% of the total activity in a control group. In contrast, the thermostability, cryostability, and pH stability properties, as well as the pH optimum (4.6), were essentially unaffected. In addition, the canine MPS type VII hepatic residual activity was unresponsive to sulfhydryl-reducing reagents and divalent cations, although incubation of normal canine β-glucuronidase with dithiothreitol and magnesium or calcium, or both, enhanced the enzymatic activity more than 15-fold.

Prevalence and Inheritance

Mucopolysaccharidosis type VII is one of the rarest of the mucopolysaccharidoses, occurring in the range of 1 in 200,000 to 1 in 500,000 births. The condition has been reported in patients from a variety of ethnogeographic origins, including Europeans,[132] Afro-Americans,[774] Mexican-Americans,[480] Latin Americans,[383] and Japanese.[828,829] No population group is known to have an especially high frequency of the condition.

The β-glucuronidase deficiency disorders are inherited in an autosomal recessive manner. The gene for β-glucuronidase has been localized to 7q11.2-7q22.[250,305,472,879]

Management

Conventional therapy. Little has been written about management of the clinical problems of pa-

tients who have the several forms of Sly syndrome. However, the types of difficulties that can be anticipated, and their management, can be extrapolated from experience with the other mucopolysaccharidoses.

Newborns who come to medical attention with nonimmune hydrops have little chance of survival, despite the range of intensive care measures that are available. Children with the infantile presentation are at risk for recurrent otitis media, progressive cardiac and respiratory disease, and skeletal abnormalities, although these complications may be relatively mild and infrequent in comparison to those in Hurler and Hunter syndromes. The mild form probably goes unrecognized, but these persons may have neurologic and behavioral disturbances for which appropriate pharmacologic treatment should be considered, with the limitations expected for individuals with organic brain disease.

Systemic treatment. Enzyme replacement therapy may be the most desirable and rational approach for the correction of enzyme deficiency disorders in humans. There has been only limited success, however, for experimental enzyme replacement strategies that involve direct administration of purified enzymes, enzyme-rich plasma or placental fractions, enzymes contained in semipermeable capsules, erythrocyte and liposome-entrapped enzymes, and enzyme preparations attached to physiologic carrier molecules. The usefulness of some of these approaches has been limited by a relatively short circulation and intracellular half-life, susceptibility to various degradation processes (possibly by the reactivity of the immune system against the foreign proteins), and the limited distribution into various cellular compartments. Clinical use of preparations of β-glucocerebrosidase[50,51] for Gaucher disease illustrates the practicability of enzyme replacement therapy for lysosomal storage diseases, especially those not affecting the central nervous system. Enzyme-producing allogeneic cells or whole organs may provide a better potential intrinsic physiologic source of deficient enzymes. Bone marrow transplantation has been attempted for Sly syndrome, but results are not yet available.

The known molecular biology of β-glucuronidase enzyme, availability of its cloned cDNA, and existence of animal models make this condition a prime candidate for continuing progress toward systemic therapy.

LABORATORY DIAGNOSIS OF THE MUCOPOLYSACCHARIDOSES

Depending on the clinical circumstances, patients enter into the diagnostic and management pathway from any one of a number of points. The following discussion is an overview of the methods, challenges and foibles of the diagnostic pathway. Erroneous tests and delayed reporting of results are common problems encountered along this route.[110] Management issues for each specific disorder have been discussed in the preceding sections.

Once the diagnosis has been established, identification of gene carriers in the family and prenatal diagnosis for subsequent pregnancies are often requested. Individuals heterozygous for these disorders have no phenotypic manifestations, and in these persons carrier identification can be accomplished, usually with good reliability, by means of quantitating enzyme activity in appropriate specimens. Molecular genetic methods are quickly evolving, however, and should provide a much higher level of diagnostic certainty in establishing heterozygosity and in providing prognostic information.

Biochemical Investigations

Urinary glycosaminoglycan excretion. Quantitation of excessive urinary glycosaminoglycan excretion has been for many years the basic diagnostic test that defines the presence of a mucopolysaccharidosis.* In normal individuals glycosaminoglycan excretion ranges from 3 to 15 mg/24 hr but varies with respect to age. Chondroitin-4-sulfate comprises about 80% of the excreted glycosaminoglycan, with dermatan sulfate and heparan sulfate accounting, in about equal parts, for the remainder.[496] Several relatively simple tests for detecting excessive glycosaminoglycan in the urine have been devised (Table 11-2). Uvebrant recommended the examination of urinary glycosaminoglycan in any child with nonspecific and unexplained mental retardation.[845] In support of this recommendation he cited the case of two sisters with Sanfilippo syndrome, type C who escaped diagnosis because of their subtle clinical and radiographic stigmata. Screening of urine led to diagnosis. Di Ferrante[205] and Di Ferrante et al.[208] have made use of the ratio between MPS of high molecular weight and MPS of low molecular weight in the urine. Since the former is raised and the latter reduced in the mucopolysaccharidoses, the ratio is particularly useful in discriminating affected persons from normal individuals and in evaluating the effects of therapy. The ratio appears to reflect the degradative defect that underlies the mucopolysaccharidoses.

The use of single-void "grab" specimens from

---

*References 205, 467, 657, 699, 700, and 754.

Table 11-2. Urine screening tests for the mucopolysaccharidoses

Testing methodology	False-positive rate (%)	False-negative rate (%)	Specimen requirement (ml)	Type of results
Direct 1, 9-dimethylmethylene blue (DMB) method	Adjustable	Adjustable	0.10	Quantitative
Toluidine blue O spot (Berry spot test)	1	31.7	0.04	Semiquantitative
Alcian blue spot test	25	0.0	10.0	Qualitative
Acid albumin turbidity test, gross	6.3	10	1.0	Semiquantitative
Acid albumin turbidity test, quantitative	17.2	10	1.0	Quantitative
Cetyltrimethylammonium bromide (CTAB) test	42	0.0	5.0	Qualitative
Cetylpyridinium chloride citrate (CPC) turbidity test	32	0.0	2.0	Quantitative
"MPS Papers" spot test	34	0.0	1 drop	Qualitative
"MPS Papers" spot test, semiquantitative modification	2.9	3.4	1 drop	Semiquantitative

From Whitley CB et al: *Clin Chem* 35:2074-2081, 1989.

normal individuals has been criticized because of sample-to-sample changes in the type of glycosaminoglycan excreted[206] and circadian periodicity in excretion.[748] False-negative results for patients with Sanfilippo and Morquio syndromes have been cited as a relatively common problem with such tests.[376,691] It is appropriate to use an aliquot of urine from a large collection, usually a 24-hour collection, to minimize the possibility of false-negative results. Wraith cites the case of a 4-year-old patient in whom the diagnosis was initially missed because of a false-negative result of a urine test; the correct diagnosis of Sanfilippo syndrome, type B was eventually made on the basis of an enzyme assay.[918] In the experience of Hopwood, screening tests measuring only urine glycosaminoglycan excretion are unreliable; 23 patients with Sanfilippo were identified by enzyme analysis, yet more than half had normal levels of urinary glycosaminoglycan.[364] The development of age-specific normative values in each laboratory is also particularly important.[372,373,895]

Most quantitative tests, including the commonly used method of Bitter and Muir[88,205,206] and some methods employing dyes,[163,195,643] rely on careful precipitation of glycosaminoglycans before analysis. In contrast, the direct 1, 9 dimethylmethylene blue (DMB) dye method[894] (vide infra) and its application to a paper matrix collection system,[895] measures all sulfated glycosaminoglycans in solution, eliminating potential loss of analyte in the precipitation step.

Henderson, McGinlay, and Cundall[336] suggested that laboratories conducting urine tests should be advised of the possibility of false-positive results; samples accidentally placed in test tubes containing the anticoagulant heparin produced an electrophoretic band that migrated in the position of heparan sulfate and resulted in an erroneous diagnosis of Sanfilippo syndrome.

Berry spot test. Berry and Spinanger[79] exploited the metachromatic color or "metachromasia" produced by glycosaminoglycan interaction with toluidine blue. In this semiquantitative method, aliquots of 5, 10, and 25 μL of urine are dotted as separate spots on a piece of Whatman No. 1 filter paper; each specimen is applied with a micropipette, 5 μL at a time, allowing each increment to dry before adding another. The paper with dried spots is then dipped in a buffered solution of 0.04 toluidine blue for 1 minute. (The toluidine blue solution is prepared by dissolving 90 mg of dye in 100 ml of Coleman certified buffer solution, pH 2.0.) The paper is drained and then rinsed in 95% ethanol. Spots with a metachromatic color read as positive, and the test result is rated from 0 to +++, depending on how many spots are positive. The test result is usually regarded as having a low false-negative rate,[78] but a high false-positive rate has been the experience in some laboratories. The individual who is reported to have a "positive Berry spot" merits further evaluation, including quantitation of urinary glycosaminoglycan excretion by means of an alternative method (not simply repeating the same test), as well as a thorough clinical evaluation. Despite the reported low false-negative rate,[78] experience reveals that diagnosis in affected individuals is occasionally missed, probably because of difficulties with the necessarily subjective assessment of color and relative inexperience with the test in laboratories that use the method infrequently.

Acid albumin turbidity test. The turbidity test[27] originally developed by Dorfman and Ott[218] and modified by Carter, Wan, and Carpenter[135] depends on the turbidity produced with acidified bovine serum albumin. A simple form of the Dorfman test consists of adding four drops of a 20% bovine albumin solution to an inch of urine in a 12.7-mm test tube. The contents of the tube are mixed, and 10% acetic acid is added drop by drop. A positive test result is indicated by a dense white precipitate. Because the reaction is sensitive to variations in salt concentration, pH, protein concentration, and other factors, some workers have preferred a more complex but standardized procedure[216] that involves dialysis of the urine specimen and determination of optical density.

Cetyltrimethylammonium bromide test. A simple procedure employing cetyltrimethylammonium bromide (CTAB), adapted from Meyer's preparative method[562] for use with glycosaminoglycan, has proved useful. Renuart[553] described this method for estimating urine glycosaminoglycan concentration by means of precipitation with a reagent consisting of a 5% solution of CTAB in one molar buffer, pH 6.0. One ml of CTAB reagent is added to 5 ml of clean, fresh urine at room temperature. It is important to be aware that any cold urine gives a positive test result. The mixture is agitated by swirling and then allowed to stand at room temperature for 30 minutes. Increased urinary glycosaminoglycan concentration is indicated by a heavy, flocculent precipitate. The reaction is almost immediate in cases of MPS type I but may be more delayed and less striking in the other mucopolysaccharidoses. A control urine specimen should be tested simultaneously. In addition to a chilled urine, pyuria can produce a false-positive test result.

Cetylpyridinium chloride–carbazole method. A procedure requiring preliminary dialysis of urine and based on the Dische carbazole reaction for uronic acid was proposed by Segni, Romano, and Tortorolo.[750] A similar method, developed by Bitter and Muir[88] and Bitter et al.[89] and modified by Di Ferrante,[205] utilizes precipitation of glycosaminoglycan with cetylpyridinium chloride (CPC) and then quantitation with the carbazole reagent. This is a labor-intensive, time-consuming approach; nevertheless, it represents a highly reliable diagnostic test and has become the standard to which all others are compared. Dorfman[214] urged caution in use of quantitative and semiquantitative screening tests in infants and young children because the normal glycosaminoglycan excretion may be comparatively high early in life.

Electrophoretic methods. A number of electrophoretic methods, in addition to identifying affected individuals, have the advantage of discriminating the specific glycosaminoglycan species.* In this way the differential diagnosis is further narrowed, thus directing laboratory evaluation to specific enzyme assays. Differential diagnosis is aided by more refined studies of urinary glycosaminoglycan with precise identification of the substance(s) that are excreted. For example, in young children with relatively severe clinical features, differentiation may be accomplished by identifying the heparan sulfate and dermatan sulfate (Hurler, Hunter, or Sly syndromes) or dermatan sulfate (Maroteaux-Lamy syndrome). A particularly high-resolution electrophoretic method is reported to be without false-negative results in identifying children with the mucopolysaccharidoses.[357]

Newborn Screening

It has been demonstrated that urinary glycosaminoglycan excretion is increased in patients with MPS, even at birth.[78] Thus the approach of evaluating newborn infants, which has become an accepted practice for other metabolic diseases, would be feasible for the mucopolysaccharidoses. A quantitative method of diagnostic testing employing the dye DMB was first described in 1988,[891,894] which surmounts many of the problems inherent in other methods. This direct DMB method

---

*References 78, 148, 327, 377, 736, and 737.

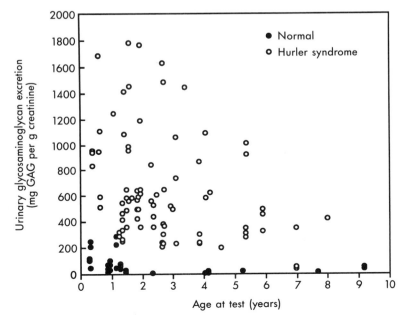

Fig. 11-63. Urinary glycosaminoglycan levels in patients with Hurler syndrome, compared to normal, determined by the automated 1,9-dimethylmethylene blue method.

has rapidly become accepted. By use of a paper matrix urine collection system,[891,895] it obviates problems of specimen transport[435] and would be feasible for mass screening of infants. The test has been automated (Fig. 11-63). Preliminary age-specific normative data, which are required by any method, have been obtained with this DMB technique. Thus the DMB method is uniquely applicable to the task of presymptomatic screening of all newborn infants for mucopolysaccharidoses.

Histochemical and Ultrastructural Diagnosis

Tissues, including peripheral blood and bone marrow, are often obtained for various reasons and may incidentally reveal the presence of an underlying MPS. For instance, vacuolization may be observed, sometimes as "reactive lymphocytes" in a routine smear prepared with Wright stain. Conjunctival biopsy and impression cytology have been used to safely obtain diagnostic tissue.[486,529]

Lagunoff and Warren[469] showed that the nitrous acid reaction for N-sulfated hexosamines is useful for detecting and measuring heparan sulfate. Alcian blue dye staining is a specific method of identifying glycosaminoglycans.[180] Only DNA interferes significantly by reacting chromogenically. Matalon et al.[535] used the method for direct assay of heparan sulfate in the amniotic fluid for the purpose of prenatal diagnosis of the Hurler syndrome. Lorincz and West[891] have preliminary experience with an interesting microspectrophotofluorometric technique. Cells from the amniotic fluid are vitally stained with acridine orange and observed immediately. The cytoplasm of cells stains metachromatically, if abnormal amounts of glycosaminoglycan are present.

After the report of Reilly[693] in 1941, the demonstration of metachromatic granules in circulating polymorphonuclear leukocytes and in bone marrow cells has been widely used as a diagnostic approach.[393,654,711] It is noteworthy that the result in bone marrow is more often positive and that Reilly granulation of the circulating polymorphs is frequently not demonstrable. Muir, Mittwoch, and Bitter[583] demonstrated a good correlation between the lymphocytic findings and the urinary excretion of glycosaminoglycan in Hurler syndrome. Maroteaux et al.[510] have described the "pink rings lymphocyte," which is a relatively specific marker for Hunter syndrome.

McKusick et al.[556] observed that metachromatic granules are not found in the cytoplasm of lymphocytes from normal persons or in patients with various disorders such as achondroplasia, the Marfan syndrome, and multiple epiphyseal dysplasia. Occasionally, however, isolated clusters of a few small, clearly defined pink granules have been found in the cytoplasm of polymorphonuclear leukocytes from normal persons. The significance of these granules is uncertain.

Scattered irregular aggregations of metachromatic granules, distinct from Reilly granules, have been noted in the cytoplasm of the majority of the polymorphs in the Morquio syndrome (MPS type IV). These characteristics of the granules may reflect the fact that, in the Morquio syndrome, a different glycosaminoglycan accumulates, namely keratan sulfate.

In the Scheie syndrome (MPS type I S) lymphocytic granules have been present in an ill-defined form in only a small proportion of cells; this probably represents a quantitative phenomenon, since these patients excrete less glycosaminoglycan than do persons with Hurler, Hunter, and Sanfilippo syndromes.

Mucopolysaccharidoses types I and II are indistinguishable on hematologic study, and inclusions may be found in neutrophils, monocytes, and lymphocytes. The diffuse distribution of granules throughout the cytoplasm of the lymphocyte is characteristic. In the bone marrow, reticulum cells contain inclusions referred to as "Gasser cells." In MPS type III, granules are clustered in restricted areas of the cytoplasm of lymphocytes. The inclusions are unusually reddish.

In the bone marrow a striking phenomenon is seen in plasma cells, which are increased in number and, often, in size. The inclusions are highly polymorphic and often enclosed in a large vacuole. These are the "Buhot cells."[338]

The peripheral blood and bone marrow show unimpressive, although definitely abnormal, metachromatic inclusions in both MPS type IV and MPS type I S. Mucopolysaccharidosis type VI, however, has the most striking inclusions of all. The neutrophils especially are choked with coarse, closely packed granules; these are "Alder-Reilly cells."[12,403,693] In MPS type VII similarly remarkable inclusions are seen in peripheral leukocytes and in bone marrow cells. Inclusions in peripheral granulocytes are typical membrane-bound lysosomes (Fig. 11-62).[76,910]

Enzymatic Diagnosis

Definitive diagnosis of a specific MPS is accomplished by quantitation of deficient enzymatic activity. If reliance is placed on plasma, multiple enzymes can be studied to exclude mucolipidosis types II and III; levels of these enzymes, by virtue of a primary defect of intracellular compartmentalization, are many-fold elevated in extracellular fluids (plasma) but are at near-normal levels in cell homogenates (leukocytes).[897] In the evaluation of any of the sulfatase deficiencies assay of several sulfatase enzymes is important in excluding multiple sulfatase deficiency, which might be confused with Hunter syndrome or, rarely, Maroteaux-Lamy syndrome. It is important that determination of enzyme activity should be undertaken in a laboratory with considerable experience. Because of the complexity of each assay, reference values or "normal range" may vary considerably from laboratory to laboratory and are not comparable. Several of the enzyme assays employ convenient, sensitive fluorogenic 4-methylumbelliferyl (MU) substrates and have largely replaced p-nitrophenyl derivative substrates in most laboratories. A number of enzyme assays require "natural" substrates, usually radiolabeled oligosaccharides or derivatives of heparin or other glycosaminoglycans.

Mucopolysaccharidosis type I (Hurler, Hurler-Scheie, and Scheie syndromes and variants). Measurement of deficient α-L-iduronidase enzyme activity is readily accomplished[254,312] with the fluorogenic MU-α-L-iduronide substrate.[365,892] Carrier testing has been performed by differentiating normal from half-normal levels of enzyme activity[878,892] but is not without error (Fig. 11-64). Clinically normal individuals with complete deficiency of α-L-iduronidase[892] or low levels of enzyme activity in these assays[362] have been identified but are relatively rare. To avoid erroneous diagnosis and termination of a normal fetus in such families, attempts at prenatal diagnosis should always be preceded by determination of enzyme levels in both parents (by means of the identical method to be used for prenatal diagnosis), thus excluding alleles with low or absent activity. Accurate prenatal diagnosis in families with parents who are carriers of a nonpathologic, low-activity α-L-iduronidase allele is difficult (Fig. 11-65). In such families in vitro measurement of radiosulfate accumulation has been used to exclude the pathologic state,[273] which might also be evaluated by means of a molecular genetic approach.

It has been proposed that radiolabeled dissac-

charide substrate derived from heparin or dermatan sulfate will discriminate between patients with Hurler syndrome and those with Scheie syndrome,* but such tests have not received general acceptance. These oligosaccharide substrates closely resemble natural glycosaminoglycans and make it possible to determine the enzyme kinetics of the small amounts of residual α-L-iduronidase activity, which might be predictive of clinical outcome.†

Mucopolysaccharidosis type II (Hunter syndrome). Determination of iduronate sulfatase activity necessitates the use of oligosaccharide substrates, chiefly disaccharides, derived from heparin or heparin.‡ Plasma has a relatively high level of enzyme activity and is a convenient diagnostic material, although other tissues have been used,

---

*References 149, 150, 210, 353, 530, 584, and 585.
†References 31, 359, 360, 361, 530, 530a, 585, and 841.
‡References 38, 254, 280, 353, 361, 490, and 492.

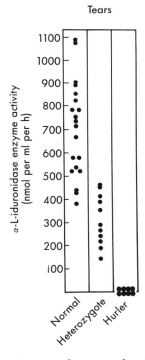

Fig. 11-64. Quantitation of enzyme levels, such as MU-α-L-iduronidase level in families with Hurler syndrome (such as in tears, as shown), may be indicative of genotype. However, it may be difficult to discriminate carrier heterozygotes with certainty because of a region of "overlap." (From Whitley CB, Krivit W, Gorlin RJ: *Am J Med Genet* 28:233-243, 1987.)

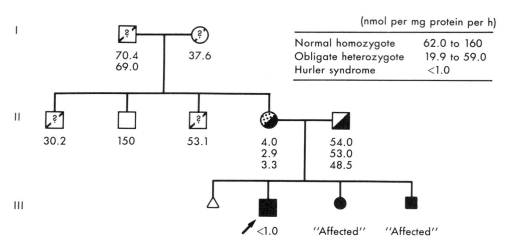

	(nmol per mg protein per h)
Normal homozygote	62.0 to 160
Obligate heterozygote	19.9 to 59.0
Hurler syndrome	<1.0

Fig. 11-65. Leukocyte MU-α-L-iduronidase enzyme activities in a family, identifying the compound heterozygote for a Hurler gene *(half-filled)* and the allele for low activity without pathologic manifestation *(stippled).* It may not be possible to distinguish the low activity allele in the presence of a normal allele on the basis of leukocyte enzyme activity. (From Whitley CB, Krivit W, Gorlin RJ: *Am J Med Genet* 28:233-243, 1987.)

including cultured fibroblasts and Epstein-Barr virus (EBV)–transformed lymphoblastoid cell lines.[571] The level of residual enzyme activity in cultured fibroblasts has not been correlated with the severity of clinical disease; thus there are no biochemical methods for distinguishing "mild" and "severe" forms of the Hunter syndrome. Molecular genetic methods are useful to distinguish some patients with major gene deletions[169,641,907] associated with severe disease. Diagnosis of Hunter carrier status by enzymatic methods[26,97,142,941] is particularly challenging insofar as random X inactivation (lyonization) is not uniform in every heterozygous female. Quantitation of enzyme in individual hair bulbs (each presumed to represent a clone of uniformly lyonized cells) has been used as a method to test for carriers.[26]

Mucopolysaccharidosis type IIIA (Sanfilippo syndrome, type A). Sulfamidase cleaves sulfate from N-sulfate groups of heparan sulfate (heparan N-sulfamidase). N-^{35}S-heparin is the most commonly used substrate; the specific activity of commercial heparin is not sufficiently high, however, for the measurement of enzyme activity in tissues or body fluids in which levels are low. In addition, it is evident that the enzyme acts specifically on

N-sulfate groups in nonreducing terminal glucosamine residues. The number of such locations on commercial heparin is not known and cannot readily be determined. Most of the radioactive sulfur is in a position such that it will not be released by the action of the enzyme, and a maximum of 5% of the label may be released by sulfamidase. Oligosaccharide substrates have been used with success.[255,826] Clear differentiation of obligate heterozygotes from normal controls is thought possible by strict temperature control during incubation[537] and rigid standardization of the amount of protein used per assay.[792,831] Nevertheless, conflicting results have been obtained when the same persons have been studied in different laboratories.

Mucopolysaccharidosis type IIIB (Sanfilippo syndrome, type B). The activity of N-acetylglucosaminidase, previously measured with p-nitrophenyl derivative,[618,868,869] is now usually quantified with MU-2-acetamido-2-α-D-glucopyranoside.[527] Carriers can be identified by assay of serum enzyme activity.[869,848]

Mucopolysaccharidosis type IIIC (Sanfilippo syndrome, type C). The activity of acetyl-CoA:α-glucosaminide N-acetyltransferase is measured by use of a complex (^{3}H) trisaccharide,[442] tetrasaccharide or disaccharide prepared from heparin or oligosaccharides[354] as a substrate, and cultured skin fibroblasts as an enzyme source. More recently evaluations have been made of a monosaccharide, (^{14}C)glucosamine.[640] In this technique leukocytes from patients showed no detectable enzyme activity even after 24 hours of incubation, and the mean activity in obligate heterozygotes was 50% that in the normal subjects. The advantages of the (^{14}C)glucosamine substrate seem to be higher levels of enzyme activity and a greater quantitative differentiation between normals, heterozygotes, and homozygotes.[640]

Mucopolysaccharidosis type IIID (Sanfilippo syndrome, type D). N-acetylglucosamine 6-sulfatase is measured using a radiolabeled trisaccharide derived from heparan sulfate as a substrate and cultured fibroblasts and leucocytes as enzyme sources.[459] The preparation of the substrate is time consuming and requires special skills. The radiolabeled monosaccharide N-acetylglucosamine (1-^{14}C)6-sulfate has been used as a substrate,[227] but the turnover rate was slow (2% to 5% conversion after 17 hours of incubation). The substrate Glc NAc6S-IdOA can be conveniently prepared from a heparin-derived disaccharide for enzyme assay.[257] Products are separated using high-voltage electrophoresis to measure the level of de-O-sulfation. This method can be used to diagnose Sanfilippo syndrome, type D and appears to distinguish obligate heterozygotes.

Mucopolysaccharidosis type IVA (Morquio syndrome type A). Galactosamine 6-sulfatase has been measured with radiolabeled oligosaccharide substrates derived from chondroitin-6-sulfate and keratan sulfate.[355,356,933] More convenient fluorogenic substrates have been described[853] and successfully used in heterozygote identification.

Mucopolysaccharidosis type IVB (Morquio syndrome, type B). Deficiency of β-galactosidase has been conveniently measured with MU-β-D-galactopyranoside.[24,285] Oligosaccharide substrates have been used to demonstrate low levels of residual activity in fibroblasts.[593] In some but not all instances the level of residual enzymatic activity was related to severity of disease and thus represents a potential prognostic indicator.

Mucopolysaccharidosis type VI (Maroteaux-Lamy syndrome). In the past, measurement of N-acetylgalactosamine 4-sulfatase was accomplished by fractionation of sulfatase isozymes measured with the chromogenic substrate p-nitrophenyl sulfate; the enzyme was frequently referred to as aryl sulfatase B. More recently the sulfatase activities have been determined with MU-sulfate substrate and differentiated by means of anion-exchange chromatography, electrophoresis, or differential inhibition or by immune capture with monoclonal antibody.[113,244,544,690,744] The 4-sulfatase enzyme activity has also been measured directly with radiolabeled oligosaccharides derived from dermatan sulfate or chondroitin-4-sulfate.[365] These methods have been used for carrier testing,[69,544] but their accuracy is problematic.

Mucopolysaccharidosis type VII (Sly syndrome). The definitive diagnosis of Sly syndrome rests on determination of deficiency of β-glucuronidase,[64,774] as in the diagnosis of the original case by means of p-nitrophenyl-β-glucuronide.[311,774] A reliable and more sensitive method currently used in many laboratories employs the fluorogenic substrate MU-β-D-glucuronide substrate.[286,636] The enzyme can also be quantitated with radiolabeled disaccharides[584] and with any of these assays proves to be virtually absent in patients when measured in plasma, leukocytes, cultured fibroblasts, or any other tissues. Intermediate activity is found in heterozygotes and has been used for carrier testing.[286,311] A pseudodeficiency allele has been demonstrated.

Prenatal Diagnosis

The Hurler and Hunter syndromes are routinely diagnosed antenatally by means of biochemical methods when mothers have shown themselves to be at risk by giving birth to an affected child in a previous pregnancy.[362,791] Fratantoni et al.[254] made use of ^{35}SO$_4$-accumulation kinetics and cytoplasmic metachromasia of amniotic fluid cells for prenatal diagnosis. Matalon et al.[535] suggested that recognition of an elevated glycosaminoglycan content of the amniotic fluid might be a valid diagnostic method. They found that normal fluid had about 0.02 mg/ml (range, 0.006 to 0.095) of glycosaminoglycan in the second trimester of pregnancy. The fluid from a 14-week pregnancy in which a baby with the Hurler syndrome was subsequently born contained 0.087 mg/ml. Furthermore, whereas the glycosaminoglycan of pooled normal amniotic fluid was about 80% hyaluronic acid and 13% dermatan sulfate, the Hurler fluid contained 63% heparan sulfate. The authors pointed out that the increased heparan sulfate could be detected directly in the amniotic fluid. Danes et al.[181] showed that the glycosaminoglycan content of amniotic fluid, as reflected by uronic acid, decreases progressively during pregnancy and is relatively high in the early stages. Matalon, Dorfman, and Nadler[533] subsequently concluded that direct chemical study of the amniotic fluid is not a reliable method for prenatal diagnosis of mucopolysaccharidoses. This conclusion is consistent with that arrived at in connection with almost all lysosomal storage diseases: prenatal diagnosis is usually not based on study of the fluid and uncultured cells; confirmation by testing of cultured amniotic cells is usually necessary. Prenatal diagnosis of Hurler syndrome[272,273,791] or Hunter syndrome[23,439,440,489,644] is now routinely accomplished on the basis of deficient enzyme activity measured in chorionic villus samples (CVS) and amniocentesis specimens. Measurement of enzyme in fetal plasma has also been undertaken.[498] Enzyme levels in maternal serum have been monitored as a possible marker for the Hunter genotype in the fetus.[942,943]

Prenatal diagnosis of Sanfilippo syndrome, types A,[441,832] B,[272,567,578] and C[211] has been shown to be highly reliable as early as the ninth or tenth week of pregnancy. The diagnosis is accomplished by measuring the activity of the appropriate enzyme in chorionic villi or cultured fetal cells from amniotic fluid. When enzyme assays were performed on 37 pregnant women at risk for Sanfilippo syndrome, type A, nine fetuses were diagnosed as being homozygous for the condition. The diagnosis was confirmed by means of enzyme tests performed on fetal fibroblasts after the termination of the pregnancies. The diagnosis of the other 28 fetuses as normal or as heterozygote carriers was confirmed when, after birth, they showed no evidence of the disease.[441] Another diagnostic indication of MPS type III in a fetus is the detection by means of electrophoresis[578] of excess heparan sulfate in the amniotic fluid. Regarding Sanfilippo syndrome, type D, Freeman and Hopwood[257] reported that N-acetylglucosamine 6-sulfatase activity has been detected in chorionic villi from a 12-week pregnancy using a radiolabeled monosul-

fated disaccharide as a substrate. A spectrophotometric assay has also been developed.[613] Such methods may prove useful for prenatal diagnosis as more experience is gained.

The Morquio syndrome, type A has been diagnosed antenatally on a regular basis by measuring enzymatic activity in fresh and cultured chorionic villus tissue and amniocytes.[23,933,939]

Successful prenatal diagnosis of MPS type VI has been accomplished by measurement of deficient enzyme activity in amniocytes[438,744,852] and chorionic villus tissue, but methods must be carefully standardized to avoid problems caused by interference from other sulfatases.

Prenatal diagnosis of MPS type VII can be accomplished by demonstrating deficiency of β-glucuronidase in amniocytes or chorionic villus biopsy specimens.[272,511]

Morphologic criteria (inclusion morphology) have not been reliable for prenatal diagnosis of any of the MPS diseases, although various methods have been studied.[375,891]

OTHER GENETIC MUCOPOLYSACCHARIDOSES AND RELATED DISEASES

It is more than likely that the entities described earlier in this chapter are not the only genetic defects of glycosaminoglycan metabolism. The following discussion concerns additional conditions in which such a disturbance is suspected.

Hopwood and Morris[358] speculated that deficiency of glucosamine-6-sulphatase should result in accumulation of heparan sulfate and predicted an additional Sanfilippo syndrome phenotype. Thus far, no affected individuals have been identified. The authors also suggested that deficiency of glucuronate-2-sulfatase should result in accumulation of heparan sulfate (and chondroitin sulfate) and produce a phenotype resembling the Sanfilippo syndrome.[256] The enzyme has been purified from normal human liver, but no person with a disorder attributable to defective activity has yet been recognized. The designation MPS type VIII was proposed, and later retracted, for this putative disorder, which is not currently recognized as an existent clinical entity.

Several other lysosomal storage diseases must be considered in the differential diagnosis of the mucopolysaccharidoses. Among these conditions are the mucolipidosis (ML) disorders originally defined by Spranger and Wiedemann[780] and more recently designated *heteroglycanoses* or *oligosaccharidoses*. Other disorders of defective lysosomal metabolism, multiple sulfatase deficiency and aspartylglycosaminuria, may also warrant consideration in the differential diagnosis.

Sialidosis (Mucolipidosis Type I, Neuraminidase Deficiency, and Cherry-Red Spot–Myoclonus Syndrome)

Clinical manifestations. Four distinct clinical forms of sialidosis have been recognized.

Neonatal sialidosis (hydropic sialidosis). In the neonatal form of sialidosis the infant is born with hydrops fetalis and either is stillborn or dies within the first few months of life.[309,835] Additional features typically include pericardial effusion, corneal clouding, hepatosplenomegaly, inguinal hernias, stippled epiphyses, and periosteal cloaking of the long bones.

Infantile sialidosis (nephrosialidosis). The infantile form becomes evident during the first year of life and is characterized by moderately severe dysostosis multiplex, hepatosplenomegaly, glomerular nephropathy,[418] hearing loss, seizures, pyramidal tract signs, and severe mental retardation. Visual loss, a macular cherry-red spot, myoclonus, and ataxia are seen in older children.[827] Affected individuals may survive into the second decade of life.

Childhood sialidosis. This form of the condition usually becomes apparent during childhood, when the patient develops features reminiscent of Hurler syndrome. There is a flat nasal bridge and anteverted nostrils, mild to moderate gingival enlargement with widely spaced teeth, enlarged tongue, a barrel-shaped chest, and, frequently, hernias. Hepatomegaly is sometimes detected, but splenomegaly is rare. Sensorineural deafness is present. The radiographic features are typical of mild to moderate dysostosis multiplex. As the disease progresses, ataxia, nystagmus, muscle wasting, and weakness develop. At this point in the course of the disease, a cherry-red spot is observable and strabismus and sometimes cataract and corneal clouding may be evident. Neither mental retardation nor seizures are present, but peripheral neurologic involvement usually manifests as sensory deficits, irregular deep tendon reflexes, and decreased nerve conduction velocities. Congenital adrenal hypoplasia may be an additional factor.[631] Patients become chairbound in adolescence, but decline is not rapid. Pneumonia and

complications related to the neurologic changes are the usual cause of death in adolescence or early adulthood.

Juvenile sialidosis (cherry-red spot–myoclonus syndrome). The descriptive name of this condition points out the main features of this disorder[14]: the presence of a macular cherry-red spot and seizure-like episodes (notably without loss of consciousness) that result from repetitive bursts of severe generalizing myoclonus. Affected individuals have a normal facial appearance and are remarkable for the lack of organomegaly, dysostosis multiplex, and corneal clouding. Psychomotor retardation and mental deficiency are not present until the later, preterminal stages of disease.

Cytoplasmic inclusions are present in peripheral lymphocytes, bone marrow macrophages, hepatocytes and Kupffer cells of liver, and neurons.[14] By electron microscopy these inclusions are seen to be membrane-bound lysosomal accumulations of reticulogranular material.[804]

Fundamental defect. The sialidosis group of disorders results from deficiency of the enzyme glycoprotein sialidase, which is responsible for degradation of $\alpha 2\text{->}3$ and $\alpha 2\text{->}6$ neuraminosyl linkages in sialoglycan moieties of glycoproteins.[859,860] As a consequence there are lysosomal accumulation and urinary excretion of undegraded sialyloligosaccharides in which sialic acid residues occupy the terminal nonreducing postion. There is also accumulation of gangliosides containing sialic acid.[842] Deficiency of the enzyme can be demonstrated in cultured fibroblasts and leukocytes, and half-normal levels are found in parents of affected individuals. Patients who lack sialidase and β-galactosidase have a different disorder, galactosialidosis (discussed later in this chapter).

Prevalence and inheritance. The childhood form of sialidosis appears to be more prevalent among Japanese, but the other forms have been observed in several different ethnogeographic populations.[835] The gene for glycoprotein sialidase has been localized to 6p21.3.[581]

Inclusion-Cell Disease (Leroy Syndrome, Mucolipidosis Type II)

Clinical manifestations. The clinically disparate disorders mucolipidosis (ML) types II and III are now recognized as relatively severe and mild forms of the same basic molecular defect.

Inclusion-cell (I-cell) disease (Leroy syndrome, ML type II) is a disorder resembling Hurler syndrome with severe clinical and radiologic features* but with normal levels of glycosaminoglycan excretion. Leroy and DeMars[482] and Leroy, DeMars, and Opitz[483] first delineated the disorder and noted striking fibroblast inclusions (hence the terminology "inclusion-cell" or "I-cell" disease) that are useful in diagnosis.[429] Congenital dislocation of the hips, thoracic abnormalities, hernia, and hyperplastic gums are evident soon after birth. Radiographic studies show that the bones exhibit changes of dysostosis multiplex similar to but more severe than those in Hurler syndrome.[649-651] Retarded psychomotor development, clear corneas, and restricted joint mobility are other features. Craniosynostosis and hydrocephalus have been reported.[919] Death usually results from infection or heart failure.[715,742] The disorder can be diagnosed prenatally.[36,65,80,646,671] Bone marrow transplantation has been accomplished,[920] but the clinical outcome remains undetermined.

Pathology. On gross and microscopic examination ML type II is quite similar to the mucopolysaccharidoses; however, I-cell disease also has features of oligosaccharidosis.[36,138,412] Subepithelial connective tissue is hypercellular, and the numerous histiocytes and fibroblasts are extensively vacuolated.[430] Electron microscopy shows that the inclusions are single-membrane limited and consist of fibrillogranular and membranous lamellar material.[315] The lipid content of cultured fibroblasts is three times that of normal.

Fundamental defect. Weismann et al.[897] found extremely high levels of lysosomal enzymes in the medium of cultured fibroblasts and postulated "leaky lysosomes" as the cause of the disorder. Hickman and Neufeld[341] later observed that lysosomal hydrolases in the media from cultured fibroblasts of patients with I-cell disease were not taken up by fibroblasts cultured from normal individuals; they suggested a defect in the synthesis of lysosomal enzymes. This postulate was subsequently modified to the current view[598] that most

lysosomal enzymes (and other lysosomal proteins[687]) are subject to defective posttranslational modifications resulting in incorrect trafficking of proteins to lysosomes. In normal cells most lysosomal enzymes undergo "maturation," which involves a two-step process in the Golgi apparatus, adding a terminal mannose-6-phosphate to the carbohydrate moiety of lysosomal enzymes. Mucolipidosis type II results from a defect in the initial step of this process, altered protein structure[67] and deficient activity of the phosphotransferase enzyme, UDP-N-acetylglucosamine:lysosomal enzyme N-acetylglucosaminyl-1-phosphotransferase. As a consequence lysosomal enzymes are not routed to the lysosome but are extruded extracellularly. Enzymes lacking terminal mannose-6-phosphate are also unavailable for reuptake by mannose-6-phosphate receptors found on the cell surface that mediate recovery of some proteins for endocytosis to lysosomes. This latter phenomenon accounts for the observation of Hickman and Neufeld[341] that lysosomal enzymes of cultured fibroblasts from patients with I-cell disease are not endocytosed by normal cells. As a consequence a variety of substrates accumulates in lysosomes, which secondarily impair normal cell functions such as neutrophil chemotaxis.[714]

Prevalence and inheritance. Male and female sibs have been observed, and consanguinity of parents is relatively common,[780] both observations indicating the autosomal recessive mode of transmission. Although no epidemiologic data are available, many cases have been reported[238,479,482,483]; however, the condition is probably more rare than 1 in 100,000 births. The gene for phosphotransferase has been localized to the long arm of chromosome 4, region 4q21-q23, although complementation studies have suggested that multiple genes may produce the ML II (and ML III) phenotype.[66,580]

Pseudo-Hurler Polydystrophy (Mucolipidosis Type III)

Clinical manifestations. Under the designation "pseudopolydystrophie de Hurler" Maroteaux and Lamy[522] in 1966 described four cases with many of the features of the Hurler syndrome but with a much slower clinical evolution and no glycosaminuria. The authors pointed out that the same disorder was probably present in a patient

---

*References 155, 294, 519, 568, 569, 630, and 671.

earlier listed among "cases defying classification" by McKusick et al.[556] The sibs reported by Steinbach et al.[786] presumably had this condition. Patients usually come to medical attention in childhood, typically at the age of about 3 years, with stiffness of joints as the main complaint. Coarse facies and short stature are features in some. The cornea shows a fine, "ground-glass" clouding.[833] Aortic valve disease, often resulting in regurgitation, is present in most. Hypoplasia of the odontoid process was noted in one instance. An early, detailed description of the radiographic changes of mild dysostosis multiplex was provided by McKusick et al.[559] Patients frequently have carpal tunnel syndrome, which has been successfully treated by means of surgical release of the transverse carpal ligament.[784]

Pathology. Spranger and Wiedemann's classification[780] of pseudo-Hurler polydystrophy as an ML was supported by electronmicroscopic studies. Danes found cytoplasmic metachromasia with toluidine blue and alcian blue staining in the cultured skin fibroblasts of several of McKusick's patients.[553] In the bone marrow Maroteaux and Lamy[522] found cells reminiscent of those of Hurler syndrome, but the vacuoles appeared empty. Fibroblasts of the conjunctiva show cytoplasmic vacuolization that is delimited by a single membrane.[679] (Metachromasia on light microscopic observation of specimens stained with toluidine blue and alcian blue suggests that the vacuoles contain glycosaminoglycans.) In addition, a rather large amount of membranous lamellar material similar to that seen in fibroblasts from patients with the sphingolipidoses is demonstrated by means of electron microscopy; its appearance is consistent with glycolipid.

Fundamental defect. Pseudo-Hurler polydystrophy results from a defect of the same phosphotransferase enzyme activity that is causative of I-cell disease; these disorders, ML II and ML III, thus can be regarded as relatively "severe" and "mild" forms of the same heritable defect in which differences probably result from the degree of the enzymatic defect.[475] The molecular defect is described in the preceding section, I-Cell Disease. Several different complementation groups of defects have been suggested to account for the spectrum of ML types II and III phenotypes.[66,580]

Prevalence and inheritance. McKusick observed two families, each with an affected brother and sister and normal parents, consistent with autosomal recessive inheritance.[553] Inclusions were not seen by means of histochemical or ultrastructural techniques in conjunctival fibroblasts of the unaffected parents,[679] but other methods have been used for heterozygote diagnosis. The disorder is inherited in an autosomal recessive manner, although multiple different genetic loci are involved.[580]

Galactosialidosis (Galactosidase-Neuraminidase Deficiency)

Clinical manifestations. In a patient with corneal clouding and macular cherry-red spot, deficiency of β-galactosidase in cultured fibroblasts and conjunctiva was demonstrated by Goldberg et al.[291] in 1971. In subsequent patients studied by Wenger Tarby, and Wharton[888] the level of glycoprotein sialidase was also shown to be reduced. The phenotype of combined galactosidase-neuraminidase deficiency ranges from mild to severe. Glycosaminoglycan excretion is normal, but abnormal urinary sialyloligosaccharides are found. Prenatal diagnosis is possible.[437] Three clinical presentations are recognized.

Neonatal (hydropic) galactosialidosis. A small number of neonates are born with a condition clinically indistinguishable from G_{M1}-gangliosidosis but with edema and ascites; the diagnosis of galactosialidosis is confirmed by measuring deficiencies of β-galactosidase and glycoprotein sialidase. The clinical features include corneal clouding, macular cherry-red spot, and telangiectasia of the conjunctiva and skin. Dysostosis multiplex of the skeleton resembles the changes found in G_{M1}-gangliosidosis or I-cell disease. Death occurs at birth or within the first few months of life.

Late infantile galactosialidosis. Another group of children with galactosialidosis comes to medical attention during the first 2 years of life, presenting with coarse facial features, hepatosplenomegaly, kyphoscoliosis, dysostosis multiplex, and developmental delay. Abnormal ophthalmologic and neurologic signs may not be present at this stage but are likely to appear as the disease advances.

Juvenile galactosialidosis (Goldberg-Wenger syndrome). Most patients with galactosialidosis have been diagnosed in late childhood or early adulthood. This later-onset form, first identified by Goldberg et al.[291] and Wenger et al.,[888] is characterized as slowly progressive disease with cerebellar ataxia, tremor and action myoclonus, pyramidal signs (without extrapyramidal signs or nystagmus), cherry-red spot with progressive loss of visual acuity, mild dysostosis multiplex, mild coarsening of facial features, and intellectual impairment.[291,888] Angiokeratoma and corneal opacification are usually present, and hearing loss sometimes develops.

Pathology. Patients with any of the galactosialidoses have vacuolated peripheral lymphocytes, although these may be difficult to demonstrate on histochemical study. Ultrastructural techniques have demonstrated the lysosomal nature of the defect.[68,804]

Fundamental defect. Studies using somatic cell hybridization with cells from mildly and severely affected patients have failed to show complementation, thus suggesting that the three clinical phenotypes result from allelic mutations at a single locus.[349] These disorders result from defects in a 32-kd noncatalytic protective glycoprotein, which is required for aggregation of 64-kd β-galactosidase monomers and their protection against lysosomal proteolytic degradation and for activation of glycoprotein sialidase.[348]

Prevalence and inheritance. Intrafamilial phenotypic variation is less common than interfamilial variation. The juvenile form has been recognized predominantly in the Japanese population. The gene has been localized to chromosome 20.[581]

Mannosidosis (Acid α-D-Mannosidase Deficiency)

In a child with clinical features suggesting the Hurler syndrome, Ockerman and Hultberg[623,624,626] found normal urinary excretion of glycosaminoglycans but increased amounts of mannose-containing compounds in tissues, accompanied by deficiency of α-mannosidase. This condition, termed mannosidosis, is a lysosomal disease that, like G_{M1}-gangliosidosis, ML II, and others, resembles Hurler syndrome in some respects.

Clinical manifestations. Mannosidosis is usually divided into two types based on the age of clinical presentation.[389]

Infantile mannosidosis (type I). Infantile mannosidosis is characterized by rapid progression of mental deterioration, obvious hepatosplenomegaly, severe dysostosis multiplex, and death between 3 and 10 years of age. Bone marrow transplantation has been accomplished but with a poor clinical outcome.[901]

Juvenile mannosidosis (type II). The milder form of juvenile-onset mannosidosis is characterized by normal early development and the appearance of mental retardation during childhood and adolescence. There is a correspondingly slower progression of other features, including hearing loss,[455] mild dysostosis multiplex, and cognitive function.[607,608] Destructive synovitis, hydrocephalus, spastic paraplegia, and pancytopenia have been reported in patients with type II disease.

The disease has been well characterized in feline* and bovine animal models.[232,330,345,400]

Pathology. Ultrastructural examination of the liver reveals vacuolated hepatocytes and Kupffer cells, often with a reticulogranular appearance, although heterogeneous inclusions are the rule.[436] A similar pathologic appearance is also seen in muscle.[421] In the central nervous system there is widespread and marked ballooning of nerve cells, with the cytoplasm being highly vacuolated or empty-appearing. Membrane-bound vacuoles with a reticulogranular appearance are evident on electron microscopy.

Fundamental defect. Deficiency of α-mannosidase enzyme is readily documented in tissues from patients with either form of mannosidosis[422]; however, some patients have relatively high residual activity. Because of the deficiency of α-mannosidase, there is systemic lysosomal accumulation of oligosaccharides,[881] including deposition in the brain tissue.[625] The enzyme can be transferred from normal lymphocytes to enzyme-deficient fibroblasts by direct cell contact.[2,515]

Prevalence and inheritance. Pedigree data from a large number of families have indicated autosomal recessive inheritance, and the gene has been localized to the pericentric region 19p13.2-q12.[528]

_____
*References 1, 17, 137, 396, 682, and 881.

β-Mannosidosis

Jones and Dawson[401] described deficiency of β-mannosidase in a strain of goats prior to recognition of the associated disorder in humans. In 1986 Wenger et al.[889] identified the disease in a child, and Cooper, Sardharwalla, and Roberts[160] and Cooper et al.[161] identified two adult siblings affected with the condition.

Clinical manifestations. The clinical phenotype resulting from deficient β-mannosidase is not well characterized because only a few patients have been identified. A boy diagnosed at 18 months of age with β-mannosidase deficiency is the youngest example; however, this child was also deficient in heparan sulfamidase (Sanfilippo syndrome, type A). The affected child had progressive coarsening of facial features, delayed acquisition of speech, hyperactivity, mental deficiency, and radiographic features of mild dysostosis multiplex. He also excreted excessive amounts of glycosaminoglycans and oligosaccharides.

The adults with β-mannosidase deficiency came to diagnosis on the basis of mental retardation but without other neurologic signs. These siblings lacked other physical stigmata and had normal hearing.[219]

Pathology. There are no pathologic studies of the human disease, but studies of the condition in goats* have revealed lysosomal storage inclusions in all tissues.

Fundamental defect. The disorder results from complete deficiency of lysosomal β-mannosidase. Partial characterization of the storage products has been accomplished.[346]

Prevalence and inheritance. The disorder appears to be extremely rare. Based on the animal model and limited human information, it is likely to be inherited in an autosomal recessive fashion (although the human disorder has not been seen in females and X-linked recessive inheritance has not been excluded).

Fucosidosis

In sibs with clinical features somewhat suggestive of Hurler syndrome who were described by

---

*References 98-100, 172, 501, 502, 653, and 694.

Durand, Borrone, and Della Cella,[223] Van Hoof and Hers[858] found deficiency of α-fucosidase activity in the liver. Thereafter Durand and Borrone[222] demonstrated accumulation of fucose in all tissues and suggested the term *fucosidosis*. The clinical features were progressive cerebral degeneration, dementia, and loss of muscle strength followed by intense spasticity, decorticate rigidity, progressive emaciation, thick skin, excessive sweating, and cardiomegaly. Early death occurred at 3 years 9 months and 5 years 2 months of age in these sibs.[223]

In a 9-year-old child with an unusual skeletal dysplasia labeled "spondylometaphyseoepiphyseal dysplasia," Schafer, Powell, and Sullivan[726] found deficiency of α-L-fucosidase in fibroblasts cultured from the skin. The patient showed no extraskeletal features. Thus the phenotype was quite different from that in the previous cases. Patel, Watanabe, and Zeman[647] described yet another phenotype with deficiency of α-L-fucosidase. Their patient survived to 16 years of age, and from the age of 4 years angiokeratoma had been present as in Fabry disease. Severe mental retardation was an additional feature.

Clinical manifestations. Fucosidosis is rarely diagnosed in infants younger than 6 months of age but should be suspected in infants with a history of frequent upper respiratory tract infection and developmental delay. Although there is considerable variation,[903] physical features include coarse facial features with thick skin, lips, and tongue. There may be mild hepatosplenomegaly and generalized hypotonia with diminished deep-tendon reflexes. Some children never learn to walk unassisted, and a neurodegenerative course has been observed.[676] Abundant sweating with increased salinity of the sweat has been noticed in young patients. Radiographic studies may show mild thoracolumbar kyphoscoliosis and cardiomegaly. Slowing of linear growth usually occurs from 2 years of age. Fucose-containing oligosaccharides are excreted in the urine and should be demonstrated to confirm the diagnosis of fucosidosis.[432] Determination of complete α-L-fucosidase deficiency is a definitive diagnostic test result; however, rare patients have unusually high levels of residual enzyme activity that is thermolabile.[92] Metabolic correction has been studied in vitro[16] and in an animal model treated by bone marrow transplantation.[812,814-819]

Pathology. Lysosomal oligosaccharide storage is widespread and peripheral lymphocytes are vacuolated. Other cells are distended by inclusions: hepatocytes, Kupffer cells, histocytes, glomerular endothelial cells, and bronchial and rectal mucosal endothelium, as well as fibrocytes of skin and conjunctiva.[259] In the brain there is loss of neuronal and myelin cells, and membrane-bound inclusions are observed in the remaining neurons. Extensive pathologic studies have been undertaken in the animal model of fucosidosis.[16,46,262,813]

Fundamental defect. Systemic deficiency of lysosomal α-L-fucosidase is the primary defect,[203,204] and deficiency of this enzyme results in accumulation of a variety of fucose-containing oligosaccharides derived from the carbohydrate moieties of glycoproteins. Dawson and Spranger[188] demonstrated that abnormal glycosphingolipid is present in high concentration in the liver. The gene for α-L-fucosidase has been identified and characterized, including some mutations.[185,461,621,902]

Prevalence and inheritance. Fucosidosis, which is quite rare, appears to be more common in southern Italians, New Mexican Spanish-Americans, and Navajo American Indians. The condition is autosomal recessive, and the gene has been localized to 1q34.

G_{M1}-Gangliosidosis (Generalized Gangliosidosis)

G_{M1}-gangliosidosis was first recognized as a distinct entity by Landing et al.[474] and has also been referred to as generalized gangliosidosis.

Clinical manifestations. G_{M1}-gangliosidosis is characterized by mild Hurler-like manifestations with moderate progressive mental retardation, the skeletal changes of dysostosis multiplex, normal glycosaminoglycan excretion, and peculiar inclusions in cultured fibroblasts. Three clinical types are distinguished based on the patient's age at presentation.[449]

The infantile form, G_{M1}-gangliosidosis, type I, is usually recognized shortly after birth. The face may resemble that of patients with Hurler syndrome. Coarsening of the facies may be present at birth or become apparent during infancy.[453] Typical features include macrocephaly with frontal

bossing, depressed nasal bridge, prominent philtrum, gingival enlargement, and full cheeks. Corneal clouding is rare, but a cherry-red spot develops in most instances.[121,234] Hepatosplenomegaly is present and hydroceles are common. The hands are short and stubby, and kyphoscoliosis is an early finding. Infants are hypotonic, with a poor suck-and-swallow reflex. The child exhibits gross motor delay and never learns to sit or crawl. Diffuse cutaneous telangiectasia[71,289] (analogous to that of Fabry disease and fucosidosis) is present. Hyperpigmented macules have also been observed.[752] Cardiomyopathy[141,767] and skeletal myopathy[141] have been noted. The radiographic appearance is that of severe dysostosis multiplex resembling Hurler syndrome or I-cell disease. Neurologic deterioration progresses, with failure to thrive, seizures, blindness, deafness, and, often, quadriplegia. Life span is limited, ranging from 6 months to 2 years of age. Bone marrow transplantations in the canine model[622] and in one child have resulted in poor outcomes.

The other forms of G_{M1}-gangliosidosis, type II (juvenile-onset) and type III (adult-onset),[306,628,844,845a] are characterized by minimal physical stigmata, with progressive neurologic deterioration.[642]

Pathology. The birefringent cytoplasmic inclusions in cultured fibroblasts stain positive with periodic acid–Schiff stain and Sudan black B fat stain. Matalon et al.[534] demonstrated that the inclusions stain metachromatically with toluidine blue after treatment with chloroform-methanol. Thus storage of both glycosaminoglycans and glycolipids in lysosomes[260] was suggested. Peripheral lymphocytes are vacuolated, and the unique appearance of eosinophils is a helpful diagnostic marker.[283] At autopsy lysosomal inclusions are found in tissues of the nervous system,[385] including the retina, and also are seen in rectal and skin biopsy specimens.[288,381] Abnormalities are already present in the fetus, indicative of the early genesis of significant disease.[83] The same biochemical defect has been identified in cats[47] and in a strain of Portuguese water dogs,[723,759] which have been the object of considerable neuropathologic study.[402,448]

Fundamental defect. O'Brien et al.[619] introduced the term generalized gangliosidosis because small but excessive amounts of G_{M1}-gangliosides were found in the liver and spleen together with a large excess in the brain. Scott, Lagunoff, and Trump[745] reported considerable accumulations of a glycosaminoglycan in the liver and spleen and suggested a relationship to the genetic mucopolysaccharidoses. Suzuki[803] tentatively identified the glycosaminoglycan as keratan sulfate. Okada and O'Brien[629] discovered deficient lysosomal β-galactosidase activity, seemingly the same enzyme as that deficient in Morquio syndrome, type B.[805] Biochemical studies later characterized the storage materials of G_{M1}-gangliosidosis to be glycosphingolipids (G_{M1}-ganglioside and asialo-G_{M1}-ganglioside) and galactose-containing oligosaccharides.[616,617,619] These accumulate primarily in the central nervous system[28,417] but can be found in viscera and can be demonstrated in cultured fibroblasts[513] and urine[806] from affected individuals. Recent studies have shown that the genetic defects of G_{M1}-gangliosidosis and Morquio syndrome, type B are, in fact, different allelic mutations resulting in altered specificities of β-galactosidase enzyme activity; there may be some overlap in clinical and biochemical phenotypes.[308]

Prevalence and inheritance. Spranger and Wiedemann[780] observed three affected siblings and noted parental consanguinity in one instance, thus suggesting an autosomal recessive mode of inheritance. Other reports have confirmed the mode of transmission for the infantile, juvenile, and adult forms[306] of the disease. There are no estimates of the frequency of this disorder, which is probably more rare than 1 in 100,000 births. The gene has been localized to the region 3p21-cen.

Aspartylglycosaminuria

Excessive urinary excretion of aspartylglycosamine was first recognized by Jenner and Pollitt[391] in 1967 in adults with mental retardation who had coarse facial features reminiscent of the mucopolysaccharidoses. Subsequent biochemical studies revealed deficiency of a lysosomal enzyme involved in the degradation of glycoprotein oligosaccharide moieties.[675]

Clinical manifestations. The disorder becomes apparent in early childhood with developmental delay and speech and language deficits. These later progress to an attention deficit (hyperactivity) disorder, and finally to more severe intellectual deterioration. There is coarsening of facial features, and hepatosplenomegaly may be found in younger patients. Radiographic features resemble the changes of typical dysostosis multiplex, with a thick calvarium, flattening and anterior beaking of some thoracolumbar vertebrae, cortical thinning of tubular bones, osteoporosis, and occasional pathologic fractures.[734] The diagnosis can be confirmed by identification of increased levels of specific oligosaccharides and by measurement of the defect in enzymatic activity.

Pathology. Lymphocytes are vacuolated and lysosomal inclusions are apparent in most tissues, especially on electron microscopic study.[384]

Fundamental defect. The disorder results from deficiency of 1-aspartamido-β-N-acetylglucosamine-aminohydrolase,[675] a lysosomal enzyme contributing to the degradation of oligosaccharides derived from various glycoproteins.[105] Elevation of serum dolichol levels is likely to be a secondary phenomenon.[716]

Prevalence and inheritance. Aspartylglycosaminuria has a relatively high frequency in the Finnish population but has also been observed in other ethnogeographic groups.[143,371,734] Inheritance is autosomal recessive, and the gene has been localized to 4q21-qter.

Sialic Acid Storage Disease (Including Salla Syndrome)

Clinical manifestations. Two clinical phenotypes have been associated with excessive intracellular accumulation and excessive urinary excretion of sialic acid, a presumed defect in lysosomal sialic acid transport.

Infantile sialic acid storage disease. Newborns with the early infantile form of sialic acid storage disease have coarsening of the facial features, axial hypotonia with hypertonia of the limbs, hypopigmentation, diarrhea, recurrent infections, and hypochromic anemia.[830] A few affected infants have neonatal hydrops. Mild dysostosis multiplex, laryngomalacia, and cardiomegaly have been reported in some instances. The disorder is lethal in infancy or early childhood as a result of infections or other problems related to profound debilitation.

Late infantile sialic acid storage disease (Salla syndrome). The later-onset disorder of excessive sialic acid excretion is named for Salla, the geographic region of northern Finland where the first kindred was recognized.[695,790] Affected children come to medical attention during late infancy or early childhood with developmental delay but with normal facial features, normal radiographic appearance of the skeleton, and equivocal organomegaly. Speech development is only minimal. The neurologic disease is progressive, with ataxia, nystagmus, pyramidal spasticity with hyperactive tendon reflexes, and seizures. A milder phenotype is also recognized.[246] Prenatal diagnosis has been accomplished based on estimation of sialic acid content in amniocytes.[645]

Pathology. Clear membrane-bound lysosomal inclusions are seen by means of electron microscopy in peripheral lymphocytes and in other tissues.[830,912]

Fundamental defect. The primary metabolic defect appears to be related to lysosomal transport of sialic acid, but it has not been precisely identified.

Prevalence and inheritance. All types appear to be autosomal recessive. The form described as Salla syndrome appears to have a higher incidence in northern Scandinavia, but it is also observed in other populations.[224,912]

Mucolipidosis Type IV

The first patient with ML type IV was described by Berman[75] in 1974. Clinical diagnosis of this disorder has been extremely challenging, and the basic defect remains unknown.

Clinical manifestations. The clinical spectrum of ML type IV and the natural history in the Ashkenazi population have been reviewed.[18] The disorder becomes evident as mild or moderate psychomotor retardation, typically during the first year of life. There are multiple ophthalmologic abnormalities, including variable degrees of corneal opacification, corneal surface irregularities, strabismus, retinal degeneration, and myopia.[3,603,821] In contrast to the mucopolysaccharidoses, organomegaly and skeletal changes are not present. Urinary glycosaminoglycan excretion is normal. Despite the early age of onset, central nervous sys-

tem involvement and the ophthalmologic abnormalities are relatively nonprogressive. In fact, improvement has been seen in some patients who have had occupational and physical therapy. This lack of deterioration is quite unusual when compared to the deterioration in other lysosomal storage diseases. Life expectancy is largely unknown: patients identified since 1974 remain alive. Because the primary defect is unknown, the diagnosis must be accomplished by correlating clinical features with ultrastructural findings (discussed later in this section) and ganglioside-loading studies.[936]

Pathology. Phase-contrast microscopy of cultured fibroblasts shows numerous 1-2 μm inclusions similar to those in ML type II. Further evidence for classifying this disorder as an ML is provided by electronmicroscopy; ultrastructural studies of a skin biopsy specimen show lamelated structures indicative of lipid storage (phospholipids and gangliosides) but also fibrillogranular material suggestive of water-soluble materials (glycosaminoglycans). Identification of these ultrastructural markers in cultured amniotic fluid cells and chorionic villi have facilitated prenatal diagnosis.[633]

Fundamental defect. The primary defect of ML type IV remains unknown, but quantitative biochemical studies have shown accumulation of phospholipids, gangliosides, and glycosaminoglycans.[37,44,45,491] In contrast to the lysosomal enzymes in ML types II and III, most lysosomal enzymes are measured at normal levels in cultured fibroblasts and in plasma, thus excluding an analogous defect in lysosomal enzyme processing.

Prevalence and inheritance. Mucolipidosis type IV is found in relatively high frequency among Ashkenazi Jews; this group accounts for about half of the known cases. Although there have been no epidemiologic studies, approximately 60 patients are known, almost all of whom belong to this ethnogeographic group.

Multiple Sulfatase Deficiency (Mucosulfatidosis, Austin Syndrome)

In 1965 Austin[32] described the first patients with this disorder, who were subsequently found to have deficiency of several lysosomal sulfatase enzymes. Consequently the initial diagnosis may be one of the other sulfatase-deficiency conditions (e.g., metachromatic leukodystrophy, Maroteaux-Lamy syndrome, and the like) but with "atypical" features.

Clinical manifestations. The disorder is usually severe, with many abnormalities leading to concern before the patient is 2 years of age.[602] The clinical phenotype includes several abnormalities attributable to specific sulfatase-deficiency states.[431] There are usually several features of Maroteaux-Lamy syndrome (hepatosplenomegaly and dysostosis multiplex), neurodegenerative signs with demyelination, as seen in infantile metachromatic leukodystrophy,[32] and ichthyosis characteristic of steroid sulfatase deficiency. Ophthalmologic examination shows loss of retinal pigment, grey maculae, and optic atrophy. Affected children progress to a vegetative state and die during the first decade of life. Clinical variants include a neonatal form with a more rapidly progressive course[117,847] and a late-onset form with slower deterioration. The diagnosis is confirmed by demonstration of excessive excretion of urinary glycosaminoglycans and significant deficiencies of several sulfatase enzymes.

Pathology. Alder-Reilly granulation of leukocytes is usually present, as well as lysosomal inclusions in other tissues.[237]

Fundamental defect. It is likely that the mutations responsible for multiple sulfatase deficiency affect a protein responsible for stabilizing several sulfatase enzymes. The enzymes deficient in this condition are heparan sulfamidase (MPS type IIIA), iduronate-2-sulfatase (MPS type II), steroid sulfatase (ichthyosis), arylsulfatase A (metachromatic leukodystrophy), and arylsulfatase B (MPS type VI).

Prevalence and inheritance. The disorder follows an autosomal recessive mode of transmission, but the genetic locus has not been identified. The disorder is extremely rare and is panethnic in distribution.[237]

PRINCIPLES OF MANAGEMENT

The management of the MPS group of conditions that have been reviewed in this chapter is not an easy matter. Although many texts still indicate that "no specific therapy is available," this fatalistic view is gradually giving way to the more humane philosophy that some measures are useful in providing comfort, a better quality of life, and some increase in longevity. In sum the attitudes that determine medical management for affected individuals are changing dramatically, despite the many hurdles to be overcome in achieving satisfactory care.

In addition to the modest but encouraging improvements that have been achieved by early attempts at bone marrow transplantation, there is a general appreciation of the difficulties and challenges for families coping with affected children. This includes a recognition that appropriate management includes a "phased" transition of care required by the patient.[168] Initially the family needs special education and counseling regarding the nature of the condition. Later the child becomes increasingly handicapped with major physical limitations and may need surgical repair of hernias, tonsillectomy, adenoidectomy, and tracheostomy, together with special attention to cardiac complications and pulmonary infections. Anesthesia is especially challenging and requires special attention; practitioners should be alerted to these issues.[41,42,63,338,771] The family needs special assistance in traversing the morass of medical care and community resources. In some instances the family may need help in dealing with the terminal stages of the disease, possibly including respite care. A clinic for children with developmental disabilities that has a multidisciplinary approach provides the optimal setting for long-term management.

At the time of diagnosis each affected child should have a thorough medical evaluation, including a review of the history of infections and respiratory symptoms and a hearing assessment. The diagnosis should be confirmed by quantitation of the appropriate enzyme(s) in blood and by measurement of urine glycosaminoglycan excretion. A formal psychometric evaluation (e.g., Bayley Scales of Infant Development) and cranial imaging (CT or MRI) should be performed to establish the extent of neurologic involvement. A cardiologist should assess the status of the heart and make recommendations based on physical examination, chest radiograph, electrocardiogram, and echocardiogram. If there is involvement of the cardiac valves, antibiotics should be administered at the time of dental and surgical procedures in order to prevent the development of subacute bacte-

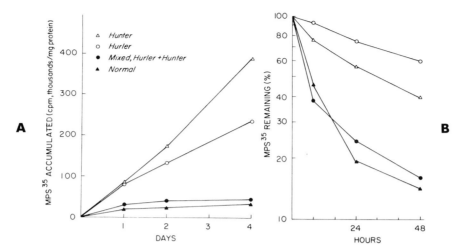

Fig. 11-66. Experiments indicate defective glycosaminoglycan degradation in fibroblast cell lines derived from individuals with Hurler and Hunter syndromes, and mutual correction of their defects by coculture. **A,** Excessive accumulation of radiolabeled glycosaminoglycan (MPS³⁵) in disease fibroblasts. **B,** Retarded clearance of radiolabeled glycosaminoglycan in disease fibroblasts. (Courtesy Dr. Elizabeth F. Neufeld, University of California at Los Angeles.)

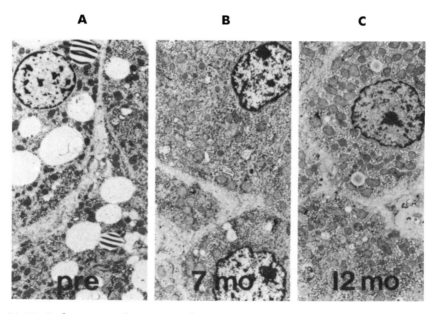

Fig. 11-67. Before transplantation, electron microscopy of liver showed the ultrastructural correlates of lysosomal glycosaminoglycan accumulation. Single membrane-bound inclusions, some the size of cell nuclei, were abundant in all hepatocytes, **A,** and in Kupffer cells (not shown). Examination at 7 and 12 months after transplantation, **B** and **C,** revealed normal morphologic appearance of liver without ultrastructural evidence of lysosomal disease. (From Whitley CB et al: *Birth Defects* 22:7-24, 1986.)

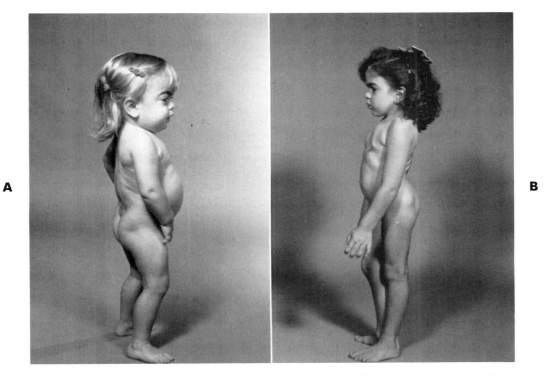

Fig. 11-68. A, General appearance of a 2-year-old girl with Hurler syndrome, before transplantation. **B,** The same child at 9½ years of age, after engraftment with marrow from her brother.

rial endocarditis. Patients with MPS should have a thorough medical evaluation annually, including follow-up laboratory tests. Children who travel by air should receive an antibiotic and a decongestant 2 days before and for 2 days after the flight. This regimen minimizes the risk of otitis media resulting from inherent eustacian tube dysfunction.

Early experiments by Neufeld et al.[600] differentiated nonallelic forms of MPS by demonstrating "corrective factors," initially by means of cocultivation (Fig. 11-66), and, later, by incubation of cells with partially purified enzyme. Such studies essentially mapped out an approach to treatment, which has evolved from strategies for enzyme replacement to the current application of allogeneic bone marrow transplantation; undoubtedly, gene therapy will become an accepted, superior method of intervention.

Bone marrow transplantation achieves considerable metabolic correction in many tissues. For example, in patients with Hurler syndrome, serial liver biopsy specimens have demonstrated small increases in α-L-iduronidase enzyme activity after donor engraftment, levels reaching 3% to 10% of normal. These relatively small increases in enzyme level are associated with reversal of hepatic glycosaminoglycan accumulation[698,902] and clearance of the morphologic correlates of lysosomal substrate accumulation (Fig. 11-67). As a consequence, there is diminution of the clinical stigmata, including attenuation of the usually progressive dysmorphic physical appearance (Fig. 11-68). Several mechanisms of metabolic correction may be operating (Fig. 11-69).

The clinical efficacy of bone marrow transplantation is limited in two respects. The physiologic "blood-brain" barrier presents a significant impediment to the treatment of the neurologic aspects of MPS. Despite this barrier, bone marrow transplantation effectively reduces lumbar spinal fluid pressure and the manifestations of hydrocephalus. The extent by which enzyme penetrates into central nervous system parenchyma and its effect on progressive metabolic brain injury continue to be

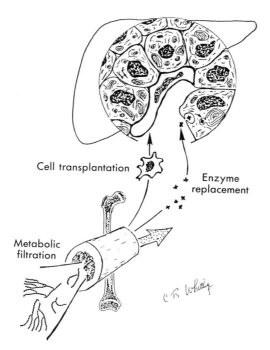

Fig. 11-69. Four mechanisms may explain metabolic correction in liver after bone marrow transplantation for mucopolysaccharidoses. *Cell transplantation* of normal stem cells for the hepatic Kupffer cell population replaces a small pool of defective cells. Endogenous *enzyme replacement* to lysosomes may occur by receptor-mediated uptake of circulating enzyme (illustrated) or by transfer of enzyme mediated by direct cell-to-cell contact. *Metabolic filtration* of blood-borne substrates by metabolically competent transplanted marrow may also decrease the circulating pool of glycosaminoglycans. In Sly syndrome (and, possibly, in other mucopolysaccharidoses) *plasma catalysis* (not shown) of glycosaminoglycan by free enzyme in the plasma compartment may be effective if the reaction occurs at plasma pH, as would be expected for β-glucuronidase. (Modified from Whitley CB et al: *Birth Defects* 22:7-24, 1986.)

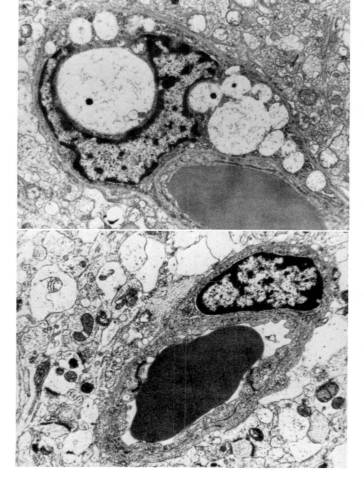

Fig. 11-70. A, Brain perithelial cell markedly distended with lysosomal inclusions from a Plott hound affected with α-L-iduronidase deficiency, a canine model for Hurler-Scheie syndrome. **B,** Perithelial cells appear normal in an affected litter mate 1 year after marrow transplantation. (Courtesy Dr. Robert Shull, College of Veterinary Medicine, Knoxville, Tenn.)

evaluated. There is some evidence from animal models to suggest that enzyme does enter the brain tissue[762,766] and reduces the accumulation of stored molecules (Fig. 11-70). Although children who have received successful transplantation are not without sequelae, longevity and quality of life for some patients is impressive, especially for those who are engrafted early in the course of the disease.

A second limitation in the achievement of effective treatment stems from the observation that the clinical outcome is limited by any preexisting tissue damage. For example, an abnormal pattern of skeletal growth established early in the course of disease will continue to cause significant disability, particularly when kyphoscoliosis, hip dysplasia, and knock-knees are part of the phenotype. Furthermore, brain damage resulting from hydrocephalus and from more direct neuron injury is not repairable. Thus a major determinant of long-term intellectual outcome appears to be the degree of brain damage present before engraftment; younger children having normal intellectual function and minimal structural damage (assessed by cranial CT scan or MRI) appear to derive the greatest benefit from transplantation. Newborn screening for MPS[895] (analogous to newborn testing for other metabolic disorders, e.g., phenylketonuria and galactosemia) and early transplantation in affected infants should result in a substantial improvement in long-term outcome.

The practice of concerned families meeting to provide mutual support goes back historically to the informal gatherings in Minneapolis of Sylvester Sanfilippo with some of his patients in the 1960s. In 1974 several families in New York formalized a group, the National MPS Society, in order to enable affected families to share concerns and solutions regarding their children. Under the vigorous leadership of its president, Marie Capobianco, this Society evolved, was incorporated as a nonprofit organization in the 1980s, and began to hold annual meetings around the country. The growth of such family-developed support groups in the United States and in other countries has served to bring together the families who otherwise develop a sense of isolation. Such family support groups also motivate clinicians and laboratory investigators toward advancing clinical and basic research.

In 1988 the First International Congress on Mucopolysaccharidosis and Related Diseases was held in Minneapolis to consolidate recent progress. At the conclusion of the meeting Victor McKusick summarized[891] the state of research:

What we need to do in this group of conditions is to go for the genes. This is not just for gene therapy, but because the ultimate goal may be, as much as anything else, for "gene diagnosis," especially because of the allelic heterogeneity on the one hand and, on the other hand, the necessity for early diagnosis in order to institute therapy in time for maximum benefit. I hope that in 20, 30, or 40 years from now we will have gene therapy and we will look back on this era as a primitive stage in development of management for these conditions.

REFERENCES

1. Abraham D et al: Structural analysis of the major urinary oligosaccharides in feline alpha-mannosidosis, *Biochem J* 233:899-904, 1986.
2. Abraham D et al: Lymphocytes transfer only the lysosomal form of alpha-D-mannosidase during cell-to-cell contact, *Exp Cell Res* 175:158-168, 1988.
3. Abraham FA et al: Retinal function in mucolipidosis IV, *Ophthalmologica* 191:210-214, 1985.
4. Adachi K, Chole RA: Management of tracheal lesions in Hurler syndrome, *Arch Otolaryngol Head Neck Surg* 116:1205-1207, 1990.
5. Adebahr G, Ritter C: Mucopolysaccharidosis II (Hunter syndrome) and III (Sanfilippo syndrome) as a cause of emaciation initially related to neglect, *Z Rechtsmed* 95:285-295, 1985.
6. Adinolfi M, Brown S: Strategies for the correction of enzymatic deficiencies in patients with mucopolysaccharidoses, *Dev Med Child Neurol* 26:404-408, 1984.
7. Adinolfi M et al: Transplantation of fetal fibroblasts and correction of enzymatic deficiencies in patients with Hunter's or Hurler's disorders, *Transplantation* 42:271-274, 1986.
8. Aegerter EE, Kirkpatrick JA Jr: *Orthopaedic diseases: physiology, pathology and radiology*, Philadelphia, 1958, WB Saunders, p 99.
9. Afifi AK et al: Computed tomography and magnetic resonance imaging of the brain in Hurler's disease, *J Child Neurol* 5:235-241, 1990.
10. Ahern-Rindell AJ, Murnane RD, Prieur DJ: Interspecific genetic complementation analysis of human and sheep fibroblasts with beta-galactosidase deficiency, *Somatic Cell Mol Genet* 15:525-533, 1989.
11. Akle C et al: Transplantation of amniotic epithelial membranes in patients with mucopolysaccharidoses, *Exp Clin Immunogenet* 2:43-48, 1985.
12. Alder A: Uber konstitutionell bedingte Granulationsveranderungen der leukozyten, *Helv Paediatr Acta* 11:165, 1944.
13. Allanson JE et al: Deletion mapping of the beta-glucuronidase gene, *Am J Med Genet* 29:517-522, 1988.
14. Allegranza A et al: Sialidosis type I: pathological study in an adult, *Clin Neuropathol* 8:266-271, 1989.

15. Allen HJ, Ahmed H, DiCioccio RA: Metabolic correction of fucosidosis lymphoid cells by galaptin-alpha-L-fucosidase conjugates, *Biochem Biophys Res Commun* 172:335-340, 1990.

16. Alroy J, Ucci AA, Warren CD: Human and canine fucosidosis: a comparative lectin histochemistry study, *Acta Neuropathol* 67:265-271, 1985.

17. Alroy J et al: Morphology of leukocytes from cats affected with alpha-mannosidosis and mucopolysaccharidosis VI (MPS VI), *Vet Pathol* 26:294-302, 1989.

18. Amir N, Zlotogora J, Bach G: Mucolipidosis type IV: clinical spectrum and natural history, *Pediatrics* 79:952-959, 1987.

19. Anderson CE et al: Morquio's disease and dysplasia epiphysealis multiplex: a study of epiphyseal cartilage in seven cases, *J Bone Joint Surg* 44A:295-306, 1962.

20. Andersson B, Tandberg O: Lipochondrodystrophy (gargoylism, Hurler syndrome) with specific cutaneous deposits, *Acta Paediatr Scand* 41:162-167, 1952.

21. Andreassi A, Andreassi A: A proposito di un case di gargoilismo: esiste nella provincia de l'Aquila inn "focolaio" di tale forma morbosal, *Minerva Pediatr* 21:1077-1082, 1969.

22. Andria G et al: Sanfilippo B syndrome (MPS III B): mild and severe forms within the same sibship, *Clin Genet* 15:500-504, 1979.

23. Applegarth DA et al: Morquio disease presenting as hydrops fetalis and enzyme analysis of chorionic villus tissue in a subsequent pregnancy, *Pediatr Pathol* 7:593-599, 1987.

24. Arbisser AI et al: Morquio-like syndrome with beta-galactosidase deficiency and normal hexosamine sulphatase activity: mucopolysaccharidosis IVB, *Am J Med Genet* 1:195, 1977.

25. Archer IM, Kingston HM, Harper PS: Prenatal diagnosis of Hunter syndrome, *Prenat Diagn* 4:195-200, 1984.

26. Archer IM et al: Carrier detection in Hunter syndrome, *Am J Med Genet* 16:61, 1983.

27. Asami T, Mito Y, Askai K: Mass-screening for acid mucopolysaccharidosis using urine samples by modified HCl-albumin turbidity method, *Rinsho Byori* 37:1247-1251, 1989.

28. Asano K et al: A case of GM1-gangliosidosis type I: glycosphingolipid profiles of urine and transformed lymphocytes, cultured skin fibroblasts and transformed lymphocytes, *Jpn J Exp Med* 60:73-79, 1990.

29. Ashby WR, Stewart RM, Watkin IH: Chondro-osteo-dystrophy of Hurler type (gargoylism): a pathological study, *Brain* 60:149-179, 1997.

30. Ashraf J et al: Transoral decompression and posterior stabilisation in Morquio's disease, *Arch Dis Child* 66:1318-1321, 1991.

31. Ashton LJ et al: Immunoquantification and enzyme kinetics of α-L-iduronidase in cultured fibroblasts from normal controls and mucopolysaccharidosis type I patients, *Am J Hum Genet* 50:787-794, 1992.

32. Austin JH: Studies in metachromatic leukodystrophy. XII. Multiple sulfatase deficiency, *Arch Neurol* 28:258-264, 1973.

33. Awwaad S: Dysostosis multiplex: review of literature and report of two cases with unusual manifestations, *Arch Pediatr* 78:184-193, 1961.

34. Aycock EK, Paul IR Jr: Gargoylism: a report of two cases in Negroes, *J S C Med Assoc* 53:128-130, 1957.

35. Aylsworth AS et al: Mannosidosis:phenotype of a severely affected child and characterization of α-mannosidase activity in cultured fibroblasts from the patient and his parents, *J Pediatr* 88:814-818, 1976.

36. Babcock DS et al: Fetal mucolipidosis II (I-cell disease): radiologic and pathologic correlation, *Pediatr Radiol* 16:32-39, 1986.

37. Bach G, Desnick RJ: Lysosomal accumulation of phospholipids in mucolipidosis IV cultured fibroblasts, *Enzyme* 40:40-44, 1988.

38. Bach G et al: The defect in the Hunter syndrome: deficiency of sulfoiduronate sulfatase, *Proc Natl Acad Sci USA* 70:2134-2138, 1973.

39. Bach G et al: The defect in the Hurler and Scheie syndromes: deficiency of α-L-iduronidase, *Proc Natl Acad Sci USA* 69:2048-2051, 1972.

40. Baines D: Suxamethonium in mucopolysaccharidosis (letter; comment), *Anaesth Intensive Care* 17:382, 1989.

41. Baines D, Keneally J: Anaesthetic implications of the mucopolysaccharidoses: a fifteen year experience in a children's hospital, *Anaesth Intensive Care* 11:198-202, 1983.

42. Baines D, Keneally J: Mucopolysaccharidoses and anaesthesia (letter), *Can J Anaesth* 35:540-541, 1988.

43. Banna M, Hollenberg R: Compressive meningeal hypertrophy in mucopolysaccharidosis (letter), *AJNR* 8:385-386, 1987.

44. Bargal R, Bach G: Phospholipids accumulation in mucolipidosis IV cultured fibroblasts, *J Inherited Metab Dis* 11:144-150, 1988.

45. Bargal R, Bach G: Phosphatidylcholine storage in mucolipidosis IV, *Clin Chim Acta* 181:167-174, 1989.

46. Barker C et al: Canine alpha-L-fucosidase in relation to the enzymatic defect and storage products in canine fucosidosis, *Biochem J* 254:861-868, 1988.

47. Barker CG et al: GM1 gangliosidosis (type 1) in a cat, *Biochem J* 235:151-158, 1986.

48. Bartman J, Blanc WA: Fibroblast cultures in Hurler's and Hunter's syndromes: an ultrastructural study, *Arch Pathol* 89:279-285, 1970.

49. Bartman J, Mandelbaum IM, Gregoire PE: Mucopolysaccharides of serum and urine in a case of Morquio's disease, *Rev Fr Etude Clin Biol* 8:250-254, 1969.

50. Barton NW et al: Therapeutic response to intravenous infusions of glucocerebrosidase in a patient with Gaucher disease, *Proc Natl Acad Sci USA* 87:1913-1916, 1990.

51. Barton NW et al: Replacement therapy for inherited enzyme deficiency: macrophage-target glucocerebrosidase for Gaucher's disease, *N Engl J Med* 324:1464-1470, 1991.

52. Barton RW, Neufeld EF: The Hurler corrective factor: purification and some properties, *J Biol Chem* 246:7773-7779, 1971.

53. Barton RW, Neufeld EF: A distinct biochemical deficit in the Maroteaux-Lamy syndrome (mucopolysaccharidosis VI), *J Pediatr* 80:114-116, 1972.

54. Bartsocas CS et al: Sanfilippo type C disease: clinical findings in four patients with a new variant of mucopolysaccharidosis III, *Eur J Pediatr* 130:251-258, 1979.

55. Beaudet AL et al: β-glucuronidase deficiency: altered enzyme substrate recognition (abstract), *Am J Hum Genet* 24:25a, 1972.

56. Beaudet AL et al: Variation in the phenotypic expression of β-glucuronidase deficiency, *J Pediatr* 86:388-394, 1975.

57. Beck M, Cole G: Disc oedema in association with Hunter's syndrome: ocular histopathological findings, *Br J Ophthalmol* 68:590-594, 1984.

58. Beck M et al: Heterogeneity of Morquio disease, *Clin Genet* 29:325-331, 1986.

59. Beck M et al: Morquio's disease type B (beta-galactosidase deficiency) in three siblings, *S Afr Med J* 72:704-707, 1987.

60. Beebe RT, Formel PF: Gargoylism: sex-linked transmission in nine males, *Bull Hist Med* 44:582-585, 1954.

61. Begany A et al: Forme fruste of Hunter's disease, *Z Hautkr* 64:228-230, 1989.

62. Begg AC: Nuclear herniations of the intervertebral disc: their radiological manifestations and significance, *J Bone Joint Surg* 96B:180-193, 1954.

63. Belani KG et al: Perioperative management, morbidity and new findings in children with the mucopolysaccharidoses, *J Pediatr Surg* (in press).

64. Bell CE, Sly WS, Brot FE: Human β-glucuronidase deficiency mucopolysaccharidosis, *J Clin Invest* 59:97, 1977.

65. Ben-Yousef Y, Mitchell DA, Nadler HL: First trimester prenatal evaluation for I-cell disease by *N*-acetyl-glucosamine 1-phosphotransferase assay, *Clin Genet* 33:38-43, 1988.

66. Ben-Yousef Y et al: Characterization of the mutant *N*-acetylglucosaminylphosphotransferase in I-cell disease and pseudo-Hurler polydystrophy: complementation analysis and kinetic studies, *Enzyme* 35:106-116, 1986.

67. Ben-Yousef Y et al: Altered molecular size of *N*-acetylglucosamine 1-phosphotransferase in I-cell disease and pseudo-Hurler polydystrophy, *Biochem J* 248:697-701, 1987.

68. Berard-Badier M: Etude ultrastructurale du parenchyme hepatique dans les mucopolysaccharidoses, *Pathol Biol* (Paris) 18:117-128, 1970.

69. Beratis NG et al: Arylsulfatase B deficiency in Maroteaux-Lamy syndrome: cellular studies and carrier identification, *Pediatr Res* 9:639-641, 1985.

70. Beratis NG et al: Sanfilippo disease in Greece, *Clin Genet* 29:129-132, 1986.

71. Beratis NG et al: Angiokeratoma corporis diffusum in GM1 gangliosidosis, type 1, *Clin Genet* 36:59-64, 1989.

72. Berg K, Danes BS, Bearn AG: The linkage relation of the loci for the Xm serum system and the X-linked form of Hurler's syndrome (Hunter's syndrome), *Am J Hum Genet* 20:398-401, 1968.

73. Berkhan O: Zwei Falle von Skaphokephalie, *Arch Anthrop* 34:8, 1907.

74. Berliner MI: Lipin keratitis of Hurler's syndrome (gargoylism or dysostosis multiplex): clinical and pathologic report, *Arch Ophthalmol* 22:97-105, 1939.

75. Berman ER: Congenital corneal clouding with abnormal systemic storage bodies: a new variant of mucolipidosis, *J Pediatr* 85:519-526, 1974.

76. Bernsen PL et al: Phenotypic expression in mucopolysaccharidosis VII, *J Neurol Neurosurg Psychiatry* 50:699-703, 1987.

77. Berry HK: Procedures for testing urine specimens dried on filter paper, *Clin Chem* 5:603-608, 1959.

78. Berry HK: Screening for mucopolysaccharide disorders with the Berry spot test, *Clin Biochem* 20:365-371, 1987.

79. Berry HK, Spinanger J: A paper spot test useful in study of Hurler's syndrome, *J Lab Clin Med* 55:136-138, 1962.

80. Besley GT et al: Prenatal diagnosis of mucolipidosis II by early amniocentesis (letter), *Lancet* 335:1164-1165, 1990.

81. Betremieux P et al: Insuffisance cardiaque aigue chez une fillette attiente de maladie de Maroteaux-Lamy, *Ann Pediatr* 32:639-641, 1985.

82. References deleted in proofs.

83. Bieber FR et al: Pathologic findings in fetal GM1 gangliosidosis, *Arch Neurol* 43:736-738, 1986.

84. Bindschedler IJ: Polydystrophie du type Hurler chez un frere et une soeur, *Bull Soc Pediatr Paris* 36:571-576, 1938.

85. Birkenmeier EH et al: Murine mucopolysaccharidosis type VII: characterization of a mouse with beta-glucuronidase deficiency, *J Clin Invest* 83:1258-1266, 1989.

86. Birkenmeier EH et al: Increased life span and correction of metabolic defects in murine mucopolysaccharidosis type VII after syngeneic bone marrow transplantation, *Blood* 78:3081-3092, 1991.

87. Bishton RL, Norman RM, Tingey A: The pathology and chemistry of a case of gargoylism, *J Clin Pathol* 9:305-315, 1956.

88. Bitter T, Muir HM: A modified uronic acid carbazole reaction, *Anal Biochem* 4:330-334, 1962.

89. Bitter T et al: A contribution to the differential diagnosis of Hurler's disease and forms of Morquio's syndrome, *J Bone Joint Surg* 48B:637-645, 1966.

90. Black SH et al: Maroteaux-Lamy syndrome in a large consanguineous kindred: biochemical and immunological studies, *Am J Med Genet* 25:273-279, 1986.

91. Blaw ME, Langer LO: Spinal cord compression in Morquio Brailsford disease, *J Pediatr* 74:599-600, 1969.

92. Blitzer MG et al: A thermolabile variant of α-L-fucosidase—clinical and laboratory findings, *Am J Med Genet* 20:535-539, 1985.

93. Böcker E: Zur Erblichkeit der Dysostosis multiplex, *Z Kinderheilk* 63:688, 1949.

94. Bona C, Stanescu V, Ionescu V: Histochemical studies of growing human cartilage in Morquio's disease, *J Pathol* 103:134-140, 1971.

95. Booth CW, Nadler HL: In vitro selection for the Hunter gene, *N Engl J Med* 288:636, 1973.

96. Booth CW, Nadler HL: Plasma infusion in an infant with Hurler's syndrome, *J Pediatr* 82:273-278, 1973.

97. Booth CW, Nadler HL: Demonstration of the heterozygous state in Hunter's syndrome, *Pediatrics* 53:396-399, 1974.

98. Boyer PJ, Lovell KL: Investigation of dysmyelinogenesis in caprine beta-mannosidosis: in vitro characterization of oligodendrocytes, *Glia* 3:222-227, 1990.

99. Boyer PJ et al: Caprine beta-mannosidosis: abnormal thyroid structure and function in a lysosomal storage disease, *Lab Invest* 63:100-106, 1990.

100. Boyer PJ et al: Regional central nervous system oligosaccharide storage in caprine beta-mannosidosis, *J Neurochem* 55:660-664, 1990.

101. Bradbury JA, Martin L, Strachan IM: Acquired Brown's syndrome associated with Hurler-Scheie's syndrome, *Br J Ophthalmol* 73:305-308, 1989.

102. Brailsford JF: Chondro-osteo-dystrophy, roentgenographic and clinical features of child with dislocation of vertebrae, *Am J Surg* 7:404-410, 1929.

103. Brama I et al: Upper airway obstruction in Hunter syndrome, *Int J Pediatr Otorhinolaryngol* 11:229-235, 1986.

104. Brante G: Gargoylism: a mucopolysaccharidosis, *Scand J Clin Lab Invest* 4:43-46, 1952.

105. Brassart D et al: Catabolism of *N*-glycosylprotein glycans: evidence for a degradation pathway of sialylglyco-asparagines resulting from the combined action of the lysosomal aspartylglucosaminidase and endo- *N*-acetyl-beta-D-glucosaminidase; a 400-MHz 1H-NMR study, *Eur J Biochem* 169:131-136, 1987.

106. Braunlin EA et al: Evaluation of coronary artery disease in Hurler syndrome by coronary artery angiography, *Am J Cardiol* (in press).

107. Braunlin EA et al: Great vessel anomaly in Hurler syndrome, (in press).

108. Breider MA, Shull RM, Constantopoulos G: Long-term effects of bone marrow transplantation in dogs with mucopolysaccharidosis I, *Am J Pathol* 134:677-692, 1989.

109. Brill CB et al: Spastic quadriparesis due to C_1-C_2 subluxation in Hurler syndrome, *J Pediatr* 92:441-443, 1978.

110. Brimble A, Pennock C, Stone J: Results of a quality assurance exercise for urinary glycosaminoglycan excretion, *Ann Clin Biochem* 27:133-138, 1990.

111. Broadhead DM et al: Full expression of Hunter's disease in a female with an X-chromosome deletion leading to nonrandom inactivation, *Clin Genet* 30:392-398, 1986.

112. Brooks DA et al: Immunoquantification of the low abundance lysosomal enzyme *N*-acetylgalactosamine 4-sulphatase, *J Inherited Metab Dis* 13:108-120, 1990.

113. Brooks DA et al: Analysis of *N*-acetylgalactosamine-4-sulfatase protein and kinetics in mucopolysaccharidosis type VI patients, *Am J Hum Genet* 48:710-719, 1991.

114. Brosius FC, Roberts WC: Coronary artery disease in the Hurler syndrome: qualitative and quantitative analysis of the extent of coronary narrowing at necropsy in six children, *Am J Cardiol* 47:649-653, 1981.

115. Brown DH: Tissue storage of mucopolysaccharides in Hurler-Pfaundler's disease, *Proc Natl Acad Sci USA* 43:789-790, 1957.

116. Brown TC: The airway in mucopolysaccharidoses (letter), *Anaesth Intensive Care* 12:178, 1984.

117. Burch M et al: Multiple sulphatase deficiency presenting at birth, *Clin Genet* 30:409-415, 1986.

118. Burillon C, Pey C, Durand L: Penetrating keratoplasty and corneal dystrophy in Scheie's syndrome, *J Fr Ophthalmol* 12:561-568, 1989.

119. Butman SM, Karl L, Copeland JG: Combined aortic and mitral valve replacement in an adult with Scheie's disease, *Chest* 96:209-210, 1989.

120. Butterworth T, Strean LP: *Clinical genodermatoses*, Baltimore, 1962, Williams & Wilkins.

121. Cabral A et al: A case of GM1 gangliosidosis type I, *Ophthalmic Paediatr Genet* 10:63-67, 1989.

122. Caffey J: Gargoylism (Hunter-Hurler disease, dysostosis multiplex, lipochondrodystrophy): prenatal and neonatal bone lesions and their early postnatal evaluation, *Am J Roentgenol* 67:715-731, 1952.

123. Cahane M et al: Glaucoma in siblings with Morquio syndrome, *Br J Ophthalmol* 74:382-383, 1990.

124. Calatroni A, Donnelly PV, DiFerrante N: The glycosaminoglycans of human plasma, *J Clin Invest* 48:332-343, 1969.

125. Callahan WP, Hackett RL, Lorincz AE: New observations by light microscopy on liver histology in the Hurler's syndrome: a needle biopsy study of 11 patients utilizing plastic embedded tissue, *Arch Pathol* 83:507-512, 1967.

126. Callahan WP, Lorincz AE: Hepatic ultrastructure in the Hurler syndrome, *Am J Pathol* 48:277-298, 1966.

127. Campbell TN, Fried M: Urinary mucopolysaccharide excretion in the sex-linked form of the Hurler syndrome, *Proc Soc Exp Biol Med* 108:529-533, 1961.

128. Cantor LB, Disseler JA, Wilson FM: Glaucoma in the Maroteaux-Lamy syndrome, *Am J Ophthalmol* 108:426-430, 1989.

129. Cantz M, Chrambach A, Neufeld EF: Characterization of the factor deficient in the Hunter syndrome by polyacrylamide gel electrophoresis, *Biochem Biophys Res Commun* 39:936-942, 1970.

130. Cantz M, Gehler J: The mucopolysaccharidoses: inborn errors of glycosaminoglycans catabolism, *Hum Genet* 32:233, 1976.

131. Cantz M et al: The Hunter corrective factor: purification and preliminary characterization, *J Biol Chem* 247:5456-5462, 1972.

132. Capdeville R et al: A new case of mucopolysaccharidosis type VII with major skeletal abnormalities, *Ann Pediatr* 30:689-692, 1983.

133. Carneiro-Sampaio MM et al: Selective IgA deficiency associated with Hunter syndrome, *Rev Hosp Clin Fac Med Sao Paulo* 43:246-249, 1988.

134. Carpenter S, Karpati G: Lysosomal storage in human skeletal muscle, *Hum Pathol* 17:683-703, 1986.

135. Carter CH, Wan AT, Carpenter DG: Commonly used tests in the detection of Hurler's syndrome, *J Pediatr* 73:217-221, 1968.

136. Caruso RC et al: Electroretinographic findings in the mucopolysaccharidoses, *Ophthalmology* 93:1612-1616, 1986.

137. Castagnaro M: Lectin histochemistry of the central nervous system in a case of feline alpha-mannosidosis, *Res Vet Sci* 49:375-377, 1990.

138. Castagnaro M et al: Lectin histochemistry and ultrastructure of kidneys from patients with I-cell disease, *Arch Pathol Lab Med* 111:285-290, 1987.

139. Chang P, Rosa NE, Davidson RB: Differential assay of arylsufatase A and B activities: a sensitive method for cultured human cells, *Anal Biochem* 117:382-389, 1981.

140. Chapman S et al: Atypical radiological features of beta-glucuronidase deficiency (mucopolysaccharidosis VII) occurring in an elderly patient from an inbred kindred, *Br J Radiol* 62:491-494, 1989.

141. Charrow J, Hvizd MG: Cardiomyopathy and skeletal myopathy in an unusual variant of GM1 gangliosidosis, *J Pediatr* 108:729-732, 1986.

142. Chase DS et al: Genetics of Hunter syndrome: carrier detection, new mutations, segregation and linkage analysis, *Ann Hum Genet* 50:349-360, 1986.

143. Chitayat D: Aspartylglucosaminuria in a Puerto Rican family: additional features of a panethnic disorder, *Am J Med Genet* 31:527-532, 1988.

144. Chou Y-C: Ocular signs in gargoylism, *Clin Med J* 78:190, 1959.

145. Christiansen SP, Smith TJ, Henslee-Downey PJ: Normal intraocular pressure after a bone marrow transplant in glaucoma associated with mucopolysaccharidosis type I-H, *Am J Ophthalmol* 109:230-231, 1990.

146. Clarke JT et al: Hunter disease (mucopolysaccharidosis type II) in a karyotypically normal girl, *Clin Genet* 37:355-362, 1990.

147. Clarke JT et al: Hunter disease (mucopolysaccharidosis type II) associated with unbalanced inactivation of the X chromosomes in a karyotypically normal girl, *Am J Hum Genet* 49:289-297, 1991.

148. Clausen J, Dyggve HV, Melchoir JC: Mucopolysaccharidosis: paper electrophoretic and infra-red analysis of the urine in gargoylism and Morquio-Ullrich's disease, *Arch Dis Child* 38:364-379, 1963.

149. Clements PR et al: Human α-L-iduronidase. 1. Purification, monoclonal antibody production, native and subunit molecular mass, *Eur J Biochem* 152:21-28, 1985.

150. Clements PR et al: Human α-L-iduronidase. II. Catalytic properties, *Eur J Biochem* 152:29-34, 1985.

151. Cockayne EA: Gargoylism (chondro-osteodystrophy, hepatosplenomegaly, deafness) in two brothers, *Proc R Soc Med* 30:104-107, 1936.

152. Colavita N et al: A further contribution to the knowledge of mucopolysaccharidosis I H/S compound: presentation of two cases and review of the literature, *Australas Radiol* 30:142-149, 1986.

153. Cole HN Jr et al: Gargoylism with cutaneous manifestations, *Arch Dermatol Syph* 66:371-383, 1952.

154. Collins MLZ, Traboulsi EI, Maumenee IH: Optic nerve head swelling and optic atrophy in the systemic mucopolysaccharidoses, *Ophthalmology* 97:1445-1449, 1990.

155. Colome MF et al: Radiological case of the month: type II mucolipidosis with neonatal disclosure, *Arch Fr Pediatr* 42:539-540, 1985.

156. Constantopoulos G, Dekaban AS, Scheie HG: Heterogeneity of disorders in patients with corneal clouding, normal intellect, and mucopolysaccharidosis, *Am J Ophthalmol* 72:1106-1117, 1971.

157. Constantopoulos G, Scott JA, Shull RM: Corneal opacity in canine MPS I: changes after bone marrow transplantation, *Invest Ophthalmol Vis Sci* 30:1802-1807, 1989.

158. Constantopoulos G et al: Neurochemical characterization of canine alpha-L-iduronidase deficiency disease (model of human mucopolysaccharidosis I), *J Neurochem* 45:1213-1217, 1985.

159. Conzelmann E, Sandhoff K: Partial enzyme deficiencies: residual activities on the development of neurological disorders, *Dev Neurosci* 6:58-71, 1983-1984.

160. Cooper A, Sardharwalla IB, Roberts MM: Human beta-mannosidase deficiency, *N Engl J Med* 315:1231, 1986.

161. Cooper A et al: Alpha- and beta-mannosidoses, *J Inherited Metab Dis* 13:538-548, 1990.

162. Coppa GV et al: Clinical heterogeneity in Sanfilippo disease (mucopolysaccharidosis type D): presentation of two new cases, *Eur J Pediatr* 140:130-132, 1983.

163. Coppa GV et al: Clinical application of a new simple method for the identification of mucopolysaccharidoses, *Helv Paediatr Acta* 42:419-423, 1987.

164. Coran AG, Eraklis AJ: Inguinal hernia in the Hurler-Hunter syndrome, *Surgery* 61:302-304, 1967.

165. Cottier H: Infantile kardiovaskuläre Sklerose bei Gargoylismus, *Schweiz Z Allg Path* 20:745-753, 1957.

166. Craig WS: Gargoylism in a twin brother and sister, *Arch Dis Child* 29:293-303, 1954.

167. Crocker AC: Therapeutic trials in the inborn errors: an attempt to modify Hurler's syndrome, *Pediatrics* 42:887-888, 1968.

168. Crocker AC, Cullinane MM: Families under stress: the diagnosis of Hurler's syndrome, *Postgrad Med* 51:223-229, 1972.

169. Crotty PL, Whitley CB: Assessment of iduronate-2-sulfatase mRNA expression in Hunter syndrome (mucopolysaccharidosis type II), *Hum Genet* (in press).

170. Crotty PL et al: Molecular genetics of Hunter syndrome: characterization of mutations in the gene encoding human iduronate-2-sulfatase, *Am J Clin Pathol* (in press).

171. Cuhadar M, Blaauw G: Carpal tunnel syndrome in childhood, *Z Kinderchir* 38:330-332, 1983.

172. Dahl DL et al: Beta-mannosidosis: prenatal detection of caprine allantoic fluid oligosaccharides with thin layer, gel permeation and high performance liquid chromatography, *J Inherited Metab Dis* 9:93-98, 1986.

173. Danes BS, Bearn AG: Hurler's syndrome: demonstration of an inherited disorder of connective tissue in cell culture, *Science* 149:987-989, 1965.

174. Danes BS, Bearn AG: Hurler's syndrome: effect of retinol (vitamin A alcohol) on cellular mucopolysaccharides in cultured human skin fibroblasts, *J Exp Med* 124:1181-1192, 1966.

175. Danes BS, Bearn AG: Cellular metachromasia: a genetic marker for studying the mucopolysaccharidoses, *Lancet* 1:241-243, 1967.

176. Danes BS, Bearn AG: The effect of retinol (vitamin A alcohol) on urinary excretion of mucopolysaccharides in the Hurler syndrome, *Lancet* 1:1029-1030, 1967.

177. Danes BS, Bearn AG: Correction of cellular metachromasia in cultured fibroblasts in several inherited mucopolysaccharidoses, *Proc Natl Acad Sci USA* 67:357-364, 1970.

178. Danes BS, Degnan M: Different clinical and biochemical phenotypes associated with β-glucuronidase deficiency, *Birth Defects* 10:251-257, 1974.

179. Danes BS, Grossman H: Bone dysplasias, including Morquio's syndrome studied in skin fibroblast cultures, *Am J Med* 47:708-720, 1969.

180. Danes BS, Scott JE, Bearn AG: Further studies on metachromasia in cultured human fibroblasts: staining of glycosaminoglycans (mucopolysaccharides) by Alcian blue in salt solutions, *J Exp Med* 132:765-774, 1970.

181. Danes BS et al: Antenatal diagnosis of mucopolysaccharidoses (letter), *Lancet* 1:946-947, 1970.

182. Danes BS et al: Different clinical and biochemical phenotypes associated with β-glucuronidase deficiency, *Birth Defects Original Article Series 10* (12):251, 1974.

183. Dangel ME, Tsou BH: Retinal involvement in Morquio's syndrome (MPS IV), *Ann Ophthalmol* 17:349-354, 1985.

184. Danks DM et al: The Sanfilippo syndrome: clinical, biochemical radiological, haematological, and pathological features of nine cases, *Aust Paediatr J* 8:174-186, 1972.

185. Darby JK et al: Restriction analysis of the structural alpha-L-fucosidase gene and its linkage to fucosidosis, *Am J Hum Genet* 43:749-755, 1988.

186. Davies DL et al: Hurler-Scheie phenotype associated with consanguinity, *J Inherited Metab Dis* 12(suppl):265-268, 1989.

187. Davis DB, Currier FP: Morquio's disease: report of two cases, *JAMA* 102:2173-2176, 1934.

188. Dawson G, Spranger JW: Fucosidosis: a glycosphingolipidosis (letter), *N Engl J Med* 285:122, 1971.

189. Dawson IM: The histology and histochemistry of gargoylism, *J Pathol Bacteriol* 67:587-604, 1954.

190. Dean MF: The iduronate sulphatase activities of cells and tissue fluids from patients with Hunter syndrome and normal controls, *J Inherited Metab Dis* 6:108-111, 1983.

191. Dean MF, Muir H: Mobilization of glycosaminoglycans by plasma infusion in mucopolysaccharidosis type III, *Nature [New Biol]* 243:143-146, 1973.

192. Dean MF et al: Enzyme replacement therapy by fibroblast transplantation: long-term biochemical study in three cases of Hunter's syndrome, *J Clin Invest* 63:138-145, 1979.

193. DeCloux RJ, Friederici HHR: Ultra-structural studies of the skin in Hurler's syndrome, *Arch Pathol* 88:350-358, 1969.

194. DeJong BP, Robertson WV, Schafer IA: Failure to induce scurvy by ascorbic acid depletion in a patient with Hurler's syndrome, *Pediatrics* 42:889-903, 1968.

195. DeJong JG et al: Dimethylmethylene blue−based spectrophotometry of glycosaminoglycans in untreated urine: a rapid screening procedure for mucopolysaccharidoses, *Clin Chem* 35:1472-1477, 1989.

196. Dekaban AS, Holden KR, Constantopoulos G: Effects of fresh plasma or whole blood transfusions on patients with various types of mucopolysaccharidosis, *Pediatrics* 50:688-692, 1972.

197. Dekaban AS, Patton VM: Hurler's and Sanfilippo's variants of mucopolysaccharidosis, *Arch Pathol* 91:434-443, 1971.

198. DeLange C: Dysostosis multiplex of the Hurler type (gargoylism), *Psychiatr Neurol* (Basel) 1-2:2-7, 1942.

199. Delleman JW, de Jong PT: Pigment epithelial pattern dystrophy: a peripheral type, *Br J Ophthalmol* 69:754-757, 1985.

200. DelMonte MA et al: Histopathology of Sanfilippo's syndrome, *Arch Opthalmol* 101:1255-1262, 1983.

201. Delvin EE, Pottier A, Glorieux FH: Comparative activity of arylsulfatases A and B on two synthetic substrates, *Biochem J* 157:353-356, 1976.

202. Desjobert A, Larget-Piet L: Variations in urinary mucopolysaccharides after injection of fibroblasts into patients with mucopolysaccharidoses, *Clin Chem* 33:1879-1882, 1987.

203. DiCioccio RA, Barlow JJ, Matta KL: Specific activity of alpha-L-fucosidase in sera with phenotypes of either low, intermediate, or high total enzyme activity and in a fucosidosis serum, *Biochem Genet* 24:115-130, 1986.

204. DiCioccio RA, Darby JK, Willems PJ: Abnormal expression of alpha-L-fucosidase in lymphoid cell lines of fucosidosis patients, *Biochem Genet* 27:279-290, 1989.

205. DiFerrante NM: The measurement of urinary mucopolysaccharides, *Anal Biochem* 21:98-106, 1967.

206. DiFerrante N, Lipscomb HS: Urinary glycosaminoglycans versus creatinine excretion: a used and abused parameter, *Clin Chim Acta* 30:69-72, 1970.

207. DiFerrante N, Nichols BL: A case of the Hunter syndrome with progeny, *Johns Hopkins Med J* 130:325-328, 1972.

208. DiFerrante N et al: Induced degradation of glycosaminoglycans in Hurler's and Hunter's syndromes by plasma infusion, *Proc Natl Acad Sci USA* 68:303-307, 1971.

209. DiFerrante N et al: Mucopolysaccharidosis VI (Maroteaux-Lamy disease): clinical and biochemical study of a mild variant case, *Johns Hopkins Med J* 135:42-54, 1974.

210. DiNatale P, Leder IG, Neufeld EF: A radioactive substrate and assay for α-L-iduronidase, *Clin Chim Acta* 77:211-218, 1977.

211. DiNatale P et al: First-trimester prenatal diagnosis of Sanfilippo C disease, *Prenat Diagn* 7:603-605, 1987.

212. Dodion J et al: Etude d'un cas d'oligophrenie polydystrophique (mucopolysaccharidose HS), *Pathol Eur* 1:50-66, 1966.

213. Donaldson MD et al: Hurler syndrome with cardiomyopathy in infancy, *J Pediatr* 114:430-432, 1989.

214. Dorfman A: Metabolism of acid mucopolysaccharides, *Biophys J* 4(suppl):155-165, 1964.

215. Dorfman A: Studies on the biochemistry of connective tissue, *Pediatrics* 22:576-589, 1958.

216. Dorfman A. In Stanbury JB, Wyngaarden JB, Frederickson DS, editors: *The metabolic basis of inherited disease*, ed 2, New York, 1966, McGraw-Hill.

217. Dorfman A, Lorincz AE: Occurrence of urinary acid mucopolysaccharides in the Hurler syndrome, *Proc Natl Acad Sci USA* 43:443-446, 1957.

218. Dorfman A, Ott ML: A turbidimetric method for the assay of hyaluronidase, *J Biol Chem* 172:367-375, 1948.

219. Dorland L et al: Beta-mannosidosis in two brothers with hearing loss, *J Inherited Metab Dis* 11:255-258, 1988.

220. Duckett S et al: The ultrastructure of metachromatic bodies in cultured fibroblasts in Hunter's syndrome, *Dev Med Child Neurol* 11:764-770, 1969.

221. Dugas M et al: Psychotic symptoms during the evolution of dementia in mucopolysaccharidosis of Hurler-Scheie phenotype, *Arch Fr Pediatr* 42:373-375, 1985.

222. Durand P, Borrone C: Fucosidosis and mannosidosis: glycoprotein and glycosylceramide storage diseases, *Helv Paediatr Acta* 26:19-27, 1971.

223. Durand P, Borrone C, Della Cella G: Fucosidosis, *J Pediatr* 75:665, 1969.

224. Echenne B et al: Salla disease in one non-Finnish patient, *Eur J Pediatr* 145:320-322, 1986.

225. Einhorn NH, Moore JR, Rountree IG: Osteochondrodystrophia deformans (Morquio's disease); observations at autopsy in one case, *Am J Dis Child* 72:536-544, 1946.

226. Einhorn NH et al: Osteochondrodystrophia deformans (Morquio's disease): report of three cases, *Am J Dis Child* 61:776-794, 1941.

227. Elliott H, Hopwood JJ: Detection of the Sanfilippo D syndrome by the use of a radiolabeled monosaccharide sulfate as the substrate for the estimation of *N*-acetylglucosamine-6-sulfate sulfatase, *Anal Biochem* 138:205-209, 1984.

228. Ellis RWB: Gargoylism (chondro-osteodystrophy, corneal opacities, hepatosplenomegaly and mental deficiency), *Proc R Soc Med* 30:158, 1936.

229. Ellis RWB, Sheldon W, Capon NB: Gargoylism (chondro-osteo-dystrophy, corneal opacities, hepatosplenomegaly and mental deficiency), *Q J Med* 5:119-139, 1936.

230. Elsner B.: Ultrastructure of the rectal wall in Hunter's syndrome, *Gastroenterology* 58:856-862, 1970.

231. Emanuel RW: Gargoylism with cardiovascular involvement in two brothers, *Br Heart J* 16:417-422, 1954.

232. Embury DH, Jerrett IV: Mannosidosis in Galloway calves, *Vet Pathol* 22:548-551, 1985.

233. Emerit I, Maroteaux P, Vemant P: Deux observations de mucopolysaccharidose avec atteinte cardio-vasculaire, *Presse Med* 74:507-510, 1966.

234. Emery JM et al: G$_{M1}$-gangliosidosis: ocular and pathological manifestations, *Arch Ophthalmol* 85:177-187, 1971.

235. Engel D: Dysostosis multiplex (Pfaundler-Hurler syndrome), two cases, *Arch Dis Child* 14:217-230, 1939.

236. Erickson RP et al: Inefficacy of fresh frozen plasma therapy of mucopolysaccharidosis II, *Pediatrics* 50:693-701, 1972.

237. Eto Y et al: MSD multiple sulfatase deficient disorder: a review of clinical, pathological, biochemical and pathogenic findings, *Acta Paediatr Jpn* 25:17-21, 1983.

238. Falk K, Gross H, Zinnganell K: Difficult intubation and anesthesia in Pfaundler-Hurler disease, *Anaesthesist* 38:208-209, 1989.

239. Fasce L et al: Problems of differential diagnosis between Scheie's syndrome (MPS I S) and Hurler-Scheie syndrome (MPS I H/S): report of a case of probable Scheie syndrome, *Minerva Pediatr* 40:247-251, 1988.

240. Feilberg V, Hejgaard N: Morquio-Brailsford disease in a refugee from Vietnam: orthopedic and social arrangements, *Ugeskr Laeger* 149:1138-1139, 1987.

241. Ferrer I et al: Focal dendritic swellings in Purkinje cells in mucopolysaccharidoses type I, II and III: a Golgi and ultrastructural study, *Neuropathol Appl Neurobiol* 14:315-323, 1988.

242. Fidzianska E et al: Assignment of the gene for human arylsulfatase B, ARSB, to chromosome region 5p11-5qter, *Cytogenet Cell Genet* 38:150-151, 1984.

243. Finlayson LA: Hunter syndrome (mucopolysaccharidosis II), *Pediatr Dermatol* 7:150-152, 1990.

244. Fluharty AL et al: Uridine diphospho-*N*-acetylgalactosamine-4-sulfate sulfohydrolase activity of human arylsulfatase B and its deficiency in the Maroteaux-Lamy syndrome, *Biochem Biophys Res Commun* 64:955-962, 1975.

245. Fong LV et al: Endocardial fibroelastosis in mucopolysaccharidosis type VI, *Clin Cardiol* 10:362-364, 1987.

246. Fontaine G et al: La sialurie: un trouble metabolique original, *Helv Paediatr Acta* 23(suppl XVII):1-32, 1968.

247. Fortuin JJH, Kleijer WF: Hybridization studies of fibroblasts from Hurler, Scheie and Hurler-Scheie compound patients: support for the hypothesis of allelic mutants, *Hum Genet* 53:155-159, 1980.

248. Fortuin JJH, Kleijer WJ: Hybridization of fibroblasts from Hurler, Scheie and Hurler-Scheie compound patients: support for the hypothesis of allelic mutations, *Hum Genet* 65:155-159, 1980.

249. Fraccaro M et al: Morquio's disease: metachromatic granules in cultured fibroblasts, *Lancet* 1:508-509, 1967.

250. Francke U: The human gene for β-glucuronidase is on chromosome 7, *Am J Hum Genet* 28:357-362, 1976.

251. Fratantoni JC, Hall CW, Neufeld EF: The defect in Hurler's and Hunter's syndromes: faulty degradation of mucopolysaccharide, *Proc Natl Acad Sci USA* 60:699-706, 1968.

252. Fratantoni JC, Hall CW, Neufeld EF: Hurler and Hunter syndromes: mutual correction of the defect in cultured fibroblasts, *Science* 162:570-572, 1968.

253. Fratantoni JC, Hall CW, Neufeld EF:The defect in Hurler and Hunter syndromes. II. Deficiency of specific factors involved in mucopolysaccharide degradation, *Proc Natl Acad Sci USA* 64:360-366, 1969.

254. Fratantoni JC et al: Intrauterine diagnosis of the Hurler and Hunter syndromes, *N Engl J Med* 280:686-688, 1969.

255. Freeman C, Hopwood JJ: Human liver sulphamate sulphohydrolase: determination of native protein and subunit M$_r$ values and influence of substrate algycone structure on catalytic properties, *Biochem J* 234:83-92, 1986.

256. Freeman C, Hopwood JJ: Human liver glucuronic acid-2-sulphatase: purification, characterization and catalytic properties, *Biochem J* 259:209-216, 1989.

257. Freeman C, Hopwood JJ: Sanfilippo D syndrome: estimation of *N*-acetylglucosamine-6-sulfatase activity with a radiolabeled monosulfated disaccharide substrate, *Anal Biochem* 176:244-248, 1989.

258. Freeman C, Hopwood JJ: Human α-L-iduronidase—catalytic properties and an integrated role in the lysosomal degradation of heparan sulfate, *Biochem J* 282:899-908, 1992.

259. Freitag F et al: Hepatic ultrastructure in fucosidosis, *Virchows Arch [B]* 7:99-113, 1971.

260. Freitag F, Blumcke S, Spranger J: Hepatic ultrastructure in mucolipidosis I (mucopolysaccharidosis), *Virchows Arch [B]* 7:189-204, 1971.

261. Friedmann I et al: Histopathological studies of the temporal bones in Hurler's disease (mucopolysaccharidosis [MPS] IH), *J Laryngol Otol* 99:29-41, 1985.

262. Friend SC, Barr SC, Embury D: Fucosidosis in an English springer spaniel presenting as a malabsorption syndrome, *Aust Vet J* 62:415-420, 1985.

263. Fujitani T et al: Pathological and biochemical study in the adenoid of mucopolysaccharidosis II, *Int J Pediatr Otorhinolaryngol* 10:205-122, 1985.

264. Fujubayashi S et al: Properties of α-L-iduronidase in cultured skin fibroblasts from α-L-iduronidase-deficient patients, *Hum Genet* 65:268-278, 1984.

265. Gardner DG: Metachromatic cells in the gingiva in Hurler's syndrome, *Oral Surg* 26:782-789, 1968.

266. Gardner DG: The oral manifestations of Hurler's syndrome, *Oral Surg* 32:46-57, 1971.

267. Gardner DG: The dental manifestations of the Morquio syndrome (MPS type IV): a diagnostic aid, *Am J Dis Child* 129:1445-1448, 1975.

268. Garn SM, Hurme VO: Dental defects in three siblings afflicted with Morquio's disease, *Br Dent J* 93:210-212, 1952.

269. Gasper PW et al: Correction of feline arylsulphatase B deficiency (mucopolysaccharidosis VI) by bone marrow transplantation, *Nature* 312:467-469, 1984.

270. Gasteiger H, Liebenam L: Beitrag zur Dysostosis multiplex unter besonderer Berüchsichtigung des Augenbefundes, *Klin Monastbl Augenheilkd* 99:433-447, 1937.

271. Gatti R et al: Sanfilippo type D disease: clinical findings in two patients with a new variant of mucopolysaccharidosis III, *Eur J Pediatr* 138:168, 1982.

272. Gatti R et al: Comparative study of 15 lysosomal enzymes in chorionic villi and cultured amniotic fluid cells: early prenatal diagnosis in seven pregnancies at risk for lysosomal storage diseases, *Prenat Diagn* 5:134-136, 1985.

273. Gatti R et al: Prenatal diagnosis of mucopolysaccharidosis I: a special difficulty arising from an unusually low en-

zyme activity in mother's cells, *Prenat Diagn* 5:149-154, 1985.

274. Gehler J et al: Mucopolysaccharidosis VII: β-glucuronidase deficiency, *Humangenetik* 23:149, 1974.

275. Gerber A, Raab AP, Sobel AE: Vitamin A poisoning in adults with description of a case, *Am J Med* 16:729-745, 1954.

276. Gibbs DA et al: A clinical trial of fibroblast transplantation for the treatment of mucopolysaccharidoses, *J Inherited Metab Dis* 6:62-81, 1983.

277. Gilbert EF, Guin GH: Gargoylism: a review, including two occurrences in the American Negro, *Am J Dis Child* 95:69-80, 1958.

278. Gills JP et al: Electroretinography and fundus oculi findings in Hurler's disease and allied mucopolysaccharidoses, *Arch Ophthalmol* 74:596-603, 1965.

279. Gills JP et al: Hurler's disease and allied mucopolysaccharidoses, *Arch Ophthalmol* 74:596-603, 1965.

280. Ginsberg LC, DiFerrante DT, DiFerrante N: A substrate for direct measurement of L-iduronic acid 2-sulfate sulfatase, *Carbohydr Res* 64:225-235, 1978.

281. Ginzburg AS et al: Successful use of nasal-CPAP for obstructive sleep apnea in Hunter syndrome with diffuse airway involvement, *Chest* 97:1496-1498, 1990.

282. Gitzelmann R et al: Unusually mild course of β-glucuronidase deficiency in two brothers (mucopolysaccharidosis VII), *Helv Paediatr Acta* 33:413-428, 1978.

283. Gitzelmann R et al: Anomalous eosinophil granulocytes in blood and bone marrow: a diagnostic marker for infantile GM1-gangliosidosis? *Eur J Pediatr* 144:82-84, 1985.

284. Giugliani R et al: G_{M1} gangliosidosis: clinical and laboratory findings in eight families, *Hum Genet* 70:347-354, 1985.

285. Giugliani R et al: Progressive mental recession in siblings with Morquio disease type B (mucopolysaccharidosis IV B), *Clin Genet* 32:313-325, 1987.

286. Glaser JH et al: β-Glucuronidase deficiency and mucopolysaccharidosis: methods for enzymatic diagnosis, *J Lab Clin Med* 82:969-977, 1983.

287. Glober GA et al: Mucopolysaccharidosis, an unusual cause of cardiac valvular disease, *Am J Cardiol* 22:133-136, 1968.

288. Goebel HH: Morphology of the gangliosidoses, *Neuropediatrics* 15:97-106, 1984.

289. Goetting MG, Dasouki MJ: Cerebral atrophy, macrosomia, and cutaneous telangiectasia in G_{M1} gangliosidosis (letter), *J Pediatr* 107:644-645, 1985.

290. Goldberg G, Grutzner P: Compound Hurler-Scheie disease in 3 siblings, *Klin Monatsbl Augenheilkd* 187:120-123, 1985.

291. Goldberg M et al: Macular cherry-red spot, corneal clouding and β-galactosidase deficiency, *Arch Intern Med* 128:387-398, 1971.

292. Goldberg MF, Duke JR: Ocular histopathology in Hunter's syndrome: systemic mucopolysaccharidosis, type II, *Arch Ophthalmol* 77:503-512, 1967.

293. Goldberg MF, Scott CI, McKusick VA: Hydrocephalus and papilledema in the Maroteaux-Lamy syndrome (mucopolysaccharidosis, type VI), *Am J Ophthalmol* 69:969-975, 1970.

294. Goodman ML, Pang D: Spinal cord injury in I-cell disease, *Pediatr Neurosci* 14:315-318, 1988.

295. Gordon BA, Haust MD: The mucopolysaccharidoses, types I, II, and III: urinary findings in 29 cases, *Clin Biochem* 3:209-215, 1970.

296. Gorlin RJ, Cohen MM, Levin LS: *Syndromes of the head and neck*, ed 3, New York, 1990, Oxford University Press.

297. Greaves MW, Inman PM: Cutaneous changes in the Morquio syndrome, *Br J Dermatol* 81:29-36, 1969.

298. Green MA: Gargoylism (lipochondrodystrophy), *J Neuropathol Exp Neurol* 7:399-417, 1948.

299. Griffiths SB, Findlay M: Gargoylism: clinical, radiological and haematological features in two siblings, *Arch Dis Child* 32:229-234, 1958.

300. Groebe H et al: Morquio syndrome (mucopolysaccharidosis IVB) associated with beta-galactosidase deficiency: report of two cases, *Am J Hum Genet* 32:258-272, 1980.

301. Gross DM et al: Echocardiographic abnormalities in the mucopolysaccharide storage diseases, *Am J Cardiol* 61:170-176, 1988.

302. Grossman H, Dorst JP: The mucopolysaccharidoses. In Kaufmann H, editor: *Progress in pediatric radiology*, vol IV, St Louis 1972, Mosby–Year Book.

303. Grumbach MM, Meyer K: Urinary excretion and tissue storage of sulfated mucopolysaccharides in Hurler's syndrome, *Am J Dis Child* 96:467-469, 1958.

304. Gschwind C, Tonkin MA: Carpal tunnel syndrome in children with mucopolysaccharidosis and related disorders, *J Hand Surg* 17A:44-47, 1992.

305. Gtzeschik KH: Assignment of human genes: β-glucuronidase to chromosome 7, adenylate kinase 1 to 9, a second enzyme with enolase activity to 12, and mitochondrial IDH to 15, Gene Mapping Conference, Baltimore 3:495, 1975.

306. Guazzi GC et al: Type 3 (chronic) G_{M1} gangliosidosis presenting as infanto-choreo-athetotic dementia, without epilepsy, in three sisters, *Neurology* 38:1124-1127, 1988.

307. Guibard P et al: Mucopolysaccharidose type VII par deficit en β-glucuronidase: etude d'une famille, *J Genet Hum* 27:29, 1979.

308. Guibaud P et al: Morquio syndrome moderated by beta galactosidase deficiency: mucopolysaccharidosis (type IV B) or oligosaccharidosis, *Ann Pediatr* 30:681-686, 1983.

309. Guibaud P et al: Fetal ascites as a manifestation of infantile sialidosis: significance of a study of oligosaccharides in amniotic fluid, *J Genet Hum* 33:317-324, 1985.

310. Guise KS et al: Isolation and expression and *Escherichia coli* of a cDNA clone encoding human β-glucuronidase, *Gene* 34:105-110, 1985.

311. Hall CW, Cantz M, Neufeld EF: A β-glucuronidase deficiency mucopolysaccharidosis: studies in cultured fibroblasts, *Arch Biochem Biophys* 155:32-38, 1973.

312. Hall CW, Neufeld EF: A α-L-iduronidase activity in cultured skin fibroblasts and amniotic fluid cells, *Arch Biochem Biophys* 158:817-821, 1973.

313. Halperin SL, Curtis GM: The genetics of gargoylism, *Am J Ment Defic* 46:298-301, 1942.

314. Hambrick GW, Scheie HG: Studies of the skin in Hurler's syndrome: mucopolysaccharidosis, *Arch Dermatol* 85:455-471, 1962.

315. Hanai J, Leroy J, O'Brien JS: Ultrastructure of cultured fibroblasts in I-cell disease, *Am J Dis Child* 122:34-38, 1971.

316. Handelman L, Menahem S, Eisenbruch IM: Transcultural understanding of a hereditary disorder: mucopolysaccharidosis VI in a Vietnamese family, *Clin Pediatr* 28:470-473, 1989.

317. Reference deleted in proofs.

318. Haskins ME et al: Mucopolysaccharide storage disease in three families of cats with arylsulfatase B deficiency: leukocyte studies and carrier identification, *Pediatr Res* 13:1203-1210, 1979.

319. Haskins ME et al: Mucopolysaccharidosis in a domestic short-haired cat—a disease distinct from that seen in the Siamese cat, *J Am Vet Med Assoc* 175:384, 1979.

320. Haskins ME et al: α-L-iduronidase deficiency in a cat: a model of mucopolysaccharidosis I, *Pediatr Res* 13:1294-1297, 1982.

321. Haskins ME et al: β-Glucuronidase deficiency in a dog: a model of mucopolysaccharidoses VII, *Pediatr Res* 18:980-984, 1984.

322. Hässler E: Die Beziehungen der Hurlerschen Krankheit (Dysostosis multiplex-dysostotische Idiotie Gargolismus) zum Kretinismus, *Mschr Kinderheilk* 86:96-110, 1941.

323. Haust MD, Gordon BA: Ultrastructural and biochemical aspects of Sanfilippo syndrome—type III genetic mucopolysaccharidosis, *Connect Tissue Res* 15:57-64, 1986.

324. Haust MD, Landing BH: Histochemical studies in Hurler's disease: a new method for localization of acid mucopolysaccharide, and an analysis of lead acetate "fixation," *J Histochem Cytochem* 9:79-86, 1961.

325. Haust MD et al: The fine structure of liver in children with Hurler's syndrome, *Exp Mol Pathol* 10:141-161, 1969.

326. Haust MD et al: Heparitin sulfate mucopolysaccharidosis (Sanfilippo disease): a case study with ultrastructural, biochemical, and radiologic findings, *Pediatr Res* 5:137-150, 1971.

327. Haust MD et al: Clinicopathological conference: an adolescent girl with severe mental impairment and mucopolysacchariduria, *Am J Med Genet* 22:1-27, 1985.

328. Hayes E, Babin R, Platz C: The otologic manifestations of mucopolysaccharidoses, *Am J Otol* 2:65-69, 1980.

329. Hayflick S et al: Acute infantile cardiomyopathy as a presenting feature of mucopolysaccharidosis VI, *J Pediatr* 120:269-272, 1992.

330. Healy PJ, Harper PA, Dennis JA: Phenotypic variation in bovine alpha-mannosidosis, *Res Vet Sci* 49:82-84, 1990.

331. Hecht JT et al: Mild manifestions of the Morquio syndrome, *Am J Med Genet* 18:368-371, 1984.

332. Helmholtz HF, Harrington ER: Syndrome characterized by congenital clouding of the cornea and by other anomalies, *Am J Dis Child* 41:793-800, 1931.

333. Helwig-Larsen HF, Morch ET: Genetic aspects of osteochondrodystrophy: Silfverskiold's and Morquio's syndromes, *Acta Pathol Microbiol Scand* 22:335-357, 1945.

334. Henderson JL: Gargoylism: review of principal features with report of five cases, *Arch Dis Child* 15:201-214, 1940.

335. Henderson JL et al: Pathology and biochemistry of gargoylism: report of three cases with review of literature, *Arch Dis Child* 27:230-256, 1952.

336. Henderson MJ, McGinlay JM, Cundall DB: Heparin and suspected Sanfilippo syndrome (letter), *Arch Dis Child* 64:633-634, 1989.

337. Herranz Jordan B et al: Mucopolysaccharidosis type III A in a girl with atrial septal defect and paroxysmal supraventricular tachycardia, *Ann Exp Pediatr* 32:85-87, 1990.

338. Herrick IA, Rhine EJ: The mucopolysaccharidoses and anaesthesia: a report of clinical experience, *Can J Anaesth* 35:67-73, 1988.

339. Hers HG: Inborn lysosomal diseases, *Gastroenterology* 48:625-633, 1965.

340. Hers HG, Van Hoof F: The genetic pathology of lysosomes, *Prog Liver Dis* 3:185-205, 1970.

341. Hickman S, Neufeld EF: A hypothesis for I-cell disease:defective hydrolases that do not enter lysosomes, *Biochem Biophys Res Commun* 49:992-999, 1972.

342. Hobaek A: *Problems of hereditary chondrodysplasias*, Oslo, 1961, Oslo University Press.

343. Hobbs JR et al: Reversal of clinical features of Hurler's disease and biochemical improvement after treatment by bone marrow transplantation, *Lancet* 2:709-712, 1981.

344. Hobbs JR et al: Lysosomal enzyme replacement therapy by displacement bone marrow transplantation with immunoprophylaxis, *Adv Clin Enzymol* 3:184, 1986.

345. Hocking JD, Jolly RD, Batt RD: Deficiency of α-mannosidase in Angus cattle, *Biochem J* 128:69-78, 1972.

346. Hokke CH et al: Novel storage products in human beta-mannosidosis, *J Inherited Metab Dis* 13:273-276, 1990.

347. Honjoh M et al: Fucosidosis type 3 with angiokeratoma corporis diffusum, *J Dermatol* 12:174-182, 1985.

348. Hoogeveen AT, Verheyen FW, Galjaard H: The relation between human lysosomal β-galactosidase and its protective protein, *J Biol Chem* 255:4937-4945, 1980.

349. Hoogeveen AT et al: Genetic heterogeneity in human neuraminidase deficiency, *Nature* 285:500-502, 1980.

350. Hoogerbrugge PM et al: Correction of lysosomal enzyme deficiency in various organs of β-glucuronidase-deficient mice by allogeneic bone marrow transplantation, *Transplantation* 43:609-614, 1987.

351. Hooper JMD: An unusual case of gargoylism, *Guy's Hosp Rep* 101:222-228, 1952.

352. Hopkins R et al: Inguinal hernia in the Hurler-Hunter syndrome, *Surgery* 61:302-304, 1973.

353. Hopwood JJ: α-L-iduronidase, β-D-iduronidase and 2-sulfo-L-iduronate-2-sulfatase: preparation and characterization of radioactive substrates from heparin, *Carbohydrate Res* 69:203-207, 1979.

354. Hopwood JJ, Elliott H: The diagnosis of Sanfilippo C syndrome, using monosaccharide and oligo-saccharide substrate to assay acetyl-CoA:2-amino-2-deoxy-a-glucoside *N*-acetyltransferase activity, *Clin Chim Acta* 112:67-75, 1981.

355. Hopwood JJ, Elliott H: Detection of Morquio A syndrome using radio-labelled substrates derived from keratan sulphate for the estimation of galactose 6-sulphate sulphatase, *Clin Sci* 65:325-332, 1983.

356. Hopwood JJ, Elliott H: Selective depolymerisation of keratan sulfate: production of radiolabelled substrates for 6-O-sulfogalactose sulfatase and β-galactosidase, *Carbohydr Res* 117:263-274, 1983.

357. Hopwood JJ, Harrison JR: High-resolution electrophoresis of urinary glycosaminoglycans, *Anal Biochem* 199:120-127, 1982.

358. Hopwood JJ, Morris CP: The mucopolysaccharidoses: diagnosis, molecular genetics and treatment, *Mol Biol Med* 7:381-404, 1990.

359. Hopwood JJ, Muller V: Biochemical discrimination of Hurler and Scheie syndromes, *Clin Sci* 57:265-272, 1979.

360. Hopwood JJ, Muller V: Diagnostic enzymology of α-L-iduronidase with special reference to a sulphated disaccharide derived from heparin, *Clin Sci* 62:193-201, 1982.

361. Hopwood JJ, Muller V: Selective depolymerisation of dermatan sulfate: production of radiolabelled substrates for α-L-iduronidase, sulfo-iduronate sulfatase and β-D-glucuronidase, *Carbohydr Res* 122:227-239, 1983.

362. Hopwood JJ, Muller V, Pollard AC: Post- and pre-natal assessment of α-L-iduronidase deficiency with a radiolabelled natural substrate, *Clin Sci* 56:591-599, 1979.

363. Hopwood JJ et al: A fluorometric assay using 4-methylumbelliferyl α-L-iduronidase for the estimation of α-L-iduronidase and the detection of Hurler and Scheie syndromes, *Clin Chim Acta* 92:257-265, 1979.

364. Hopwood JJ et al: Enzymatic diagnosis of the mucopolysaccharidoses: experience of 96 cases diagnosed in a five year period, *Med J Aust* 1:257-265, 1982.

365. Hopwood JJ et al: Diagnosis of Maroteaux-Lamy syndrome by the use of radiolabelled oligosaccharides as substrates for the determination of arylsulphatase B activity, *Biochem J* 234:507-514, 1986.

366. Hors-Cayla MC, Maroteaux P, deGrouchy J: Fibroblastes en culture au cours de mucopolysaccharidosis influence du serum sur la metachromasie, *Ann Genet* 11:265-266, 1968.

367. Horstmann G, Lullmann-Rauch R: Mucopolysaccharidosis-like alterations in cardiac valves of rats treated with tilorone, *Virchows Arch* 48:33-45, 1985.

368. Horton WA, Schimke RN: A new mucopolysaccharidosis, *J Pediatr* 77:252-258, 1970.

369. Hoshino M et al: Fucosidosis: ultrastructural study of the eye in an adult, *Graefes Arch Clin Exp Ophthalmol* 227:162-171, 1989.

370. Hoyme HE et al: Presentation of mucopolysaccharidosis VII (beta-glucuronidase deficiency) in infancy, *J Med Genet* 18:237-239, 1981.

371. Hreidarsson S et al: Aspartylglucosaminuria in the United States, *Clin Genet* 23:427-435, 1983.

372. Huang K-C, Sukegawa K, Orii T: Glycosaminoglycan excretion in random samples of urine, *Clin Chim Acta* 151:141-146, 1985.

373. Huang K-C, Sukegawa K, Orii T: Screening test for urinary glycosaminoglycans and differentiation of various mucopolysaccharidoses, *Clin Chim Acta* 151:147-156, 1985.

374. Hubeny MJ, Delano RJ: Dysostosis multiplex, *Am J Roentgenol* 46:336-342, 1941.

375. Hug G et al: Antenatal diagnosis of mucopolysaccharidosis type I (Hurler's disease) is not possible by electron microscopy of uncultured amniotic fluid cells, *J Med Genet* 21:359-363, 1984.

376. Humbel R, Etringer S: A colorimetric method for the determination of sulfated glycosaminoglycans, *Rev Roum Biochim* 11:21-24, 1974.

377. Humbel R, Marchal C, Fall M: Differential diagnosis of mucopolysaccharidosis by means of thin-layer chromatography of urinary acidic glycosaminoglycans, *Helv Paediatr Acta* 24:648, 1969.

378. Hunter C: A rare disease in two brothers: evaluation of scapula, limitation of movement of joints and other abnormalities, *Proc R Soc Med* 10:104-116, 1917.

379. Hurler G: Ueber einen Typ multipler Abartungen, vorwiegend am Skelettsystem, *Z Kinderheilk* 24:220-234, 1919.

380. Hussels IE et al: Treatment of mucopolysaccharidoses, *Birth Defects* 10:212-225, 1972.

381. Ikeda S et al: Ultrastructural findings of rectal and skin biopsies in adult G_{M1}-gangliosidosis, *Acta Pathol Jpn* 36:1823-1831, 1986.

382. Inuzuka S et al: A case of chronic intestinal pseudo-obstruction complicated by mucopolysaccharidoses I Scheie type, *Nippon Shokakibyo Gakkai Zasshi* 83:2429-2434, 1986.

383. Irani D et al: Postmortem observations on β-glucuronidase deficiency presenting as hydrops fetalis, *Ann Neurol* 14:486-490, 1983.

384. Isenberg JN, Sharp HL: Aspartylglucosaminuria: unique biochemical and ultrastructural characteristics, *Hum Pathol* 7:469-481, 1976.

385. Iwamasa T et al: Demonstration of G_{M1}-ganglioside in nervous system in generalized G_{M1}-gangliosidosis using cholera toxin B subunit, *Acta Neuropathol* 73:357-360, 1987.

386. Iwamoto M et al: Ocular histopathology and ultrastructure of Morquio syndrome (systemic mucopolysaccharidosis IV A), *Graefes Arch Clin Exp Ophthalmol* 228:342-349, 1990.

387. Jackson WPU: Clinical features, diagnosis and osseous lesions of gargoylism exemplified in 3 siblings, *Arch Dis Child* 26:549-557, 1951.

388. Jacobsen AW: Hereditary osteochondrodystrophia deformans: a family with twenty members affected in five generations, *JAMA* 113:121-124, 1939.

389. Jansen PH et al: Mannosidosis: a study of two patients, presenting clinical heterogeneity, *Clin Neurol Neurosurg* 89:185-192, 1987.

390. Jellinger K et al: New phenotype of adult alpha-L-iduronidase deficiency (mucopolysaccharidosis I) masquerading as Friedreich's ataxia with cardiopathy, *Clin Neuropathol* 9:163-169, 1990.

391. Jenner FA, Pollitt RJ: Large quantities of 2-acetamido-1-(β-L-aspartamido)-1, 2-dideoxyglucose in the urine of mentally retarded siblings, *Biochem J* 103:48-49, 1967.

392. Jensen OA et al: Hurler/Scheie phenotype: report of an inbred sibship with tapetoretinal degeneration and electron-microscopic examination of the conjunctiva, *Ophthalmologica* 176:194-204, 1978.

393. Jermain LF, Rohn RJ, Bond WH: Studies on the role of the reticuloendothelial system in Hurler's disease, *Am J Med Sci* 239:612-621, 1960.

394. Jervis GA: Gargoylism: (lipochondrodystrophy) study of 10 cases with emphasis on formes frustes, *Arch Neurol Psychiatry* 63:681-712, 1950.

395. Jewesbury RC, Spence JC: Two cases: (1) oxycephaly and (2) acrocephaly, with other congenital deformities, *Proc R Soc Med* 14:270, 1921.

396. Jezyk PF, Haskins ME, Newman LR: Alpha-mannosidosis in a Persian cat, *J Am Vet Med Assoc* 189:1483-1485, 1986.

397. Jezyk PF et al: Mucopolysaccharidosis in a cat with arylsulfatase B deficiency: a model of Maroteaux-Lamy syndrome, *Science* 198:834-836, 1977.

398. John RM, Hunter D, Swanton RH: Echocardiographic abnormalities in type IV mucopolysaccharidosis, *Arch Dis Child* 65:746-749, 1990.

399. Johnson GL et al: Echocardiographic mitral valve deformity in the mucopolysaccharidoses, *Pediatrics* 67:401-406, 1981.

400. Johnson MA et al: Magnetic resonance imaging of the brain in Hurler syndrome, *AJNR* 5:816-819, 1984.

400a. Jolly RD et al: Mannosidosis: ocular lesions in the bovine model, *Curr Eye Res* 6:1073-1078, 1987.

401. Jones MZ, Dawson G: Caprine β-mannosidosis: inherited deficiency of β-D-mannosidase, *J Biol Chem* 256:5185-5188, 1981.

402. Jope RS, Baker HJ, Conner DJ: Increased acetylcholine synthesis and release in brains of cats with G$_{M1}$ gangliosidosis, *J Neurochem* 46:1567-1572, 1986.

403. Jordans GHW: Hereditary granulation anomaly of leucocytes (Alder), *Acta Med Scand* 129:348-351, 1947.

404. Kabnick EM et al: Diagnosis of Hurler's syndrome with chest roentgenogram, *J Natl Med Assoc* 76:515-518, 1984.

405. Kaendler S et al: Cervical myelopathy in mucopolysaccharidosis type II (Hunter's syndrome): neuroradiologic, clinical and histopathologic findings, *Dtsch Med Wochenschr* 115:1348-1352, 1990.

406. Kagalwala TY et al: The mucopolysaccharidoses: a study of 48 cases, *Ind J Pediatr* 55:919-925, 1988.

407. Kaibara N et al: Hurler-Scheie phenotype: a report of two pairs of inbred sibs, *Hum Genet* 53:37-41, 1979.

408. Kaibara N et al: Hurler-Scheie phenotype with parental consanguinity: report of an additional case supporting the concept of genetic heterogeneity, *Clin Orthop* 175:233-236, 1983.

409. Kajii T et al: Hurler/Scheie genetic compound (mucopolysaccharidosis 1H/1S) in Japanese brothers, *Clin Genet* 6:394-400, 1974.

410. Kakaiya RK et al: Characteristics and natural history of alloimmunization following HLA-matched leukocyte transfusion in Hunter's syndrome, *Ann Clin Lab Sci* 14:276-284, 1984.

411. Kakaiya RM et al: HLA alloimmunization with leukocyte concentrates from HLA-matched and HLA-non-matched donors in patients with Hunter's syndrome, *Ann Clin Lab Sci* 15:435-440, 1985.

412. Kamiya M et al: I-cell disease: a case report and review of the literature, *Acta Pathol Jpn* 36:1679-1692, 1986.

413. Kaplan D: Classification of the mucopolysaccharidoses based on the pattern of mucopolysacchariduria, *Am J Med* 47:721-729, 1969.

414. Kaplan D et al: Keratosulfate-chondroitin sulfate peptide from normal urine and from urine of patients with Morquio syndrome (mucopolysaccharidosis IV), *J Lab Clin Med* 71:48-55, 1968.

415. Kaplan P, Wolfe LS: Sanfilippo syndrome type D, *J Pediatr* 110:267-271, 1987.

416. Karpati G et al: Multiple peripheral nerve entrapments: an unusual phenotype variant of the Hunter syndrome (mucopolysaccharidosis II) in a family, *Arch Neurol* 31:418, 1974.

417. Kasama T, Taketomi T: Abnormalities of cerebral lipids in G$_{M1}$-gangliosidoses, infantile, juvenile, and chronic type, *Jpn J Exp Med* 56:1-11, 1986.

418. Kashtan CE et al: Proteinuria in a child with sialidosis: case report and histological studies, *Pediatr Nephrol* 3:166-174, 1989.

419. Kato S et al: Bone marrow transplantation in children, *Tokai J Exp Clin Med* 11:54-57, 1986.

420. Kaufman HH et al: Cervical myelopathy due to dural compression in mucopolysaccharidosis, *Surg Neurol* 17:404-410, 1982.

421. Kawai H et al: Skeletal muscle pathology of mannosidosis in two siblings with spastic paraplegia, *Acta Neuropathol* 68:201-204, 1985.

422. Kawai H et al: Isozyme pattern of leukocyte alpha-D-mannosidase in patients with mannosidosis, *Jinrui Idengaku Zasshi* 33:1-7, 1988.

423. Keith O, Scully C, Weidmann GM: Orofacial features of Scheie (Hurler-Scheie) syndrome (alpha-L-iduronidase deficiency), *Oral Surg Oral Med Oral Pathol* 70:70-74, 1990.

424. Kelemen G: Hurler's syndrome and the hearing organ, *J Laryngol* 80:791-803, 1966.

425. Keller C et al: Mukopolysaccharidose Typ VI-A (Morbus Maroteaux-Lamy): Korrelation der klinischen und pathologisch-anatomischen, Befunde bei einen 27 jahrigen Patienten, *Helv Paediatr Acta* 42:317-333, 1987.

426. Kempthorne PM, Brown TEK: Anaesthesia and the mucopolysaccharidoses: a survey of techniques and problems, *Anaesth Intensive Care* 11:203-207, 1983.

427. Kennealy FV: The ocular manifestations of gargoylism, *Am J Ophthalmol* 36:663-674, 1953.

428. Kenyon KR, Maumenee AE: The histological and ultrastructural pathology of congenital hereditary corneal dystrophy: a case report, *Invest Ophthalmol* 7:475-500, 1968.

429. Kenyon KR, Sensenbrenner JA: Mucolipidosis II (I-cell disease): ultrastructural observations of conjunctiva and skin, *Invest Ophthalmol* 10:355-367, 1971.

430. Kenyon KR et al: Ocular pathology of the Maroteaux-Lamy syndrome: a histologic and ultrastructure report of two cases, *Am J Ophthalmol* 73:718-741, 1972.

431. Kepes JJ, Berry A, Zacharias DL: Multiple sulfatase deficiency: bridge between neuronal storage diseases and leukodystrophies [published erratum appears in *Pathology* 20(4), 1988, following p 411], *Pathology* 20:285-291, 1988.

432. Kin NM: Comparison of the urinary glycoconjugates excreted by patients with type I and type II fucosidosis, *Clin Chem* 33:44-47, 1987.

433. King DH, Jones RM, Barnett MB: Anaesthetic considerations in the mucopolysaccharidoses, *Anaesthesia* 39:26-131, 1984.

434. King JH: Personal communication, 1964.

435. Kirk JM: Anomalous mucopolysaccharide screening result due to bacterial contamination of urine, *Clin Chem* 36:386-387, 1990.

436. Kjellman B et al: Mannosidosis: a clinical and histopathologic study, *J Pediatr* 75:366-373, 1969.

437. Kleijer WJ: Prenatal diagnosis of sialidosis with combined neuraminidase and β-galactosidase deficiency, *Clin Genet* 16:60-61, 1979.

438. Kleijer WJ et al: Prenatal diagnosis of Maroteaux-Lamy syndrome, *Lancet* 2:50, 1976.

439. Kleijer WJ et al: Prenatal monitoring for the Hunter syndrome: the heterozygous female fetus, *Clin Genet* 15:113-117, 1979.

440. Kleijer WJ et al: First trimester diagnosis of Hunter syndrome on chorionic villi (letter), *Lancet* 2:472, 1984.

441. Kleijer WJ et al: First trimester diagnosis of mucopolysaccharidosis IIIA (Sanfilippo A disease), *N Engl J Med* 314:185-186, 1986.

442. Klein U et al: Sanfilippo syndrome type C: assay for acetyl-CoA; α-glucosaminide N-acetyltransferase in leukocytes for detection of homozygous and heterozygous individuals, *Clin Genet* 20:55-59, 1981.

443. Knecht J, Cifonelli JA: Studies on heparitin sulfate of normal and Hurler tissues, *J Biol Chem* 242:4652-4661, 1967.

444. Knecht J, Dorfman A: Structure of heparitin sulfate in tissues of the Hurler syndrome, *Biochem Biophys Res Commun* 21:509-515, 1965.

445. Knudson AG Jr, DiFerrante N, Curtis JE: The effect of leukocyte transfusion in a child with type II mucopolysaccharidosis, *Proc Natl Acad Sci USA* 68:1738-1741, 1971.

446. Kny W: Zur Kenntnis der Dysostosis multiplex Typ Pfaundler-Hurler, *Z Kinderheilkd* 63:366-377, 1942.

447. Kobayashi N: Acid mucopolysaccharide granules in the glomerular epithelium in gargoylism, *Am J Pathol* 35:591-605, 1959.

448. Koenig ML et al: Reduced Ca2+ flux in synaptosomes from cats with G_{M1} gangliosidosis, *Brain Res* 424:169-176, 1987.

449. Kohlschutter A: Clinical course of G_{M1} gangliosidoses, *Neuropediatrics* 15:71-73, 1984.

450. Kohn G et al: A new phenotypic variant of α-L-iduronidase deficiency, *Monogr Hum Genet* 10:7-10, 1978.

451. Kopits SE, Steingass MH: Experience with the "halo-cast" in small children, *Surg Clin North Am* 50:935-943, 1970.

452. Kopits SE et al: Congenital atlantoaxial dislocations in various forms of dwarfism, *J Bone Joint Surg* 54-A:1349, 1972.

453. Kordysz E, Wozniewicz B: Landing disease, G_{M1} generalized gangliosidosis, and malabsorption syndrome, *Pediatr Pathol* 9:467-473, 1989.

454. Koskenoja M, Suvanto E: Gargoylism: report of adult form with glaucoma in two sisters, *Acta Ophthalmol* 37:234-240, 1954.

455. Kraft E, Zorowka P: Pediatric audiologic-phoniatric aspects of mannosidosis, *HNO* 38:99-101, 1990.

456. Kresse H: Mucopolysaccharidosis IIIA (Sanfilippo A disease): deficiency of heparin sulfamidase in skin fibroblasts and leucocytes, *Biochem Biophys Res Commun* 54:111, 1973.

457. Kresse H, Neufeld EF: The Sanfilippo A corrective factor: purification and mode of action, *J Biol Chem* 247:2164-2170, 1972.

458. Kresse H et al: Biochemical heterogeneity of the Sanfilippo syndrome: preliminary characterization of two deficient factors, *Biochem Biophys Res Commun* 42:892-898, 1971.

459. Kresse H et al: Sanfilippo disease type D: deficiency of N-acetylglucosamine-6-sulfate sulfatase required for heparan sulfate degradation, *Proc Natl Acad Sci USA* 77:6822-6826, 1980.

460. Kressler RJ, Aegerter EE: Hurler's syndrome (gargoylism): summary of literature and report of case with autopsy findings, *J Pediatr* 12:579-591, 1938.

461. Kretz KA et al: Characterization of EcoRI mutation in fucosidosis patients: a stop codon in the open reading frame, *J Mol Neurosci* 1:177-180, 1989.

462. Krivit W et al: Bone marrow transplantation in the Maroteaux-Lamy syndrome (mucopolysaccharidosis type VI): biochemical and clinical status 24 months after transplantation, *N Engl J Med* 311:1606-1611, 1984.

463. Krovetz LJ, Lorincz AE, Schiebler GL: Cardiovascular manifestations of the Hurler syndrome: hemodynamic and angiocardiographic observations in 15 patients, *Circulation* 31:132-141, 1965.

464. Krovetz LJ, Schiebler GL: Cardiovascular manifestations of the genetic mucopolysaccharidoses. In Bergsma, D, editor: *Clinical delineation of birth defects, vol 13. Cardiovascular system*, Baltimore, 1972, Williams & Wilkins.

465. Kyle JW et al: Correction of murine mucopolysaccharidosis VII by a human beta-glucuronidase transgene, *Proc Natl Acad Sci USA* 87:3914-3918, 1990.

466. Lagunoff D, Gritzka TL: The site of mucopolysaccharide accumulation in Hurler's syndrome: an electron microscopic and histochemical study, *Lab Invest* 15:1578-1588, 1966.

467. Lagunoff D, Pritzl P, Scott CR: Urinary N-sulfate glycosaminoglycan excretion in children: normal and abnormal values, *Proc Soc Exp Biol Med* 126:34, 1967.

468. Lagunoff D, Ross R, Benditt EP: Histochemical and electron microscopic study in a case of Hurler's disease, *Am J Pathol* 41:273-288, 1962.

469. Lagunoff D, Warren G: Determination of 2-deoxy-2-sulfoaminohexose content of mucopolysaccharides, *Arch Biochem* 99:396-400, 1962.

470. Lahdensuu S: Fälle der sogenannten Pfaundler-Hulersche Krankheit (Dysostosis multiplex), *Mschr Kinderheilkd* 92:340, 1943.

471. Lahey ME, Lomas RD, Worth TC: Lipochondrodystrophy (gargoylism), *J Pediatr* 31:220-226, 1947.

472. Lalley PA et al: Assignment of the gene for β-glucuronidase (β-GUS) to chromosome 7 in man, Gene Mapping Conference, Baltimore, 3:184, 1975.

473. Lamon JM et al: Bone cysts in mucopolysaccharidosis I-S (Scheie syndrome), *Johns Hopkins Med J* 146:73-74, 1980.

474. Landing BH et al: Familial neurovisceral lipidosis: an analysis of eight cases of a syndrome previously reported as "Hurler-variant," "pseudo-Hurler," and "Tay-Sachs disease with visceral involvement," *Am J Dis Child* 108:503-522, 1964.

475. Lang L et al: Lysosomal enzyme phosphorylation in human fibroblasts: kinetic parameters offer a biochemical rationale for two distinct defects in the uridine diphospho-N-acetylglucosamine: lysosomal enzyme precursor N-acetylglucosamine-1-phosphotransferase, *J Clin Invest* 76:2191-2195, 1985.

476. Langer LO, Carey LS: The radiologic manifestations of the HS-mucopolysaccharidosis of Sanfilippo, *Ann Radiol* 7:315-325, 1964.

477. Langer LO, Carey LS: The roentgenographic features of the KS-mucopolysaccharidosis of Morquio (Morquio-Brailsford's disease), *Am J Roentgenol* 97:1-20, 1966.

478. Langer LO Jr, Kronenberg RS, Gorlin RJ: A case simulating Hurler syndrome of unusual longevity, without abnormal mucopolysacchariduria: a proposed classification of the various forms of the syndrome and similar diseases, *Am J Med* 40:448-457, 1966.

479. Lapeer GL, Shanks GL: Mucolipidosis type III (pseudo-Hurler polydystrophy): conservative treatment of myofascial pain dysfunction syndrome with the sterling silver splint, *Oral Surg Oral Med Oral Pathol* 61:448-452, 1986.

480. Lee LE et al: β-Glucuronidase deficiency, *Am J Dis Child* 139:57, 1985.

481. LeGuern E et al: More precise localization of the gene for Hunter syndrome, *Genomics* 7:358-362, 1990.

482. Leroy JG, DeMars RI: Mutant enzymatic and cytological phenotypes in cultured human fibroblasts, *Science* 157:804, 1967.

483. Leroy JG, DeMars RI, Opitz JM: I-cell disease. In Bergsma D, editor: *The clinical delineation of birth defects. IV. Skeletal dysplasia*, New York, 1969, National March of Dimes Foundation, pp 174-185.

484. Levin LS et al: Oral findings in the Morquio syndrome (MPS IV), *Oral Surg* 39:390-395, 1975.

485. Levy LA et al: Ultrastructure of Reilly bodies (metachromatic granules) in the Maroteaux-Lamy syndrome (mucopolysaccharidosis VI): a histochemical study, *Am J Clin Pathol* 73:416-422, 1980.

486. Liberti J: Diagnosis of lysosomal storage diseases by the ultrastructural study of conjunctival biopsies, *Pathol Ann* 15(part 1):37-66, 1980.

487. Lichtenstein JR, Bilbrey GL, McKusick VA: Clinical and probable genetic heterogeneity within mucopolysaccharidosis II: report of a family with the mild form, *Johns Hopkins Med J* 131:425-435, 1972.

488. Lie SO et al: Bone marrow transplantation in metabolic diseases, *Transplant Proc* 20:499-500, 1988.

489. Liebaers I, DiNatale P, Neufeld EF: Iduronate sulphatase in amniotic fluid: an aid in the prenatal diagnosis of the Hunter syndrome, *J Pediatr* 90:423, 1977.

490. Liebaers I, Neufeld EF: Iduronate sulfatase activity in serum, lymphocytes, and fibroblasts—simplified diagnosis of the Hunter syndrome, *Pediatr Res* 10:733-736, 1976.

491. Lieser M et al: Ganglioside G_{M3} sialidase activity in fibroblasts of normal individuals and of patients with sialidosis and mucolipidosis IV: subcellular distribution and some properties, *Biochem J* 260:69-74, 1989.

492. Lim TW et al: An assay for iduronate sulfatase (Hunter corrective factor), *Carbohydr Res* 37:103-109, 1974.

493. Lindsay S: Cardiovascular system in gargoylism, *Br Heart J* 12:17-32, 1950.

494. Lindsay S et al: Gargoylism: study of pathologic lesion and clinical review of twelve cases, *Am J Dis Child* 76:239-306, 1948.

495. Linker A, Evans LR, Langer LO: Morquio's disease and mucopolysaccharide excretion, *J Pediatr* 77:1039-1047, 1970.

496. Linker A, Terry KD: Urinary acid mucopolysaccharides in normal man and in Hurler's syndrome, *Proc Soc Exp Biol Med* 11:743-746, 1963.

497. Lipson SJ: Dysplasia of the odontoid process in Morquio's syndrome causing quadriparesis, *J Bone Joint Surg* 59A:340, 1977.

498. Lisson W et al: Prenatal diagnosis of Hunter syndrome using fetal plasma, *Prenat Diagn* 8:59-62, 1988.

499. Litjens T et al: Chromosomal localisation of ARSB, the gene for human *N*-acetyl-galactosamine-4-sulphatase, *Hum Genet* 82:67-68, 1989.

500. Loeb H et al: Biochemical and ultrastructural studies in Hurler's syndrome, *J Pediatr* 73:860-874, 1968.

501. Lovell KL: Caprine beta-mannosidosis: development of glial and myelin abnormalities in optic nerve and corpus callosum, *Glia* 3:26-32, 1990.

502. Lovell KL, Boyer PJ: Dysmyelinogenesis in caprine beta-mannosidosis: ultrastructural and morphometric studies in fetal optic nerve, *Int J Dev Neurosci* 5:243-253, 1987.

503. Lowry RD, Renwick DHG: The relative frequency of the Hurler and Hunter syndromes (letter), *N Engl J Med* 284:221-222, 1971.

504. Lowry RB et al: Morquio syndrome (MPS IVA) and hypophosphatasia in a Hutterite kindred, *Am J Med Genet* 22:463-475, 1985.

505. Lowry RB et al: An update on the frequency of mucopolysaccharide syndrome in British Columbia (letter), *Hum Genet* 85:389-390, 1990.

506. Lustmann J et al: Dentigerous cysts and radiolucent lesions of the jaw associated with Hunter's syndrome, *J Oral Surg* 33:679-685, 1975.

507. Madsen JA, Linker A: Vitamin A and mucopolysaccharidosis: a clinical and biochemical evaluation, *J Pediatr* 75:843-952, 1969.

508. Magee KR: Leptomeningeal changes associated with lipochondrodystrophy (gargoylism): report of case, *Arch Neurol Psychiatry* 63:282-297, 1950.

509. Magrini U et al: Mucopolysaccharidoses: autoradiographic study of sulphate ^{35}S uptake by cultured fibroblasts, *Ann Hum Genet* 31:231-236, 1968.

510. Maier-Redelsperger M, Stern MH, Maroteaux P: Pink rings lymphocyte: a new cytologic abnormality characteristic of mucopolysaccharidosis type II (Hunter disease) (letter), *Pediatrics* 82:286-287, 1988.

511. Maire I et al: β-Glucuronidase deficiency: enzyme studies in an affected family and prenatal diagnosis, *J Inherited Metab Dis* 2:29-34, 1979.

512. Malone BN et al: Resolution of obstructive sleep apnea in Hurler syndrome, *Int J Pediatr Otorhinolaryngol* 15:23-31, 1988.

513. Mancini GM et al: Ganglioside G_{M1} metabolism in living human fibroblasts with beta-galactosidase deficiency, *Hum Genet* 73:35-38, 1986.

514. Mapes CA et al: Enzyme replacement in Fabry's disease, an inborn error of metabolism, *Science* 169:987-989, 1970.

515. Margollicci M et al: Direct transfer in vitro of alpha-D-mannosidase activity from normal lymphocytes to fibroblasts of a patient with alpha-mannosidosis, *J Inherited Metab Dis* 13:277-279, 1990.

516. Markesbery WR: Mucopolysaccharidoses: ultrastructure of leukocyte inclusions, *Ann Neurol* 8:332-336, 1980.

517. Markicheva NA: Lamellar keratoplasty in congenital mucopolysaccharidosis of the Maroteaux-Lamy type, *Vestn Oftalmol* 101:63-65, 1985.

518. Maroteaux P: Differentiation biochemique des maladies de Hurler et de Hunter par fractionnement de l'heparitine sulfate, *Rev Eur Etud Clin Biol* 15:203-205, 1970.

519. Maroteaux P, Hors-Cayla MC, Pont J: La mucolipidose de type II, *Presse Med* 78:179-181, 1970.

520. Maroteaux P, Lamy M: Opacites corneennes et trouble metabolique dans la maladie de Morquio, *Rev Fr Etud Clin Biol* 6:481-483, 1961.

521. Maroteaux P, Lamy M: Hurler's disease, Morquio's disease, and related mucopolysaccharidoses, *J Pediatr* 67:312-323, 1965.

522. Maroteaux P, Lamy M: La pseudopolydystrophie de Hurler, *Presse Med* 74:2889-2892, 1962.

523. Maroteaux P, Lamy M, Foucher M: La maladie de Morquio: etude clinique, radiologique et biologique, *Presse Med* 71:2091-2094, 1963.

524. Maroteaux P, Spranger J, Wiedemann HR: Der metatropische Zwergwuchs, *Arch Kinderheilk* 173:211-226, 1966.

525. Maroteaux P et al: Une observation familiale d'oligo-phrenie polydystrophique, *J Genet Hum* 15:99-102, 1966.

526. Maroteaux P et al: Une nouvelle dysostose avec elimination urinaire de chondroitine-sulfate B, *Presse Med* 71:1849-1852, 1969.

527. Marsh J, Fensom AH: 4-Methylumbelliferyl alpha-*N*-acetylglucosaminidase activity for diagnosis of Sanfilippo B disease, *Clin Genet* 27:258-262, 1985.

528. Martiniuk F et al: Further regional localization of the genes for human acid alpha glucosidase (GAA), peptidase D (PEPD) and alpha-mannosidase B (MANB) by somatic cell hybridization, *Hum Genet* 69:109-111, 1985.

529. Maskin SL, Bode DD: Electron microscopy of impression-acquired conjunctival epithelial cells, *Ophthalmology* 93:1518-1523, 1986.

530. Matalon R, Deanching M: The enzymic basis for the phenotypic variation of Hurler and Scheie syndrome, *Pediatr Res* 11:519, 1977.

530a. Matalon R, Deanching M, Omura K: Hurler, Scheie and Hurler/Scheie "compound": residual activity of α-L-iduronidase toward natural substrates suggesting allelic mutations, *J Inherited Metab Dis* 6(suppl):133-134, 1983.

531. Matalon R, Dorfman A: Hurler's syndrome, an α-L-iduronidase deficiency, *Biochem Biophys Res Commun* 47:959-964, 1972.

532. Matalon R, Dorfman A: Sanfilippo A syndrome: sulfamidase deficiency in cultured skin fibroblasts and liver, *J Clin Invest* 54:907-912, 1974.

533. Matalon R, Dorfman A, Nadler HL: A chemical method for the antenatal diagnosis of mucopolysaccharidoses (letter), *Lancet* 1:798-799, 1972.

534. Matalon R et al: Lipid abnormalities in a variant of the Hurler syndrome, *Proc Natl Acad Sci USA* 59:1097, 1968.

535. Matalon R et al: A chemical method for the antenatal diagnosis of mucopolysaccharidoses, *Lancet* 1:83-84, 1970.

536. Matalon R et al: Morquio's syndrome: deficiency of a chondroitin sulfate *N*-acetylhexoamine sulfate sulfatase, *Biochem Biophys Res Commun* 61:759-765, 1974.

537. Matalon R et al: Carrier detection for Sanfilippo A syndrome, *J Inherited Metab Dis* 11:158-60, 1988.

538. Mathur PS: Gargoylism, *Ind J Pediatr* 24:372, 1957.

539. Maumenee AE: Congenital hereditary corneal dystrophy, *Am J Ophthalmol* 50:1114-1124, 1960.

540. Maynard, JA et al: Morquio's disease (mucopolysaccharidosis type IV), ultrastructure of epiphyseal plates, Lab. Invest. 28:194-205, 1973.

541. McClure J et al: The histological and ultrastructural features of the epiphyseal plate in Morquio type A syndrome (mucopolysaccharidosis type IVA), *Pathology* 18:217-221, 1986.

542. McCormick WF: Rupture of the stomach in children: review of the literature and a report of seven cases, *Arch Pathol* 67:416, 1959.

543. McDonnell JM, Green WR, Maumenee IH: Ocular histopathology of systemic mucopolysaccharidosis, type II-A (Hunter syndrome, severe), *Ophthalmology* 92:1772-1779, 1985.

544. McGovern MM et al: An improved method for heterozygote identification in feline and human mucopolysaccharidosis VI, arylsulfatase B deficiency, *Enzyme* 26:206-210, 1981.

545. McGovern MM et al: Animal model studies of allelism: characterization of arylsulfatase B mutations in homoallelic and heteroallelic (genetic compound) homozygotes with feline mucopolysaccharidosis VI, *Genetics* 110:733-749, 1985.

546. McGovern MM et al: Bone marrow transplantation in Maroteaux-Lamy syndrome (MPS type VI): status 40 months after BMT, *Birth Defects* 22(1):41-53, 1986.

547. McKusick VA: *Heritable disorders of connective tissue*, ed 1, St Louis, 1956, Mosby–Year Book, pp 153-183.

548. McKusick VA: Hereditary disorders of connective tissue, *Bull NY Acad Med* 35:143-156, 1959.

549. McKusick VA: *Heritable disorders of connective tissue*, ed 2, St Louis, 1960, Mosby–Year Book, pp 242-384.

550. McKusick VA: On the X chromosome of man, *Ann Intern Med* 56:991-996, 1962.

551. McKusick VA: *Heritable disorders of connective tissue*, ed 3, St Louis, 1966, Mosby–Year Book, pp 325-399.

552. McKusick VA: The nosology of the mucopolysaccharidoses, *Am J Med* 47:730-747, 1969.

553. McKusick VA: *Heritable disorders of connective tissue*, ed 4, St Louis, 1972, Mosby–Year Book, pp 521-686.

554. McKusick VA: Personal observation, 1988.

555. McKusick VA, Neufeld EF: The mucopolysaccharide storage diseases. In Stanbury JB et al, editors: *The metabolic basis of inherited diseases*, ed 5, New York, 1983, McGraw-Hill, pp 751-777.

556. McKusick VA et al: The genetic mucopolysaccharidoses, *Medicine* 44:445-483, 1965.

557. McKusick VA et al: Allelism, non-allelism and genetic compounds among the mucopolysaccharidoses: corrective factors in nosology, genetics and therapy, *Trans Assoc Am Phys* 85:151-171, 1972.

558. McKusick VA et al: Allelism, non-allelism and genetic compounds among the mucopolysaccharidoses: hypotheses, *Lancet* 1:993-996, 1972.

559. Melhem R et al: Roentgen findings in mucolipidosis III (pseudo-Hurler polydystrophy), *Radiology* 106:153-160, 1973.

560. Meyer K: Abstracts of 130th American Chemical Society meetings, *Am Chem Soc* Sept, 1956, p 150.

561. Meyer K et al: Excretion of sulfated mucopolysaccharides in gargoylism (Hurler's syndrome), *Proc Soc Exp Biol Med* 97:275-279, 1958.

562. Meyer K et al: Sulfated mucopolysaccharides of urine and organs in gargoylism (Hurler's syndrome). II. Additional studies, *Proc Soc Exp Biol Med* 102:587-590, 1959.

563. Meyer SJ, Okner HB: Dysostosis multiplex with special reference to ocular findings, *Am J Ophthalmol* 22:713, 1939.

564. Michail J et al: Maladie de Morquio (osteochondrodystrophie polyepiphysaire deformante) chez deux freres, *Helv Paediatr Acta* 11:403-413, 1956.

565. Michalski JC et al: The structure of six urinary oligosaccharides that are characteristic for a patient with Morquio syndrome type B, *Carbohydr Res* 1:351-363, 1982.

566. Millman G, Whittick JW: Sex-linked variant of gargoylism, *J Neurol Neurosurg Psychiatry* 15:253-259, 1952.

567. Minelli A et al: First-trimester prenatal diagnosis of Sanfilippo disease (MPSIII) type B, *Prenat Diagn* 8:47-52, 1988.

568. Miwa Z et al: Dental characteristics of a patient with I-cell disease (mucolipidosis II), *Shoni Shikagaku Zasshi* 23:233-242, 1985.

569. Mogle P et al: Calcification of intervertebral disks in I-cell disease, *Eur J Pediatr* 145:226-227, 1986.

570. Moore KJ, Paigen K: Genome organization and polymorphism of the murine β-glucuronidase region, *Genomics* 2:25-31, 1988.

571. Morabito E et al: Biochemical diagnosis of Hunter syndrome on Epstein-Barr virus-transformed lymphoblastoid cell lines, *Clin Chem Acta* 181:125-133, 1989.

572. Moreno JA et al: Mucopolysaccharidosis VII: familial study, *Arch Neurobiol (Madr)* 51:147-153, 1988.

573. Morquio L: Sur une forme de dystrophie osseuse familiale, *Bull Soc Pediatr de Paris* 27:115, 1929.

574. Morquio L: Sur une forme de dystrophie osseuse familiale, *Arch Med d'Enf* 38:5-24, 1935.

575. Morreau H et al: Vitamin A intoxication as a cause of pseudotumor cerebri, *J Biol Chem* 264:20655-20663, 1989.

576. Moser HW et al: Infusion of normal HLA-identical leukocytes in Sanfilippo disease type B. *Arch Neurol* 31:329, 1974.

577. Mossman J et al: Hunter's disease in a girl: association with X:5 chromosomal translocation disrupting the Hunter gene, *Arch Dis Child* 58:911-915, 1983.

578. Mossman J et al: Prenatal tests for Sanfilippo disease type B in four pregnancies, *Prenat Diagn* 3:347-350, 1983.

579. Mueller OT, Shows TB, Opitz JM: Apparent allelism of the Hurler, Scheie, and Hurler/Scheie syndromes, *Am J Med Genet* 18:547-556, 1984.

580. Mueller OT et al: Mucolipidosis II and III: the genetic relationship between two disorders of lysosomal enzyme biosynthesis, *J Clin Invest* 72:1016, 1983.

581. Mueller OT et al: Sialidosis and galactosialidosis: chromosomal assignment of two genes associated with neuraminidase-deficiency disorders, *Proc Natl Acad Sci* 83:1817-1821, 1986.

582. Muenzer J et al: Attempted enzyme replacement using human amnion membrane implantations in mucopolysaccharidoses, *J Inherit Metab Dis* 15:25-37, 1992.

583. Muir H, Mittwoch V, Bitter T: The diagnostic value of isolated urinary mucopolysaccharides and of lymphocytic inclusions in gargoylism, *Arch Dis Child* 38:358-363, 1963.

584. Muller VJ, Hopwood JJ: Radiolabelled disaccharides for the assay of β-D-glucuronidase activity and the detection of mucopolysaccharidosis type VII, *Clin Chim Acta* 123:357-360, 1982.

585. Muller VJ, Hopwood JJ: Alpha-L-iduronidase deficiency in mucopolysaccharidosis type I against a radiolabelled sulfated disaccharide substrate derived from dermatan sulfate, *Clin Genet* 26:414-421, 1984.

586. Murata R et al: MR imaging of the brain in patients with mucopolysaccharidosis, *AJNR* 10:1165-1170, 1989.

587. Mutoh T et al: Atypical adult G_{M1}-gangliosidosis: biochemical comparison with other forms of primary beta-galactosidase deficiency, *Neurology* 36:1237-1241, 1986.

588. Mutoh T et al: A family with beta-galactosidase deficiency: three adults with atypical clinical patterns, *Neurology* 36:54-59, 1986.

589. Mutoh T et al: Purification and characterization of human liver beta-galactosidase from a patient with the adult form of G_{M1}-gangliosidosis and a normal control, *Biochim Biophys Acta* 964:244-253, 1988.

590. Nanba E et al: G_{M1} gangliosidosis: abnormalities in biosynthesis and early processing of beta-galactosidase in fibroblasts, *Biochem Biophys Res Commun* 152:794-800, 1988.

591. Naumann G: Clearing of cornea after perforating keratoplasty in mucopolysaccharidosis type VI (Maroteaux-Lamy syndrome) *New Engl J Med* 312:(letter)995, 1985.

592. Nelson A et al: Mucopolysaccharidosis VII (β-glucuronidase deficiency) presenting as a nonimmune hydrops fetalis, *J Pediatr* 101:574-576, 1982.

593. Nelson J, Broadhead D, Mossman J: Clinical findings in 12 patients with MPS IV A (Morquio's disease): further evidence for heterogeneity. I. Clinical and biochemical findings, *Clin Genet* 33:111-120, 1988.

594. Nelson J, Carson D: Pituitary function studies in a case of mild Hunter's syndrome (MPS IIB), *J Med Genet* 26:731-732, 1989.

595. Nelson J, Grebbell FS: The value of computed tomography in patients with mucopolysaccharidosis, *Neuroradiology* 29:544-549, 1987.

596. Nelson J, Kinirons M: Clinical findings in 12 patients with MPS IV A (Morquio's disease). Further evidence for heterogeneity. II. Dental findings, *Clin Genet* 33:121-125, 1988.

597. Nelson J, Thomas PS: Clinical findings in 12 patients with MPS IV A (Morquio's disease). Further evidence for heterogeneity. III. Odontoid dysplasia, *Clin Genet* 33:126-130, 1988.

598. Neufeld EF: Lysosomal storage diseases, *Ann Rev Biochem* 60:257-280, 1991.

599. Neufeld EF, Muenzer J: The mucopolysaccharidoses. In Scriver CR et al: *The metabolic basis of inherited disease,* New York, 1989, McGraw-Hill, pp 1565-1587.

600. Neufeld EF et al: The Hunter syndrome in females: is there an autosomal recessive form of iduronate sulfatase deficiency? *Am J Hum Genet* 29:455-461, 1977.

601. Neuhauser EB et al: Arachnoid cysts in the Hurler-Hunter syndrome, *Ann Radiol* 11:453-469, 1968

602. Nevsimalova S et al: Multiple sulfatase deficiency in homozygous twins, *J Inherit Metab Dis* 7:38-40, 1984.

603. Newman NJ et al: Corneal surface irregularities and episodic pain in a patient with mucolipidosis IV (clinical conference), *Arch Ophthalmol* 108:251-254, 1990.

604. Nidiffer FD, Kelly TE: Developmental and degenerative patterns associated with cognitive, behavioral and motor difficulties in the Sanfilippo syndrome: an epidemiological study, *J Ment Defic Res* 27:185-203, 1983.

605. Nishimura Y et al: Nucleotide sequence of rat preputial gland β-glucuronidase cDNA and in vitro insertion of its encoded polypeptide into microsomal membranes, *Proc Natl Acad Sci* 83:7292-7296, 1986.

606. Njå A: Sex-linked type of gargoylism, *Acta Paediat* 93:267-286, 1946.

607. Noll RB, Kulkarni R, Netzloff ML: Follow-up of language and cognitive development in patients with mannosidosis, *Arch Neurol* 43:157-159, 1986.

608. Noll RB, Netzloff ML, Kulkarni R: Long-term follow-up of biochemical and cognitive functioning in patients with mannosidosis, *Arch Neurol* 46:507-509, 1989.

609. Noller F: Dysostosis multiplex (Hurler) und verwandte Krankheitsbilder, *Deutsch Z Chir* 258:259, 1943.

610. Nonne M: Familiares Verkommen (3 Geschwister) einer Kombination von imperfekter Chondrodystrophie mit imperfekten Myxoedema infantile, *Deutsch Z Nervenheilk* 899:263, 1925.

611. Novacyzk MJ et al: Glaucoma as an early complication in Hurler's disease, *Arch Dis Child* 63:1091-1093, 1988.

612. Novoa F et al: Non-surgical macrocephaly, *Rev Child Pediatr* 55:78-85, 1984.

613. Nowakowski RW, Thompson JN, Taylor KB: Sanfilippo syndrome, type D: a spectrophotometric assay with prenatal diagnostic potential, *Pediatr Res* 26:462-466, 1989.

614. Nussbaum BL: Dentistry for the at-risk patient: mucopolysaccharidosis III (Sanfilippo syndrome): a nine-year case study, *ASDC J Dent Child* 57:466-469. 1990.

615. Nwokoro N, Neufeld EF: Detection of Hunter heterozygotes by enzymatic analysis of hair roots, *Am J Hum Genet* 31:42-49, 1979.

616. O'Brien J: Generalized gangliosidosis, *J Pediatr* 75:167-186, 1969.

617. O'Brien JS: Five gangliosidosis, Lancet 2(letter):805, 1969.

618. O'Brien JS: Sanfilippo syndrome: profound deficiency of alpha-acetylglucosaminidase activity in organs and skin fibroblasts from type B patients, *Proc Natl Acad Sci* 69:1720-1722, 1972.

619. O'Brien JS et al: Generalized gangliosidosis: another inborn error of ganglioside metabolism? *J Pediatr* 67(abstract):949, 1965.

620. O'Brien JS et al: Generalized gangliosidosis: another inborn error of ganglioside metabolism? *Am J Dis Child* 109:338-346, 1965.

621. O'Brien JS et al: Molecular biology of the alpha-L-fucosidase gene and fucosidosis, *Enzyme* 38:45-53, 1987.

622. O'Brien JS et al: Bone marrow transplantation in canine G_{M1} gangliosidosis, *Clin Genet* 38:274-280, 1990.

623. Ockerman PA: Deficiency of beta-galactosidase and alpha-mannosidase: primary enzyme defects in gargoylism and a new generalized disease, *Acta Paediat Scand* 177(suppl):35-36, 1967.

624. Ockerman PA: A generalized storage disorder resembling Hurler's syndrome, Lancet 2:239, 1967.

625. Ockerman PA: Mannosidosis: isolation of oligosaccharide storage material from brain, *J Pediatr* 75:360-365, 1969.

626. Ockerman PA, Hultberg B: Fractionation of 4-methylumbellifery-β-galactosidase activities in liver in gargoylism, *Scand J Clin Lab Invest* 22:199-202, 1968.

627. Oda H et al: Hunter's syndrome: an ultrastructural study of an autopsy case, *Acta Pathol Jpn* 38:1175-1190, 1988.

628. Ohta K et al: Type 3 (adult) G_{M1} gangliosidosis: case report, *Neurology* 35:1490-1494, 1985.

629. Okada S, O'Brien JS: Generalized gangliosidosis: β-galactosidase deficiency, *Science* 160:1002-1004, 1968.

630. Okada S et al: I-cell disease: clinical studies of 21 Japanese cases, *Clin Genet* 28:207-215, 1985.

631. Oohira T et al: The infantile form of sialidosis type II associated with congenital adrenal hyperplasia: possible linkage between HLA and the neuraminidase deficiency gene, *Hum Genet* 70:341-343, 1985.

632. Orii T et al: Late onset N-acetylgalactosamine-6-sulfate sulfatase deficiency in two brothers, *Connect Tissue* 13:169-175, 1981.

633. Ornoy A: Early prenatal diagnosis of mucolipidosis IV, *Am J Med Genet* 27:983-985, 1987.

634. Ortega Aramburu JJ et al: Transplante de medula osea en mucopolisacaridos tipe I, variedad de Hurler-Scheie: correccion metabolica y efectos clinicos, *An Esp Pediatr* 33:368-375, 1990.

635. Oshima A et al: Cloning, sequencing, and expression of cDNA for human β-glucuronidase, *Proc Natl Acad Sci USA* 84:685-689, 1987.

636. Oshima A et al: Cloning, sequencing, and expression of cDNA for human beta-galactosidase, *Biochem Biophys Res Commun* 157:238-244, 1988.

637. Osler W: Sporadic cretinism in America, *Trans Cong Am Phys* 4:169, 1897.

638. Paigen K: The genetic control of enzyme realization during differentiation. In Fishbein M, editor: *Congenital malformations*, New York, 1963, International Medical Congress, pp 181-190.

639. Paigen K: The genetics of enzyme realization. In Rechcigl M, editor: *Enzyme synthesis and degradation in mammalian systems*, Basel, 1971, S Karger, pp 1-46.

640. Pallini R et al: Sanfilippo type C diagnosis: assay of acetyl-CoA:alpha-glucosamine N-acetyltransferase using [^{14}C]glucosamine as substrate and leukocytes as enzyme source, *Pediatr Res* 18:543-545, 1984.

641. Palmieri G et al: The iduronate sulfatase gene: isolation of a 1.2-Mb YAC contig spanning the entire gene and identification of heterogeneous deletions in patients with Hunter syndrome, *Genomics* 12:52-57, 1992.

642. Pampiglione G, Harden A: Neurophysiological investigations in G_{M1} and G_{M2} gangliosidoses, *Neuropediatrics* 15:74-84, 1984.

643. Panin G et al: A simple spectrophotometric method for the quantitative determination of urinary glycosaminoglycan excretion, *Clin Chem* 32:2073-2076, 1986.

644. Pannone N et al: Prenatal diagnosis of Hunter syndrome using chorionic villi, *Prenat Diagn* 6:207, 1986.

645. Parfrey NA, Hutchins GM: Hepatic fibrosis in the mucopolysaccharidoses, *Am J Med* 81:825-829, 1986.

646. Parvathy MR, Mitchell DA, Ben-Yoseph Y: Prenatal diagnosis of I-cell disease in the first and second trimesters, *Am J Med Sci* 297:361-364, 1989.

647. Patel V, Watanabe I, Zeman W: Deficiency of α-L-fucosidase, *Science* 176:426-427, 1972.

648. Paterson DE et al: Maroteaux-Lamy syndrome: mild form-MPS VIB, *Br J Radiol* 55:805-812, 1982.

649. Pazzaglia UE et al: Mucolipidosis II: correlation between radiological features and histopathology of the bones, *Pediatr Radiol* 19:406-413, 1989.

650. Pazzaglia UE et al: Neonatal mucolipidosis II, the spontaneous evolution of early bone lesions and the effect of vitamin D treatment: report of two cases, *Pediatr Radiol* 20:80-84, 1989.

651. Pazzaglia UE et al: Study of the bone pathology in early mucolipidosis II (I-cell disease), *Eur J Pediatr* 148:553-557, 1989.

652. Pearce RD et al: Induction of hemopoietic chimerism in the caprine fetus by intraperitonal injection of fetal liver cells, *Experientia* 45:307-308, 1989.

653. Pearce RD et al: Caprine beta-D-mannosidosis: characterization of a model lysosomal storage disorder, *Can J Vet Res* 54:22-29, 1990.

654. Pearson HA, Lorincz AE: A characteristic bone marrow finding in the Hurler syndrome, *Pediatrics* 34:280-282, 1964.

655. Peck JE: Hearings loss in Hunter's syndrome, mucopolysaccharidosis II, *Ear Hear* 5:243-246, 1984.

656. Pedrini V, Lenuzzi L, Zambotti V: Isolation and identification of keratosulfate in urine of patients affected by

Morquio-Ullrich disease *Proc Soc Exp Biol Med J* 10:847-849, 1962.

657. Pennock CA: A review and selection of simple laboratory methods used for the study of glycosaminoglycan excretion and the diagnosis of the mucopolysaccharidoses, *J Clin Pathol* 29:111-123, 1976.

658. Pennock CA, Barnes IC: The mucopolysaccharidoses, *J Med Genet* 13:169-181, 1976.

659. Pennock CA, Mott MG, Batstone GF: Screening for mucopolysaccharidoses, *Clin Chem Acta* 27:93-97, 1970.

660. Perkins DG, Haust MD: Ultrastructure of myocardium in the Hurler syndrome: possible relation to cardiac function, *Virchows Arch* 394A:195-205, 1982.

661. Perks WH et al: Sleep apnoea in Scheie's syndrome, *Thorax* 35:85-91, 1980.

662. Peters ME et al: Narrow trachea in mucopolysaccharidoses, *Pediatr Radiol* 15:225-228, 1985.

663. Peters C et al: Phylogenetic conservation of arylsulphatases: cDNA cloning and expression of human arylsulphatase B, *J Biol Chem* 265:3374-3381, 1990.

664. Petersen EM: Sanfilippo's syndrome type C: the first known case, *S Afr Med J* 69:63-68, 1986.

665. Peterson DI et al: Myelopathy associated with Maroteaux-Lamy syndrome, *Arch Neurol* 32:127-129, 1975.

666. Pfaundler M: Demonstrationen uber einen Typus kindlicher Dysostose, *Jahrb Kinderheilk*, 92:420, 1920.

667. Pfeiffer RA et al: Beta-glucuronidase deficiency in a girl with unusual clinical features, *Eur J Pediatr* 126:155, 1977.

668. Pilz H et al: Deficiency of arylsulfatase B in two brothers ages 40 and 38 years (Maroteaux-Lamy syndrome type B), *Ann Neurol* 6:315-325, 1979.

669. Pizzutillo PD et al: Atlantoaxial instability in mucopolysaccharidosis type VII, *J Pediatr Orthop* 9:76-78, 1989.

670. Poenaru L et al: A variant of mucolipidosis. II. Clinical, biochemical and pathological investigations, *Eur J Pediatr* 147:321-327, 1988.

671. Poenaru L et al: Prenatal diagnosis of mucolipidosis type II on first-trimester amniotic fluid, *Prenat Diagn* 10:231-235, 1990.

672. Pohl JF: Chondro-osteodystrophy (Morquio's disease): progressive kyphosis from congenital wedge-shaped vertebrae, *J Bone Joint Surg* 21:187-192, 1939.

673. Poilvache P et al: Carpal tunnel syndrome in childhood: report of five new cases, *J Pediatr Orthop* 9:687-690, 1989.

674. Poinlet J: Maladie de Hurler authentique avec intelligence normale chez une adulte et ses deux germains, *Bull Mem Soc Med Hôp Paris* 19:457-473, 1968.

675. Pollitt RJ, Jenner FA, Merskey H: Aspartylglucosaminuria: an inborn error of metabolism associated with mental defect, Lancet 2:253-255, 1968.

676. Portoian-Shuhaiber S et al: Siblings with a progressive neurodegenerative condition associated with basal ganglia calcifications, retinitis pigmentosa and decreased levels of fucosidase: a new presentation? *J Inherit Metab Dis* 10:397-398, 1987.

677. Pronicka E et al: Carpal tunnel syndrome in children with mucopolysaccharidosis: needs for surgical tendons and median nerve release, *J Ment Defic Res* 32:79-82, 1988.

678. Putnam MC, Pelkan KF: A case of scaphocephaly with

malformations of skeleton and other tissues, *Am J Dis Child* 29:51-58, 1925.

679. Quigley HA, Goldberg MF: Conjunctival ultrastructure in mucolipidosis III (pseudo-Hurler polydystrophy), *Invest Ophthalmol* 10:568-580, 1971.

680. Quigley HA, Goldberg MF: Scheie syndrome and macular corneal dystrophy: an ultrastructural comparison of conjunctiva and skin, *Arch Ophthalmol* 85:553-564, 1971.

681. Quigley HA, Kenyon KR: Ultrastructural and histochemical studies of a newly recognized form of systemic mucopolysaccharidosis (Maroteaux-Lamy syndrome, mild phenotype), *Am J Ophthalmol* 77:809-818, 1974.

682. Raghavan S et al: Characterization of alpha-mannosidase in feline mannosidosis, *J Inherit Metab Dis* 11:3-16, 1988.

683. Rampini S: Der Spat Hurler: Ullrich-Scheie syndrome, mucopolysacharidosis V, *Schweiz Med Wschr* 99:1769-1778, 1969.

684. Rampini S, Maroteaux P: Ein ungewohnliche Phanotyp des Hurler-Syndrome, *Helv Paediatr Acta* 21:376-386, 1966.

685. Rampini S et al: Mukopolysaccharidose VI-A (Morbus Maroteaux-Lamy, schwere Form), *Helv Paediatr Acta* 41:515-530, 1986.

686. Rampini S et al: Mucopolysacharidosis IV-A (Maroteaux-Lamy disease, severe form): incipient compressive myelopathy, cerebrospinal fluid fistula and tracheal stenosis in an adult patient, *Helv Paediatr Acta* 41:515-530, 1987.

687. Ranieri E, Paton B, and Poulos A: Preliminary evidence for a processing error in the biosynthesis of Gaucher activator in mucolipidosis disease types II and III, *Biochem J* 233:763-772, 1986.

688. Rao BM et al: Rare multivalvular involvement in a family of Scheie syndrome, *Indian J Pediatr* 55:317-322, 1988.

689. Rask MR: Morquio-Brailsford osteochondrodystrophy and osteogenesis imperfecta: report of a patient with both conditions, *J Bone Joint Surg* 45A:561-570, 1963.

690. Rattazzi MC et al: Electrophoresis of arylsulfatase from normal individuals and patients with metachromatic leukodystrophy, *Am J Hum Genet* 25:310-316, 1973.

691. Rattenbury JM, Worthy E, Allen JC: Screening tests for glycosaminoglycans in urine: experience from regional interlaboratory surveys, *J Clin Pathol* 41:936-939, 1988.

692. Rauch RA, Friloux LA, Lott IT: MR imaging of cavitary lesions in the brain with Hurler/Scheie, *AJNR* 10(suppl 5):1-3, 1989.

693. Reilly WA: The granules in leucocytes in gargoylism, *Am J Dis Child* 62:489-491, 1941.

694. Render JA, Lovell KL, Jones MZ: Otic pathology of caprine beta-mannosidosis, *Vet Pathol* 25:437-442, 1988.

695. Renlund M: Clinical and laboratory diagnosis of Salla disease in infancy and childhood, *J Pediatr* 104:232-236, 1984.

696. Rennert OM: Disk electrophoresis of acid mucopolysaccharides, *Nature* 213:1133, 1967.

697. Renteria VG, Ferrans VJ, Roberts WC: The heart in the Hurler syndrome: gross, histologic and ultrastructural observations in five necropsy cases, *Am J Cardiol* 38:487-501, 1976.

698. Resnick JM et al: Pathology of the liver in mucopolysaccharidoses: light and electron microscopic assessment before and after bone marrow transplantation, *Bone Marrow Transplantation* (in press).

699. Rezvani I, Collipp PJ, Di George AM: Evaluation of screening tests for urinary mucopolysaccharides, *Pediatrics* 57:64-68, 1973.

700. Rezvani I et al: Screening tests for the detection of mucopolysaccharide (MPS) disorders: evaluation of a new test, *Pediatr Res* 6:401, 1972.

701. Rich C, DiFerrante N, Archibald RM: Acid mucopolysaccharide excretion in the urine of children, *J Lab Clin Med* 50:686-691, 1957.

702. Riggio S et al: Radiologic aspects of a severe form of Maroteaux-Lamy syndrome, *Radiol Med (Torino)* 70:629-630, 1984.

703. Roberts MW et al: Occurrence of multiple dentigerous cysts in a patient with the Maroteaux-Lamy syndrome (mucopolysaccharidosis, type VI), *Oral Surg* 58:169-175, 1984.

704. Roberts SH et al: Further evidence localizing the gene for Hunter's syndrome to the distal region of the X chromosome long arm, *J Med Genet* 26:309-313, 1989.

705. Robertson DA et al: Human glucosamine 6-sulphatase cDNA reveals homology with steroid sulphatase, *Biochem Biophys Res Commun* 157:218-224, 1988.

706. Robertson DA et al: Chromosomal location of the gene for human glucosamine-6-sulphatase to 12q14, *Hum Genet* 79:175-178, 1988.

707. Robins MM, Stevens HF, Linker A: Morquio's disease: an abnormality of mucopolysaccharide metabolism, *J Pediatr* 62:881-889, 1963.

708. Rome LH, Garvin AJ, Neufeld EF: Human kidney α-L-iduronidase: purification and characterization, *Arch Biochem Biophys* 189:344-353, 1978.

709. Rosen DA et al: Keratoplasty and electron microscopy of the cornea in systemic mucopolysaccharidosis (Hurler's disease), *Can J Ophthalmol* 3:218-230, 1968.

710. Roubicek M, Gehler J, Spranger J: The clinical spectrum of alpha-iduronidase deficiency, *Am J Med Genet* 20:471, 1985.

711. Royer P: La cellile de Buhot et le diagnostic d'un gargoylisme, *Sang* 30:37-40, 1959.

712. Ruggles HE: Dwarfism due to disordered epiphyseal development, *Am J Roentgenol* 25:91-94, 1931.

713. Russell DS: Observations on the pathology of hydrocephalus: special report series, *Med Res Council* no 265, London, 1948, p 52.

714. Sakaguchi T et al: Impaired neutrophil chemotaxis in two patients with mucolipidosis II, *Acta Paediatr Scand* 77:608-609, 1988.

715. Sakura N et al: Asymmetric ventricular septal hypertrophy in I-cell disease, *J Inherit Metab Dis* 9:401-402, 1986.

716. Salaspuro M et al: Elevated levels of serum dolichol in arspartylglucosaminuria, *Life Sci* 47:627-632, 1990.

717. Sanfilippo SJ, Good RA: A laboratory study of the Hurler syndrome, *Am J Dis Child* 102:(abstract)140, 1964.

718. Sanfilippo S et al: Mental retardation associated with acid mucopolysacchariduria (heparitin sulfate type), *J Pediatr* 63:837, 1969.

719. Sanguinetti N et al: The arylsulfatases of chorionic villi: potential problems in the first-trimester diagnosis of metachromatic leucodystrophy and Maroteaux-Lamy disease, *Clin Genet* 30:302-308, 1986.

720. Sasaki CT et al: Hunter's syndrome: a study in airway obstruction, *Laryngoscope* 97:280-285, 1987.

721. Sataloff RT, Schiebel BR, Spiegel JR: Morquio's syndrome, *Am J Otolaryngol* 8:443-449, 1987.

722. Saul RA et al: Atypical presentation with normal stature in Maroteaux-Lamy syndrome (MPS VI), *Proc Greenwood Ctr* 3:49-52, 1984.

723. Saunders GK et al: G_{M1} gangliosidosis in Portuguese water dogs: pathologic and biochemical findings, *Vet Pathol* 25:265-269, 1988.

724. Scaap T, Bach G: Incidence of mucopolysaccharidosis in Israel: is Hunter disease a "Jewish disease?" *Hum Genet* 56:221-226, 1980.

725. Schachern PA et al: Mucopolysaccharidosis I-H (Hurler's syndrome) and human temporal bone histopathology, *Ann Otol Rhinol Laryngol* 93:65-69, 1984.

726. Schafer IA, Powell DW, Sullivan JC: Lysosomal bone disease, *Pediatr Res* 5(abstract):391-392, 1971.

727. Schafer IA et al: Vitamin C–induced increase of dermatan sulfate in cultured Hurler's fibroblasts, *Science* 153:1008-1010, 1966.

728. Scheie HG: Personal communication, 1988.

729. Scheie HG: Personal communications, 1989.

730. Scheie HG, Hambrick GW Jr, Barness LA: A newly recognized forme fruste of Hurler's disease (gargoylism), *Am J Ophthalmol* 53:753-769, 1962.

731. Schenk EA, Haggerty J: Morquio's disease: a radiologic and morphologic study, *Pediatrics* 34:839-850, 1964.

732. Schinz HR, Furtwrangler A: Zur Kenntnis einer hereditaren Osteo-Arthropathie mit rezessivem Erbgang, *Deutsch Z Chir* 207:309-416, 1928.

733. Schmidt H et al: Radiological findings in patients with mucopolysaccharidosis I H/S (Hurler-Scheie syndrome), *Pediatr Radiol* 17:409-414, 1987.

734. Schmidt H et al: Skeletal changes in two German children with aspartylglycosaminuria, *ROFO* 149:143-146, 1988.

735. Schmidt MB: Die anatomischen Veranderungen des Skeletts bei der Hurlerschen Krankheit, *Zbl Allg Path* 79:113-123, 1942.

736. Schuchman EH, Desnick RJ: A new, continuous monodimensional electrophoretic system for the separation and quantification of individual glycosaminoglycans, *Anal Biochem* 117:419-423, 1981.

737. Schuchman EH, Desnick RJ: Mucopolysaccharidosis type I and subtypes: presence of immunologically cross-reactive material and in vitro enhancement of the residual alpha-L-iduronidase activities, *J Clin Invest* 81:98-105, 1988.

738. Schuchman EH, Jackson CE, Desnick RJ: Human arylsulphatase B: MOPAC cloning, nucleotide sequence of a full-length cDNA, and regions of amino acid identity with arylsulphatase A and C, *Genomics* 6:149-158, 1990.

739. Schuchman EH et al: Human α-L-iduronidase. I. Purification and properties of the high uptake (higher molecular weight) and the low uptake (processed) forms, *J Biol Chem* 259:3132-3138, 1984.

740. Schuchman EH et al: Human α-L-iduronidase. II. Comparative biochemical and immunologic properties of the purified low and high uptake forms, *Enzyme* 31:166-175, 1984.

741. Schuchman EH et al: Characterization of the defective beta-glucuronidase activity in canine mucopolysaccharidosis type VII, *Enzyme* 42:174-180, 1989.

742. Schulz R et al: Mucolipidosis type II (I-cell disease) with unusually severe heart involvement, *Monatsschr Kinderheilkd* 135:708-711, 1987.

743. Schwartz MF, Werblin TP, Green WR: Occurrence of mucopolysaccharide in corneal grafts in the Maroteaux-Lamy syndrome, *Cornea* 4:58-66, 1985-1986.

744. Schwartz M et al: Arylsulphatase B studies in skin fibroblasts from patients with Maroteaux-Lamy syndrome with special reference to elecrophoretic mobility and prenatal diagnosis, *J Inherit Metab Dis* 3:99-100, 1980.

745. Scott CR, Lagunoff D, Trump BF: Familial neurovisceral lipidosis, *J Pediatr* 71:357-366, 1967.

746. Scott HS et al: Chromosomal localization of the human α-L-iduronidase gene (IDUA) to 4p16.3, *Am J Hum Genet* 47:802-807, 1990.

747. Scott HS et al: Human alpha-L-iduronidase: cDNA isolation and expression, *Proc Natl Acad Sci USA* 81:9695-9699, 1991.

748. Scott JE, Newton DJ: The recovery and characterization of acid glycosaminoglycans in normal human urine: influence of a circadian rhythm, *Connect Tissue Res* 3:157-164, 1975.

749. Scully RE et al: Case 4, 1991: presentation of case, *New Engl J Med* 324:251-259, 1991.

750. Segni G, Romano C, Tortorolo G: Diagnostic test for gargoylism, *Lancet* 2(letter):420, 1964.

751. Sela M et al: Oral manifestations of Morquio's syndrome, *Oral Surg* 39:583-589, 1975.

752. Selsor LC, Lesher JL Jr: Hyperpigmented macules and patches in a patient with G_{M1} type 1 gangliosidosis, *J Am Acad Dermatol* 20:878-882, 1989.

753. Semenza GL, Pyreitz RE: Respiratory complications of mucopolysaccharide storage disorders, *Medicine* 67:209-219, 1988.

754. Sewell AC: Urinary screening for disorders of heteroglycan metabolism: results of 10 years' experience with a comprehensive system, *Klin Wochenschr* 66:48-53, 1988.

755. Sewell AC, Pontz BF, Benischek G: Mucopolysaccharidosis type IIIC (Sanfilippo): early clinical presentation in a large Turkish pedigree, *Clin Genet* 34:116-121, 1988.

756. Sewell AC et al: Mucopolysaccharidosis type VII (β-glucuronidase deficiency): a report of a new case and a new survey of those in the literature, *Clin Genet* 21:366-373, 1982.

757. Shapiro J, Stome M, Crocker A: Airway obstruction and sleep apnea in Hurler and Hunter syndromes, *Ann Otol Rhinol Laryngol* 94:458-461, 1985.

758. Shapiro LJ et al: The relationship of α-L-iduronidase and Hurler corrective factor, *Arch Biochem Biophys* 172:156-161, 1976.

759. Shell LG et al: Neuronal-visceral G_{M1} gangliosidosis in Portuguese water dogs, *J Vet Intern Med* 3:1-7, 1989.

760. Shih VE: Mucopolysaccharidoses. In Shih V, editor: *Laboratory techniques for the detection of hereditary metabolic disorders*, Cleveland, 1973, CRC, pp 103-106.

761. Shimoda-Matsubayashi S et al: MRI findings in the mild type of mucopolysaccharidosis II (Hunter's syndrome), *Neuroradiology* 32:328-330, 1990.

762. Shull RM, Breider MA, Constantopoulos GC: Long-term neurological effects of bone marrow transplantation in a canine lysosomal storage disease, *Pediatr Res* 24:347-352, 1988.

763. Shull RM, Hastings NE: Fluorometric assay of alpha-L-iduronidase in serum for detection of affected and carrier animals in a canine model of mucopolysaccharidosis I, *Clin Chem* 31:826-827, 1985.

764. Shull RM, Walker MA: Radiographic findings in a canine model of mucopolysaccharidosis I: changes associated with bone marrow transplantation, *Invest Radiol* 23:124-130, 1988.

765. Shull RM et al: Canine α-L-iduronidase deficiency: a model of mucopolysaccharidosis I, *Am J Pathol* 109:244-248, 1982.

766. Shull RM et al: Bone marrow transplantation in canine mucopolysaccharidoses I: effects within the central nervous system, *J Clin Invest* 79:435-443, 1987.

767. Simma B, Sperl W, Hammerer I: G_{M1} gangliosidosis and dilated cardiomyopathy, *Klin Padiatr* 202:183-185, 1990.

768. Singh J et al: N-acetylgalactosamine-6-sulphatase in man: absence of the enzyme in Morquio disease, *J Clin Invest* 57:1036-1040, 1976.

769. Singh S, Petrie JG, Pirozynski WJ: Clinicopathological review of ten cases of Morquio's disease, *Can J Surg* 5:404-410, 1962.

770. Sjogren P, Pedersen T: Anaesthetic problems in Hurler-Scheie syndrome: report of two cases, *Acta Anaesthesiol Scand* 30:484-486, 1986.

771. Sjogren P, Pederson T, Steinmetz H: Mucopolysaccharidoses and anaesthetic risks, *Acta Anaesthesiol Scand* 31:214-218, 1987.

772. Sly WS: Multiple recognition forms of human β-glucuronidase and their pinocytosis receptors: implications for gene therapy, *Birth Defects* 16:115, 1980.

773. Sly WS: Personal communication, 1991.

774. Sly WS et al: Beta-glucuronidase deficiency: report of clinical, radiologic, and biochemical features of a new mucopolysaccharidosis, *J Pediatr* 82:249-257, 1973.

775. Smith R, McCort JJ: Osteochondrodystrophy (Morquio-Brailsford type): occurrence in three siblings, *Calif Med* 88:55-59, 1959.

776. Spranger JW: Biochemical definition of the mucopolysaccharidoses: the range of hereditary anomalies, *Z Kinderheilk* 108:17-31, 1970.

777. Spranger JW: The systemic mucopolysaccharidoses, *Ergebn Inn Med Kinderheilkunde*, 32:165, 1972.

778. Spranger JW: The systemic mucopolysaccharidoses, *Ergebn Inn Med Kinderheilk* 32:185-265, 1972.

779. Spranger JW: Beta-galactosidase and the Morquio syndrome, *Am J Med Genet* 1:207-209, 1977.

780. Spranger JW, Wiedemann HR: The genetic mucolipidoses: diagnosis and differential diagnosis, *Humangenetik* 9:113-139, 1970.

781. Spranger JW et al: Die HS mucopolysaccharidose von Sanfilippo (polydystrophie oligophrenie): Bericht uber 10 patienten, *Z Kinderheilk* 101:71-84, 1967.

782. Spranger JW et al: Mucopolysaccharidosis VI (Maroteaux-Lamy's disease), *Helv Paediatr Acta* 25:337-302, 1970.

783. Spranger JW et al: Mucopolysaccharidosis II (Hunter disease) with corneal opacities, *Eur J Pediatr* 129:11-16, 1978.

784. Starreveld E, Ashenhurst EM: Bilateral carpal tunnel syndrome in childhood: a report of two sisters with mucolipidosis III (pseudo-Hurler polydystrophy), *Neurology* 25:234-238, 1975.

785. Stauffer NR et al: Echocardiographic follow-up in Hurler syndrome after bone marrow transplantation, *Circulation* 84 (suppl 2):462, 1991.

786. Steinbach HL et al: The Hurler syndrome without abnormal mucopolysacchariduria, *Radiology* 90:472-478, 1968.

787. Steiness I: Acid mucopolysaccharides in urine in gargoylism, *Pediatrics* 27:112-117, 1961.

788. Stephan HL et al: Mucopolysaccharidosis I presenting with endocardial fibrolastosis of infancy, *Am J Dis Child* 143:782-784, 1989.

789. Steven IM: Domiciliary use of nasopharyngeal intubation for obstructive sleep apnoea in a child with mucopolysaccharidosis, *Anaesth Intensive Care* 16:493-494, 1988.

790. Stevenson RE et al: Sialic acid storage disease with sialuria: clinical and biochemical features in the severe infantile type, *Pediatrics* 72:441-449, 1983.

791. Stirling LJ et al: Fluorimetric assay for prenatal detection of Hurler and Scheie homozygotes and heterzygotes, *Lancet* 1:147-148, 1978.

792. Stone J, Brimble A, Pennock CA: Carrier detection for Sanfilippo A syndrome, *J Inherit Metab Dis* 13:184-186, 1990.

793. Storm B et al: Bone marrow allograft in Hurler's disease: clinical and biological results after a 1 year's development, *Ann Pediatr (Paris)* 35:117-120, 1988.

794. Strains R, Merliss R, Reiser R: Gargoylism: review of literature and report of sixth autopsied case with chemical studies, *Am J Clin Pathol* 17:671-694, 1947.

795. Stramm L et al: Disease expression in cultured pigment epithelium: feline mucopolysaccharidosis VI, *Invest Ophthalmol Vis Sci* 26:182-192, 1985.

796. Stramm LE et al: Arylsulfatase B activity in cultured retinal pigment epithelium: regional studies in feline mucopolysaccharidoses VI, *Invest Ophthalmol Vis Sci* 27:1050-1057, 1986.

797. Strauss L: The pathology of gargoylism: report of case and review of literature, *Am J Pathol* 24:855-887, 1948.

798. Strauss L, Platt R: Endocardial sclerosis in infancy associated with abnormal storage (gargoylism): report of a case in an infant, age 5 months, and review of the literature, *J Mt Sinai Hosp NY* 24:1258-1271, 1957.

799. Sturmer J: Mucopolysaccharidose type VI-A (Morbus Maroteaux-Lamy syndrome), *Klin Mbl Augenheilk* 194:273-281, 1989.

800. Stumpf DA, Austin JH: Sulfatase B deficiency in the Maroteaux-Lamy syndrome (mucopolysaccharidosis VI), *Trans Am Neurol Assoc* 97:29-32, 1972.

801. Summers CG et al: Ocular changes in the mucopolysaccharidoses after bone marrow transplantation: a preliminary report, *Ophthalmology* 96:977-984, 1989.

802. Suthers GK et al: Genetic mapping of new RFLPs at Xq27-Xq28, *Genomics* 9:37-43, 1991.

803. Suzuki K: Cerebral G_{M1}-gangliosidosis: chemical pathology of visceral organs, *Science* 159:1471-1472, 1968.

804. Takahashi K, Naito M, Suzuki Y: Genetic mucopolysaccharidoses, mannosidosis, sialidosis, galactosialidosis, and I-cell disease: ultrastructural analysis of cultured fibroblasts, *Acta Pathol Jpn* 37:385-400, 1987.

805. Takahashi Y, Orri T: Diagnosis of subtypes of G_{M1} gangliosidosis in vitro and in vivo: using urinary oligosaccharides as substrates, *Clin Chim Acta* 179:219-227, 1989.

806. Takahashi Y, Orri T: Severity of G_{M1} gangliosidosis and urinary oligosaccharide excretion, *Clin Chim Acta* 179:153-162, 1989.

807. Tamagawa et al: Neuropathological study and chemicopathological correlation in sibling cases of Sanfilippo syndrome type B, *Brain Dev* 7:599-609, 1985.

808. Tamaki N et al: Myelopathy due to diffuse thickening of the cervical dura mater in Maroteaux-Lamy syndrome: report of a case, *Neurosurgery.* 21:416-419, 1987.

809. Taylor HR et al: Report of mucopolysaccharidosis occurring in Australian aborigines, *J Med Genet* 15:455-461, 1978.

810. Taylor J et al: Nephrotic syndromes and hypertension in two children with Hurler syndrome, *J Pediatr* 108:726-629, 1986.

811. Taylor JA et al: Human N-acetylgalactosamine-4-sulphatase biosynthesis and maturation in normal, Maroteaux-Lamy and multiple-sulphatase-deficient fibroblasts, *Biochem J* 268:379-386, 1990.

812. Taylor RM, Farrow BR, Stewart GJ: Correction of enzyme deficiency by allogeneic bone marrow transplantation following total lymphoid irradiation in dogs with lysosomal storage disease (fucosidosis), *Transplant Proc* 18:326-329, 1986.

813. Taylor RM, Martin IC, Farrow BR: Reproductive abnormalities in canine fucosidosis, *J Comp Pathol* 100:369-380, 1989.

814. Taylor RM, Stewart GJ, Farrow BR: Improvement in the neurologic signs and storage lesions of fucolipidosis in dogs given marrow transplant at an early age, *Transplant Proc* 21:3818-3819, 1989.

815. Taylor RM et al: Enzyme replacement in nervous tissue after allogeneic bone-marrow transplantation for fucosidosis in dogs, *Lancet* 2:772-774, 1986.

816. Taylor RM et al: Lysosomal enzyme replacement in neural tissue by allogeneic bone marrow transplantation following total lymphoid irradiation in canine fucosidosis, *Transplant Proc* 19:2730-2734, 1987.

817. Taylor RM et al: The clinical effects of lysosomal enzyme replacement by bone marrow transplantation after total lymphoid irradiation on neurologic disease in fucosidase deficient dogs, *Transplant Proc* 20:89-93, 1988.

818. Taylor RM et al: The effect of bone marrow–derived cells on lysosomal enzyme activity in the brain after marrow engraftment, *Transplant Proc* 21:3822-3823, 1989.

819. Taylor RM et al: Histological improvement and enzyme replacement in the brains of fucosidosis dogs after bone marrow engraftment, *Transplant Proc* 21:3074-3075, 1989.

820. Tellez-Nagel I: Mucolipidosis IV: clinical, ultrastructural, histochemical and chemical studies of a case including brain biopsy, *Arch Neurol* 33:828-835, 1976.

821. Terry K, Linker A: Distinction among four forms of Hurler's syndrome, *Proc Soc Exp Biol Med* 115:394-402, 1964.

822. Teyssier G et al: Mucopolysaccaridose de type VII a revelation neonatale, *Arch Fr Pediatr* 38:603-604, 1981.

823. Thomas JE: Gargoylism in the African; report of a case, *Cent Afr J Med* 4:112-114, 1958.

824. Thomas SL, Childress MH, Quinton B: Hypoplasia of the odontoid with atlanto-axial subluxation in Hurler's syndrome, *Pediatr Radiol* 15:353-354, 1985.

825. Thompson GR, Nelson NA, Grobelny SL: A new mucopolysaccharidosis with increased urinary excretion of chondroitin sulfate A, *Arthritis Rheum* 11(abstract):516, 1968.

826. Thompson JN, Rodén L, Reynertson R: Oligosaccharide substrates for heparin sulfamidase, *Anal Biochem* 152:412-422, 1986.

827. Till JS, Roach ES, Burton BK: Sialidosis (neuraminidase deficiency) types I and II: neuro-ophthalmic manifestations, *J Clin Neurol Ophthalmol* 7:40-44, 1987.

828. Tomatsu S et al: Molecular basis of mucopolysaccharidosis type VII: replacement of Ala^{619} in beta-glucuronidase with Val, *Gene* 89:283-287, 1990.

829. Tomatsu S et al: Mucopolysaccharidosis type VII: characterization of mutations and molecular heterogeneity, *Am J Hum Genet* 48:89-96, 1991.

830. Tondeur M et al: Infantile form of sialic acid storage disorder: clinical, ultrastructural and biochemical studies in two siblings, *Eur J Pediatr* 139:142-147, 1982.

831. Toone JR, Applegarth DA: Carrier detection in Sanfilippo A syndrome, *Clin Genet* 33:401-403, 1988.

832. Torok O et al: Prenatal diagnosis of Sanfilippo A disease (mucopolysaccharidosis III A), *Orv Hetil* 127:2385-2387, 1986.

833. Traboulsi EI, Maumenee IH: Ophthalmologic findings in mucolipidosis III (pseudo-Hurler polydystrophy), *Am J Ophthalmol* 15:592-597, 1986.

834. Tsuzaki S et al: An unusually mild variant of Hunter's syndrome in a 14-year-old boy: normal growth and development, *Acta Pediatr Scand* 76:844-846, 1987.

835. Tsvetkova IV et al: Biochemical study of sialidosis type I in a Russian family, *J Inherit Metab Dis* 10:18-23, 1987.

836. Turki I et al: Sanfilippo disease, type C: three cases in the same family, *Neuropediatrics* 20:90-92, 1989.

837. Tuthill CR: Juvenile amaurotic idiocy: marked adventitial growth associated with skeletal malformations and tuberculomas, *Arch Neurol Psychiatr* 32:198-209, 1934.

838. Tylki-Szymanska A et al: Amniotic tissue transplantation as a trial of treatment in some lysosomal storage diseases, *J Inherit Metab Dis* 8:101-104, 1985.

839. Ullrich O: Die Pfaundler-Hurlersche Krankheit: ein Beitrag zinm Problem pleiotroper Genwirkinng in der Erbpathologie des Menschen, Ergebn, *Inn Med Kinderheilk* 63:929, 1943.

840. Ullrich O, Wiedemann HR: Zur Frage der konstitintionellen Granulationsanomalien der Leukocyten in ihrer Beziehung zin enchondralen Dysostosen, *Klin Wschr* 31:107, 1953.

841. Ullrich K et al: Late onset form of mucopolysaccharidosis type I: clinical aspect and biochemical characterization of residual α-L-iduronidase activity, *J Inherit Metab Dis* 4:171-172, 1981.

842. Ullrich-Bott B et al: Lysosomal sialidase deficiency: increased ganglioside content in autopsy tissues of a sialidosis patient, *Enzyme* 38:262-266, 1987.

843. Upadhyaya M et al: Localization of the gene for Hunter syndrome on the long arm of X chromosome, *Hum Genet* 74:391-398, 1986.

844. Ushiyama M et al: Type III (chronic) G_{M1}-gangliodosis: histochemical and ultrastructural studies of rectal biopsy, *J Neurol Sci* 71:209-223, 1985.

845. Uvebrant P: Sanfilippo type C syndrome in two sisters, *Acta Paediatr Scand* 74:137-139, 1985.

845a. Uyama E et al: Three siblings with type III G_{M1}-gangliodosis: pathophysiology of dystonia and MRI findings, *Rinsho Shinkeigaku* 30:819-827, 1990.

846. Uzman LL: Chemical nature of the storage substance in gargoylism: Hurler-Pfaundler's disease, *Arch Pathol* 60:308-318, 1955.

847. Vamos E et al: Multiple sulfatase deficiency with early onset, *J Inherit Metab Dis* 4:103-104, 1981.

848. Vance JM et al: Carrier detection in Sanfilippo syndrome type B: report of six families, *Clin Genet* 20:135-140, 1981.

849. Van de Kamp JJP: *The Sanfilippo syndrome: a clinical and genetical study of 75 patients in the Netherlands*, doctoral thesis, S-Gravenhage, 1979, JH Pasmans.

850. Van de Kamp JJP et al: Genetic heterogeneity and clinical variability in the Sanfilippo syndrome (types A, B, and C), *Clin Genet* 20:152-60, 1981.

851. Van der Horst GT et al: Morquio B syndrome: a primary defect in beta-galactosidase, *Am J Med Genet* 16:261-275, 1983.

852. Van Dyke DL et al: Prenatal diagnosis of Maroteaux-Lamy syndrome, *Am J Med Genet* 8:235-242, 1981.

853. van Diggelen OP et al: A fluorimetric enzyme assay for the diagnosis of Morquio disease type A (MPS IV A), *Clin Chim Acta* 187:131-139, 1990.

854. Van Gemund JJ et al: Electron microscopy of intestinal suction–biopsy specimens as an aid in the diagnosis of mucopolysaccharidoses and other lysosomal storage diseases, *Maandschr Kindergeneesk* 39:211-217, 1971.

855. Van Gemund JJ et al: Morquio B disease, spondylepiphyseal dysplasia associated with acid β-galactosidase deficiency: report of three cases in one family, *Hum Genet* 64:50-54, 1983.

856. Van Hoof F, Hers HG: L'ultrastructure des cellules hepatiques dans la maladie de Hurler (gargoylisme), *CR Acad Sci* 259:1281-1283, 1964.

857. Van Hoof F, Hers HG: The abnormalities of lysosomal enzymes in mucopolysaccharidoses, *Eur J Biochem* 7:34-44, 1968.

858. Van Hoof F, Hers HG: Mucopolysaccharidosis by absence of a fucosidase, *Lancet* 1 (letter):1198, 1968.

859. Van Pelt J et al: Isolation and structural characterization of sialic acid–containing storage material from mucolipidosis I (sialidosis) fibroblasts, *Biochim Biophys Acta* 965:36-45, 1988.

860. Van Pelt J et al: Structural analysis of O-glycosidic type of sialyloligosaccharide-alditols derived from urinary glycopeptides of a sialidosis patient, *Eur J Biochem* 174:183-187, 1988.

861. Van Schrojenstein-de Valk HMJ, van de Kamp JJP: Follow-up on seven adult patients with mild Sanfilippo B–disease, *Am J Med Genet* 28:125-129, 1987.

862. Veasy CA: Ocular findings associated with dysostosis multiplex and Morquio's disease, *Arch Ophthalmol* 25:557-563, 1941.

863. Vestermark S et al: Mental retardation in a patient with Maroteaux-Lamy syndrome, *Clin Genet* 31:114-117, 1987.

864. Vinals Torras M et al: Manifestation of Scheie mucopolysaccharidosis I: carpal tunnel syndrome in childhood, case report, *Arch Neurobiol* 48:113-123, 1985.

865. Vine AK: Uveal effusion in Hunter's syndrome: evidence that abnormal sclera is responsible for the uveal effusion syndrome, *Retina* 6:57-60, 1986.

866. Vogler C et al: A murine model of mucopolysacchridosis VII: gross and microscopic findings in beta-glucuronidase-deficient mice, *Am J Pathol* 136:207-17, 1990.

867. Voisin J, Voisin R: Un cas d'achondroplasie, *Encephale (Paris)* 4:221-227, 1909.

868. Von Figura K, Kresse H: The Sanfilippo B corrective factor: an N-acetyl-α-D-glucosaminidase, *Biochem Biophys Res Commun* 48:262, 1972.

869. Von Figura K et al: Sanfilippo B disease: serum assays for detection of homozygous and heterozygous individuals in three families, *J Pediatr* 83:607-611, 1973.

870. Von Noorden GK, Zellweger H, Ponseti IV: Ocular findings in Morquio-Ullrich's disease, *Arch Ophthalmol* 64:585-591, 1960.

871. Waheed A et al: Deficiency of UDP-N-acetylglucosamine: lysosomal enzyme N-acetylglucosamine-1-phosphotransferase in organs of I-cell patients, *Biochem Biophys Res Commun* 105:1052-1058, 1982.

872. Wakai S et al: Skeletal muscle involvement in mucopolysaccharidosis type IIA: severe type of Hunter syndrome, *Pediatr Neurol* 4:178-180, 1988.

873. Wald SL, Schmidek HH: Compressive myelopathy associated with type VI mucopolysaccharidosis (Maroteaux-Lamy syndrome), *Neurosurgery* 14:83-88, 1984.

874. Walkley SU, Baker HJ, Rattazzi MC: Initiation and growth of ectopic neurites and meganeurites during postnatal cortical development in ganglioside storage disease, *Brain Res Dev Brain Res* 51:167-178, 1990.

875. Walkley SU, Haskins ME, Shull RM: Alterations in neuron morphology in mucopolysaccharidosis type I: a Golgi study, *Acta Neuropathol (Berlin)* 75:611-620, 1988.

876. Wallace BJ et al: Mucopolysaccharidosis type III: morphologic and biochemical studies of two siblings with Sanfilippo syndrome, *Arch Pathol* 82:462-473, 1966.

877. Wallace SP, Prutting CA, Gerber SE: Degeneration of speech, language, and hearing in a patient with mucopolysaccharidosis VII, *Int J Pediatr Otorhinolaryngol* 19:97-107, 1990.

878. Wapner RS, Brandt IK: Hurler syndrome: α-L-iduronidase activity in leukocytes as a method for heterozygote detection, *Pediatr Res* 10:629-632, 1976.

879. Ward JC et al: Regional gene mapping of human β-glucuronidase (GUSB) by dosage analysis: assignment to region 7q11.23-7q21, *Am J Hum Genet* 35:56A, 1983.

880. Warkentin PI et al: Bone marrow transplantation in Hunter syndrome, *Birth Defects* 22:31-39, 1986.

881. Warren CD et al: The accumulation of oligosaccharides in tissues and body fluids of cats with alpha-mannosidosis, *Carbohydr Res* 180:325-338, 1988.

882. Washington JA: Lipochondrodystrophy. In *Brennemann's practice of pediatrics*, vol 4, Hagerstown, Md, 1937, WF Prior.

883. Wassman ER et al: Postmortem findings in the Hurler-Scheie syndrome (mucopolysaccharidosis I-H/S), *Birth Defects* 18(3B):13-18, 1982.

884. Watts RW, Spellacy E, Adams JH: Neuropathological and clinical correlations in Hurler disease, *J Inherit Metab Dis* 9:261-272, 1986.

885. Webman MS et al: Obliterated pulp cavities in the Sanfilippo syndrome (mucopolysaccharidosis III), *Oral Surg* 734-738, 1977.

886. Wehnert M, Machill G, Petruschka L: Genetic complementation analysis in somatic cell hybrids of alpha-L-iduronidase deficient cells, *Hum Genet* 69:287, 1985.

887. Weissmann B, Santiago R: α-L-iduronidase in lysosomal extracts, *Biochem Biophys Res Commun* 46:1430-1433, 1972.

888. Wenger DA, Tarby TJ, Wharton C: Macular cherry-red spots and myoclonus with dementia: coexistent neuraminidase and β-galactosidase deficiencies, *Biochem Biophys Res Commun* 82:589-595, 1978.

889. Wenger DA et al: Human β-mannosidase deficiency, *New Engl J Med* 315:1201, 1986.

890. Whiteside JD, Cholmeley JA: Morquio's disease: review of literature with description of four cases, *Arch Dis Child* 27:487-497, 1952.

891. Whitley CB: Conference report: first international congress on mucopolysaccharidosis and related diseases: 70 years of research, *Am J Med Genet* 32:372-373, 1989.

892. Whitley CB, Krivit W, Gorlin RG: A non-pathologic allele (I^W) for low alpha-L-iduronidase enzyme activity vis-a-vis prenatal diagnosis of Hurler syndrome, *Am J Med Genet* 28:233-243, 1987.

893. Whitley CB et al: Bone marrow transplantation for Hurler syndrome: assessment of metabolic correction, *Birth Defects* 22:7-24, 1986.

894. Whitley CB et al: Diagnostic test for mucopolysaccharidosis. I. Direct method for quantifying excessive urinary glycosaminoglycan excretion, *Clin Chem* 35:374-379, 1989.

895. Whitley CB et al: Diagnostic test for mucopolysaccharidosis. II. Rapid quantification of glycosaminoglycan in urine samples collected on a paper matrix, *Clin Chem* 35:2074-2081, 1989.

896. Wiedemann HR: Ainsgedehnte und allgemeine erblich bedingte Bildungs: und Wachstumsfehler des fronchengerlistes, *Mschr Kinderheilk* 102:136-148, 1954.

897. Wiesmann UN et al: Multiple lysosomal enzyme deficiency due to enzyme leakage? New Engl J Med 284 (letter):109-110, 1971.

898. Wiesmann UN, Rampini S: Mild form of the Hunter syndrome: identity of the biochemical defect with the severe type, *Helv Paediatr Acta* 29:73-78, 1974.

899. Wiesmann V, Neufeld EF: Scheie and Hurler syndromes: apparent identity of the biochemical defect, *Science* 169:72-74, 1970.

900. Wilder RT, Belani KG: Fiberoptic intubation complicated by pulmonary edema in a 12-year-old child with Hurler syndrome, *Anesthesiology* 72:205-207, 1990.

901. Will A et al: Bone marrow transplantation in the treatment of alpha-mannosidosis, *Arch Dis Child* 62:1044-1049, 1987.

902. Willems PJ et al: Identification of a mutation in the structural alpha-L-fucosidase gene in fucosidosis, *Am J Hum Genet* 43:756-763, 1988.

903. Willems PJ et al: Intrafamilial variability in fucosidosis, *Clin Genet* 34:7-14, 1988.

904. Wilson CS et al: Aortic stenosis and mucopolysaccharidosis, *Ann Intern Med* 92:496-498, 1980.

905. Wilson D et al: Neonatal beta-glucuronidase deficiency mucopolysaccharidosis (MPS VII): autopsy findings, J *Neuropathol Exp Neurol* 41:344-349, 1982.

906. Wilson PJ et al: Hunter syndrome: isolation of an iduronate-2-sulfatase cDNA clone and analysis of patient DNA, *Proc Natl Acad Sci USA* 87:8531-8535, 1990.

907. Wilson PJ et al: Frequent deletions at Xq28 indicate genetic heterogeneity in Hunter syndrome, *Hum Genet* 86:505-508, 1991.

908. Winters PR et al: Alpha-iduronidase deficiency and possible Hurler-Scheie genetic compound, *Neurology* 26:1003-1007, 1976.

909. Wislocki GB, Sognnaes RF: Histochemical reactions of normal teeth, *Am J Anat* 87:239-275, 1950.

910. Wisniewski K et al: Sanfilippo disease, type A with some features of ceroid lipofuscinosis, *Neuropediatrics* 16:98-105, 1985.

911. Woessner S et al: Type VII mucopolysaccharidosis (Sly disease), *Sangre (Barc)* 34:153-155, 1989.

912. Wolburg-Buchholz K et al: Familial lysosomal storage disease with generalized vacuolization and sialic aciduria: sporadic Salla disease, *Neuropediatrics* 16:67-75, 1985.

913. Wolfe JH et al: Restoration of normal lysosomal function in mucopolysaccharidosis type VII cells by retroviral vector-mediated gene transfer, *Proc Natl Acad Sci* 87:2877-2881, 1990.

914. Wolff D: Microscopic study of temporal bones in dysostosis multiplex (gargoylism), *Laryngoscope* 52:218-223, 1942.

915. Worth HM: Hurler's syndrome: a study of radiologic appearances in the jaws, *Oral Surg* 22:21-35, 1966.

916. Wraith JE, Alani SM: Carpal tunnel syndrome in the mucopolysaccharidoses and related disorders, *Arch Dis Child* 65:962-963, 1990.

917. Wraith JE, Danks DM, Rogers JG: Mild Sanfilippo syndrome: a further cause of hyperactivity and behavioural disturbance, *Med J Aust* 147:450-451, 1987.

918. Wraith JE, Rogers JG, Danks DM: The mucopolysaccharidoses, *Aust Paediatr J* 23:329-334, 1987.

919. Yamada H et al: Craniosynostosis and hydocephalus in I-cell disease (mucolipidosis II), *Childs Nerv Syst* 3:55-57, 1987.

920. Yamaguchi K et al: Improvement of tear lysosomal enzyme levels after treatment with bone marrow transplantation in a patient with I-cell disease, *Ophthalmic Res* 21:226-229, 1989.

921. Yamamoto Y et al: Isolation, characterization, and mapping of a human acid beta-galactosidase cDNA, *DNA Cell Biol* 9:119-127, 1990.

922. Yatziv S, Erickson RP, Epstein CJ: Mild and severe Hunter syndrome (MPS II) within the same siblings, *Clin Genet* 11:319, 1977.

923. Yatsiv S et al: The therapeutic trial of fresh plasma infusions over a period of 22 months in two siblings with Hunter syndrome, *Isr J Med Sci* 11:802-808, 1975.

924. Yeager AM et al: A therapeutic trial of amniotic epithelial cell implantation in patients with lysosomal storage diseases, *Am J Med Genet* 22:347-355, 1985.

925. Young ID, Harper PS: Long-term complications in Hunter's syndrome, *Clin Genet* 16:125-132, 1979.

926. Young ID, Harper PS: Mild form of Hunter's syndrome: clinical delineation based on 31 cases, *Arch Dis Child* 57:828-836, 1982.

927. Young ID, Harper PS: The natural history of the severe form of Hunter's syndrome: a study based on 52 cases, *Dev Med Child Neurol* 25:481-489, 1983.

928. Young ID, Hunter PS: Incidence of Hunter's syndrome, *Hum Genet* 60:391-392, 1982.

929. Young ID et al: A clinical and genetic study of Hunter's syndrome. I. Heterogeneity, *J Med Genet* 10:408-411, 1982.

930. Young ID et al: A clinical study of Hunter's syndrome. II. Differences between the mild and severe forms, *J Med Genet* 10:408-411, 1982.

931. Young R et al: Compressive myelopathy in Maroteaux-Lamy syndrome: clinical and pathologic findings, *Ann Neurol* 8:336-340, 1980.

932. Yutaka T et al: Iduronate sulfatase analysis of hair roots for identification of Hunter syndrome heterozygotes, *Am J Hum Genet* 30:575, 1978.

933. Yven M, Fenson AH: Diagnosis of classical Morquio's disease: N-acetylgalactosamine 6-sulfate sulfatase activity in cultured fibroblasts, leukocytes, amniotic cells and chorionic villi, *J Inherit Metab Dis* 8:80-86, 1985.

934. Zabel RW et al: Scheie's syndrome: an ultrastructural analysis of the cornea, *Ophthalmology* 96:1631-1638, 1989.

935. Zechner G, Moser M: Osteosclerosis and mucopolysaccharidosis, *Acta Otolaryngol* 103:384-386, 1987.

936. Zeigler M, Bach G: Internalization of exogenous gangliosides in cultured fibroblasts for the diagnosis of mucolipidosis IV, *Clin Chim Acta* 157:183-189, 1986.

937. Zellweger H, Giaccai L, Firzli S: Gargoylism and Morquio's disease, *Am J Dis Child* 84:421-435, 1952.

938. Zellweger H et al: Morquio-Ullrich's disease: report of two cases, *J Pediatr* 59:549-561, 1961.

939. Zhao H et al: Prenatal diagnosis of Morquio disease type A using a simple fluorometric enzyme assay, *Prenat Diagn* 10:85-91, 1990.

940. Zimmermann B et al: Severe aortic stenosis in systemic lupus erythematosus and mucopolysaccharidosis type II (Hunter's syndrome), *Clin Cardiol* 11:723-725, 1988.

941. Zlotogora J, Bach G: Heterozygote detection in Hunter syndrome, *Am J Med Genet* 17:661-665, 1984.

942. Zlotogora J, Bach G: Hunter's syndrome: activity of iduronate sulfate sulfatase in the serum of pregnant heterozygotes, *New Engl J Med* 311(letter):331-332, 1984.

943. Zlotogora T, Bach G: Hunter syndrome: prenatal diagnosis in maternal serum, *Am J Hum Genet* 38:253-260, 1986.

944. Zlotogora J, Zeigler M, Bach G: Selection in favor of lysosomal storage disorders? *Am J Hum Genet* 42:271-273, 1988.

945. Zlotogora J et al: Hunter syndrome among Ashkenazi Jews in Israel: evidence for prenatal selection favoring the Hunter allele, *Hum Genet* 71:329-332, 1985.

12

Fibrodysplasia Ossificans Progressiva

Peter Beighton

Fibrodysplasia ossificans progressiva (FOP) is a bizarre disorder in which affected persons are immobilized by progressive soft tissue ossification. The basic defect is unknown, but in view of the predominant involvement of connective tissues, FOP qualifies for inclusion in this book.

HISTORICAL NOTE

The name *myositis ossificans progressiva*[97] is said to have been assigned to this condition by von Dusch in 1868. The designation in which fibrositis is substituted for myositis has been used more frequently in recent decades,[42,76,116] since the primary change is in the connective tissues, specifically, the aponeuroses, fasciae, and tendons, and the muscles are only secondarily affected. It is not entirely improper to refer to the condition as fibrositis, since the lesions may appear to be inflammatory during early stages. However, *fibrodysplasia*, the term suggested by Bauer and Bode,[2] is probably the most valid.[30] The condition has been referred to as Munchmeyer disease,[65] but the use of this eponym seems inappropriate in view of Rosenstirn's report[97] that Munchmeyer's article of 1869 concerned only the fifteenth reported case. Indeed, the first case may have been described by Guy Patin as early as 1692.[87] Extraordinarily clear descriptions of the end stages of the disease were provided in the *Philosophical Transactions of the Royal Society of London* in the first half of the eigh-teenth century by John Freke and others.[34,35] John Freke (1688-1756), a London surgeon and a man of wide culture, was a friend of the author Joseph Fielding, who mentions him twice in *Tom Jones*. Freke saw his patient with FOP at St. Bartholomew's Hospital[34,35]:

April 14, 1736, there came a Boy of healthy Look and 14 Years of Age, to ask of us at the Hospital, what should be done to cure him of many large Swellings on his Back, which began about 3 Years since, and have continued to grow as large on many Parts as a Penny-loaf, particularly on the left side. They arise from all the vertebrae of the Neck, and reach down to the Os sacrum; they likewise arise from every Rib of his Body, and joining together in all Parts of his Back, as the Ramifications of Coral do, they make, as it were, a fixed bony Pair of Bodice.

Abernethy, Hawkins, Hutchinson,[58] Volkmann, Kronecker, Virchow, Paget, Rolleston,[96] Garrod,[37] Parkes Weber, Opie, and many others added cases. In a review of the subject in 1918 Rosenstirn[97] abstracted 119 case reports, thereafter, further reviews appeared.[28,74,75,84] Lutwak estimated that about 260 individuals with the condition had been documented up to 1963.[74] In a drug trial reported in 1972 Geho and Whiteside[39] treated the condition in 52 affected persons for more than 6 months. The total group of patients called to their attention or receiving treatment for less than 6 months was appreciably larger. More recently, additional series of FOP patients have been published,* and in 1983 FOP was extensively reviewed by Michael Connor of Glasgow in his classic monograph, *Soft Tissue Ossification*.[10] By 1990 about 600 cases could be identified in the world literature.

CLINICAL MANIFESTATIONS

Fibrodysplasia ossificans progressiva is evident at birth in shortening of the great toes and to a lesser extent the thumbs.[50,89,97] The condition is otherwise innocuous at this stage and may remain unrecognized until soft tissue ossification commences in late childhood.[36] The great toe is affected in most instances, but the thumb is involved in less than half the cases. Abnormalities of other digits are much less common.[29] Hallux valgus frequently results, and it is often this feature rather than shortening of the digit that impresses the observer. The shortening is the result of changes in the phalangeal bones; the proximal phalanx may be completely suppressed, although synostosis of the phalanges of the great toe is perhaps the most characteristic change. Clinodactyly or radial curvature of the fifth finger may also occur.

In midchildhood transient localized cystic swellings appear first in the subcutaneous tissues of the neck and back and, later, in the limbs. Their development may be spontaneous or precipitated by trauma, and their resolution may be accompanied by discharge of serosanguineous fluid. At times fever is associated with the tumors, and acute rheumatic fever may be simulated.[98] As the swelling subsides, ectopic ossification forms at the affected sites. The dorsal aspect of the trunk and the proximal portions of the extremities are usually affected,[57] although plantar and palmar fascia may also be involved. Bony bars and bridges cause progressive deformity and limitation of joint movement. Fracture may occur in the ectopic bone,[82] but the skeleton is not otherwise unduly fragile. It is not uncommon for exostoses to develop at the attachments of fibrous structures to bones, for instance, in the occipital region of the skull or as an anterior calcaneal spur.

Columns and plates of bone eventually replace the tendons, fasciae, and ligaments. The spine may become completely rigid and malaligned.[82] Koontz' patient[63] "was completely unable to sit down . . . she either had to lie down or stand up.

She had enough motion in one of her knee joints so that she could walk with a very halting, mincing step. She was of slight build, weighing very little, and it was simple to carry this plank-like girl around."[64] Fairbank[29] presented drawings of skeletons showing extensive changes. Often a ridge of bone on the back appears like a handle by which the patient can literally be lifted.[114] A girl with severe FOP is depicted in Fig. 12-1.

Stature and mentality are usually normal. Conductive deafness develops after adolescence in about 25% of affected persons.* Baldness, greasy skin, and irregular menses represent additional minor features of the disorder, and cardiac valvular defects have been documented in isolated cases.[60] A few women with FOP have had successful pregnancies, producing both normal and affected offspring,[111] but the management of pregnancy in patients with FOP poses many problems.[22,32] For instance, if movements of the hip joints are restricted by soft tissue ossification, cesarean section may be necessary. Prenatal diagnosis is not yet possible.

The process of ectopic ossification slows in adulthood,[104] but most persons with FOP are seriously handicapped by 30 years of age.[15] The tongue, heart, diaphragm, abdominal wall, perineum, eyes, and sphincters usually enjoy immunity from the process, but in the later stages movement may be possible only in the jaw, tongue, eyes, and digits.[14,83,91] Involvement of the masseter muscle and ankylosis of the temporomandibular joint may create difficulties during anesthesia, feeding, and dental care.† Nevertheless, despite the eventual severity of the disablement, persons with FOP may survive beyond middle age.[29,63,64] Pneumonia consequent on restricted respiratory excursion is often the cause of death.

Radiographs reveal widespread but mild changes in the osseous skeleton.[17,20,31] In particular, the cervical vertebral bodies are small, with large pedicles and spines,[17,110] whereas the spinal canal is narrow in the lumbar region. Vertebral fusion occurs in the later stages.[16,48] The femoral necks are broad and short, and the acetabula are shallow.

The ectopic bone in the soft tissues becomes apparent on radiographic examination a few months after the development of the tumors. It often be-

---

*References 11, 14, 15, 95, 99, 104, and 113.

*References 15, 19, 66, 73, 74, 78, 95, and 106.
†References 16, 51, 59, 70, 102, 112, and 124.

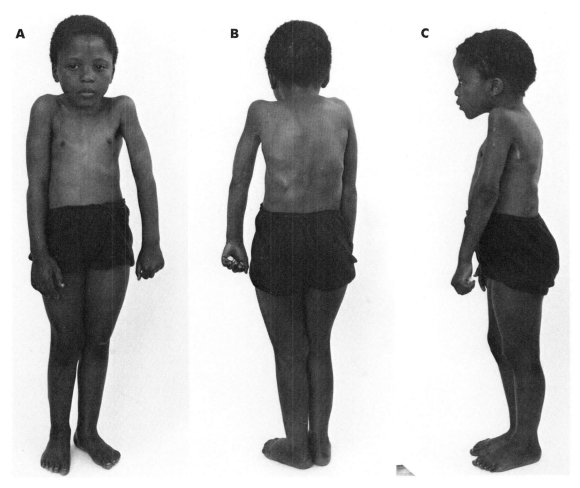

Fig. 12-1. A 6-year-old Zulu girl with FOP. **A,** The child is severely disabled, with fixation of the shoulders and spine. **B,** Ossifying swellings are present in the posterior thorax. **C,** Ectopic bone has formed at excision sites on the left thoracic and lumbar regions. (From Connor JM, Beighton P: *S Afr Med J* 61:404-406, 1982.)

comes attached to the skeleton, thereby contributing to the immobility (Fig. 12-2). Ossification at the sites of the tumors can be recognized by means of computed tomography and isotopic scans before it is visible on conventional radiographs.[7,47,56,69,90] Computerized tomographic scanning is the best method currently available for demonstrating the extent of the ectopic ossification (Fig. 12-3). Magnetic resonance imaging is also a useful means of assessing soft tissue changes.[6]

Diphosphonate therapy, which has been used in a number of younger patients, leads to disorganized metaphyseal growth.[123] In addition, osteo-

porosis consequent on long-standing immobility contributes to the radiographic changes in the later stages of the disorder.

Laboratory investigations of routine hematologic and biochemical values yield normal results, and urinary hydroxyproline concentrations are not perturbed.[104,105] Electrocardiographic abnormalities[12] have been documented, but these are inconsistent and of uncertain significance. As would be expected, pulmonary function studies show reduced lung volumes and restricted ventilation.[12] In patients with FOP, obtaining biopsy specimens of connective tissue elements for histopathologic studies is contraindicated, since pro-

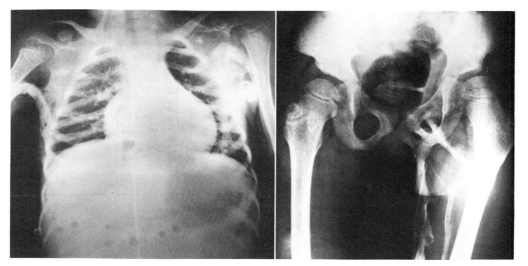

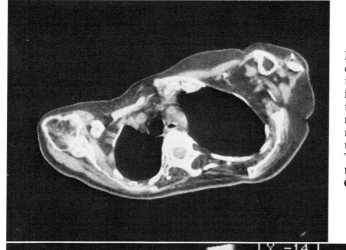

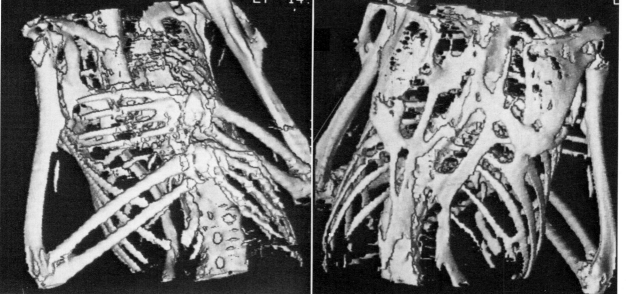

Fig. 12-2. A 5-year-old Xhosa girl with FOP. **A,** Chest radiograph showing well-formed struts of ectopic bone that unite both humeri to the ribs. In adolescence this girl had a painful fracture of one of these bony struts. **B,** Anteroposterior radiograph of the pelvis and hips. Extensive ectopic ossification in the left thigh has anchored the femur to the pubis. (From Cremin B, Connor JM, Beighton P: *Clin Radiol* 33:499-508, 1982.)

Fig. 12-3. A woman of British stock at 53 years of age. The condition developed in this patient in midchildhood; for the past decade she has been totally immobilized except for residual movements in her jaw and fingertips. Despite this extreme handicap, her morale and general health have remained good. **A,** Computerized tomographic scan of the midthoracic region. This transverse view demonstrates ectopic bone and gross distortion of the thoracic cage. **B,** Three-dimensional computerized tomographic scan of the thorax and upper limbs. Extensive ectopic bone is evident. **C,** Back view. (Courtesy Professor B. Cremin).

cedures of this type can exacerbate the process of ossification.[13,53]

The diagnosis of FOP is easily made, once the ectopic bone has appeared. In the early stages the presenting symptom of apparent stiffness of the muscles in the back of the neck has been misinterpreted as "fibrositis," "myalgia," and idiopathic torticollis. The transient soft tissue swellings can be mistaken for a pyogenic inflammatory process[118] or for soft tissue tumors such as lymphadenopathy or sarcoma. In tropical environments infestation with exotic parasites such as Loa loa and Guinea worm enter into the differential diagnosis of the swellings. Localized ectopic calcification may follow trauma[24,86] or may develop in conditions such as tumoral calcinosis and dermatomyositis. The nonspecific term *myositis ossificans,*

which loosely pertains to disorders of this type, is a source of semantic confusion.

REVIEW OF CASES

In the fourth edition of this book McKusick[80] gave summaries of 12 patients with FOP who had been seen at the Johns Hopkins Hospital between 1931 and 1971. He commented as follows:

All but two were still living in 1971. One had been reported by Koontz,[63] and two were briefly referred to by Geschickter and Maseritz.[40] In none of these 12 families has another case of FOP been known. All the patients have abnormalities of the toes or fingers, or both. One patient (described in Case 5) did not have any problems until the age of 25 years, when lumps appeared above one knee. In another patient [described in Case 3] torticollis was noted at 1 month of age, and ad-

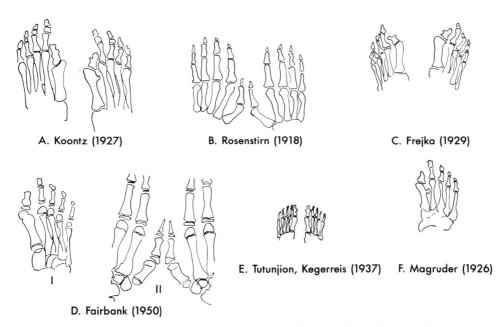

A. Koontz (1927)   B. Rosenstirn (1918)   C. Frejka (1929)

D. Fairbank (1950)   E. Tutunjion, Kegerreis (1937)   F. Magruder (1926)

Fig. 12-4. Tracings of radiographs of hands and feet in selected reported cases (not reproduced to the same scale). **A,** Hands little affected. In feet, monophalangeal first digit and biphalangeal fifth digit. On the right, the fourth toe is also biphalangeal. Exostosis on the first right metatarsal and a bone bridge between metatarsals on the left are evident. **B,** The short, pointed terminal phalanx of the thumb is typical. The first metacarpal on the left is abnormal in shape. (Frequently the first metacarpal and metatarsal have a disorganized trabecular pattern.) The terminal phalanges of the other digits, especially, the second and third, are also short and pointed. **C,** The fingers were not discussed. The first toe is monophalangeal, and the others are biphalangeal at the most. Typical hallux valgus is present. **D,** *I,* Seven years of age. First metatarsal appears to have been lengthened by fusion with the proximal phalanx. The other toes are all biphalangeal. *II,* Ten years of age. The characteristic short, pointed terminal phalanx is seen. Microdactyly of the great toes was also present. **E,** No comment was made on the state of the hands. A monophalangeal first toe can be present without microdactyly or hallux valgus. **F,** Typical monophalangy of first toe and biphalangy of others. Exostosis like that in Koontz's patient is evident. *Continued.*

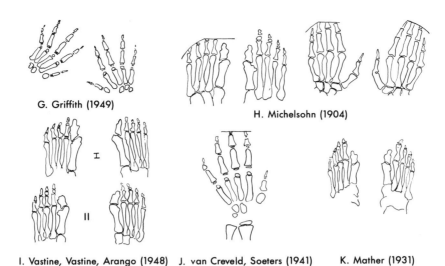

G. Griffith (1949)

H. Michelsohn (1904)

I

II

I. Vastine, Vastine, Arango (1948)   J. van Creveld, Soeters (1941)   K. Mather (1931)

Fig. 12-4, cont'd. G, Typically short, pointed terminal phalanx of thumbs and of other fingers. The fifth fingers were curved (clinodactylous) on clinical examination. The great toes were monophalangeal. **H,** First toes are monophalangeal; fifth toes are biphalangeal. Typical thumbs. **I,** *I* and *II*, Identical twins. Monophalangy of first toes. Biphalangy of fourth and fifth toes. **J,** Five years of age. Typical thumb. **K,** Monophalangeal first toe. Biphalangeal fifth toe. In the feet of many patients in the illustrated cases of FOP, sesamoid bones have been conspicuous by their absence. In their place, projections similar to exostoses occur, particularly at the distal end of the first metatarsal. It is likely that these "exostoses" are synostoses of sesamoid bones with the metatarsal. (**A** from Koontz AR: *Am J Med Sci* 174:406-412, 1927. **B** from Rosenstirn J: *Ann Surg* 68:485-520, 591-637, 1918. **C** from Frejka B: *J Bone Joint Surg* 11:157-166, 1929. **D** from Fairbank HAT: *An atlas of general affections of the skeleton*, Baltimore, 1951, Williams & Wilkins. **E** from Tutunjian KH, Kegerreis R: *J Bone Joint Surg* 19:503-510, 1937. **F** from Magruder LF: *Am J Roentgenol* 15:328-331, 1926. **G** from Griffith G: *Arch Dis Child* 24:71-74, 1949. **H** from Michelsohn J: *Z Orthop Chir* 12:424-443, 1904. **I** from Vastine JH II, Vastine MF, Arango O: *Am J Roentgenol* 59:204-212, 1948. **J** from van Creveld S, Soeters JM: *Am J Dis Child* 62:1000-1013, 1941. **K** from Mather JH: *Br J Radiol* 4:207-210, 1931.)

vanced FOP was present when he was seen at the age of 16 months.

Abstracts of these 12 cases with relevant illustrations are presented for their historical value and to provide a perspective of the manifestations and natural history of the disorder (Fig. 12-4).

CASE 1

The case of N.J., born in 1908, was reported by Koontz[63] in 1927, with excellent illustrations of the gross appearance and radiologic changes, including those of the thumbs and great toes. The maternal grandfather and his two brothers developed late in life what apparently were Dupuytren contractures. A cousin on the maternal side apparently had a deformity of the toes similar to the patient's. The patient's first symptom was stiffness at the age of 9 years. Menstruation never occurred. Both great toes and thumbs were short and malformed. Concentrations of calcium and phosphorus in the blood were normal. I examined the patient in April, 1956. She was then 48 years of age. The disease had progressed slowly but steadily. The jaw was partially fixed, she could not sit, and the arms were in an absolutely fixed position, with a minimum of wrist motion present. Using a long-handled fork and standing up, the patient was able to feed herself. This patient died in 1964 (at 56 years of age) of heart failure. Autopsy showed moderate coronary arteriosclerosis and pulmonary fibrosis. The mechanism of the heart failure was not entirely clear.

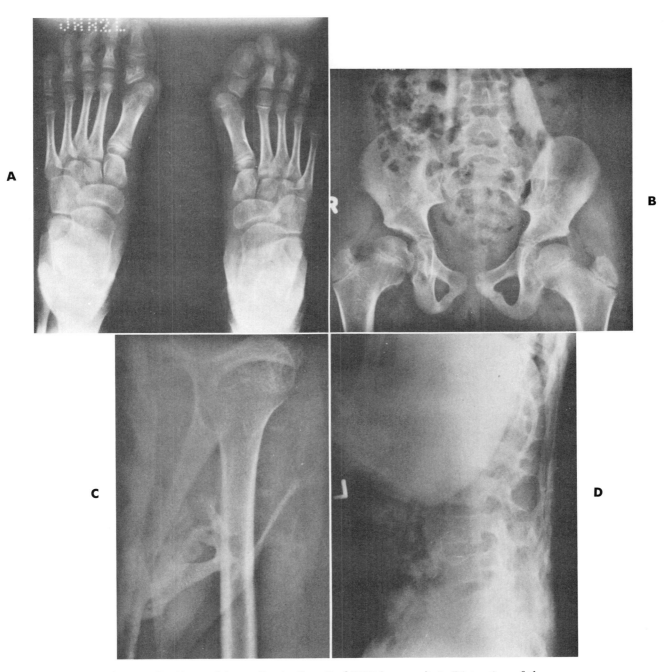

Fig. 12-5. Radiographic studies in Case 2 of FOP (see text). **A,** Distortion of the contour of the distal tip of the first metatarsal and of the proximal phalanges results in the hallux valgus deformity seen on clinical examination. A normal number of phalangeal bones are present in all toes. This, as seen from inspection of Fig. 12-4, is the exception; as a rule, monophalangy of the great toes, at least, is present. It will be interesting to see whether synostosis occurs in the future, as was observed to occur in Michelsohn's patient.[81] The hands were normal. As demonstrated in **B,** the neck of the right femur is slightly widened and blunted; immediately adjacent to the epiphyseal line the left femur is normal. Anomalous bone is seen on each side of the lower lumbar spine, especially the left. Ossification in the axillary areas, **C,** has the appearance of cortical bone. In places, it resembled the ribs in contour. At least one false joint was identified. In the lateral view of the lumbar spine, **D,** plates of bone are clearly demonstrated on the back. (Radiographs shown in **A** to **D** were made when the patient was 8 years of age.)   *Continued.*

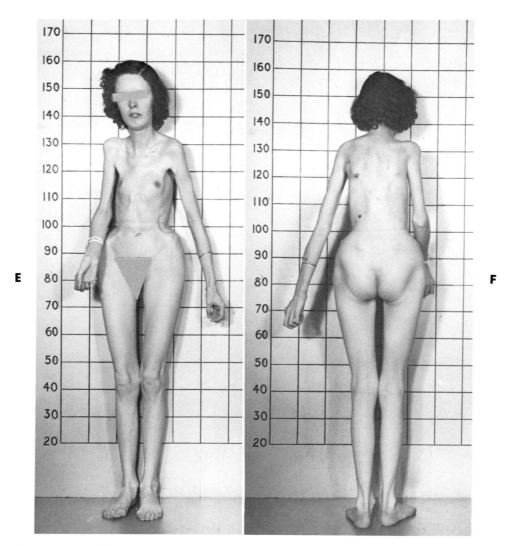

Fig. 12-5, cont'd. **E** and **F,** At 19 years of age the patient shows relatively fixed position of the arms, involvement of the anterior abdominal musculature by ossification, and short great toes. (By 19 years of age, fusion of the phalanges of the great toe was complete, creating monophalangy.)

CASE 2

B.W., a 7½-year-old white girl, has a normal brother and sister. The father had stunting of the great toes similar to the patient's, but no other instance of FOP is known in the family. At the age of 10 months, when the patient began to sit up, the head leaned to the left. At the age of 6½ years she developed an exostosis on the right knee after trauma. However, she remained apparently well otherwise until the age of about 7 years, when she began to complain of pain in the left side of her neck and firmness and tenderness were discovered

there. Thereafter, swelling and induration developed on the back, abdomen, and shoulder. There was marked limitation of motion of the neck, arms, and spine, and the head was held to the left. Dermatomyositis was the initial diagnosis. Fig. 12-5 shows radiographic studies of this patient.

Follow-up (1971, 27 years of age). After 4 years without a flare-up the patient developed lesions at many sites and stiffness in both elbows, so that it became impossible for her to feed herself. An adrenal steroid (Medrol) has been administered for the last 6

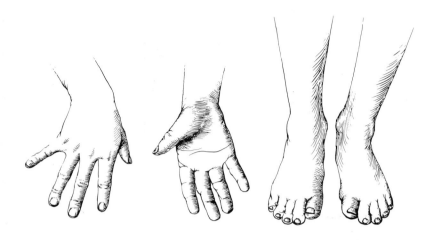

Fig. 12-6. Drawings of the hands and feet of the patient described in Case 4 of the FOP series (see text). Microdactyly of the thumbs and toes is strikingly demonstrated.

months with apparent benefit. She is able to get about well and has no recognized hearing loss. Her jaw has limited motion. She is able to feed herself with a long-handled fork and drink with a long straw.

CASE 3

R.W. at birth was found to have hallux valgus and short thumbs. At 1 month the head was noted to be bent to the left and there was a firm mass in the sternocleido-mastoid muscle. Thereafter asymmetry of the face developed. Lumps appeared in many areas over the back and scalp. These masses never appeared inflamed. There were, however, frequent bouts of unexplained fever. Examination revealed atrophy of the left side of the face. The sternocleidomastoid muscle on the left was converted into a stony hard mass. The nuchal ligament was similarly affected. Extensive involvement about the scapulae (which were attached to the ribs) and the trapezius muscle formed a yoke on the back.

Follow-up (1971, 24 years of age). The disorder appeared to become quiescent at puberty. The patient was graduated from architectural school but encountered difficulty obtaining a job because of his disability. He walks without aids, dresses himself, and eats regular food, although jaw motion is moderately limited. He is unable to sit and must recline because of fixation of the pelvic girdle. Hearing is defective, and he uses a hearing aid in the ear to which he is able to reach his hand.

CASE 4

V.W. has seven siblings, but none has either microdactyly or FOP. She was presumably well until the age of 6 years, when she fell from a swing, striking her back. Swelling and discoloration resulted. Radiographic films at that time revealed "a spider's web on the spine." Thereafter, there was a steadily progressive increase in stiffness and limitation of motion of joints. The thumbs and toes had always been small. It is of note that the fa-

cial muscles were involved in this case. By the age of 25 years the jaws became locked and the upper teeth had to be removed to permit alimentation. Fig. 12-6 presents drawings of this patient.

Follow-up (1971). The patient died in 1965 at the age of 57 years, after a severe respiratory infection.

CASE 5

F.K. was well until the age of 25 years, when a "bump" developed above one knee after trauma. During the following year there were several episodes of soreness and swelling in the left side of the neck, with difficulty in swallowing. There are six siblings. No other members of the family had microdactyly or ossification. The patient's thumbs were small, with fusion of the interphalangeal and metacarpophalangeal joints (Fig. 12-7). All the terminal phalangeal joints of the second and fourth fingers were fused. Hearing was impaired bilaterally. As long as the patient could remember, he had had restriction of motion of the head, mandible, both shoulders, right elbow, both thumbs, both hips, left knee, left ankle, and toes of the left foot. Supposedly, poliomyelitis affecting mainly the left leg had occurred at 5 years of age, but suspicion is cast on the diagnosis by later developments. When restudied in 1963 this patient was found to be remarkably little changed from the state described and photographed 30 years previously. Review of the history indicated that in childhood he was never very active and that severe incapacitation probably began in his teens. As had been true 30 years earlier, he was rendered almost immobile by his disease and showed striking changes in the thumbs and great toes. The thumb was monophalangeal. The distal two phalanges of the index fingers were also fused, as were some of the proximal row of the carpal bones. In the feet a single blocklike bone replaced the first metatarsal and phalanges of the first toe. The second, third, and fourth metatarsals were fused with the proximal phalanges.

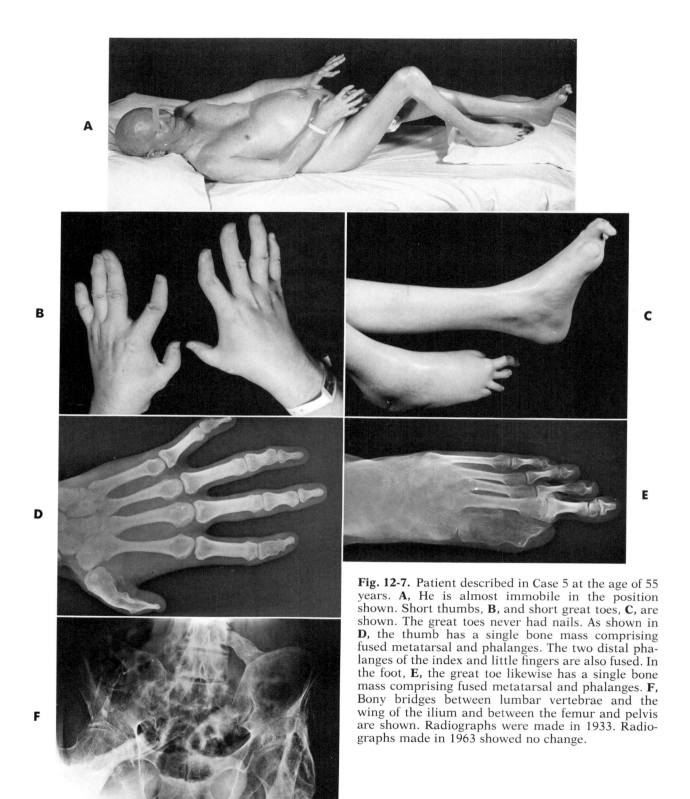

Fig. 12-7. Patient described in Case 5 at the age of 55 years. **A,** He is almost immobile in the position shown. Short thumbs, **B,** and short great toes, **C,** are shown. The great toes never had nails. As shown in **D,** the thumb has a single bone mass comprising fused metatarsal and phalanges. The two distal phalanges of the index and little fingers are also fused. In the foot, **E,** the great toe likewise has a single bone mass comprising fused metatarsal and phalanges. **F,** Bony bridges between lumbar vertebrae and the wing of the ilium and between the femur and pelvis are shown. Radiographs were made in 1933. Radiographs made in 1963 showed no change.

The tarsal bones showed striking fusion with one another and with the metatarsals. The ankle joints were completely fused, as was also the spine, both the vertebral bodies and the apophyseal joints being affected. This is the most severe instance of bony fusions in this series. The deafness was of mixed conductive and nerve type. Although old otitis media was proposed as the cause, ossicle fusion seems possible.

Follow-up (1971, 63 years of age). The patient's condition continues unchanged and on the whole he "gets along" remarkably well. Chronic constipation is a problem. Vomiting spells appear to be related to it. This man probably holds a record for survival with this disease.

CASE 6

M.W. was seen at the age of 14 years, and a diagnosis of calcinosis of the muscles of both hips was rendered. However, on retrospect there can be no question that FOP was actually present. The boy had always been stiff, and after a blow on the back at the age of 5 years, a lump on the left scapula was noted. The mass was biopsied and called sarcoma. The boy was given only 3 months to live; he is still alive, although disabled, at the age of 27 years. Other lumps appeared, and flexion contracture of the hips and right knee gradually developed. The left great toe was short and deformed.

CASE 7

P.H., born October 4, 1951, had as his first manifestation of FOP the appearance (in 1954) of transient, nontender "bumps" in the posterior part of the scalp. A biopsy diagnosis of neurofibromatosis was made. The correct diagnosis was made in October 1956, by which time typical ossifying changes in the aponeuroses of the back had developed. A striking feature at that time was local heat over the involved areas of the back. The thumbs and toes were characteristically short. Two older siblings, born in 1947 and 1949, are normal, and no definite abnormality has been detected in members of the family. Other features of note include short, broad femoral necks and exostosis-like spurs on the upper end of each tibia at the site of muscle attachments (Fig. 12-8). Steroid therapy undoubtedly suppresses acute inflammatory phases in this patient. It probably had no effect on the ossification process. (See Lutwak[74] for further details on this patient.)

Follow-up (1971). The patient is a prelaw student and does well academically. He is able to care for himself completely, can sit in a chair, and lives in a dormitory. His hearing is unimpaired. Occasional small lumps appear on his back. He no longer takes cortisone but for several years has been on continuous tetracycline therapy.

CASE 8

C.A.B., born May 22, 1960, was noted at birth to have "bunions" on both feet. At approximately 2 weeks of age

the mother noted that the infant's head could not be turned to one side. A physician rendered a diagnosis of wryneck. Heat, swelling, and firmness of the sternocleidomastoid and other neck muscles were progressive, and right sternocleidomastoid myomectomy was performed at the age of 1 year. Between 2 and 3 years of age bony protuberances began to develop over the posterior chest wall. A characteristic evolution beginning with erythema, swelling, and warmth characterized the lesions. By 4½ years of age marked immobilization of the head and shoulder girdle with restriction of thoracic expansion had developed. As well as an extensive posterior truncal development of bone, the anterior abdominal wall contained firm lumps and plates. Mobility of the lower extremities was little if at all reduced. The great toes were monophalangeal and short, with hallux valgus. The thumbs appeared normal and were normal on radiographic study. As in Case 7, ossified tendinous insertions suggesting exostoses of diaphyseal aclasis were seen in the distal femur, radius, and ulna and in the proximal humerus.

Follow-up (1971). The patient is severely incapacitated with involvement of the masseter, cervical,

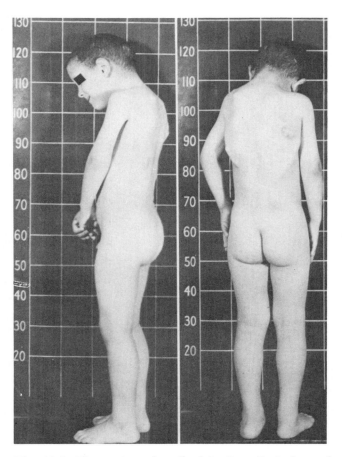

A, B

Fig. 12-8. The patient described in Case 7. **A,** Lateral view (June 1958). **B,** Rear view (June 1958).   *Continued.*

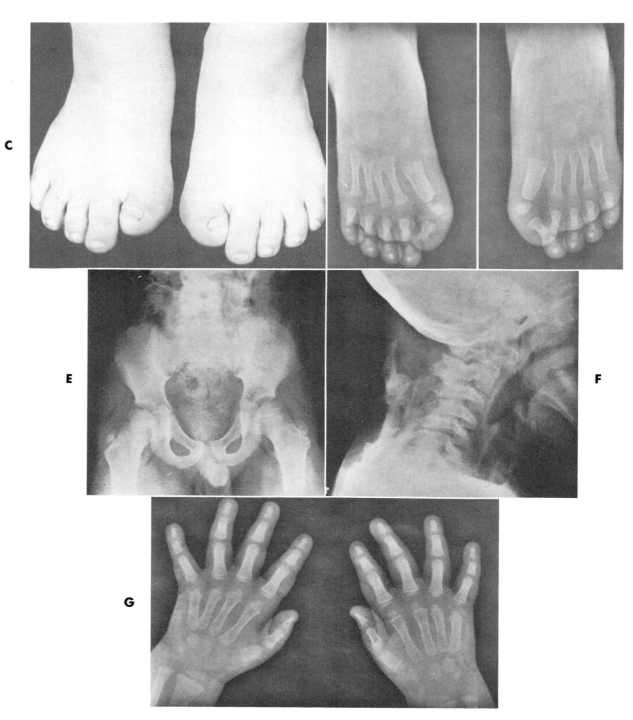

Fig. 12-8, cont'd. **C,** Feet, showing microdactyly of great toes. **D,** Radiograph of feet (April 1957). **E,** The neck of the femur is short and broad. **F,** Extensive ossification of nuchal ligament and adjacent ligaments. **G,** Short thumbs, mainly because of short first metacarpals.

paraspinal, and abdominal muscles and ankylosis of the shoulders and hips. An ossific contracture of the right hip was accompanied by subluxation. Several teeth were removed to facilitate feeding. In 1969 exostoses were removed from the spine and both scapulae. Ulceration had developed over the bony prominences.

CASE 9

J.U., born in December 1959, first developed "lumps" in the scalp above the ears at 18 months of age. The thumbs and first toes were noted to be small at birth. Progressive involvement of the back, axillae, and arms led to complete immobility of the upper trunk, neck, shoulders, and elbows. At 5½ years of age he was still able to feed himself and, because of relatively little involvement of the legs, to play actively. The arms were small. The knees and ankles were prominent. No new lesions had appeared for over a year, the last one being on the bottom of the left foot. Lesions on the back had ulcerated with extrusion of calcific material but then healed satisfactorily. The patient is the youngest of four children of normal parents who were 41 (father) and 35 years of age at the time of his birth. The oldest of the four children died of brain tumor at 6 years of age.

Follow-up (1971). The patient has marked shoulder-girdle limitation. Although surgical mobilization by excision of bony bridges was considered, no such procedures have been performed. He has a chronically ulcerated area over the left ankle.

CASE 10

D.S., a white boy born June 6, 1967, was noted at birth to have short first toes. The thumbs were normal. At the age of 2 weeks a left sternomastoid tumor was noted, and at 1 month a hard, movable subcutaneous nodule about 3 cm in diameter was seen over the sixth thoracic vertebra. By 3 months of age this nodule had begun to calcify. The diagnosis of FOP was made in October 1967, when calcification of the sternocleidomastoid muscle was noted. By the age of 8 months motion of the head, especially to the left, was limited and nodules were present on the back of the head. At 5 months of age a fall resulted in right occipital skull fracture. Salaam-type seizures began about that time. The electroencephalogram was abnormal, evolving into a typical hypsarrhythmia pattern by February 1968. Neurologic examination suggested left-sided hemiparesis. At this writing (1971) the disorder appears to be quiescent. The parents were 41 (father) and 36 years of age at the time of his birth.

CASE 11

D.C.H., a white boy born October 17, 1967, was noted at birth to have short first toes that turned inward and were loose-jointed. In the first week of life a nodule was noted on his back. This was removed at 6 weeks of age. Two more growths were removed from above the scar,

and a larger mass, which extended almost to the crest of the ilium, was excised in February 1968. Thereafter a generalized firm thickening over the entire back developed, with limitation of spinal motion. Excised masses were described as showing, on microscopic examination, interlacing strands of "tumor cells" replacing muscle and dermis. The "tumor cells" were spindle shaped and had central nuclei with a scanty amount of cytoplasm. A few scattered mitotic figures were seen. Radiographic films showed an extensive plate of ossification extending from the sacral to the thoracic areas of the back. An exostosis was demonstrated on the medial aspect of the proximal tibial metaphysis at a site of muscle attachment. The parents were 32 (father) and 34 years of age at the time of his birth. On a diet low in calcium and vitamin D the patient has grown normally and has shown no radiologic evidence of rickets, but the FOP process has continued to progress.

CASE 12

S.E., a white boy, was born November 20, 1969, to a 21-year-old mother and a 40-year-old father. The parents were unrelated. A child born in March 1972, is normal. Bilateral hallux valgus was noted at birth. No trauma to the neck during delivery was recalled. At 3 months of age a pea-sized swelling appeared over the occiput. By 4½ months of age it was the size of a hen's egg. The second swelling noted was behind the left ear. Several swellings over the calvaria appeared and regressed spontaneously. Limitation of head motion as a result of restriction in the left side of the neck progressed to frank torticollis by the age of 4 months. Strabismus was first noted at about the same time but may have been present from birth. Facial asymmetry resulting from torticollis was evident from the age of 6 months. At the age of 8 months FOP was diagnosed on the basis of radiographically demonstrated ossification in the left sternocleidomastoid muscle, with associated phalangeal anomalies and hallux valgus. Fracture of the ossified sternomastoid occurred with a fall at the age of 18 months.

Examination (October 1971) showed left torticollis, left facial hypoplasia, and left convergent strabismus resulting from left rectus palsy. The head was tilted to the left and forward with rotation of the face to the right. Well-circumscribed nodules were palpable over the parietal area of the skull, and a rocky protuberance was palpable over the left mastoid area. Much of the left sternocleidomastoid was replaced by a bony mass. Both first toes were small, with valgus deformity. The fifth fingers showed clinodactyly. The thumbs were biphalangeal but small, especially the left.

Radiologic studies showed no paraspinal ossification. The femoral necks were broad. Exostoses were seen at the site of muscle attachment at the lateral aspect of each tibia proximally.

Forced duction of the eye globes, performed with the

patient under anesthesia, showed full movements, and the result of histologic examination of the ocular muscles was normal, thus excluding FOP at that site.

The patient was treated with disodium editronate 20 mg/kg of body weight, and after 6 weeks the ossified mass of the left sternomastoid was excised. Maintenance in a halo cast was continued for 8 weeks after operation. At ten weeks after operation, passive extension and left lateral flexion of the neck were measured as 20 degrees, both having been 10 degrees before operation.

PREVALENCE AND INHERITANCE

In the past it was suggested that FOP is appreciably more frequent in men and boys, in a ratio as high as 4:1.[98] In Rosenstirn's collection of cases,[97] 62% were male (68 males and 40 females, of cases clearly described as to diagnosis and sex). On the other hand, two thirds of the large series of patients on the treatment program of Geho and Whiteside[39] were women and girls. It is now generally accepted that the sex ratio is equal.

In reports in the last two decades of the nineteenth century Sympson[109] and Stonham[107] each documented microdactyly in a father and son and FOP in the son. Drago[23] made a similar observation in a mother and son. The full syndrome has been described in both father and son,[5] in five male members of three generations,[38] and in identical twins.[26,116] Instances of involvement of successive generations, including male-to-male transmission, have been assembled and documented.[14] There is little doubt that FOP is inherited as an autosomal dominant trait with a particularly wide range of phenotypic expression. The chromosomal locus of the faulty gene is unknown.[10]

Because of the severity of the physical handicap in adulthood, reproduction is unusual, and almost all cases are the result of new dominant mutation. Viparelli[117] documented increased parental age in sporadic cases, and Tunte, Becker, and Knorre[113] confirmed the paternal-age effect on the basis of 23 sporadic cases that they collected anew,[3] together with 16 found in the literature. The mean paternal age was 36.3 years, a value similar to that found in sporadic cases of Marfan syndrome and of achondroplasia. This paternal-age effect was subsequently reconfirmed by Rogers and Chase.[93] A mutation rate for the FOP gene of 1.8 per million and a minimum prevalence in the population of Great Britain of one affected person per 1.64 million have been calculated.[14] The karyotype has been found to be normal in a number of

patients,[66,67,113] including several in McKusick's series.[80]

Most reports of FOP have emanated from Europe and North America, but the condition has also been documented in other regions, including Africa,[11,27,65] India,[9,25] Japan,[108] and the West Indies.[18] It is probable that apparent discrepancies in population frequencies are the consequence of circumstances influencing ascertainment and survival rather than representative of anomalous mutation rates.

PATHOLOGY

The pathologic process in FOP has not been fully elucidated. In 1901 Rolleston[96] expressed the opinion that the disease was a defect of the mesoblast, and in 1929 Hirsch and Löw-Beer[55] called the condition an "exceedingly unusual anomaly of the mesenchyme." Nevertheless, as early as 1926, Gruber[44] had determined that skeletal muscle was fundamentally normal. Other investigators have postulated that FOP was primarily a myopathy,[8,103] and the observation that ossification develops in the heart muscle of a rat after ligation of the ventricles has been regarded as supporting this hypothesis.[101] It has also been suggested that the primary defect might lie in the small blood vessels and that the initial lesion is a hemorrhage, which is followed by organization and ossification of the hematoma.[97] Another theory proposes that there might be defective activity of an inhibitor mechanism that controls the orderly crystalization of bone minerals on collagen fibers.[41,74] It is also possible that the fundamental defect resides in the connective tissues and that an abnormal collagen capable of supporting ossification is present at the sites of disease activity.

In the initial stages of the disorder connective tissue proliferates between muscle fiber bundles and in the soft tissues, whereas fibroblasts aggregate around blood vessels. There are high levels of alkaline phosphatase in these regions.[13,54,58,71,122] Electron microscopic studies of the inflammatory swellings have revealed active fibroblasts with an extensive endoplasmic reticulum and enlarged Golgi bodies.[52] These fibroblasts have a morphologic and cytochemical resemblance to osteoblasts.[79]

In 1938 Geschickter and Maseritz[40] depicted cartilage and young osteoid tissue surrounded by osteoblasts in the affected soft tissues. These changes may closely resemble those of osteogenic sarcoma,[88] and although the apparent occurrence of this malignant tumor in FOP has been documented,[85] it is unlikely that a propensity to neoplasia is a genuine complication of FOP. The ectopic cartilage, which contains high levels of collagen type II, is resorbed and replaced by calcified bone matrix containing collagen type I, as in normal enchondromal ossification. The histologic appearances are identical to those of normal bone.[108]

Sporadic instances of FOP have been documented in cats, a setter dog, and a horse.[97,100,119,120] The condition is transmitted as an autosomal dominant trait in pigs; in an impressive demonstration of this mode of inheritance a boar with FOP sired 34 affected piglets out of a total of 115 offspring.[100] It seems clear that, as in the human, porcine FOP is the consequence of heterozygosity for a single mutant gene.

MANAGEMENT

No specific treatment for FOP exists, although a wide range of therapeutic agents have enjoyed popularity at one time or another. Beryllium[45,46,62,114] has been used in the past because of its inhibitory effect on alkaline phosphatase. Androgens, corticosteroids,[72,92] vitamins B and E, penicillamine, EDTA (disodium ethylenediaminetetraacetic acid),[52,68,74] and isoretinoin[21] have also been employed, as has a diet low in calcium and phosphorus; all have proved to be ineffective.

Diphosphonates (disodium-ethane-1-hydroxy-1, 1-diphosphate or ethane-1-hydroxy-1, 1-diphosphate [EHDP]) have been in vogue.[1,39] In 1972 Geho and Whiteside[39] reported treatment with EHDP of 52 patients for at least 6 months and for a mean time of 1½ years. The majority of these patients seemed to be "stabilized" or somewhat improved while on a regimen of EHDP. In several, withdrawal of EHDP resulted in exacerbation of the disease process, whereas reinstitution of EHDP therapy was accompanied by symptomatic relief. Despite these encouraging results, the long-term benefits are problematic. EHDP inhibits calcification of ectopic bone matrix but does not interfere with its production; it also has a detrimental effect on normal skeletal development.[94,123]

Surgical excision of bone bridges for the purpose of joint mobilization has been performed;[49] as with any operative intervention in FOP, however, there is an ever-present danger of exacerbating the process of soft tissue ossification.[15,121] Operations performed to place limbs in a position of function, whereby the affected person can achieve independent feeding and personal hygiene, may be a valuable component of management. In the late stages of the disorder, when the patient is virtually immobile, specialized nursing techniques may be required.[61]

In the absence of any efficacious therapy and in view of the fluctuant but progressive course and ultimately severe handicap, modification of lifestyle is necessary. Trauma, venipuncture, intramuscular injections, tooth extraction, and surgical operations can all cause ossification and should be avoided, whenever possible. General measures include provision of wheelchairs, power beds, and long-handled utensils. Because pneumonia is a common cause of death, prophylactic antiinfluenzal and antipneumococcal vaccination and vigorous oral antibiotic therapy for chest infection have an important role. Genetic counseling is based on the conventional autosomal dominant recurrence risks; cognizance must be taken of the magnitude of the "burden of the disease."

REFERENCES

1. Bassett CA et al: Diphosphonates in the treatment of myositis ossificans (letter), *Lancet* 2:845 only, 1969.
2. Bauer KH, Bode W: *Erbpathologie der Stützgewebe beim Menschen. Handbuch der Erbbiologie des Menschen*, vol 3, Berlin, 1940, Julius Springer, p 105.
3. Becker PE, von Knorre G: Myositis ossificans progressiva, *Ergebn Inn Med Kinderheilk* 27:1-31, 1968.
4. Bona C et al: Histochemical and cytoenzymological studies in myositis ossificans, *Acta Histochem (Jena)* 27:207-224, 1967.
5. Burton-Fanning FW, Vaughan AL: A case of myositis ossificans, *Lancet* 2:849-850, 1901.
6. Caron KH et al: MR imaging of early fibrodysplasia ossificans progressiva, *J Comput Assist Tomogr* 14(2):318-321, 1990.
7. Carter SR et al: Value of bone scanning and computed tomography in fibrodysplasia ossificans progressiva, *Br J Radiol* 62(735):269-272, 1989.
8. Chaco J: Myositis ossificans progressiva, *Acta Rheum Scand* 13:235-240, 1967.
9. Chopra K, Saha MM and Saluja S: Fibrodysplasia ossificans progressiva, *Indian Pediatr* 24(8):677-680, 1987.
10. Connor JM: *Soft tissue ossification*, Berlin, 1983, Springer-Verlag, pp 54-74.
11. Connor JM, Beighton P: Fibrodysplasia ossificans progressiva in South Africa: case reports, *S Afr Med J* 61(11):404-406, 1982.
12. Connor JM, Evans CC, Evans DAP: Cardiopulmonary function in fibrodysplasia ossificans progressiva, *Thorax* 36:419-423, 1981.
13. Connor JM, Evans DA: Quantitative and qualitative studies on skin fibroblast alkaline phosphatase in fibrodysplasia ossificans progressiva, *Clin Chim Acta* 117(3):355-360, 1981.

14. Connor JM, Evans DA: Genetic aspects of fibrodysplasia ossificans progressiva, *J Med Genet* 19(1):35-39, 1982.

15. Connor JM, Evans DA: Fibrodysplasia ossificans progressiva: the clinical features and natural history of 34 patients, *J Bone Joint Surg* 64(1):76-83, 1982.

16. Connor JM, Evans DA: Extra-articular ankylosis in fibrodysplasia ossificans progressive, *Br J Oral Surg* 20(2):117-121, 1982.

17. Connor JM, Smith R: The cervical spine in fibrodysplasia ossificans progressiva, *Br J Radiol* 55(655):492-496, 1982.

18. Cooles P, Favot I, Madhavan R: Fibrodysplasia (myositis) ossificans progressiva in Dominica, *West Indian Med J* 38(1):48-50, 1989.

19. Cottafava F et al: Fibrodysplasia ossificans: presentation of a case of exceptional severity, *Minerva Pediatr* 38(1-2):344-351, 1986.

20. Cremin B, Connor JM, Beighton P: The radiological spectrum of fibrodysplasia ossificans progressiva, *Clin Radiol* 33(5):499-508, 1982.

21. Crofford LJ et al: Failure of surgery and iso-retinoin to relieve jaw immobilization in fibrodysplasia ossificans progressiva: report of two cases, *J Oral Maxillofac Surg* 48(2):204-208, 1990.

22. Davidson BN, Bowerman RA, LaFerla JJ: Myositis ossificans progressiva and pregnancy: a therapeutic dilemma, *J Reprod Med* 30(12):945-947, 1985.

23. Drago A: Contributo allo studio della moisite ossificente progressive multipla, *Pediatria* 27:715-753, 1919.

24. Ducloyer P et al: Circumscribed non-traumatic myositis ossificans: apropos of 14 cases and a general review, *Rev Chir Orthop* 74(7):659-668, 1988.

25. Dwivedi R: Myositis ossificans progressiva, *J Indian Med Assoc* 41:558 only, 1963.

26. Eaton WL, Conkling WS, Daeschner CW: Early myositis ossificans progressiva occurring in homozygotic twins: a clinical and pathologic study, *J Pediatr* 50:591-598, 1957.

27. Ebrahim GJ, Grech P, Slavin G: Myositis ossificans progressiva in an African child, *Br J Radiol* 39:952-953, 1966.

28. Fairbank HAT: Myositis ossificans progressiva, *J Bone Joint Surg* 32B:108-116, 1950.

29. Fairbank HAT: *An atlas of general affections of the skeleton*, Baltimore, 1951, Williams & Wilkins, pp 150-158.

30. Falls HF: Skeletal system, including joints. In Sorsby A: *Clinical genetics*, St Louis, 1953, Mosby–Year Book.

31. Fang MA et al: Technetium-99m MDP demonstration of heterotopic ossification in fibrodysplasia ossificans progressiva, *Clin Nucl Med* 11(1):8-9, 1986.

32. Fox S et al: Myositis ossificans progressiva and pregnancy. II. *Obstet Gynecol* 69(3):453-435, 1987.

33. Frejka B: Heterotopic ossification and myositis ossificans progressiva, *J Bone Joint Surg* 11:157-166, 1929.

34. Freke J: A case of an extraordinary exostosis on the back of a boy, *Philos Trans R Soc Lond 1735-1743* 41:413, 1736.

35. Freke J: *Philos Trans R Soc Lond 1740*. Quoted by Major RH: *Classic descriptions of disease, with biographical sketches of the authors*, ed 3, Springfield, Ill, 1945, Charles C Thomas, p 304.

36. Friend J: Myositis ossificans progressiva, *Arch Middlesex Hosp* 1:208-212, 1951.

37. Garrod AE: The initial stage of myositis ossificans, *St Bartholomew's Hosp Rep* 43:43-49, 1907.

38. Gaster A: Discussion in meeting of West London Medico-Chirurgical Society, Oct 7, 1904, *West London Med J* 10:37, 1905.

39. Geho WB, Whiteside JA: Experience with disodium etidronate on diseases of ectopic calcification. In Frame B, Parfitt AM, Duncan H, editors: *Clinical aspects of metabolic bone disease: proceedings of the International Symposium on Clinical Metabolic Bone Diseases*, New York, 1972, American Elsevier, pp 506-511.

40. Geschickter CF, Maseritz IH: Myositis ossificans, *J Bone Joint Surg* 20:661-674, 1938.

41. Glimcher MJ: Specificity of the molecular structure of organic matrices in mineralization. In Sognnaes RF, editor: *Calcification in biological systems*, Washington, DC, 1960, American Association for the Advancement of Science, p 421.

42. Greig DM: *Clinical observations of the surgical pathology of bone*, Edinburgh, 1931, Oliver & Boyd, p 170.

43. Griffith G: Progressive myositis ossificans: report of a case, *Arch Dis Child* 24:71-74, 1949.

44. Gruber GB: Anmerkungen zur Frage der Weichteilverknöcherungen, besonders der Myopathia osteoplastica, *Virchows Arch* 260:457-465, 1926.

45. Gutman AB, and Yü TF: A further consideration of the effects of beryllium salts on in vitro calcification of cartilage: metabolic interrelations, *Trans Josiah Macy Jr Found* 3:90, 1950.

46. Guyatt BL, Kay HD, Branion HD: Beryllium "rickets," *J Nutr* 6:313-324, 1933.

47. Gwinn JL: Radiological case of the month: progressive myositis ossificans, *Am J Dis Child* 116:655-656, 1968.

48. Hall CM, Sutcliffe J: Fibrodysplasia ossificans progressiva, *Ann Radiol* 22:119-123, 1979.

49. Harris NH: Myositis ossificans progressiva, *Proc Roy Soc Med* 54:70-71, 1961.

50. Helferich H: Ein Fall von sogenannter Myositis ossificans progressiva, *Aerztl Intelligenz-Blatl* 26:485-489, 1879.

51. Hellinger MJ: Myositis ossificans of the muscles of mastication, *Oral Surg* 19:581-587, 1965.

52. Hentzer B, Jacobsen HH, Asboe-Hansen G: Fibrodysplasia (myositis) ossificans progressiva treated with disodium etidronate, *Clin Radiol* 29(1):69-75, 1978.

53. Hentzer B, Kobayasi T, Asboe-Hansen G: Ultrastructure of dermal connective tissue in fibrodysplasia ossificans progressiva, *Acta Derm Venereol* 57(6):477-485, 1977.

54. Herrmann J et al: Fibrodysplasia ossificans progressiva and the XXXXY syndrome in the same sibship. In Bergsma D, editor: *Clinical delineation of birth defects. V. Phenotypic aspects of chromosomal aberrations*, New York, 1969, National Foundation, March of Dimes.

55. Hirsch F, Löw-Beer A: Ueber einen Fall von Myositis ossificans progressiva, *Med Klin* 25:1661-1664, 1929.

56. Holan J, Galanda V, Buchanec J: Isotopenuntersuchungen bei der Fibrodysplasia ossificans progressiva im Kindersalter mittels Radiostrontium, *Radiol Diagn (Berlin)* 14:719-726, 1973.

57. Hsu LC, Hsu KY, Leong JC: Severe scoliosis associated with fibrodysplasia ossificans progressiva: a report of two cases, *Spine* 11(6):643-644, 1986.

58. Hutchinson J: Case of multiple exostoses with ossification of fascia in various parts and ichthyosis, *Med Times Gazette* 1:317 only, 1860.

59. Iriarte JI, Coulon JP, Reychler H: Temporomandibular ankylosis and progressive ossifying myositis: review of the literature apropos of a case report, *Rev Stomatol Chir Maxillofac* 91(1):51-55, 1990.

60. Jaworski RC, Gibson M: Mitral and aortic valve abnormalities in a patient with fibrodysplasia ossificans progressiva, *Pathology* 15(3):325-328, 1983.

61. Jones B, Love B, Crosbie D: The patient with myositis ossificans progressiva, *Nurs Clin North Am* 4:189-196, 1969.

62. Klemperer FW, Miller JM, Hill CJ: The inhibition of alkaline phosphatase by beryllium, *J Biol Chem* 180:281-288, 1949.

63. Koontz AR: Myositis ossificans progressiva, *Am J Med Sci* 174:406-412, 1927.

64. Koontz AR: Personal communication to McKusick.

65. Lalugue P et al: Réflexions à propos d'un cas de myosite ossifiante progressiva non traumatique ou maladie de Munchmeyer, *Presse Méd* 71:2098 only, 1963.

66. Letts RM: Myositis ossificans progressiva: a report of two cases with chromosome studies, *Can Med Assoc J* 99:856-862, 1968.

67. Letts RM: Myositis ossificans progressiva, *Can Med Assoc J* 100:133 only, 1969.

68. Liberman UA, Barzel U, DeVries A: Myositis ossificans traumatica with unusual course: effect of EDTA on calcium, phosphorus and manganese excretion, *Am J Med Sci* 254:35-47, 1967.

69. Lindhout D, Golding RP, Taets van Amerongen AH: Fibrodysplasia ossificans progressiva: current concepts and the role of CT in acute changes, *Pediatr Radiol* 15(3):211-213, 1985.

70. Lininger TE, Brown EM, Brown M: General anesthesia and fibrodysplasia ossificans progressiva, *Anesth Analg* 68(2):175-176, 1989.

71. Lins FM, Abath GM: Doenca ossificante progressiva, *Pediat Prát* 30:131-144, 1959.

72. Lockhart JD, Burke FG: Myositis ossificans progressiva: report of case treated with corticotropin (ACTH), *Am J Dis Child* 87:626-635, 1954.

73. Ludman H, Hamilton EB, Eade AW: Deafness in myositis ossificans progressiva, *J Laryngol Otolaryngol* 82:57-63, 1968.

74. Lutwak L: Myositis ossificans progressiva: mineral, metabolic and radioactive calcium studies of the effects of hormones, *Am J Med* 37:269-293, 1964.

75. Magruder LF: Myositis ossificans progressiva: case report and review of the literature, *Am J Roentgenol* 15:328-331, 1926.

76. Mair WF: Myositis ossificans progressiva, *Edinburgh Med J* 39:13-36, 1932.

77. Mather JH: Progressive myositis ossificans, *Br J Radiol* 4:207-210, 1931.

78. Maudsley RH: Case of myositis ossificans progressiva, *Br Med J* I:954-956, 1952.

79. Maxwell WA et al: Histochemical and ultrastructural studies in fibrodysplasia ossificans progressiva (myositis ossificans progressiva), *Am J Pathol* 87(3):483-498, 1977.

80. McKusick VA: *Heritable disorders of connective tissue*, ed 4, St Louis, 1972, Mosby–Year Book, pp 687-702.

81. Michelsohn J: Ein Fall von Myositis ossificans progressiva, *Z Orthop Chir* 12:424-443, 1904.

82. Nerubay J, Horoszowski H, Goodman RM: Fracture in progressive ossifying fibrodysplasia: a case report, *Acta Orthop Scand* 58(3):289-291, 1987.

83. Nunnelly JF, Yussen PS: Computed tomographic findings in patients with limited jaw movement due to myositis ossificans progressiva, *J Oral Maxillofac Surg* 44:818-821, 1986.

84. Nutt JJ: Report of a case of myositis ossificans progressiva with bibliography, *J Bone Joint Surg* 5:344-359, 1923.

85. Pack GT, Braund RR: Development of sarcoma in myositis ossificans: report of three cases, *JAMA* 119:776-779, 1942.

86. Parnes EI, Hinds EC: Traumatic myositis ossificans of the masseter muscle: report of case, *J Oral Surg* 23:245-250, 1965.

87. Patin G: Letter of 27 August 1648 written to AF. In *Lettres choisies de feu M. Guy Patin*, Cologne, 1692, P du Laurens, p 28.

88. Paul JR: A study of an unusual case of myositis ossificans, *Arch Surg* 10:185-195, 1925.

89. Pol: "Brachydaktylie," "Klinodaktylie," Hyperphalangie und ihre Grundlagen: Form und Entstehung der meist unter dem Bild der Brachydaktylie auftretenden Varietäten, Anomalien und Missbildungen der Hand und des Fusses, *Virchows Arch* 229:388-530, 1920.

90. Reinig JW et al: Fibrodysplasia ossificans progressiva: CT appearance, *Radiology* 159(1):153-157, 1986.

91. Renton P, Parkin SF, Stamp TC: Abnormal temporomandibular joints in fibrodysplasia ossificans progressiva, *Br J Oral Surg* 20:31-38, 1982.

92. Riley HD Jr, Christie A: Myositis ossificans progressiva, *Pediatrics* 8:753-767, 1951.

93. Rogers JG, Chase GA: Paternal age effect in fibrodysplasia ossificans progressiva, *J Med Genet* 16(2):147-148, 1979.

94. Rogers JG, Dorst JP, Geho WB: Use and complications of high-dose disodium etidronate therapy in fibrodysplasia ossificans progressiva, *J Pediatr* 91(6):1011-1014, 1977.

95. Rogers JG, Geho WB: Fibrodysplasia ossificans progressiva: a survey of forty-two cases, *J Bone Joint Surg* 61:909-914, 1979.

96. Rolleston HD: Progressive myositis ossificans, with references to other developmental diseases of the mesoblast, *Clin J* 17:209-214, 1901.

97. Rosenstirn J: A contribution to the study of myositis ossificans progressiva, *Ann Surg* 68:485-520, 591-637, 1918.

98. Ryan KJ: Myositis ossificans progressiva: review of the literature with report of case, *J Pediatr* 27:348-352, 1945.

99. Schroeder HW, Zasloff M: The hand and foot malformations in fibrodysplasia ossificans progressiva, *Johns Hopkins Med J* 147:73-78, 1980.

100. Seibold HR, Davis CL: Generalized myositis ossificans (familial) in pigs, *Vet Pathol* 4:79-88, 1967.

101. Selye H, Mahajan S, Mahajan RS: Histogenesis of experimentally induced myositis ossificans in the heart, *Am Heart J* 73:195-201, 1967.

102. Shipton EA et al: Anaesthesia in myositis ossificans progressiva: a case report and clinical review, *S Afr Med J* 67(1):26-28, 1985.

103. Smith DM et al: Myositis ossificans progressiva: case report with metabolic and histochemical studies, *Metabolism* 15:521-528, 1966.

104. Smith R: Myositis ossificans progressiva: a review of current problems, *Semin Arthritis Rheum* 4:369-380, 1975.

105. Smith R, Russell RGG, Woods CG: Myositis ossificans progressiva: clinical features of eight patients and their response to therapy, *J Bone Joint Surg (Br)* 58:48-57, 1976.

106. Sorensen MS: Fibrodysplasia ossificans progressiva and hearing loss, *Int J Pediatr Otorhinolaryngol* 14(1):79-82, 1987.

107. Stonham C: Myositis ossificans, *Lancet* 2:1485-1491, 1892.

108. Suzuki T et al: Myositis ossificans progressiva with parathyroid hyperplasia and polycystic ovary, *Acta Pathol Jpn* 26:251-262, 1976.

109. Sympson T: Case of myositis ossificans, *Br Med J* 2:1026-1027, 1886.

110. Thickman D et al: Fibrodysplasia ossificans progressiva, *AJR* 139(5):935-941, 1982.

111. Thornton YS, Birnbaum SJ, Lebowitz N: A viable pregnancy in a patient with myositis ossificans progressiva, *Am J Obstet Gynecol* 156(3):577-578, 1987.

112. Trester PH et al: Myositis ossificans, circumscripta and progressiva, with surgical correction of the masseter muscle: report of two cases, *J Oral Surg* 27:201-205, 1969.

113. Tünte W, Becker PE, Knorre GV: Zur Genetik der Myositis ossificans progressiva, *Humangenetik* 4:320-351, 1967.

114. Tutunjian KH, Kegerreis R: Myositis ossificans progressiva, with report of case, *J Bone Joint Surg* 19:503-510, 1937.

115. Van Creveld S, Soeters JM: Progressive myositis ossificans, *Am J Dis Child* 62:1000-1013, 1941.

116. Vastine JH II, Vastine MF, Arango O: Myositis ossificans progressiva in homozygotic twins, *Am J Roentgenol* 59:204-212, 1948.

117. Viparelli V: La miosite ossificante progressiva, *Ann Neuropsichiat Psicoanal* 9:297, 1962.

118. Voynow JA, Charney EB: Fibrodysplasia ossificans progressiva presenting as osteomyelitis-like syndrome, *Clin Pediatr* 25(7):373-375, 1986.

119. Waldron D et al: Progressive ossifying myositis in a cat, *J Am Vet Med Assoc* 187(1):64-65, 1985.

120. Warren HB, Carpenter JL: Fibrodysplasia ossificans in three cats, *Vet Pathol* 21(5):495-499, 1984.

121. Weiss IW, Fisher L, Phang JM: Diphosphonate therapy in a patient with myositis ossificans progressiva, *Ann Intern Med* 74:933-936, 1971.

122. Wilkins WE, Reagan EM, Carpenter GK: Phosphatase studies on biopsy tissue in progressive myositis ossificans with report of a case, *Am J Dis Child* 49:1219-1221, 1935.

123. Wood BJ, Robinson GC: Drug induced bone changes in myositis ossificans progressiva, *Pediatr Radiol* 5:40-43, 1976.

124. Woolley MM, Morgan S, Hays DM: Heritable disorders of connective tissue: surgical and anesthetic problems, *J Pediatr Surg* 2:325-331, 1967.

CHAPTER 13

Other Heritable and Generalized Disorders of Connective Tissue

Peter Beighton

In addition to the entities discussed in detail earlier in this book, a few others may qualify as heritable disorders of connective tissue and thus deserve mention. The following are briefly reviewed in this chapter:

Osteopoikilosis
Fibromatoses
   Dupuytren contracture
   Léri pleonosteosis
   Peyronie disease
   Other fibromatoses
Paget disease of bone
Epidermolysis bullosa
Occipital horn syndrome
Menkes syndrome
Miscellaneous disorders
   Generalized arterial calcification of infancy
   Werner syndrome
   Progeria
   Wrinkly Skin syndrome
   Connective tissue nevi
   Keloid
   Pachydermoperiostosis
Osteochondroses

OSTEOPOIKILOSIS
Nomenclature

Although earlier references can be found,[45] osteopoikilosis, like osteopetrosis, was first de-

scribed definitively by H. Albers-Schönberg* in 1915.[1] It is sometimes referred to as "spotted bones," an appropriate designation, as is evident in Fig. 13-1. *Osteopoikilosis* is derived from Greek words meaning "mottled bones," and the bone lesion is also referred to as "osteitis condensans generalisata," "osteosclerosis disseminata," or "osteodysplasia enostotica." The skin lesions were first described in 1928 by Buschke and Ollendorff[10] (and, later, by Helen Ollendorff, using her married name, Curth[16]) as "dermatofibrosis lenticularis disseminata." It has been suggested that osteodermatopoikilosis might be a satisfactory designation for the entire syndrome, but this term has not found its way into general use. There is now a trend toward using the conjoined eponym "Buschke-Ollendorf" for the complete syndrome.[19,26,50]

Manifestations

Neither the osseous nor the cutaneous changes have any known clinical significance; they are usually discovered incidentally, since the bone lesions are asymptomatic and the skin lesions, inconspicuous (Fig. 13-2). The practical importance of the disorder lies in the potential for confusion

---

*Heinrich Albers-Schönberg (1865-1915) was the doyen of German radiologists. He made many contributions to academic radiology, but his career was curtailed as a result of radiation-induced neoplasia in his hands and arms.

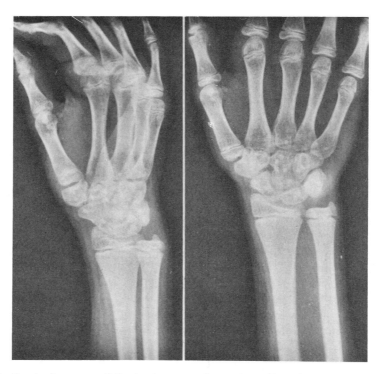

Fig. 13-1. Typical osteopoikilosis discovered incidentally when radiologic studies for wrist injury were performed in a 13-year-old boy.

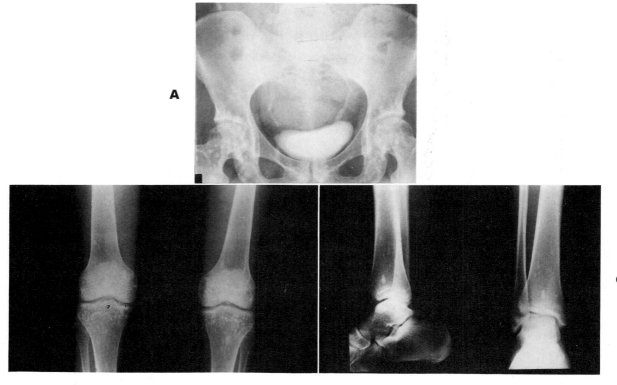

Fig. 13-2. Osteopoikilosis. **A,** Osteopoikilosis was first diagnosed in middle age in this patient when characteristic multiple sclerotic foci were recognized in the femoral heads and adjacent pelvic regions after radiographic contrast studies for unrelated urinary tract problems. **B,** Radiographic skeletal survey revealed sclerotic foci around the knee joint. **C,** Foci were scant at the ankles.

with osteoblastic metastases to the skeleton.[39] Distinction may not be easily made; indeed, circumscribed bony lesions detected in a middle-aged woman after mastectomy for the treatment of carcinoma were initially thought to represent osteopoikilosis.[22] Their true neoplastic nature was recognized only after biopsy and histopathologic studies.

The bone lesions are circumscribed, round areas of increased bone density, usually less than 1 cm in diameter, situated particularly at the ends of the bones of the extremities (but not necessarily in the epiphyses) and in the small bones of the feet and wrists. The foci can be demonstrated by computerized tomography and nuclear magnetic resonance imaging, as well as by conventional radiographic examination.[17] The sclerotic foci may be bilaterally symmetric, and at times they are linear (striate) in distribution.[56] For example, Voorhoeve[52] found vertical striae parallel to the long axis of the bones and as a fan shape in the wings of the ilia, but no sclerotic spots, in two children whose father had typical spots and no striae. In the context of this condition it is noteworthy that osteopoikilosis, as well as melorheostosis, osteopathia striata, and osteopetrosis, is a component of mixed-sclerosing-bone dystrophy[35] syndrome.

The skull has been spared in most cases, although Bistolfi[5] described involvement of the occipital bone. In all three patients investigated by Funstein and Kotschiew[21] sclerotic foci were present in the skull; indeed, the calvarial lesions were the predominant manifestation in Erbsen's patient.[20] Involvement of the lumbar spine,[31,47] ribs, and vertebrae[12] has been documented in isolated cases. The characteristic distribution of the bone lesions is shown in Fig. 13-3. As was nicely demonstrated by Funstein and Kotschiew,[21] in pronounced cases the sclerotic islands tend to be oriented along the "traction and pressure lines,"[31] especially at points of crossing of these lines.

The skin lesions, always inconspicuous, are located most often on the posterior aspect of the thighs and buttocks, occasionally on the arms and trunk, but never on the face. Their location bears no constant relation to that of the bone changes, although the head is usually unaffected by either skin or bone lesions. The skin lesions are compact, slightly elevated, whitish yellow, and usually oblong or oval in outline. Like the bone foci, they sometimes occur in longitudinal streaks. They are usually about the size of a lentil or a pea, from

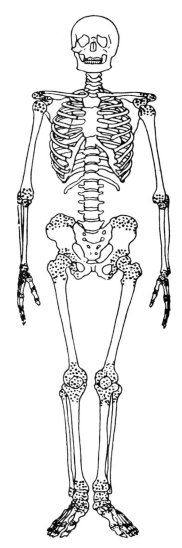

Fig. 13-3. Typical location of bone lesions in osteopoikilosis.[14] (From Cocchi V. In Schinz HR et al [Case JT, editor]: *Roentgendiagnostics,* New York, 1951, Grune & Stratton.)

which their name (dermatofibrosis lenticularis disseminata) is in part derived. Both skin and bone are usually involved,[18,28,46,56] but in several instances, only one or other of these syndromic components have been present in persons with osteopoikilosis.

Information concerning the age of onset and the subsequent evolution of both the osseous and cutaneous changes is meager, but it is clear that both sites may be involved in the first years of life. Furthermore, it appears that once formed, the bone lesions remain static for many years. The skin changes may regress with time[53]; the longest reported follow-up, 17 years, concerned a woman first observed in adolescence.[34]

Keloids may occur with increased frequency in persons with osteopoikilosis.[16] The only internal ramification that has even been suggested is that of fibrous nodules of the peritoneal lining, discovered during laparotomy in a 13-year-old patient who had severe abdominal pains.[44] It can fairly be stated that this was not a "clear case," since the gross appearance of the nodules suggested tuberculosis. Other conditions that have occurred with osteopoikilosis include scleroderma beginning at the age of 7 months[51] and rheumatoid arthritis.[13,15] Exostoses were present in the patients reported by Albers-Schönberg,[1] Albronda,[2] and Risseeuw.[38]

The condition is conventionally considered incapable of producing symptoms and prognostically insignificant. This optimism may not be fully warranted, however, since reports have been made of persons with osteopoikilosis who have had osteosarcoma,[33] chondrosarcoma,[23] and giant cell tumor.[3] Basal cell nevus syndrome[6] and spinal canal stenosis[54] have also been recorded in association with osteopoikilosis.

Pathology

Histologic studies of the bone lesions in an 18-year-old boy who died of a seemingly unrelated cause were made by Schmorl.[40] He found that each "island" is a clump of osseous trabeculae that are thicker at the periphery than at the center. The trabeculae at the center form a complex network with ordinary marrow in the intervening space. Lagier, Mbakop, and Bigler [27] correlated radiographic and histopathologic findings in two adults and concluded that the nature and distribution of the bone lesions were the consequence of interaction between a generalized abnormality of connective tissue and mechanical stresses in bone.

The skin lesions consist of collagenous fibrosis with preservation of the elastic fiber elements.[9,10] They represent connective tissue nevi,[42] and in both clinical and histologic appearance they may be distinguished only with difficulty from the nevi found in tuberous sclerosis. Cairns[11] termed the skin disorder "familial juvenile elastoma"; however, although elastic tissue dominates the histologic picture in some instances, it seems likely that the basic defect does not reside in this tissue.[36] A mother and three offspring with familial elastic nevi were studied by Macedo et al.[29]; none of these patients had bone changes, and the authors proposed that this particular condition was a *forme fruste* of Buschke-Ollendorf syndrome. The heritable skin disorders in which collagen or elastin is abnormal have been reviewed in detail by Uitto and Shamban.[48]

Genetics

More than 400 cases have now been reported, and a perspective of the frequency of the disorder is provided by the data of Jonaseh,[25] who identified 12 cases among 211,000 radiographic studies undertaken for unrelated purposes.

The disorder is inherited as an autosomal dominant mendelian trait with considerable variation in phenotypic expression. Busch[9] found 14 cases in three generations of one family; the condition probably extended further back in the ancestry, since there were three affected siblings in the first generation studied. Hinson[24] identified the disorder in two generations and Verbov,[49] in three generations; Melnick[32] documented involvement in 17 persons in four generations. Considerable intrafamilial variation often is present in the phenotype; for instance, in radiographic studies of the entire skeleton Bloom[7] found only a single spot in the sister of a patient with widespread involvement. Schönenberg[41] recorded the bone changes in eight persons in three generations; six of these individuals also had skin involvement. Wilcox[55] documented the bone condition in a father and daughter and Voorhoeve,[52] in a father, son, and daughter. Risseeuw[38] saw the disorder in a man, six of his children, and a grandson. Albronda[2] reported the bone condition in a woman and one son and daughter; there were no skin changes. Berlin et al.[4] observed two extensively affected kindreds. Many family members had osteopoikilosis without skin lesions, whereas some had skin changes without bone involvement. Raque and Wood[36] described skin and bone lesions in a brother and sister and in the son of the former. The combination of skin and bone lesions occurred in two or more family members mentioned in several additional reports.[8,11,43,56,57] Marshall[30] described skin and bone changes in a mother and son, and Reymond et al.[37] documented the presence of osteopoikilosis in identical twins.

Basic Defect

The basic defect appears to be a spotty hyperplasia of collagen in the corium and bone matrix; However, this is little more than a restatement of the histologic findings. What is basically involved in this condition and why there is the peculiar spotty distribution are obscure. Voorhoeve[52] thought the bone lesions originate in cartilage. He based this theory on his observation in two children of striated lesions extending a variable distance into the diaphysis from the epiphyseal line. The relative immunity of the skull and clavicle ("membranous bones") may be supporting evidence for an endochondral origin.

FIBROMATOSES

The fibromatoses are a group of disorders that share the common characteristic of fibrous proliferation. They differ from each other in the anatomic distribution and clinical consequences of the fibrous lesions. In most of these conditions the genetic background is uncertain and the pathogenesis is obscure.

The following fibromatoses form the subject of this section: Dupuytren contracture, Léri pleonosteosis, Peyronie disease, and other fibromatoses.

Dupuytren Contracture

Dupuytren* contracture involves the palmar fascia and causes progressive flexion of the digits, especially the fourth and fifth. (Fig. 13-4). Onset is usually in adulthood and progression is slow. Knuckle pads[65,66,70,76,79] and plantar nodules[62] often are associated with Dupuytren contracture; possible relationships with epilepsy[63,70,76] and diabetes mellitus[75] are less clear-cut. Although diagnosis is usually easily made, there is some phenotypic overlap with the familial fibromatoses[80] and congenital digital contractural syndromes.

Dupuytren contracture occurs predominantly in men. Geographic distribution is patchy; for instance, it is rare in blacks[71,72] and Orientals[78] but present in 15% of the men on the isolated island of Tristan da Cunha.[60] Numerous examples of familial clustering have been reported, and a genetic basis seems likely.[64,66,67-69,76] Autosomal dominant inheritance with partial sex-limitation and frequent nonpenetrance is possible, although environmental influences also seem to have a role in the pathogenesis.[77] These exogenous agents include alcohol consumption[59,61] and cigarette smoking.[58] Because of narrowing of the fascia microvessels[73,74] it has been suggested that the localized fibroblastic proliferation, which represents a precursor of the palmar fascial contracture, is stimulated by oxygen free-radical release.

Léri Pleonosteosis

In 1921 Léri* described a previously unrecognized condition in a 35-year-old man, his 4-year-old daughter, and his infant son.[85] The disorder was not present at birth and became evident

---

*Guillame Dupuytren (1777-1825) was the doyen of French surgeons in his day. He had outstanding intellectual abilities, and he became a baron and a millionaire. His abrasive personality earned him the nickname "the Napoleon of surgery."

*André Léri (1875-1930), a distinguished Parisian physician, made significant contributions in diverse fields, including neurology, psychiatry, and ophthalmology. He published extensively on the subject of skeletal disorders, and his name is sometimes eponymously attached to melorheostosis and dyschondrosteosis.

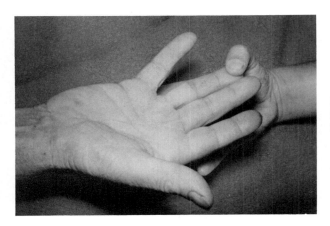

Fig. 13-4. Dupuytren contracture. Flexion of the fifth finger resulting from fibrous contracture of the palmar fascia.

sooner or later in extrauterine life. The father was only 62 inches tall and had short, broad hands and feet with thickened palmar pads and accentuated creases; limitation of motion was present in the wrists, elbows, hips, and knees. The toes, and presumably the thumbs as well, were broad and stiff. Léri termed the condition "pleonosteosis" on an incorrect assumption that the basic abnormality was excessive ossification.[86] Fairly numerous cases have since been described in the French literature,[81,83,87,93–96] including one report from Russia,[83] and some in the German literature[88]; there have also been reports in journals from Brazil and Argentina,[98] but only a few cases are known in Britain[84,90] and North America.[89]

The clinical characteristics of Léri pleonosteosis are broadening and deformity of the thumbs and great toes, flexion contractures of the interphalangeal joints, and limitation of motion in other joints, including the spine. A form of "hammertoe" may develop. Mongoloid facies has been described[98] but is by no means an invariable feature. Intelligence is usually normal, although there are at least two reports of impairment of the intellect.[92,96]

Semifixed internal rotation of the upper limbs and external rotation of the lower limbs are usually present. In general the limbs are short. The joints of the hands, in particular, may appear to be swollen. The hands are short, square, and thick. Involvement of the lower extremities seems to be less striking, possibly because less intricate movements are required of the feet and ankles.

A complication of the fibrous hyperplasia in the hands and feet can be nerve compression, notably, carpal tunnel syndrome involving the median nerves and Morton metatarsalgia resulting from involvement of the digital nerves of the feet. Compression of the spinal cord and nerve roots as a result of generalized vertebral enlargement and joint facet disease has been documented in a 20-year-old man by means of myelographic and computerized tomographic studies.[90]

Watson-Jones[98] described the dense fibrous tissue removed from the wrist and consisting essentially of a highly hyperplastic anterior carpal ligament. The specimen consisted of greatly increased, dense collagenous tissue, which in portions was actually fibrocartilage. Elastic fibers were conspicuous in their absence. Mucinous material was present and numerous "tissue mast

cells" in tissue removed from the foot were described.

Léri thought the fundamental abnormality was one of excessive and perhaps precocious ossification of the epiphyses. It seemed more likely to Watson-Jones[98] that the joint deformities are due to capsular contractures, that in general the abnormality resides in the fibrous tissues, and that the "thickening of the bones may be due to periosteal traction at their metaphyseal attachments."

All evidence suggests that pleonosteosis is inherited as a mendelian autosomal dominant trait. Multigenerational families with pleonosteosis have been documented,[92,97] including an impressive kindred from Manchester, Great Britain, in which seven persons had the disorder.[84]

In the differential diagnosis the familial multiple articular contractural syndromes, especially, autosomal dominant distal arthrogryposis, warrant consideration. A mucopolysaccharidosis (MPS) (especially, MPS I S, or the Scheie syndrome) and arthritis, either rheumatoid or degenerative, come in for consideration. One would suspect that the case thought by Rocher and Pesme[93] to be one of pleonosteosis with corneal opacification was in fact a mucopolysaccharidosis. This diagnosis is also likely in Case 4 of Watson-Jones[98] and in some other reported cases reviewed by Rukavina et al.[97] Other disorders associated with stiff joints and short stature include the Weill-Marchesani syndrome (Chapter 5), the "stiff skin syndrome" reported by Esterly and McKusick,[82] and the dominantly inherited dwarfing disorder described by Moore and Federman.[91]

Peyronie Disease

Peyronie* disease (induratio penis plastica) has the initial manifestation in middle age of painless, slowly progressive curvature of the penis as a result of fibrous induration. The condition is comparatively common: Horton, Sadove, and Devine had personal experience of more than 1000 cases in a 16-year period.[104] Ultrasonography has proved a useful tool in evaluation of the extent and progression of the disorder.[99,103,109] A variety of techniques are used for surgical correction of the penile deformity.[102,106]

The cause of Peyronie disease is unknown, but

---

*Francois de la Peyronie (1678-1747) was a founder of the Royal Academy of Paris and surgeon to King Louis XIV.

an association with Dupuytren contracture exists.[101,108] Also a disturbing report has been made of the occurrence of Peyronie disease as a side effect of therapy with adrenergic blocking agents.[105] Familial aggregation is well documented.[107,110] After a study of three multigenerational families Bias et al.[100] concluded that the condition was a male-limited autosomal dominant trait.

Other Fibromatoses

Monostotic and polyostotic fibrous dysplasia of bone are well recognized disorders in which a variety of orthopedic complications result from localized skeletal fibrosis. These conditions are conventionally regarded as nongenetic, but Happle[113] has advanced the interesting hypothesis that they might represent the consequence of somatic mutation. If this concept is correct, it might also be applicable to other, similar conditions. A few other uncommon heritable conditions exist in which soft tissue fibrosis or bony fibrosis is a major feature and in which a clear-cut mode of inheritance has been established.

Cherubism is a fibrous disorder that predominantly involves the maxilla and mandible[115] and has the initial manifestation of bilateral swelling of the cheeks and jaws (Fig. 13-5). The fanciful name of the condition is derived from the resemblance of individuals with the condition to biblical cherubs. The disorder usually develops in childhood and progresses slowly, until it becomes quiescent in midadulthood. Autosomal dominant inheritance is well documented[116]; phenotypic expression is variable,[115] and the question of possible heterogeneity is unresolved.

The association of cherubism with gingival fibromatosis, mental retardation, epilepsy, hypertrichosis, stunted growth, and juvenile arthritis has been documented in two affected sibs with consanguineous parents[118] and in four other sibs from a consanguineous Brazilian family.[117] It seems likely that this condition is inherited as an autosomal recessive trait.

Proliferation of fibrous tissue is the major feature of a number of poorly delineated disorders such as aggressive fibromatosis[112] and familial fibromatosis.[120] The association of soft tissue nodules and metaphyseal lesions characterizes multiple fibromatosis.[119] Congenital generalized fibromatosis[114] may be the same disorder. Heterogeneity is likely, and there is good evidence for an autosomal recessive form of this condition inasmuch as two sets of siblings with unaffected consanguineous parents have been recorded.[111]

PAGET DISEASE OF BONE

In Paget's original case report[175] published in 1877, Paget* described the clinical and histopathologic features of a man who had progressive enlargement of the skull, curving of the spine, and bowing of the legs in association with retinal hemorrhage and deafness. Since that time numerous cases have been reported, and it has become apparent that the disorder is common. Indeed, it has been estimated that as many as 10% of all persons in the eighth decade of life may have Paget disease.[143]

Paget disease can become evident initially with the manifestation of localized bone pain or enlargement. More frequently Paget disease is clinically silent and often is diagnosed by chance radiographic recognition of the characteristic areas of bony sclerosis and lucency (Fig. 13-6). Unexplained elevation of serum alkaline phosphatase levels is another common mode of presentation.

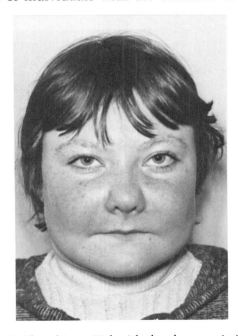

Fig. 13-5. Cherubism. Girl with the characteristic swelling of cheeks and jaws. (Courtesy Professor R. Gorlin.)

*James Paget (1814-1899) was a prominent nineteenth-century surgeon at St. Bartholomew's Hospital in London. He became the president of the Royal College of Surgeons and was made a baronet for his services to Queen Victoria and the royal family.

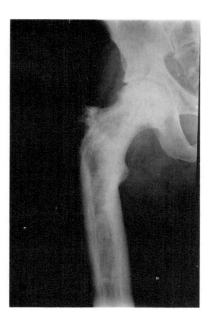

Fig. 13-6. Radiograph of the upper end of an affected femur showing the characteristic irregular sclerosis of Paget disease.

Paget disease may be confined to a single bone, but it is sometimes widespread. The pelvis, spine, skull, and proximal long bones are the sites of predilection, and in symptomatic patients the affected bones may be painful and tender. Pathologic fractures are common,[128] whereas sarcomatous change is well documented but infrequent.[164] Deafness may develop as a result of compression of the eighth cranial nerve and involvement of the bony structures of the middle ear.[156] Vascularity of the bony lesions occasionally precipitates high-output cardiac failure, whereas excessive bone turnover may lead to hypercalcemia and nephrocalcinosis. Angioid streaks in the retina provide an interesting parallel with pseudoxanthoma elasticum (PXE).

The management of Paget disease centers around therapy with calcitonin[138,182] and phosphonates,[124,127,136,161,196] both of which are efficacious to some extent. Prosthetic replacement of the knee[130] and hip joints[174] has been successfully accomplished, although vascularity of affected bone can pose problems during surgery. Computerized tomography and nuclear magnetic resonance imaging have proved of value in the assessment of the severity and extent of bone involvement.[183]

Because Paget disease clusters in families, it is possible that there is a genetic component in the pathogenesis. In the fourth edition of this book

McKusick posed the following question: "Is Paget disease of bone a generalized heritable disorder of connective tissue?" The gist of his discussion, which was based on a review of historical data, is as follows:

The evidence that Paget disease of bone can legitimately be considered a heritable abiotrophy, probably of the collagen matrix of bone, can be summarized in the way indicated in the following paragraphs. None of the pieces of evidence is by itself conclusive, but taken together, they make a rather convincing argument.

1. The hereditary nature of the process appears to be established. However, it is worthwhile to examine the evidence, since one review,[185] which is otherwise comprehensive, makes no mention of the genetic factor in discussing etiology. In 1889 Paget himself[176] wrote: "I have tried in vain to trace any hereditary tendency to the disease. I have not found it twice in the same family." However, the observations of familial aggregation reported from even before that time (beginning with Pick[178] in 1883) are fairly numerous (see Fig. 13-7).

In 1946 Koller[158] could find in the literature 28 families in which more than one case was described. Since then, other reports* of familial aggregation have appeared. Stemmermann[193] identified Paget disease in members of three successive

---
*References 122, 123, 134, 153, 155, 167, 171, 189, and 193.

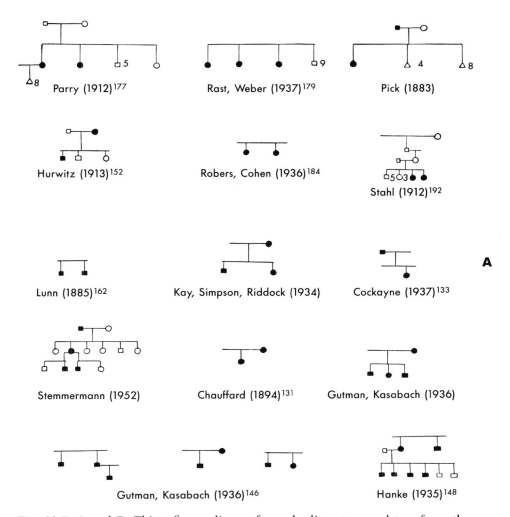

Fig. 13-7. A and **B,** Thirty-five pedigrees from the literature and two from the unpublished data of Brayshaw and McKusick, showing familial aggregation of Paget disease. Moehlig,[166] Ashley-Montagu,[123] and probably others reported Jewish pedigrees. Concordance in identical twins was reported by Koller,[158] Mozer,[170] and Dickson, Camp, and Ghormley.[136] In the last instance there was a striking similarity of distribution in the twins, both having, for example, tibial involvement. In the twins observed by Mozer[170] onset of clinically evident abnormalities occurred at the age of 48 years in both. In Irvine's pedigree[153] the affected man died of malignant osteoclastoma of the jaw, and both daughters had onset of Paget disease of the skull and jaw at the age of 18 years. In the pedigree of Brayshaw and McKusick, the first individual in the second generation, a female, had so-called osteitis pubis and changes in the skull compatible with Paget disease. The alkaline phosphatase level, however, was always normal. The other two individuals had Paget disease in entirely typical form and were discovered on study of the records of the hospital; if a more detailed study of the family were made, other members with Paget disease would probably be found. *Continued.*

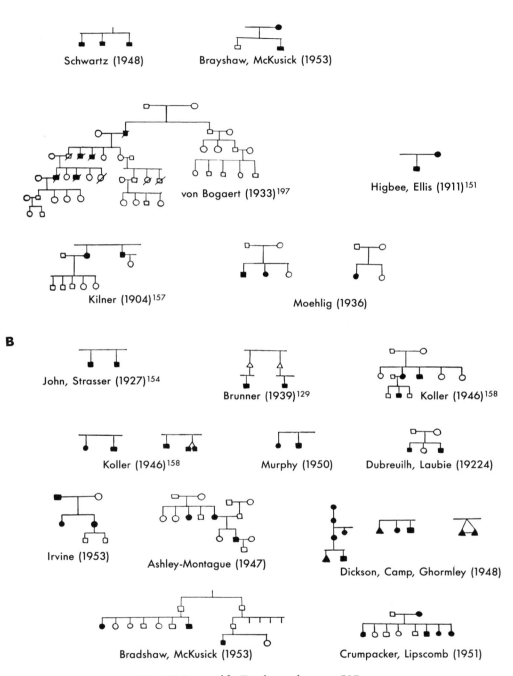

Schwartz (1948)

Brayshaw, McKusick (1953)

von Bogaert (1933)[197]

Higbee, Ellis (1911)[151]

Kilner (1904)[157]

Moehlig (1936)

B

John, Strasser (1927)[154]

Brunner (1939)[129]

Koller (1946)[158]

Koller (1946)[158]

Murphy (1950)

Dubreuilh, Laubie (19224)

Irvine (1953)

Ashley-Montague (1947)

Dickson, Camp, Ghormley (1948)

Bradshaw, McKusick (1953)

Crumpacker, Lipscomb (1951)

Fig. 13-7, cont'd. For legend see p. 527.

generations. It appears to have occurred in four generations of a Jewish family known to me and also in two other kinships, as indicated in Fig. 13-7. Aschner, Hurst, and Roizin[122] described it in monozygous twin brothers and claimed that by 1952 a total of 57 families with multiple cases had been described. Martin[163] as well as others also described the disease in both of identical twins. Galbraith[144] found 77 reported families and added four. In 1968 Evens and Bartter[141] concluded that at least 87 families with multiple affected members had been described. They added a kindred with affected members in three sibships related as cousins through the mothers, who were sisters.

When one undertakes to study the heredity of a condition such as Paget disease, one encounters several difficulties. In the first place, the disease has some of the earmarks of an abiotrophy. That it is an abiotrophy remains, of course, to be established. At any rate, the disease usually has its onset late in life, by which time the parents are likely to have died, the siblings may be widely scattered geographically, and the children will probably not yet be old enough to have the condition. In the second place, Paget disease is often subtle in its manifestations. A high proportion of affected persons are asymptomatic, and the change in bone is discovered only incidentally on radiologic examination made for unrelated purposes or possibly in search for an explanation of an otherwise obscure elevation of serum alkaline phospatase activity. In the course of a detailed study of 7941 individuals over 61 years of age, 85 cases of Paget disease were found, but of these patients only three had complaints referable to the disorder of bone.[168]

In general the data accumulated are consistent with the view that the trait for Paget disease is controlled by a simple medelian autosomal dominant gene. However, Ashley-Montagu[123] suggested that Paget disease is inherited as an incompletely dominant gene, carried on an X-chromosome.

Considering how frequently Paget disease occurs in at least mild form (in 3% of all persons over 40 years of age, according to Schmorl[188]), it could be argued that it would be extraordinary if 30 or 40 families with more than one case could not be discovered. Along the same line it may be noted that Sabatini[187] found Paget disease in two married couples in which the marital partners were unrelated. There seems to be a significant familial aggregation of cases, and the evidence in the pedigrees with more than two cases is particularly convincing. The frequency of Paget disease

in the general population is roughly 0.013%,[158] and it can be estimated that the probability of two or more cases occurring in the same family by chance alone is very slight indeed.

2. Angioid streaks of the retina are associated with only two conditions with any regularity. These conditions are pseudoxanthoma elasticum (PXE) and Paget disease of bone.[160,169,195] Angioid streaks of the fundus of the eye, PXE in the skin, and Paget disease in the bones have been observed in the same patient.[200] There may be reasons for believing that there is no fundamental relationship between Paget disease and PXE: the fact that angioid streaks, which are an integral part of a definite disorder of connective tissue (PXE), occur also in Paget disease suggests that this condition may likewise be a disorder of connective tissue with abnormalities much more widespread than the bone lesions alone would suggest. Also, in Paget disease there occur other ocular abnormalities such as corneal degeneration,[198] cataract,[159] and choroiditis[132] independent of angioid streaks, which further raise the question of whether a generalized abiotrophy of connective tissue may be present.

3. A quality of reasonableness, although not constituting proof, makes it attractive to persons familiar with bone and with the clinical behavior of Paget disease to speculate that the disease is fundamentally an abiotrophy of the collagen matrix of bone, which breaks down with the passage of years. Albright and Reifenstein[121] present evidence that Paget disease is primarily a destruction or, perhaps it is permissible to say, a degeneration of bone with secondary reparative overproduction of bone.

In general the involvement of the skeleton follows a pattern of localization consistent with the view that "wear-and-tear" is a contributing factor in the development of the lesions. Weight-bearing structures are usually involved primarily. The bones of the upper extremity are, for example, much less often involved than those of the legs. Persons with Paget disease in severe form are often obese. The high incidence of obesity and tallness in the families of patients with Paget disease was emphasized by Moehlig.[166,167]

In his classic necropsy study Schmorl[188] determined that the femur is one of the most commonly affected bones (more than 30% of cases) and the humerus, one of the least (less than 5%). The most frequently affected bone is the sacrum (57% of cases). The vertebrae are affected in half the cases, and the incidence of involvement, in descending frequency, is lumbar, thoracic, and cervical spine. In brief, beginning with the sacrum there is a progressive decrease in frequency of involvement as one progresses craniad. An amazing finding[188] is that the right femur is involved by Paget disease more than twice as often as is the left femur (31% as against 15%). Undoubtedly people are right-legged or left-legged, just as they are right-handed or left-handed. Albright and Reifenstein[121] have documented an instance of predominant involvement in the skull laterally at the attachment of the masseter and temporal muscles. Involvement of other areas of the skull, often a striking feature, is more difficult to explain on a wear-and-tear basis. However, wear-and-tear is probably only a contributing factor in the development and localization of the disorder, the primary factor being, perhaps, a hereditary weakness. Schmorl[188] noted that changes tend to be most pronounced at the attachments of tendons and ligaments to bones. Kay et al.[155] made the important observation that in a brother and sister with Paget disease, both with unilateral involvement of the radius, the left radius was involved in the left-handed individual and the right radius in the right-handed one. This appears to be a nice demonstration of the interaction of genetic and postnatal factors.

4. Vascular disease has been thought to occur prematurely and with increased incidence in Paget disease[191] and to be independent of the "high-output" heart failure, which may occur as a result of the vascular peculiarities that functionally resemble arteriovenous fistulae.[140,194] Medial sclerosis of the Mönckeberg type is regarded as being frequent in affected persons. Harrison and Lennox[149] found valvular calcification in 39% of their patients with Paget disease, an incidence five times that in a control group of comparable age distribution. Vascular calcification may be related merely to the periodic hypercalcemia to which those persons are subjected, and the elevation of levels of circulating alkaline phosphatase may contribute. Extraskeletal calcification occurs commonly,[173,190,199] possibly for the reasons mentioned but also, perhaps, because of an abnormality of connective tissue. Urinary calculi, which are frequent, would seem to be explained by the urinary excretion of high levels of calcium. Salivary calculi, which were identified in 20 of 111 cases,[185] may have a somewhat similar basis. This fourth bit of evidence is by far the weakest of the points bearing on the possible nature of Paget disease as an abiotrophy of the collagen matrix of bone.

Hitherto, a principal view of the pathogenesis of Paget disease has implicated vascular changes. This view would consider that intimately related to the primary defect is the increased vascularity of the bones. This vascular involvement may represent a significant and at times intolerable burden to the heart similar to that of arteriovenous fistulae,[191] may represent a problem in hemostasis to surgeons,[135] and may result in the skin overlying bones severely affected by Paget disease being warmer than elsewhere. In the present state of ignorance it is probably at least equally valid to suspect that Paget disease of bone may be an abiotrophy of the collagen matrix and that the vascular phenomena are secondary developments.

In the three decades since McKusick's review, evidence has accumulated to indicate that viral infection plays a significant role in Paget disease.[150,165,180,181] This contention is based on the observation that the geographic and ethnic distribution is patchy[126,147,172,186] and is supported by the recognition of viral inclusions in osteoclasts obtained from affected persons.[165,180] Nevertheless, the well-documented instances of apparent generation-to-generation transmission of Paget disease and an unconfirmed report of linkage to the human lymphocyte antigen system[142] are suggestive of a strong genetic component. Uncertainties remain, however, since localized geographic clustering, as in Lancashire[125] and Australia,[145] may be indicative of the activity of an environmental factor. In the last analysis it is possible that the pathogenesis of Paget disease concerns a complex interaction of viral infection, genetic susceptibility, and unknown environmental influences.

Epidermolysis Bullosa

Ingrid Winship

Epidermolysis bullosa (EB) is a descriptive term for the hereditary blistering disorders. This designation, introduced by Koebner in 1886, is now regarded as a misnomer, since lysis of the epidermis occurs only in one type of the disease. Epidermolysis bullosa is divided into the following major subgroups according to the level of blister formation in the skin and the consequent presence or absence of scarring: simplex (nonscarring), atrophicans (junctional), and dystrophic (scarring). Each of these may be further subdivided on the basis of clinical, genetic, ultrastructural, and

Table 13-1. Subtypes of dystrophic (scarring) epidermolysis bullosa

Subtype	Age of onset	Teeth	Mode of inheritance	Distribution of lesions	Clinical concomitants	Electron microscopic features
EBD Cockayne Touraine	0-5 yr	—	AR	Dorsum of extremities	Malignancy noted in scars	Dermolytic blisters below basal lamina anchoring fibrils; changes only in predilection sites
EBD Pasini	First week	—	AD	Mainly limbs; oral mucosa	Albopapuloid patches present in adolescence	As in EBD Cockayne Touraine but with changes in all sites
EBD pretibial	11-24 yr	—	AD	Pretibial	Occasional albopapular lesions	
EBD inversa	Birth	—	AR	Perianal, perivulvar	Anal and esophageal strictures; sideropenic anemia	Dermolytic blistering
EBD progressiva	Late childhood or adolescence	—	AR	Hands, feet, knees, elbows; oral mucosa	Progressive perceptive deafness	Widened lamina vara with amorphous deposits; normal hemidesmosomes
EBD Hallopeau-Siemens	Birth or infancy	Hypoplastic enamel	AR	Hands, feet, knees, elbows; oral esophageal and corneal	Syndactyly, contractures	Dermolytic blisters with dissolution of collagen fibrils; secondary absence of anchoring fibrils
EBD fine	Birth	—	AR	Limbs only	Slow centripetal progression of symmetric blistering	Focal widening of intracellular spaces in lower epidermis; absence of anchoring fibrils
EBD Winship	Birth	Aplastic enamel	AR? XL?	Generalized	Alopecia; short stature	Dermolytic blistering with absence of anchoring fibrils

EBD, Epidermolysis bullosa dystrophica; *AR,* autosomal recessive; *AD,* autosomal dominant; *XL,* X-linked.

biochemical features, and at least 26 subtypes are known to exist.[201,202,203,206,207]

In the dystrophic or scarring forms of EB the changes are beneath the basal lamina and the connective tissues are involved. In the simplex and atrophicans (junctional) subgroups the pathologic changes are superficial to the basal lamina. In EB simplex, Koebner type, keratin production by epidermal cells is apparently delayed, with resultant weakness of the basal cells and susceptibility to trauma.[205] Since there is no alteration of connective tissue in simplex and atrophicans EB, these disorders are not considered further in this review.

Epidermolysis Bullosa Dystrophica

Epidermolysis bullosa dystrophica (EBD) is a heterogeneous group of disorders that are subcategorized on a basis of the pattern of genetic transmission and the anatomic distribution of the skin lesions (Table 13-1). The condition is characterized by blistering of the skin, which heals with scarring and atrophy (Figs. 13-8 and 13-9). The lesions have their onset at birth or in the prenatal

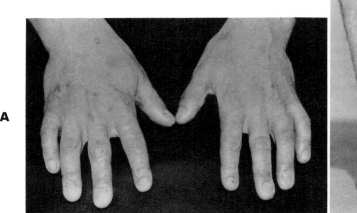
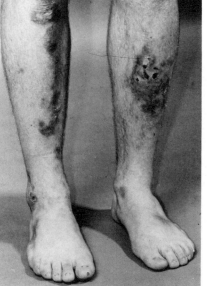

Fig. 13-8. **A,** Hands of a man with an autosomal recessive form of EBD. The skin is blistered and scarred, and the fingernails are dystrophic. **B,** The legs of the patient in **A.** Episodes of spontaneous blistering have led to widespread scarring, producing an appearance resembling that of EDS (see Chapter 6).

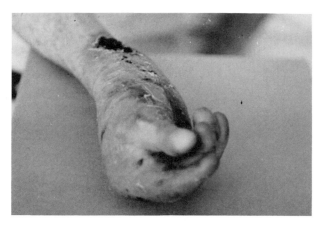

Fig. 13-9. The classic "mitten" appearance of the hand in a young man with EBD, Hallopeau-Siemens (mutilans) type. The skin is dystrophic and scarred, and soft tissue syndactyly has resulted from blistering and its sequelae.

period; thereafter they persist throughout life. The mucous membranes, as well as the skin, are fragile; blistering results in scarring and may lead to strictures within the mucosal linings of the gastrointestinal and urogenital tracts and damage to the eye. Subungual blistering may cause partial or complete loss of nails, and abnormalities of dental enamel also can occur.

Conventional light microscopy of the affected skin reveals subepidermal bullae in the absence of any significant cellular infiltration. The bullae develop below the basal lamina of the dermoepidermal junction, with the basal lamina forming the roof of the blister. The floor of the blister cavity is dermal collagen. The most significant ultrastructural changes in most subtypes of EBD are a reduction in the number and size of the anchoring fibrils and a loss of their pattern of crossstriations.[202,207] In this regard electron microscopic examination is the definitive investigation in the diagnosis of EBD. Details of the structure of the dermoepidermal junction are shown in Fig. 13-10.

The pathogenesis of EBD is uncertain. However, since type VII collagen is a major structural component of the anchoring fibrils, which are abnor-mal in the condition, the type VII collagen gene is a possible candidate for the site of the causative mutation.

Prenatal diagnosis has been accomplished in the autosomal recessive forms of EBD by means of electron microscopic investigation of biopsy specimens of fetal skin, with the use of immunofluorescence labeling of specific monoclonal antibodies.[204]

OCCIPITAL HORN SYNDROME

The occipital horn syndrome (OHS) has been the subject of considerable semantic confusion, since it previously has been termed "X-linked cutis laxa" and also has been given the numerical designation "IX" in the classification of Ehlers-Danlos syndrome (EDS). To avoid further problems, the condition has now been withdrawn from the EDS nosology, in which the category "IX" remains vacant and the use of the term "X-linked cutis laxa" also has been abandoned. The OHS is now classified with Menkes syndrome as a condition in which secondary changes in connective tissue are caused by faulty copper metabolism.

Occipital horn syndrome is characterized by

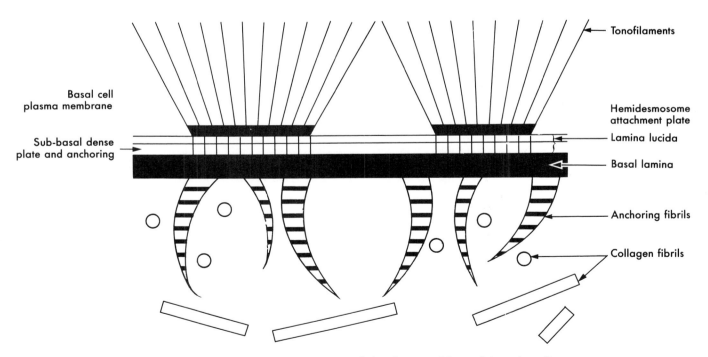

Fig. 13-10. Diagram of the ultrastructure of the dermoepidermal junction. Dystrophic forms of EB involve the connective tissues, which are situated beneath the basal lamina.

varying combinations of chronic diarrhea, bladder neck obstruction, thoracic malformation, fusions in the carpus, and personality abnormalities. Bony protuberances, or "horns," on the occiput, which develop in late childhood, are a pathognomonic radiographic feature.[220] The joints are sometimes hypermobile[213] (hence the initial categorization with EDS), the nose is hooked, and the philtrum is long (as in patients with Cutis Laxa).

The condition was delineated by Lazoff et al.,[217] when they reported a prepubescent boy and his two maternal uncles who all had a skeletal dysplasia, occipital horns, intestinal malabsorption, and obstructive uropathy. Thereafter Byers et al.[210] demonstrated a deficiency of lysyl oxidase in three males with a familial disorder, which the authors termed "X-linked cutis laxa"; these affected males were from separate branches of the family, and they were connected by obligate heterozygous females who had mild articular hypermobility during childhood. Two additional families with occipital horns, short broad clavicles, and fused carpal bones were documented by MacFarlane et al.[218] in a report entitled "A New Form of the Ehlers-Danlos Syndrome with Skeletal Dysplasia." The semantic confusion was resolved when Hall[212] recognized that the patients reported by Byers et al.[211] and MacFarlane et al.[218] had the same entity. Thereafter the designation *occipital horn syndrome* was formalized and promulgated in the Berlin nosology.[208]

Decreased serum concentrations of copper and ceruloplasmin were noted in the early cases,[211,218] and diminished lysyl oxidase activity was subsequently demonstrated in the medium of cultured skin fibroblasts.[216] It was also shown that copper concentrations were elevated in cultured skin fibroblasts but diminished in hair and serum.[216] Many similarities exist between OHS and Menkes disease, and it seems probable that these conditions are closely related. Indeed, Kaitila et al.[214] suggested that the disorders might be allelic, and Peltonen et al.[219] produced evidence from studies of collagen and copper metabolism to support this viewpoint. Kiuvaniemi, Peltonen, and Kivirikko,[215] after studying cultured cells, suggested that synthesis of the lysyl oxidase protein might be impaired. Minor abnormalities of copper storage have been observed in the fibroblasts obtained from a woman who was a potential carrier of the faulty gene.[209]

Menkes Syndrome (Kinky Hair Syndrome)

D.M. Danks

Historical Note

Like homocystinuria, the Menkes syndrome has been described and elucidated within the last decade. Menkes et al.[253] observed a kindred in which five males in an X-linked recessive pedigree pattern (Fig. 13-11) had the neurologic and hair changes that are now considered typical. Other clinical features were added on the basis of cases observed in various parts of the world.[224,225,231] The description of arteriographic and skeletal changes[261] was particularly noteworthy in the delineation of Menkes syndrome as a heritable disorder of connective tissue.[235]

The elucidation of Menkes syndrome as a genetic defect in intestinal absorption of copper was an achievement of Danks et al.[230,236,237] in Melbourne. The work was first published in 1972, 10 years after the first clinical report of the disorder.

Menkes et al.[253] termed the syndrome "a sex-linked recessive disorder with retardation of growth, peculiar hair and focal cerebral and cerebellar degeneration." O'Brien suggested that "kinky hair syndrome"[255] is a particularly useful designation for the detection of cases because the hair change thus becomes an easily remembered feature. On the other hand, Danks, Cartwright, and Stevens[234] pointed out that alopecia totalis, not kinky hair, may be the finding, and detection of cases, they suggested, may actually be hampered by the name. French et al.[239] and Kapur et al.[249] referred to the disorder as trichopoliodystrophy, meaning dystrophy of the hair and gray matter. As with several other syndromes discussed in this book, the eponymic designation seems preferable for the present. A precise designation based on the defect in copper absorption may be possible in the near future.

Clinical Manifestations

Premature birth is frequent, but birth weight is appropriate for the length of gestation. In the neonatal period infant boys with Menkes syndrome often display instability of temperature, transient jaundice, and poor feeding but otherwise seem to be progressing satisfactorily. Lethargy and failure to feed well have their onset at 4 to 8 weeks of age.

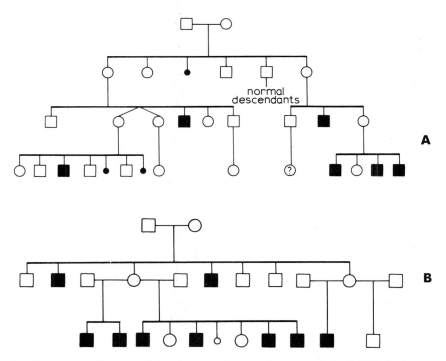

Fig. 13-11. Two pedigrees of Menkes syndrome showing typical X-linked recessive inheritance. **A,** Family of Menkes et al.,[253] restudied by French et al.[239] **B,** Family of Aguilar et al.[221]

Hypothermia and peripheral circulatory failure (with or without septicemia) may divert attention from the serious brain disorder. Seizures develop early in some cases. Usually the seizures are myoclonic and become difficult to control.

With the passage of time the evidence of brain disorder increases steadily, and the seizures become persistent. Muscle tone varies at different stages in the same patient. Severe spasticity is unusual. Hypothermia may be a recurrent problem. Subdural hematoma, a manifestation of the disorder of blood vessels, may be an initial feature in the first 6 months of life or may be a terminal event. Survival in diagnosed cases has varied from 6 months to 14 years, but it is likely that some infants die without recognition of the specific disorder.

Danks et al.[236,237] suggested that the facial appearance is characteristic (Fig. 13-12, *A*) and consists of "pallid skin, pudgy tissues, horizontal tangled eyebrows, and a 'cupid's bow' upper lip." The hair is usually normal in the neonate, but postnatal growth produces lackluster, hypopigmented

hair that stands up in a tangled disarray on the vertex and breaks off to leave a palpable stubble in the occipital and temporal areas where it has rubbed on the bed. Microscopic examination of the hair shows pili torti (Fig. 13-12, *B*) and clinches the diagnosis.

Radiographic studies (Fig. 13-12, *C* and *D*) of the skeleton show wormian bones of the skull and metaphyseal spurs of the femurs and, less often, of the humerus and radius. Subperiosteal calcification may occur along the shafts of the long bones.[261]

Arteriography (Fig. 13-13) shows widespread elongation, tortuosity, and luminal irregularity in all arteries of the body. Arterial occlusion can develop.

Notable negative findings include normal thyroid function studies, absence of anemia, normal white blood cell counts, and normal urinary excretion of amino acids. Plasma levels of lactate and pyruvate may be elevated.

Main findings of necropsy have been in the

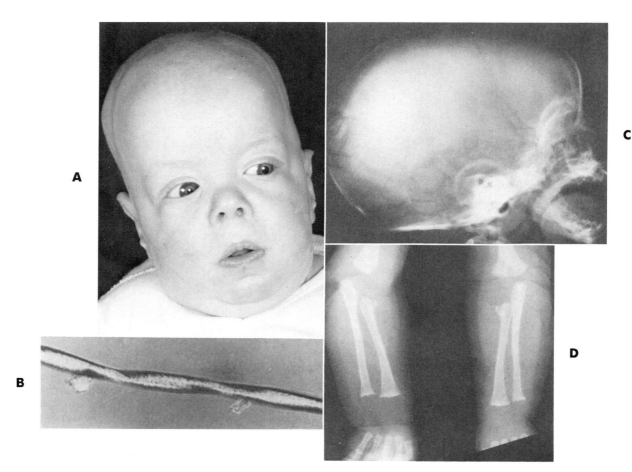

Fig. 13-12. Menkes syndrome. P. M. was admitted to the hospital at 3 months of age for investigation of suspected visual loss. The infant was born at 37 weeks' gestation. The parents were not related. Of four sibs one had a lumbar meningocele and one had an unexplained convulsion at 10 years of age. In the newborn nursery the baby showed persistent hypothermia and lethargy. In addition, unexplained hyperbiliru-binemia occurred, with peaking of the bilirubin level on the fifth day. The parents noted that at 6 weeks of age the infant did not smile or follow objects. Head control was poor, and spontaneous movements diminished. Examination showed a promi-nent forehead and short, sparse, course hair of the scalp and eyebrows, **A.** A large right inguinal hernia was readily reducible. Several minor motor seizures occurred during the examination. Although opticokinetic nystagmus was demonstrated, the patient did not follow bright objects consistently. The optic disks were dysplastic. The infant was generally hypotonic with hypoactive deep tendon reflexes. The diag-nosis of Menkes syndrome was confirmed by microscopic demonstration of pili torti, **B,** and chemical finding of low levels of serum ceruloplasmin and serum copper. Furthermore, the findings of radiographic studies were entirely consistent. Skull ra-diograph, **C,** showed multiple wormian bones along the lambdoidal and squamosal sutures. **D,** Irregular bony fragments extended laterally from the proximal metaphy-ses of the radii. The distal ends of the radius, ulna, tibia, and fibula showed cupping bilaterally. Electroencephalogram showed multiple spike discharge consistent with a diffuse cerebral disturbance. (Patient seen through courtesy of Dr. Robert H. A. Haslum. Biochemical studies were performed by Dr. N. A. Holtzman.)

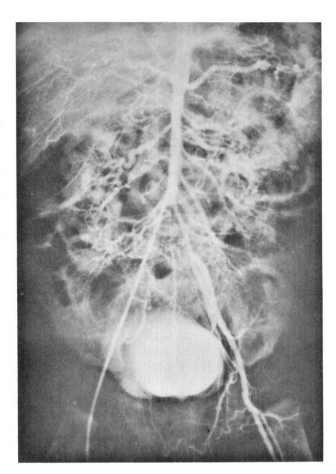

Fig. 13-13. Arteriogram in a 4-month-old infant with Menkes syndrome showing widespread arterial changes. The right renal artery is narrowed proximally and dilated and tortuous distally. The left common iliac artery is narrowed. (Courtesy Dr. David M. Danks, Melbourne).

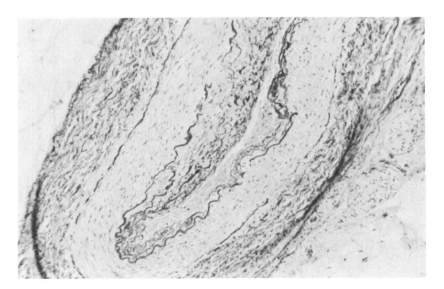

Fig. 13-14. Histopathologic study of large artery in Menkes syndrome. Disruption, fragmentation, and reduplication of the internal elastic lamina and thickening of the intima are demonstrated (magnification × 130). (Courtesy Dr. David M. Danks, Melbourne.)

brain and blood vessels. The brain shows extensive neuronal degeneration, gliosis, and cystic degeneration. Indeed, the cerebral histopathologic features and the changes in the cerebral lipids were, until recently, focused on, to the exclusion of the important arterial changes.[221,241,257] The ocular histopathologic manifestations have been described.[257] In arteries of all parts of the body, fragmentation and reduplication of the internal elastic lamina (Fig. 13-14), as well as fragmentation of elastic fibers throughout the media, are evident.[254]

Genetics and Incidence

X-linked recessive inheritance is well documented (Fig. 13-11). The gene is located at or close to the long arm of chromosome X, band 13 (Xq13).[249] Some heterozygous females show mild pili torti or patchy lack of pigmentation. Serum copper levels are normal in heterozygotes, and a proportion of heterozygotes can be detected by demonstration of the copper retention phenotype (discussed in the section, Basic Defect) in cultured fibroblasts. Full expression of the disease has been described in a female with an X-autosome translocation, breakpoint Xq13.[249] As with all X-linked conditions, the biopsy specimen may be taken from a patch of skin in which only the normal X chromosome is expressed, giving a false-negative result. The gene locus may be homologous with the X-chromosomal *mottled* (Mo) locus in mice.

The incidence is of the order of 1 in 70,000 live births.[231]

Variant Forms

Two patients have been described with a form of Menkes disease that is clearly different from the classic variety.[229,256,262] The initial manifestations in one of these patients were ataxia and moderately delayed motor development at the age of 2 years.[256] In the second the initial manifestations were recurrent urinary tract infections and hernias, as well as delayed development.[262] These patients must be distinguished from long-surviving patients with classic manifestations who have had profound brain damage by the age of 6 months but who have survived with severe mental impairment for much longer than usual, up to 14 years of age.[240]

Occipital horn syndrome (see p. 533) is closely related to Menkes syndrome and has considerable overlap with the second of the two mild cases just mentioned. Unfortunately the neurologic and in-tellectual status has never been well documented in patients with OHS, nor have extensive skeletal surveys been described in long-surviving patients with Menkes syndrome. The Australian patient does not have occipital horns or the typical changes in clavicles or scapulae.[233] Studies of copper transport in cultured cells fail to distinguish between classic Menkes syndrome, mild Menkes syndrome, and OHS.[250] A similar situation exists in the various strains of mice that have X-linked inherited disturbances of copper transport and show differences that are not entirely explicable on the basis of differing severity of the same disturbance.[227,231] For instance, the male mice with the brindled mutation die of a rapidly progressive neurologic disorder by the age of 15 days without significant connective tissue abnormalities, whereas the blotchy males live many months without neurologic abnormalities but develop a progressive set of connective tissue abnormalities. In neither species can one be sure whether there is one series of allelic mutations of differing severity or two or more closely linked loci concerned with different steps in intracellular copper transport. The similarities between the human and murine conditions are strong enough to use the results of studies in mice when considering the nature of the basic defect in humans.

Basic Defect

It is quite clear that the clinical effects of Menkes syndrome are caused by deficiency of available copper within cells. Most of the symptoms and signs can be directly explained by the deficient function of copper enzymes. For example, lysyl oxidase deficiency accounts for the arterial, skin, and connective tissue abnormalities,[232,250] tyrosinase deficiency accounts for pigmentary disturbance,[246] and deficiency of copper-dependent disulphide bonding of keratin explains pili torti.[236,242] The features differ from the effects of nutritional copper deficiency[230] inasmuch as they are generally much more severe, especially in connective tissues and brain, and in that anemia and neutropenia are absent. The problem is not a simple copper deficiency but rather a disturbance of the intracellular copper transport processes. Although the normal intracellular copper transport processes are not understood, it is clear that the mutation causes copper to accumulate within the cells bound to metallothionein and deprives the copper enzymes of this essential element. A number of hypotheses have been put forward, but no firm evidence permits distinction among the many possible explanations.[222,227,231]

The mutation is expressed in most body cells, with the possible exception of hepatocytes. Given adequate access to copper within the blood stream, nearly all tissues except liver accumulate copper to abnormal levels. Although there is some reduction in placental transport of copper,[252] the supply of copper is still sufficient to allow accumulation of copper to abnormally high levels in all organs of the fetus except the liver, which shows abnormally low levels.[226,245] The brain is included among the organs with elevated levels of copper. Postnatally the process of sequestration of copper in an inaccessible form involves the intestinal mucosa[238] and leads to gross copper malabsorption.[237] The same process occurring in renal tubular epithelium further increases the copper deficiency. Thus deficiency of available copper in the circulation compounds the diversion of copper to accessible sites within cells.

Copper adminstered by injection is taken up by the liver and quickly corrects the low levels of ceruloplasmin (therefore of copper) found in the blood of untreated humans or mice.[231] This prompt response supports the notions that the liver is not affected by the mutation and that the low levels of copper found in the liver of untreated individuals reflect the combination of malabsorption and the avidity of other tissues for any copper that is absorbed. Cultured fibroblasts, lymphocytes, or renal epithelial cells show a copper accumulation phenotype.[228,243] The initial uptake of copper is normal, but the copper accumulates to abnormal levels over some hours and the recently uptaken copper is released much more slowly than normal.[244] These findings are compatible with the presence of a defect in some aspect of the excretion of copper from the cells or with the diversion of copper to a slow-turnover intracellular pool.[228,251] This phenotype in cultured cells can be used for prenatal diagnosis[259] and for carrier detection, although carrier detection is hampered by the consequence of X-chromosomal inactivation.[247,248]

Treatment with copper injections is ineffectual if commenced once substantial brain damage has occurred, at least in regard to neurologic progress. At the time of writing, four patients in various countries are making good progress after receiving injections of copper histidine that were commenced soon after birth.[223,233,258] None of these children is completely normal but all have intelligence quotients in the low normal range and exhibit only hair abnormalities and mild connective tissue disturbance at ages ranging from 3 to 12 years. The experience with treatment of brindled mice suggests that prenatal treatment may give an even better result,[260] although one of the four children, who was delivered at 35 weeks' gestation and received treatment from 2 days after birth,[233] is not doing noticeably better in performance than the other three.

MISCELLANEOUS DISORDERS
Generalized Arterial Calcification of Infancy

Generalized arterial calcification of infancy has been noted in multiple sibs[263,264,266,268,270] (Fig. 13-15). The justification for mentioning this condition in a discussion of heritable disorders of connective tissue is provided by the evidence suggesting that fundamentally the disorder is a degeneration of the elastic fibers. The calcification shows a remarkable predilection for the internal elastic lamina. Fine calcium incrustation of the lamina is the minimal lesion. Later, the lamina is ruptured and occlusive changes of the tunica intima take place. Spontaneous regression of calcification and long-term survival have been documented in a sporadic case.[269] Since calcification is probably a secondary feature, it has been suggested that a more apt designation for the condition would be "occlusive infantile arteriopathy."[271] After detailed ultrastructural studies of a neonate with the disorder Anderson et al.[263] proposed that inflammation or infection together with abnormal iron metabolism might be involved in the pathogenesis.

Death as a result of myocardial infarction usually occurs in the first 6 months after birth,[265] and hypertension is a major problem in survivors.[267] The clinical diagnosis is suggested by the discovery of calcification in a peripheral vessel in an infant with electrocardiographic evidence of coronary artery disease. Idiopathic infantile hypercalcemia, of which there may be more than one etiologic variety, is probably unrelated.

Werner Syndrome

In a doctoral dissertation in 1904 Werner* documented four German sisters with cataracts and

---

*Otto Werner (1879-1936) was a general practitioner in northern Germany during the first three decades of the twentieth century. His description of the condition that bears his name represents his only known contribution to academic medicine.

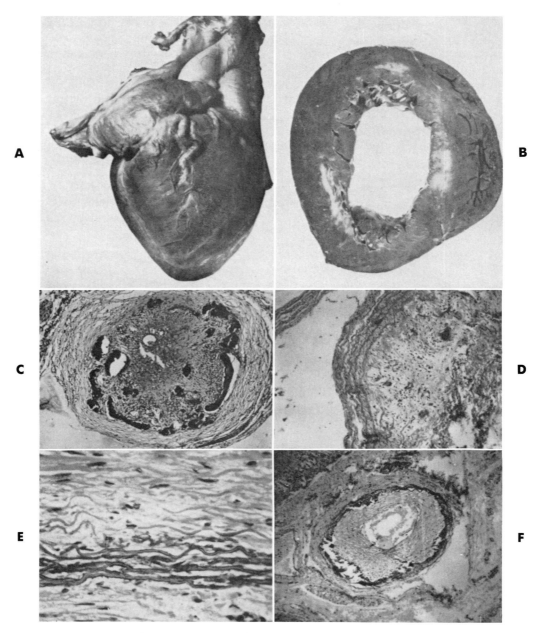

Fig. 13-15. Generalized arterial calcification of infancy. M.W. died of heart failure at 4 months of age. Beginning at the age of 3 weeks he appeared to have a respiratory infection with cough and dyspnea. He was pale and had episodes of sweating. On several occasions he had attacks in which he cried out suddenly and stiffened his body. Peripheral cyanosis, cardiac and hepatic enlargement, and ST-segment and T-wave changes in the electrocardiogram were found. The striking feature was the presence of calcified, tortuous coronary arteries, **A.** When the heart was sectioned, evidence of old and recent myocardial infarction was discovered, **B.** Calcification was seen in small arteries of the omentum. On histologic study many arteries, including the aorta and pulmonary artery, showed calcification around elastic laminae, which appeared fragmented, **C.** In the outer part of the pulmonary artery, granuloma formation was demonstrated in the area of interruption of the elastic fibers, **D.** Aorta, **E,** stained by the periodic acid-Schiff technique, showed deeply stained margins of abnormal elastic fibers contrasting with the weakly staining edges of normal fibers. In the coronary artery, **F,** after calcium was removed by dilute nitric

scleroderma.[286] In addition to the eye and skin changes, the main clinical features of the syndrome are a large torso with thin limbs, a beaked nose, premature aging with early graying of the hair, diabetes mellitus, arteriosclerosis, and susceptibility to malignancy.[278,281,284] On histologic study the corium is atrophic, and Mönckeberg calcification is present in the arteries.

The premature aging in patients with Werner syndrome is reminiscent of progeria (see p. 543), and the skin changes resemble those of the Rothmund-Thomson syndrome.[285] McKusick has pointed out that Werner syndrome also enters into the differential diagnosis of conventional scleroderma and that the presence of cataracts represents an important diagnostic indicator.

Werner syndrome is comparatively common: in a literature survey in 1966 Epstein et al.[275] were able to recognize reports of 125 affected persons in 94 kindreds. Localized geographic areas of increased prevalence seem to exist; in Japan Goto et al.[276] observed 80 cases in 42 families (i.e., three per one million of the population), whereas Cerimele et al.[274] documented a high frequency in Sardinia.

Cell lines derived from cultured skin fibroblasts often comprise several clones, each of which has a different balanced chromosomal translocation[282] ("variegated translocation mosaicism"[277]). In keeping with the phenotypic features of premature aging, the life span of cell lines is shortened[283] and cultured fibroblast responses to growth factors are diminished.[273]

The autosomal recessive mode of transmission in Werner syndrome was well demonstrated in pedigrees published in 1963 by McKusick et al.[279]

(Fig. 13-16). The clinical details of the cases of family members with Werner syndrome, which are given in the following paragraphs, provide a clear perspective of the manifestations of the disorder. Briefly the characteristics of the patients with the Werner syndrome were as follows:

CASE 1

L.S. had bilateral cataract extraction at 37 years of age. At 39 years of age he was noted to have premature graying of the hair, sclerodermatous changes of the extremities with extensive subcutaneous calcification and ulcers about the ankles, testicular atrophy, and short stature (60½ inches) with large torso. Tendons were also calcified, and there was striking crepitus on motion of most joints. It is noteworthy that macular degeneration resembling that usually considered senile was observed in the patient at the age of 39 years. The patient died of sarcoma arising in the right thigh. On histologic study the appearance of the tumor suggested nerve sheath origin.

CASE 2

M.S.K. was first discovered to have stigmata of Werner syndrome when the kindred was restudied in 1962. Diminished vision began at the age of 11 years. Cataracts were removed at the ages of 21 years and 52 years. At the latter time mild diabetes was discovered. By 25 years of age she was strikingly gray-haired. She is 62 inches tall, with thin white hair and the characteristic facies of Werner syndrome. The facial skin was tight and the nose beaked, but the extremities were spared. Three years previously, "central and disseminated patches of healed chorioretinitis" were described and interpreted as an aftermath of toxoplasmosis. However, in view of the retinal changes described in her brother, L.S., it seems possible that these changes were directly related to Werner syndrome.

---

acid, material staining with periodic acid-Schiff reagent was demonstrated surrounding the elastic lamellae. The association of calcium deposition with abnormal elastic fibers was demonstrated in the stains of the aorta. Histologic findings suggest that accumulation of mucopolysaccharide is a consequence of degenerative change in elastic fibers. Similar evidence is available in Erdheim's cystic medial necrosis, in the Marfan syndrome, and in experimental lathyrism. That alteration in the mucopolysaccharide of ground substance is followed by deposition of calcium salts is well recognized. In generalized arterial calcification of infants, the "basic defect" may reside in the elastic fibers. Accumulation of mucopolysaccharide and deposition of calcium may be secondary and tertiary phenomena. C.W., brother of M.W., died at the age of 7 months after an illness identical to that in M.W. Serum calcium concentration and alkaline phosphatase activity were normal. Autopsy revealed widespread arterial calcification and myocardial infarction. (Photographs and information courtesy Dr. Alan L. Williams, Melbourne.)

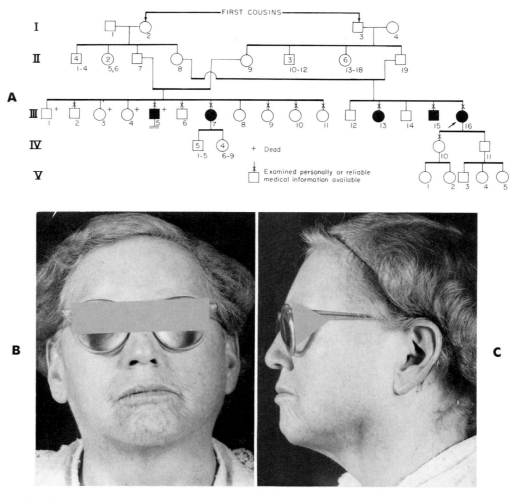

Fig. 13-16. Werner syndrome. In two sibships of the kindred diagrammed in **A**, five cases of the Werner syndrome were observed. The two sibships are related to each other as double third cousins. Coefficient of relationship of the parents of the affected persons in both sibships is $\frac{1}{64}$, since the parents are second cousins. **B** and **C**, The face of an affected woman showed tightness of the skin around the mouth and beaking of the nose. Bilateral cataracts were discovered when she was in her thirties, and below-knee amputations were carried out at the ages of 38 and 45 years, after sympathectomy and skin grafting had failed.

CASE 3

O.A. was reported by Boatwright, Wheeler, and Cawley.[272] Bilateral cataracts were discovered at 35 years of age. Scleroderma of the feet and legs with ulceration and subcutaneous calcification began at the age of 40 years. She was 59 inches tall, and the extremities were spindly, especially in comparison with the stocky trunk. The facies were birdlike. Esophageal changes suggestive of scleroderma were subsequently demonstrated by means of radiographic studies. Amputation of both legs was performed because of chronic ulcers, and osteogenic sarcoma was discovered in the right first metatarsal and cuneiform bones. The patient died 7 months later. Because of the rarity of reported autopsies in cases of Werner syndrome, the findings in this case are of note. Death was the result of widespread metastases of osteogenic sarcoma arising in the leg. In addition, the aorta and coronary arteries showed extensive artherosclerosis. The mitral ring was extensively calcified.

CASE 4

E.L.R. was first reported by Boatwright, Wheeler, and Cawley.[272] Bilateral cataracts were discovered at the age of 34 years. Soon afterward the hair became gray, and sclerodermatous changes developed in the feet and ankles, with painfully disabling callosities and ulcers. The voice was high pitched. The patient was found to have diabetes. The case was later reported in more detail, with autopsy findings, by Perloff and Phelps.[280] Autopsy revealed extensive atherosclerosis and vessel calcification but no abnormality of endocrine glands.

CASE 5

K.E., the proband, shown in Fig. 13-16, *B* to *D*, was referred to also by Boatwright, Wheeler, and Cawley[272] and by Perloff and Phelps.[280] Radiographic studies showed generalized osteoporosis and calcification at the root of the aorta, extending into the myocardium. A systolic ejection murmur in the aortic area was interpreted as indicative of aortic valve sclerosis with mild stenosis. Esophageal motility was normal. The chromosomes of this patient were found to be normal. Radiographs, for example, of the hand, showed pronounced osteoporosis. There was subcutaneous calcification over the elbow.

It is noteworthy that sarcoma occurred in at least two affected persons in this family. The increased frequency of neoplasia has been noted in the literature. The occurrence of aortic valve sclerosis is illustrated by K.E. (Family studied by Dr. R.M. Goodman.)

Progeria

Progeria is a remarkable disorder in which premature aging is the major feature. Children with progeria have a senile appearance, with sparse hair and thin subcutaneous tissues. The skeleton is gracile and osteoporotic, and mild generalized dysplastic changes are present. Coxa valga and attenuation and shortening of the terminal phalanges are the most obvious radiographic features (Fig. 13-17). Death resulting from the complications of "old age," notably, myocardial infarction or cerebrovascular accidents, usually occurs by the end of the second decade. Survival into the third and fourth decades has been reported in Indo-Nepalese brothers.[293] There is no effective treatment for progeria, although there are proponents of coronary artery bypass surgery in appropriate cases.[289]

Hopkin Hopkins, a famous fairground exhibitionist of the nineteenth century and son of the Welsh poet Lewis Hopkins, is said to have had progeria. His younger sister Joan was also af-

fected, and McKusick has suggested that these sibs might have had some other progeroid disorder, such as Cockayne syndrome.

Although more than 60 cases have been reported, there is uncertainty concerning the genetic basis of progeria. Most cases have been sporadic, and there is an equal sex ratio. There are far too few familial cases for the condition to be autosomal recessive. Nevertheless, sibs with progeria have been reported[290,291,294] and affected monozygous twin brothers with progeria have been documented.[295] In a comprehensive review of early reports parental consanguinity was noted only in three of 19 patients.[288] A paternal-age effect has been recorded,[288,292] and new dominant mutation is possible.[287] In these circumstances the familial cases could be explained on a basis of gonadal mosaicism.

Wrinkly Skin Syndrome

The Wrinkly Skin syndrome (WSS) is a rare autosomal recessive disorder in which wrinkling of the skin of the dorsal surfaces of the hands and feet is associated with microcephaly and mental retardation. The skin changes are present at birth, together with increased palmar and plantar creases. Other variable syndromic components include stunted stature, joint laxity, and developmental delay. About 10 cases have been reported; all have been children, and the long-term natural history is unknown.

A decrease in the length and number of elastin fibers in affected skin has been documented by Casamassima et al.[296] The elastin was not fragmented, and no significant abnormalities were revealed on electron microscopic study.

All reports of WSS have concerned children with origins in the Middle East, and in every instance the parents have been unaffected. The WSS was first reported by Israeli workers, when they documented sibs with WSS in an Iraqi Jewish family.[297] Sisters with WSS in an Iranish Jewish family[298] and Saudi Arabian sibs with WSS[300] have since been recorded.

There is little doubt that WSS is an autosomal recessive trait. The occurrence in the Middle East in both non-Ashkenazi Jewish and Arab populations might reflect either a common ancestor or a process of gene flow.[299]

Connective Tissue Nevi

The connective tissue nevi are a group of conditions characterized by aggregation of elastin or

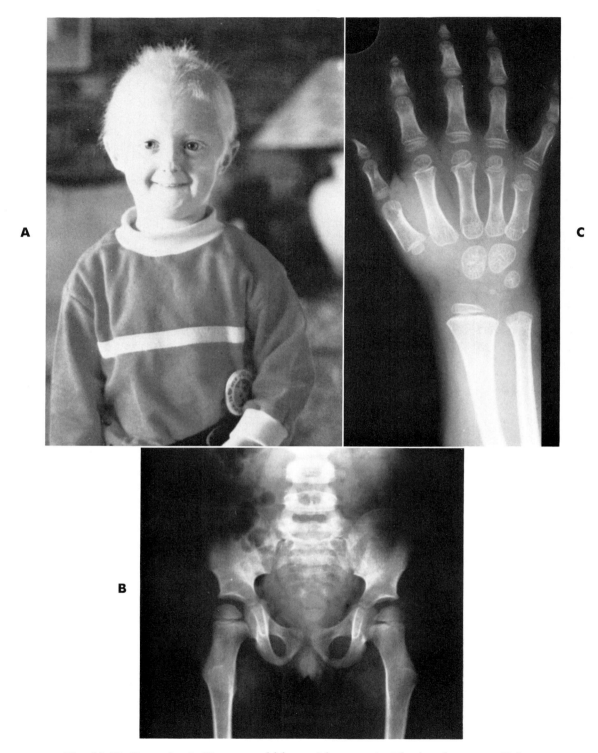

Fig. 13-17. Progeria. **A,** Five-year-old boy with progeria. The boy has a small face, narrow nose, sparse, fuzzy hair and absent eyebrows. Subcutaneous fat is scanty, and veins on the forehead are prominent. **B,** Radiograph of the hips and pelvis showing characteristic coxa valga. Tubular bones are gracile and osteoporotic. **C,** Radiograph of the hand showing shortening and tapering of the terminal phalanges.

collagen into nodular skin lesions. The nevi may occur in persons with otherwise normal health or as components of multisystem genetic syndromes. Connective tissue nevi have been extensively reviewed by Uitto, Santa-Cruz, and Eisen.[310]

Elastin nevi. The skin lesions of dermatofibrosis lenticularis disseminata, which accompany osteopoikilosis (see p. 519), are elastin nevi, as are the indurated changes in the skin flexures in PXE (see Chapter 10).

Elastosis perforans serpiginosa or Miescher elastoma is an elastic tissue nevus that becomes evident as reddish raised annular skin lesions. The nodules can occur in isolation, either sporadically or as an autosomal dominant trait.[301] They are also encountered as infrequent concomitants of Down syndrome,[302] and they can be precipitated by penicillamine therapy.[305,308,311] The elastoma occasionally occurs in the major heritable connective tissue disorders, notably, Marfan syndrome, OI, and EDS; whether its occurrence is confined to any specific subtypes of these conditions remains to be determined.

The name "Miescher" is applied to actinic granuloma, as well as to elastosis perforans serpiginosa. To avoid confusion, the descriptive terms rather than the eponym are now in general use.

Collagen nevi. The rough indurated "shagreen," or "shark skin," patch that occurs in tuberous sclerosis is a collagen nevus (Fig. 13-18). The embryologic mechanism that localizes this unusual lesion to the lumbar region and the reasons for its presence as a pleiotropic manifestation of the tuberous sclerosis gene are as yet unknown.

Familial cutaneous collagenomata are small nodules of densely packed collagen tissue, which usually occur on the back. They are innocuous and are inherited as an autosomal dominant trait.[309] They can also occur with cardiomyopathy and hypogonadism,[307] but it is not known whether this association is an autonomous genetic entity.

Familial reactive collagenosis is characterized by recurrent crops of umbilicated nodules.[304,306] These lesions are precipitated by trauma and cold,[303] and they are the result of extrusion of collagen fibers through the dermis. Sibs with these lesions have been documented, and autosomal recessive inheritance seems likely. In some persons the skin lesions are associated with renal failure and diabetes mellitus.

Keloid

Keloid results from proliferation of connective tissue (Fig. 13-19). It almost always occurs in scars, although familial occurrence in the absence of trauma has been documented. Blacks are notoriously susceptible to keloid formation,[313] but a strong tendency to keloid has also been observed

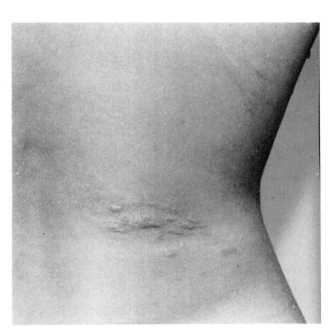

Fig. 13-18. Connective tissue nevi. A characteristic "shagreen" patch is present over the lumbar region in a young man with tuberous sclerosis. The raised, uneven, indurated lesion is composed of irregular, densely packed collagen fibers. "Shagreen" has the connotation of "shark skin" and denotes the rough texture of the patch.

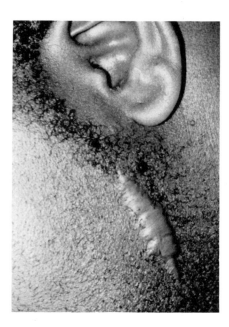

Fig. 13-19. Keloid. Young man sustained a laceration in the skin over the mandible, below the ear. During wound healing, heaped-up keloid developed in the scar.

in some white families.[312] Cosman et al.[314] found that 3% of persons with keloid had a positive family history. The pathogenesis of keloid formation is unknown.

Pachydermoperiostosis

The main features of pachydermoperiostosis are clubbing and thickening of the digits and oiliness of the face, forehead, and scalp.[318] Transverse ridging of the scalp known as cutis verticus gyrata is sometimes an additional feature. The condition develops at puberty and boys are much more severely affected than are girls.[320] Radiographs reveal that the cortices of the tubular bones of the extremities are widened and dense, with distal periostial thickening. The clinical importance of pachydermoperiostosis lies in distinguishing this benign disorder from the digital clubbing that is associated with neoplasia or cardiopulmonary disease.

Familial aggregation is well recognized, and considerable evidence exists that pachydermoperiostosis is usually an autosomal dominant trait.[320] It is also possible that a less common autosomal recessive type exists, since sibs with pachydermoperiostosis and unaffected consanguineous parents have been documented.[316] Familial digital clubbing with skin involvement may be a separate disorder.[319]

Pachydermoperiostosis must be distinguished

from a form of familial acromegaly.[317] It also differs from familial idiopathic arthropathy of children, in which periosteal new-bone formation in the shafts of the tubular bones is associated with cranial ossification defects.[315]

OSTEOCHONDROSES

In many members of the osteochondroses, epiphysitis, or *aseptic necrosis* group of disorders, eponyms abound and confound. These conditions are defined as noninflammatory, noninfectious derangements of the normal process of bony growth occurring at various ossification centers at the time of their greatest developmental activity. They usually become evident in childhood or young adulthood and their course is self-limiting. They differ in terms of their anatomic localization and natural history, and they are important by virtue of their orthopedic implications.[321,331]

The osteochondroses are distinctive entities inasmuch as no clinical overlap exists, and different forms do not occur in the same person or family. Family clustering has been observed, and although there is presumably a genetic component in their pathogenesis, they are not simple mendelian disorders.

The following osteochondroses (anatomic site of skeletal involvment is italicized) are briefly reviewed in this section: Perthes disease (Legg-Calvé-Perthes disease), *femoral capital epiphyses;*

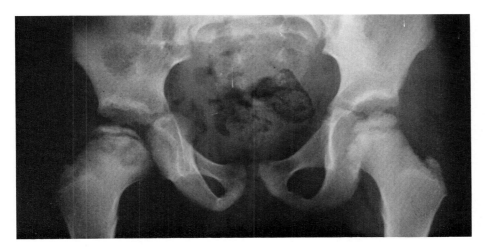

Fig. 13-20. Perthes disease. Radiograph of the hips showing flattening and irregularity of the femoral capital epiphyses with cystic changes in the adjacent metaphyses. Perthes disease is bilateral in about 5% of cases, and in this situation several heritable bone dysplasias enter into the differential diagnosis.

Osgood-Schlatter disease, *tibial tubercle;* and Scheuermann disease, *vertebral bodies.*

Other, rare osteochondroses and the anatomic sites of involvement are the following:

Thiemann disease, *phalangeal epiphyses*
Köhler disease, *tarsal navicular bone*
Kienböck disease, *carpal semilunar bone*
Freiberg disease, *head of second metatarsal*
Sever disease, *calcaneus*
Johannsson-Larsen syndrome, *patella*

Perthes Disease

The designation *Perthes** has been the source of some semantic confusion, since it is sometimes not realized that the terminal *s* is part of the name, not the possessive form of the eponym.

Perthes disease is the most common of the osteochondroses. It is usually unilateral and is predominant in males.[322] Onset occurs toward the end of the first decade, with slowly progressive pain in the hip joint and disturbance of gait. The condition eventually becomes quiescent, but if it is inadequately managed, secondary osteoarthritis may develop in the affected joint.

Perthes disease is an idiopathic aseptic necrosis of the femoral capital epiphysis, and on radiographic examination there is flattening and fragmentation, with areas of sclerosis and lucency[323] (Fig. 13-20). These changes can be mimicked by sickle-cell disease, hypothyroidism, and many bone dysplasias; in the atypical familial or bilateral Perthes disease, skeletal survey and other appropriate investigations should be undertaken to exclude these disorders. Isotopic or nuclear magnetic resonance imaging is currently favored as a diagnostic approach, especially in the early stages of the condition.

Although familial aggregation of Perthes disease has been recorded, the vast majority of cases are sporadic. After large-scale epidemiologic surveys were undertaken in Canada[324] and Great Britain,[326] it was suggested that the condition might have a multifactorial origin with a comparatively small genetic component.

Osgood-Schlatter Disease

Osgood-Schlatter* disease or osteochondritis of the tibial tubercle usually develops at the beginning of the second decade. Involvement is unilateral, and boys are predominantly affected.[328,330] The prime etiologic factor is thought to be exces-

---

*Georg Clemens Perthes (1869-1927) was a professor of surgery at Tübingen. His name is sometimes associated with those of Arthur Thornton Legg (1874-1939) and Jacques Calvé (1875-1954) as a designation for this disorder.

*Robert Bayley Osgood (1873-1956) was a professor of orthopedic surgery at Harvard University and chief of staff at the Massachussetts General Hospital. Carl Schlatter (1864-1934) was a professor of surgery in Zurich, Switzerland.

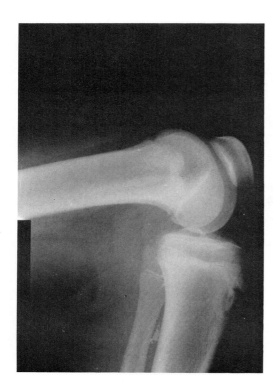

Fig. 13-21. Osgood-Schlatter disease. Lateral radiograph of the knee in an adolescent boy who had spontaneous localized pain and tenderness. Fragmentation of the tibial tubercule is evident. Treatment was conservative, and recovery was complete.

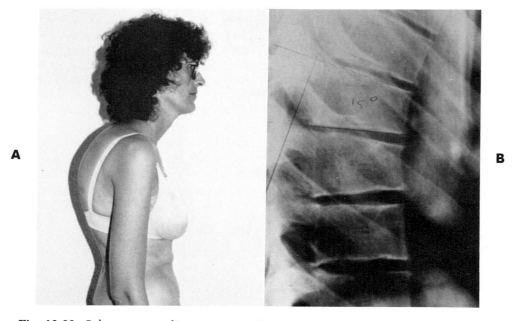

Fig. 13-22. Scheuermann disease. **A,** An affected woman with long-standing dorsal kyphosis. The condition developed insidiously after puberty; the deformity became static after progressing slowly for several years, but discomfort has persisted. **B,** Lateral radiograph of the upper thoracic spine showing kyphosis caused by anterior vertebral wedging. Disk spaces are narrow, and the vertebral end plates are sclerotic.

sive traction on the immature epiphyseal insertion of the patella tendon.

The initial manifestations are pain and tenderness over the tibial tubercle. There is no systemic disturbance, and the symptoms usually resolve spontaneously within a few weeks of onset. Long-term orthopedic sequelae are rare.[327] Radiographs reveal fragmentation of the tibial tubercle (Fig. 13-21); these appearances are pathognomonic, and diagnosis is easily made.

Scheuermann Disease

In 1921 Scheuermann* documented a large series of patients with anterior wedging of the vertebral bodies associated with "round shoulders" and backache.[329] The thoracic spine was mainly involved, and most persons with the condition were adolescent boys. The condition, which now bears Scheuermann's name, follows a prolonged course; mild but persistent backache is the major symptom. The disorder eventually becomes quiescent, but minor spinal malalignment may persist (Fig. 13-22). Trauma resulting from heavy lifting has been incriminated in the pathogenesis, but since the condition has often been observed in sedentary persons, other etiological factors must be operative.

Most cases of Scheuermann disease are sporadic, although generation-to-generation transmission has been documented in a few instances.[325] It seems probable that Scheuermann disease is heterogeneous, but the various forms await delineation.

---

*Holger Werfel Scheuermann (1877-1960) was a radiologist in Copenhagen, Denmark. Scheuermann twice submitted his findings in the form of a doctoral thesis at the University of Copenhagen, but it was rejected on both occasions. In 1959, when Scheuermann was 82 years of age, the degree was finally conferred upon him, *hons causa*.

REFERENCES
Osteopoikilosis

1. Albers-Schönberg H: Eine seltene, bisher nicht bekannte Strukturanomalie des Skelettes, *Fortschr Roentgenstr* 23:174 only, 1915.
2. Albronda J: Familiale osteopoikilie, *Ned Tijdschr Geneeskd* 100:3533-3542, 1956.
3. Ayling RM, Evans PE: Giant cell tumour in a patient with osteopoikilosis, *Acta Orthop Scand* 59(1):74-76, 1988.
4. Berlin R et al: Osteopoikilosis; a clinical and genetic study, *Acta Med Scand* 181:305-314, 1967.
5. Bistolfi: Cited by Curth HO, reference 16.
6. Blinder G et al: Widespread osteolytic lesions of the long bones in basal cell nevus syndrome, *Skeletal Radiol* 12:196-198, 1984.
7. Bloom AR: Osteopoecilia, *Am J Surg* 22:239-243, 1933.
8. Briottet J, Dechelotte J, Rivot G: Familial osteopoikilosis, *J Radiol Electr* 47:789-793, 1966.
9. Busch KFB: Familial disseminated osteosclerosis, *Acta Radiol Scand* 18:693-714, 1937.
10. Buschke A Ollendorff H: Ein Fall von Dermatofibrosis lenticularis disseminata und Osteopathia condensans disseminata, *Derm Wschr* 86:257-262, 1928.
11. Cairns RJ: Familial juvenile elastoma; osteopoikilosis (two cases), *Proc R Soc Med* 60:1267-1270, 1967.
12. Castellano E, Piotti F: A case of spotty osteopecilia with unusual costal and vertebral localization, *Minerva Med* 58:4082-4090, 1967.
13. Cazzola M et al: Rheumatoid arthritis associated with osteopoikilosis: a case report, *Clin Exp Rheumatol* 7(4):423-426, 1989.
14. Cocchi U. In Schinz HR et al (Case JT, editor): *Roentgen-diagnostics*, New York, 1951, Grune & Stratton, p 744.
15. Copeman WSC, editor: *Textbook of rheumatic diseases*, Edinburgh, London, 1955, E & S Livingstone, p 307.
16. Curth HO: Dermatofibrosis lenticularis disseminata and osteopoikilosis, *Arch Dermatol Syph* 30:552-560, 1934.
17. Dahan S et al: Iconographie du syndrome de Buschke-Ollendorff: étude tomodensitometrique et en résonance magnetique nucleaire de l'ostéopoecilie, *Ann Dermatol Venereol* 116(3):225-230, 1989.
18. Danielsen L, Midtgaard K, Christensen HE: Osteopoikilosis associated with dermatofibrosis lenticularis disseminata, *Arch Dermatol* 100:465-470, 1969.
19. Ehlers G, Mayerhausen W: Buschke-Ollendorff-Syndrom, *Z Hautkr* 64(10):869-874, 1989.
20. Erbsen H: Die Osteopoikilie (Osteopathia condensans disseminata), *Ergebn Med Strahlenforsch* 7:137-174, 1936.
21. Funstein L, Kotschiew K: Ueber die Osteopoikilie, *Fortschr Roentgenstr* 54:595-603, 1936.
22. Ghandur-Mnaymneh L, Broder LE, Mnaymneh WA: Lobular carcinoma of the breast metastatic to bone with unusual clinical, radiologic, and pathologic features mimicking osteopoikilosis, *Cancer* 53(8):1801-1803, 1984.
23. Grimer RJ et al: Chondrosarcome chez un patient porteur d'osteopoikilie. A propos d'un cas, *Rev Chir Orthop* 75(3):188-190, 1989.
24. Hinson A: Familial osteopoikilosis, *Am J Surg* 45:566-573, 1939.
25. Jonaseh E: 12 Fälle von Osteopoikilie, *Fortschr Roentgenstr* 82:344-353, 1955.
26. Kobus RJ, Lubbers LM, Coleman CR: Connective tissue nevus and osteopoikilosis in the hand: the Buschke-Ollendorff syndrome, *J Hand Surg (Am)* 14(3):535-538, 1989.
27. Lagier R, Mbakop A, Bigler A: Osteopoikilosis: a radiological and pathological study, *Skeletal Radiol* 11(3):161-168, 1984.
28. Llado Blanch A, Covas Planells I, Estrach Planella T: Alteraciones del metabolismo fosfocalcico en la osteopoiquilia (sindrome de Buschke-Ollendorf), *An Esp Pediatr* 31(2):139-141, 1989.

29. Macedo N et al: Nevos elasticos de caracter familiar. Sindrome de Buschke-Ollendorf. Forma frustra? *Med Cutan Ibero Lat Am* 17(3):189-192, 1989.

30. Marshall J: Osteopoikilosis and connective tissue naevi; a syndrome of hereditary polyfibromatosis, *S Afr Med J* 44:775-777, 1970.

31. Martincic N: Osteopoikilie (spotted bones), *Br J Radiol* 25:612-614, 1952.

32. Melnick JC: Osteopathia condensans disseminata (osteopoikilosis): study of a family of 4 generations, *Am J Roentgenol* 82:229-238, 1959.

33. Mindell ER, Northup CS, Douglass HO: Osteosarcoma associated with osteopoikilosis: case report, *J Bone Joint Surg (Am)* 60:406-408, 1978.

34. Nichols BH, Shiflett EL: Osteopoikilosis; report of an unusual case, *Am J Roentgenol* 32:52-63, 1934.

35. Pacifici R et al: Mixed-sclerosing-bone-dystrophy; 42-year follow-up of a case reported as osteopetrosis, *Calcif Tissue Int* 38(3):175-185, 1986.

36. Raque CJ, Wood MG: Connective-tissue nevus: dermatofibrosis lenticularis disseminata with osteopoikilosis, *Arch Dermatol* 102:390-396, 1970.

37. Reymond JL et al: Buschke-Ollendorf syndrome. An electron microscopic study, *Dermatologica* 166(2):64-68, 1983.

38. Risseeuw J: Familiäre osteopoikilosis, *Ned Tijdschr Geneeskd* 80:3827-3834, 1936.

39. Ritterhoff RJ, Oscherwitz D: Osteopoikilosis associated with bronchogenic carcinoma and adenocarcinoma of stomach, *Am J Roentgenol* 48:341-346, 1942.

40. Schmorl G: Anatomische Befunde bei einem Fall von Osteopoikilie, *Fortschr Roentgenstr* 44:1-8, 1931.

41. Schönenberg H: Osteopoikilia with dermofibrosis lenticularis disseminata (Buschke Ollendorf syndrome), *Klin Paediatr* 187(2):123-133, 1975.

42. Schorr WF, Opitz JM, Reyes CN: The connective tissue nevus−osteopoikilosis syndrome, *Arch Dermatol* 106:208-218, 1972.

43. Smith AD, Waisman M: Connective tissue nevi: familial occurrence and association with osteopoikilosis, *Arch Dermatol* 81:249-252, 1960.

44. Steenhuis DJ: About a special case of osteitis condensans disseminata, *Acta Radiol* 5:373-374, 1926.

45. Stieda A: Ueber umschriebene Knochenverdichtungen im Bereich der Substantia spongiosa im Röntgenbilde, *Beitr Klin Chir* 45:700-703, 1905.

46. Sváb V: A propos de l'ostéopoecilie héréditaire, *J Radiol Electr* 16:405-415, 1932.

47. Tong EC, Samii M, Tchang F: Bone imaging as an aid for the diagnosis of osteopoikilosis, *Clin Nucl Med* 13(11):816-819, 1988.

48. Uitto J, Shamban A: Heritable skin diseases with molecular defects in collagen or elastin, *Dermatol Clin* 5(1):63-84, 1987.

49. Verbov J: Buschke-Ollendorff syndrome (disseminated dermatofibrosis with osteopoikilosis), *Br J Dermatol* 96:87-90, 1977.

50. Verbov J, Graham R: Buschke-Ollendorf syndrome: disseminated dermatofibrosis with osteopoikilosis, *Clin Exp Dermatol* 11:17-26, 1986.

51. Von Bernuth F: Ueber Sklerodermie, Osteopoikilie und Kalkgicht im Kindesalter, *Z Kinderheilk* 54:103-116, 1932.

52. Voorhoeve N: A hitherto undescribed roentgen picture of abnormality of the skeleton, *Ned Tijdschr Geneeskd* 68:869-879, 1924.

53. Walpole IR, Manners PJ: Clinical considerations in Buschke-Ollendorff syndrome, *Clin Genet* 37(1):59-63, 1990.

54. Weisz GM: Lumbar spinal canal stenosis in osteopoikilosis, *Clin Orthop* 166:89-92, 1982.

55. Wilcox LF: Osteopoikilosis (disseminated condensing osteopathy), *Am J Roentgenol* 27:580-584, 1932.

56. Windholz F: Ueber Familiäre Osteopoikilie und Dermatofibrosis lenticularis disseminata, *Fortschr Roentgenstr* 45:566-582, 1932.

57. Young LW, Gershman I, Simon PR: Osteopoikilosis: familial documentation, *Am J Dis Child* 134:415-416, 1980.

Dupuytren contracture

58. An HS et al: Cigarette smoking and Dupuytren's contracture of the hand, *J Hand Surg (Am)* 13(6):872-874, 1988.

59. Attali P et al: Dupuytren's contracture, alcohol consumption, and chronic liver disease, *Arch Intern Med* 147(6):1065-1067, 1987.

60. Beighton P, Valkenburg HA: Bone and joint disorders on Tristan da Cunha, *S Afr Med J* 48:734-747, 1974.

61. Bradlow A, Mowat AG: Dupuytren's contracture and alcohol, *Ann Rheum Dis*, 45(4):304-307, 1986.

62. Conway H: Dupuytren's contracture, *Am J Surg* 87:101-119, 1954.

63. Early PF: Dupuytren's contracture, *J Bone Joint Surg* 44(B):602-613, 1962.

64. Early PF: Genetics of Dupuytren's contracture, *Br Med J* 1:908 only, 1964.

65. Garrod AE: On an unusual form of nodule upon the joints of the fingers, *St Bartholomew's Hosp Rep* 29:157, 1893.

66. Garrod AE: Concerning pads upon the finger joints and their clinical relationship, *Br Med J* 2:8 only, 1904.

67. Kipikasa A: The share of hereditary in the formation of Dupuytren's contracture, *Acta Chir Plast* 14:52-59, 1972.

68. Kostia J: A Dupuytren contracture family, *Ann Chir Gynaec Fenniae* 46:351-358, 1957.

69. Ling RSM: The genetic factor in Dupuytren's disease, *J Bone Joint Surg* 45(B):709-718, 1963.

70. Lund M: Dupuytren's contracture and epilepsy. Clinical connection between Dupuytren's contracture, fibroma plantae, periarthrosis humeri helodermia, induratio penis plastica and epilepsy with attempt at pathogenetic valuation, *Acta Psychiatr Neurol* 16:465-492, 1941.

71. Makhlouf MV, Cabbabe EB, Shively RE: Dupuytren's disease in blacks, *Ann Plast Surg* 19(4):334-336, 1987.

72. Mennen U: Dupuytren's contracture in the Negro, *J Hand Surg (Br)* 11(1):61-64, 1986.

73. Murrell GA, Francis MJ, Howlett CR: Dupuytren's contracture. Fine structure in relation to aetiology, *J Bone Joint Surg (Br)* 71(3):367-373, 1989.

74. Murrell GA, Hueston JT: Aetiology of Dupuytren's contracture, *Aust New Z J Surg* 60(4):247-252, 1990.

75. Ruffino C et al: An elevated incidence in the association of diabetes mellitus and Dupuytren's disease, *Minerva Med* 80(4):371-375, 1989.

76. Skoog T: Dupuytren's contraction with special reference to etiology and improved surgical treatment; its occurrence in epileptics; note on knuckle pads, *Acta Chir Scand* 96(suppl)139:1-190, 1948.

77. Teleky L: Dupuytren's contraction as occupational disease, *J Indust Hyg* 21:233-235, 1939.

78. Vathana P, Setpakdi A, Srimongkol T: Dupuytren's contracture in Thailand, *Bull Hosp Jt Dis Orthop Inst* 50(1):41-47, 1990.

79. Weber FP: A note on Dupuytren's contraction, camptodactylia and knuckle pads, *Br J Dermatol Syph* 50:26-31, 1938.

80. Young IW, Forth RW: Familial fibromatosis, *Clin Genet* 20:211-216, 1981.

Léri pleonosteosis

81. Cohen, de Herdt: Pléonostéose familiale, *J Neurol Psychiatr* 28:395, 1928.

82. Esterly NB, McKusick VA: Stiff skin syndrome, *Pediatrics* 47:360-369, 1971.

83. Feiguine E, Tikhodéeff S: Un cas rare d'osteopathie systematisée: un cas de pléonostéose, *Arch Méd Enf* 35:654-663, 1932.

84. Hilton RC, Wentzel J: Léri's pleonosteosis, *Quart J Med* 29:419-429, 1980.

85. Léri A: Une maladie congénitale et héréditaire de l'ossification: la pléonostéose familiale, *Bull Soc Méd Hop Paris* 45:1228-1230, 1921.

86. Léri A: Dystrophie osseuse généraliséе congénitale et heréditaire: la pléonostéose familiale, *Presse Méd,* 30:13-16, 1922.

87. Léri A: Sur la pléonostéose familiale, *Bull Soc Méd Hop Paris* 48:216-220, 1924.

88. Materna A: Zur Pathologie der Pléonostéose (Léri), *Beitr Path Anat* 112:112-136, 1952.

89. McKusick VA: Unpublished observations.

90. Metcalfe RA, Butler P: Spinal cord compression in Léri's pleonosteosis, *Br J Radiol* 58:1117-1119, 1985.

91. Moore WT, Federman DD: Familial dwarfism and "stiff joints"; report of a kindred, *Arch Intern Med* 115:398-404, 1965.

92. Neel JV, Schull WJ: *Human heredity,* Chicago, 1954, The University of Chicago, p 309.

93. Rocher HL, Pesme P: Un cas de pléonostéose (maladie de Léri) avec cornées opalescentes, *J Méd Bordeaux* 123:121-125, 1946.

94. Rocher HL, Roudil G: La pléonostéose (maladie de Léri). Étude anatomoclinique et radiographique, *Bordeaux Chir* 3:359-384, 1932.

95. Rothea M: *La pléonostéose familiale (maladie d'André Léri),* Theses, Paris and Nancy, No 421.

96. Rouillard J, Barreau P: Un nouveau cas de pléonostéose héréditaire avec atteintes graves des grosses articulations, *Bull Soc Méd Hop Paris* 51:794-802, 1927.

97. Rukavina JG et al: Léri's pleonosteosis; a study of a family with a review of the literature, *J Bone Joint Surg* 41(A):397-408, 1959.

98. Watson-Jones R: Léri's pleonosteosis, carpal tunnel compression of the medial nerves and Morton's metatarsalgia, *J Bone Joint Surg* 31(B):560-571, 1949.

Peyronie disease

99. Balconi G et al: Ultrasonic evaluation of Peyronie's disease, *Urol Radiol* 10(2):85-88, 1988.

100. Bias WB et al: Peyronie's disease: a newly recognized autosomal-dominant trait, *Am J Med Genet* 12:227-235, 1982.

101. Desai KM, Gingell JC: Penile corporeal fibrosis complicating papaverine self-injection therapy for erectile impotence, *Eur Urol* 15(1-2):132-133, 1988.

102. Fallon B: Cadaveric dura mater graft for correction of penile curvature in Peyronie disease, *Urology* 35(2):127-129, 1990.

103. Hamm B, Friedrich M, Kelami A: Ultrasound imaging in Peyronie disease, *Urology* 28(6):540-545, 1986.

104. Horton CE, Sadove RC, Devine CJ Jr: Peyronie's disease, *Ann Plast Surg* 18(2):122-127, 1987.

105. Kristensen BO: Labetalol-induced Peyronie's disease? A case report, *Acta Med Scand* 206:511-512, 1979.

106. Mufti GR et al: Corporeal plication for surgical correction of Peyronie's disease, *J Urol* 144(2 Pt 1):281-282, 1990.

107. Murley RS: Peyronie's disease, *Br Med J* 1:908 only, 1964.

108. Nyberg LM et al: Identification of an inherited form of Peyronie's disease with autosomal dominant inheritance and association with Dupuytren's contracture and histocompatibility B7 cross-reacting antigens, *J Urol* 128:48-51, 1982.

109. Princivalle M et al: Echographic diagnosis of Peyronie's disease, *Radiol Med (Torino)* 78(1-2):74-78, 1989.

110. Schourop K: Plastic induration of penis, *Acta Radiol* 26:313-323, 1945.

Other fibromatoses

111. Baird PA, Worth AJ: Congenital generalised fibromatosis: an autosomal recessive condition? *Clin Genet* 9:488-494, 1976.

112. Griffiths HJ, Robinson K, Bonfiglio A: Aggressive fibromatosis, *Skel Radiol* 9:179-184, 1983.

113. Happle R: The McCune-Albright syndrome: a lethal gene surviving by mosaicism, *Clin Genet* 29:321-324, 1986.

114. Heiple KG, Perrin E, Aikawa M: Congenital generalised fibromatosis: a case limited to osseous lesions, *J Bone Joint Surg* 54(A):663-669, 1972

115. Jones WA: Cherubism; a thumbnail sketch of the diagnosis and a conservative method of treatment, *Oral Surg* 20:648-653, 1965.

116. Peters WJ: Cherubism: a study of 20 cases in one family, *Oral Surg* 47:307-311, 1979.

117. Pina-Neto JM et al: Cherubism, gingival fibromatosis, epilepsy and mental deficiency (Ramon syndrome) with juvenile rheumatoid arthritis, *Am J Med Genet* 25:433-441, 1986.

118. Ramon Y, Berman W, Bubis JJ: Gingival fibromatosis combined with cherubism, *Oral Surg* 24:436-448, 1967.

119. Stout AP: Juvenile fibromatoses, *Cancer* 7:953-978, 1984.

120. Young ID, Fortt RW: Familial fibromatosis, *Clin Genet* 20:211-216, 1981.

Paget disease of bone

121. Albright F, Reifenstein EC Jr: *The parathyroid glands and metabolic bone disease: selected studies,* Baltimore, 1948, Williams & Wilkins, pp 284-301.

122. Aschner BM, Hurst LA, Roizin L: Genetic study of Paget's disease (osteitis deformans) in monozygotic twin brothers, *Acta Genet Med* 1:67-79, 1952.

123. Ashley-Montagu MF: Paget's disease (osteitis deformans) and heredity, *Am J Hum Genet* I:94-95, 1949.

124. Audran M et al: Treatment of Paget's disease of bone with (4-chlorophenyl) thiomethylene bisphosphonate, *Clin Rheumatol* 8(1):71-9, 1989.

125. Barker DJP et al: Paget's disease of bone: the Lancashire focus, *Br Med J* 280:1105-1107, 1980.

126. Barry HC: *Paget's disease of bone*, Edinburgh, London, 1969, E & S Livingstone.

127. Bickerstaff DR et al: Improvement in the deformity of the face in Paget's disease treated with diphosphonates, *J Bone Joint Surg* 72(1):132-136, 1990.

128. Bidner S, Finnegan M: Femoral fractures in Paget's disease, *J Orthop Trauma* 3(4):317-322, 1989.

129. Brunner W: Osteodystrophia deformans Paget unter besonderer Berücksichtigung unserer annex Erfahrungen der letzten 10 Jahre, *Deutsch Z Chir* 52:585, 1939.

130. Cameron HU: Total knee replacement in Paget's disease, *Orthop Rev* 18(2):206-208, 1989.

131. Chauffard A: Discussion of paper by Gilles de la Tourette and Marinesco, *Bull Soc Méd Hop Paris* 11(series 3):426, 1894.

132. Clegg JT: Paget's disease with mental symptoms and choroiditis, *Lancet* 2:128-131, 1937.

133. Cockayne EA: Quoted by Rast and Weber.[60]

134. Crumpacker EL, Lipscomb PR: Familial incidence of Paget's disease of bone (osteitis deformans): report of occurrence in three siblings, *Med Clin North Am* 35:1203-1208, 1951.

135. Dandy WE: Personal communication to McKusick.

136. Dickson DD, Camp JD, Ghormley RK: Osteitis deformans (Paget's disease of bone), *Radiology* 44:449-470, 1945.

137. Dodd GW et al: Radiological assessment of Paget's disease of bone after treatment with the bisphosphonates EHDP and APD, *Br J Radiol* 60(717):849-860, 1987.

138. Dokoh S et al: Evaluation by using radionuclide uptake of bone in Paget's disease of bone: special reference to treatment with calcitonin, *Radioisotopes* 37(6):339-342, 1988.

139. Dubreuilh W, Laubie: Maladie osseuse de Paget chez deux fréres, *Bull Soc Dermatol Fr* 31:87-89, 1924.

140. Edholm OG, Howarth S, McMichael J: Heart failure and bone blood flow in osteitis deformans, *Clin Sci* 5:249-260, 1945.

141. Evens RG, Bartter FC: The hereditary aspect of Paget's disease (osteitis deformans), *JAMA* 205:900-902, 1968.

142. Fotino M, Haymovits A, Falk CT: Evidence for linkage between HLA and Paget's disease, *Transplant Proc* 9:1867-1868, 1977.

143. Freeman DA: Paget's disease of bone, *Am J Med Sci* 295(2):144-158, 1988.

144. Galbraith HJB: Familial Paget's disease of bone, *Br Med J* 2:29 only, 1954.

145. Gardner MJ, Guyer PB, Barker DJP: Radiological prevalence of Paget's disease of bone in British migrants to Australia, *Br Med J* 1:1655-1657, 1978.

146. Gutman AB, Kasabach HH: Paget's disease (osteitis deformans): analysis of 116 cases, *Am J Med Sci* 191:361-380, 1936.

147. Guyer PB, Chamberlain AT: Paget's disease of bone in South Africa, *Clin Radiol* 39(1):51-52, 1988.

148. Hanke H: Osteodystrophische Erkrankungen und ihre Begrenzung, *Deutsch Z Chir* 245:641-691, 1935.

149. Harrison CV, Lennox B: Heart block in osteitis deformans, *Br Heart J* 10:167-176, 1948.

150. Harvey L et al: Ultrastructural features of the osteoclasts from Paget's disease of bone in relation to a viral aetiology, *J Clin Pathol* 35:771-779, 1982.

151. Higbee WS, Ellis AG: A case of osteitis deformans, *J Med Res* 24:43-68, 1911.

152. Hurwitz SH: Osteitis deformans, Paget's disease: a report of six cases occurring in the Johns Hopkins Hospital and Dispensary, *Bull Johns Hopkins Hosp* 24:263-274, 1913.

153. Irvine RE: Familial Paget's disease with early onset, *J Bone Joint Surg* 35(B):106-112, 1953.

154. John E, Strasser U: Zur Aetiologie, Klinik und Therapie der Ostitis fibrosa deformans (Paget), *Deutsch Z Nervenheilk* 97:81-94, 1927.

155. Kay HD et al: Osteitis deformans, *Arch Intern Med* 53:208-248, 1934.

156. Khetarpal U, Schuknecht HF: In search of pathologic correlates for hearing loss and vertigo in Paget's disease: a clinical and histopathologic study of 26 temporal bones, *Ann Otol Rhinol Laryngol* 145(suppl):1-16, 1990.

157. Kilner WJ: Two cases of osteitis deformans in one family, *Lancet* I:221-223, 1904.

158. Koller F: Ueber die Heredität der Ostitis deformans Paget, *Helv Med Acta* 13:389, 1946.

159. Laederich L, Mamon H, Beuchesne H: Un cas de maladie osseuse de Paget avec cataracte de type endocrinien, *Bull Soc Méd Hop Paris* 65:529, 1938.

160. Lambert RK: Paget's disease with angioid streaks of the retina, *Arch Ophthalmol* 22:106-109, 1939.

161. Lando M, Hoover LA, Finerman G: Stabilization of hearing loss in Paget's disease with calcitonin and etidronate, *Arch Otolaryngol Head Neck Surg* 114(8):891-894, 1988.

162. Lunn JR: Four cases of osteitis deformans, *Trans Clin Soc London* 18:272-277, 1885.

163. Martin E: Considérations sur la maladie de Paget, *Helv Med Acta* 14:319-333, 1947.

164. Mehta RC, Wilson MA, Perlman SB: Osteosarcoma arising in Paget's disease of the calvarium, *J Nucl Med* 29(3):414-416, 1988.

165. Mills BG, Singer FR: Nuclear inclusions in Paget's disease of bone, *Science* 194:201-203, 1976.

166. Moehlig RC: Paget's disease (osteitis deformans) and osteoporosis: similarity of the 2 conditions as shown by familial background and glucose tolerance studies, *Surg Gynecol Obstet* 62:815-822, 1936.

167. Moehlig RC: Osteitis deformans: familial constitutional hereditary background as etiological factors, *J Mich Med Soc* 51:1004-1007, 1027, 1952.

168. Monroe RT: *Diseases of old age*, Cambridge, 1951, Harvard University, p 304.

169. Morrison WH: Osteitis deformans with angioid streaks: report of a case, *Arch Ophthalmol* 26:79-84, 1941.

170. Mozer JJ: Discussion of Koller's published pedigree, reference 158.

171. Murphy W: Osteitis deformans in a brother and sister, *Med J Aust* 1:507 only, 1950.

172. Nagant de Deuxchaisnes C, Krane SM: Paget's disease of bone: clinical and metabolic observations, *Medicine* 43:233-266, 1964.

173. Narins L, Oppenheimer GD: Calcification of vas deferens associated with Paget's disease of bone, *J Urol* 67:218-221, 1952.

174. Nerubay J, Caspi I: Total hip replacement in two patients with Paget's disease, *Orthop Rev* 15(9):605-606, 1986.

175. Paget J: On a form of chronic inflammation of bones (osteitis deformans), *Med Chir Tr* 60:37-64, 1877.

176. Paget J: Remarks on osteitis deformans, *Illust Med News* 2:181, 1889.

177. Parry TW: A case of osteitis deformans in which fracture of a femur took place as the result of stooping, *Br Med J* 1:879 only, 1912.

178. Pick: Osteitis deformans, *Lancet* 2:1125-1126, 1883.

179. Rast H, Weber FP: Paget's bone disease in three sisters, *Br Med J* 1:918 only, 1937.

180. Rebel A, Malkan K, Basle M: Particularites ultra structurales des osteoclasts de la maladie de Paget, *Rev Rhum Mal Osteoartic* 41:767-773, 1974.

181. Rebel A et al: Contribution of modern research technique to the identification of a virus in Paget's disease of bone, *Bull Assoc Anat* 70(209):15-20, 1986.

182. Reginster JY et al: One year's treatment of Paget's disease of bone by synthetic salmon calcitonin as a nasal spray, *J Bone Miner Res* 3(3):249-252, 1988.

183. Roberts MC et al: Paget disease: MR imaging findings, *Radiology* 173(2):341-345, 1989.

184. Roberts RE, Cohen MJ: Osteitis deformans (Paget's disease of bone), *Proc R Soc Med* 19:13, 1936.

185. Rosenkrantz JA, Wolf J, Kaicher JJ: Paget's disease (osteitis deformans); review of 111 cases, *Arch Intern Med* 90:610-633, 1952.

186. Ryan EG: Paget's disease of bone, *Ann Rev Med* 28:143-152, 1977.

187. Sabatini G: "Ostitis fibrosa" di Paget in due coppie di coniugi, *Minerva Med* 1:607-611, 1948.

188. Schmorl G: Ueber Ostitis deformans Paget, *Virchows Arch* 283:694-751, 1932.

189. Schwartz LA: Paget's disease in 3 male siblings: clinical report, *J Mich Med Soc* 47:1244-1247, 1948.

190. Seligman B, Nathanson L: "Metastatic" calcification in the soft tissues of the legs in osteitis deformans, *Ann Intern Med* 23:82-91, 1945.

191. Sornberger CF, Smedal MI: Mechanism and incidence of cardiovascular changes in Paget's disease (osteitis deformans): critical review of literature with case studies, *Circulation* 6:711-726, 1952.

192. Stahl BF: Osteitis deformans, Paget's disease, with reports of two cases and autopsy in one, *Am J Med Sci* 143:525-539, 1912.

193. Stemmermann W: Die Ostitis deformans Paget unter Berücksichtigung ihrer Vererbung, *Ergebn Inn Med* 3(ns):185-219, 1952.

194. Storsteen KA, Janes JM: Arteriography and vascular studies in Paget's disease of bone, *JAMA* 154:472-474, 1954.

195. Terry TL: Angioid streaks and osteitis deformans, *Trans Am Ophthalmol Soc* 32:555-573, 1934.

196. Thiebaud D et al: A single infusion of the bisphosphonate AHPrBP (APD) as treatment of Paget's disease of bone, *Am J Med* 85(2):207-12, 1988.

197. Van Bogaert L: Ueber eine hereditäre und familiäre Form der Pagetschen Ostitis deformans mit Chorioretinitis pigmentosa, *Z Ges Neur* 147:327-345, 1933.

198. Von der Heydt R: Osteitis deformans with pigmented corneal degeneration, second case on record, *Am J Ophthalmol* 20:1139-1141, 1937.

199. Wells HG, Holley SW: Metastatic calcification in osteitis deformans (Paget's disease of bone), *Arch Pathol* 34:435-442, 1942.

200. Woodcock CW: Transactions of the Cleveland Dermatological Society, *Arch Dermatol Syph* 65:623 only, 1952.

Epidermolysis bullosa

201. Eady RAJ, Tidman MJ: Diagnosing epidermolysis bullosa, *Br J Dermatol* 108:621-626, 1983.

202. Fine JD: Epidermolysis bullosa: clinical aspects, pathology and recent advances in research, *Int J Dermatol* 25:143-157, 1986.

203. Gedde-Dahl TJ, Anton-Lamprecht I: Epidermolysis bullosa. In Emery A, Rimoin D, editors: *Principles and practices of medical genetics*, Edinburgh, 1983, Churchill Livingstone.

204. Heagerty AHM et al: Identification of an epidermal basement membrane defect in recessive forms of dystrophic epidermolysis bullosa by LH7:2 monoclonal antibody: use in diagnosis, *Br J Dermatol* 117:271-275, 1987.

205. Ito M et al: Epidermolysis bullosa simplex (Koebner) is a keratin disorder, *Arch Dermatol* 127:367-372, 1991.

206. Priestley GC et al: *Epidermolysis bullosa: a comprehensive review of classification, management and laboratory studies*, London, 1990.

207. Winship IM: *Epidermolysis bullosa*, doctoral thesis, University of Cape Town, 1986.

Occipital horn syndrome

208. Beighton P et al: International nosology of heritable disorders of connective tissue, Berlin, 1986, *Am J Med Genet* 29:581-594, 1988.

209. Blackston RD, Hirschhorn K, and Elsas LJ: Ehlers-Danlos syndrome (EDS), type IX: biochemical evidence for X-linkage. *Am J Hum Genet* 41(abstract):A49 only, 1987.

210. Byers PH et al: An X-linked form of cutis laxa due to deficiency of lysyl oxidase, *Birth Defects Orig Art Ser* 12(5):293-298, 1976.

211. Byers PH et al: X-linked cutis laxa: defective collagen crosslink formation due to decreased lysyl oxidase activity, *New Engl J Med* 303:61-65, 1980.

212. Hall JG: Personal communication to McKusick, 1980.

213. Hollister DW: Clinical features of Ehlers-Danlos syndrome types VIII and IX. In Akeson W, Glimcher MJ, and Bornstein P, editors: *Proceedings of workshop on inherited connective tissue disorders*, New York, 1981, Elsevier-North Holland.

214. Kaitila II et al: A skeletal and connective tissue disorder associated with lysyl oxidase deficiency and abnormal copper metabolism. In Papadatos CJ, Bartsocas CS editors: *Skeletal dysplasias*, New York, 1982, Alan R Liss, pp. 307-316.

215. Kuivaniemi H, Peltonen L, Kivirikko KI: Type IX Ehlers-Danlos syndrome and Menkes syndrome: the decrease in lysyl oxidase activity is associated with a corresponding deficiency in the enzyme protein, *Am J Hum Genet* 37:798-808, 1985.

216. Kuivaniemi H et al: Abnormal copper metabolism and deficient lysyl oxidase activity in a heritable connective tissue disorder, *J Clin Invest* 69:730-733, 1982.

217. Lazoff SG et al: Skeletal dysplasia, occipital horns, intestinal malabsorption, and obstructive uropathy: a new hereditary syndrome, *Birth Defects Orig Art Ser* XI(5):71-74, 1975.

218. MacFarlane JD et al: A new Ehlers-Danlos syndrome with skeletal dysplasia, *Am J Hum Genet* 32(abstract):118A only, 1980.

219. Peltonen L et al: Alterations in copper and collagen metabolism in the Menkes syndrome and a new subtype of the Ehlers-Danlos syndrome, *Biochemistry* 22:6156-6163, 1983.

220. Sartoris DJ, Resnick D: The horn: a pathognomonic feature of paediatric bone dysplasias, *Aust Paediatr J* 23(6):347-349, 1987.

Menkes syndrome (kinky hair syndrome)

221. Aguilar MJ et al: Kinky-hair disease. I. Clinical and pathological features, *J Neuropathol Exp Neurol* 25:507-522, 1966.

222. Al-Rashid RA, Spangler J: Neonatal copper deficiency, *New Engl J Med* 285:841-843, 1971.

223. Baerlocher KE et al: Menkes' disease: clinical, therapeutic and biochemical studies, *J Inherited Metab Dis* 6(suppl 2):87-88, 1983.

224. Billings DM, Degnan M: Kinky hair syndrome: a new case and a review, *Am J Dis Child* 121:447-449, 1971.

225. Bray PF: Sex-linked neurodegenerative disease associated with monilethrix, *Pediatrics* 36:417-420, 1965.

226. Camakaris J, Mann JR, Danks DM: Copper metabolism in mottled mouse mutants: copper concentration in tissues during development, *Biochem J* 180:597-604, 1979.

227. Danks DM: Of mice and men, metals and mutations, *J Med Genet* 23:99-106, 1986.

228. Danks DM: Copper deficiency in infants with particular reference to Menkes' disease. In Howell JMcD, Gawthorne M, editors: *Copper in man and animals*, Boca Raton, 1987, CRC.

229. Danks DM: The mild form of Menkes disease: progress report on original case, *Am J Med Genet* 30:859-864, 1988.

230. Danks DM: Copper deficiency in humans, *Ann Rev Nutr* 8:235-257, 1988.

231. Danks DM: Disorders of copper transport. In Scriver CR et al, editors: *The metabolic basis of inherited disease*, ed 6, New York, 1989, McGraw-Hill.

232. Danks DM: Disorders of copper transport: Menkes disease and the occipital horn syndrome. In Royce PM, Steinmann B, editors: *Extracellular matrix and inheritable disorders of connective tissue*, 1990, Alan R Liss.

233. Danks DM: personal communication to McKusick.

234. Danks DM, Cartwright E, Stevens BJ: Menkes' steely-hair (kinky-hair disease), *Lancet* 1:891 only, 1973.

235. Danks DM et al: Is Menkes' syndrome a heritable disorder of connective tissue? Lancet 2(letter):1089 only, 1971.

236. Danks DM et al: Menkes' kinky hair syndrome: an inherited defect in copper absorption with widespread effects, *Pediatrics* 50:188-201, 1972.

237. Danks DM et al: Menkes' kinky-hair syndrome: an inherited defect in intestinal absorption with widespread consequences, *Lancet* 1:1100-1102, 1972.

238. Danks DM et al: Menkes' kinky hair disease: further definition of the defect in copper transport, *Science* 179:1140-1141, 1973.

239. French JH et al: Trichopoliodystrophy. I. Report of a case and biochemical studies, *Arch Neurol* 26:229-244, 1972.

240. Gerdes AM et al: Variability in clinical expression of Menkes syndrome, *Eur J Pediatr* 148:132-135, 1988.

241. Ghatak NR et al: Trichopoliodystrophy. II. Pathological changes in skeletal muscle and nervous system, *Arch Neurol* 26:60-72, 1972.

242. Gillespie JM: The isolation and properties of some soluble proteins from wool. VIII. The proteins of copper-deficient wool, *Aust J Biol Sci* 17:282, 1964.

243. Goka TJ et al: Menkes disease: a biochemical abnormality in cultured human fibroblasts, *Proc Natl Acad Sci USA* 73:604-606, 1976.

244. Herd SM et al: Uptake and efflux of copper-64 in Menkes' disease and normal continuous lymphoid cell line, *Biochem J* 247:341-347, 1987.

245. Heydorn K et al: Extra-hepatic storage of copper. A male foetus suspected of Menkes disease, *Humangenetik* 29:171-175, 1975.

246. Holstein TJ et al: Effect of altered copper metabolism induced by mottled alleles and diet on mouse tyrosinase, *Proc Soc Exp Biol Med* 162:264-268, 1979.

247. Horn N: Menkes X-linked disease: heterozygous phenotype in cloned fibroblast cultures, *J Med Genet* 17:257-261, 1980.

248. Horn N, Mooy P, McGuire VM: Menkes' X-linked disease, two clonal cell populations in heterozygotes, *J Med Genet* 17:262-266, 1980.

249. Kapur S et al: Menkes syndrome in a girl with X-autosome translocation, *Am J Med Genet* 26:503-510, 1987.

250. Kuivaniemi H, Peltonen L, Kivirikko KI: Type IX Ehlers-Danlos syndrome and Menkes syndrome: the decrease in lysyl oxidase activity is associated with a corresponding deficiency in the enzyme protein, *Am J Hum Genet* 37:798-808, 1985.

251. Leone A, Pavlakis GN, Hamer DH: Menkes' disease: abnormal metallothionein gene regulation in response to copper, *Cell* 40:301-309, 1985.

252. Mann JB, Camakaris J, Danks DM: Copper metabolism in mottled mouse mutants: defective placental transfer of ^{64}Cu to foetal brindled (Mo^{br}) mice, *Biochem J* 186:629-631, 1980.

253. Menkes JH et al: A sex-linked recessive disorder with retardation of growth, peculiar hair and focal cerebral and cerebellar degeneration, *Pediatrics* 29:764-779, 1962.

254. Oakes BW, Danks DM, Campbell PE: Human copper deficiency: ultrastructural studies of the aorta and skin in a child with Menkes' syndrome, *Exp Mol Pathol* 25:82-98, 1976.

255. O'Brien JS, Sampson EL: Kinky hair disease. II. Biochemical studies, *J Neuropathol Exp Neurol* 25:523-530, 1966.

256. Procopis P, Camakaris J, Danks DM: A mild form of Menkes' syndrome, *J Pediatr* 98:97-99, 1981.

257. Seelenfreund MH, Gartner S, Vinger PF: The ocular pathology of Menkes' disease (kinky hair disease), *Arch Ophthalmol* 80:718-720, 1968.

258. Sherwood G, Sarkar B, Sasskortsak A: Copper histidine therapy in Menkes' disease: prevention of progressive neurodegeneration, *J Inherited Metab Dis* 12(suppl 2):393-396, 1989.

259. Tonnesen T, Horn N: Prenatal and postnatal diagnosis of Menkes disease, an inherited disorder of copper metabolism, *J Inherited Metab Dis* 12(suppl):207-214, 1989.

260. Wenk G, Suzuki K: The effect of copper supplementation on the concentration of copper in the brain of the brindled mouse, *Biochem J* 205:485-487, 1982.

261. Wesenberg RL, Gwinn JL, Barnes GR Jr: Radiological findings in the kinky-hair syndrome, *Radiology* 92:500-506, 1969.

262. Westman JA et al: Atypical Menkes steely hair disease, *Am J Med Genet* 30:853-858, 1988.

Generalized arterial calcification of infancy

263. Anderson KA et al: Idiopathic arterial calcification of infancy in newborn siblings with unusual light and electron microscopic manifestations, *Arch Pathol Lab Med* 109:838-842, 1985.

264. Hunt AC, Leys DG: General arterial calcification of infancy, *Br Med J* 1:385-386, 1957.

265. Maayan C et al: Idiopathic infantile arterial calcification: a case report and review of the literature, *Eur J Pediatr* 142:211-215, 1984.

266. Meradjo M et al: Idiopathic infantile arterial calcification in siblings: radiologic diagnosis and successful treatment, *J Pediatr* 92:401-405, 1978.

267. Milner LS et al: Hypertension as the major problem of idiopathic arterial calcification of infancy, *J Pediatr* 105:934-938, 1984.

268. Raphael SS, Horne WI, Hyde TA: Arterial medial calcification of infancy in brothers, *Can Med Assoc J* 103:290-293, 1970.

269. Sholler GF et al: Generalized arterial calcification of infancy: three case reports, including spontaneous regression with long-term survival, *J Pediatr* 105:257-260, 1984.

270. Williams AL: *The pathology of cardiac failure in infancy*, thesis for degree of Doctor of Medicine, University of Melbourne, 1958.

271. Witzleben CL: Idiopathic infantile arterial calcification—a misnomer? *Am J Cardiol* 26:305-309, 1970.

Werner syndrome

272. Boatwright H, Wheeler CE, Cawley EP: Werner's syndrome, *Arch Intern Med* 90:243-249, 1952.

273. Bauer EA et al: Diminished response of Werner's syndrome fibroblasts to growth factors PDGF and FGF, *Science* 234:1240-1243, 1986.

274. Cerimele D et al: High prevalence of Werner's syndrome in Sardinia: a description of six patients and estimate of the gene frequency, *Hum Genet* 62:25-30, 1982.

275. Epstein CJ et al: Werner's syndrome; a review of its symptomatology, natural history, pathologic features, genetics and relationship to the natural aging process, *Medicine* 45:177-221, 1966

276. Goto M et al: Family analysis of Werner's syndrome: a survey of 42 Japanese families with a review of the literature, *Clin Genet* 19:8-15, 1981.

277. Hoehn H et al: Variegated translocation mosaicism in human skin fibroblast cultures, *Cytogenet Cell Genet* 15:282-298, 1975.

278. Irwin GW, Ward PB: Werner's syndrome, with a report of two cases, *Am J Med* 15:266-271, 1953.

279. McKusick VA et al: Medical genetics 1962, *J Chronic Dis* 16:457-634, 1963.

280. Perloff JK, Phelps ET: A review of Werner's syndrome, with a report of the second autopsied case, *Am Intern Med* 48:1205-1220, 1958.

281. Reed R, Seville RH, Tattersall RN: Werner's syndrome, *Br J Dermatol* 65:165-176, 1953.

282. Scappaticci S, Cerimele D, Fraccaro M: Clonal structural chromosomal rearrangements in primary fibroblast cultures and in lymphocytes of patients with Werner's syndrome, *Hum Genet* 62:16-24, 1982.

283. Schonberg S et al: Werner's syndrome proliferation in vitro clones of cells bearing chromosome translocations, *Am J Hum Genet* 36:387-397, 1984.

284. Smith RC, Winer LH, Martel S: Werner's syndrome; report of two cases, *Arch Dermatol* 71:197-204, 1955.

285. Thannhauser SJ: Werner's syndrome (progeria of the adult) and Rothmund's syndrome; two types of closely related heredofamilial atrophic dermatoses with juvenile cataracts and endocrine features; critical study with five new cases, *Ann Intern Med* 23:559-626, 1945.

286. Werner O: *Über Katarakt in Verbindung mit Sklerodermie*, doctoral dissertation, University of Kiel, 1904, Schmidt and Klaunig.

Progeria

287. Brown WT: Human mutations affecting ageing: a review, *Mech Ageing Dev* 9:325-336, 1979.

288. De Busk FL: The Hutchinson-Gilford progeria syndrome, *J Pediatr* 80:697-724, 1972.

289. Dyck JD et al: Management of coronary artery disease in Hutchinson-Gilford syndrome, *J Pediatr* 111:407-410, 1987.

290. Franklyn PP: Progeria in siblings, *Clin Radiol* 27(3):327-333, 1976.

291. Gabr M et al: Progeria, a pathologic study, *J Pediatr* 57:70-77, 1960.

292. Jones KL et al: Older paternal age and fresh gene mutation: data on additional disorders, *J Paediatr* 86:84-88, 1975.

293. Parkash H: Hutchinson-Gilford progeria: familial occurrence, *Am J Med Genet* 36:431-433, 1990.

294. Rava G: Su un nucleo familiare di progeria, *Minerva Med* 58:1502-1509, 1967.

295. Viegas J, Souza PLR, Salzano FM: Progeria in twins, *J Med Genet* 11(4):384-386, 1974.

Wrinkly Skin syndrome

296. Cassamassima AC et al: Wrinkly skin syndrome: phenotype and additional manifestations, *Am J Med Genet* 27:885-893, 1987.

297. Gazit E et al: The wrinkly skin syndrome: a new heritable disorder of connective tissue, *Clin Genet* 4:186-192, 1973.

298. Goodman RM et al: The wrinkly skin syndrome and cartilage hair hypoplasia in sibs of the same family. In Papadatos CJ, Bartsocas CS, editors: *Progress in clinical and biological research, vol 104, skeletal dysplasias*, New York, 1982, Alan J Liss, pp 205-214.

299. Hurvitz SA, Baumgarten A, Goodman RM: The wrinkly skin syndrome: a report of a case and review of the literature, *Clin Genet* 38:307-313, 1990.

300. Karrar ZA et al: The wrinkly skin syndrome: a report of two siblings from Saudi Arabia, *Clin Genet* 23:308-310, 1983.

Connective tissue nevi

301. Ayala F, Donofrio P: Elastosis perforans serpiginosa: report of a family, *Dermatologica* 166:32-37, 1983.
302. Diaz F: Elastosis perforans serpiginosa associated with Down's syndrome and sex-linked ichthyosis. Treatment with 13-cia-retinoic acid, *Med Cutan Ibero Lat Am* 17(4):209-214, 1989.
303. Kanan MW: Familial reactive perforating collagenosis and intolerance to cold, *Br J Dermatol* 91:405-414, 1974.
304. Mehregan AH, Schwartz OD, Livingood CS: Reactive perforating collagenosis, *Arch Dermatol* 96:277-282, 1967.
305. Meyrick TRH, Kirby JD: Elastosis perforans serpiginosa and pseudothanxoma elasticum-like skin changes due to D-penicillamine, *Clin Exp Dermatol* 10(4):386-391, 1985.
306. Nair BKH et al: Reactive perforating collagenosis, *Br J Dermatol* 91:399-403, 1974.
307. Sacks HN et al: Familial cardiomyopathy, hypogonadism and collagenoma, *Ann Intern Med* 93:813-817, 1980.
308. Sahn EE et al: D-penicillamine-induced elastosis perforans serpiginosa in a child with juvenile rheumatoid arthritis: report of a case and review of the literature, *J Am Acad Dermatol* 20:279-288, 1989.
309. Uitto J, Santa-Cruz DJ, Eisen AZ: Familial cutaneous collagenoma: genetic studies on a family, *Br J Dermatol* 101:185-189, 1979.
310. Uitto J, Santa-Cruz DJ, Eisen AZ: Connective tissue nevi of the skin, *J Am Acad Dermatol* 3:441-461, 1980.
311. van Jooste T et al: Elastosis perforans serpiginosa: clinical, histomorphological and immunological studies, *J Cutan Pathol* 15(2):92-97, 1988.

Keloid

312. Bloom D: Heredity of keloids: review of the literature and report of a family with multiple keloids in five generations, *J Med* 56:511-519, 1956.
313. Bohrod MG: Keloids and sexual selection: a study in the racial distribution of disease, *Arch Dermatol Syph* 36:19-25, 1937.
314. Cosman B et al: The surgical treatment of keloids, *Plast Reconstr Surg* 27:335-358, 1961.

Pachydermoperiostosis

315. Cremin BJ: Familial idiopathic osteoarthropathy of children: a case report and progress, *Br J Radiol* 43:568-570, 1970.

316. Findlay GH, Oosthuizen WJ: Pachydermoperiostitis: syndrome of Touraine, Solente and Gole, *S Afr Med J* 25:747-752, 1951.
317. Gray PI, Steyn AF: Touraine-Solenti-Gole syndrome: a case report, *S Afr Med J* 54:1071-1072, 1978.
318. McKusick VA: Pachydermoperiostosis. In Fitzpatrick TB et al, editors: *Dermatology in internal medicine*, New York, 1971, McGraw-Hill, pp 1227-1228.
319. McKusick VA: *Mendelian inheritance in man*, ed 4, Baltimore, 1975, Johns Hopkins University, pp 246.
320. Rimoin DL: Pachydermoperiostosis (idiopathic clubbing and periostosis): genetic and physiologic considerations, *New Engl J Med* 272:923-931, 1965.

Osteochondroses

321. Apley AG, Solomon LS: *Apley's system of orthopaedics and fractures*, ed 6, London, 1982, Butterworth Scientific.
322. Burwell RG: Perthes' disease: growth and aetiology, *Arch Dis Child* 63:1408-1412, 1988.
323. Caffey JP: The early roentgenographic changes in essential coxa plana: their significance in pathogenesis, *Am J Roentgenol* 103:620-634, 1968.
324. Gray IM, Lowry RB, Renwick DHG: Incidence and genetics of Legg-Perthes disease (osteochondritis deformans) in British Columbia: evidence of polygenic determination, *J Med Genet* 9:197-202, 1972.
325. Halal, F Gledhill RB, Fraser FC: Dominant inheritance of Scheuermann's juvenile kyphosis, *Am J Dis Child* 132:1105-1107, 1978.
326. Hall DJ: Genetic aspects of Perthes' disease: a critical review, *Clin Orthop* 209:100-114, 1986.
327. Jeffreys TE: Genu recurvatum after Osgood-Schlatter's disease: report of a case, *J Bone Joint Surg* 47B:298-299, 1965.
328. Osgood RB: Lesions of the tibial tubercle occurring during adolescence, *Bost Med Surg J* 148:114-117, 1903.
329. Scheuermann H: Kyphosis dorsalis juvenilis, *Z Orthop Chir* 41:305-317, 1921.
330. Schlatter C: Verletzungen des schnabel-förmigen Fortsatzes der oberen Tibiaepiphyse, *Beitr Klin Chir* 38:874, 1903.
331. Sharrard WJW: *Paediatric orthopaedics and fractures*, Oxford, Edinburgh, 1971, Blackwell Scientific Publications.

14

Genetic Disorders of the Osseous Skeleton

David L. Rimoin
Ralph S. Lachman

The osseous skeleton, the largest specialized connective tissue, participates in many of the generalized heritable disorders of connective tissue previously discussed in this book. In addition, it is subject to a large number of gene-determined derangements, with primary effects often limited to bone and cartilage. Several comprehensive reviews of these disorders have been published that may be helpful in supplementing the survey undertaken in this book.*

The bone dysplasias represent a difficult category of hereditary disease because the types are legion; most are rare or fairly rare, so most physicians, even specialists such as orthopedists and radiologists, encounter them infrequently and until recently almost nothing was known of their pathogenesis. With the recent explosion of knowledge in the biochemistry and molecular biology of connective tissue, rapid progress should occur in the delineation of the basic defects in these disorders. Indeed, mutations in the type II collagen gene have now been delineated in the spondyloepiphyseal dysplasia (SED) family of disorders.†

The principal method of nosologic study has been radiologic, complemented by observations of the clinical natural history, familial (i.e., genetic) characteristics, and chondroosseous pa-

thology. Discovery of the basic biochemical and molecular defects in these disorders will lead to further nosologic clarification.

HISTORICAL NOTE

Early important nosologic and genetic studies of skeletal dysplasias were published by Morch of Copenhagen in 1941,[406] Grebe of Frankenburg, Germany, in 1955,[170] Hoback of Norway in 1961,[227] Rubin of the United States in 1964,[486] and Lamy and Maroteaux of Paris.[318-321,368-384] In addition, Spranger in Germany,[543-560] Kozlowski in Australia,[297-303] Giedeon in Switzerland,[148,149,151] and Gorlin,[160-166] Hall,[182-190] Horton,[232-242] Silence,[526-531] Langer,[326-335] McKusick,[391-398] and Rimoin and Lachman* in North America have contributed extensively to this field.

Morch recognized the occurrence of "different degrees of chondrodystrophy" but overlooked the heterogeneity in his series. A survey of the cases illustrated in Morch's monograph[406] indicates that several have a skeletal dysplasia distinct from achondroplasia.

Grebe[170] recognized heterogeneity in the broad group of skeletal dysplasias and divided them into *Mopstyp* (pug-dog–like) and *Dackeltyp* (dachshund-like). The former group consisted of cases of classic achondroplasia; the latter group, characterized by normal head and face, included mainly pseudoachondroplasia. A survey of the cases in

---

*References 30, 33, 53, 118, 227, 231, 318, 319, 369, 434, 470, 471, 476, 486, 549, 550, 588, 633, and 642.

†References 3, 70, 294, 341, 412, 436, 591, and 612.

*References 48-50, 311-317, 470-478, and 514-518.

Grebe's monograph permits identification of a number of distinct entities, some of which Grebe recognized as separate from either the *Mopstyp* or the *Dackeltyp*.

Lamy and Maroteaux[318] gave a useful synthesis of their own experience and that recorded by other authors up to 1960 in their monograph *Les Chondrodystrophies Genotypiques.* The brief historical sketches are useful. The authors pointed out that achondroplasia, then called fetal rickets, was recognized as a distinct entity by Depaul in 1851. However, the distinction is generally accredited to Parrot, perhaps because in 1878 he introduced the new term, "achondroplasia." Pierre Marie contributed to the nosography of achondroplasia in the adult (he pointed out the trident hand), and Porak also gave early descriptions and pointed out the similarities as well as the distinctness of achondroplasia and osteogenesis imperfecta congenita (OI). Kaufmann[276,277] described the anatomicopathologic characteristics of achondroplasia, although his "chondrodystrophia foetalis hypertrophica" appears to have been metatropic dwarf-

ism. The disorder described as "foetus achondroplasie" by Lamy and Maroteaux[318] (see Fig. 4-5) was clearly an example of thanatophoric dwarfism, which they first delineated and named in a publication 7 years later.[375] They delineated the X-linked form of SED tarda on genetic and radiographic study.[318] Hypochondroplasia was recognized as an entity distinct from achondroplasia, and it was concluded that the inheritance is probably dominant. Maroteaux has published extensively on the delineation of the skeletal dysplasias and has reviewed his findings in his textbook, *Bone Diseases of Children.*[369]

The monograph by Hobaeck[227] presented a collection of 43 Norwegian families studied in detail from a clinical, genetic, and radiographic point of view. A large number of illustrations were provided. The discussion of genetics was often weak. It seems that Hobaeck found a remarkably large number of families with recessive disorders. The fjord geography of Norway, with resulting inbreeding, was probably responsible.

Rubin[486] reviewed earlier classifications of bone

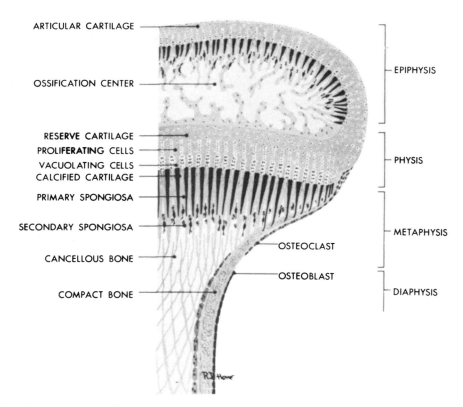

Fig. 14-1. Anatomicohistologic correlation of bone structure. (From Rubin P: *Dynamic classification of bone dysplasias,* St Louis, 1964, Mosby—Year Book.)

dysplasias, namely, those of Brailsford,[53] Fairbank,[118,119] and Jaffe (as communicated to Hirsch[224]), Jackson,[256] Sear,[503] Lamy and Maroteaux,[318] and Hobaeck.[227] Rubin[486] classified generalized hereditary dysplasias of the osseous skeleton according to whether the major site of abnormality was epiphyseal, physeal, metaphyseal, or diaphyseal (Fig. 14-1). (Rubin's proposal of the term *physis* and its adjectival form *physeal* to refer to the growth zone seems both useful and logical.) Each class of dysplasia had, by this system, subclasses of hypoplasias and hyperplasias, and in most of the subclasses more than one genus of disorder was recognized. In 1974 Spranger, Langer, and Wiedemann[548] published their classic atlas on bone dysplasias, which is still a useful guide to the radiographic diagnosis of these disorders.

Since the fourth edition of *Heritable Disorders of Connective Tissue* was published in 1972, hundreds of papers have been published on the clinical delineation of the skeletal dysplasias and numerous attempts have been made to create meaningful classifications and standard nomenclature.

CLASSIFICATION AND NOMENCLATURE

The current nomenclature for these disorders is most confusing and is based on the part of the skeleton that is affected on radiographic examination (e.g., the epiphyseal dysplasias and the metaphyseal dysplasias); on a Greek term that describes the appearance of the bone or the course of the disease (e.g., diastrophic (twisted) dysplasia or thanatophoric (death bringing) dysplasia); on an eponym (e.g., Kniest dysplasia or Ellis-van Creveld syndrome); or on a term that attempts to describe the pathogenesis of the condition (e.g., achondroplasia or osteogenesis imperfecta).[476]

The extent of the heterogeneity in these disorders and the variety of methods used for their classification have resulted in further confusion. Clinical classification has divided the skeletal dysplasias into those with short-limbed dwarfism and those with short-trunk dwarfism. The short-limbed varieties have been further subdivided on the basis of the segment of the long bones that is most severely involved. Other clinical classifications have been based on the age of onset of the disorder, for example, those disorders that manifest themselves at birth (achondroplasia) versus those that first manifest in later life (e.g., pseudoachondroplasia). Associated clinical abnormalities

have also been used to subdivide these disorders. Examples are the myopia of SED congenita, the cleft palate of Kniest dysplasia, the fine hair of cartilage-hair hypoplasia, and the polydactyly and congenital heart disease of the Ellis-van Creveld syndrome. Still other disorders have been classified on the basis of their apparent mode of inheritance, for example, the dominant and X-linked varieties of SED.

The most widely used method of differentiating the skeletal dysplasias has been the detection of skeletal radiographic abnormalities. Radiographic classifications are based on the different parts of the long bones that are abnormal (epiphyses, metaphyses, or diaphyses) (Figs. 14-2 and 14-3). Thus epiphyseal and metaphyseal dysplasias can be further divided depending on whether the spine is also involved (e.g., SED and spondylometaphyseal dysplasias). Furthermore, each of these groups can be further divided into several distinct disorders based on a variety of other clinical and radiographic differences.

Thus both the classification and the nomenclature of the skeletal dysplasias have evolved in a haphazard fashion; frequently several different names have been used for the same disorder and similar names have been used for clearly distinct disorders by different authors. Furthermore, no obvious correlation between the classification cri-

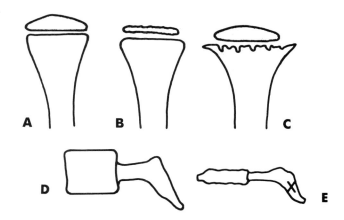

Fig. 14-2. Classification of the chondrodysplasias based on radiographic involvement of, **A** to **C**, long bones and, **D** and **E**, vertebrae. Bone involvement and disease categories are, **A** and **D**, normal; **B** and **D**, epiphyseal dysplasia; **C** and **D**, metaphyseal dysplasia; **B** and **E**, spondyloepiphyseal dysplasia; **C** and **E**, spondylometaphyseal dysplasia; and, **B**, **C**, and **E**, spondyloepimetaphyseal dysplasia. (From Rimoin D, Shohat M: *Endocrinologist* 1:240-248, 1991.)

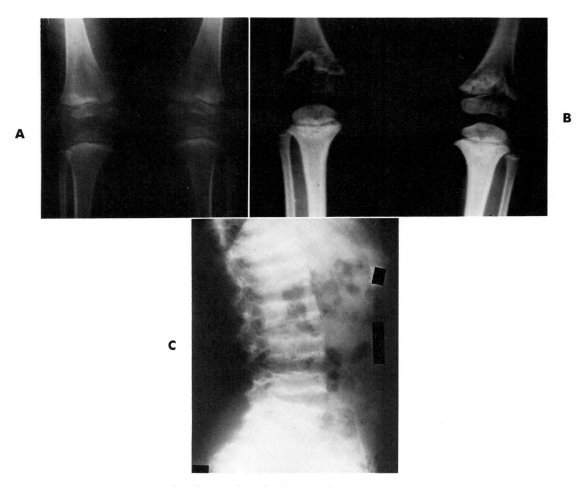

Fig. 14-3. Radiographs of, **A** and **B,** the knee and, **C,** spine in patients with a variety of skeletal dysplasias. **A,** Epiphyseal dysplasia. Small, irregular epiphyses and normal metaphyses are evident in a patient with spondyloepiphyseal dysplasia. **B,** Metaphyseal dysplasia. Normal epiphyses and splayed irregular metaphyses can be seen in a patient with metaphyseal dysplasia. **C,** Platyspondyly. The flattened, irregularly shaped vertebrae are evident in a patient with spondyloepiphyseal dysplasia. (From Rimoin D, Shohat M: *Endocrinologist* 1:240-248, 1991.)

teria and potential pathogenetic mechanisms is usually apparent.[475,476,550] In an attempt to develop a uniform nomenclature for these syndromes the International Nomenclature of Constitutional Diseases of Bone was proposed in 1970 and updated in 1977, 1983, and 1991 (see Appendix C). This International Nomenclature originally divided the constitutional disorders of the skeleton into five major groups: the osteochondrodysplasias (abnormal growth or development of cartilage or bone, or both); the dysostoses (malforma-

tions of individual bones, singly or in combination); the idiopathic osteolyses (a group of disorders associated with multifocal resorption of bone); the skeletal disorders associated with chromosomal aberrations; and primary metabolic disorders.

The osteochondrodysplasias were further divided into (1) defects of growth of tubular bones or spine, or both (e.g., achondroplasia), which are frequently referred to as chondrodysplasias; (2) disorganized development of cartilage and fibrous components of the skeleton (e.g., multiple cartilaginous exostoses), and (3) abnormalities of density or cortical diaphyseal structure or metaphyseal modeling, or both (e.g., osteogenesis imperfecta).

The chondrodysplasias were further subdivided into those disorders evident at birth and those that first become apparent in later life. This division may be purely artificial, since identical pathogenetic mechanisms of differing degrees of severity may occur in allelic disorders, resulting in differences in the age of manifestation. For example, both congenital and infantile presentations of osteogenesis imperfecta are seen within the same families manifesting dominant inheritance. On the other hand, many disorders that share common radiographic features and have thus been classified into one group, such as the metaphyseal dysplasias, may result from different pathogenetic mechanisms.

Because short stature is a frequent finding in these disorders, the term "dwarfism" has been historically used for them. However, "dwarfism" is thought to result in social stigmatization and is popularly unappealing; for these and other reasons the term "dwarfism" was dropped from the nomenclature and replaced by the term "dysplasia." This latter term, which means "disordered growth," reflects the probable pathogenesis of the majority of the chondrodysplasias. In contrast, malformations of single bones or groups of bones, which presumably do not reflect a generalized disorder of the skeleton, have been referred to as "dysostoses."

Although the International Nomenclature provides a uniform standard for referring to specific disorders so that the same disease is called the same thing by all authors, many of the names are inaccurate. For example, achondroplasia and achondrogenesis are inaccurate terms in defining the pathogenesis of these conditions but are so well entrenched in the literature that they persist. As the morphology, pathogenesis, and especially the basic biochemical and molecular defect in each of these disorders is unraveled, this nomenclature should be changed to refer to the specific pathogenetic or metabolic defect. The etiologic or pathogenetic nomenclature is now used for certain skeletal dysplasias, such as the mucopolysaccharidoses, mucolipidoses, and disorders of mineralization (e.g., beta-glucuronidase deficiency, fucosidosis, and hypophosphatasia).

The nomenclature is still far from complete, since new heterogeneity within the skeletal dysplasias is continuously being discovered. Furthermore, some disorders once thought to be distinct are now being recognized as one disorder with marked clinical variability.[48,472,544,545] Spranger[544,545] has classified the skeletal dysplasias into "families of disorders" that are believed to share common pathogenetic mechanisms. Recent discoveries of the biochemical and molecular defects of type II collagen in achondrogenesis II, hypochondrogenesis, and the SEDs have confirmed this concept, at least in this one family of skeletal dysplasias.[341,414,591]

The Fourth International Nomenclature committee, which met in Germany in 1991, not only updated the nomenclature with the addition of a number of newly described syndromes but also totally revised the organization of these disorders into a clinically and pathogenetically based classification[560] (Appendix C). Thus disorders that share clinical, radiographic, or morphologic features, suggesting that they may fall into a family of disorders that share common pathogenetic mechanisms, were grouped together. This classification will certainly undergo constant revision as the basic defect in each of these disorders is discovered.

CHONDROOSSEOUS MORPHOLOGY

In recent years morphologic studies of chondroosseous tissue have revealed specific abnormalities in many of the skeletal dysplasias.* In certain of these disorders histologic examination of chondroosseous tissue may be useful in making an accurate diagnosis of the specific skeletal disorder. In other disorders, no histopathologic alterations are present or they are nonspecific; in these cases pathologic examination is useful in ruling out a diagnosis.

On morphologic grounds the chondrodysplasias can be broadly divided into the following categories: (1) those disorders that show no qualitative abnormality in endochondral ossification, (2) those in which there are morphologic abnormalities in chondrocytes, (3) those with morphologic

---

*References 48-50, 147, 150, 232, 234, 237, 242, 292, 378, 383-384, 433, 457, 470, 516, 527, 550, 561-566, 645, 646, 649, and 651.

abnormalities in matrix, and (4) those in which the abnormality is primarily localized to the area of chondroosseous transformation. In certain disorders abnormalities in two or more of these areas can be seen.

Conditions with minimal disturbance of endochondral ossification include achondroplasia and hypochondroplasia, in which endochondral ossification is qualitatively normal but abnormalities are present in the height and arrangement of proliferative columns, particularly in the center of the large growth plates.[478,564] Ultrastructural studies show an increased number of dead chondrocytes and increased levels of cytoplasmic glycogen. In asphyxiating thoracic dysplasia, in which several workers have shown prominent lipid inclusions in chondrocytes, the growth plate organization is also essentially normal.[470,564]

In the achondrogenesis syndromes, defects in the appearance of the cells, matrix, or chondroosseous transformation, or a combination of these can be seen. In achondrogenesis IA (Houston-Harris) the chondrocytes are large and contain prominent inclusions.[50] Endochondral ossification is markedly disturbed, with absence of columns of proliferative cells and lack of cellular hypertrophy. In achondrogenesis II (Langer-Saldino) there is complete disruption of endochondral ossification with large chondrocytic lacunae and little intervening matrix.[48] These changes suggested a metabolic defect leading to reduced synthesis of a matrix component. Dilation of the rough endoplasmic reticulum of the chondrocytes is found on ultrastructural examination. Indeed, achondrogenesis II is now known to be due to a defect in type II collagen synthesis, the abnormal type II collagen accumulating in the rough endoplasmic reticulum.[156]

In thanatophoric dysplasia[433] and short-rib polydactyly (SRP) syndromes type I and type II there appears to be defective maturation of chondrocytes with reduced and disorganized columnization.[112,470] Consequently, vascular invasion is irregular and chondroosseous trabeculae are short and deformed, with bridging between the trabeculae. Hypertrophic chondrocytes are irregularly arranged at the zone of chondroosseous transformation and lack columnization.[470,564] Bands of mesenchymal-like fibrous tissue extend from the perichondral area into the growth plate.

Matrix abnormalities are seen in diastrophic dysplasia, chondrodysplasia punctata (various

types), and the Dyggve-Melchior-Clausen syndrome.[470,564] In diastrophic dysplasia the matrix of the reserve zone cartilage develops a particularly fibrillar appearance and shows areas of microscar formation.[237] Chondrocytes as seen both by light microscopy and by electron microscopy are surrounded by dense corona of large collagen fibers. In Dyggve-Melchior-Clausen syndrome, chondrocytes studied by means of light microscopy appear to be arranged around relatively large common lacunae with up to 10 clustered chondrocytes.[470] In chondrodysplasia punctata of both the rhizomelic recessive and Conradi-Hünermann varieties there appears to be an alteration in epiphyseal and reserve zone cartilage matrix with areas of dystrophic (nonendochondral) ossification and fibrous dysplasia and areas of mucoid degeneration.[470,564]

New chondrodysplasias are constantly being reported, and morphologic studies have often played an integral part in their investigation and nosology. For example, dyssegmental dysplasia, type Silverman-Handmaker, and dyssegmental dysplasia, type Rolland-Desbuquois, appear to represent distinct syndromes showing large coronal vertebral clefts but differing in other radiographic and morphologic features. Syndromes with striking histopathologic abnormalities have been reported, for example, fibrochondrogenesis[564] and the syndrome reported by Greenberg et al.[171] Achondrogenesis IA (Houston-Harris) and IB (Fraccaro) have been distinguished from each other by morphologic as well as radiographic differences, whereas achondrogenesis type II (Langer-Saldino) and hypochondrogenesis have identical chondroosseous morphologic features and appear to represent variability in a single disorder.[48]

Chondroosseous histopathologic study can help in reaching a specific diagnosis when skeletal radiographs are inadequate. This has been especially true for the lethal neonatal chondrodysplasias such as thanatophoric dysplasia and achondrogenesis, which are often misdiagnosed as achondroplasia and may come to autopsy without radiographs being obtained. Provision of an accurate diagnosis by these studies can lead to significant changes in the genetic counseling given to these families. Histologic studies negated the previously held concept that thanatophoric dysplasia was inherited as an autosomal recessive trait, by demonstrating that chondroosseous tissue obtained from the three reported families[168,200,487] with multiple affected sibs with "thanatophoric dwarfism" was completely different from the histopathologic appearance of true thanatophoric dwarfism and similar to that which we have observed in achondrogenesis type I and Schneckenbecken dysplasia, known autosomal recessive disorders.[49,50,292] Thus for the parents of a child with thanatophoric dysplasia the risk of having another affected child is quite low rather than the previously quoted 25%.

Thus pathologic analysis of chondroosseous tissue can be of great help in the diagnostic evaluation of the chondrodysplasias, can lead to the delineation of new syndromes, and can provide clues to the pathogenetic mechanism operative in these disorders.

BIOCHEMICAL AND MOLECULAR STUDIES

In recent years great progress has been made in our knowledge of the basic biology of collagen and proteoglycans, and a search for biochemical defects in certain of the skeletal dysplasias has been performed. Nevertheless, except for the mucopolysaccharidoses and mucolipidoses and certain of the mineralization defects, such as hypophosphatasia, hypophosphatemic rickets, and vitamin D–dependency rickets, until recently the basic defect had not been uncovered in any of this large group of disorders.

Abnormalities in proteoglycan chemistry have been suggested in pseudoachondroplasia.[223,563,565] The cellular inclusion bodies that have been demonstrated in the chondrocytes in this disorder would suggest an abnormality in proteoglycan chemistry, since immunohistochemic staining of these inclusion bodies with antibodies directed against the proteoglycan core protein has been demonstrated.[223] Specific abnormalities in cartilage proteoglycans have also been demonstrated in several of the mouse chondrodysplasias, such as the sulfate donor defect in the brachymorphic mouse[432,500] and an absence of proteoglycan core protein in the cartilage matrix deficiency mutant (Cmd) mouse.[289] Similar defects may well exist in certain of their human counterparts.

A specific defect in collagen chemistry has been suggested in several skeletal dysplasias.[61,413,414] Type II collagen, however, appears to be qualitatively and quantitatively normal in human achondroplasia, and previously reported abnormalities in the type II collagen gene in this disorder have

not held up to further scrutiny.[109,133] Likewise the suggested abnormality in type II collagen in diastrophic dysplasia[561] may be due to an artifact in the segment long spacing collagen preparations.[412] Well-documented type II collagen defects have now been demonstrated in achondrogenesis type II (Langer-Saldino), hypochondrogenesis, the SEDs, Kniest dysplasia, some cases of Stickler syndrome, and precocious familial osteoarthropathy, suggesting that these disorders all represent a family of dysplasias caused by different mutations along the type II collagen gene.*

The rhizomelic form of chondrodysplasia punctata has been shown to be the result of a peroxisomal defect, as is Zellweger syndrome, another disorder associated with epiphyseal stippling.[220,459] In other forms of chondrodysplasia punctata, however, peroxisomal metabolism has been found to be normal.

There are now numerous clues to possible biochemical defects in several of the other skeletal dysplasias. The rapid increase in the knowledge of the basic biology and technology of collagen and proteoglycan chemistry should pave the way for an exciting era in the detection of the basic defect in many of the skeletal dysplasias. However, biochemical studies must take into account the known and potential heterogeneity in this group of disorders, if a single and consistent defect is to be found in any one disorder. Furthermore, the biochemist should take advantage of the numerous pathogenetic clues suggested by the morphologic studies in deciding which disorders might be due to defects in collagen or proteoglycan chemistry or to other defects in chondrocyte metabolism. The multiple defects in type I collagen found in osteogenesis imperfecta and in type II collagen in the SEDs and achondrogenesis type II support Spranger's concept of families of bone dysplasias that have defects in a common metabolic pathway.[544,545] Thus phenotypic variability may reflect intramolecular as well as intermolecular heterogeneity.

ANIMAL MODELS OF THE HUMAN SKELETAL DYSPLASIAS

A large number of mouse mutants with skeletal dysplasias or dysostoses have been described over the years. The mouse mutants can be classified in

---

*References 3, 70, 294, 341, 413, 414, 436, 591, and 612.

a format similar to that used for the International Nomenclature for Constitutional Diseases of Bone.[474] Most of these rodent models are inherited as autosomal recessive traits. The cartilage matrix deficiency mutant (Cmd/Cmd)[289] and brachymorphic mutants (Bm/Bm)[432,500] have been found to have defects in proteoglycan metabolism. The mouse osteopetrotic mutants have also been extensively studied, and observations in the mouse[622] led to the success of bone marrow transplantation in human osteopetrosis (precocious recessive variety).[126]

Disproportionate forms of dwarfism, which may represent models of the human chondrodysplasias, have been reported in numerous species, such as the mouse, rat, rabbit, dog, cat, ox, sheep, goat, chicken, and quail.[172,179,373,470,492] The classification of these disproportionate forms of dwarfism, however, has been most confusing, The difficulty in the classification of animal forms of skeletal dysplasia has been due to two major deficiencies in our past understanding of the human skeletal dysplasias. First, lack of recognition of the heterogeneity among the human chondrodysplasias led to the use of the term "achondroplasia" for a variety of dwarfed animals with differing pathogenetic mechanisms and modes of inheritance. Second, because of the previous misconception that human achondroplasia was associated with disorganized ossification, only those dwarfed animals that had disorganized endochondral ossification were considered analogous to human achondroplasts. Various breeds of dwarfed dogs, such as basset, pekinese, and bulldog, which possess well-organized endochondral growth zones, were subsequently named "chondrodystrophoid" rather than chondrodystrophic.[195] Thus in attempting to find animal models for the human chondrodysplasias, attention should be paid to matching the human disease to the animal model not only in terms of gross skeletal abnormalities but also in their modes of inheritance, extra skeletal anomalies, histopathologic appearance of cartilage, and biochemical defects.

The dwarfed breeds of dogs such as the bulldog and basset, which inherit their dwarfism as a dominant trait and have normal endochondral ossification, may thus be models of human achondroplasia. In contrast, a recessive form of dwarfism in the poodle and the deerhound, which had been named "achondroplasia," differs quite markedly from human achondroplasia in terms of

mode of inheritance, skeletal radiographs, and endochondral histopathologic appearance.[8,54,145] This condition actually bears a great deal of similarity to human pseudoachondroplasia, with anterior beaking of the vertebrae, epiphyseal and metaphyseal abnormalities, and enlarged chondrocytes containing inclusion bodies.[470] Thus this form of "achondroplasia" in the poodle and deerhound may prove to be a model for the study of human pseudoachondroplasia.

A recessive mutant of the rabbit, which results in disproportionate short stature, has also been called "achondroplasia."[509] These animals die in the neonatal period and on histopathogic study have disordered endochondral appearance, and they have been postulated to represent a model of human thanatophoric dwarfism rather than achondroplasia. We have been able to examine histopathologic tissue sections from these animals and have determined that the cartilage does not resemble that seen in human thanatophoric dwarfism. Mackler, Bargman, and Shepard[359] have described a defect in oxidative phosphorylation in the liver of the "achondroplastic" rabbit and have postulated that a similar defect in chondrocytes would account for their skeletal deformity. Similar abnormalities in oxidative phosphorylation should, therefore, be sought in the recessively inherited human chondrodysplasias. Abnormal endochondral ossification has also been described in Ancon sheep,[71] Creeper fowl,[322] and a variety of mouse mutants.[179,474]

It is thus apparent that there are a large number of animal forms of skeletal dysplasia, many of which may prove to be valuable models of the human chondrodysplasias or may contribute greatly to our understanding of chondroosseous development, or both. The classification and nomenclature of these animal models must be completely revised, however, since there are frequently no clinical or pathologic similarities between an animal mutant and the human disorder bearing the same name. Before an animal mutant can be said to be a model of a particular human skeletal dysplasia, a tight correlation should be found in terms of the clinical disease, extra skeletal abnormalities, mode of inheritance, radiographic skeletal abnormalities, histologic and ultrastructural appearance of cartilage, and, eventually, the basic biochemical defect. Not until such a tight correlation is found can the animal mutant be considered a true model of a specific human disorder.

On the basis of rigorous criteria, only a few of the mouse mutations have been established as analogous to human conditions. These are hypophosphatemia *(Hyo)* with X-linked hypophosphatemic rickets,[104] mottled *(Mo)* with Menkes syndrome,[461] bare patches *(Bpa)* with X-linked chondrodysplasia punctata,[198] and cleidocranial dysplasia *(Ccd)* with the human condition of the same name.[528] The use of transgenic mice and homologous recombination by means of human COL2A1 mutations and others will lead to the production of true animal models of the human skeletal dysplasias, which should be extremely valuable in delineating the pathogenesis of these disorders.[604]

DESCRIPTION OF INDIVIDUAL SKELETAL DYSPLASIAS

In the following account the skeletal dysplasias are discussed in groups according to the Fourth International Nomenclature.[560] This classification attempts to place syndromes that appear to have similar clinical and radiographic features and potentially common pathogenetic mechanisms into groups or families of disorders. Because of space limitations, some disorders in the nomenclature are excluded, especially those that do not appear to be primary heritable disorders of connective tissue, and only a limited number of references are included. For a more complete reference list the reader is referred to McKusick's *Mendelian Inheritance in Man (MIM)*; the specific MIM number for each syndrome is listed in the nomenclature (Appendix C).

Defects of Tubular (and Flat) Bones and Axial Skeleton

Achondroplasia Group

The disorders in the achondroplasia group have similar radiographic changes that appear to be due to a reduced rate of endochondral ossification. They range from severe neonatally lethal thanatophoric dysplasia through achondroplasia to mild hypochondroplasia. Although their basic defects are unknown, they are probably all secondary to allelic mutations of the same gene.

Thanatophoric dysplasia. Thanatophoric dysplasia, taking its name from the Greek word for "death bearing," was delineated and named by Maroteaux, Lamy, and Robert in 1967.[375] A number of cases previously reported as achondroplasia can be recognized as examples of thanatophoric dysplasia. This is the most common of the neonatally lethal skeletal dysplasias. Thanatophoric dysplasia has been subclassified into two categories based on the presence or absence of a "cloverleaf" skull *(kleeblattschadel)*. The skull deformity is usually associated with straight rather than curved femurs.[334] However, Horton, Harris, and Collins[233] reported monozygotic twins with thanatophoric dysplasia who were discordant for the *kleeblattschadel* anomaly; thus it may not be possible to really divide thanatophoric dysplasia into two distinct types based on the presence or absence of "clover-leaf" skull.

Clinical manifestations include marked short-limb dwarfism, curvature of the limbs, a large head, and nearly normal length of the trunk[331,375] (Fig. 14-4, *A*). Marked respiratory distress is present because of the severely restricted rib cage, leading to early death. Foramen magnum and spinal stenosis with compression of the spinal cord may contribute to the respiratory distress.[121] By means of constant life support, survival to over 4 years of age has occurred in the odd case.[357,595] Associated malformations of the brain, including megalocephaly, highly characteristic temporal lobe manifestations, abnormal cells with polymicrogyria, and neuronal heterotopia have been described.[89,512,291] There is marked hypoplasia of the middle and posterior cranial fossa, depending on the degree of craniosynostosis.

On radiographic examination the trunk appears long and narrow with short ribs, wide cupped costochondral junctions, posterior rib scalloping, and small, abnormally formed scapulae[331] (Fig. 14-4, *B*). The vertebral bodies are rounded anteriorly with severe platyspondyly, apparently wide disk spaces, and diffuse interpediculate narrowing (Fig. 14-4, *C*). On anteroposterior view, the thoracolumbar vertebrae have the appearance of an inverted letter "U" or the letter "H." The iliac bones are characteristically short and small with horizontal acetabular roofs, small sacroiliac notches, and medial and lateral spikes. The tubular bones of the hands and feet are extremely short and broad, with metaphyseal cupping. In those cases without *kleeblattschadel*, the calvarium appears large with frontal bossing and the base of the skull is extremely narrow with a depressed nasal bridge. The cases without "clover-leaf" skull have short and bowed long bones and characteristic femora

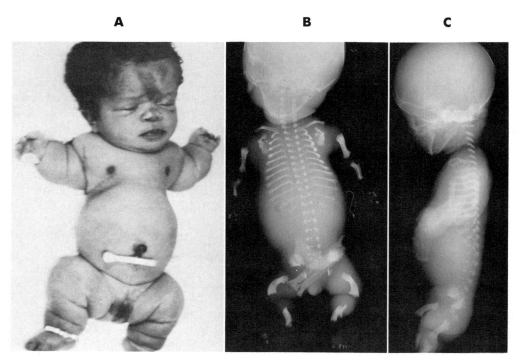

Fig. 14-4. Thanatophoric dysplasia. **A,** A newborn with prominent forehead, depressed nasal bridge, midline hemangioma, and small face with bulging eyes. The chest is small and the abdomen, protuberant. A low thoracic gibbus and short limbs with striking skin folds and limitation of elbow extension are evident. The infant died 36 hours after birth. **B,** Anteroposterior view of stillborn with thanatophoric dysplasia without *kleeblattschadel*, demonstrating "handlebar" clavicles, short anteriorly and posteriorly cupped ribs, U and H configurations of spine, abnormally conformed scapulae, trident acetabulum, decreased height and flaring of iliac wings, and micromelia with "French telephone receiver"–shaped femurs. **C,** Lateral view of thanatophoric dysplasia without "clover-leaf" skull, showing flat, anteriorly rounded vertebrae, relatively enlarged skull, and micromelia.

associated with hyperlucency of the proximal metaphyseal area (telephone-receiver–shaped). In addition, all the metaphyses are irregular and flared. In cases with "clover-leaf" skull the femora tend to be straight rather than curved but still have the characteristic fade-out of the proximal femoral neck (Fig. 14-4, *D* to *F*).

The chondroosseous morphologic appearance is characteristic, with an irregular growth plate and few proliferative and hypertrophic cells.[241,433] There are small areas with a few hypertrophic cells forming fairly normal-appearing primary trabeculi, but in most of the growth plate the hypertrophic zone is replaced by fibrous-appearing mesenchymal tissue, leading to abnormal bone formation. These "fibrous bands" are particularly prominent at the periphery of the growth plate. They are more severe and occupy more of the growth plate area in cases of thanatophoric dysplasia with "clover-leaf" skull.

Polyhydramnios is frequent in pregnancies associated with thanatophoric fetuses. Prenatal diagnosis can be made easily in the second trimester of pregnancy by means of the ultrasonographic findings of short limbs and platyspondyly.[311]

Although a number of papers have described familial aggregation of thanatophoric dysplasia with multiple affected sibs, these cases turn out not to be true thanatophoric dysplasia but rather to be cases of achondrogenesis and Schneckenbecken dysplasia.[73,168,200,470,487] The only possible exceptions are sibs with thanatophoric dysplasia

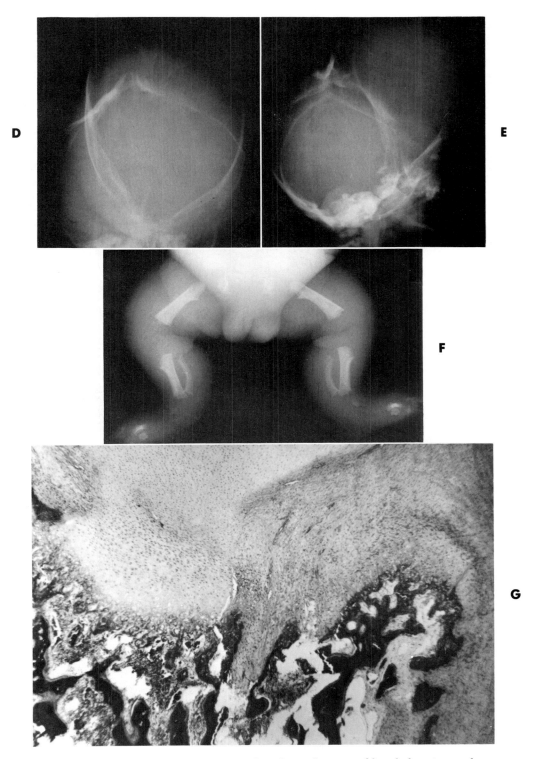

Fig. 14-4, cont'd. D, Anteroposterior and, **E,** lateral views of head showing a clover-leaf–shaped skull. **F,** Anteroposterior view of the pelvis showing the straight femora with short necks and proximal, faded out, rounded metaphyses. **G,** Micrograph of distal femoral cartilage from neonate with thanatophoric dysplasia (Goldner's stain, magnification × 55). The short, irregular columns on the left of the growth plate and the "fibrous" mesenchymal-like band on the right, which surrounds the abnormal bone formation (*black*), can be seen.

associated with *kleeblattschadel* described by Partington et al.[438] and a sib pair described by Bouvet, Maroteaux, and Feingold.[51] (Only one of these sibs, however, was carefully examined.) Concordant identical twins have been described on several occasions.[653] Several studies have examined parental age in thanatophoric dysplasia and, at least in the large study in Spain by Martinez-Frias, Ramos-Arroyo, and Salvador,[386] paternal age was definitely increased. Thus the finding of increased parental age and the large number of

cases with infrequent recurrence that have been described would suggest that thanatophoric dysplasia represents a new autosomal dominant mutation and that parents of an affected child can be reassured that the risk for recurrence is quite low.

Achondroplasia. Achondroplasia is the prototype chondrodysplasia or, at least, the prototype of short-limb dwarfism and of those forms evident at birth. Achondroplasia can be definitively diagnosed in the neonate because of characteristic

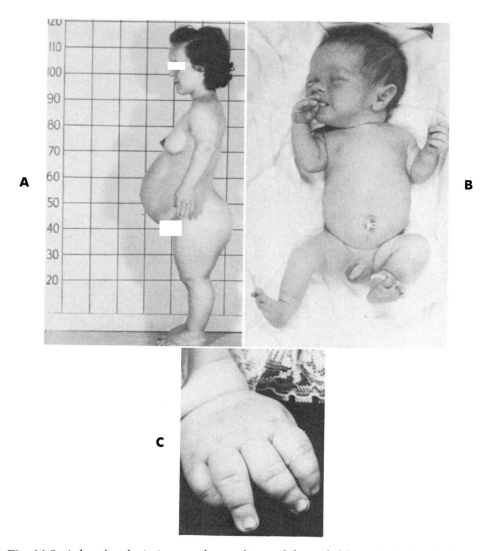

Fig. 14-5. Achondroplasia in a mother and two of three children. **A,** Mother is shown during third pregnancy. Unlike the patients affected by pseudoachondroplastic dysplasia, the bridge of the nose is "scooped out" and the forehead is bulging. **B,** Newborn achondroplastic son. **C,** Trident appearance of hands in the 3-year-old daughter. The fingers, when apposed, do not touch over their entire length.

findings on clinical and radiographic examination[330,331,373,424] (Figs. 14-5 to 14-7). In infancy these patients have a large head with depressed nasal bridge, short limbs with excessive redundant skin folds ("Michelin man" appearance), short trident hands, and a thoracolumbar gibbus. Standard growth curves for achondroplasia have been prepared and are available in chart form.[236] They are based on measurements performed on

several hundred individuals with achondroplasia and chart the variance in cumulative height, growth velocity, upper-segment to lower-segment ratio (US/LS), and head circumference in achondroplastic children from infancy to adulthood.

Infants with achondroplasia are usually hypotonic and have difficulty supporting their heads because of both the hypotonia and the large, heavy head. Milestones in motor development are

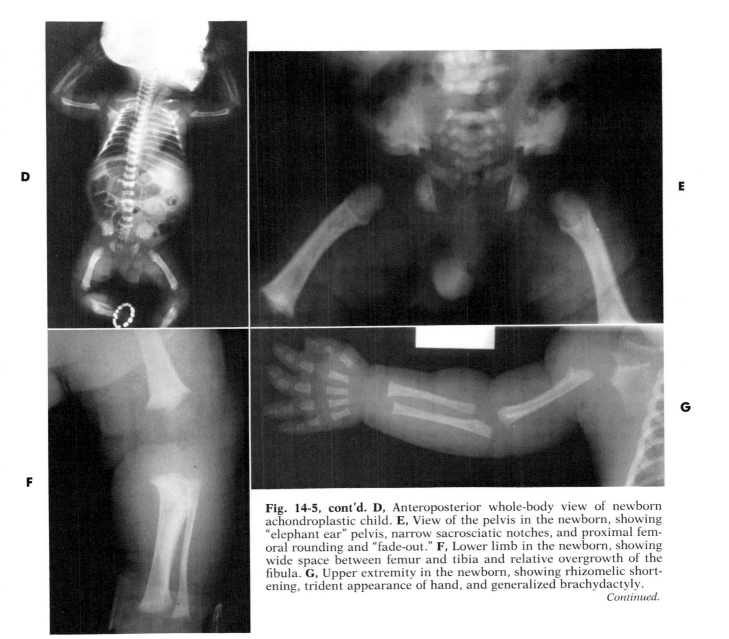

Fig. 14-5, cont'd. D, Anteroposterior whole-body view of newborn achondroplastic child. **E,** View of the pelvis in the newborn, showing "elephant ear" pelvis, narrow sacrosciatic notches, and proximal femoral rounding and "fade-out." **F,** Lower limb in the newborn, showing wide space between femur and tibia and relative overgrowth of the fibula. **G,** Upper extremity in the newborn, showing rhizomelic shortening, trident appearance of hand, and generalized brachydactyly.

Continued.

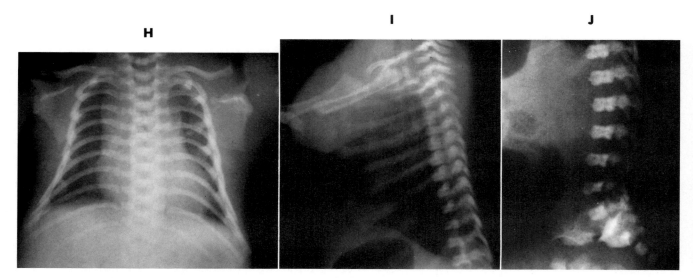

Fig. 14-5, cont'd. H, Anteroposterior and, **I,** lateral views of newborn chest showing short ribs with anterior splaying and narrowed thorax. **J,** Lateral views of lumbar spine showing mild platyspondyly with anterior rounding of the vertebrae.

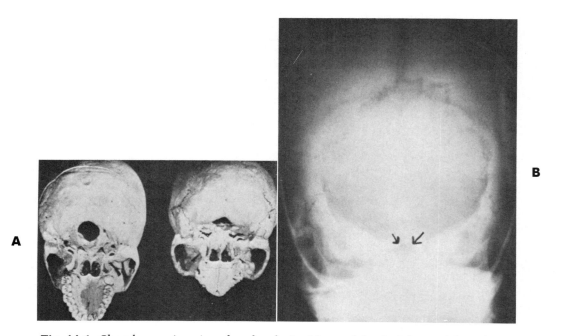

Fig. 14-6. Chondrocranium in achondroplasia. Many of the facial, cranial, and neurologic features of achondroplasia are the result of involvement of the chondrocranium but not of the calvaria, which is membrane bone. **A,** A comparison of the base of the skull in a 1-year-old child with achondroplasia, showing small, misshapen foramen magnum. **B,** Radiograph of skull showing flattened foramen magnum *(arrows).* (From Stockard CR: *The physical basis of personality,* New York, 1931, WW Norton.)

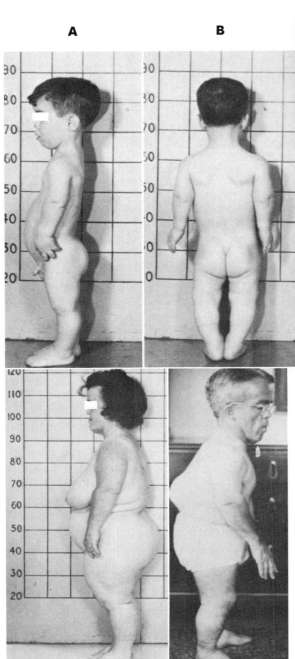

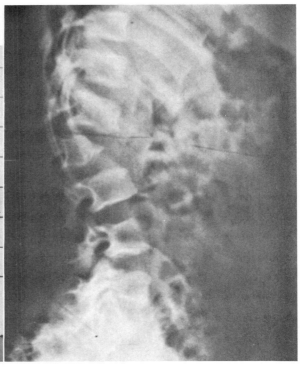

Fig. 14-7. Lumbar gibbus in achondroplasia. **A** to **C,** Child, shown at 4½ years of age, was first noted to have lumbar gibbus at 3 months of age. Because of steady increase in the upper lumbar kyphos, a fusion operation was performed at 6 years of age. **A,** Side and, **B,** rear views showing thoracolumbar kyphosis, genu varum, and other features of achondroplasia. **C,** Lateral radiographic view of lumbar spine showing marked scalloping of the posterior margin of the vertebral bodies, wedging of the L2 vertebra, and subluxation. **D,** This woman at 46 years of age had typical features of achondroplasia. An unusually severe thoracolumbar kyphosis extended from T11 to L3 and formed almost a right angle. Spontaneous anterior fusion had developed between the vertebral bodies from T12 to L3. Neurologic examination was completely normal. She has successfully completed two pregnancies, giving birth each time to an infant with achondroplasia. **E,** At 47 years of age this man is 100 cm tall. He works as a statistical clerk and is asymptomatic except for aching legs at night. As indicated, he has a severe lumbar gibbus.

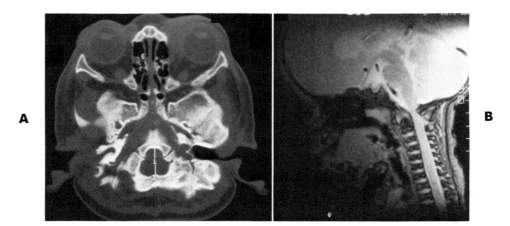

Fig. 14-8. Achondroplasia in a 6-month-old infant. **A,** Computed tomographic scan through the foramen magnum demonstrates a decrease in both the anteroposterior and the lateral dimension, exaggerated in its anterior portion. **B,** Magnetic resonance imaging at the same age; sagittal cut through the brain stem and upper cord region, demonstrating encroachment and bony pinching of the medullary cervical cord interface region, primarily from the posterior aspect.

usually delayed, although there is marked variability in degree of muscle tone and development. Standard charts for developmental milestones in infants with achondroplasia have been published.[190] The large head has been claimed to be due both to true megencephaly and to hydrocephalus. The increased fluid accumulation in the brain is thought to be due to narrowing of all of the foramina leaving the base of the skull, including the foramen magnum and the venous channels.[95,206,454] (Figs. 14-6 and 14-8). Infants may have respiratory difficulties with sleep apnea, which appears to be secondary both to central (cervical medullary compression due to the narrow foramen magnum) and to peripheral (choanal stenosis, small nasopharynx, small trachea, and small chest) causes.[423,442] Sudden infant death syndrome has been described at an increased frequency. This appears to occur at a later age than usual (after 6 months of age), and it may occur with the infant in the upright position, when the heavy head suddenly slumps over and severe cervical medullary compression of the cord is found. Craniocervical decompression can relieve the cord compression resulting from foramen magnum stenosis and reduce or abolish neurologic and respiratory complaints.[252] The indications for this surgery, however, are controversial. Surgical decompression of the jugular foramina has been shown

to relieve symptoms by reducing cerebrospinal fluid formation and outflow resistance.[355] The majority of infants with achondroplasia, however, gain normal muscle tone by 1 to 2 years of age and quickly catch up on all motor development milestones. Magnetic resonance imaging (MRI) of the skull in infants with achondroplasia demonstrates enlarged ventricles, increased fluid in the subarachnoid space, especially in the frontal areas, and compression of the emerging cord at the level of the foramen magnum (Fig. 14-8). With time, the size of the foramen magnum outgrows the cord and the posterior notching of the cord disappears. It is our opinion that the foramen magnum compression is the proximate cause of the hypotonia. Standards for foramen magnum size in achondroplasia have been published based on computed tomographic views of the base of the skull.[207,209]

In infancy and childhood, otitis media is a common complication that leads to an increased incidence of conductive hearing loss in the child and adult.[154] Abnormalities in the shape and size of the middle-ear ossicles are present in achondroplastic dwarfism, but the degree of foreshortening of the auditory canals does not appear to correlate with the severity of hearing loss.[81,518] The degree of hearing loss appears to be more directly correlated with the frequency and severity of otitis media in childhood. Careful attention to prophylaxis against middle-ear infections is important, and adenoidectomies and tympanic membrane tube installation are frequently required.

The shortness of the limbs is predominately rhizomelic ("root of limb") as opposed to mesomelic (i.e., the shortening is especially striking in the humerus and femur) (Fig. 14-5). During early childhood marked genu varum is frequently present. Loose-jointedness is usually striking in the knees of the child with achondroplasia and contributes to the bowed legs. A valgus deformity of the knees may be present in young children, which later converts to a varus deformity. The fibula is relatively long compared with the tibia, especially proximally, and also contributes to the knee deformity. It appears that the bowing in later childhood is secondary to fibular overgrowth; this bone is attached at both ends to the shorter tibia, and this causes the fibula to bow outward (similar to the frame of the bow of an archer's bow and arrow). Ponseti[457] suggested that proximal fibular epiphysiodesis or removal of the proximal end of the fibula in midchildhood would allow the tibia to catch up in length with the fibula, with subsequent reduction in the degree of genu varum. The bowed legs may result in abnormal angulation of the ankle mortice, which frequently leads to difficulties in ambulation later in life. Osteotomies of the tibia and removal of a section of the fibula are frequently necessary to correct the leg deformities. In recent years bilateral extended limb lengthening has been used to increase the length of the legs and the arms in individuals with achondroplasia. This procedure has achieved a great deal of success in some centers.[254,424,609] Achondroplasts are the ideal candidates for this surgery because of the ligamentous laxity, excess soft tissues, and dwarfism, which is entirely secondary to shortened limbs. Correction of the varus deformity can also be accomplished during the extended limb-lengthening procedure.

Incomplete extension and limitation in pronation and supination at the elbows are the rule in achondroplasia. As pointed out by Pierre Marie and by other early writers, the hand is usually trident: a wedge-shaped gap between the third and fourth fingers creates this appearance, the three prongs of the trident being fingers 4 and 5, fingers 2 and 3, and the thumb. The fingers usually cannot be placed in parallel apposition because of the large proximal segments.

The child and adult with achondroplasia have a characteristic facies and general appearance. Because of the defective development of the chondrocranium, the nose is "scooped out" and the maxilla is hypoplastic. The calvarium is bulging, and the mandible is relatively prognathic. After infancy the thoracolumbar gibbus usually gives way to lumbar lordosis (Fig. 14-7). The exaggerated lumbar lordosis results in a pelvic tilt such that the sacrum lies almost horizontal and the buttocks are prominent. The gait is ducklike. In approximately 10% of individuals with achondroplasia the lumbar gibbus persists and is associated with a wedged-shaped vertebra in the thoracolumbar junctional region. If progressive thoracolumbar gibbus occurs after the age of weight bearing, vertebral fusion may have to be performed to prevent severe deformity. In late adolescence and adulthood, spinal stenosis can become a major problem. Because of the decreased size of the spinal canal and the increased lordosis, little space is available surrounding the cord and cauda equina.[521] Symptoms of claudication of the cord with pain and paresthesias in the lower limbs frequently develop in individuals with achondroplasia.[110,269,498,613] These symptoms are induced by walking progressively shorter distances and are relieved by assuming a squatting position. Symptoms of cervical cord compression can also be found with paresthesias and weakness in the upper limbs. When objective signs occur, wide laminectomies are necessary to prevent permanent paresis.[463,578] Great care must be given in manipulating the vertebral canal in these individuals because of the severe diminution of the subarachnoid space.

We have found MRI to be an excellent tool in evaluating these individuals. Frequently, however, myelograms are necessary to pinpoint the exact site of the block proximally. Because of the risk of posterior fossa herniation, it has been recommended that all myelograms should be performed by means of cysternal puncture in persons with achondroplasia. The degree of lumbar lordosis can contribute to the frequency of spinal stenosis, since it has been shown that the achondroplastic spinal canal loses approximately 30% of its volume when placed in the lordotic position.[521] Correction of the lumbar lordosis in the Vilarrubias type of extended leg lengthening may well decrease the frequency and severity of the symptoms of cord or nerve root compression in these individuals.[609] Occasionally symptoms of spinal stenosis develop acutely with mild to moderate disk protrusion in a narrowed spinal canal.

Obesity is a common problem in achondroplasia and, when present, aggravates the morbidity associated with lumbar stenosis and contributes to nonspecific joint problems and possible early cardiovascular mortality.[209,435] The cause of the obesity is unknown but is probably associated with markedly decreased height and decreased physical activity associated with normal-sized internal organs and normal appetite.

Radiographic manifestations of achondroplasia include a large skull with relatively small base, small foramen magnum, upward tilt of the petrous pyramid, low position of the mastoid process, small posterior face resulting from craniosynostosis at the base of the skull, and small angle at the base of the skull (85 to 120 degrees compared with the normal angle of 110 to 125 degrees). Computed tomography (CT) scans reveal megalencephaly, dilation of the lateral ventricles, and at times, cochlear rotation. The size of the foramen magnum is markedly reduced both in transverse and in sagittal dimension[207,209] (Fig. 14-8, *A*). The vertebral bodies are short, flat, and bullet shaped in early life. They demonstrate a lack of the normal increase in interpediculate distance from the upper lumbar vertebrae caudally.[534] They have short pedicles, resulting in a narrow spinal canal. The pelvis has a "champagne glass" appearance with squared-off iliac wings resembling elephant ears, short, narrow sciatic notches, and flat acetabular roofs. The limbs are short with short, thick tubular bones, notched growth plates (V-shaped), circumflex-like insertions of the epiphyses into the metaphyses, flared metaphyses, and a characteristic proximal lucency of the femoral necks in infancy. The phalanges and metacarpals are short. Fibular overgrowth is present, especially proximally. The sternum appears to be thick and stubby, and the ribs are short with deep concave ends.

Chondroosseous morphologic study reveals regular, well-organized endochondral ossification in many growth plates, but in the centers of certain primarily weight-bearing joints there can be focal disruption of the growth plate[56,478,564] (Fig. 14-9). The columns are short and the septa can be somewhat wide. These changes suggest a quantitative decrease in the rate of endochondral ossification.

The prevalence of achondroplasia is uncertain; previous estimates are undoubtedly incorrect because of misdiagnosis. Using modern diagnostic criteria, Gardner[146] estimated a mutation rate of 0.000014 (1.4 per 100,000 gametes per generation). Orioli, Castilla, and Barbosa-Neto[431] reported on

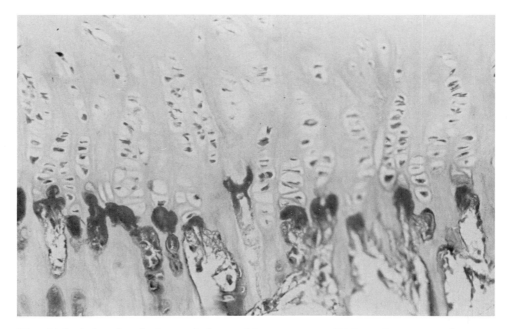

Fig. 14-9. Achondroplasia, pathology of heterozygote. Light microscopy of costochondral junction showing regular column formation (Mission trichome).

the frequency of skeletal dysplasias among 349,470 births (live and stillbirths). The prevalence rate for achondroplasia was between 0.5 and 1.5 per 10,000 births. The mutation rate was estimated to be between 1.72 and 5.57 × 10⁻⁵ per gamete per generation. The stated range is a consequence of the uncertainty of diagnosis in some cases. In Denmark, Anderson and Hauge[10] determined the prevalence of generalized bone dysplasias by means of a study of all children born in a county during a 14-year period. The figures showed that achondroplasia was less common than generally thought (1.3 per 100,000), as opposed to the frequency of thanatophoric dysplasia (3.8 per 100,000). Stoll et al.[573] found a mutation rate of 3.3 × 10⁻⁵ per gamete per generation.

Achondroplasia is inherited as an autosomal dominant trait with essentially complete penetrance. Although it had previously been said that there is little variability in achondroplasia, there appears to be marked variability, with the coefficient of variance of height being as great as that in the general population.[473] About 80% of the cases of achondroplasia are a result of new mutations, there being a considerable reduction in effective reproductive fitness.[406] Paternal-age effect on mu-

tation rate has been noted.[411,445] A few cases of achondroplasia have been described in sibs who are the offspring of normal parents; in several instances cousins have been described.* Gonadal mosaicism may be the explanation for such families. Numerous cases of homozygous achondroplasia in offspring of two achondroplastic parents have been described.[187,154] These infants have severe dwarfism and marked changes in the cranium resulting in early death (Fig. 14-10). The histologic appearance seems to be similar to that seen in thanatophoric dysplasia, with short columns of cells and fibrous ingrowth.[562] These infants die of early respiratory embarrassment resulting from the neurologic deficit[206] and a small thoracic cage. Yang[647] reported upper cervical myopathy in such a homozygote. Prenatal diagnosis of homozygous achondroplasia can be achieved by finding decreased femoral lengths by 18 weeks of gestation. Prenatal diagnosis of heterozygous achondroplasia, however, is not possible in the second trimester, since femur length is within normal limits and does not drop off until 24 weeks of gestation.[188,311]

---

*References 52, 99, 428, 430, 452, and 617.

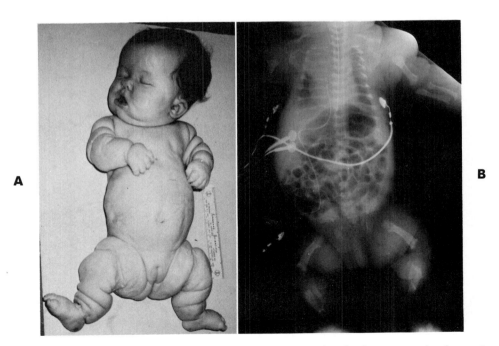

Fig. 14-10. Infant with homozygous achondroplasia who died at 1 month of age. **A,** Postmortem photograph showing severe changes of achondroplasia. **B,** Anteroposterior full-trunk and extremity radiograph shows a remarkable similarity to the radiographic appearance of thanatophoric dysplasia without *kleeblattschadel* (see Fig. 14-4, **B**).

As of 1991, the basic defect in achondroplasia was unknown. Strom[579] and Eng et al.[109] reported finding abnormalities of the type II collagen gene in achondroplasia. The report by Eng, Pauli, and Strom[109] was later withdrawn because "the figures which were generated in the laboratory of Strom and Eng were improperly assembled and therefore could not be used to support the conclusions of the article." Normal cartilage biochemistry has since been found in achondroplastic cartilage, and linkage analysis has excluded COL2A1 as the site of the mutation.[133,425] Although there appears to be an increased number of cases of achondroplasia associated with neurofibromatosis, suggesting potential linkage between these two loci, Pulst et al.[462] demonstrated that the achondroplasia locus does not map close to the neurofibromatosis gene on human chromosome 17.

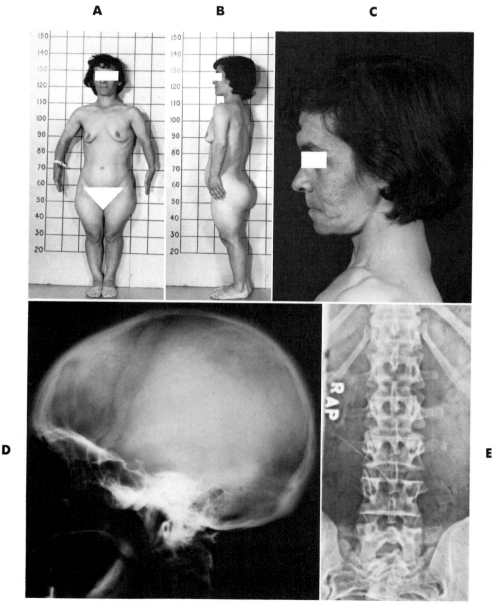

Fig. 14-11. Hypochondroplasia in a mother and son. **A,** Frontal and, **B,** lateral views of the mother at the age of 34 years. **C,** Normal profile in the mother. **D,** The skull shows minimal shortening of the base. **E,** Lower spine in the mother showing narrow interpediculate distance and low articulation of the sacrum on the iliac bones.

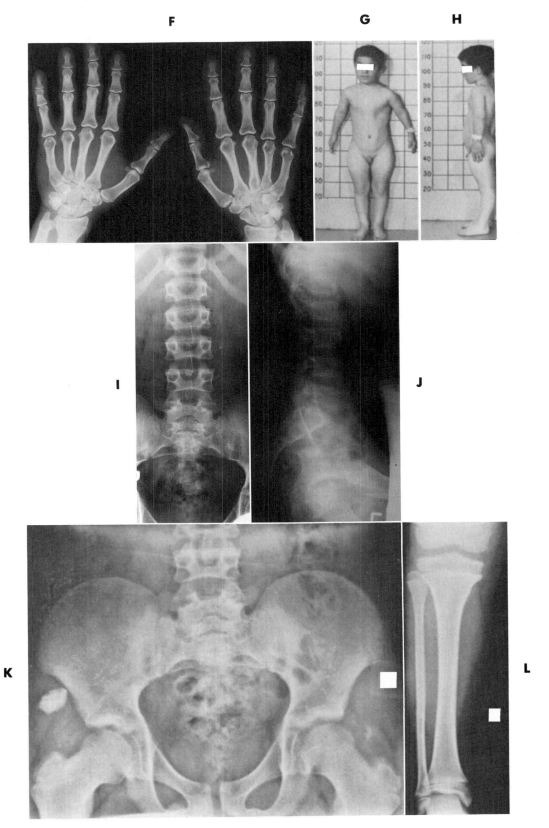

Fig. 14-11, cont'd. F, The mother's hands, showing bones that are short but not as strikingly short as hands in persons with achondroplasia. **G,** Frontal and, **H,** lateral views of the 11-year-old son. The Harrison grooves are evident. **I,** Frontal and, **J,** lateral views of the spine in the son, showing caudad narrowing of the spinal canal in both dimensions and increased space between the vertebral bodies. **K,** Pelvis in the son, demonstrating the lack of the usual signs of achondroplasia. The calcified mass on the left is at an injection site. **L,** Bones of the leg, showing relatively long fibula.

Hypochondroplasia. Hypochondroplasia resembles achondroplasia, but all the features are much milder.[25,618,182] Birth weight and length may be within the lower limit of normal, and short stature is usually not recognized until 2 to 3 years of age. The head and face are almost normal, although there may be mild frontal bossing. Mild short-limb dwarfism is present, with heights ranging into the low normal range. The body build is broad and muscular. The hands are broad and stubby, as are the feet, but the trident appearance of the hands is not as apparent as in achondroplasia.

Radiographic features of hypochondroplasia are similar to but milder than those of achondroplasia. (Fig. 14-11). The skull is fairly normal except for some frontal bossing and midface hypoplasia. There can be slight shortening of the base of the skull and mild narrowing of the foramen magnum, but these seldom cause any clinical abnormalities. There is either no change or a decrease in the interpediculate distance from the first through the fifth lumbar vertebrae, as well as some posterior scalloping and mild platyspondyly. The iliac bones are short with a flat acetabular roof, small sacrosciatic notches, and small posteriorly tilted sacrum. Mild lumbar lordosis may be present. The long bones are short with wide-appearing diaphyses, mild flaring of the metaphyseal epiphyseal junctions, slight shortening of the ulna relative to the radius, elongation of the ulna styloid, elongation of the proximal fibula, shortened broad femoral neck, and rectangular proximal tibial epiphysis. Mild to moderate brachydactyly is present, with a characteristic pattern profile. All these radiographic changes are variable and may be almost normal in mildly affected individuals, except for the lack of interpediculate caudal flaring. Chondroosseous morphologic appearance in hypochondroplasia appears to be relatively normal with, perhaps, somewhat shortened columns of cells and some thickening of the matrix between columns.[470]

Numerous cases fall somewhere in the spectrum between the clinical and radiographic appearances of achondroplasia and hypochondroplasia. However, these disorders appear to breed true within families. It is quite likely that achondroplasia and hypochondroplasia are allelic disorders. As in achondroplasia, hypochondroplasia is inherited as an autosomal dominant trait. There has been a suggestion that mild mental retardation may be associated with hypochondroplasia, but the majority of individuals with hypochondroplasia have normal intelligence.[618] Evidence for allelism between hypochondroplasia and achondroplasia was claimed because of a family in which a severely affected offspring appeared to have inherited the achondroplasia gene from the father and the hypochondroplasia gene from the mother.[392,539] Although such a severe phenotype could occur as a result of a genetic compound (compound heterozygous state), it could also be the result of the combined manifestations of two nonallelic disorders.

Achondrogenesis Group

The term "achondrogenesis" has been used for a variety of distinct chondrodysplasias over the years, ranging from severe neonatally lethal dwarfism, which has now been found to be quite heterogeneous, and a severe nonlethal disorder of the limbs described by Grebe.[170] This latter disorder bears no relationship to the neonatal lethal forms and is now referred to as "Grebe dysplasia" and classified within the acromelic and acromesomelic dysplasias. The lethal forms of achondrogenesis had long been considered to consist of two well-defined chondrodysplasias (achondrogenesis type I, Parenti-Fraccaro and achondrogenesis type II, Langer-Saldino[132,437,645]). Achondrogenesis type II (Langer-Saldino) is now known to represent the severe end of the spondyloepiphyseal dysplasia (SED) family of disorders and is associated with defects in the type II collagen gene. It is therefore discussed with the SED congenita group. Achondrogenesis type I has been referred to as the Parenti-Fraccaro type. However, Borochowitz et al.[50] pointed out that this term had been used to designate cases with wide clinical variability, and they were able to delineate two distinct forms of achondrogenesis type I: type IA (the Houston-Harris form) and type IB (the Fraccaro type). Indeed, their reanalysis of Parenti's case[437] suggested the diagnosis of achondrogenesis type II.

Achondrogenesis type IA (Houston-Harris). Achondrogenesis type IA was first described in two cases by Harris, Patton, and Barson[201] and Houston, Gerrard, and Ives.[243] Borochowitz et al.[50] were able to define seven cases of their own and culled others from the literature. Both consanguinity and multiple affected sibs have been described, suggesting autosomal recessive inheritance. Polyhydramnios is common, and most individuals with achondrogenesis type IA are born prematurely. This syndrome can be readily detected early in the second trimester of pregnancy by means of ultrasonographic measurement of the limbs.[157] More than 50% of the affected infants are stillborn and the remainder die within minutes after delivery. Birth length is extremely small, ranging from 22 to 30 cm. There is an abnormal male-to-female ratio of 15 to 7. These infants have severe short-limb dwarfism with short trunk, disproportionately large cranium, and small thorax. Fetal hydrops is common. Various other congenital anomalies have been reported, including cardiac and renal abnormalities.

On radiographic examination the major feature distinguishing type IA from type IB is the presence of short, cupped flared ribs with multiple healing fractures[50] (Fig. 14-12, *A*). The skull is poorly ossified, and no vertebral ossification is present. The iliac bone is hypoplastic and inferiorly positioned.

The femur has a wedgelike configuration with spike formation on the proximal metaphyseal end. The tibia, fibula, radius, and ulna are always ossified, although quite short. Metaphyseal changes are present in both proximal and distal ends of the long bones. The pubis, talus, and calcaneus are not ossified. In older fetuses the ischium may be ossified.

Chondroosseous morphologic appearance is distinctive in this disorder and quite different from that seen in type IB and type II. The cartilaginous matrix is normal except for hypervascularity.[50] The resting zone is hypercellular. Chondrocytes lie in large lacuni with a round, centrally located nucleus (bull's-eye appearance). Unusual cytoplasmic inclusion bodies are present in chondrocytes. The growth plate lacks regular chondrocytic columns. The bone is hypercellular, and woven, calcified cartilage persists into the metaphysis. At the periphery of the section there is sometimes abnormal fibrous mesenchymal-like tissue forming ab-

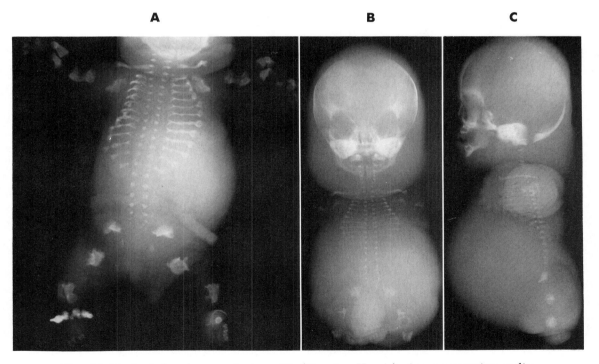

Fig. 14-12. A, Achondrogenesis type IA (Houston-Harris). Anteroposterior radiograph of trunk and extremities showing short, beaded ribs with anterior and posterior cupping; pediculate but not vertebral-body ossification; arched iliac wings; and stellate femurs with micromelic long bones. **B,** Achondrogenesis type IB (Fraccaro). **B,** Anteroposterior and, **C,** lateral full-body radiographs of fetus at 33 weeks of gestation, revealing short, thin ribs without fractures, no vertebral body ossification, hypoplastic iliac wings with cupped acetabulae, extremely short femurs with distal metaphyseal widening and cupping, and generalized micromelia.

normal hypercellular bone. On ultrastructural examination chondrocytes contain dilated cisterns of rough endoplasmic reticulum containing amorphic material.

Achondrogenesis type IB (Fraccaro). The achondrogenesis type IB form of severe micromelic dwarfism cannot be distinguished on clinical examination from type IA.[50,132] Polyhydramnios is present in the majority of pregnancies, as is premature delivery. Affected infants either are stillborn or die within minutes of birth. Birth length is severely reduced, whereas head circumference is normal for gestational age, resulting in the appearance of short-limb, short-trunk dwarfism with a disproportionately large cranium. Hydrops is common, and cleft palate has been described.

On radiographic examination these patients have a poorly ossified skull and lack of ossification of the vertebral bodies (Fig. 14-12, *B*). Some punctate posterior pedicles can be seen in many cases. The ribs are short with cupped and flared ends, but there are no fractures. The ilia are hypoplastic with some medial spikes. In contrast to type IA, the ischium in type IB is not ossified at any gestational age. The femurs are short, with a trapezoid configuration, and the tibiae and humeri are stellate. The fibula, pubis, talus, and calcaneus are not ossified.

Chondroosseous morphologic appearance is distinctive in type IB. The interterritorial cartilaginous matrix is markedly devoid of collagen fibrils.[50] A dense ring, which stains intensely with silver methenamine, surrounds the chondrocytes and appears to consist of collagen fibrils. The growth plate lacks chondrocytic columns and proliferating and hypertrophic cells. Instead, there is a fibrous mesenchymal band between cartilage and bone. Woven bone appears to arise directly from this fibrous area, resulting in trabeculi with wide osteoid lines. Lumbar vertebral bodies are unossified, although adjacent pedicles manifest exuberant woven bone formation. Ultrastructural examination reveals cartilaginous matrix that is sparse except for fibrils of collagen surrounding the chondrocytes in a ringlike manner.

Type IB has been documented in multiple sibs, and probable consanguinity has been described in one instance; these findings are suggestive of autosomal recessive inheritance. In achondrogenesis type IB, there appears to be an excess of females, as opposed to the excess of males in IA.

Spondylodysplastic Group (Perinatally Lethal)

The spondylodysplastic group of disorders consists of a number of entities that are characterized by perinatal lethality and severe platyspondyly. They differ from achondrogenesis in having vertebral bodies that are ossified, although quite small. They have been referred to as "lethal platyspondylic dwarfism" or "thanatophoric variants." Two types were defined by Horton et al.[238] and were given the names of the "Torrance" (Fig 14-13, *A* and *B*) and "San Diego" (Fig. 14-13, *C* to *E*) types, after the cities in which the individuals with these disorders were born. A third type was described from Great Britain and termed "Luton" type, following the same convention.[635] It is not clear whether these forms represent clinical variability or genetic heterogeneity. We have observed a number of forms of severe short-limbed platyspondylic dwarfism that do not fit exactly into any of the previously defined categories.

On clinical examination all types are characterized by perinatal lethality, large head, short neck, coarse facies, tiny chest, protruding abdomen, and very short arms and legs. On radiographic study these persons have decreased ossification of the cranial base; short, thin ribs; waferlike platyspondyly; hypoplastic ilia, ischia, and pubic bones; wide sacrosciatic notches; flat acetabular roofs; and short, relatively straight long bones, which are frequently widened, with metaphyseal cupping or rounding.

The three well-defined types differ in their chondroosseous morphologic appearance.[238] The Torrance type has hypercellular resting cartilage with large chondrocytes.[270] The growth plate is normal. In the San Diego type the resting cartilage appears normal with larger round chondrocytes and normal column formation. In the Luton type the resting cartilage is hypercellular, with normal to large cells, normal column formation, focal degenerating chondrocyte incorporation, and focal disorganization.[635] All cases to date have been sporadic.

Opsismodysplasia. The term "opsismodysplasia" was coined by Maroteaux et al.[383] for what they considered to be a new chondrodysplasia recognized at birth on the basis of short stature, short hands, and facial abnormalities with short nose and depressed nasal bridge. The short limbs are primarily rhizomelic, and there is a narrow thorax. Hypotonia is common, and undue susceptibil-

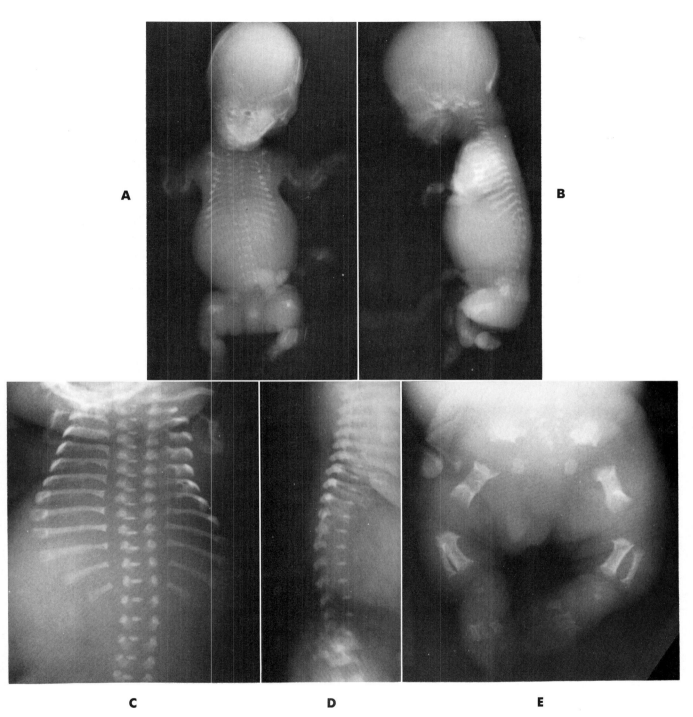

Fig. 14-13. Spondylodysplastic perinatal lethal (SDPL) group, (thanatophoric variant). **A,** Anteroposterior and, **B,** lateral radiographs of San Diego type. The wafer-thin platyspondyly, short ribs, micromelia, and bent long bones are evident. **C,** SDPL group, Torrance type. **C,** Anteroposterior and, **D,** lateral views of the spine. **E,** Anteroposterior view of the pelvis and lower extremities, revealing dense, wafer-thin vertebral bodies; short ribs with anterior and posterior cupping; flat, cupped acetabulum, hypoplastic ischium and pubis; and short, wide long bones with cupped metaphyses.

ity to respiratory infections is present. Subluxation of the first cervical vertebra (C1) on the second cervical vertebra (C2) can result in severe neurologic sequelae. Affected children die within the first few years of life, but opsismodysplasia is not lethal in the neonatal period. The condition appears to be a severe disorder of endochondral ossification.

On radiographic examination this disorder is characterized by a severe generalized delay in endochondral ossification.[657] There is absent to marked hypoplasia of vertebral body ossification with severe platyspondyly. The long bones are short and stocky, with exaggerated metaphyseal cupping and markedly delayed epiphyseal ossification. The unossified epiphyseal cartilagenous anlage is normally shaped but appears to be enlarged. The short tubular bones are short with cupping at both ends. The iliac bones are squared with horizontal acetabular roofs and medial and lateral spurs, and the ischium and pubis are hypoplastic. A large ossification defect is present at the base of the skull. The term "opsismodysplasia" was suggested by Maroteaux et al.[383] from the Greek for "delayed maturation." Chondroosseous morphologic study reveals a large and widened hypertrophic area and wide connective tissue septa surrounding the hypertrophic cells. Maroteaux et al.[383] reported that type I collagen was present in the hypertrophic zone. The description of two affected sibs with first-cousin parents suggests autosomal recessive inheritance.

Metatropic Dysplasia Group

Fibrochondrogenesis. Fibrochondrogenesis is a neonatally lethal short-limb skeletal dysplasia associated with normal head size, frontal bossing, wide sutures, flat base of the nose, small palpebral fissures, and short neck[114,340,629] (Fig. 14-14). The thorax is narrow and bell shaped, and the abdomen protuberant. The lower limbs are short and bowed, but the hands and feet are of relatively normal size. Omphalocele, cleft palate, microstomia, and small, abnormal ear pinnae have been seen in a few cases. On radiographic study the skull is undermineralized. The clavicles are long and thin with short cupped ribs and small scapulae. There is platyspondyly with posterior vertebral body hypoplasia, giving the vertebral bodies a pinched appearance. The pelvic bones are hypo-

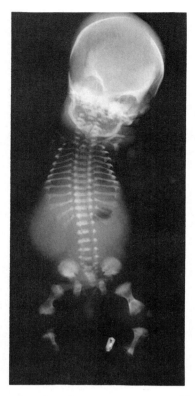

Fig. 14-14. Fibrochondrogenesis in a stillborn infant. Anteroposterior whole-body radiograph showing normal skull, "handlebar" clavicles, short, anteriorly cupped ribs, round iliac wings with narrow sacrosciatic notches, large vertical ischia, short "dumbbell" femurs with extraneous ossification (left patella?), and generalized micromelia.

plastic with squared iliac wings and a trident (three-pronged) acetabular roof. The long bones are short and dumbbell shaped with flared metaphyses. The fibulae are short, and in some cases paraosseous ectopic ossification has been present around the long bones.

The characteristic histologic feature of this condition, from whence it derives its name, is a fibrous matrix surrounding spindle-shaped chondrocytes in hyaline cartilage. Although the chondrocytes appear fibroblastic, the collagen present in this cartilage has been demonstrated to be type II. Multiple affected sibs, twins, and consanguinity have been reported in families with this disorder, suggesting autosomal recessive inheritance.[21]

Schneckenbecken dysplasia. Schneckenbecken dysplasia is a neonatally lethal skeletal dysplasia

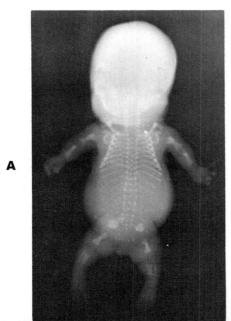

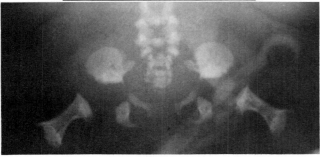

Fig. 14-15. Schneckenbecken dysplasia. Radiographs of **A,** the whole body of a fetus at 19 weeks of gestation and, **B,** the pelvis of a sibling, revealing micromelia, moderately shortened ribs, hypoplastic flat vertebrae, snail-shaped pelvis (ilia), and short splayed femurs.

associated with a hypoplastic iliac bone with a medial projection resembling a snail (hence the term *Schneckenbecken* from the German, for "snail pelvis")[49] (Fig. 14-15). Polyhydramnios is often present, and affected infants die within the newborn period. They have a large head, short neck, flat midface, and generalized edema. On radiographic examination the long bones are extremely short and dumbbell shaped with metaphyseal irregularity. The fibula is wide. The vertebral bodies are rounded with only anterior vertebral body ossification and normal posterior elements. The ribs are short and splayed, the clavicles are handlebar

shaped, and the scapulae are hypoplastic. The ilium is characteristic, with a medial projection resembling the shape of a snail's head. The acetabular roofs are flat, the sacrum is narrow, and the ischium is precociously ossified. There is brachydactyly with precociously ossified carpal and tarsal bones. Prenatal diagnosis by means of ultrasound has been accomplished in a fetus of 18 weeks' gestation.

Chondroosseous morphologic study reveals hypervascularity of the hyaline cartilage, normal-sized chondrocytes with central nuclei, little lacunar space, and hypercellularity. Knowles, Winter, and Rimoin[292] reported a first-cousin marriage that resulted in 13 pregnancies: four of the offspring were normal and five were stillborn, short-limbed dwarfs; of the latter, three were miscarried and one was terminated because of prenatally detected dwarfism. This family had been previously reported as a case of achondrogenesis.[339] The multiple affected sibs reported by Chemke, Graff and Lancet[73] and Graff, Chemke, and Lancet[168] as having thanatophoric dysplasia appear to have had Schneckenbecken dysplasia. The presence of consanguinity and multiple affected sibs suggests autosomal recessive inheritance.

Metatropic dysplasia. Metatropic dysplasia was often mislabeled "Morquio disease" in the past because of the short-trunk dwarfism. Maroteaux, Spranger, and Wiedemann[377] pointed out the characteristic features of this syndrome and gave it the name "metatropic (changing)," which refers to the change in body proportions with age. At birth a long, narrow torso with relatively short limbs suggests achondroplasia. Later, rapidly progressing scoliosis results in short-trunk dwarfism, suggesting the Morquio syndrome (Fig. 14-16, *A* and *B*). Some patients have a double fold of skin over the sacrum, which resembles a tail.

At birth the length is actually normal or even excessive, with a long, narrow torso and a cylindric thorax. Severe progressive scoliosis or kyphoscoliosis develops in early childhood. There is limitation of extension of some joints such as the hips and knees and progressive joint enlargement. Odontoid hypoplasia and C1-2 vertebral subluxation with early infant death is a major problem in this syndrome.[514] Hydrocephalus has also been reported.

In the neonatal period radiographic manifesta-

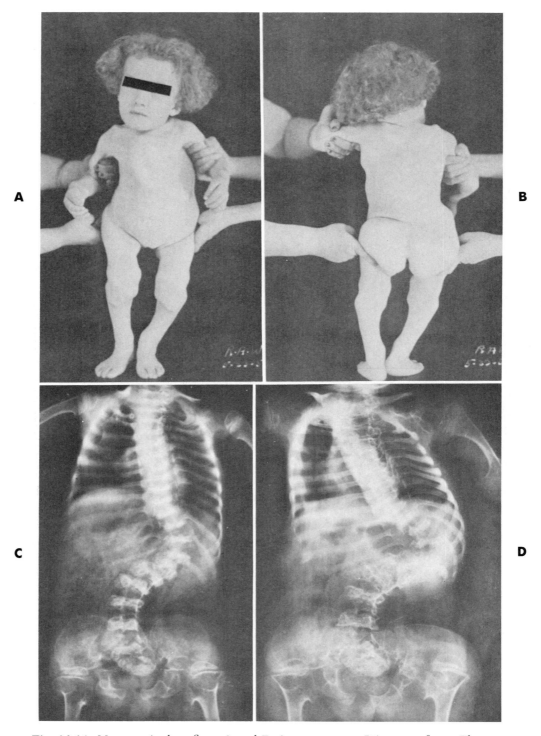

Fig. 14-16. Metatropic dwarfism. **A** and **B**, Appearance at 5½ years of age. The protuberance below the knees corresponds to the tibial heads shown in **H** and **I. C,** Frontal view of the spine at 2½ years of age. **D**, Frontal view of the spine at 5½ years of age.

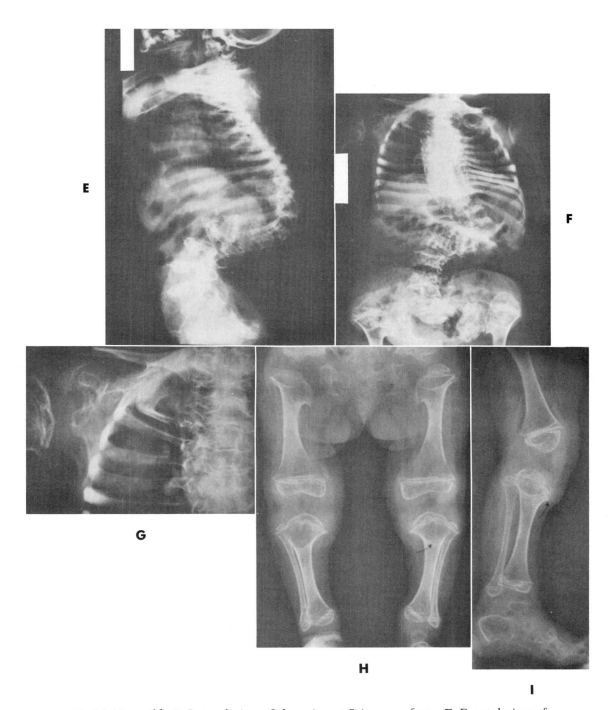

Fig 14-16 cont'd. E, Lateral view of the spine at 5½ years of age. **F,** Frontal view of the spine at 10½ years of age. **G,** Shoulder at 10½ years of age. The medial end of the clavicle is broad, whereas the lateral portion is unusually narrow. **H,** Frontal and, **I,** lateral views of lower limbs at 2½ years of age. The metaphyses are flared, especially at the knees. The arrows indicate a beak on the anterior surface of the proximal tibia.   *Continued.*

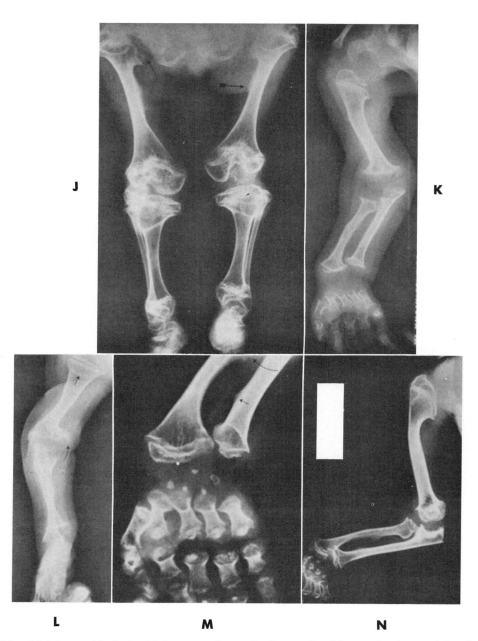

Fig. 14-16, cont'd. J, At 10½ years of age. Radiograph of legs. The femoral heads and necks are just beginning to ossify (*upper arrow*). Hyperostoses project medially from the diaphysis of each femur (*lower arrow*). **K** and **L,** Right upper limb at the age of 2½ years. The metaphyses flare markedly. At the distal humerus the flaring is so marked that an exostosis is simulated. **M,** Wrist and hand at 7½ years of age. The hand bones are square. Carpal ossification is markedly delayed. Well-formed hyperostoses project into the interosseous space from both the radius and the ulna (*arrows*). **N,** Upper limb at 10½ years of age.

tions consist of dumbbell-shaped femurs and humeri, a halberd (battle-ax) proximal femoral shape, generalized shortening of all tubular bones including the hands and feet, dense, waferlike vertebral bodies, elongated clavicles, short ribs with anterior and posterior flaring, increased distance between the posterior end of the ribs and the spine, short squared scapulae, short squared iliac wings, flat acetabular roofs, and narrow sacrosciatic notches. In childhood and adult life there are trumpetlike metaphyses of the long bones, marked epiphyseal delay, elongated fibulae, dumbbell-shaped tubular bones in the hands and feet, delayed carpal ossification, unusual sharply etched carpal and tarsal bones, increasingly severe kyphoscoliosis, hypoplastic odontoid with C1-2 vertebral dislocation on flexion, hydrocephalus, and anterior wedged vertebrae (Figs. 14-16, *C* to *N*).

Chondroosseous morphologic studies have been limited but show an absence of normal primary spongiosa, a thin seal of bone at the chondroosseous junction, and arrest of endochondral growth, suggesting uncoupling of endochondral and perichondrial growth.[46,470] Beck et al.[28] proposed that the following types of metatropic dwarfism exist: (1) a nonlethal autosomal recessive form, (2) a nonlethal dominant form, and (3) a lethal form resulting in death before or shortly after birth, possibly autosomal recessive. In the past, metatropic dysplasia had been confused with the Morquio syndrome, Kniest dysplasia, and certain forms of SED.

Short-Rib Dysplasia Group (With or Without Polydactyly)

The International Nomenclature lists four distinct types of short-rib polydactyly (SRP) syndrome (types I to IV), as well as asphyxiating thoracic dysplasia and the Ellis-van Creveld dysplasia. We think that all these disorders may represent intragenic (i.e., allelic) heterogeneity and phenotypic variability, since we have observed cases that phenotypically fall between each of these groups, creating a spectrum of disorders.

Short-Rib polydactyly syndrome type I (Saldino-Noonan type). Short-rib polydactyly syndrome type I results in death within the perinatal period.[489,557] There has been a predominance of females with this disorder. The infants are hydropic at birth with dolichocephaly, natal teeth, and mi-

crognathia.[580] They have an extremely short, narrow thorax and a protuberant abdomen. There is marked micromelia with flipperlike extremities and postaxial, and occasionally, preaxial polydactyly. In addition, the hands are small with severe brachydactyly. Renal and genital anomalies are common, and sex reversal has been described. Cardiovascular anomalies and gastrointestinal anomalies, including imperforate anus, are frequent. Hypoplastic lungs have been noted.

On radiographic examination there is dolichocephaly with poor mineralization of the frontal bones and mandibular hypoplasia (Fig. 14-17, *A* and *B*). The ribs are short and horizontally oriented. The scapulae are small, and the clavicles are superiorly located. The vertebral bodies are misshapen and squared, with coronal clefts. The iliac bones are small, and the acetabular roof flattened and trident in shape, resembling those seen in the Ellis-van Creveld syndrome and asphyxiating thoracic dysplasia (small ilia with osseous spurs projecting medially and laterally from the acetabular roofs). The tubular bones are extremely short and misshapen with ragged ends, particularly distally, and metaphyseal spurs are present. The femurs are pointed on both ends. The fibulae may be absent, and there is deficiency of ossification of the metacarpals, metatarsals, and phalanges. Early prenatal diagnosis can be readily accomplished by means of ultrasonography.[174]

On morphologic study there is absence of the zone of proliferation and loss of columnization with irregularly dispersed hypertrophic cells, separated by areas of fibrous tissue.[176,531] Fibrous overgrowth is frequently present peripherally. These changes resemble those seen in thanatophoric dysplasia. The costochondral junction is malformed and prematurely sealed with a horizontal strip of bone. Ultrastructural analysis has revealed increased calcospherite size, as opposed to the normal calcospherites in SRP type II.[175,176]

Multiple affected sibs and consanguinity have been reported. Mild cases of SRP type I merge with severe cases of SRP type III (Verma-Naumoff), and features of both type I and type III have been seen in the same patient; they may well represent one entity with significant phenotypic variability.[526,531] Erzen et al.[112] studied the histopathologic appearance of growth cartilage in one case of SRP I and found it relatively normal as compared with what they observed in three cases

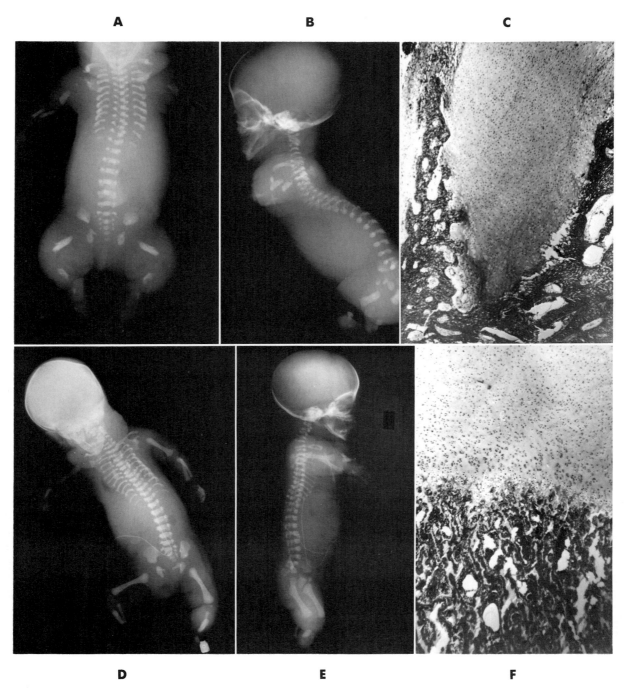

Fig. 14-17. Short-rib polydactyly dysplasias. **A** to **C,** Type I (Saldino-Noonan). **A,** Anteroposterior and, **B,** lateral full-body radiographs showing mild vertebral abnormalities, extremely short ribs, micromelia with pointed femoral bone ends, and absent fibulae. **C,** Histopathologic appearance of costochondral junction (Goldner stain, magnification × 80). The sealed growth plate with overgrowth of dysplastic bone (*dark staining*) around the cartilage (*light staining*) can be seen. **D** to **F,** Type II (Majewski). **D,** Anteroposterior and, **E,** lateral full-body radiographs revealing extremely short ribs flared anteriorly, well-formed femurs with rounded ends, and small ovoid tibias. **F,** Histopathologic appearance of costochondral junction (toluidine blue, magnification × 60). The short growth plate with few hypertrophic cells is evident.

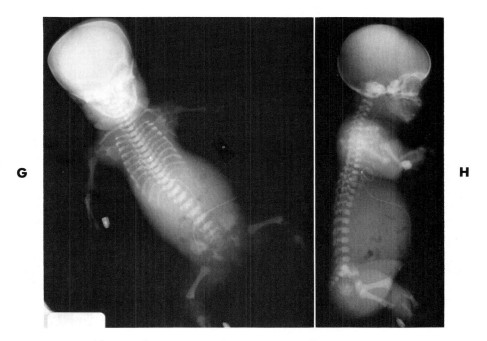

Fig. 14-17, cont'd. G and **H,** Type III (Verma-Naumoff). **G,** Anteroposterior and, **H,** lateral full-body radiographs revealing short ribs, "handlebar" clavicles, relatively normal spine, and characteristic spurs at the distal femoral metaphyses.

of SRP III; they suggested that SRP type I and type III were distinct entities. However, we have observed typical SRP type III growth-plate changes in numerous cases of SRP type I and think that types I and III represent variability rather than heterogeneity.

Short-rib polydactyly syndrome type II (Majewski type). Short-rib polydactyly syndrome type II is a perinatally lethal disorder associated with a hydropic appearance at birth, prominent forehead, and low-set, malformed ears.[84,364,557] A lobulated tongue, tight frenulum, micrognathia, midline cleft lip and palate, and short, flat nose may be present, resembling those seen in orofaciodigital syndrome type II (Mohr syndrome).[525] The thorax is extremely short and narrow with a protuberant abdomen. There is marked micromelia, particularly distally, preaxial or postaxial polydactyly or both, brachydactyly, and hypoplasia or aplasia of the nails. The larynx has been reported to be malformed, with hypoplastic epiglottis. Pulmonary hypoplasia, glomerular and renal tubular cysts, ambiguous genitalia, pachygyria, and small cerebellar vermis have also been reported.[75]

On radiographic examination the mandible is underdeveloped (Fig. 14-17, *D* and *E*). The ribs are extremely short and horizontal. The long bones are short, with rounded metaphyseal ends. The middle segments are particularly affected, especially the tibias, which are extremely short, with an ovoid configuration. Precocious ossification of the proximal femoral epiphyses is often present, as well as a decreased space between the distal femoral epiphyses and metaphyses. Polydactyly is present with distal phalangeal hypoplasia. The pelvis seems to be more normal appearing than that seen in the other forms of SRP.

Chondroosseous morphologic study shows a short growth plate with decreased proliferating and hyperplastic cells.[75] (Fig. 14-17, *F*). Calcospherite size is normal, in contrast to SRP I.[175,176]

Multiple affected sibs and consanguinity are indicative of autosomal recessive inheritance.[84] The presence of central cleft lip and palate and ovoid configuration of the tibias has led to the suggestion that orofaciodigital syndrome type II (Mohr syndrome) and SRP type II (Majewski type) are mild and severe expressions of the same autosomal recessive disorder.[401,525] The radiographic and morphologic features of SRP type II are identical to those seen in SRP type IV (Beemer form), the only major difference being the presence of polydactyly.[212] It is likely that SRP types II and IV represent the same disorder with and without polydactyly.

Short-rib polydactyly syndrome type III (Verma-Naumoff type). Infants with SRP type III die in the neonatal period as a result of thoracic asphyxia. The first patients were reported by Verma, Bhargava, and Agarwal[608] and Naumoff et al.,[420] who suggested that this condition is a distinct disorder. Sillence et al.[531] and Bernstein et al.[44] suggested that SRP types I and III are allelic disorders. Changes are similar to but milder than those of SRP type I, with micromelic dwarfism, polydactyly of the hands and feet, narrow thorax with hypoplastic lungs, cleft lip or palate or both, and a variety of other anomalies, including renal, genital, cardiovascular, and intestinal malformations.

On radiographic examination there is a short cranial base, bulging forehead, flat occiput, and sunken root of the nose (Fig. 14-17, *G* and *H*). The ribs are short with hypoplastic thin vertebrae and increased intervertebral disk spaces. The tubular bones are severely shortened with rounded metaphyseal ends and lateral spikes, often having a three-pronged ball within a V-groove appearance. Prenatal diagnosis can be readily accomplished by means of midgestational ultrasonography.[311]

Although Ezren et al.[112] found more normal growth plate on histopathologic study in a case of SRP type I than in SRP type III, we have found identical changes in both types. One case of SRP type III with cytoplasmic inclusion bodies in the chondrocytes has been reported.[648]

The major distinguishing features from SRP type I include a more rounded and fully ossified appearance of the long bones, normal to hypoplastic fibulae, and less severe involvement of the acetabulum. Sex reversal has been seen in both type I and type III.[44] Inheritance is autosomal recessive, as in other types of SRP.

Short-rib polydactyly syndrome type IV (Beemer type). Beemer et al.[29] reported what they considered to be a new SRP syndrome in two infants dying shortly after birth. Hydropic appearance, ascites, medium cleft of the upper lip, a narrow chest, and short bowed limbs were the primary features. The clinical, radiographic and morpho-

logic manifestations are identical to those of SRP type II (Majewski type) except for the polydactyly.[212] We consider that this situation represents clinical variability in SRP type II rather than a separate disorder.

Asphyxiating thoracic dysplasia. Asphyxiating thoracic dysplasia was originally dubbed "asphyxiating thoracic dystrophy of infancy" by Jeune et al.,[264] when they described two sibs who died of respiratory distress in early infancy. The central feature of this disorder is the thorax, which is small in both anteroposterior and lateral dimensions, appearing long and narrow (Fig. 14-18, *A*). Some patients die of respiratory distress; others seem to "outgrow" the respiratory problems and survive. The limbs are short. Postaxial polydactyly of the hands and feet can be present, but it rarely is symmetric as in the Ellis-van Creveld syndrome and the feet as well as the hands are likely to be affected (Fig. 14-18, *B*). (In Ellis-van Creveld syndrome the hands are always affected and the feet have polydactyly in 10% or less of the cases.) Dysplasia of the fingernails, a feature of Ellis-van Creveld syndrome, is not present in this disorder. Renal disease with death resulting from renal failure is a major development in survivors of the respiratory disease.[214,519] Intestinal malabsorption has been reported. The respiratory distress can be of varying degrees of severity in the neonatal period. The other reported anomalies have included situs inversus, abdominal muscle dysplasia, and reduced visual acuity with tapetoretinal degeneration, which resembles Leber congenital amaurosis.[634]

The major radiographic manifestations are a small bell-shaped thoracic cage with handle-bar–shaped clavicles and horizontally directed ribs with bulbous and irregular rib ends[329] (Fig. 14-18, *C*). The pelvis is small, with short flared iliac bones and a typical trident appearance of the acetabular margin. The proximal femoral ossification center is present at birth in about two thirds of the cases. The hands manifest cone-shaped epiphyses with premature fusion and shortened phalanges.

Chondroosseous morphologic appearance has been variable, ranging from a fairly normal growth plate to severely affected costochondral junctions with marked decrease in the physeal growth plate.[470,651] In most cases calcified cartilage rests in the trabeculae, deep in the metaphy-

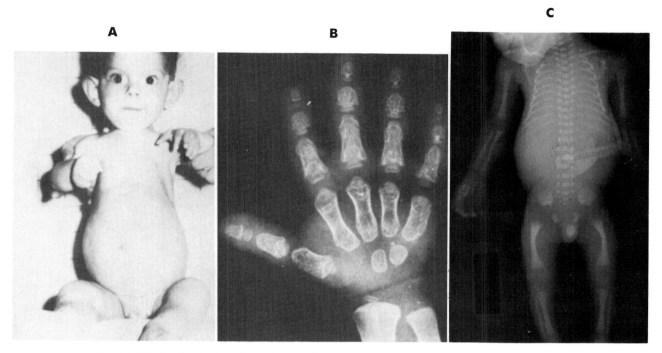

Fig. 14-18. Asphyxiating thoracic dysplasia. **A,** Appearance of a child with severe restrictive thoracic dysplasia. **B,** The hand of another child at 26 months of age. Polydactyly was not present. Otherwise, the similarity of the radiograph of the hand to that in the Ellis-van Creveld syndrome (see Fig. 14-21) is evident. **C,** Anteroposterior view of trunk and extremities showing short horizontal ribs with a bell-shaped chest; trident acetabular roof with narrow greater sacrosciatic notches; bowed, mildly shortened, normally formed femurs; and generalized mild long-bone shortening. Although the configuration of the pelvis in these cases is indistinguishable from that in the Ellis-van Creveld syndrome (see Fig. 14-22), distinction is usually possible because the proximal tibia is normally formed.

ses, have been described. Pulmonary hypoplasia has been recognized, as well as periportal fibrosis, bile duct proliferation and pancreatic fibrosis, cystic changes in the liver, pancreas, and kidney, and glomerulosclerosis.[231,325,600]

Asphyxiating thoracic dysplasia is inherited as an autosomal recessive trait. Langer[329] pointed out that radiographic differentiation of asphyxiating thoracic dysplasia and Ellis-van Creveld syndrome may not be possible in some cases. Furthermore, we have noted that on radiographic examination severe cases of asphyxiating thoracic dysplasia blend into mild forms of SRP syndrome type III, and the question of phenotypic variability or allelic mutations must be seriously considered.

Ellis-van Creveld dysplasia (chondroectodermal dysplasia). The Ellis-van Creveld syndrome is manifested by the presence of dwarfism, polydac-

tyly, dysplastic fingernails, and in about 50% of the cases, by malformations of the heart, usually a single atrium or a large ostium primum type of atrial septal defect[62,280] (Figs. 14-19 to 14-21). The condition has been described in many ethnic groups, but the greatest number of cases has been reported in a large religious isolate, the Old Order Amish of Lancaster County, Pennsylvania.[395,396] McKusick has compiled a detailed account of the condition in this population.[396]

The clinical manifestations present at birth are disproportionate, short-limb dwarfism with centrifugal shortening, postaxial polydactyly of the hands and, less commonly, of the feet, and hypoplasia and dysplasia of the nails and teeth, which may be erupted at birth (natal teeth) and which exfoliate prematurely (Figs. 14-19 to 14-21). A variety of changes are found in the mouth, where the upper lip and gum appear to be fused or attached

A   B

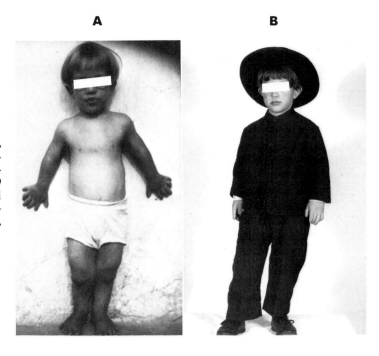

Fig. 14-19. Ellis-van Creveld syndrome. **A** and **B,** Amish boy at 5 and 9 years of age, respectively. Polydactyly, knock-knees, and short extremities are demonstrated. The extra digits had been amputated by 9 years of age. Closure of an ostium secundum atrial septal defect was performed at that age. (From McKusick, VA et al: *Trans Assoc Am Physicians* 77:154, 1964.)

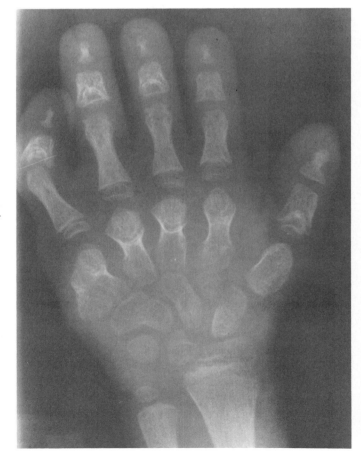

Fig. 14-20. Hand of a child with Ellis-van Creveld syndrome. The boy is shown in Fig. 14-19 at the age of 9 years. The terminal phalanges are hypoplastic. Many of the epiphyses are cone shaped and set into "wine-bottle" metaphyses. The sixth digit has been amputated. The capitate and hamate are severely deformed.

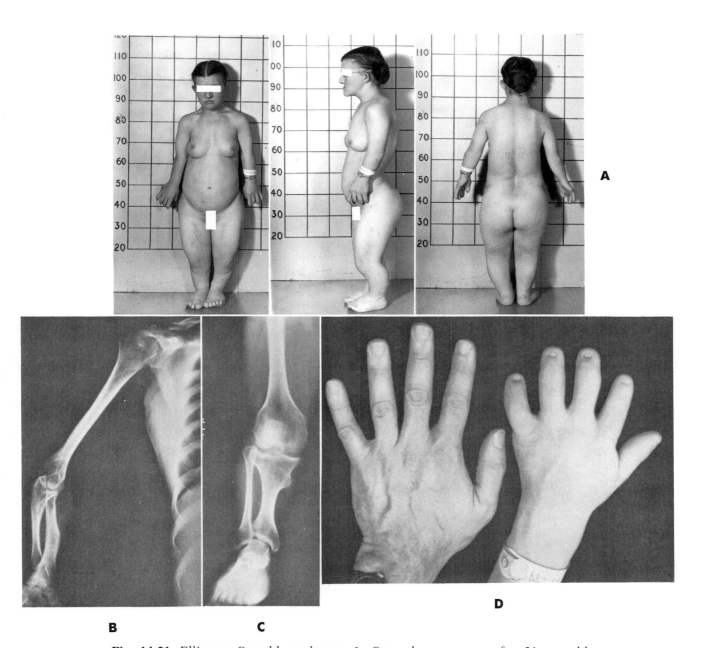

Fig. 14-21. Ellis-van Creveld syndrome. **A,** General appearance of a 21-year-old woman. The upper lip is retracted and sunken, in part due to early loss of teeth, in part due to "partial harelip." Signs of large atrial septal defect are present. The distal portion of the extremities is particularly short. **B,** Radiograph of the arm, showing shortening and malformation of the radius and ulna. **C,** Radiograph of the tibial condyles is characteristic, and the medial tibial exostosis is a common finding. **D,** The fingernails are dystrophic, and extra fingers have been amputated. Normal hand is shown for comparison.

with a short frenulum. The coexistence of the Ellis-van Creveld syndrome and the Dandy-Walker malformation has been described in several cases.[656]

The radiographic features consist of markedly shortened ribs, short and widened tubular bones, bowed femurs, premature ossification of the capital femoral epiphyses, and hypoplasia of the proximal tibial ossification center (Fig. 14-21, *B* and *C*, and Figs. 14-20, 14-22, and 14-23). The slope of the tibial metaphysis is shortened medially and longer laterally, and the fibula is short, resulting in genu valgum. The trident appearance of the acetabulum is similar to that seen in asphyxiating thoracic dysplasia. Fusion of the capitate and hamate bones is a characteristic feature, along with an os centralis and other carpal fusions (Fig. 14-22). There appears to be a delay in the maturation of the carpal bones and accelerated maturation of the phalanges. Cone-shaped epiphyses of the middle phalanges can occur. The spine and the skull are usually normal. The progressive shortening of the tubular bones of the hands distally can result in the inability to make a firm fist.[395,396]

The large Amish pedigree published by McKusick et al.[395,396] clearly documents the autosomal recessive inheritance of the Ellis-van Creveld syndrome. This disorder is difficult to differentiate on radiographic examination from asphyxiating thoracic dysplasia,[329] and we have seen cases that, on radiographic and clinical examination, fit between the Ellis-van Creveld syndrome and SRP syndrome type III. This evidence suggests the possibility that all the syndromes in this group may represent allelic disorders.

Atelosteogenesis and Diastrophic Dysplasia Group

The group of disorders described in this section consists of two types of entities. The atelosteogenesis syndromes are a group of rare disorders characterized by hypoplastic humeri or femurs, or both, and absence of ossification of several bones. Diastrophic dysplasia and "pseudodiastrophic" dysplasia are also included in this group.

Atelosteogenesis dysplasias. There are several forms of atelosteogenesis, some of which are lethal in the newborn period.[380,529,571] They are characterized by hypoplasia of the femurs and humeri,

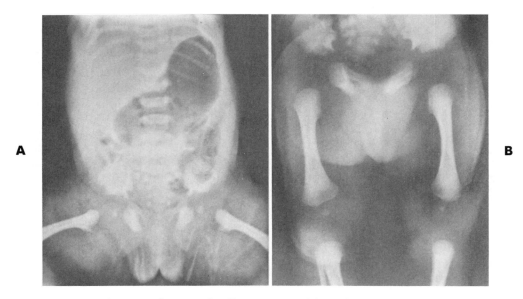

Fig. 14-22. Pelvis in infants with Ellis-van Creveld syndrome. **A,** Radiograph made on the day of birth. Unusual excrescences from the proximal femora may represent large lesser trochanters. **B,** Radiograph of the pelvis and lower limbs in another infant, 19 days old. The acetubular roof is flat and characterized by a spicule at both the medial and the lateral margin.

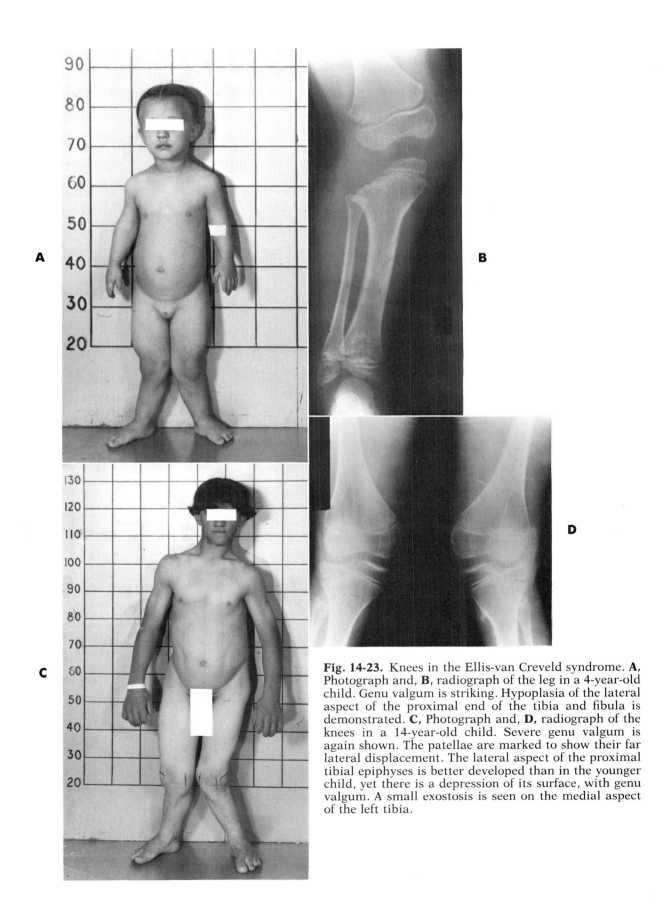

Fig. 14-23. Knees in the Ellis-van Creveld syndrome. **A,** Photograph and, **B,** radiograph of the leg in a 4-year-old child. Genu valgum is striking. Hypoplasia of the lateral aspect of the proximal end of the tibia and fibula is demonstrated. **C,** Photograph and, **D,** radiograph of the knees in a 14-year-old child. Severe genu valgum is again shown. The patellae are marked to show their far lateral displacement. The lateral aspect of the proximal tibial epiphyses is better developed than in the younger child, yet there is a depression of its surface, with genu valgum. A small exostosis is seen on the medial aspect of the left tibia.

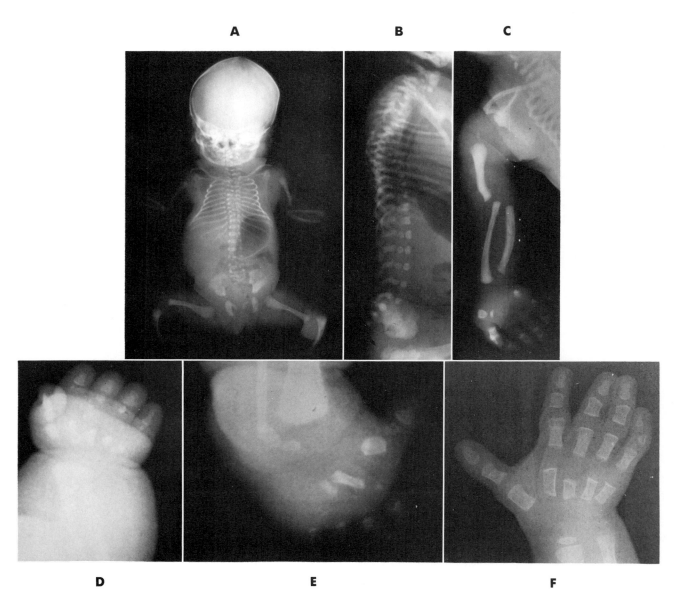

Fig. 14-24. A to C, Atelosteogenesis type I. Anteroposterior views of, **A,** the body, **B,** the lateral spine, and, **C,** the upper extremity, showing marked thoracic vertebral hypoplasia, coronal cleft vertebrae, absent fibulae, hypoplastic distally tapered humeri, and distal tuft ossification (*only*), with a hypoplastic first ray. **D** and **E,** Atelosteogenesis type II. Anteroposterior view of, **D,** the hand and, **E,** the foot, revealing large-tuft ossification, metacarpal hypoplasia, absent proximal phalanges, round middlephalangeal ossification, and a "hitchhiker" great toe. **F,** Atelosteogenesis type III. Anteroposterior radiograph of the hand in a 1-year-old infant, showing hypoplastic rectangular metacarpals, tombstone-shaped proximal phalanges, hypoplastic middle phalanges, and hypoplasia of the thumb.

particularly in their distal ends, occasionally with absence of ossification. The fibula can be unossified, and there are a variety of peculiar defects of ossification of the hands. The best characterized of these disorders is atelosteogenesis type I, which has also been called "giant cell chondrodysplasia" or "spondylo-humero-femoral hypoplasia."[382,529] This disorder is lethal in the neonatal period and is associated with a flat nasal root, midface hypoplasia, cleft palate, significant limb shortening, and deviation of the fingers.

On radiographic examination the major features are coronal and sagittal clefts of the vertebrae; platyspondyly; scoliosis; absent, short, or distally tapered humeri; shortened femur with rounded metaphyses and proximal flaring; shortened bowed radius and ulna; and shortened bowed tibia and absence of the fibula (Fig. 14-24, A to C). The hands are characteristic, with short, well-ossified distal phalanges and markedly decreased or absent ossification of the other short tubular bones. This disorder is associated with peculiar enlarged cells scattered in resting cartilage, hence the term "giant cell chondrodysplasia." This designation has not, however, gained acceptance, since giant cells of various types can be found in other disorders. Similar changes in chondroosseous tissue have been observed in patients with "boomerang dysplasia" who have atelosteogenesis-like radiographs and a boomerang-shaped

tibia.[251,302] This situation raises the question of heterogeneity versus variability.

The other disorders in this group include atelosteogenesis type II, which has fewer vertebral anomalies, short dumbbell-shaped humeri that are bifid distally, and short, dumbbell-shaped femurs[218,530] (Fig. 14-24, D and E). The fibula is hypoplastic but well formed. On histologic study the collagen in cartilage is clumped and deficient, similar to that in the diastrophic dysplasia group of disorders. A condition known as "de la Chapelle dysplasia" may be the same entity as atelosteogenesis II.[93,630]

Atelosteogenesis type III, as opposed to the other two types, is compatible with survival past infancy.[571] Segmentation defects of the cervical spine are present, and the long bones are similar to those seen in atelosteogenesis type I. The major difference occurs in the hands, where the proximal phalanges have a characteristic shape with biconvex ends (Fig. 14-24, F). In contrast to atelosteogenesis I, all the bones of the hands are ossified.

Otopalatodigital syndrome type II is an X-linked recessive disorder that resembles the atelosteogenesis syndromes in having short long bones and digital abnormalities.[55,127] The digital abnormalities in otopalatodigital syndrome type II consist of flexed overlapping fingers with syndactyly. Affected individuals have characteristic facies with large anterior fontanelles, low-set ears,

A   **B**

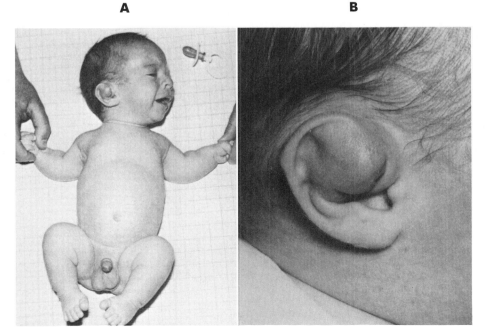

Fig. 14-25. A and **B,** Diastrophic dysplasia in an infant at the stage of acute swelling of the ear. (Courtesy Dr. Dick Hoefnagel, Hanover, N.H.)

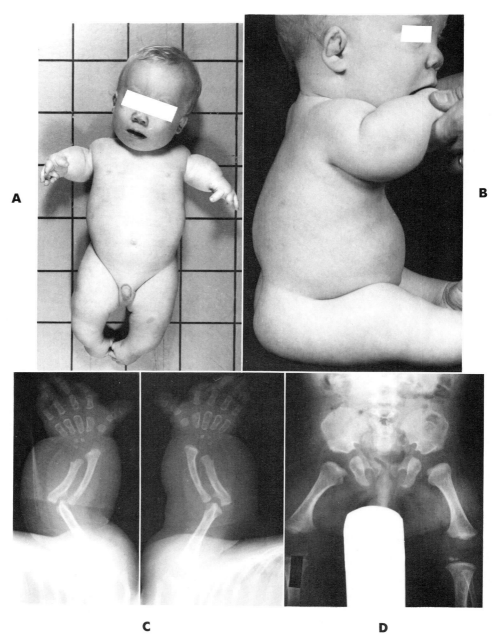

Fig. 14-26. Diastrophic dysplasia. Infant boy is shown at 6 months of age. At birth, multiple skeletal abnormalities, including cleft palate and bilateral clubfoot, were noted. At 6 months of age he was also noted to have "hitchhiker" thumbs, capillary hemangiomas of the face, kyphoscoliosis, and thick, deformed pinnae. **A,** Overall view. **B,** The deformity of the spine and ears is evident. **C,** The upper limbs at 6 months of age. All bones are short. The radii and ulnae are bowed. The proximal end of each humerus is wide and flat. The radial heads are dislocated, and the ulnae are relatively short distally. The first metacarpals are particularly short, and the thumbs are everted. Clinodactyly of the second and fourth fingers is evident. **D,** Pelvis and femora at 6 months of age. The lower spinal canal is narrow, as is the sacrum. The greater sciatic notches are short and the acetabular roofs, flat. The long bones are short and massive.

prominent forehead and hypertelorism with flat nasal bridge, micrognathia, and cleft palate.

Atelosteogenesis types I and III are sporadic disorders, whereas type II may be autosomal recessive. Otopalatodigital syndrome type II, on the other hand, is an X-linked recessive trait.

Diastrophic dysplasia. Diastrophic dwarfism derives its name from the Greek word for "bent" or "twisted"[618] (Figs. 14-25 to 14-28). ("Diastrophism" is a term used in geology to refer to the process of bending in the earth's crust, by which mountains and ocean basins are formed.) Affected persons are often diagnosed as having chondrod-

ystrophy (or achondroplasia) with clubfoot or arthrogryposis. As with so many of the skeletal dysplasias, Lamy and Maroteaux[318] delineated the entity and assigned its name.

Diastrophic dysplasia is recognizable at birth by the severe, rigid clubfoot deformity and "hitchhiker" thumb (Fig. 14-26). In about 85% of the patients the pinna of the external ear becomes acutely inflamed and swollen in the first 2 or 3 weeks of life (Fig. 14-25). Inflammation subsides, leaving the ears "cauliflowered." Later, calcification and ossification can be demonstrated[394,587] (Fig. 14-27). Precocious calcification of the tracheolaryngeal and costal cartilages is also common.

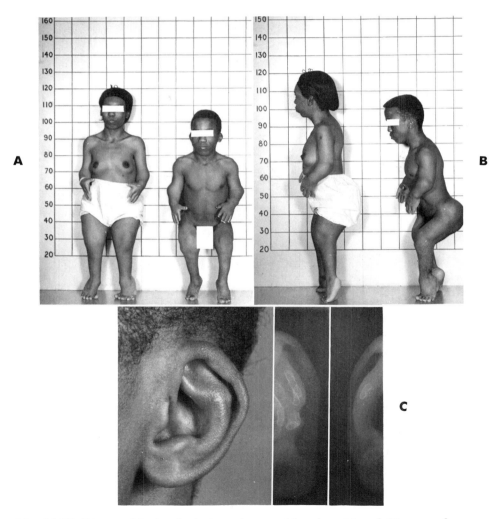

Fig. 14-27. Diastrophic dysplasia in a sister and brother, 19 and 15 years of age, respectively. Clubbed hands and feet and marked dwarfism are shown in **A** and **B.** The ears are rigid and deformed and show ossification of pinnal cartilages, **C.**

Continued.

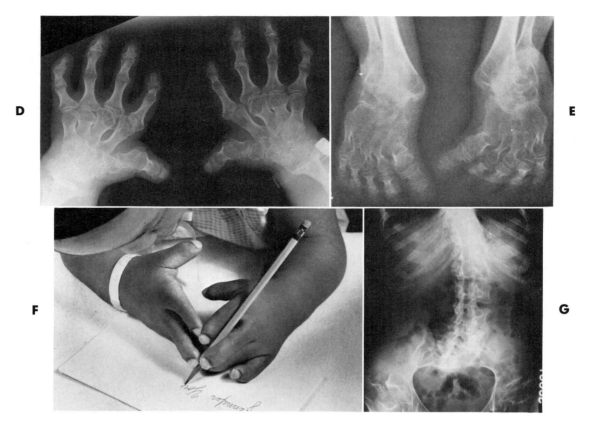

Fig. 14-27, cont'd. The severe deformity of the hands, **D,** and feet, **E,** is demonstrated. The position of the "hitchhiker" thumb is characteristic; its metacarpal is short. Ankylosis of the proximal interphalangeal joints in the second, third, and fourth fingers of both hands is also demonstrated. Because of the stiff fingers, the patient's method of writing, **F,** is awkward. **G,** Severe derangement of the hip, scoliosis, and precocious ossification of costal cartilages are shown.

Cleft palate occurs in about one fourth of the cases. In addition to the "hitchhiker" thumb, which results from an abnormality of the first metacarpal, the fingers develop symphalangism, that is, fusion of the proximal interphalangeal joints.[575] The clubfoot deformity is notoriously difficult to treat, but acceptable results have been achieved with early and persistently applied therapy. Progressive scoliosis may also develop. Neonatal death caused by collapse of the airway resulting from the abnormal tracheal, laryngeal and bronchial cartilages has been described.[139] Gustavson et al.[181] studied 14 cases of diastrophic dwarfism and suggested that there was a specific lethal variety of the disease. On the other hand, a group of patients who seemed phenotypically to have a mild form of diastrophic dwarfism were termed "diastrophic variants." A study of a large number of patients and sibships with diastrophic dysplasia suggested that the lethal severe form, typical diastrophic dysplasia, and the diastrophic variant represented phenotypic variability of the same mutation[235,317] (Fig. 14-28).

Radiologic manifestations include short, thick, clubbed tubular bones with delay in the appearance of epiphyses, fragmentation of ossifying epiphyseal centers, and epiphyseal invagination[327] (Figs. 14-26 and 14-27). In addition, the metacarpals are irregular in length and form, as are the metatarsals and phalanges. The first metacarpal is short and often oval, resulting in a proximally located "hitchhiker" thumb. Severe talipes equino-

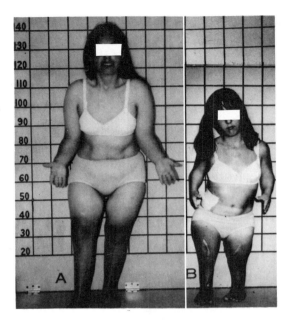

Fig. 14-28. Two girls of similar age with diastrophic dysplasia, showing the marked phenotypic variability in this disorder.

varus with metatarsal fusions is present. The carpal and tarsal bones are irregular, and there are accessory carpal centers. Carpal center development appears to be accelerated. There is hypoplasia of the acetabulum and glenoid. Scoliosis and kyphosis are progressive, and frequently hypoplasia of cervical vertebrae, narrowed interpediculate distances in the lumbar region, and cervical kyphosis are present.[306] Clefting of the posterior processes of the cervical and sacral vertebrae is a characteristic feature. Premature precocious costochondral, tracheal, and laryngeal cartilage calcification can be seen.

Chondroosseous morphologic study shows a "drop out" of chondrocytes within the matrix resulting in cystic areas that fill with fibrovascular tissue,[237,470] which results in intracartilaginous ossification. There are dense staining collagen rings around the chondrocytes. On electron microscopy numerous degenerative cells are seen with large, banded type II collagen fibrils.[237]

It has been reported that in cartilage from patients with diastrophic dysplasia there is abnormal banding of segment long spacing collagen.[561] Murray, Hollister, and Rimoin[412] have studied a number of cases and have not been able to detect this abnormality; they have provided evidence that the abnormal bands may be due to overlapping of fibers. Biochemical studies of type II collagen in this disorder have been normal.[412] The Finnish group has mapped the diastrophic dysplasia gene to 5q, whereas the COL2A1 gene is located on chromosome 12.[204] Multiple cases of affected sibs with parental consanguinity have been described, indicating autosomal recessive inheritance.

Pseudodiastrophic dysplasia. Pseudodiastrophic dysplasia was first described in two infant sisters by Burgio et al.[60] Although the condition showed some similarities to diastrophic dysplasia, specifically, rhizomelic shortening of the limbs and severe clubfoot deformity, other features were different, including proximal phalangeal joint dislocations, platyspondyly, and characteristic facies.[115] The cystic enlargement of the ear does not occur in pseudodiastrophic dysplasia, and the clubfoot deformity, unlike that in diastrophic dysplasia, responds well to physical and surgical therapy. The morphologic appearance of cartilage is also different. The autosomal recessive entity, pseudodiastrophic dysplasia, is clearly a distinct disorder, which appears to represent a primary connective tissue disease rather than a true skeletal dysplasia.[64,115]

Kniest-Stickler Dysplasia Group

Dyssegmental dysplasias (Silverman-Handmaker and Rolland-Desbuquois types). The dyssegmental dysplasias are severe neonatal dwarfing syndromes associated with segmentation defects of the vertebrae (anisospondyly).[120,163,192] Aleck et al.[5] proposed that there are two distinct forms of the disorder, the Silverman-Handmaker type, which is more severe and always results in death during the neonatal period, and the Rolland-Desbuquois form, in which survival beyond the newborn period is frequent, the radiographic changes resemble Kniest dysplasia, and the phenotype is much less severe. Both of these disorders are inherited as autosomal recessive traits.

In the severe Silverman-Handmaker type, patients are stillborn or die within 48 hours of birth (Fig. 14-29, *D* and *E*). Encephalocele or occipital defects are frequently present, and micrognathia, ear abnormalities, orbital hypoplasia, a short neck, a narrow chest, and severe microcampomelia are also features. On radiographs the segmentation defects of the spine are severe, can be seen on both anteroposterior and lateral views, and result in clefted "butterfly" or "oversized" block vertebrae. The long tubular bones are short and broad, and the femur is angulated. Chondroosseous morphologic study reveals a disorganized growth plate with failure of aggregation of calcospherites and mucoid degeneration of cartilage.[5]

The Rolland-Desbuquois type is milder than the Silverman-Handmaker type and is compatible with survival to at least 3 years of age.[5,482] This disorder resembles severe Kniest dysplasia. The extraskeletal malformations are not as common as in the Silverman-Handmaker type. On radiographic examination the major differences are in the type of segmentation defect; these segmentation defects are seen primarily on lateral views of the spine, not on anteroposterior views, and result in absent, clefted, or oversized vertebral bodies (Fig 14-29). The long tubular bones are short and broad, and the femur is angulated. The short tubular bones are

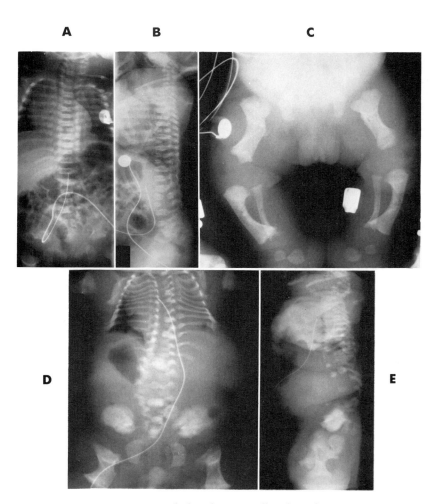

Fig. 14-29. A to **C** , Dyssegmental dysplasia, Rolland-Desbuquois type. **A,** Anteroposterior and, **B,** lateral views of the spine and, **C,** anteroposterior view of the pelvis, revealing platyspondyly, sagittal clefting, relatively normal pelvis with hypoplastic acetabular roofs, coronal clefting, and dumbbell-shaped long bones (femurs and tibia). **D** and **E,** Dyssegmental dysplasia, Silverman-Handmaker type. **D,** Anteroposterior and, **E,** lateral radiographs of the trunk, including pelvis and femurs with round amorphously dense iliac bones, anisospondyly, and short femora with splayed ends.

short and broad. Chondroosseous morphologic appearance is characterized by a relatively normal growth plate with extensive patches of broad collagen fibers in resting cartilage.[5]

Kniest dysplasia. Kniest dysplasia has some radiographic similarities to metatropic dysplasia and has been called metatropic dwarfism type II, pseudometatropic dysplasia, or "Swiss cheese" cartilage dysplasia.[523] It is associated with disproportionate dwarfism, a round face, prominent eyes, a flat midface, and cleft palate (Fig. 14-30, A). Significant myopia is present from infancy, which

can lead to vitreoretinal degeneration and retinal detachment.[387] Frequent otitis media can lead to progressive conductive deafness. The joints are large, with metaphyseal flaring, and joint motion may be limited. The hands have long fingers with prominent joints and limited flexion. Kyphoscoliosis and lordosis are progressive.

Radiographic changes include short, dumbbell-like long bones as a result of splaying of the metaphyses and irregular, punctate epiphyses with fluffiness and irregularity on both sides of the growth plate[315] (Fig. 14-30, B to I). The epiphyses of the tubular bones in the hands are flattened and

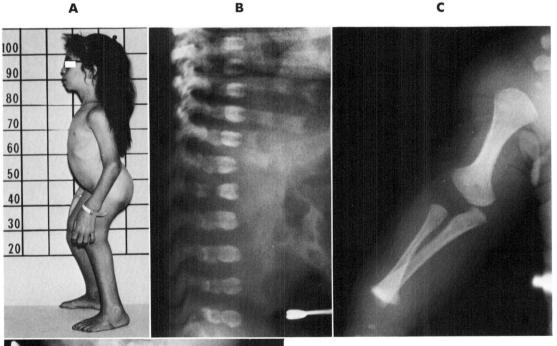

Fig. 14-30. Kniest dysplasia. **A** Twelve-year-old girl. The short-trunk dwarfism, flexion contractures of joints, and flat midface are evident. **B,** Lateral radiograph of the spine in a newborn, showing coronal clefts. **C,** Anteroposterior radiograph of upper extremity and, **D,** Anteroposterior radiograph of pelvis and lower extremities showing the dumbbell-shaped humerus and femurs, unformed acetabular roofs, and narrow greater sacrosciatic notches. *Continued.*

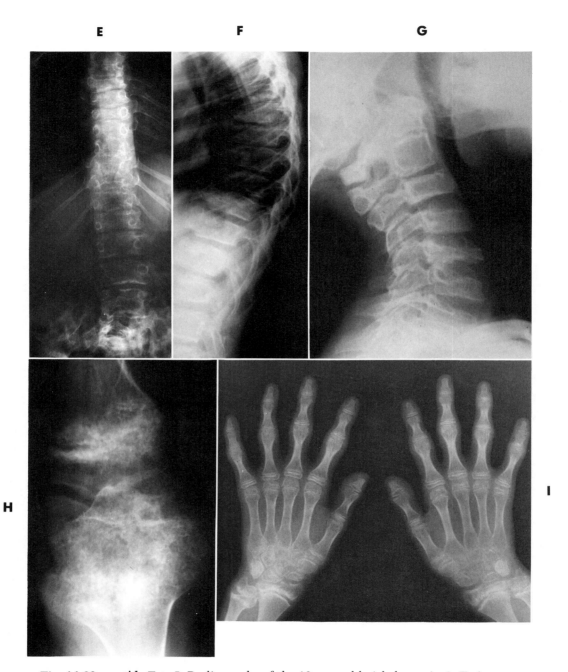

Fig. 14-30, cont'd. **E** to **I**, Radiographs of the 12-year-old girl shown in **A**. **E**, Antero-posterior and, **F**, lateral views of thoracic and, **G**, cervical spine, revealing platy-spondyly of the thoracic spine with beginning clouding effect and ununited body of C2 to odontoid, which is enlarged. Anteroposterior view of, **H**, knee and, **I**, hands, showing clouding effect on both sides of the epiphyseal plate with megaepiphyses, epimetaphyseal changes in the wrists, metaphyseal changes in the wrists, bulbous phalangeal metaphyses, and intercarpal narrowing.

squared off, with narrow joint spaces. The pelvis is abnormal in shape and marked coxa vara is present. There is platyspondyly with irregular end plates, and during infancy coronal clefting of the vertebrae can be seen. The odontoid is enlarged, and anterior fusion of the first and second cervical vertebrae has been described.

The cartilage is soft; by light microscopy it appears filled with holes and foamy lacunar changes and resembles Swiss cheese.[234,470] On electron microscopy the chondrocytes can be seen to contain large cisterns of rough endoplasmic reticulum and thin, abnormal, clumped collagen fibrils.[234,565] Excessive urinary excretion of keratan sulfate has been noted in this disorder.[138,288] Poole et al.[458] extracted cartilage from persons with Kniest dysplasia and found marked deficiency of the C propeptide of type II collagen in the extracellular matrix. Immunohistologic studies revealed that the C propeptide was clearly present in chondrocytes, corresponding to the areas of dilated rough endoplasmic reticulum. Normally, the entire procollagen peptide is secreted from the chondrocyte and the C and N propeptides are cleaved extracellularly. It is believed that the propeptides are required for normal fibril formation. Poole et al.[458] hypothesized that in Kniest dysplasia the C propeptide is cleaved intracellularly, resulting in poor fibril formation. Kniest dysplasia has been described in an affected parent and child, suggesting autosomal dominant inheritance.

Stickler syndrome (arthroophthalmopathy). In 1965 Stickler et al.[572] described an autosomal dominant disorder consisting of progressive myopia beginning in the first decade of life and resulting in retinal detachment and blindness, hearing deficits, and premature degenerative changes in various joints with abnormal epiphyseal and vertebral radiographic changes. The patients had dishlike, concave faces. This disorder has received considerable attention. The means of ascertainment have been quite different among various authors, depending on the specialty of the observer. Some have suggested that most cases of Pierre Robin sequence are cases of Stickler syndrome, whereas others use the designation for any patient with early-onset severe myopia or dominantly inherited myopia.[217,429] In general these patients have severe progressive myopia, retinal detachment, depressed nasal bridge, maxillary hypopla-

sia, cleft palate, micrognathia, and a marfanoid body build. Progressive sensoroneural hearing loss develops. Mitral valve prolapse is found in almost 50% of patients.[348] Radiographic manifestations range from a fairly normal skeleton to mild irregularity of the end plates of the vertebrae and flattening and underdevelopment of some epiphyses.[543]

Much confusion exists as to the homogeneity of the Stickler syndrome. Cases with only the facial and ocular abnormalities have been referred to as the Marshall syndrome and the Wagner syndrome.[637] Some question also exists as to whether these cases blend into the Weissenbacher-Zweymuller syndrome.[283]

In view of the differences in the diagnostic criteria for Stickler syndrome it is not surprising that homogeneity on the molecular level has not been found. Some families have been found to cosegregate with the type II collagen gene, whereas in others segregation was discordant.[135,293] A point mutation resulting in a stop codon in the type II collagen gene has now been described in at least one patient with the Stickler syndrome.[2] (The Stickler syndrome is also discussed in Chapter 3, pp. 98 and 99.)

Spondyloepiphyseal Dysplasia Congenita Group

Achondrogenesis type II—hypochondrogenesis (Langer-Saldino dysplasia). The term achondrogenesis, as discussed previously, has been used for a number of distinct entities. Achondrogenesis type II (Langer-Saldino dysplasia) appears to represent the most severe end of the SED spectrum of disorders, which range through hypochondrogenesis to SED, Stickler syndrome, and precocious osteoarthropathy at the mildest end of the spectrum[49] (Fig. 14-31). Recent studies have demonstrated that these disorders share defects in type II collagen secondary to mutations in the COL2A1 gene.[3,341,414,591]

Achondrogenesis type II is characterized by marked micromelic dwarfism, fetal hydrops, distended abdomen with barrel-shaped chest, short trunk, and large cranium, with or without cleft palate.[48,74,] This syndrome results in death within the perinatal period. The radiologic manifestations include lack of mineralization of all or many vertebral bodies, nonossified sacrum, ischium, pubis, talus, and calcaneus, markedly short long bones and tubular bones of the hands and feet, concave metaphyses, and a large, normally ossi-

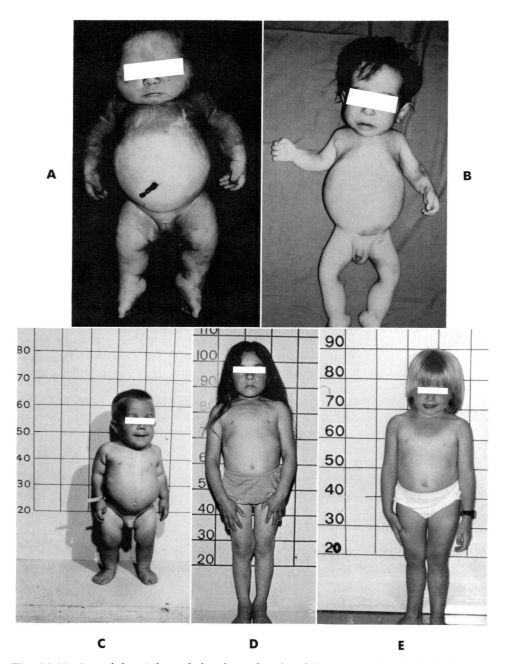

Fig. 14-31. Spondyloepiphyseal dysplasia family of disorders, all of which share a defect in type II collagen. **A,** Achondrogenesis II, hypochondrogenesis (stillborn). **B,** Spondyloepiphyseal dysplasia congenita with severe respiratory restriction in a 2-year-old. **C** to **E,** Spondyloepiphyseal dysplasia congenita in decreasing levels of severity. Short limbs and trunk, short neck, and Harrison grooves in the chest can be seen.

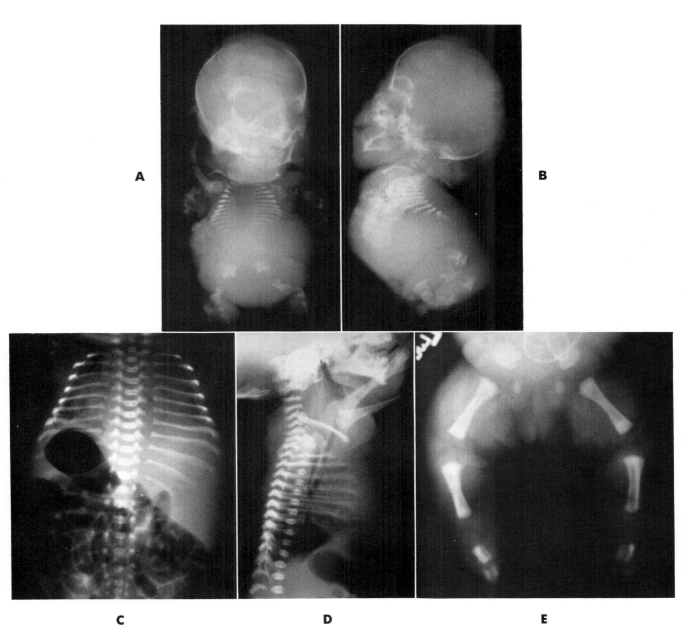

Fig. 14-32. Spondyloepiphyseal dysplasia family of disorders. Severe end of the spectrum. **A** and **B,** Achondrogenesis II. **A,** Anteroposterior and, **B,** lateral full-body radiographs show absent vertebral ossification, short ribs, micromelia with cupped metaphyses, characteristic pelvis with absent pubic bones, ischia, and concave margins medially and inferiorly of the iliac wings. **C** to **E,** Hypochondrogenesis. **C,** Anteroposterior and, **D,** lateral views of trunk and, **E,** anteroposterior view of the pelvis and lower extremities show hypoplastic, platyspondylic vertebral bodies and deficient cervical vertebral ossification, moderately short ribs, absent pubic bones, hypoplastic ischia, rounded ends of shortened long bones, absent talus, and calcaneal ossification.   *Continued.*

F   G   H

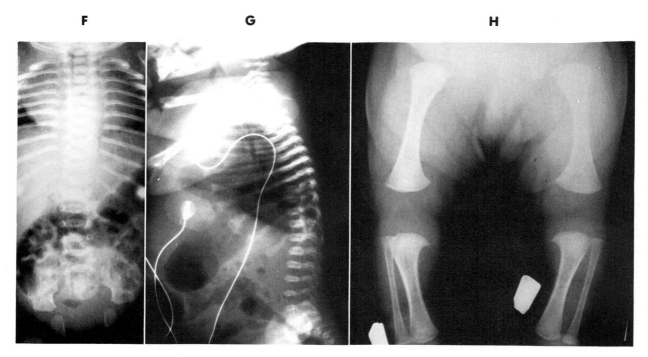

Fig. 14-32, cont'd. F to **H,** Spondyloepiphyseal dysplasia congenita. **F,** Anteroposterior and, **G,** lateral views of trunk and, **H,** anteroposterior view of pelvis and lower extremities reveal platyspondyly in well-formed vertebrae, slightly short ribs, well-formed vertical ischia, absent pubic bones, and slightly short long bones with broad, round ends.

fied calvarium with an ossification defect in the base of the skull behind the foramen magnum (Fig. 14-32, *A* and *B*). The iliac wings are small, with concave inferior and medial margins. There is variable shortening of the ribs with anterior and posterior flaring.

Hypochondrogenesis and achondrogenesis type II appear to be part of a spectrum of severity of the same disorder.[48] They would correspond to types II, III, and IV in the Whitley-Gorlin classification.[628] The clinical and radiographic features of hypochondrogenesis are identical to but less severe than those of achondrogenesis II and run a continuous spectrum of severity (Fig. 14-32, *C* to *E*). In addition, mild hypochondrogenesis type II merges into severe SED congenita.[362] Although hypochondrogenesis may be associated with perinatal death, affected individuals may live for weeks to months.[378] The spine is ossified in the lower thoracic and upper lumbar areas, but there is frequently lack of ossification, or at least severe

hypoplasia, in the cervical region and sacrum. The long bones are less shortened and have a lesser degree of cupping and flaring than in achondrogenesis type II.

Chondroosseous morphologic appearance is similar throughout the achondrogenesis type II–hypochondrogenesis spectrum.[48,155,156,240] The cartilage is quite hypervascular and the chondrocytes are surrounded by large lacunae. The columns are irregular, and hypertrophic chondrocytes may extend into the calcified cartilage spicules. The amount of cartilage matrix is reduced, and on electron microscopy cisterns of dilated rough endoplasmic reticulum are evident. Immunochemical studies by Godfrey and Hollister[155] suggested that in a case of hypochondrogenesis there was decreased to absent type II collagen in the matrix, whereas type II collagen accumulated within the cisterns of rough endoplasmic reticulum.[156] Type I collagen was also found in the vascular areas with extension into the matrix. Horton et al.[240] also documented the presence of type I and type II collagen in the cartilage of a patient with achondrogenesis II.

In 1986 Eyre et al.[116] found that cartilage in one case in the achondrogenesis type II–hypochondrogenesis spectrum had an abnormal gelatinous texture and a translucent appearance. Type II collagen could not be detected throughout the cartilage, and the predominant collagen present was type I. A number of cases in the achondrogenesis type II–hypochondrogenesis spectrum have now been studied biochemically, and all demonstrate reduced or totally absent type II collagen in the cartilage matrix.[124,155,240,413] Type I collagen is almost uniformly present. The amount of type I collagen decreases with decreasing severity of the disease. Modified type II collagen appears in the hypochondrogenesis end of the spectrum. Toward the mild SED end of the spectrum, type I collagen is not found in cartilage and all the collagen present appears to be overmodified type II collagen similar to that seen in typical cases of SED congenita. Molecular studies have now demonstrated a variety of mutations in the type II collagen gene in these patients.[70,612] Although achondrogenesis type II was considered an autosomal recessive disorder because of the occasional presence of affected sibs with normal parents, molecular studies have indicated that the mutations are present in one allele only, indicating autosomal dominant inheritance.[612]

Spondyloepiphyseal dysplasia congenita. Spranger and Weidemann[555] suggested the designation "spondyloepiphyseal dysplasia (SED) congenita" for a disorder affecting particularly the vertebrae and juxtatruncal epiphyses. Four of Spranger and Weidemann's six patients had progressive myopia. Platyspondyly, short limbs, and cleft palate can be evident at birth.[16] The term "spondyloepiphyseal dysplasia (SED)" is now used for a widely variable and heterogeneous group of disorders that affect the spine and the epiphyses. When the metaphyses are involved as well, the term "spondyloepimetaphyseal dysplasia" is used. Spondyloepiphyseal dysplasia congenita appears to be a fairly distinct entity that has marked clinical variability. On its severe side it merges into mild hypochondrogenesis, and on the mild side it can resemble severe Stickler syndrome. All cases studied to date have turned out to have a defect in type II collagen.

Short stature with a short trunk is present at birth. The face is flattened, and hypertelorism and cleft palate can be present. Myopia is present in more than 50% of the cases.[136] Vitreoretinal degeneration can lead to retinal detachment.[191] The neck is short, and there is odontoid hypoplasia, which can lead to C1-2 vertebral instability and cervical myopathy. The chest is barrel shaped and pectus carinatum can be present. The thoracic kyphosis is exaggerated, and there can be marked lumbar lordosis and a short spine. The limbs are short, but the hands and feet are relatively normal, with fingers of normal length and prominent joints. Muscular hypotonia, a waddling gait, and genu varum or valgum are frequently present. With age, degenerative arthrosis, especially in the hips, is common, often necessitating early hip replacement.[295] Wide variability in phenotypic severity exists in this disorder, ranging from infantile lethality to mild short stature and precocious degenerative arthritis in adulthood.

Radiologic manifestations in infancy include ovoid or pear-shaped vertebrae, generalized long-bone shortening with normal modeling and absent pubic ossification[547] (Fig. 14-32, F to H, and Fig. 14-33, A to C). There is no ossification of the epiphyses of the knees at birth and, usually, no talar or calcaneal ossification. The metaphyses appear normal at birth. In childhood and later life, platyspondyly develops; this can be quite variable in severity (Fig. 14-32, D and E). The odontoid is hypoplastic, with C1-2 vertebral dislocation. Epiphyseal ossification delay and irregularity are marked. When the epiphyses do ossify, they do so centrally, resulting in a small, irregularly ossified epiphysis. Arthrographic studies and MRI have demonstrated a normal anlage of the femoral head, indicating a defect in secondary ossification.[312] The long bones are short but otherwise appear normal. Prenatal diagnosis by means of ultrasonography can be made in the second trimester on the basis of shortened long bones.[311]

The major complications of this disorder are (1) myopia, vitreous degeneration, and retinal detachment; (2) C1-2 vertebral subluxation with the propensity to compression of the cervical cord; and (3) early degenerative arthrosis. Evaluation of the C1-2 subluxation should be undertaken by means of lateral radiographs obtained with the cervical vertebrae in flexion and extension. Evaluation of the spinal cord by means of MRI and of neurophysiologic function by means of somatic sensory evoked potentials is then carried out. If significant

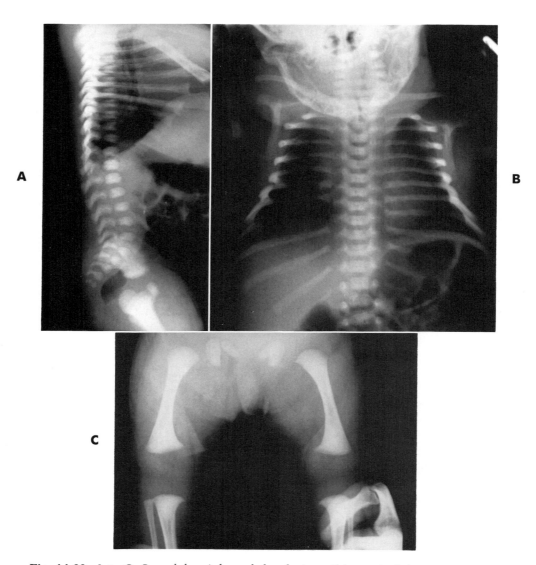

Fig. 14-33. A to **C,** Spondyloepiphyseal dysplasia, milder end of the spectrum. Radiographs in newborn period. **A,** Lateral view of spine; **B,** anteroposterior view of thorax; and, **C,** lower extremities. Platyspondyly, short splayed ribs, a narrow thorax, hypoplastic ischia, and pubic ossification are shown.

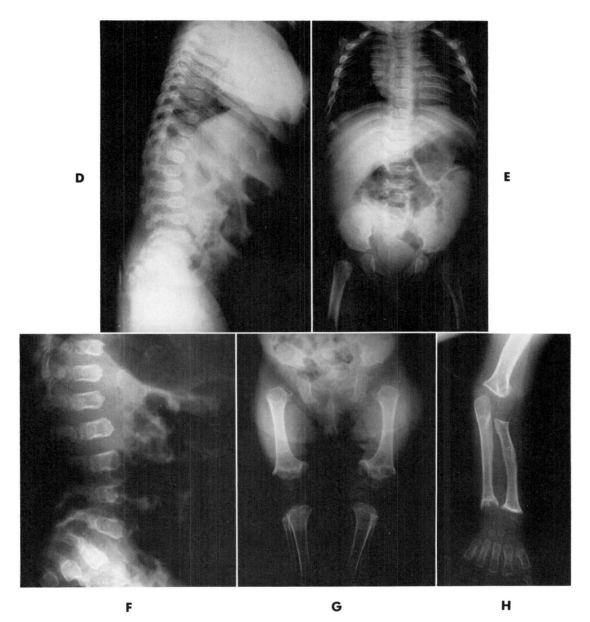

Fig. 14-33, cont'd. **D** and **E,** Same patient at 9 months of age. **D,** Lateral and, **E,** anteroposterior views of trunk, showing growth of vertebrae with persistence of platyspondyly, a mild rib cupping, and rounded proximal femurs. **F** to **H,** Spondyloepimetaphyseal dysplasia, Strudwick type. Radiographs of a 1-year-old. **F,** Lateral view of lumbar spine; **G,** anteroposterior view of pelvis and lower extremities; and, **H,** anteroposterior view of upper extremity revealing platyspondyly, flattened acetabulae, rounded proximal femurs with characteristic "dappling" (metaphyseal infractions), tiny proximal ossification centers, and significant metaphyseal involvement at the knees, with characteristic increased ulnar metaphyseal cupping and irregularity as opposed to the milder changes in the radius.

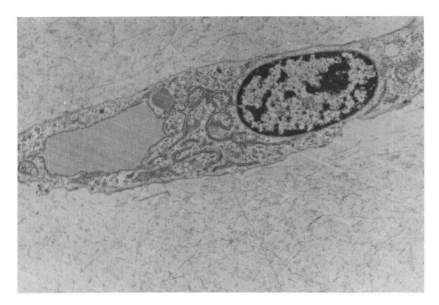

Fig. 14-34. Spondyloepiphyseal dysplasia congenita. Electron micrograph of costal cartilage showing characteristic large cistern of rough endoplasmic reticulum (magnification × 5250).

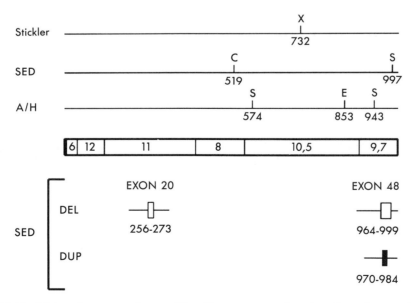

Fig. 14-35. Molecular map of type II collagen genes showing the nine mutations known in early 1992. *A/H*, achondrogenesis II, hypochondrogenesis; *DEL*, deletion; *DUP*, duplication; *SED*, spondyloepiphyseal dysplasia. (Courtesy Dr. Dan Cohn, Los Angeles.)

subluxation or neurologic symptoms are found, posterior vertebral fusion of C1-2 should be performed.[295]

Pathologic examination of chondroosseous tissue shows mild growth plate disorganization with large inclusion bodies in the chondrocytes of many of these patients.[470,649] By means of ultrastructural examination[527] (Fig. 14-34) these chondrocytic inclusions are found to be dilated cisterns of rough endoplasmic reticulum.[530] Murray et al.[416] found that the collagen of the vitreous had a smaller than normal fiber diameter and that the vitreous had central liquefaction, was attached in multiple areas, and exerted traction on the retina. Because of the presence of both cartilaginous and vitreous abnormalities, which are the major normal locations of type II collagen in the body, Murray and Rimoin[413] postulated that the basic defect in SED congenita would be in type II collagen. They demonstrated that in a large number of patients cartilage collagen exhibited electrophoretic mobility abnormalities, suggesting that the collagen was overmodified.[413,414] The supposition was that the triple-helical formation of the type II collagen molecule would stop at the point of mutation and overglycosylation would occur to the amino side of the mutation. Linkage studies have documented cosegregation of the COL2A1 gene with SED in a number of families.[9,510] Lee et al.[341] and Tiller et al.[591] demonstrated deletions and insertions in the carboxyl terminal end of the COL2A1 gene. A number of point mutations have since been found.[3,70] Correlation of the severity of the disease with the site of the mutation, however, has not yet been possible. A variety of mutations have thus been described in the type II collagen gene, ranging from single base-pair substitutions to deletions and insertions (Fig. 14-35). These abnormalities result in clinical phenotypes ranging from achondrogenesis type II through hypochondrogenesis, SED congenita, Stickler syndrome, and precocious osteoarthropathy. What had been thought to be a separate group of disorders with metaphyseal and epiphyseal radiographic changes (SEMD) may also be due to allelic mutations in the type II collagen gene, for example, spondyloepimetaphyseal dysplasia, Strudwick type (Fig. 14-32, *F* to *H*). However, several cases of spondyloepimetaphyseal dysplasia with additional nonskeletal defects have been described, and it is likely that these represent a widely heterogeneous group of disorders.[588] Spondyloepiphyseal dysplasia congenita is inherited as an autosomal dominant trait.

Other Spondyloepi-(Meta)-Physeal Dysplasias

X-linked spondyloepiphyseal dysplasia tarda. The condition discussed in this section went by a number of designations, including "Morquio's disease,"[259] before being delineated by Maroteaux and colleagues in 1957 (Fig. 14-36). Short stature, which becomes evident between the ages of 5 and 10 years, is primarily truncal. Pain in the backs and hips and limitation of motion in these joints are frequent by the teen years. Adult height varies from 130 to 155 cm.[50] Disabling polyarthrosis of the hips occurs by the fourth or fifth decade. Dorsal kyphosis and lumbar hyperlordosis may develop. The patient appears to have a short neck. Intrafamilial variability in presenting signs and symptoms can occur.[253]

The radiographic features, especially those in the spine, are distinctive.[326] Mild to moderate platyspondyly is generalized, and a hump-shaped mound of bone is present in the central and posterior portions of both superior and inferior end plates of lumbar vertebrae, with delayed ossification or nonossification of the ring epiphyses; the platyspondyly and humping of the thoracic and cervical segments is of lesser severity. The disk spaces are narrowed and scoliosis may be evident. A hypoplastic, cone-shaped odontoid process has been described. In SED tarda a fish-mouth–shaped area in the anterior parts of the lumbar vertebrae is evident on lateral view, since the involvement seen centrally and posteriorly is lacking in this area. The epiphyses in the bones of the limbs, especially the proximal parts of the limbs, are small, irregular, and dysplastic. The age at which these epiphyses become ossified is delayed. The pelvis is small, the femoral neck is short, and coxa vara may be present. Premature osteoarthritic changes occur in young adults, especially in the hips and the spine.

Several large kindreds have been reported showing the classic pattern of X-linked recessive inheritance. Heterozygotes show no major abnormality such as short stature; however, several females in the kindred studied by Bannerman, Ingall, and Mohn[22] (the same family as that studied by Jacobsen[259]) had arthritic complaints (Fig. 14-36, *A*). Cosegregation of SED tarda and deutan

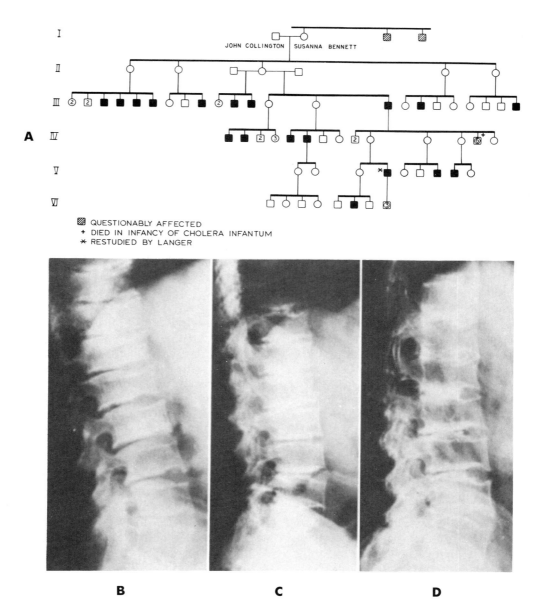

A

QUESTIONABLY AFFECTED
+ DIED IN INFANCY OF CHOLERA INFANTUM
* RESTUDIED BY LANGER

B   **C**   **D**

Fig. 14-36. X-linked spondyloepiphyseal dysplasia tarda. **A,** Pedigree of family reported by Bannerman.[22] **B** to **E,** Radiographic findings show graded changes in the lumbar spine. Heaping up of the posterior portion of the superior vertebral plate is pathognomonic, **B.** Progressive changes are shown in **C** and **D.** The changes are caused by severe eburnation of the humps on the superior and inferior vertebral end plates.

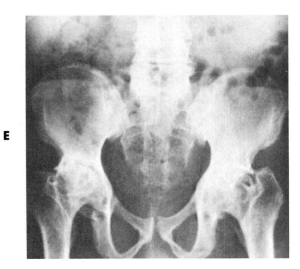

Fig. 14-36, cont'd. E, Late degenerative "arthritis" of the hips. The deep acetabula are evident. (Courtesy Dr. Leonard O. Langer, Jr, Minneapolis.)

color blindness suggested to Kousseff et al.[296] that the SED tarda locus was on the Xq28 band. Szpiro-Tapia et al.[585] were able to exclude the entire Xq region and proximal Xp regions and concluded that the SED tarda locus may be in Xp22.

Other late-onset spondyloepiphyseal dysplasias. A number of families have been reported in which pedigree data are consistent with either autosomal recessive[385,548] or autosomal dominant inheritance.[24,494,548] On radiographic examination affected persons have changes in the spine that are distinct from those in the X-linked form but show, in addition to platyspondyly, the same tendency to precocious degenerative joint disease, especially in the hips. It is likely that many of the autosomal late-onset forms of SED and SEMD represent mutations in the COL2A1 gene and fall within the SED family of disorders. The cases of precocious familial osteoarthropathy in which COL2A1 mutations have been documented could also be classified into this SED tarda–like group.[3]

Progressive pseudorheumatoid dysplasia (spondyloepiphyseal dysplasia tarda with progressive arthropathy). The disorder discussed in this section is characterized by progressive arthropathy resembling rheumatoid arthritis.[558,641] The on-

set occurs in children from 3 to 8 years of age, and patients come to medical attention with difficulties in walking, easy fatigability, and muscular weakness. Joint stiffness first affects the hips. Morning stiffness and decreased mobility of the cervical spine suggest rheumatoid arthritis. Swelling of the finger joints is primarily caused by osseous distention of the metaphyseal ends of the phalanges. The joints may appear large and prominent, and contractures may occur at the large joints. Kyphoscoliosis may develop. Rheumatoid arthritis can be readily ruled out by the presence of a normal erythrocyte sedimentation rate, a negative rheumatoid factor, and a normal synovium.

On radiographic examination there is platyspondly with anterior end-plate erosions and gouge defects, which resembles Scheuermann disease.[298] In the hands the joint spaces are narrow, the metaphyses widened, and the epiphyses flattened. The hips show enlarged femoral heads, joint-space narrowing, and acetabular irregularity. Articular spaces may be narrowed throughout the skeleton, but characteristic rheumatoid arthritic bone changes are not present.[481] Chondroosseous morphologic study shows abnormal clustering of chondrocytes with pyknotic nuclei and defective column formation.[558] The synovium is normal at biopsy. Parental consanguinity and the presence of multiple affected sibs are indicative of autosomal recessive inheritance of this disorder.

Dyggve-Melchior-Clausen dysplasia. The unusual disorder of Dyggve-Melchior-Clausen dysplasia was first described in a consanguineous family from Greenland, in which three sibs were said to have a condition resembling the mucopolysacchridoses.[102] The original patients were mentally retarded, and mucopolysaccharides were found in their urine. As other families have been described, it has become apparent that mental retardation is a variable feature of this disorder.[545,594] The patients are small at birth and develop short stature. There may be microcephaly. The trunk appears short, with scoliosis, kyphosis, and lordosis (Fig. 14-37, *A*). Joint motion becomes restricted, and a waddling gait is evident. Spranger, Bierbaum, and Herrmann[546] suggested that patients with the skeletal features of Dyggve-Melchior-Clausen dysplasia who were not mentally retarded had a distinct entity, which they called "Smith-McCort" dwarfism. The determination of whether this situation represents heterogeneity or variability will have to await demonstration of the basic defect in this recessive disorder.

The characteristic and diagnostic radiographic changes are an irregular, lacey iliac crest border and double-humped, centrally indented vertebral bodies[551] (Fig. 14-37, *B*). The vertebral body changes consist of platyspondyly with anterior beaking and a notchlike ossification defect of the end plates, producing an anteroposterior humped appearance. There can be posterior scalloping of the vertebral bodies, elongation of the vertebral laminae, and a hypoplastic odontoid process, as well as C1-2 vertebral dislocation. Costochondral junctions are widened. The actabular roof is flat, with irregular ossification, and the pubic rami and ischiopubic synchondroses are wide. The long bones are short, with irregular metaphyses, multicentric ossification, and deformity of the epiphyses, especially the proximal humeral and femoral epiphyses. The carpal bones are small, as are the metacarpals and metatarsals, and cone-shaped epiphyses can be present. There is an unusual clustering of chondrocytes in resting cartilage.[470]

Dyggve-Melchior-Clausen dysplasia has been reported in multiple sibs and consanguineous matings indicative of autosomal recessive inheritance.

The gene may have a relatively high frequency in the Lebanese.[47,417]

Wolcott-Rallison dysplasia (spondyloepiphyseal dysplasia with diabetes mellitus). The unique disorder discussed in this section is characterized by diabetes mellitus that becomes evident in infancy, together with spondyloepiphyseal dysplasia.[167,639] Small stature and difficulty in walking are features; joint pain can be a presenting symptom after 1 to 2 years of age. Patients have been reported with renal insufficiency and hepatosplenomegaly. Radiographic manifestations include generalized epiphyseal ossification delay with small, fragmented epiphyses, resorption of the capital femoral epiphyses with dislocation, and mild generalized platyspondyly. Chondroosseous morphologic study shows a paucity of chondrocytes with lack of columnization, and electron microscopy reveals dilated rough endoplasmic reticulum and thick, irregular collagen fibers, suggesting a defect in collagen synthesis or processing.[576] Biochemical and molecular analysis of collagens has not yet been reported in Wolcott-Rallison dysplasia. This disorder appears to be inherited as an autosomal recessive trait.

Pseudoachondroplasia. Pseudoachondroplasia was one of the first disorders to be distinguished

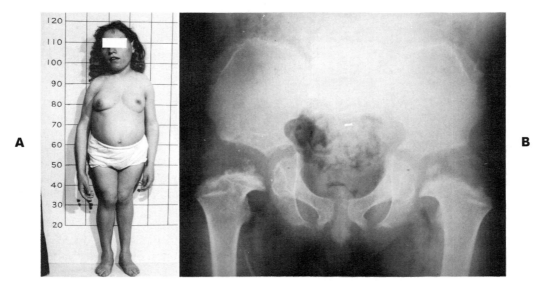

Fig. 14-37. Dyggve-Melchior-Clausen syndrome, **A,** in a 20-year-old woman. The short-trunk dwarfism can be seen. **B,** Anteroposterior view of pelvis and the hips with marked femoral epiphyseal hypoplasia, short femoral necks, and a characteristic "lacy" pattern in the apophyseal region of the iliac crests.

from achondroplasia by Maroteaux and Lamy.[371] They originally called the disorder "pseudoachondroplastic spondlyloepiphyseal dysplasia" because of its clear distinction from achondroplasia and the presence of radiographic changes in the spine and epiphyses. It is one of the more frequent skeletal dysplasias. The patients appear normal at birth, and growth retardation is seldom recognized until the second year of life or later, at which time the body proportions resemble those of persons with achondroplasia (Fig. 14-38). The head and face are normal. Indeed, the facies of persons with pseudoachondroplasia are similar and attractive. Thus in pseudoachondroplasia, dysplastic craniofacial development can result in an appearance that might be considered more aesthetically appealing than the normal. The fingers are short and do not show the trident configuration typical of achondroplasia.[130] They are hyperlax and can be pulled out in a telescoping fashion. There may be hyperlordosis, scoliosis, and kyphosis, but in many patients the back appears relatively normal. In affected individuals a waddling gait develops, and these persons have a variety of deformities of the lower limbs. These may range from genu varum to genu valgum, to a "windswept" deformity; ligamentous laxity contributes greatly to the leg deformities. Frequently, multiple osteotomies are required throughout childhood. There may be ulnar deviation of the wrists and flexion contractures of the hips, knees, and elbows in adulthood. Diminished flexion and external rotation of the hips may lead to difficulties during sexual intercourse in women.

The radiographic manifestations involve the spine, metaphyses, and epiphyses[219,641] (Fig. 14-38, C to I). The craniofacial bones appear normal. All tubular bones are quite short, with widened metaphyses and fragmentation and irregularities of the developing epiphyses. Indeed, the epiphyses of the hips and phalanges appear quite small, that is, as "miniepiphyses." The proximal ends of the metacarpals are rounded, and the carpal bones appear hypoplastic and irregular in shape. The distal metacarpals have a typical ball-in-cup appearance. In childhood, platyspondyly is characteristic, with anterior tonguing due to delayed ossification of the annular epiphyses; after puberty the vertebrae become more normal in appearance. The ribs have a spatulate appearance. The acetabula are irregular, and coxa vara is usually present.

Chondroosseous morphologic appearance in pseudoachondroplasia is characteristic. On light microscopy one can see chondrocytes containing large inclusion bodies, which on electron micro-

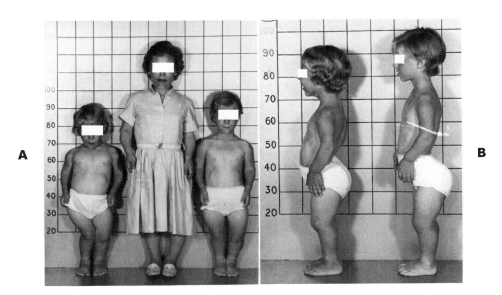

Fig. 14-38. Pseudoachondroplastic dysplasia. **A,** The 35-year-old mother and both children, 8 and 11 years of age, are affected. The size and shape of their heads are normal. The skull radiograph is normal. **B,** Both girls show exaggerated lumbar lordosis. *Continued.*

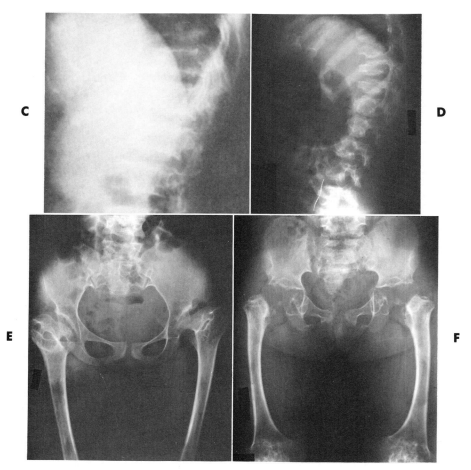

Fig. 14-38, cont'd. C, Lumbar spine in the mother, showing some flattening of vertebral bodies with irregularity of the end plates, which is, however, not diagnostic. **D,** Lumbar spine in the 11-year-old daughter, showing an anterior projection of the vertebral bodies that is due to abnormally large notches for the annular cartilages, as well as striking irregularity of the end plates. The lumbar spine, as viewed in frontal projection, does not show caudad narrowing of the interpedunculate distance, which is characteristic of achondroplasia. **E,** Hips and pelvis of the mother. **F,** Drastic changes are shown in the hips and knees of the 11-year-old daughter. **G** to **I,** Hands of the mother and the older daughter. The mother, **G,** shows short fingers, bowed forearms, and prominence on the radial aspect of the right wrist. Radiograph, **H,** shows this prominence to be produced by displacement of the distal end of the radius past the first row of carpal bones. Radiograph, **I,** of the hand of the older daughter shows evidence of marked disturbance in ossification of the carpal bones and the metaphyses and epiphyses of all bones. **J,** Pedigree. The mother is indicated by the arrow. Since continuation of the pedigree, she has had an unaffected child by her second husband. **K,** Two brothers with pseudoachondroplasia. Severe genu varum in the brother, *left,* and genu valgum in the brother, *right,* demonstrate significant intrafamilial phenotypic variability. **L,** Transmission electron micrograph of resting cartilage from a patient with pseudoachondroplasia, demonstrating the large cisterns of rough endoplasmic reticulum that contain the characteristic lamellar "onion skin" inclusion body.

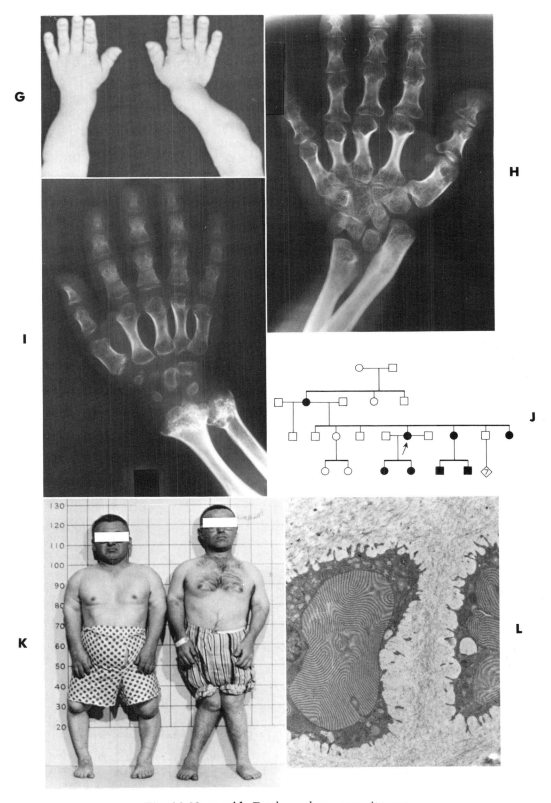

Fig. 14-38, cont'd. For legend see opposite page.

scopy show a unique "onion skin" lamellar type of pattern.[86,388,470,564] Stanescu, Stanescu and Maroteaux[561] found accumulation of a noncollagenous protein in the rough endoplasmic reticulum of the chondrocytes and absence of a proteoglycan "population" in cartilaginous tissue. The accumulated material stained with antibodies against the core proteins of proteoglycans. The authors suggested that an abnormally synthesized or processed core protein is not properly transferred to the Golgi system. We have demonstrated similar inclusion bodies in chondrocytes that stain with antibodies directed against both the proteoglycan core and link proteins. Hirata, Rimoin, and Poole[223] found that the extent of chondroitin-4,6-sulfation in the linkage region of the proteoglycans is consistently reduced in pseudoachondroplasia. The authors postulated alterations in the posttranslational processing of cartilage proteoglycan after the synthesis of the core protein and during the assembly of the glycosaminoglycan chains. It has been suggested that the defect in pseudoachondroplasia is a structural mutation in one of the proteoglycan core proteins. Lack of cosegregration of pseudoachondroplasia with the proteoglycan core protein "aggrecans" gene has been reported.[125]

Pseudoachondroplasia has in the past been suggested to represent four distinct disorders, two dominant and two recessive.[185] The vast majority of cases fit into what has previously been called "pseudoachondroplasia type III," which is the classic form described by Maroteaux and Lamy[371] and referred to in this section. This disorder can demonstrate marked phenotypic variability.[381,472] The milder dominant and recessive forms (I and II) really appear to be forms of SEMD rather than true pseudoachondroplasia. In addition, the type IV recessive form was based on a family in which a brother and sister had pseudoachondroplasia and normal parents.[184] The brother subsequently married a normal unrelated woman and fathered two daughters, one of whom had typical changes of pseudoachondroplasia.[189] Germinal cell mosaicism in one of the parents of the brother and sister was proposed to explain the presence of the condition in these affected sibs. Thus typical pseudoachondroplasia is an autosomal dominant trait (Fig. 14-38, *J*).

Dysostosis Multiplex Group

The term *dysostosis multiplex* refers to the radiographic characteristics of the mucopolysaccharidoses and mucolipidoses, that is, lysosomal storage disorders. These are discussed in Chapter 11.

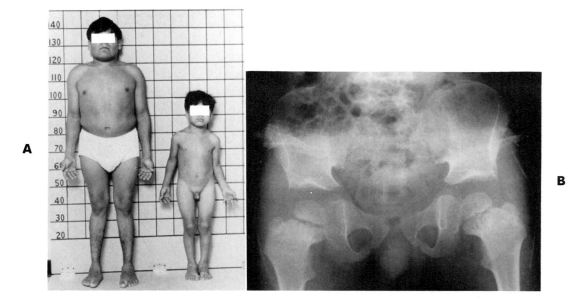

Fig. 14-39. Spondylometaphyseal dysplasia, Kozlowski type in, **A,** father and son. The short trunk is evident. **B,** Anteroposterior radiograph of pelvis and hips shows narrow greater sciatic notches, flat acetabulae, and hemispheric capital femoral epiphyses with irregularities on both sides of the growth plate (more severe on the metaphyseal side).

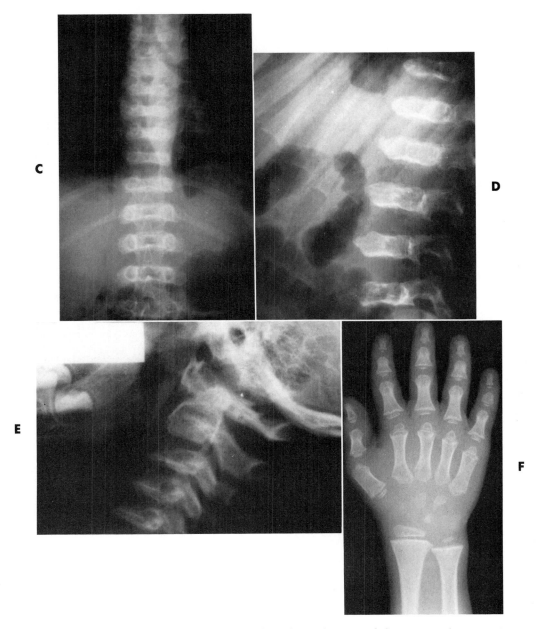

Fig 14-39, cont'd. C, Anteroposterior and, **D,** lateral views of thoracic and, **E,** cervical spine, showing the "open staircase" vertebrae with anterior rounded and pointed vertebral bodies and odontoid hypoplasia. **F,** Anteroposterior view of left hand and wrist, showing the shortening of the tubular bones of the hands with marked carpal delay and metaphyseal irregularity.

Spondylometaphyseal Dysplasia

The spondylometaphyseal dysplasias constitute a complex group of disorders characterized by the association of spondylo-(i.e., vertebral) dysplasia and metaphyseal abnormalities of the tubular bones.[376] The best known and by far the most common type was described by Kozlowski, Maroteaux, and Spranger.[299] Individuals with this type of disorder are usually normal at birth; short stature is detected in early childhood (Fig. 14-39, A). Moderate dwarfism is present, most markedly in the trunk region and in a short neck. Scoliosis or kyphosis, or both, can develop. The limbs are mildly curved in a varus position, and the hands and feet are short and stubby. There may be limitation of joint motion with some gait disturbance. The craniofacies are normal.

On radiographic examination there is generalized severe platyspondyly with an increase in height of the intervertebral disk spaces.[316] The pedicles are medially placed, giving the vertebral bodies an unusual "open staircase" appearance on anteroposterior view (Fig. 14-39, C to E). Kyphosis or kyphoscoliosis is present, as well as early degenerative spine changes. The metaphyses of the tubular bones are widened, sclerotic, and irregular. The physeal surfaces of the femoral epiphyseal ossification centers are irregular (Fig. 14-39, B). The coxa vara are characteristic. The iliac bones are short and flared. There is marked retardation of skeletal maturation, especially in the carpals (i.e., no carpal centers are seen until 5 to 6 years of age) (Fig. 14-39, F). The sphenoid and basioccipital bones are hypoplastic.

Chondroosseous morphologic study shows short irregular columns and wide septae. There can be metachromatic inclusions, and Stanescu et al.[565] have suggested that this condition is a lysosomal disorder involving proteoglycans. Although Kozlowski, Maroteaux, and Spranger[299] originally suspected autosomal recessive inheritance, affected parents and offspring have been reported, suggesting autosomal dominant inheritance.

A large number of cases with alterations in the spine and metaphyses do not fit into the Kozlowski type of spondylometaphyseal dysplasia.[301,376,588] A variety of classifications have been proposed for the spondylometaphyseal dysplasias, including a number of distinct entities such as the Schmidt type[496] and the Algerian type.[303] Maroteaux and Spranger[376] recently proposed a tentative classification of this group of disorders. On the basis of the severity of changes in the femoral

neck and a variety of other manifestations, they divided the spondylometaphyseal dysplasias into nine subgroups. It is clear that the extent of the heterogeneity in this group of disorders is still not fully resolved, and biochemical and molecular studies will be required to accurately distinguish discrete forms of SMD.

Langer et al.[335] have recently described what appears to be a distinct form of spondylometaphyseal dysplasia, which they call "the corner fracture type." This is a dominant disorder associated with short stature and developmental coxa vara. On radiographs changes in the long tubular bones simulating corner fractures and characteristic vertebral anomalies are observed.

Spondyloenchondrodysplasia. An apparently distinct form of spondylometaphyseal dysplasia is the autosomal recessive disorder known as spondyloenchondrodysplasia. First described by Schorr, Legum, and Ochshorn[497] in two sons of first-cousin parents of Iraqi Jewish background, this disorder consists of enchondromatosis similar to that of Ollier disease, in association with platyspondyly. Several other families have since been described, as well as a child who was the product of an incestuous union, indicating autosomal recessive inheritance.[140,180,366] Affected individuals have short stature, rhizomelia, genu valgum, increased anteroposterior diameter of the chest, thoracic kyphosis, lumbar lordosis, prominent joints, and bulbous ends of the ribs. Radiographs show enchondromatosis-like lesions involving the long bones and flat bones, with sparing of the hands and feet. There is severe platyspondyly with marked end-plate irregularity due to enchondromata. The proximal fibula and distal ulna appear to be more severely affected than the corresponding areas of the tibia and radius. There is some question as to whether this disorder should be classified with the spondylometaphyseal dysplasias or with other forms of enchondromatosis.

Epiphyseal Dysplasias

Multiple epiphyseal dysplasia. The term "multiple epiphyseal dysplasia" is used for a group of disorders associated with epiphyseal dysplasia of the long and short tubular bones and relatively normal vertebrae[250,403] (Fig. 14-40). The disorder may not become evident until 5 to 10 years of age, when a waddling gait or difficulty in climbing stairs or running is noted. Joint pain and limitation of motions in various joints such as knees,

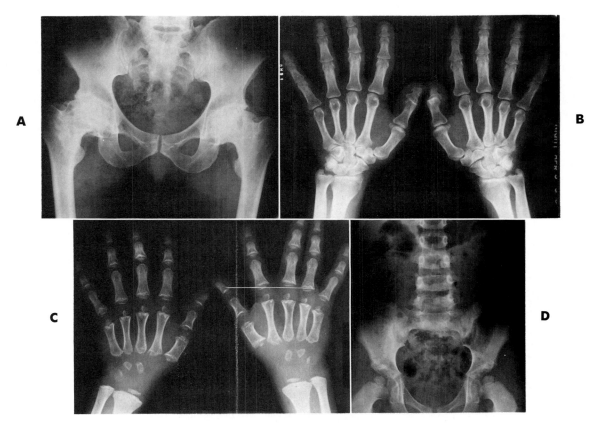

Fig. 14-40. Multiple epiphyseal dysplasia in father and son. The father, **A** and **B**, 40 years of age, is moderately short of stature and has short fingers and severe osteoarthrosis of the hips. The son, **C** and **D**, 9 years of age, shows the characteristic findings of multiple epiphyseal dysplasia, thus indicating the "cause" of the precocious osteoarthrosis in the father. The boy's sister is also affected. Inheritance is autosomal dominant. The father's father and brother and several children of the brother are similarly affected.

hips, and shoulders, are also common. In young patients a diagnosis of bilateral Legg-Perthes disease is often made, and older patients may be diagnosed as having precocious osteoarthritis of the hips.[440] Dwarfing usually is not severe, and adult heights are usually in the range of 135 to 150 cm; some affected persons are over 5 feet tall. The hands may be slightly short and stubby, as are the feet. The first manifestation of this disorder may be mild short stature associated with epiphyseal ossification delay. The abnormalities in gait and joint motion, as well as the characteristic radiographic changes, may not occur until midchildhood. Premature osteoarthropathy of the hips develops well before 30 years of age.[597]

The radiographic findings consist of bilateral symmetric irregularity and underdevelopment of epiphyseal ossification centers. Changes in the hips, knees, and ankles are most severe; changes in the upper limbs are milder. Deficiency in the lateral part of the distal tibial epiphyses, demonstrable in children, is expressed in adults as a sloping distal tibial articular surface.[343] There is delay in appearance of all secondary ossification centers of the tubular bones, hands, and wrists. With time the epiphyseal centers appear small, irregular, fragmented, and flattened as they ossify. The carpal and tarsal bones are irregular in shape and ossification. The short tubular bones of the hands and feet are short, with irregular epiphyses that may appear small and dense (ivory epiphyses). The vertebrae are usually normal but may show mild irregularity of the end plates with anterior wedging and Schmorl nodes by the second and third decades. This disorder has frequently been confused with bilateral avascular necrosis of the capital femoral epiphyses (Legg-Perthe disease) and Meyer dysplasia. Magnetic resonance imaging studies have shown that most patients do have changes compatible with avascular necrosis superimposed on the dysplastic femoral heads.[358,365] Arthrography and MRI show normal anlage of the capital femoral epiphyses with decreased joint space volume.[268,312]

The severe form of the disease, known as multiple epiphyseal dysplasia, Fairbank type, is inherited as an autosomal dominant trait. A milder form of the disease, in which the hips are primarily involved, has been termed the Ribbing form of multiple epiphyseal dysplasia.[467] It is not clear

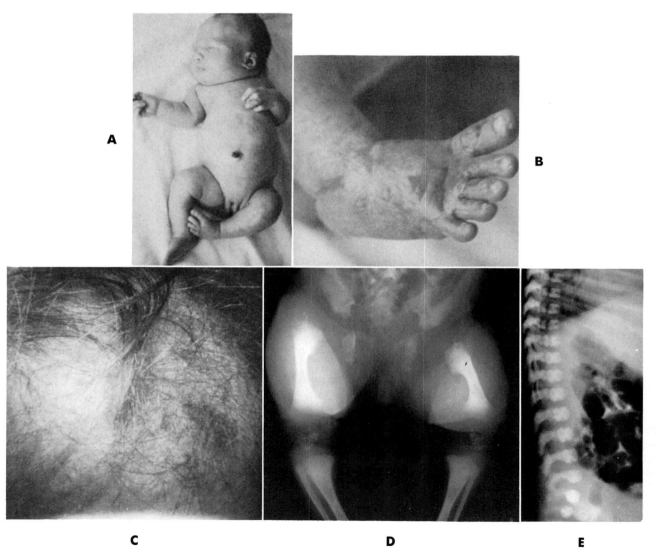

Fig. 14-41. Chondrodysplasia punctata, rhizomelic form. **A** and **B,** Appearance at birth. Extensive skin lesions and contractures of the fingers are shown. **C,** Appearance at the age of 2¾ years of age. Stringy hair and scaly skin of the scalp are shown. **D,** Anteroposterior view of the pelvis and lower extremities revealing multiple stippled calcifications in areas of epiphyses and apophyses with significant rhizomelia (short femurs). **E,** Lateral view of spine in an infant, showing coronal clefting without punctate calcification in vertebrae.

whether these two disorders represent phenotypic variability or heterogeneity. Rare, apparently autosomal recessive forms of multiple epiphyseal dysplasia associated with other clinical features have also been reported.[354]

Chondrodysplasia Punctata (Stippled Epiphyses) Group

Chondrodysplasia punctata is the term used for a group of disorders that had been variously termed Conradi-Hünermann syndrome, chondrodystrophia calcificans congenita, epiphyseal dysplasia punctata, or stippled epiphyses. A variety of distinct genetic disorders with stippled epiphyses have been described and fall under this classification. In addition, stippled and fragmented epiphyses can occur with other disorders such as the cerebrohepatorenal syndrome of Zellweger, the Smith-Lemli-Opitz syndrome, cretinism, trisomy 18, and fetal exposure to warfarin. Features common to many of these entities include stippled epiphyses, hypoplastic nasal bridge, cataracts, and icthyosiform dermatosis.[552]

Chondrodysplasia punctata, rhizomelic type. The rhizomelic type, also known as the recessive form of chondrodysplasia punctata, is associated with symmetric rhizomelic short-limb dwarfism, craniofacial dysmorphism with flat face, upward-slanting palpebral fissures, microcephaly, micrognathia, and depressed to absent bridge of the nose[552] (Fig. 14-41, *A* to *C*). Cataracts are present in approximately 70% of these individuals, and they frequently have an icthyosiform skin lesion and alopecia. Joint contractures are common. Affected infants are quite irritable, and we have found that this irritability can be ameliorated by analgesics, suggesting that there may be significant bone pain. The disorder is usually fatal in the first year of life, but survival past 10 years of age has been documented. In patients who survive, there is a high frequency of spastic tetraplegia, in addition to psychomotor retardation, growth failure, seizures, thermoregulatory instability, feeding difficulties, recurrent otitis media, and pneumonia.[625] Optic atrophy has also been described.[128]

Radiographic features include symmetric shortening of the proximal long bones (especially the femurs) and other long bones[150] (Fig. 14-41, *D* and *E*). There are punctate calcific deposits in the infantile cartilaginous skeleton and periarticular re-

gions, mild to absent stippling of the axial skeleton, and infrequently, laryngeal and tracheal calcification. Stippling gradually disappears in the first year of life, and the residual changes evident on radiographs resemble those of an epiphyseal dysplasia. Coronal clefts of the vertebrae are present.

The rhizomelic form of chondrodysplasia punctata has been reported in multiple sibs, often with parental consanguinity, indicating autosomal recessive inheritance. This disorder has been found to be associated with peroxisomal abnormalities.[220,459] In contrast to the other peroxisomal defects, in which peroxisomes are either abnormal or deficient or have a single enzyme deficiency, the rhizomelic form of chondrodysplasia punctata has been associated with multiple enzyme deficiencies, abnormalities in plasmalogen synthesis, and phytanic acid oxidation.[20,535,586] Peroxisomal structure appears to be normal by electron microscopy.[210] Thus the basic defect that results in the peroxisomal dysfunction is still unclear.

Chondrodysplasia punctata, Conradi-Hünermann type. The Conradi-Hünermann type is a less severe form of chondrodysplasia punctata than the rhizomelic form, but it is also associated with the peculiar facies resulting from the severe hypoplastic nasal bridge (koala-bear appearance), ichthyosiform erythroderma, and cataracts[524,552] (Fig. 14-42, *A*). Limb asymmetry is the major distinguishing feature of this skeletal dysplasia from other hereditary skeletal dysplasias. This disorder had long been considered to be inherited as an autosomal dominant trait, but it is now clear that it represents the X-linked dominant form of chondrodysplasia punctata.[196,274,410]

The major clinical features are the craniofacial dysmorphism, especially the frontal bossing and flat nasal bridge. Skin changes are characterized by icthyosiform erythroderma in a linear blotchy pattern and alopecia. The nails may be flattened and split. The limbs are asymmetrically shortened, and foot contractures or foot deformities may be present. Scoliosis is secondary to the limb asymmetry or vertebral anomalies, or both.

Radiographic manifestations include mild, frequently asymmetric shortening of all long bones and punctate calcific deposits in the infantile cartilaginous skeleton, including the spinal column, sternum, rib ends, coracoid processes and glenoid fossa of the scapulae, the carpal and tarsal bones,

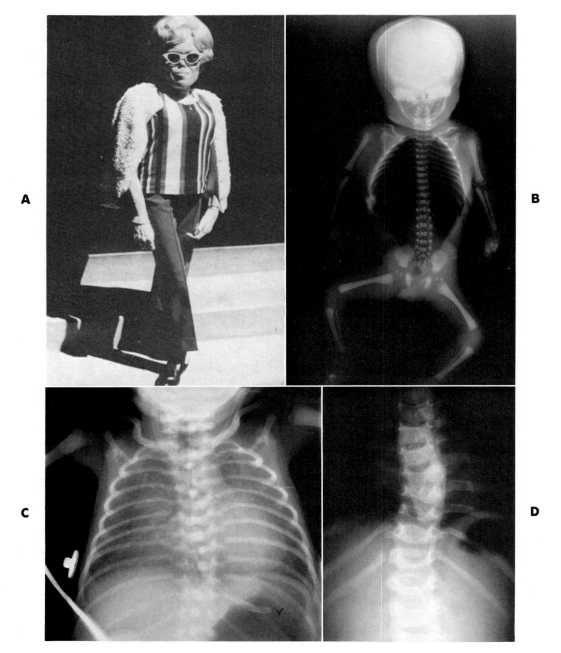

Fig. 14-42. Chondrodysplasia punctata, Conradi-Hünermann type. **A,** In a 33-year-old woman. She showed a short left femur, unusual facies, lesions of the skin (described at birth as red, thick, and covered with cream-covered horny plaques), and cataracts. The woman, who is of normal intelligence, is wearing a wig (the hair is sparse), is concealing her short left leg, and shows characteristic "koala bear" facies. She has considerable scoliosis and generalized ichthyosiform skin lesions. This is the X-linked dominant form of chondrodysplasia punctata. **B,** Anteroposterior full-body postmortem radiograph of newborn revealing multiple stippled ossification centers at the hips and in the sacrum, sagittal clefted vertabrae, and femurs and humeri of normal length. Anteroposterior view of throracic spine and chest, **C,** in the newborn period and, **D,** at 7 years of age, revealing vertebral ossification defects and clefting that later developed into vertebral body hypoplasia defects and secondary scoliosis. (Patient in **A** studied by Dr. Charles I. Scott, Jr.)

ischium, pubis, iliac bone and hyoid, as well as in the soft tissues surrounding joints, the epiphyseal centers, and the cartilage of the trachea and larynx (Fig. 14-42, *B* to *D*). There can be multiple dense calcifications of the vertebrae in infancy, in contrast to the coronal clefts and lack of calcification in the rhizomelic form of the disease. Chondroosseous morphologic study shows pathologic calcification foci in areas of chondrocyte clusters and fibrous scarring of the growth plate.[470]

The X-linked form of chondrodysplasia punctata appears to be homologous to the bare patches (Bpa) mutant in the mouse, which maps between G6PD and MDX.[196] The bare patches trait is tightly linked to the murine X-linked visual pigment genes, lending support for the idea that this disorder in humans is located on Xq28.[216] Whether abnormalities in peroxisomal function have been found in any true cases of this syndrome is controversial.[460]

Chondrodysplasia punctata, X-linked recessive type. Chondrodysplasia punctata, X-linked recessive type is a rare disorder that maps to the distal end of the short arm of the X chromosome. Curry et al.[91] observed a kindred in which two affected brothers and one of their maternal uncles were affected. Hypoplasia of the distal phalanges appears to be a distinctive feature. At birth the skin is bright red with generalized scales that desquamate in large sheets. The skin lesion subsequently has the appearance of ichthyosis. Radiographic manifestations resemble Conradi-Hünermann type, with diffuse stippling of epiphyseal, paravertebral, laryngeal, and tracheal areas and rapid disappearance of the stippling. There is hypoplasia of the distal phalanges. Carrier females have normal radiographs. Petit et al.[448] described a four-generation family with this disorder with an interstitial deletion in Xp22.3. Maroteaux[370] described four cases of chondrodysplasia punctata with hypoplasia of the distal phalanges of the fingers and moderate growth disturbances. All of his cases were males, suggesting that the distal phalangeal hypoplasia may represent a marker of the X-linked recessive form of the disorder.

Other forms of chondrodysplasia punctata. Various different genetic and acquired forms of chondrodysplasia punctata have been defined. Rittler et al.[479] described seven patients with an apparently distinct form of chondrodysplasia punctata

associated with flat midface and nose, short limbs, and otherwise normal development. Consistent radiologic manifestations were discrete calcific stippling, coronal clefts of the vertebral bodies, short tibiae, and shortness of the second and third metacarpals. The shortening of the metacarpal bones and tibiae suggests a distinct form of this disease (M-T type). Sheffield et al.[508] described a relatively mild form of chondrodysplasia punctata that may represent yet another distinct type.

Warfarin embryopathy has been well defined as a form of chondrodysplasia punctata associated with nasal bone hypoplasia in infants whose mothers had received warfarin therapy for anticoagulation.[449,507] Harrod and Sherrod[203] demonstrated that warfarin embryopathy can show familial aggregation; two sibs exposed to prenatal warfarin for treatment of thrombophlebitis showed signs, whereas a third sib from a pregnancy not exposed to intrauterine warfarin was unaffected. Stippled or fragmented epiphyses can be found in a variety of other syndromes, including the Zellweger syndrome, Smith-Lemli-Opitz syndrome, cretinism, trisomies, and the like.

Metaphyseal Dysplasias

The metaphyseal dysplasias group of disorders is associated with irregular, widened, and frayed metaphyses with relatively normal vertebrae. A variety of distinct disorders have been described, several of which are well defined; a group of less well-defined and less frequent disorders were reviewed by Taybi and Lachman.[588]

Metaphyseal dysplasia, Jansen type. Metaphyseal dysplasia, Jansen-type, which is quite rare, has severe abnormalities of all metaphyses, including those of the hands and feet.[72,262] The patients are severely dwarfed and have enlarged joints (Figs. 14-43 and 14-44). The arms are less shortened than the legs. The facial appearance, characterized by receding chin, hypertelorism, and prominent eyes, is striking.[169] Affected persons have a waddling gait, and contractural deformities of their joints develop, in particular, flexion of the hips and knees. There is gradual swelling of the joints, and the fingers are short and clubbed. The bowing of the legs results in a semisquatting stance in childhood. Hypercalcemia unassociated with parathyroid hyperplasia has been reported.

On radiographs the base of the skull is undeveloped and sclerotic, with brachycephaly and prom-

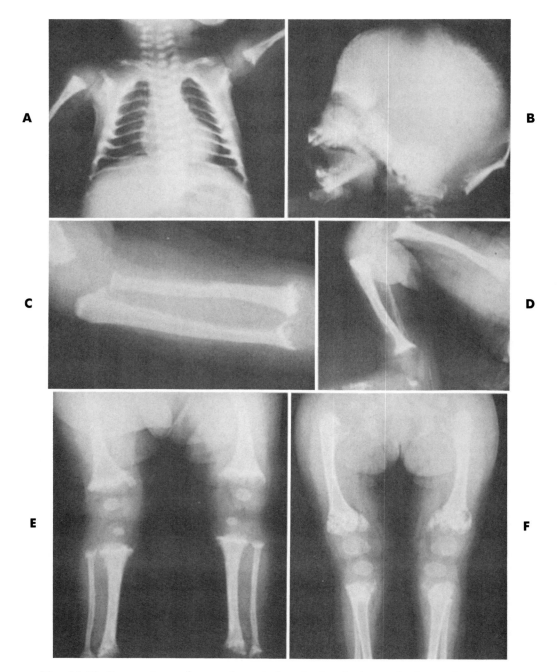

Fig. 14-43. Jansen type of metaphyseal chondrodysplasia. **A,** Radiograph of an infant at the age of 4 days. Irregularity of metaphyses, spindly, deformed ribs with fractures, and fetal demineralization are shown. **B,** At the age of 4 days the calvaria shows a peculiar reticular pattern. **C** and **D,** At the age of 4 days rachitiform changes and subperiosteal new bone formation and resorption are demonstrated. **E,** At 6 months of age the changes are suggestive of rickets, except that bone density is increased. **F,** At 5 years of age the gross changes in the metaphyses are typical of those described for this disorder. This patient had hypercalcemia and was twice explored for parathyroid abnormality, with negative results. (Courtesy Dr. John F. Holt, Ann Arbor, Mich.)

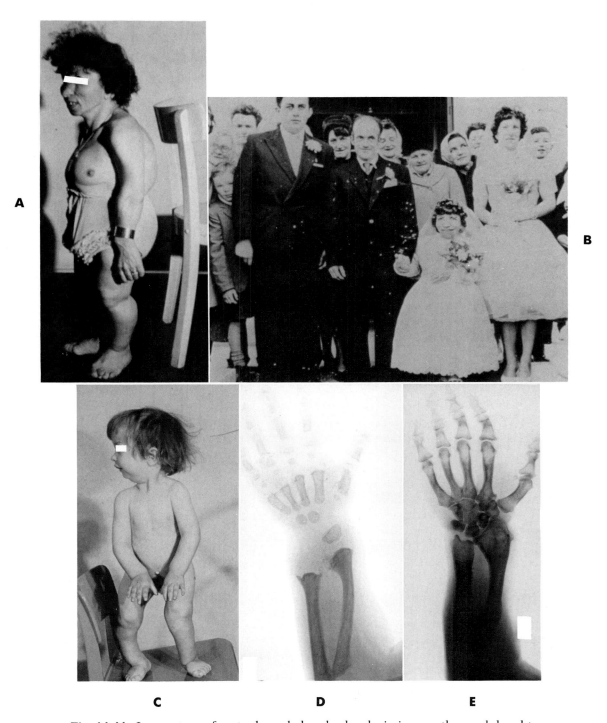

Fig. 14-44. Jansen type of metaphyseal chondrodysplasia in a mother and daughter. **A,** General appearance of the mother, who had a height of 102 cm. **B,** Wedding picture showing the mother with spouse of normal stature. **C,** Affected daughter. The small chin is characteristic. **D,** Radiograph of the arm and the hand of the daughter. **E,** Radiograph of the arm and the hand of the mother.   *Continued.*

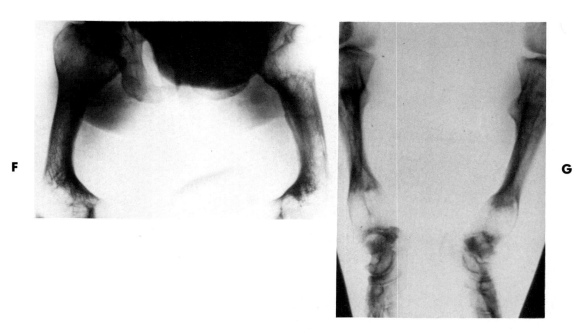

Fig. 14-44, cont'd. F, Radiograph of the femora of the mother. **G,** Radiograph of the legs of the mother. Remarkable "healing" of the metaphyseal lesions is demonstrated. The areas of bones that were previously the sites of striking lesions are now expanded and abnormally radiolucent. (From Lenz WD. In Bergsma D, editor: *Clinical delineation of birth defects. IV. Skeletal dysplasias,* New York, 1969, National Foundation, March of Dimes.)

inent supraorbital ridges and zygomatic arches (Figs. 14-43 and 14-44). Hypoplasia and irregular mineralization of the mandibles have been reported. The metaphyses are markedly expanded and cupped, with extensive irregularity of mineralization. Later, they appear to show large areas of nonossified cartilage mixed with scattered islands of bone and calcification. The epiphyses are relatively normal. The diaphyses are short and broadened. There is bowing of the lower limbs and short tubular bones, with wide distances between the epiphyses and the metaphyses. Irregular mineralization can also be seen in the anterior rib ends, acetabular and glenoid areas, and other areas of the shoulder and pelvic girdles. Dwarfism and skeletal deformities persist in adult life, but there is marked improvement in the appearance of bone texture in the metaphyseal regions.[94,532] Sclerosis in the cranial bones leads to deafness in some cases. This disorder has been found in an affected parent and child, indicating autosomal dominant inheritance.[345]

Metaphyseal dysplasia, Schmid type. The autosomal dominant disorder discussed in this section has been described in several families with multiple affected members, including the large Mormon kindred with dwarfism reported by Stephens[570] as having achondroplasia. The patients come to medical attention with short stature, bowed legs, and waddling gait in the second year of life[313,495] (Fig. 14-45, *A*). The degree of short stature relative to norms increases with age. Affected women have achieved successful vaginal delivery.

The radiographic manifestations include diffuse metaphyseal flaring and growth plate irregularity and widening, most severe at the knees[313] (Fig. 14-45, *B*). The capital femoral epiphyses appear enlarged, and coxa vara, femoral bowing, and an irregular acetabular roof are present. In contrast to cartilage-hair hypoplasia, the proximal femoral metaphyses are dysplastic. There is anterior cupping, splaying, and sclerosis of the ribs. The hands and vertebrae are normal.

Chondroosseous morphologic study shows clusters of hypertrophic cells surrounded by dense collagen with extension into the metaphyses, similar to that seen in the other metaphyseal dysplasias. Dilation of the rough endoplasmic reticulum containing a granular material has been reported,[85]

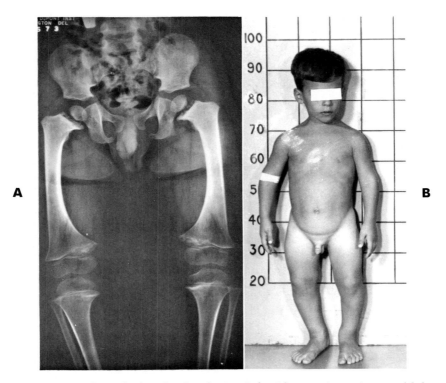

Fig. 14-45. Metaphyseal chondrodysplasia, Schmid type in a 6-year-old boy. **A,** Marked changes are seen at both ends of the femora, tibiae, and fibulae. The epiphyseal ossification centers are well formed; however, asymmetric, wedgelike medial involvement of the distal femur and proximal tibia results in genu varum. **B,** Appearance of the patient at the age of 6 years. The Harrison grooves are evident. (**A** courtesy Dr. G. Dean MacEwen, Wilmington, Del. From McKusick VA et al: *Bull Hopkins Hosp* 116:285, 1965.)

but this condition may have represented a form of spondylometaphyseal dysplasia.

Lachman, Rimoin, and Spranger[313] analyzed 20 cases and reviewed the literature. They suggested that metaphyseal dysplasia, Schmid type was often overdiagnosed. On radiographic and clinical examination this disorder has been confused at times with vitamin D–resistant rickets.[96] Advanced paternal age in sporadic cases has been noted, supporting autosomal dominant inheritance.[483]

An autosomal recessive form of metaphyseal chondrodysplasia that clinically resembles the Schmid type may exist. Spahr and Spahr-Hartmann[541] reported a family with radiographic changes closely similar to those of the Schmid type but with multiple affected sibs and consanguinity, indicating autosomal recessive inheritance.

Metaphyseal dysplasia, McKusick type (cartilage-hair hypoplasia). Metaphyseal dysplasia, McKusick type was first described by McKusick et al.[398] in the Old Order Amish. It is characterized by sparse, light-colored, fine hair and dwarfism, hence the term "cartilage-hair hypoplasia" (Fig. 14-46, *A*). The degree of dwarfism varies markedly, ranging from extremely short (under 105 cm) to close to 150 cm tall. The hair on microscopic study has abnormally small caliber.[282] In individuals born to families with dark, thick hair and dark complexion, the hair may appear brown and fairly normal in texture, but it does differ markedly from the parents' hair. The head and face are unaffected. The hands and feet are pudgy, with loose jointedness and foreshortened fingernails. Separation of the metacarpal phalangeal joints can be accomplished readily by pulling at the ends of the fingers (telescoping of the fingers). The elbows cannot be fully extended. Harrison grooves are present in the chest wall. Ankle deformity results from the excessive length of the fibula distally relative to the tibia. Bowed legs occur frequently but are less consistently present than in the Schmid type and are due to tibial-fibular rather than femoral curvature. Congenital intestinal malabsorption and megacolon may be present.

Susceptibility to severe and sometimes fatal varicella infection and a tendency to leukopenia have been reported, with impairment of thymus-derived cell (T-cell) function and defective bone marrow–derived cell (B-cell) proliferation.[202,356,453,455,611] There is some evidence that the frequency of malignancy, especially lympho-proliferative disease such as Hodgkin disease, is

increased in these patients.[134] Because of this propensity to severe varicella, the provision of varicella-zoster immune globin to patients exposed to chickenpox is important. It is our experience that patients who have normal immune function test results do not have an increased propensity to severe varicella.

Radiographic manifestations include flaring, cupping, fragmentation, and scalloping of the metaphyses of the tubular bones, most prominently in the knees (Fig. 14-46, B). Irregular cyst-like radiolucencies of the metaphyses may extend into the diaphyses. The shape of the epiphyses may be altered, corresponding to the deformed metaphyseal zones. Carpal and tarsal bones are small and irregular in contour. There is marked

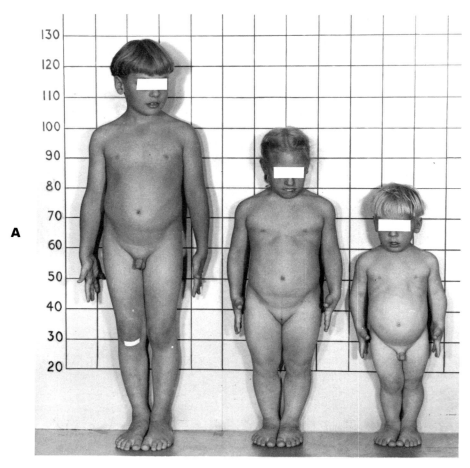

Fig. 14-46. Cartilage-hair hypoplasia. **A,** Three Amish children. *Left* to *right,* Unaffected 7-year-old boy; affected 9-year-old girl; affected 5-year-old boy. The affected children have Harrison grooves of the chest resembling those of rickets and have thin hair, which is lighter than that of the unaffected sibs.

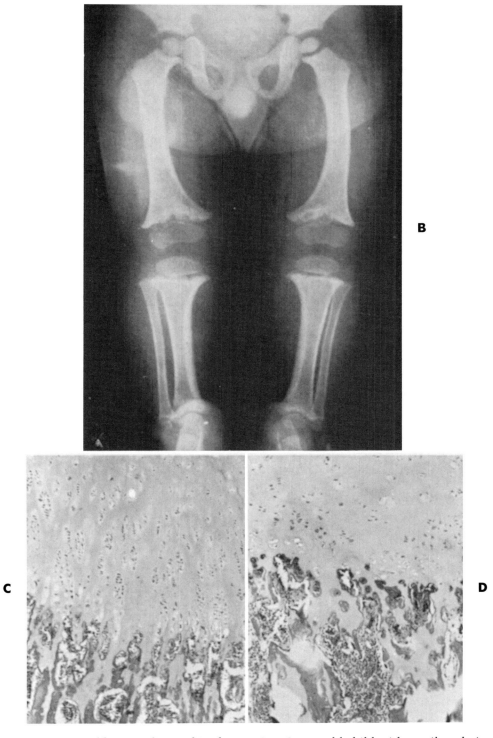

Fig. 14-46, cont'd. B, Radiographic changes in a 2-year-old child with cartilage-hair hypoplasia. The proximal femora are relatively spared. **C** and **D,** The finding of cartilage-hair hypoplasia on rib biopsy in a 5-year-old affected child, **D,** is contrasted with the normal findings, **C,** in a 5-year-old child with congenital heart disease. (From McKusick VA et al: *Trans Assoc Am Physicians* 77:51, 1964.)

shortening of the metacarpals, metatarsals, and phalanges. There may be metaphyseal cupping and mild cone-shaped epiphyses in the short tubular bones. The costochondral junctions are cupped and have cystlike radiolucencies. There is mild flaring of the lower rib cage and a short sternum. The vertebrae are often normal but may be somewhat small, with mild irregularity of the end plates. C1-2 vertebral subluxation has been described in this syndrome. We have observed one affected individual in whom quadriplegia developed after a fall. The femoral heads are small, and the femoral metaphyses are normal or only mildly involved, as compared with their significant involvement in the Schmid type. Chondroosseous morphologic study has demonstrated the same clustering of hypertrophic chondrocytes with extension into the metaphyses as that seen in the other metaphyseal dysplasias[398] (Fig. 14-46, *C* and *D*). Occurrence in multiple affected sibs with parental consanguinity indicates the autosomal recessive inheritance of this disorder.

Metaphyseal dysplasia with exocrine pancreatic insufficiency and cyclic neutropenia (Shwachman type). The syndrome discussed in this section is associated with growth retardation, metaphyseal dysplasia, and pancreatic insufficiency.[513,520,598] The onset of symptoms is in infancy, with low birth weight and growth retardation leading to short-limb dwarfism of moderate degree.[1] Malabsorption syndrome results from exocrine pancreatic insufficiency. Recurrent infections are frequent, associated with leukopenia or neutropenia, or both, and defective neutrophil chemotaxis. Respiratory distress has been described in the newborn.

On radiographs metaphyseal changes may be present in hips and knees, in particular, changes consisting of small lucent patches and sclerotic serrations at or adjacent to the provisional zone of calcification.[399] There is irregularity in the ossification of the anterior rib ends. Coxa vara and slipping of the capital femoral epiphyses may develop. The exocrine pancreas is replaced by fat, whereas the islets of Langerhans are normal. It is of interest that malabsorption and hematologic changes are also present in cartilage-hair hypoplasia, another form of metaphyseal dysplasia. Immune deficiencies and metaphyseal dysplasia are also found in adenosine deaminase deficiency.

Adenosine deaminase deficiency. Adenosine deaminase deficiency is the cause of one form of severe combined immunodeficiency disease in which there is dysfunction of both B and T lymphocytes with impaired cellular immunity and decreased production of immunoglobulins.[225] Metaphyseal dysplasia, especially of the ribs and long bones, has been described in adenosine deaminase deficiency. This would suggest that adenosine deaminase deficiency may be the defect in many cases reported as "achondroplasia and Swiss type agammaglobulinemia." These individuals have recurrent infections and failure to thrive and often die by 2 years of age. They exhibit a ricketic rosary, and their costochondral junctions appear widened and cupped. The long bone metaphyses are flared. Low levels of adenosine deaminase activity are found in peripheral blood cells and fibroblasts. Chondroosseous morphologic study demonstrates absence of the zone of proliferating cells, absent column formation, and irregular calcified cartilage with poor trabecular formation.[69,464] Reversal of both the immune defect and the metaphyseal changes can occur after treatment by means of bone marrow transplantation or red blood cell infusion.[285,456,654] This deficiency was the first disorder to be treated by means of somatic-cell gene therapy in the United States.

Brachyrachia (Short-Spine Dysplasia)

Brachyolmia. The brachyolmias are associated with short-trunk dwarfism; the major radiographic changes are present in the spine.[129,232] Affected individuals all have normal birth length, and marked short-trunk dwarfism first becomes apparent in early childhood. Scoliosis is frequent. The extremities appear relatively normal, but careful measurement may reveal shortening. At least three distinct types of brachyolmia have been defined[515] (Fig. 14-47). Type I (Hobaeck type) is inherited as an autosomal recessive trait and is associated with squared-off platyspondyly, narrow intervertebral spaces, marked end plate irregularity, and close-set pedicles on anteroposterior view. Toledo et al.[593] described a family with similar radiographic changes, but the affected patients also had corneal opacities and precocious anterior rib calcification. Whether this family represents a distinct entity or variability within the Hobaeck type is unknown. Type II, the Maroteaux type, differs

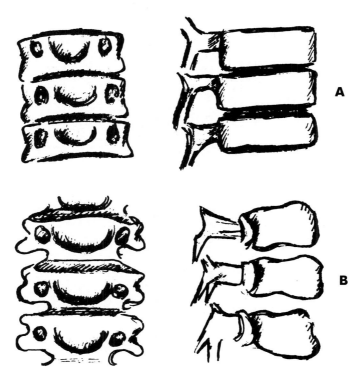

Fig. 14-47. Brachyolmia. Schematic representation of the characteristic radiographic features (anteroposterior and lateral views). **A,** Hobaeck type. Rectangular and elongated vertebral bodies are seen on lateral views. **B,** Maroteaux type. Rounding of the anterior and posterior vertebral borders with less elongation on lateral view. Both types show universal platyspondyly, reduced intervertebral spaces, and extension of the lateral margins of the vertebrae. (From Shohat M et al: *Am J Med Genet* 33:209-219, 1989.)

from type I in having rounded vertebral edges, mild end plate irregularity, and normal intervertebral disk spaces. Precocious falx cerebri calcification can be seen. Type III has been described in one family in which there was severe involvement of the vertebrae similar to that in type II, as well as severe cervical platyspondyly.[515] Type III was described in a mother and son, suggesting autosomal dominant inheritance.

Kozlowski et al.[301] stated that pure brachyolmia does not exist and that metaphyseal involvement may be minimal and scattered but is always present; the authors grouped these disorders with the spondylometaphyseal dysplasias. We consider that although minimal metaphyseal changes can be seen in some patients with brachyolmia, numerous persons have been documented in whom the metaphyses and epiphyses appear to

be perfectly normal. Chondroosseous morphologic appearance is nonspecific, with an irregular growth plate, somewhat short columns, and wide septae.[232,515]

Mesomelic Dysplasias

Mesomelic dysplasias are a heterogeneous group of bone dysplasias with disproportionate shortening of the middle segments of the limbs, with or without hand and foot involvement. Several of the well-characterized forms of the disease are illustrated in Fig. 14-48 and presented in Table 14-1. These forms can be differentiated from each other on the basis of the size and shape of the radius, ulna, tibia, and fibula and by the presence of involvement in the hands and feet or the type of involvement present. A variety of other syndromes associated with mesomelic shortening of the long

Table 14-1. Classification of mesomelic dysplasia

Feature	Dyschondrosteosis	Langer type	Nievergelt	Rheinhardt-Pfeiffer type	Werner type	Robinow type	Ellis-van Creveld type
Mode of inheritance	AD	AR	AD	AD	AD	AD	AR
Age at onset	Late childhood	Birth	Birth	Birth	Birth	Birth	Birth
Extent of short stature	Mild	Dwarfed	Dwarfed	Mild	Dwarfed	Mild	Moderate
Degree of shortening in upper and lower extremities	++/+	+++/+++	++/+++	+/+	-/+++	++/+/-	++/++
Acromelia	—	—	—	—	—	—	++
Radiologic changes							
Ulnae	Madelung deformity	Distal hypoplasia	Rhomboid	Distal hypoplasia	—	Distal hypoplasia	Short
Radii	Short and curved	Short and deformed; proximal hypoplasia	Rhomboid proximal dislocation	Flat and curved; proximal dislocation	—	Short; proximal dislocation	Short
Tibiae	Short	Short; proximal hypoplasia	Rhomboid	Short	Rudimentary	—	Short; proximal erosion
Fibulae	Short	Proximal hypoplasia; rudimentary	Rhomboid	Proximal hypoplasia; curved	Proximal dislocation	—	Short
Metacarpals and tarsals	(?)Short	—	Tarsal synostosis	—	(?)Fusion	—	Short
Phalanges	(?)Short	—	—	—	Polysyndactyly; thumb aplasia	—	Short and stubby
Other radiologic and clinical changes	Cubitus valgus; coxa valga; (?) exostoses; elbow contracture	Mandibular hypoplasia; ulnar deviation of hands	Radioulnar synostosis; elbow contracture; clubfoot	Bowing of forearm; ulnar deviation of hands; cutaneous dimple	Thick humerus; hypoplastic patella	Craniofacial dysmorphism; hypoplastic external genitalia; vertebral rib abnormalities	Acetabular changes; genu valgum; heart defect; narrow chest; ectodermal abnormalities

From Kaitila I et al: *Clin Orthop* 114:94, 1976.

Symbols signify marked (+++), moderate (++), and slight (+) shortening and proportionately normal size (−). *AD*, autosomal dominant: *AR* autosomal recessive.

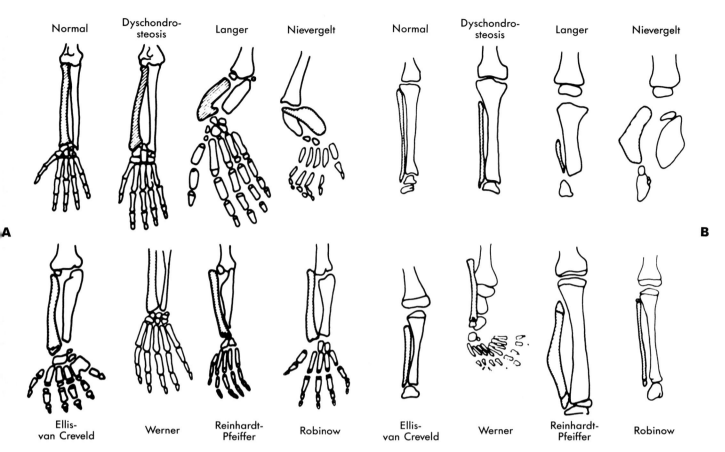

A

B

Fig. 14-48. Mesomelic dysplasias. A schematical presentation of the characteristic radiographic features of the various forms of mesomelic skeletal dysplasias. The drawings are from original case reports, which were of patients of various ages and therefore present developmental stages for each dysplasia. **A,** Right forearm and hand: normal adult; dyschondrosteosis, adult; Langer type, 4 years of age; Nievergelt type, 2½ years of age; Werner type, adult; Ellis-van Creveld type, 6 years of age; Reinhardt-Pfeiffer type, 14 years of age; and Robinow type, 5½ years of age. **B,** Right leg: normal, adult; dyschondrosteosis, adult; Langer type, 2½ years of age; Nievergelt type, 2 years of age; Werner type, 10 months of age; Ellis-van Creveld type, 6 years of age; Reinhardt-Pfeiffer type, 14 years of age; and Robinow type, 5½ years of age. (From Kaitilla et al: *Clin Orthop Rel Res* 114:94-106, 1976.)

bones has been reported.[588] Because of space limitations, only the most common of these disorders (dyschondrosteosis) are described in detail.

Dyschondrosteosis (Léri-Weill disease). Dyschondrosteosis is the mildest and most common form of mesomelic dysplasia. Characteristic of dyschondrosteosis are mesomelic dwarfism and a typical malformation of the distal radius and ulna (Madelung deformity)[26,215] (Fig. 14-49). The distal end of the ulna is hypoplastic and dorsally dislo-

cated; the distal radius is bowed.[14] The disorder was described and named by Léri and Weill in 1929. Langer[327] has postulated that most or all persons with bilateral congenital Madelung deformity have dyschondrosteosis. On the other hand, Felman and Kirkpatrick[122] concluded that patients with Madelung deformity who are above the 25th percentile for height probably do not have dyschondrosteosis, that isolated Madelung deformity occurs as a distinct genetic trait, and that marked shortening of the tibia relative to the fe-

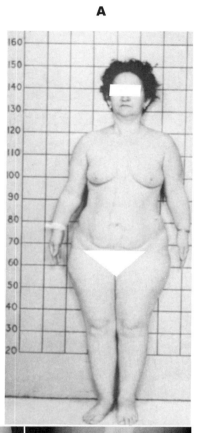

Fig. 14-49. Dyschondrosteosis, **A,** in 42-year-old woman. She is 145 cm tall and has a Madelung deformity of the distal forearms. Her mother and maternal grandmother and three of her five daughters are likewise short and have Madelung's deformity. **B,** Arms of her daughter, 21 years of age. Madelung's deformity is demonstrated. **C,** Anteroposterior radiograph of the forearm in a teenage girl, showing mesomelia with radial bowing and a Madelung-like deformity at the wrist.

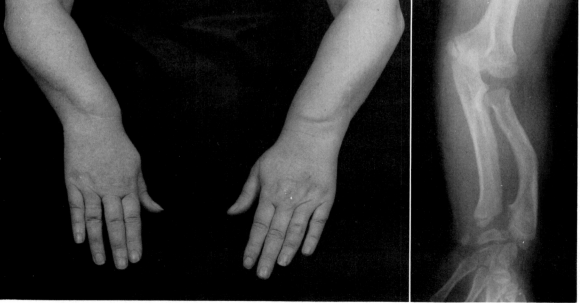

mur suggests dyschondrosteosis. These individuals have mild to moderate mesomelic dwarfism with shortness of the forearms and lower legs.[92] In addition to the Madelung deformity, there is limitation of motion of the elbow and wrist.

Radiographs show shortening and bowing of the radius, triangulation of the distal radial epiphyses, widening of the distance between the radius and ulna, wedging of carpal bones between the distal radius and ulna, and subluxation or posterior dislocation of the distal ulna (Fig. 14-49, *B* and *C*). Compared with the fibula, the tibia is shortened and mildly curved. Dyschondrosteosis must be distinguished from other disorders with Madelung-like deformity such as multiple exostoses, Turner syndrome, and acromesomelic dysplasia.

Dyschondrosteosis appears to be more common in females. Whether the inheritance is autosomal dominant or X-linked dominant is controversial, but clear instances of male-to-male transmission have been described.[349] McKusick[392] postulated that the apparent paucity of males may be due to incomplete ascertainment as a result of the milder clinical phenotype in males.

The homozygous state of the dyschondrosteosis gene apparently leads to a more severe condition known as "mesomelic dwarfism of the hypoplastic ulna, fibula, and mandible type" (Langer type).[113,141,308,330] There is severe hypoplasia of the ulna and fibula and a thick, curved radius and tibia. In several families reported with this disorder the parents were short and had various minor signs of dyschondrosteosis, variable degrees of Madelung deformity, and mesomelic shortening.[158] A large three-generation family has been described in which multiple members had mesomelic dysplasia; however, some had typical dyschondrosteosis, one had typical Reinhardt-Pfeiffer type, and a fetus had a severe form compatible with the Langer type.[596] These authors suggested that the various types of mesomelic dysplasia may not be distinct in origin.

Acromelic and Acromesomelic Dysplasias

The group of acromelic and acromesomelic dysplasias is associated with shortening of the limbs, primarily affecting the hands and feet (Figs. 14-50 to 14-52). The term "peripheral dysostosis" has been used in the past for this general group of disorders. Various distinct syndromes have now been defined in which distal (acro-) or a combination of

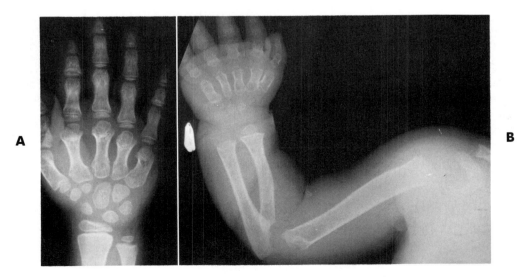

Fig. 14-50. Acromelic and acromesomelic dysplasias. **A,** Acrodysostosis. Anteroposterior view of hand and wrist, with generalized shortening of the tubular bones of the hand, some cone-shaped epiphyses, and otherwise normal epiphyseal development and ossification. **B,** Acromesomelic dysplasia. Anteroposterior radiograph of upper extremity, revealing changes similar to those in Fig. 14-50, **A,** as well as significant mesomelia.

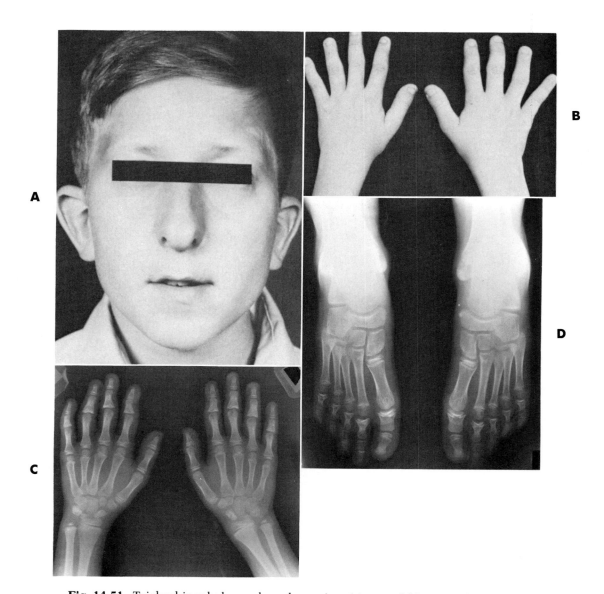

Fig. 14-51. Trichorhinophalangeal syndrome in a 14-year-old boy. **A,** The face shows sparse lateral eyebrows and characteristic nasal configuration. **B,** Photograph and, **C,** radiograph of hands. Cone-shaped epiphyses and crooked fingers are demonstrated. **D,** Radiograph of feet showing cone-shaped epiphyses.

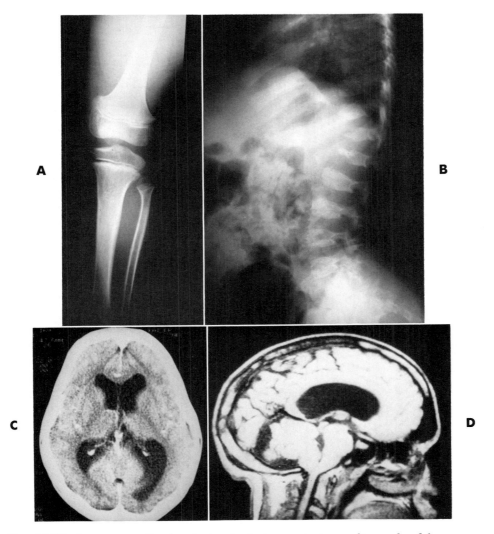

Fig. 14-52. Acromesomelic dysplasia. **A,** Anteroposterior radiograph of lower extremity, revealing mesomelia with normal epiphyses and metaphyses (see Fig. 14-50, **B**). **B,** Lateral radiograph of spine showing upper lumbar anterior vertebral body hypoplasia, pointing, and posterior wedging and scalloping. **C,** Computed tomographic scan and, **D,** magnetic resonance imaging of the brain, showing significant communicating hydrocephalus with bony intrusion of the posterior lip of the foramen magnum up into the posterior fossa.

distal and mesomelic (middle-segment) shortening of the limbs occurs (Fig. 14-50). The clinical radiographic, pathologic, and genetic features of these conditions are outlined in Table 14-2. The conditions can be differentiated primarily on the basis of the type of radiographic abnormality in the hand and wrist (Fig. 14-50), the presence of long bone and vertebral abnormalities, and a variety of

extra skeletal manifestations, in particular, peculiar facies. The trichorhinophalangeal dysplasias have received a great deal of attention because of the presence of a cytogenetic abnormality in the long arm of chromosome 8 and are discussed separately. Geleophysic dysplasia is associated with lysosomal vacuolization of numerous organs, including the liver, heart, and bronchi.[516,559] Geleo-

Table 14-2. Acromelic and acromesomelic dysplasias

Disorder	Clinical features			
	Stature	Hands	Feet	Other
Acromicric dysplasia	Short after 2 years	Small; limited finger flexion	Small	Unusual facies
Geleophysic dysplasia	Short	Small; tight skin; small nails	Small	"Happy" facies; hepatosplenomegaly; cardiac failure; tracheal narrowing; joint contractures
Acrodysostosis	Short	Short	Small (+/−)	"Saddle" nose; hypertelorism; MR (+/−); hypogonadism
Trichorhinophalangeal I	Short	Short, crooked fingers	Short; polydactly, (+/−)	Sparse hair; lateral thin eyebrows; pear-shaped nose; long philtrum
Trichorhinophalangeal II (Langer-Giedion)	Short	Short	Short	Pear-shaped nose; long philtrum; sparse hair; microcephaly; MR; redundant skin
Saldino-Mainzer (acrodysplasia with RP and nephropathy)	Short	Short, especially, middle phalanges	Short	Nephropathy with renal failure; retinitis pigmentosa; ataxia
Albright hereditary osteodystrophy (pseudohypoparathyroidism)	Mild shortening	Short fourth metatarsal	Short fourth metacarpal	Round face; MR (+/−); subcutaneous calcification; hypocalcemia (+/−); PTH unresponsiveness; impaired olfaction (+/−)
Acromesomelic dysplasia	Very short	Short, stubby fingers	Short; large first toe	Prominent head; short nose; short limbs; thoracic kyphosis; lumbar lordosis
Grebe dysplasia	Very short; tiny limbs	Very short, broad, toe-like fingers	Very short, rudimentary toes	Valgus deformity of forearms and feet

CFE, Capital femoral epiphyses; *MR,* mental retardation; *PTH,* parathyroid hormone; *RP,* retinitis pigmentosa.

physic dysplasia appears to be a lysosomal storage disorder, although the biochemical defect has not yet been defined.

Trichorhinophalangeal dysplasias. Trichorhinophalangeal dysplasias have been categorized into types I and II, primarily on the basis of the latter syndrome being associated with exostoses. Giedion[147] first delineated this syndrome, which has abnormalities of the hair (sparse and slow growing on the head and entire body, with early balding and sparse, lateral eyebrows), the nose (pear shaped, with a long philtrum), and the fingers (crooked, with cone-shaped epiphyses) (Fig. 14-51). Giedion's patient had two supernumerary incisors. Gidion confirmed two previous reports; in each report two sibs were affected, and the parents were consanguineous in one, suggesting autosomal recessive inheritance.[148] In the fourth edition of this book, McKusick[391] reported two af-

Radiographic features				Pathologic features	Mode of inheritance
Phalanges	**Metacarpals**	**Long bones**	**Other**		
Short; cone-shaped epiphyses	Short proximal pointing; first pseudoepiphysis	Short; flat CFE		Abnormal growth plate	AD
Short; broad proximal	Short; proximal pointing (+/−)	Short	J-shaped sella	Lysosomal vacuolization	AR
Short; cone epiphyses	Short, especially, first		Brachycephaly; hypoplastic nasal bone		AD
Cone-shaped epiphyses; "ivory" epiphyses	Short	Legg Perthes (+/−)	Midface hypoplasia		AD; AR; 8q deletion
Short; cone-shaped epiphyses; exostoses	Short exostoses	Exostoses; Legg Perthes (+/−)	Cerebral atrophy		Sporadic; 8q24 deletion
Cone-shaped short middle phalanges	Short, especially, middle phalanges	Flat CFE			AR
	Short fourth metacarpal and metatarsal		Reduced renal size and concentrating ability		AD; (?)XL;AR
Very short; cone-shaped epiphyses; large first toes	Very short; cone-shaped epiphyses	Short, especially, radius and ulna; dislocated radial head	Beaked vertebrae; scaphocephalic skull		AR
Very hypoplastic or absent	Hypoplastic	Short to absent			AR

fected families. In one, occurrence in a grandfather, son, and grandson with no consanguinity seems to make autosomal dominant inheritance a certainty. In the other, a brother and sister were affected and the parents were consanguineous. All these cases fit into trichorhinophalangeal dysplasia type I without exostoses.

Trichorhinophalangeal dysplasia type II is also known as the Langer-Giedion syndrome.[149,333] This disorder has similarities to TRP I, particularly with regard to the facies, the bulbous nose, sparse hair, and cone-shaped epiphyses. Distinguishing features are multiple exostoses, mental retardation, microcephaly, and redundant skin. Inconsistent features include hyperextensible joints, recurrent upper respiratory tract infections, and delayed speech development. Affected infants may be "floppy." The exostoses can be quite striking.

All cases have been sporadic, and the majority have been in males. In 1980 Beuhler et al.[57] reported the case of a teen-aged girl with features suggestive of Langer-Giedion syndrome associated with terminal deletion of 8q (the band q24 was missing from one chromosome 8). Pfeiffer[450] described deletion of segment q13-22 of the long arm of chromosome 8 in a mentally retarded boy with Langer-Giedion syndrome. In addition, this patient had colobomata of the iris and a defect of the fourth and fifth fingers. Since then, a variety of chromosomal abnormalities involving the region of 8q2-8q24 has been described. Buhler et al.[59] concluded that the Langer-Giedion syndrome was due to a deletion extending from 8q24.11 to 8q24.13. Abnormalities in this region have also been described in patients with trichorhinophalangeal dysplasia type I.[142] It has been speculated that the Langer-Giedion syndrome is a consequence of a deletion or other mutation of two or more independent adjacent loci, one of which causes exostoses and the other, trichorhinophalangeal dysplasia.[59] The area postulated to be involved in the trichorhinophalangeal phenotype is a small segment, 8q24.12.[123] It has also been postulated that this region must, therefore, be responsible for the dominant syndrome of multiple exostoses. Apparently, cosegregation of multiple exostoses syndrome with 8q has been documented in some families, but discordance has been claimed in others, suggesting genetic heterogeneity.

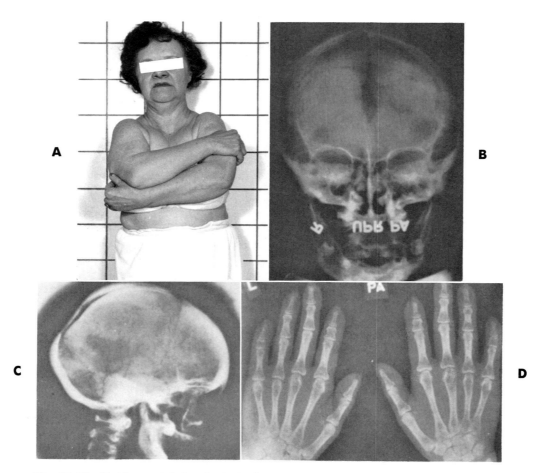

Fig. 14-53. Cleidocranial dysplasia in four generations of a kindred studied by Dr. Raymond Pearl and his colleagues in 1929 (unpublished). Demonstrated here are findings in a 58-year-old woman. **A,** Rather prominent forehead and ease of adduction of shoulders are shown. **B** and **C,** Wide sutures, especially the sagittal, patent anterior fontanelle, and occipital wormian bones are evident. She is almost edentulous. **D,** Short second and fifth middle phalanges are shown, as in Fig. 14-54. The mother of this woman was affected, and she has an affected son and grandson. Affected members of this kindred are short in stature.

Dysplasias with Significant (But Not Exclusive) Membranous Bone Involvement

Cleidocranial dysplasia. Cleidocranial dysplasia, previously known as cleidocranial dysostosis, is characterized by defective development of the skull, with multiple wormian bones and delay in closure of the sutures; the clavicles and pubic bones are hypoplastic or absent, and the symphysis pubis is wide[131,255,273] (Figs. 14-53 and 14-54). Spina bifida occulta in the lower cervical and upper thoracic spine and wide sacroiliac joints are frequent findings.[262] The acetabula may be hypoplastic and associated with hip dislocation. There may be respiratory distress in the newborn due to thoracic cage deformity. The head is large and brachycephalic with large fontanelles and wide sutures in infancy and delay of suture closure. The face is small, and there is a saddle-type nose. Dental eruption is delayed, there is dental impaction, and supernumerary teeth may be present. The teeth can have multiple caries, which can lead to early loss of the permanent teeth. Mobility of

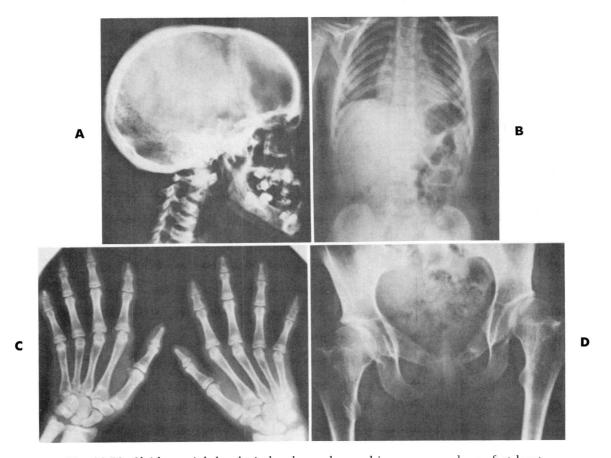

Fig. 14-54. Cleidocranial dysplasia has been observed in many members of at least three generations. **A,** Wide lambdoidal sutures with multiple wormian bones are demonstrated. **B,** Hypoplasia of the clavicles, which are in two parts, is evident in this 7-year-old child. Some affected members of the family have a severe anomaly of the lower cervical and upper thoracic spine. **C,** Short middle phalanges in the second and fifth fingers and tapered terminal phalanges in this 19-year-old patient are evident. **D,** Hypoplasia of the pubis and ischium with separation at the pubic symphysis can be seen in this 17-year-old patient. The acetabula, especially the left, are shallow. Dislocation of the hip has occurred in several affected members of the family.

shoulders is marked as a result of absence or hypoplasia of the clavicles, permitting excessive facility in opposing the shoulders. The chest is narrow. An abnormal gait and mild shortness of stature may be features.

Radiographic manifestations include a brachycephalic skull with increased biparietal diameter, frontal bossing, widely spaced sutures, multiple wormian bones, absent parietal bone ossification, and an anterior fontanel that remains open into adulthood. The posterior occipital synchondrosis can persist until 4 to 5 years of age. A variety of facial bone abnormalities may occur. There is persistence of the synchondrosis between the vertebral bodies and neural arches and posterior wedging of the thoracic vertebrae. Spina bifida and kyphoscoliosis may develop. The ribs are short, with a prominent downward slope, and only 11 pairs of ribs may be present. There is total aplasia or partial aplasia of the clavicles with small scapulae. Various abnormalities of the bones of the hands occur, including unequal size of the metacarpals, short middle phalanges, pseudoepiphyses, and cone-shaped epiphyses. There is absent or delayed ossification of pubic bones, wide symphysis pubis, and underdeveloped vertical hypoplastic iliac wings. This abnormality in the pelvis can result in cephalopelvic disproportion and can cause severe dystocia. There is delay in deciduous dentition with slow appearance of permanent teeth, some remaining unerupted.

Cleidocranial dysplasia has been well documented as a dominant trait in several large, extensively affected families.[256] Apparent autosomal recessive cleidocranial dysplasia, sometimes associated with abnormalities of the thumbs and a variety of unusual hand malformations, has been reported.[159,451,655] Sillence et al.[528] have described cleidocranial dysplasia in mice, which appears to be a true model of the human disease. The mutation was radiation induced and inherited as an autosomal dominant trait with variable expressivity. The homozygous state was lethal in utero.

Osteodysplasty (Melnick-Needles syndrome).
Melnick and Needles[402] described families with individuals in multiple generations who had a severe congenital bone disorder characterized by typical facies (exophthalmos, full cheeks, micrognathia, and malalignment of the teeth), flaring of the metaphyses of the long bones, S-like curvature of the bones of legs, irregular constrictions in the

ribs, and sclerosis of the base of the skull. The term "osteodysplasty" was suggested by Coste, Maroteaux, and Chourakii[88] for this condition. The radiographic features of this syndrome include sclerosis of the base of the skull and mastoids; delay in closure of the anterior fontanelle; micrognathia; tall vertebrae with anterior concavity of the thoracic vertebrae; cortical irregularity and ribbonlike appearance of the ribs; cortical irregularity and flaring of the clavicles; flared iliac wings with flat acetabular roofs; metaphyseal flaring of short and long bones with long femoral necks; and a delay in general ossification.[162] The majority of cases reported have been in females, and apart from one doubtful instance, no male-to-male transmission has been reported.[34] Krajewska-Walasek, Winkielman, and Gorlin[304] found six examples of this syndrome in males: there were three well-documented lethal examples of this disorder among the offspring of affected females and three in males born to normal parents, presumably representing new mutations. The supposition is that this syndrome is inherited as an X-linked dominant trait lethal in males.[101] Beighton and Hamersma[34] speculated that frontometaphyseal dysplasia and Melnick-Needles syndrome may be due to mutations in the same gene.

Bent-Bone Dysplasia Group

The bent-bone dysplasia group of disorders is characterized by bending of the long bones. A number of cases have been described in which simple congenital bowed bones can occur without other features.[12] In addition, bending of the long bones can be seen in a variety of syndromes that result in decreased strength of the bones, such as osteogenesis imperfecta and hypophosphatasia.[287,517] At least three distinct genetic syndromes associated with bending of the long bones have been described; differentiation is based on whether the bones are short or long and on associated malformations.

Campomelic dysplasia (long-limb type). The disorder discussed in this section is the classic form of campomelic dysplasia associated with congenital bowing and angulation of the long bones, together with other skeletal and extraskeletal defects.[183,246] The designation "campomelic" or "camptomelic dwarfism" was proposed by Maroteaux et al.[379] because of the bowing of the legs, especially the tibias. Cleft palate, micrognathia, flat face, and hypertelorism are frequently present. Most patients die of respiratory distress in the neonatal period. Lee, Issacs, and Strauss[342] described three cases, emphasizing tracheobronchial hypoplasia as a significant factor in the neonatal respiratory deaths. Limbs are bent, and there can be a deep dimple over the apex of the bend. Generalized hypertonia and central nervous system abnormalities have been described. Polyhydramnios during pregnancy is a frequent feature. A variety of renal and cardiac defects have been encountered in some patients. This disorder is characterized by an excess of phenotypic females, which appears to be due to the frequent sex reversal in this condition, that is, XY individuals with female genitalia.[228,247]

Radiographic manifestations include an elongated skull with a high, flat forehead; hypoplasia and poor ossification of the cervical vertebrae; bell-shaped thorax with only 11 pairs of ribs; hypoplastic scapulae; contracted pelvis with narrow, tall iliac wings and a vertical-appearing pelvic outlet; and significant angulation and bending of the long bones, especially the femurs and tibias (Fig. 14-55, *A*). The fibula can be hypoplastic. There may be lack of ossification of the talus associated with talipes equinovarus. A case of campomelic dysplasia in a family with a balanced t5;8 translocation[83] has been described, leading to the speculation that the campomelic dysplasia gene may be at either 5q33.1 or 8q21.4. However, a case of campomelic dysplasia has been reported with a 17q paracentric inversion.[367] Multiple affected sibs have been described, which, together with parental consanguinity, indicates autosomal recessive inheritance.[144,246]

Kyphomelic dysplasia (campomelic dysplasia, short-limb normocephalic type). Kyphomelic dysplasia is associated with congenital bowing of short, broad bones, in contrast to the bowing of the longer, thinner bones associated with classic campomelic dysplasia.[182,287,361,590] The proximal parts of the limbs are most severely affected, particularly the femurs (Fig. 14-55, *B*). Significant skin dimples can be found over the apex of the

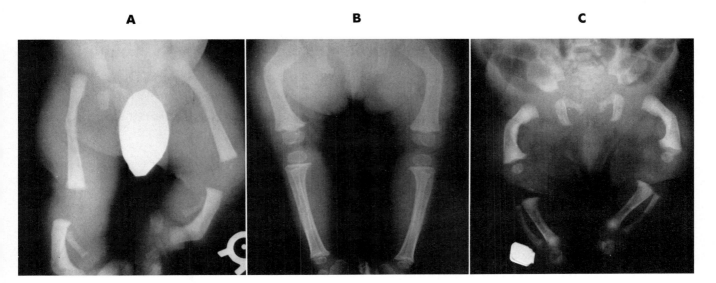

A   **B**   **C**

Fig. 14-55. Campomelic dysplasias. **A,** Classic campomelic dysplasia. Anteroposterior radiograph of pelvis and lower extremities, showing narrow, high iliac wings; long, bent femurs; short, bent tibiae; and hypoplastic fibulae. **B,** Kyphomelic dysplasia. Anteroposterior radiograph of hips and lower extremities shows short, bent femurs with mild distal femoral metaphyseal irregularity and relatively straight tibiae and fibulae. **C,** Stuve-Wiedemann type. Anteroposterior radiograph of pelvis and lower extremities, revealing normal pelvis, hypoplastic acetabular roofs, severe generalized micromelia with bent femurs, and relatively longer bowed fibulae and straight tibiae.

bends. In infancy the metaphyses are moderately flared and irregular, but they improve dramatically during childhood.[466] The ribs can be short, resulting in a narrowed chest and "pigeon breast." The peripheral joints show some limitation in motion. Mental development is normal. Disproportionate short stature persists as affected children get older. Although these patients can die in the neonatal period, survival is possible and leads to a relatively mild phenotype. Similar long-bone changes have been described in persons with craniosynostosis, who probably represent the Antley-Bixler syndrome.[13]

The first cases of short-limb campomelic dysplasia were described by Stuve and Wiedemann[581] in affected sisters (Fig. 14-55, *C*). These individuals had significantly shortened femurs, and the apex of the bend was toward the metaphyseal area, not the diaphyseal area as in campomelic and kyphomelic forms. The Stuve-Wiedemann type appears to represent a distinct disorder. All these various forms of campomelic dysplasia are apparently inherited as autosomal recessive traits.

Multiple Dislocations with Dysplasias

The group of disorders discussed here are characterized by severe loose-jointedness and short stature. These enter into the differential diagnosis of the Ehlers-Danlos syndrome, and they are discussed in Chapter 6.

Larsen syndrome. Larsen syndrome is characterized by severe loose-jointedness with multiple dislocations and a typical flat face.[245,337] The joint laxity is even more marked than that found in the severe forms of Ehlers-Danlos syndrome. This joint laxity can result in dislocated elbows and hips, as well as knees with severe genu recurvatum and a Z-shaped foot. The tibia is frequently dislocated anteriorly on the femur. The fingers are somewhat cylindric, with spatulate thumbs and short, broad fingertips. The severe dislocation of the ankle is often resistant to surgery for clubfoot. Dysmorphism of the cervical and thoracic spine leading to severe neurologic impairment has been reported. Hearing loss secondary to abnormality of the joint between the incus and stapes, as well as fixed stapes foot plates, has been described.[567] The major radiographic features are joint dislocations; accessory ossicles of the wrists and ankles; double or triple calcaneal ossification centers; short metacarpals, metatarsals, and distal phalan-

ges; spatulate thumb tufts; and abnormal segmentation of vertebrae. The frontal and facial bones are flattened, with shallow orbits, hypertelorism, and micrognathia. Both autosomal dominant[199,581] and autosomal recessive[568] forms of Larsen syndrome have been described. We have observed numerous cases of Larsen syndrome without characteristic facies. Several cases of Larsen syndrome associated with neonatal death have been described.[76,80,409] Whether these represent variability or heterogeneity remains to be determined.

Desbuquois syndrome. Desbuquois syndrome is a rare disorder associated with severe loose-jointedness and extra ossification centers in the hands, which produce extra phalanges and result in deviation of the fingers.[97] Coronal clefts of the vertebrae may be present; these and the extra ossification centers disappear with age. On radiographs the proximal femur has a characteristic "Swiss key" appearance associated with an enlarged trochanter.

Other features of Desbuquois syndrome may include generalized hypotonia and mental retardation. The syndrome has been reported in multiple affected sibs, suggesting autosomal recessive inheritance. Grischke et al.[173] described prenatal diagnosis of this syndrome by means of ultrasound in the 24th week of gestation, and Golbus[156a] has observed a case in which the characteristic hand malformations were detected by means of fetoscopy early in pregnancy.

Spondyloepimetaphyseal dysplasia with joint laxity. Spondyloepimetaphyseal dysplasia with joint laxity, first described in South Africa, is associated with short stature, joint laxity, and severe scoliosis.[37] The short stature is present at birth. The facies are characteristic, with an oval shape, prominent eyes, long upper lip, small mandible, and bluish sclerae. Cleft palate is present in some cases. Joint laxity is especially striking in the hands, which have short fingernails and spatulate terminal phalanges. Kyphoscoliosis develops at an early age and is progressive. Clubfoot and dislocated hips can be present. Death may occur in infancy because of congenital heart disease; in later childhood, intractible spinal malalignment can lead to fatal cardiorespiratory embarrassment. The skin may be soft, doughy, and stretchy, resembling that in Ehlers-Danlos syndrome.

Radiographic manifestations include platyspondyly with ovoid vertebrae and end plate irregularities.[37,297] Flared iliac wings, coxa valga, and delayed ossification of the capital femoral epiphyses are features, along with generalized epiphyseal ossification delay, radial head dislocations, widened metaphyses of long bones, and short tubular bones with metaphyseal irregularity. Multiple affected sibs and consanguinity have been reported, indicative of autosomal recessive inheritance.[37]

Osteodysplastic Primordial Dwarfism Group

This group of disorders is characterized by microcephaly and severe proportionate dwarfism.

Since the disorders do not appear to represent heritable disorders of connective tissue, they are not discussed here.

Syndromes Associated with Osteoporosis

The disorders associated with osteoporosis appear to be associated with defects in the osseous matrix. They are discussed in Chapter 8.

Dysplasia with Defective Mineralization

Dysplasias with defective mineralization are inborn errors of mineral metabolism resulting in osteomalacia and ricketlike changes. Since the disorders are not heritable disorders of connective

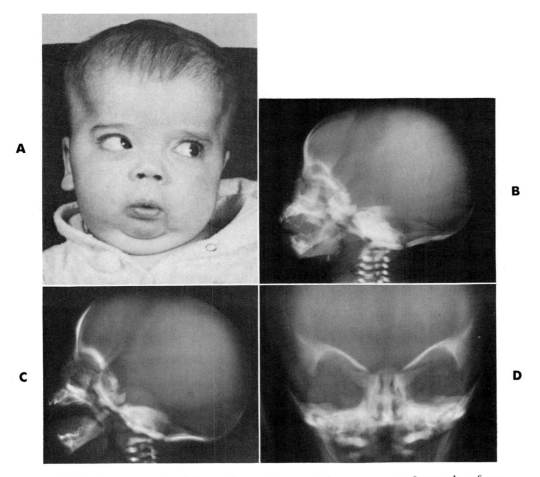

Fig 14-56. Osteopetrosis of the malignant type. **A,** Appearance at 9 months of age, showing frontal bossing. **B** and **D,** Skull at 12 days of age. The sutures are abnormally wide, and the density of all bones is increased, most particularly in the face, orbital roofs, base of the skull, and cervical vertebrae. **C,** Skull at about 3½ months of age. **D,** As seen in the frontal view, the orbits are harlequin-shaped, as in hypophosphatasia. *Continued.*

E   F   G   H

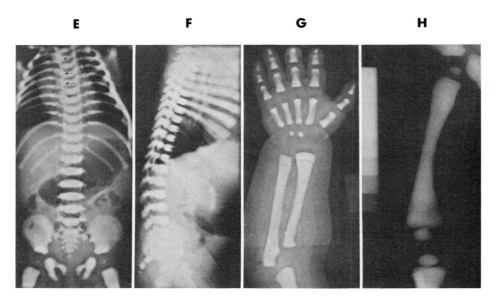

Figure 14-56, cont'd. **E** and **F,** Views of the trunk, taken of infant at 4 months of age, showing greatly increased bone density. The oval radiodensities indicated by the arrows are sternal ossification centers. In the lateral view, **F,** the vertebral bodies show prominent anterior vascular notches. **G,** The hand and forearm at about 10 months of age show classic changes of osteopetrosis, including the bone-within-bone appearance in metacarpals and phalanges. **H,** At 10 months of age the femur, like the distal radius and ulna, shows alternating zones of increased and decreased density. (From Avery ME, Dorst JP, Walker DG. In Bergsma D, editor: *Clinical delineation of birth defects. IV. Skeletal dysplasias,* New York, 1969, National Foundation, March of Dimes.)

tissue, they are not discussed here, the reader is referred to general reviews such as that by Scriver et al.[502]

Dysplasias with Increased Bone Density

Osteopetrosis. Osteopetrosis (also called "marble bones," "osteosclerosis fragilis generalisata," and "Albers-Schönberg disease,"[106] occurs in the following forms:

1. Autosomal recessive form, which is also termed the "malignant form" because of early death[389,592] (Fig. 14-56)
2. Relatively benign autosomal dominant form[222,400] (Fig. 14-57)
3. Autosomal recessive form associated with renal tubular acidosis and mental retardation, secondary to carbonic anhydrase II deficiency[537]
4. Less well-defined autosomal recessive forms, including a mild disease resembling the

dominant disorder[275] and a lethal form associated with markedly reduced osteoclasts in bone[105]

Autosomal dominant form. The main clinical features of the autosomal dominant form of osteopetrosis are fractures and osteomyelitis, especially of the mandible.[265,490] The bone shows dramatic changes on radiologic and pathologic study (Fig. 14-57). The vertebral bodies have a characteristic "sandwich" (rugger jersey) appearance because of excessive sclerosis in upper and lower portions, with an intervening area of lesser density. All bones, especially the short tubular and round bones of the extremities, may have a "bone-within-bone" appearance. The bones are described by some authors as being hard enough to turn the edge of a steel chisel, whereas others claim the bones to be more like chalk. Usually they are excessively brittle and susceptible to spontaneous pathologic fractures. The original patient of Al-

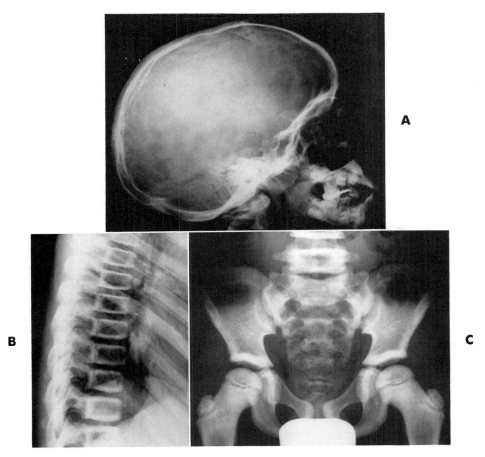

Fig. 14-57. Osteopetrosis (dominant form). **A,** Lateral radiograph of skull, revealing increased density of the skull base. **B,** Lateral radiograph of thoracic spine, showing "rugger jersey" vertebrae and increased rib density. **C,** Anteroposterior radiograph of pelvis, showing sclerosis of the epimetaphyseal and apophyseal regions of the pelvic bones and femurs.

bers-Schönberg* in 1907 was 26 years of age and is said to have been alive 10 years later at reexamination by Reiche. Alexander's patient[6] (in 1923) was 43 years of age.

Elevated acid phosphatase levels have been described,[265] and some have suggested benefit from treatment with calcitriol[286] but this has not been

*Albers-Schönberg was one man; the syndrome is not named for two persons, as is the Ehlers-Danlos syndrome or the Grönblad-Strandberg syndrome. Care should be taken not to confuse osteopetrosis with osteopoikilosis, which was also first described in a definitive manner by Albers-Schönberg; some writers have evidenced this confusion.

well documented. Patients with the autosomal dominant form of osteopetrosis can be relatively asymptomatic, and the disorder may become evident only by means of chance radiography. Walpole et al.[623] described a kindred in which the phenotypic spectrum varied from an asymptomatic condition in adults to a severely affected infant who came to medical attention with symptoms of anemia, hepatosplenomegaly, hydrocephalus, and blindness. The temporal bone in this condition contains dense lamellar bone and areas of residual calcified cartilage.[405] Narrowing of the ear canals and obliteration of the mastoid air cells are features. In addition to hearing loss resulting from the compression of the auditory nerve, conductive hearing loss due to bone deposition on the ossicles also can occur.

Reverse transcriptase activity has been described in cultured mononuclear blood cells isolated from a patient with the autosomal dominant form of osteopetrosis.[309,310] This enzyme was found to be similar to the reverse transcriptase purified from human lymphotropic viruses. Since reverse transcriptase is the hallmark of retroviruses, the authors postulated that historically a retrovirus may have been involved in the origin of autosomal dominant osteopetrosis.

Autosomal recessive or malignant form. The recessive or malignant form (Fig. 14-56) appears early in life; indeed, it may be detected in utero. It involves the entire skeleton and may result in such encroachment on the hematopoietic tissue of the bone marrow that pancytopenia is a leading clinical feature.[108,353,389,592] A disorder like that in humans has been observed in the rabbit,[443] the mouse,[620] domestic fowl,[324] and white-tailed deer.[538] The major features of the human disease are macrocephaly, progressive deafness and blindness, hepatosplenomegaly, and severe anemia that begins in early infancy or fetal life. The condition results from defective resorption of immature bone. Fractures are common, as are choanal atresia and osteomyelitis. Radiographs demonstrate a narrowness of the neural and vascular foramina with thick, dense skull, most markedly at the base; generalized increased density of the long bones with alternate radiolucent bands in the metaphyses and diaphyses; splaying of the metaphyses; a bone-within-bone appearance of the long and short tubular bones; and dense, normal-sized vertebrae with prominent anterior vascular notches.

Based on the observation that temporary parabiosis with normal mice resulted in the permanent cure of the disease in the gray lethal osteopetrotic mouse,[621,622] bone marrow transplantation has been undertaken with success in the human recessive disorder.[82,126,522,540] Bone lesions and hematopoietic abnormalities resolve after therapy, but neurosensory deficits observed before the transplantation can persist.[126] Transient hypercalcemia has been described after successful engraftment.[465] The basic defect in autosomal recessive osteopetrosis is unknown, but impairment of macrophage colony stimulating factor production ap-

pears to be a key event in the pathogenesis of the osteopetrotic (op/op) mouse.[419] Indeed, the murine mutation of osteopetrosis has been found to be in the coding region of the macrophage colony stimulating factor gene.[652]

Osteopetrosis with renal tubular acidosis. Osteopetrosis with renal tubular acidosis is a distinct autosomal recessive disorder.[426,632] It becomes evident in the first 2 years of life because of fractures. Short stature, mental retardation, dental malocclusion, and visual impairment from optic nerve compression are also features. Mild anemia can be present in infancy but usually improves with time. Serum acid phosphatase levels can be elevated, and electrolyte changes are suggestive of a mild tubular acidosis. Electron microscopic study of bone suggests that osteoclasts fail to form "ruffled" membranes, characteristic of active bone-resorbing cells.[632] Sly et al.[536,537] studied a number of patients with this disorder and found low levels of carbonic anhydrase II (CA II) in affected persons and intermediate levels in obligatory heterozygotes, suggesting that CA II has a distinct role in osteoclast function and bone resorption. Renal tubular acidosis in this disorder falls between that of the mild proximal and the prominent distal types. Mental retardation is present in some cases, and because of the diffuse, dense cerebral calcifications, Ohlsson et al.[426] referred to this disorder as "marble brain" disease. Consanguinity was present in nine of 12 pedigrees reported by Sly et al.,[537] establishing this disorder as a rare autosomal recessive trait.

Dysosteosclerosis. Dysosteosclerosis is characterized by osteosclerosis and platyspondyly[244,556] (Fig. 14-58). Affected individuals are short, and their bones have a tendency to fracture. Cranial nerve compression can occur. Macular atrophy of the skin has been reported, as well as flattened fingernails and poorly calcified or chalky tooth enamel. The facies can be unusual, with a narrow midface and a narrow, beaklike nose with micrognathia. There may be progressive motor retardation. Cranial nerve involvement results in decreased visual acuity, optic atrophy, blindness, and facial palsy. Radiographs show sclerosis of the vault, base of the skull, and mastoids, with failure of pneumatization of the paranasal sinuses.[244,556] The optic and auditory canals and other foramina are narrowed. The vertebrae are charac-

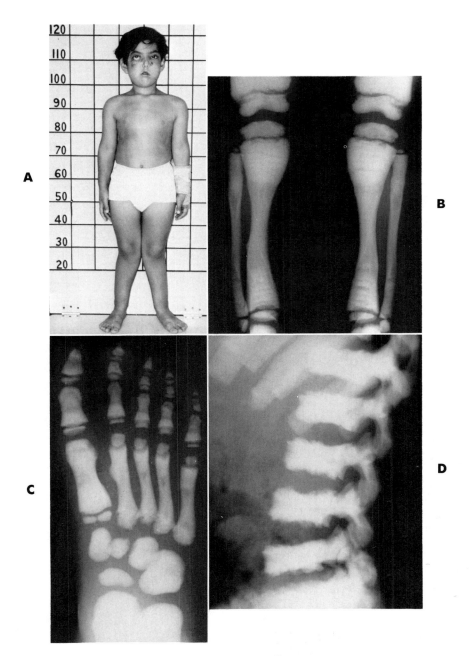

Fig. 14-58. Dysosteosclerosis. **A,** Ten-year-old affected boy. Exophthalmos, strabismus, and genu valgum are evident. **B,** Anteroposterior radiograph of lower extremities, showing metaphyseal and diaphyseal modeling defects (Erlenmeyer-flask deformities) with alternating lines of normal and increased density and dense epiphyses. **C,** Anteroposterior radiograph of foot, showing tapering resorption of the tufts and, **D,** lateral radiograph of lumbar spine with platyspondyly and punctate densities throughout the vertebral bodies, producing end-plate irregularity.

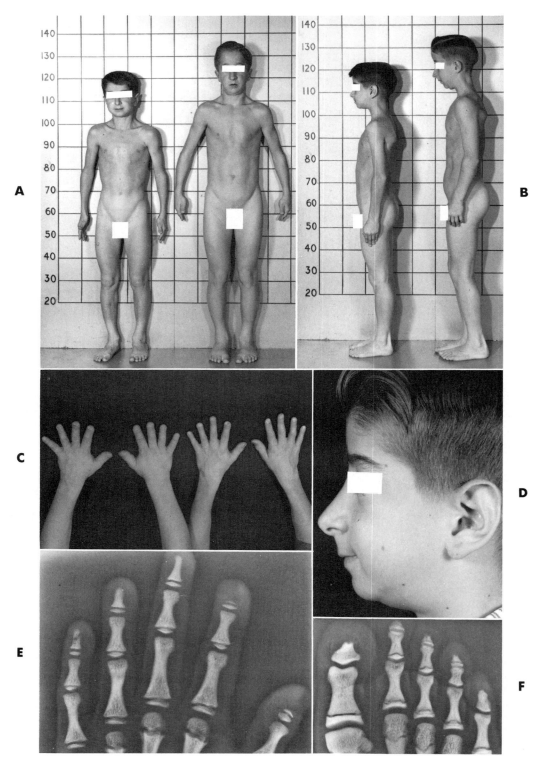

Fig. 14-59. For legend see opposite page.

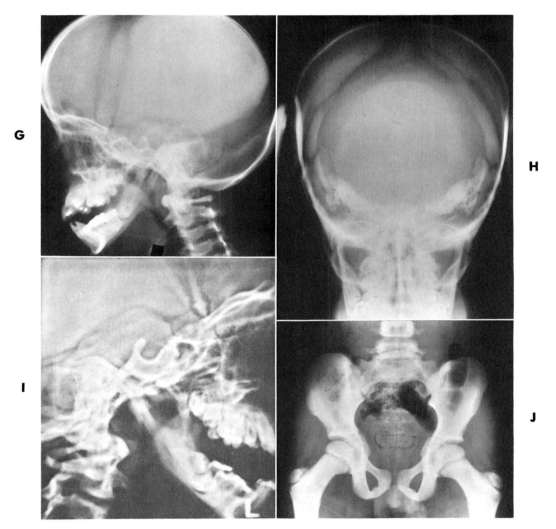

Fig. 14-59, cont'd. Pyknodysostosis in two second cousins. These two males, 13 and 16 years of age, have short stature, generalized osteosclerosis with bone fragility, multiple wormian bones, delayed closure of the sutures and fontanelles of the skull, and hypoplasia of the terminal phalanges and of the distal ends of the clavicles. The mandible has no angle, and several teeth are missing or malpositioned. Neither set of parents is known to be consanguineous. **A** and **B,** Cousins at the ages of 12 and 16 years. The short stature is evident. **C,** The terminal phalanges and fingernails are foreshortened, and several of the nails are spooned. **D,** Receding chin and lack of mandibular angle are demonstrated in the younger cousin. **E** and **F,** Radiographs of the fingers and toes show osteosclerosis and hypoplasia of the terminal phalanges, with fragmentation in the fifth finger. **G** to **I,** The skull of the younger cousin at the age of 13 years shows wide sutures that contain a few wormian bones. The mandibular angle is nearly 180 degrees. The bones rival in density the teeth (exclusive of the fillings). The teeth, poorly detailed because of the sclerosis of the jawbones, are irregularly positioned. **J,** Radiograph of pelvis in the younger cousin at the age of 13 years, showing osteosclerosis and mild protrusion of the acetabulum.

teristic, with progressive platyspondyly and irregular punctate sclerosis. The ribs are short, thick, and sclerotic, as are the sternum, clavicles, and scapulae. The tubular bones are club-shaped with an Erlenmeyer-flask configuration of the widened distal femoral shaft and metaphyses. Dense metaphyseal lines lie adjacent to relatively transparent diaphyses. There may be resorption of phalangeal tufts.

Pathologic bone displays dense, unresorbed calcified cartilage with little bone formation and narrowed fibrotic marrow spaces.[271] We have observed similar histologic changes in patients with lead intoxication, suggesting that this autosomal recessive disorder may be secondary to a defect in a lead-dependent enzyme involved in the resorption of calcified cartilage.[271] Multiple affected sibs and parental consanguinity have been reported, indicating the autosomal recessive inheritance of this disorder.[543]

Pyknodysostosis. Pyknodysostosis, a unique disorder associated with deformity of the skull, fragility of bones, short stature, and osteosclerosis, was first described by Maroteaux and Lamy[372] and Andren et al.[11] This syndrome bears some resemblance to cleidocranial dysplasia: both the cranium and other parts of the skeleton are involved, there are multiple wormian bones, and there is delayed closure of the cranial sutures, particularly the lambdoid and sagittal[396,404] (Fig. 14-59). The ramus of the mandible is short and the angle is missing, so this bone is essentially straight and the jaw appears to be receding. As in osteopetrosis, the dense bones are fragile and fractures are frequent. Acroosteolysis (hypoplasia) of the terminal phalanges is a characteristic feature that is manifested clinically by the presence of short ends of the fingers. The calvarium appears prominent, with smallness of the facial features, prominent nose, and micrognathia. Dental abnormalities include delayed eruption, persistent deciduous teeth, irregular permanent teeth, partial anodontia, and dental infections.

Radiographs show frontal and occipital bossing with wormian bones, significantly delayed closure of the fontanelle, dense skull, underdeveloped mastoid cells and sinuses, and an obtuse or absent angle of the mandible (Fig. 14-59, *C* to *J*). Generalized osteosclerosis is present, with hypoplasia or resorption of the acromial end of the clavicle. There is partial or total resorption of the distal

phalanges, often with fragmentation. Brittle bones result in pathologic fractures of the long bones and the vertebral arches. On pathologic study the growth plates contain narrow, small islands of cells instead of columns, and short primary trabeculae and inclusions in the chondrocytes.[565]

Maroteaux and Lamy[373] suggested that the French artist Toulouse-Lautrec (1864-1901) had this condition (Fig. 14-60). His features, which were noted to be consistent with pyknodysostosis, were dwarfing, parental consanguinity, bone frac-

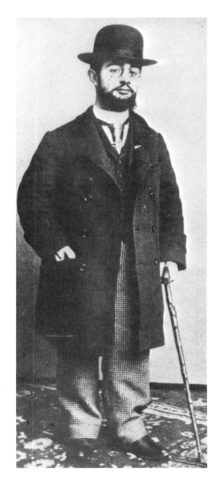

Fig. 14-60. Toulouse-Lautrec (1864-1901) was previously thought to have had osteogenesis imperfecta. On review of the evidence in light of the delineation of the "new" skeletal dysplasia, pyknodysostosis, Maroteaux and Lamy concluded that this was the condition from which he suffered. Parental consanguinity, fragility of bones leading to fractures on minor trauma, a receding chin, and possibly, open fontanelles, which prompted the artist to wear a hat most of the time, are features pointed out as suggesting pyknodysostosis.

ture after relatively mild trauma and probably, a large fontanelle, which prompted him to wear a hat much of the time. Pyknodysostosis shows a high frequency of parental consanguinity, indicating a rare autosomal recessive trait.[504]

Osteosclerosis, dominant type of Stanescu. The rare disorder of osteosclerosis, dominant type of Stanescu, is associated with short stature, craniofacial malformations with brachycephaly, small face, and proptosis, as well as a beaked nose, short neck, brachydactyly, rhizomelia, dental decay, and malocclusion.[98,566] Radiographic manifestations include brachyturricephaly, decreased sinuses and mastoid air cells, obtuse mandibular angle, dense, thick cortices of the long bones, and generalized brachydactyly with normal distal phalanges. This disorder appears to be inherited as an autosomal dominant trait.

Osteomesopyknosis (axial osteosclerosis). Osteomesopyknosis is a rare disorder characterized by sclerosis of the pelvis and spine, with sparing of the skull, tubular bones, hands, feet, ribs, and clavicles.[381,574] The femoral heads are also sclerotic. Affected individuals are of normal stature. They may have low back pain or pelvic pain. Sclerosis of the vertebral bodies occurs along the end plates, and on CT scans patchy sclerotic lesions are evident. This disorder is inherited as an autosomal dominant trait.[533]

Osteopoikilosis (Buschke-Ollendorff syndrome). The term "osteopoikilosis" means "spotted bones." Circumscribed sclerotic areas of different sizes and shapes (round, oval, or lenticular) are located in the spongiosa of the skeleton, particularly in the pelvis, metaphyses, epiphyses of the long bones, tarsals, and carpals.[336,623] This condition is usually of no clinical consequence. Spotty skin lesions (connective tissue nevi) are also found in many cases.[607] This disorder is fairly common and has been reported in large pedigrees that demonstrate autosomal dominant inheritance. There is intrafamilial variability, and the bone or skin lesions may be present separately in members of the same family.[43] Osteopoikilosis is further reviewed in Chapter 13.

Melorheostosis (Léri disease). The term "melorheostosis" is derived from the Greek *melos*, a limb, and *rheos*, a stream. The basic radiographic le-

sions are linear, dense cortical hyperostotic areas following the long axis of bone, which resemble melted wax dripping down the side of a candle.[27,408] This hyperostosis can extend into the medullary cavity, and small bone deposits can be found within surrounding soft tissues. It can affect one or more bones involving the limbs, shoulder girdles, and pelvis and, less commonly, the spine, ribs, and skull. There may be premature closure of the epiphyseal growth plate. These changes may extend across joints. Frequently bone pain and joint stiffness are present. Skin and soft tissue abnormalities may occur in conjunction with these bone abnormalities. Symptomatic relief after vasodilator therapy has been reported.[505] Pathologic study shows irregularly arranged haversian systems with dense, thick trabeculae. Melorheostosis occurs sporadically and is probably not genetic. Because the bony lesions follow sclerotomes, it has been postulated that they may represent an acquired postnatal neuropathy of sensory nerves.[414] Melorheostosis may be associated with osteopoikilosis and osteopathia striata (mixed sclerosing bone dysplasia).

Osteopathia striata. Osteopathia striata takes its name from the longitudinal osteosclerotic streaks seen in the long bones on radiography.[118,613] It can occur in an isolated fashion in the asymptomatic sporadic form as vertical, fine, dense, linear striations, especially at the ends of the long tubular bones. Osteopathia striata can also occur in an autosomal dominant disorder associated with cranial sclerosis. The osteosclerosis in the cranial and facial bones can lead to disfigurement and disability resulting from pressure on cranial nerves, notably, facial palsy and deafness. Cleft palate has occurred. Horan and Beighton[230] established this disorder as an autosomal dominant trait. They emphasized the association of the basal skull thickening and sclerosis resulting in hearing deficit. Winter et al.[636] observed this disorder in a family over three generations with marked variability in expression, ranging from mild cranial enlargement to cranial anomaly with severe Pierre Robin sequence. In the most severe case this disorder was diagnosed prenatally by observation of increased biparietal diameter of the fetal head on ultrasound. Osteopathia striata has also been described in the X-linked dominant condition known as Goltz syndrome (focal dermal hypoplasia), mixed sclerosing bone dysplasia, and

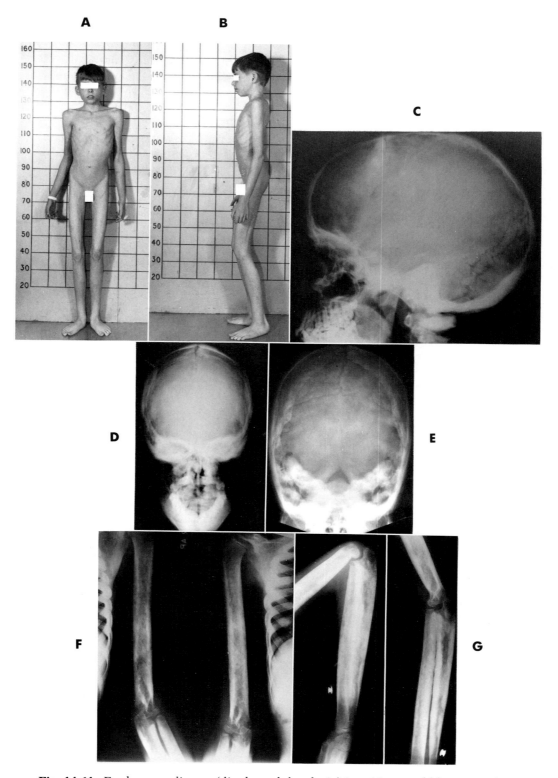

Fig. 14-61. Englemann disease (diaphyseal dysplasia) in a 12-year-old boy. **A** and **B,** The physical findings include debility, generalized reduction in muscle mass, semi-flexed position of the knees and hips, and lack of the normal tapering in the lower femora. **C** to **E,** Skull radiographs showing thickening and sclerosis of the chondro-cranium, mandible, and orbits. **F** and **G,** Radiographs of upper limbs show swelling of the diaphyses of the long bones. The cortices are irregularly thickened and scle-rotic.

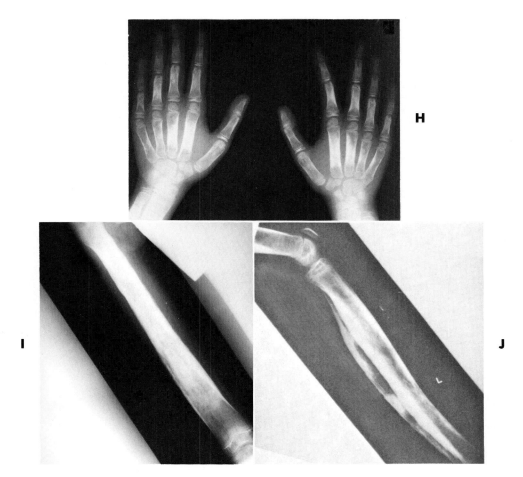

Fig. 14-61, cont'd. H, Modeling of the bones of the hands is less disturbed. Considerable sclerosis and cortical thickening, however, are evident. The ribs, clavicles, vertebrae, and pelvis showed relatively little change. **I** and **J,** The lower limbs, like the upper limbs, show irregular internal and external cortical thickening leading to irregular diaphyseal swelling.

sponastrime dysplasia. Whyte and Murphy[631] described a woman and her two daughters with osteopathia striata associated with a macular dermopathy and white forelock, suggesting an X-linked dominant syndrome.

Diaphyseal dysplasia (Camurati-Engelmann syndrome, Engelmann disease). Diaphyseal dysplasia is characterized by expansion and sclerosis of the diaphyses of the long bones, which lack the normal modeling, and by muscular hypoplasia and generalized weakness[153,542] (Fig. 14-61). Pains in the legs are a conspicuous symptom. Involvement of the cranium occurs only to a mild degree

but as a rule is evident on radiologic study. Onset is often before the age of 10 years and always before 30 years of age. The children who come to medical attention with this disease have a waddling gait, muscular weakness, pain in the extremities, asthenic habitus, decreased muscle mass, and genu valgum and may have shiny, tightly stretched skin over the tibiae and maxilla.[421,422] Various ocular and systemic manifestations such as anemia and hepatosplenomegaly have been described.[90] A remarkable response of the bone pain to corticosteroid therapy has been observed.[7,485]

On radiographic study progressive cortical thickening is present on both the periosteal and

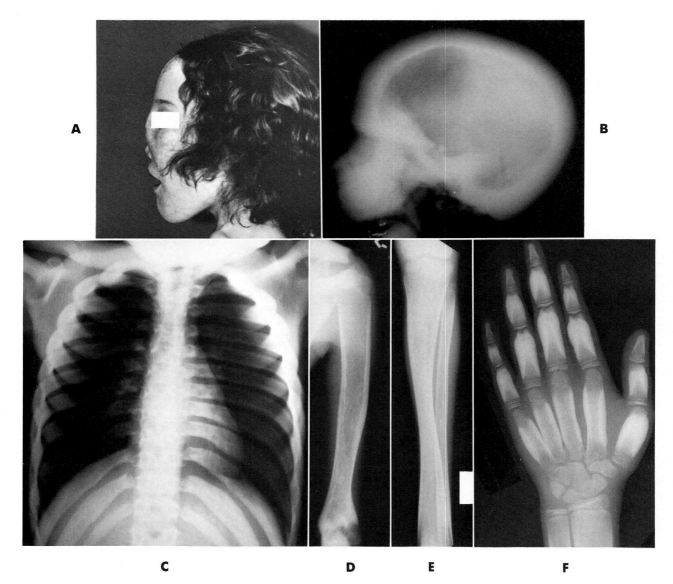

Fig. 14-62. Craniodiaphyseal dysplasia. **A,** A 16-year-old affected boy. Severe malar overgrowth, large head, and engulfed nose can be seen. **B,** Lateral skull radiograph showing severe diffuse calvarial midface sclerosis (especially of the diploe). **C,** Anteroposterior radiograph of thorax, showing diffusely widened and sclerotic ribs. **D,** Upper and, **E,** lower extremities showing generalized sclerosis and diaphyseal modeling abnormality of the long bones. **F,** Anteroposterior view of hand, showing characteristic short-bone modeling abnormalities and flamelike cortical sclerosis of metacarpals and phalanges.

the endosteal surfaces of the limb bones, leading to narrowing of the medullary canals. The process usually begins with the shaft of the femur or tibia but may involve all long bones. There is frontal and occipital bossing with sclerotic changes of the base of the skull, which may also involve the cranial vault and facial bones. Narrowing of the cranial foramina can be symptomatic. Computed tomography scans have demonstrated that the endosteal bone thickening is greater than the periosteal involvement. Morphological examination reveals rapid new bone formation with woven osteoid and lack of harversian system development.[638] Large pedigrees have been described with this syndrome with lack of penetrance and marked variability in expression.[542] The condition described by Ribbing[468] and sometimes referred to as "Ribbing disease" is clearly a milder form of diaphyseal dysplasia (not to be confused with the Ribbing type of multiple epiphyseal dysplasia).

Craniodiaphyseal dysplasia. Craniodiaphyseal dysplasia is associated with cranial and facial hyperostosis that results in a grossly distorted face, with hyperostosis of the frontal bone and progressive hypertelorism[267,272,599] (Fig. 4-62). The cranial vault thickening results in nasal obstruction, increasing deafness and loss of vision. Occlusion of the vascular foramina can lead to seizures and sudden death.[290] Radiographic study shows marked thickening and sclerosis of the calvarium and facial bones that produce a "leontiasis ossium" appearance. The cranial foramina and the paranasal sinuses can become narrowed or obliterated. There is moderate widening and sclerosis of the ribs and extensive thickening and sclerosis of the clavicles. The long-bone diaphyses are straight and slender, with hyperostotic diaphyseal widening. The cortex of the short tubular bones is widened. The long bones do not show metaphyseal flaring. The majority of cases appear to be inherited as an autosomal recessive trait.[165] One family has been described by Schaffer et al.[493] in which a mother and son had craniodiaphyseal dysplasia, a greater degree of hyperostosis and sclerosis than is seen in the recessive form, and some metaphyseal modeling defect.

Lenz-Majewski hyperostotic dwarfism. Lenz-Majewski hyperostotic dwarfism is a rare syndrome characterized by intrauterine growth retardation, delayed closure of the fontanels, hypertelorism, choanal stenosis with nasal obstruction, dental and enamel dysplasia, hyperextensible joints, proximal symphalangism, interdigital webbing, loose skin with prominent cutaneous veins, an emaciated appearance, and mental retardation.[346,480] Radiologic features include progressive sclerosis of the skull, facial bones, and vertebrae; broad clavicles and ribs; diaphyseal undermodeling and midshaft cortical thickening; metaphyseal and epiphyseal hyperostosis; short middle phalanges; and retarded skeletal maturation. Chondroosseous morphologic study showed increased bone formation and defective coupling of formation and resorption.[177] All reported cases have been sporadic, although there is some hint of increased paternal age, suggesting dominant inheritance.[392]

Endosteal hyperostosis, Van Buchem type (hyperostosis corticalis generalisata). The rare hyperostotic disorder discussed in this section has onset of symptoms around puberty.[103,602,603] The chin becomes widened and thickened, head size is normal, and mild exophthalmos, facial nerve palsy, optic atrophy, and deafness are present. Serum alkaline phosphatase levels are increased. There may be increased intracranial pressure. On radiologic study endosteal diaphyseal hyperostosis of the tubular bones and narrowing of the medullary cavity are present; as well as normal or widened diaphyses of the long bones and periosteal excrescences (Fig. 14-63). Endosteal sclerosis of the neurocranium with loss of diploe and involvement of the cranial nerve foramina is a major feature. The mandible is hyperostotic and sclerotic, as are the ribs and clavicles. Milder sclerosis of the pelvis and vertebrae is present. Fryns and Van den Berghe[143] described a young boy with this syndrome who developed facial nerve problems by 2 months of age, suggesting that narrowing around the cranial nerves may occur before sclerosis of the skull is visible on radiographs. This syndrome was described in members of an inbred Dutch kindred, indicative of autosomal recessive inheritance.[602]

Sclerosteosis. Sclerosteosis differs from van Buchem disease primarily on the basis of earlier onset, greater severity of the bone dysplasia, and the presence of syndactyly of the fingers.[38,40,193]

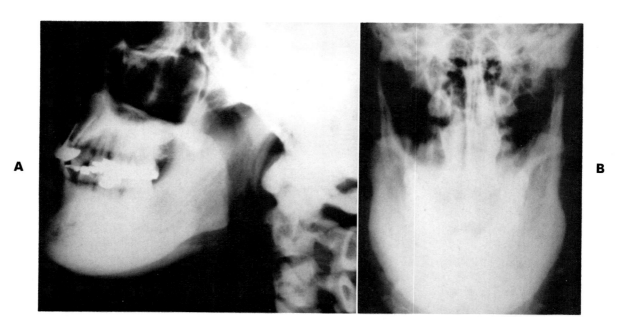

Fig. 14-63. Van Buchem dysplasia. **A,** Lateral and, **B,** anteroposterior views of the mandible, revealing diffuse sclerosis of the mandible with a modeling abnormality.

The jaw has an unusually square appearance. These patients are excessively tall. The hyperostosis of the skull, which can begin in infancy, can lead to anosmia, facial asthesia, strabismus, and exophthalmos.[418] Increased intracranial pressure may result in sudden death.[569] This condition has been described in large kindreds in the Afrikaner population of South Africa and in a highly inbred Brazilian community, which was of Dutch extraction.[137] The occurrence of both sclerosteosis and van Buchem disease in individuals of Dutch ancestry argues for their having a fundamental genetic identity. Phenotypic differences may be due to the epistatic effect of modifying genes.[40] Sclerosteosis is inherited as an autosomal recessive trait.

Endosteal hyperostosis, Worth type. The Worth type of endosteal hyperostosis is inherited as an autosomal dominant trait, in contrast to van Buchem disease.[161,380] The onset of the disease is usually in late childhood, and affected persons often remain asymptomatic. In addition to a prominent forehead, their features are a progressive asymmetric enlargement of the mandible associated with an increased gonial angle, with some widening of the cranial sutures. As in other hyperosto-

sis disorders, torus palatinus is often present, but cranial nerve involvement is uncommon. Serum alkaline phosphatase concentrations are normal.

Radiographic changes include endosteal sclerosis of the cranium, loss of diploe, mandibular hyperostosis and sclerosis, and an increased mandibular angle. There is endosteal sclerosis of the diaphyses of the long tubular bones with mild involvement of the bones of the hands and feet. There are mild changes in the vertebrae, ribs, clavicles, and pelvis. Most cases of this autosomal dominant variety of hyperostosis are benign, but Perez-Vicente et al.[446] described a Spanish family with severe involvement that resulted in neurologic damage with hearing loss, intracranial hypertension, and long tract signs.

Pachydermoperiostosis. Pachydermoperiostosis, which is associated with coarse facial features, clubbing of the hands and feet, and periosteal new bone formation, is not a primary defect of connective tissue (see Chapter 13).

Frontometaphyseal dysplasia. Frontometaphyseal dysplasia is associated with extreme frontal hyperostosis that causes prominence of the supraciliary ridges. Other features include a wide nasal bridge, antimongoloid palpebral fissures, and a small, pointed chin.[34,160] Malocclusion and dental anomalies are present. Various extraskeletal manifestations have been reported in individual cases. Radiographs reveal a thick frontal ridge, often with absence of pneumatization of the frontal sinuses, antegonial notching of the body of the mandible, and marked hypoplasia of the angle and condylar process of the mandible. Dentition is defective. The rib contours can be irregular. There is increased density and lack of modeling of the diaphyses of the long bones with some flaring of the metaphyses. In some instances the long bones may be mildly affected or almost unaffected. A variety of anomalies of the carpal bones and phalanges may exist. Frontometaphyseal dysplasia appears to be inherited as an X-linked recessive trait.[166] This syndrome may be confused with otopalatodigital syndrome, and it has been suggested that since they both appear to be X-linked disorders, they may represent the same entity.[584]

Craniometaphyseal dysplasia. Both autosomal dominant and autosomal recessive forms of the craniometaphyseal dysplasias have been identified.[165] In general the autosomal recessive form is more severe. Both are characterized by hyperostosis of the cranial and facial bones with compression of cranial nerves at the foramina and by changes in the metaphyses of the long bones. Fig. 14-64 shows the changes in a family with the dominant form of the disease. Although this disorder was reported as an instance of Pyle disease, this designation is appropriately reserved for metaphyseal dysplasia with little or no craniofacial involvement and with autosomal recessive inheritance.[477] Other case reports on Pyle disease are better categorized as autosomal dominant craniometaphyseal dysplasia.[553] The metaphyseal flaring is less abrupt than in Pyle disease, producing a clublike rather than an Erlenmeyer-flask deformity. Features include a large, broad head with frontal bossing, hypertelorism, flat nasal root, and large mandible, frequently with the mouth held open because of choanal obstruction. From early in life a ridge of bone can be seen running from the bridge of the nose to the zygomatic arch. Neurologic manifestations are due to stenosis of foramina and result in cranial nerve involvement that causes optic atrophy, progressive deafness,

and facial nerve paralysis. Dentition may be affected. Vascular occlusion can occur. There can be considerable variability in clinical severity.[35,67,477]

Radiographic study shows progressive diffuse hyperostosis of the cranial vault and base and of the facial bones, with cranial foraminal narrowing and accentuated bands of ossification along the cranial sutures.[35,229,477] The paranasal sinuses and mastoid air cells are usually obliterated. The metaphyses of the tubular bones are flared and widened. In early life the metaphyses may appear relatively lucent compared with the diaphyses.

In the recessive form, nasal obstruction is usually complete and involvement of multiple cranial nerves is invariable.[258,444] Deafness and facial paralysis are the rule in this entity.

The facies are leonine in craniometaphyseal dysplasia and craniodiaphyseal dysplasia; these disorders are among the "causes" of the old "wastebasket" diagnosis of "leontiasis ossea."[351] Multiple affected sibs with parental consanguinity and multiple affected members in multiple generations have been reported, indicative of either autosomal recessive (less common) or autosomal dominant (more common) forms of the disease, respectively.

Pyle disease (metaphyseal dysplasia). Despite bizarre radiographic changes, Pyle disease has few clinical findings other than genu valgum.[31,249,511] The craniofacial bones are at the most only mildly affected, thus distinguishing Pyle disease from the craniometaphyseal dysplasias.[165] The term "Pyle disease" has been misused to refer to a variety of conditions. Spranger and Langer[547] reviewed the skull radiographic film of Pyle's original case and failed to find the changes characteristic of craniometaphyseal dysplasia. The femora show an Erlenmeyer-flask deformity. The humerus is abnormally broad and undermodeled in its proximal two thirds, as are the radius and ulna in their distal portion. The metacarpals are broad distally, as are the phalanges in their proximal portions. The metaphyseal flaring is usually more abrupt and more marked in Pyle disease than in the craniometaphyseal dysplasias.

Backwin and Krida[19] restudied Pyle's original patient and on finding similar changes in the patient's sister, claimed the term "familial metaphyseal dysplasia." Others have also reported affected sibs, as well as parental consanguinity. Beighton[31] found about 20 reported cases with affected sibs of

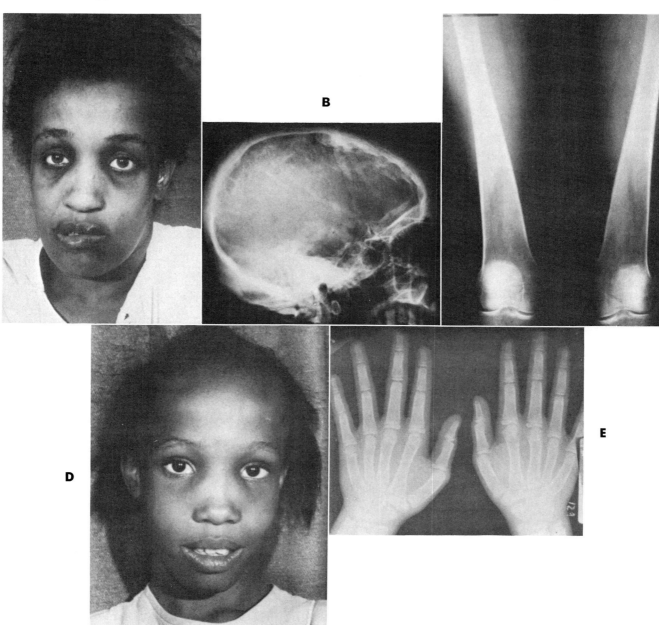

Fig. 14-64. Autosomal dominant craniometaphyseal dysplasia. A kindred that contains seven documented and two probable cases. The proband had left facial weakness from the age of 5 years; progressive hearing loss was first noted at 9 years of age. Examination at 44 years of age, **A,** showed a broad nasal bridge with an elevated wing of bone extending to the zygoma bilaterally, left peripheral facial palsy, diminished hearing bilaterally, and weakness and hypoesthesia of the left side of the body. As demonstrated by means of radiographic examination, **B,** the calvaria was found to be markedly thickened, especially in the occipital area. The frontal and maxillary sinuses were opacified, and the mastoid air cells were poorly aerated. Narrowing of the foramen magnum and internal auditory canals was thought to account for the left-side neurologic deficit and deafness, respectively. The long bones, especially the femora, **C,** were club-shaped as a result of metaphyseal flaring. **D,** A 12-year-old affected daughter of the proband had noticeably decreased hearing and tinitus in the right ear for 1 year and several episodes of vertigo on awakening. The appearance of the nasal bridge is similar to that in her mother. **E,** The bones of her hands showed defective modeling, in addition to radiographic changes similar to those seen in her mother.

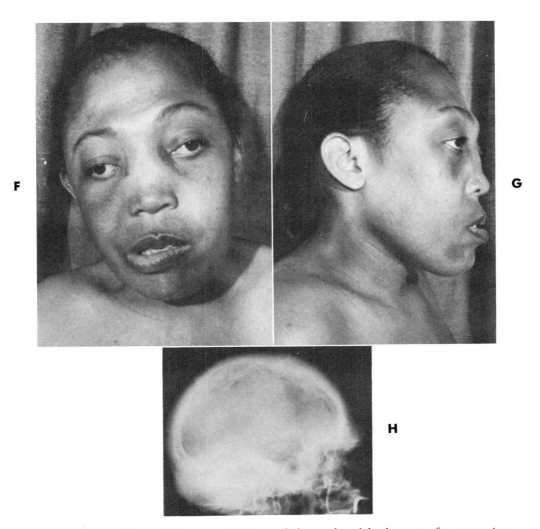

Fig. 14-64, cont'd. F, A 42-year-old sister of the proband had onset of progressive visual impairment at the age of 2 years. The findings at examination included, in addition to obvious craniofacial deformity, left total facial palsy, blindness, and deafness. **H,** Radiographic changes in the skull were marked.

Continued.

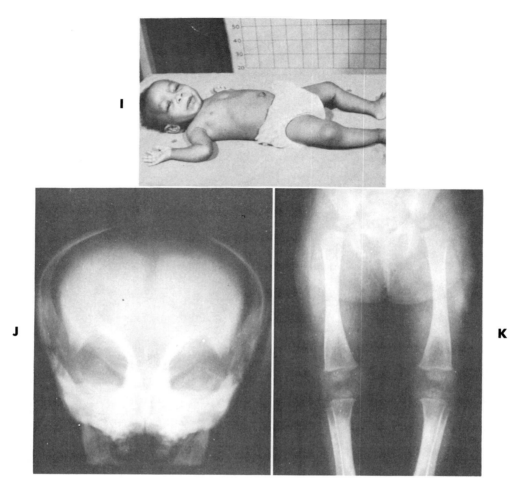

Fig. 14-64, cont'd. **I,** An 8-month-old daughter of the woman shown in **F** to **H** already had typical facial features and typical radiographic findings of craniometaphyseal dysplasia in the skull, **J,** and long bones, **K.** (From Rimoin DL, Woodruff SL, Holman BL. In Bergsma D, editor: *Clinical delineation of birth defects. IV. Skeletal dysplasia,* New York, 1969, National Foundation, March of Dimes.)

normal parents, and in two instances, parental consanguinity. Urteaga et al.[601] described an ancient skeleton from the Mochica culture of Peru (200 A.D. to 800 A.D.) with Pyle disease.

Osteoectasia with hyperphosphatemia (hyperphosphatasia, juvenile Paget disease). Osteoectasia with hyperphosphatemia manifests in infancy with a large head and expanded and bowed extremities.[18,111] The patients are dwarfed and have "pigeon breast" deformity, premature shedding of deciduous teeth, and significant muscle weakness.

High levels of acid and alkaline phosphatase and of leucine aminopeptidase have been found. Urinary excretion of hydroxyproline is elevated.[117,305] On radiographs progressive skeletal deformity with enlargement and thickening of the skull, widening of the diploic space, and uneven mineralization of the calvarium are evident. The spine shows platyspondyly and kyphoscoliosis with concave vertebral bodies. There is an osteomalacia-like deformity of the pelvis with protrusio acetabuli. The long bones are curved and thickened with cylindric transverse trabeculae, narrowed or dilated medullary canal, and unusual radiolucent bone texture. The short tubular bones are thickened. Some improvement after calcitonin therapy has been reported.[627] This syndrome has been reported in sibs, indicative of autosomal recessive inheritance.

Oculodentoosseus dysplasia. Oculodentoosseus dysplasia has characteristic facial features, including microphthalmus, thin nose with a long, prominent nasal bridge, anteverted nostrils, and hypoplastic alae nasi.[36,164,441] The teeth are small, with generalized enamel hypoplasia. Various digital anomalies, including syndactyly, camptodactyly, and clinodactyly, as well as malformations of other organs, have been reported. Radiographs show bilateral syndactyly and camptodactyly of the fourth and fifth fingers, clinodactyly of the fifth finger, hypoplasia of the middle phalanx of the index finger, and hypoplasia or absence of the middle phalanges of some toes. The orbits are small, with orbital hypertelorism; the mandible is wide and thickened; and there is undertubulation of the long bones. Autosomal dominant inheritance has been well documented. A severe autosomal recessive form of the disorder has been documented in a pair of siblings and a cousin who were members of a large consanguineous Afrikaner kindred.[36]

Caffey disease (infantile cortical hyperostosis). Caffey disease, which rarely, if ever, appears after 5 months of age, is sometimes present at birth and has even been identified in utero.[42] The acute manifestations are inflammatory, with fever and hot, tender swelling of the involved bones (for example, mandible and ribs).[63,107] Despite striking radiographic changes in the acute stages, the affected bones often revert to normal. These patients have irritability, fever, and palor during the acute episodes and soft tissue swelling adjacent to the involved bones. Erythrocyte sedimentation rates are elevated, as are C-reactive protein and immunoglobulin levels. Radiographs show subperiosteal cortical hyperostosis, whereas the epiphyses of the long bones are spared. The mandible, clavicle, and ribs are most often involved. Although classically Caffey disease has been regarded as a sporadic disease and thought to be inflammatory and perhaps infectious, autosomal dominant inheritance has now been documented in a number of families.[107,360] The tibia is most often involved in the familial cases. It has been claimed that the sporadic form of this disorder is decreasing in incidence.[360]

Disorders Associated with Disorganized Development of Cartilaginous and Fibrous Components of the Skeleton

Dysplasia epiphysealis hemimelica (Trevor disease). Dysplasia epiphysealis hemimelica is characterized by overgrowth of one side of an epiphysis, resulting in unilateral, asymmetric hard swellings, especially of the knee or ankle, or both, with or without pain or restriction of motion[15,66,598] (Fig. 14-65). Various valgus deformities of the legs may occur, depending on the site of involvement. There may be a painful flatfoot. The talus is the most common site of involvement, followed by the distal femoral epiphysis, the distal tibial epiphysis, and the carpal bones and scapula. The upper extremities are less commonly involved. After epiphyseal plate fusion the disorder becomes quiescent. On radiographs overgrowth of one side of the epiphyses with irregular contour and ossification is apparent. Overgrowth of the adjacent bones and advanced bone age in their epiphyses are present. The adjacent metaphyses and growth plates may be involved secondary to the primary disorder. Chondroosseous morphologic study shows an exostosis with a cartilaginous cap arising from an epiphysis, apophysis, or round bone.

Dysplasia epiphysealis hemimelica is fairly common and has a male-to-female ratio of 3:1. No familial cases have yet been described, and an unaffected monozygotic twin has been reported.[100] Hensinger et al.[213] described a kindred in which multiple members had dysplasia epiphysealis hemimelica, intracapsular or periarticular chondromas of the knee, extraskeletal chondromas, and osteochondromas. This unique syndrome appeared to be inherited as an autosomal dominant trait in that family.

Multiple cartilaginous exostoses (osteochondromatosis, diaphyseal aclasis). Multiple cartilaginous exostoses are manifested by the presence of cartilaginous excrescences on the ends of the dia-

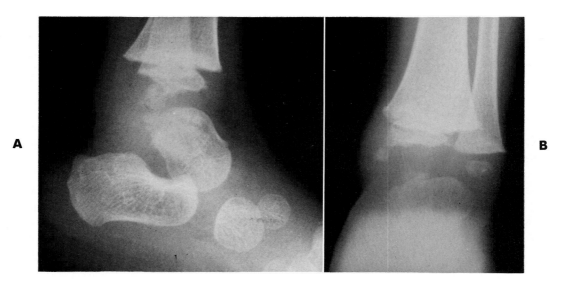

Fig 14-65. Dysplasia epiphysealis hemimelica (Trevor disease). **A,** Lateral and, **B,** anteroposterior views of the ankle, revealing irregularity of the distal tibial epiphysis with overgrowth and similar involvement of the roof of the talus.

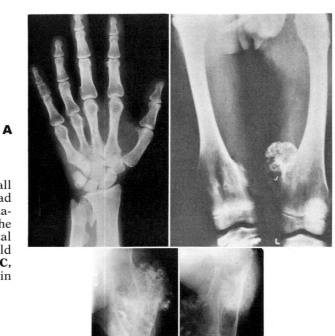

Fig. 14-66. Multiple cartilaginous exostoses. **A,** Small exostoses in a 16-year-old girl whose father also had multiple exostoses. The shortening of the fourth metacarpal was probably caused by an exostosis, but the short middle phalanx of the little finger is an incidental abnormality. **B,** Exostoses of the femur in a 10-year-old boy. That on the right has been partially removed. **C,** Two views of enormous exostoses of the left humerus in a 40-year-old man.

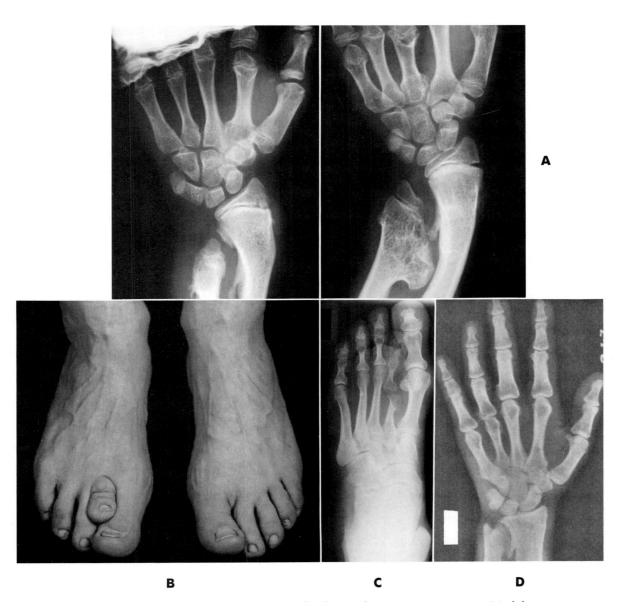

Fig. 14-67. Deformity resulting from multiple cartilaginous exostoses. **A,** Madelung-like deformity of forearm. **B** and **C,** Short second metatarsal on the right. **D,** Short fourth metacarpal.

physes of bones of the extremities,[211,260,279,307] (Figs. 14-66 and 14-67). The ribs and the scapulae may also be affected, but the calvarium is not involved. Deformity of the legs, the forearms (resembling Madelung deformity), and the hands (for example, short metacarpal) is frequent. The patients are usually of reduced stature. Neurologic complications occur in some patients as a result of pressure on the spinal cord or peripheral nerves.[338,610]

Onset may be in infancy or early childhood, but some patients are recognized incidentally as adults, indicative of the wide variability of expressivity in this syndrome. The lumps and bumps are usually not tender. Genu valgum, coxa vara, and Madelung-like deformity may occur secondary to the exostoses. In order of frequency the sites commonly affected are in the regions of the shoulders, knees, and ankles. Large protrusions over the thighs may interfere with thigh apposition and result in discomfort caused by bumping while walking. Malignant transformation to an osteochondrosarcoma may occur in adulthood. Variable incidences ranging from 0.5% to 20% to 40% have been described. It is quite likely that the higher figures result from bias of ascertainment and that the frequency of osteosarcomatous degeneration is well under 5%.[615] Potential malignancy should be suspected when the growth of a lesion follows closure of the epiphyses, since these lesions resemble normal growth plates and fuse at the time of puberty. Surgical removal of the exostoses should be performed for correction or prevention of deformity, for nerve or vessel compression, and for cosmetic reasons. There is no need to remove the lesions unless they are symptomatic or grow after epiphyseal closure.

On radiographs the exostotic growths originate from the metaphyseal edge, with the apex directed away from the epiphyses. The exostoses can result in abnormality of tubulation of the bone and the disproportionate shortening of affected bones, especially the ulna and fibula. Any endochondral bone may be involved, including the flat bones, short tubular bones, ribs, spine, and base of the skull.

The disorder is inherited as an autosomal dominant trait. It has been postulated that the gene for multiple exostoses may be located in the region of 8q24, since similar exostoses can be seen in the Langer-Giedion syndrome (trichorhinophalangeal dysplasia type II), which has been found to be associated with deletions in this region.[57] Indeed, the gene for multiple exostoses has been localized to the region 8q23-24.1, but not all families have been found to cosegregrate with markers in this region, suggesting genetic heterogeneity.[427]

The disease is said to be more severe and frequent in males than in females. This is probably due to diminished expression in a minority of females, since a marked male predominance is found only in a few families.[211] The disorder has a high frequency in the Chamarros of the island of Guam.[307] A similar disorder has been described in horses.[407]

Enchondromatosis (Ollier disease). Enchondromatosis is characterized by abnormal growth of unossified cartilage in the diaphyses of the long bones.[363,506] Involvement is usually asymmetric.

The cartilaginous tumors cause expansion of the shaft of the involved bones and may impede longitudinal growth. In cases of severe involvement all fingers, for example, may be remarkably enlarged. These defects result in asymmetry in length and shape of the involved limbs, with enlargement of metaphyseal regions and lumps and bumps on the hands and feet. The carpals, tarsals, base of skull, and the spine are rarely involved. The iliac crest is frequently involved, with a ragged-appearing edge seen on radiographs. Kyphoscoliosis, pathologic fractures, or gait disturbance may rarely result. These lesions may evolve into chondrosarcomas, but the frequency of the malignant transformation is really unknown and has probably been overemphasized in the literature as a result of ascertainment bias.[499] Granulosa cell tumors of the ovary have been described in several instances.[606] Many of the cases resulting in malignancy may well have been Maffucci syndrome, in which hemangiomata are present.

The genetic basis of Ollier disease is unknown. Most cases are sporadic, and there have been a few instances of familial occurrence.[65,321,484] Dominant inheritance with reduced penetrance is possible.

Maffucci syndrome. Maffucci syndrome consists of enchondromatosis with hemangiomata[352,583] (Fig. 14-68). The disorder can become evident at all ages, even in infancy. Asymmetry in length and shape of the involved limbs is present, with enlarged metaphyseal regions and lumps and bumps on the hands and feet. These can become quite large and grotesque. Multiple cutaneous and subcutaneous hemangiomas are seen. They are often cavernous and can result in arteriovenous shunts and platelet trapping. The enchondromas may occur in the head and neck, involve the base of the skull, extend down into the pharynx, and compress cranial nerves. Maffucci syndrome has been associated with multiple malignant tumors, including chondrosarcomas, angiosarcomas, adenocarcinomas, gliomas, and the like. Sun et al.[583] reported that chondrosarcoma developed in nine patients with the Maffucci syndrome seen at the Mayo Clinic. From a review of the English literature, the authors concluded that the incidence of chondrosarcoma in this disorder is 17.8%; however, the same reservations previously mentioned, concerning bias of ascertainment in arriving at

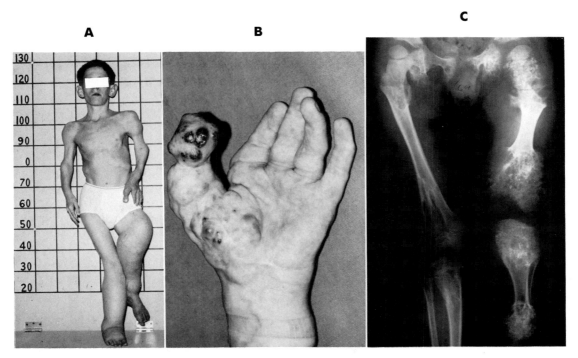

Fig. 14-68. Maffucci syndrome. **A,** Affected 15-year-old boy with marked asymmetry of the limbs, hemangiomata, and lymphedema. **B,** His hand, at 21 years of age. The severe hemangiomata can be seen. **C,** Anteroposterior radiograph of his lower extremities with marked enchondral abnormalities (greater on the left than on the right) and phleboliths in the soft tissues.

these figures, are justified. Maffucci syndrome occurs sporadically and has no known genetic basis. Somatic cell mutation of a type inconsistent with a viable zygote, if it occurs in a germ cell, is at least a remote possibility.

Metachondromatosis. Metachondromatosis is a disorder that combines the radiographic features of both multiple exostoses and Ollier disease (enchondromatosis).[224,314,368] The exostoses occur at the metaphyseal region and point toward the growth plate, in contrast to those in multiple exostoses, in which they point away from the growth plate. Again, unlike multiple exostoses, in metachondromatosis the exostoses are most common in the tubular bones of the hands and feet.[284] Enchondromatosis lesions can occur in the iliac crest, proximal femur, and other areas. Abnormalities may be present in the vertebrae. Differentiation of metachondromatosis from multiple exostoses is important because of the regression

of the lesions in the former, with little or minimal residual deformity. Metachondromatosis has been reported in multiple generations of several families, suggesting autosomal dominant inheritance.[24,284,605]

Osteoglophonic dysplasia. Osteoglophonic dysplasia is associated with craniofacial abnormalities and fibrous metaphyseal defects.[32] The term "osteoglophonic (hollowed out)" is based on the radiographic appearance of the metaphyses. Individuals with osteoglophonic dysplasia have rhizomelic dwarfism with short stubby extremities. Their facial features are abnormal, with acrocephaly, frontal bossing, hypertelorism, mandibular prognathism, unerupted teeth, highly arched palate, and anteverted nares. The neck is short, and lumbar lordosis may be a feature. Radiographic examination reveals craniosynostosis, midface hypoplasia, prognathism, and cystic changes of the mandibular ramus. Platyspondyly with anterior projections and a narrow spinal canal with posterior scalloping of the lumbar vertebral bodies can be seen. There are gross dysplastic changes in the metaphyses and epiphyses of the long bones, with irregular areas of radiolucency. The short bones of the hands may be shortened and broadened. Radiolucent areas can also be seen in the ilium. The metaphyseal lesions consist of benign whorls of fibrous tissue.[278] The disorder appears to be inherited as an autosomal dominant trait.[281]

Polyostotic fibrous dysplasia (Jaffe-Lichtenstein syndrome, McCune-Albright syndrome). Polyostotic fibrous dysplasia can occur with lesions isolated to the skeletal system (Jaffe-Lichtenstein syndrome), or in association with café-au-lait macules and endocrinopathy (McCune-Albright syndrome).[4,350,390] The bony lesions appear in childhood or adolescence and become evident on clinical examination by the presence of limb deformity, pain, and leg length discrepancy or pathologic fractures, or both. Facial asymmetry and a leontiasis osseum appearance can be present. Scoliosis, lordosis, and chest deformity can also occur. The lesions tend to be unilateral. On radiographs they appear as lacunar or mixed, somewhat opaque lesions with thinning and expansion of the cortex (Fig. 14-69). They can result in bowing of the long bones and pathologic fractures. Hyperostosis of the skull, in particular, at the base, can occur with

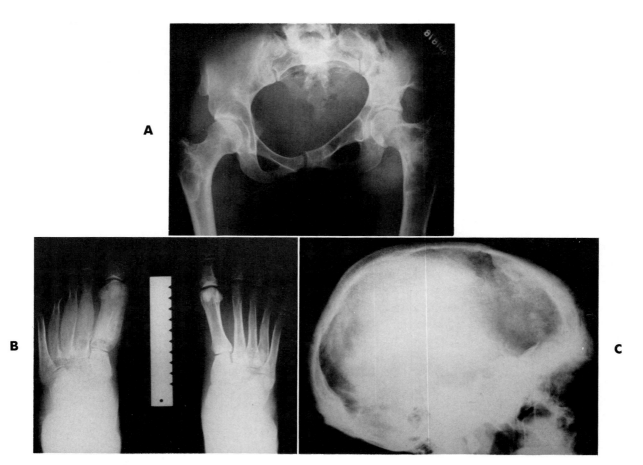

Fig. 14-69. Fibrous dysplasia (McCune-Albright syndrome). **A,** Anteroposterior radiograph of the pelvis and hips, revealing mixed lucent and sclerotic lesions that involve the left ileum, left pubis and ischium, left femoral neck and shaft, and right proximal femur. **B,** Similar lesions involve the shafts of the left metatarsals. **C,** The skull shows increased density of the base with "cotton-wool" changes in the frontal and parietal bones.

obliteration of the paranasal sinuses. A "shepherd's crook" deformity of the femoral neck is characteristic. The café-au-lait patches associated with Mc-Cune-Albright syndrome are often unilateral and on the same side as the bony lesions; they are darker than the café-au-lait spots in neurofibromatosis and have an irregular outline, giving them a "coast of Maine" shape rather than the smooth "coast of California" configuration of the neurofibromatosis lesions. The major endocrinologic feature is precocious puberty, which occurs in more than half of the cases that occur in females.[439] Precocious puberty can also occur in males.[152] Hyperthyroidism, excess secretion of growth hormone with gigantism, Cushing syndrome, and gynecomastia have also been observed.[79] Hypophosphatemic rickets occurs occasionally.

Radiographic examination may show advanced skeletal maturation and premature closure of the epiphyseal plates. The fibrous dysplasia is often unilateral, with the pelvis and upper portion of the femur being the most common sites, as well as dense skull lesions. Upward convexity of the intracellular contents and increased height of the pituitary fossa are features.[469] Calvarial "doughnut" lesions and diploic widening can occur.

There are few convincing instances of the familial occurrence of polyostotic dysplasia, with the exception of concordant monozygotic twins.[344,392] Happle[197] hypothesized that polyostotic fibrous dysplasia was caused by an autosomal dominant lethal gene that is compatible with viability only when it is in a mosaic state. This disorder is now known to be due to a mosaic state of an activating mutation in the GNAS1 gene, which codes for a stimulatory adenosinetriphosphate (ADT)–dependent G protein.[626] Interestingly, inactivating mutations in the same gene result in another disorder named for Fuller Albright, which is known as Albright hereditary osteodystrophy, or pseudohypoparathyroidism.

Cherubism (familial fibrous dysplasia of the jaw). Cherubism is associated with swelling of the lower face beginning in the first 2 to 4 years of life.[300] These changes progress, then subside after puberty. The jaw swelling appears to be hard and painless and is often symmetric. The lips may be everted and thickened and the eyes appear to be down-turned. Lymphangiopathy in some patients can increase the appearance of swelling of the

lower face. Various problems in dentition and speech are present; problems with swallowing and chewing may occur.

Radiologic manifestations include expansion of the mandible in children, with well-defined multilocular, soap-bubble–appearing radiolucencies extending from the malar region to the mandibular notch.[45,87,616] The maxilla is less often involved, as are the anterior rib and proximal femoral areas. In adults granular and sclerotic changes remain at the site of previous disease activity. Cherubism is a benign, self-limiting condition. The early lesions contain well-vascularized areas rich in giant cells; later the lesions become fibrotic, and finally, bone formation occurs.[77] Cherubism has variability in expressivity, and because of its subsidence after the third decade, care must be taken to rule out the disease in parents of affected individuals.[266] This disorder appears to be inherited as an autosomal dominant trait.[447,491]

Myofibromatosis (congenital generalized fibromatosis). Myofibromatosis is a rare disorder characterized by multiple fibroblastic tumors involving the skin, striated muscles, bones, and viscera.[68,577] The tumors may be present at birth or develop during the first weeks of life. The radiographic changes are somewhat similar to those in endochondromatosis, with multiple cystic lesions involving the metaphyses and adjacent diaphyses. Multiple soft tissue nodules are present. The prognosis is poor when several internal organs are affected; of such infants, 80% are said to die within the first 4 months of life.[78] However, complete spontaneous regression has also been observed. Myofibromatosis has been observed in multiple sibs of consanguineous matings, indicative of autosomal recessive inheritance.[17] Several exceptions, however, such as the presence of affected half-sisters[248] and an affected father and daughter,[263] have complicated the interpretation of the genetics in this disorder.

Idiopathic Osteolyses

The group of idiopathic osteolyses involves resorption of bone at the ends of the digits, in the carpals and tarsals, or at multiple sites. The disorders are classified on the basis of the area of resorption and the associated malformations. Since these disorders do not appear to represent primary heritable disorders of connective tissue, they are not discussed here.

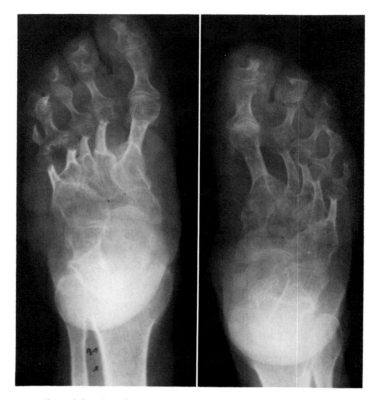

Fig. 14-70. Results of footbinding in early life. Radiograph of the feet of a Canton-reared Chinese woman, showing short bones with broad ends and possible fusion of the right fourth and fifth proximal phalanges at their bases.

CONCLUSION

The wide variety of skeletal dysplasias that result from gene mutation does not permit summarization. Although the classification and nomenclature of these diseases are mainly descriptive at the phenotypic and primary radiographic level, recent advances have led to the delineation of the basic gene mutation in several of the skeletal dysplasias. We can look forward to a time when the understanding of each disorder at the molecular level will be sufficiently advanced to allow logical classification, prevention, and, we hope, specific treatment.

From the viewpoint of entity delineation, phenocopies (exogenously induced mimics of genetic disorders) are relatively uncommon among the skeletal dysplasias. Examples of phenocopies include individuals with the fetal warfarin syndrome and chondrodysplasia punctata and young persons with thalassemia in whom enchondroma-tosis develops after desferoximine therapy. Fig. 14-70 presents radiographs of the feet, which, per se, might be thought to represent some genetic skeletal dysplasia. However, this appearance is the result of long-term binding of the feet in a Chinese woman, thus representing another phenocopy.

REFERENCES

1. Aggett PJ et al: Shwachman's syndrome: a review of 21 cases, *Arch Dis Child* 55:331-347, 1980.
2. Ahmad NN et al: Stop codon in the procollagen II gene (COL2A1) in a family with the Stickler syndrome (arthro-ophthalmopathy), *Proc Natl Acad Sci USA* 88:6624-6627, 1991.
3. Ala-Kokko L et al: Single base mutation in the type II procollagen gene (COL2A1) as a cause of primary osteoarthritis associated with a mild chondrodysplasia, *Proc Natl Acad Sci USA* 87:6565-6568, 1990.
4. Albright F et al: Syndrome characterized by osteitis fibrosa disseminata, areas of pigmentation and endocrine dysfunction, with precocious puberty in females: report of five cases, *New Engl J Med* 216:727-746, 1937.

5. Aleck KA et al: Dyssegmental dysplasia: clinical, radiographic, and morphologic evidence of heterogeneity, *Am J Med Genet* 27:295-312, 1987.

6. Alexander WG: Report of a case of so-called "marble-bones" with a review of the literature and a translation of article, *Am J Roentgenol* 10:280-301, 1923.

7. Allen DT et al: Corticosteroids in the treatment of Englemann's disease: progressive diaphyseal dysplasia, *Pediatrics* 46:523-531, 1970.

8. Amlof J: On achondroplasia in the dog, *Zbl Veterinaermed* 8:43, 1961.

9. Anderson IJ et al: Spondyloepiphyseal dysplasia, mild autosomal dominant type is not due to primary defects of type II collagen, *Am J Med Genet* 37:272-276, 1990.

10. Anderson PE Jr, Hauge M: Congenital generalized bone dysplasias: a clinical, radiological and epidemiological survey, *J Med Genet* 26:37-44, 1989.

11. Andren L et al: Osteopetrosis acro-osteolytica: a syndrome of osteopetrosis, acro-osteolysis and open sutures of the skull, *Acta Chir Scand* 124:496-550, 1962.

12. Angle CR: Congenital bowing and angulation of the long bones, *Pediatrics* 13:257-268, 1954.

13. Antley RM, Bixler D: Trapezoidocephaly, midface hypoplasia and cartilage abnormalities with multiple synostoses and skeletal fractures, *Birth Defects (Original Article Series)* 11(2):397-401, 1975.

14. Anton JI, Reitz GB, Spiegel MB: Madelung's deformity, *Ann Surg* 108:411-439, 1938.

15. Azouz EM et al: The variable manifestations of dysplasia epiphysealis hemimelica, *Pediatr Radiol* 15:44-49, 1985.

16. Bach C et al: Dysplasia spondylo-epiphysaire congenitale avec anomalies multiples, *Arch Fr Pediatr* 24:23-34, 1967.

17. Baird PA, Worth AJ: Congenital generalized fibromatosis: an autosomal recessive condition? *Clin Genet* 9:488-494, 1976.

18. Bakwin H, Eiger MS: Fragile bones and macrocranium, *J Pediatr* 49:558-564, 1956.

19. Bakwin H, Krida A: Familial metaphyseal dysplasia, *Am J Dis Child* 53:1521-1527, 1937.

20. Balfe A et al: Aberrant subcellular localization of peroxisomal 3-ketoacyl-CoA thiolase in the Zellweger syndrome and rhizomelic chondrodysplasia punctata, *Pediatr Res* 27:304-310, 1990.

21. Bankier A et al: Fibrochondrogenesis in male twins at 24 weeks gestation, *Am J Med Genet* 38:95-98, 1991.

22. Bannerman RM, Ingall GB, Mohn JF: X-linked spondyloepiphyseal dysplasia tarda: clinical and linkage data, *J Med Genet* 8:291-301, 1971.

23. Barber KE, Gow PJ, Mayo KM: A family with multiple musculoskeletal abnormalities, *Ann Rheum Dis* 43:275-278, 1984.

24. Basset GS, Cowell HR: Metachondromatosis: report of four cases, *J Bone Joint Surg* 67(A):811-814, 1985.

25. Beals RK: Hypochondroplasia: a report of five kindreds, *J Bone Joint Surg* 51(A):728-736, 1969.

26. Beals RK et al: Dyschondrosteosis and Madelung's deformity: report of three kindreds and review of the literature, *Clin Orthop* 116:24-28, 1976.

27. Beauvais P et al: Léri's melorheostosis: three pediatric cases and a review of the literature, *Pediatr Radiol* 6:153, 1977.

28. Beck M et al: Heterogeneity of metatropic dysplasia, *Eur J Pediatr* 140:231-237, 1983.

29. Beemer FA et al: A new short rib syndrome: report of two cases, *Am J Med Genet* 14:115-123, 1983.

30. Beighton P: *Inherited disorders of the skeleton*, ed 2, Edinburgh, 1988, Churchill Livingstone.

31. Beighton P: Pyle disease (metaphyseal dysplasia), *J Med Genet* 24:321-324, 1987.

32. Beighton P: Osteoglophonic dysplasia, *J Med Genet* 26:572-576, 1989.

33. Beighton P, Cremin B: *Sclerosing bone dysplasias*, Berlin, 1980, Springer-Verlag.

34. Beighton P, Hamersma H: Frontometaphyseal dysplasia: autosomal dominant or X-linked? *J Med Genet* 17:53-56, 1980.

35. Beighton P, Hamersma H, Horan F: Craniometaphyseal dysplasia: variability of expression within a large family, *Clin Genet* 15:252-258, 1979.

36. Beighton P, Hamersma H, Raad M: Oculodentoosseous dysplasia: heterogeneity or variable expression? *Clin Genet* 16:169-177, 1979.

37. Beighton P, Kozlowski K: Spondylo-epi-metaphyseal dysplasia with joint laxity and severe, progressive kyphoscoliosis, *Skeletal Radiol* 5:205-212, 1980.

38. Beighton P et al: Sclerosteosis: an autosomal recessive disorder, *Clin Genet* 11:1-7, 1977.

39. Beighton P et al: The manifestations and natural history of spondylo-epi-metaphyseal dysplasia with joint laxity, *Clin Genet* 26:308-317, 1984.

40. Beighton P et al: The syndromic status of sclerosteosis and van Buchem disease, *Clin Genet* 25:175-181, 1984.

41. Benacevraf B et al: Achondrogenesis type I: ultrasound diagnosis in utero, *J Clin Ultrasound* 12:357-359, 1984.

42. Bercau G et al: La difficulte du diagnostic de la maladie de Caffey in utero: a propos d'un cas simulant l'osteogenese imparfaite letale, *Ann Pediatr* 38:15-18, 1991.

43. Berlin R et al: Osteopoikilosis: a clinical and genetic study, *Acta Med Scand* 181:305-314, 1967.

44. Bernstein R et al: Short rib polydactyly syndrome: a single or heterogeneous entity? A re-evaluation prompted by four new cases, *J Med Genet* 22:46-53, 1985.

45. Bianchi SD: The computed tomographic appearances of cherubism, *Skeletal Radiol* 16:6-10, 1987.

46. Boden SD et al: Metatropic dwarfism: uncoupling of endochondral and perichondral growth, *J Bone Joint Surg* 69(A):174-184, 1987.

47. Bonafede RP, Beighton P: The Dyggve-Melchior-Clausen syndrome in adult siblings, *Clin Genet* 14:24-30, 1978.

48. Borochowitz Z et al: Achondrogenesis II, hypochondrogenesis: variability vs. heterogeneity, *Am J Med Genet* 24:273-288, 1986.

49. Borochowitz Z et al: A distinct lethal neonatal chondrodysplasia with snail-like pelvis: Schneckenbecken dysplasia, *Am J Med Genet* 25:47-59, 1986.

50. Borochowitz Z et al: Achondrogenesis type I: delineation of further heterogeneity and identification of two distinct subgroups, *J Pediatr* 112:23-31, 1988.

51. Bouvet JP, Maroteaux P, Feingold J: Etude genetique du nanisme thanatophore, *Ann Genet* 17:181-188, 1974.

52. Bowen P: Achondroplasia in two sisters with normal parents, *Birth Defects (Original Article Series)* 10(2):31-36, 1974.

53. Brailsford JF: *Radiology of bones and joints*, ed 5, Baltimore, 1953, Williams & Wilkins.

54. Breur G et al: Clinical, radiographic, pathologic and genetic features of osteochondrodysplasia in Scottish deerhounds, *J Am Vet Med Assoc* 195:606, 1989.

55. Brewster TG et al: Oto-palato-digital syndrome, type II: an X-linked skeletal dysplasia, *Am J Med Genet* 20:249-254, 1985.

56. Briner J, Giedion A, Spycher MA: Variation of quantitative and qualitative changes of enchondral ossification in heterozygous achondroplasia, *Pathol Res Pract* 187:271-278, 1991.

57. Buhler EM, Malik NJ: The tricho-rhino-phalangeal syndrome(s), chromosome 8 long arm deletion: is there a shortest region of overlap between report cases? TRP I and TRP II syndromes: are they separate entities? *Am J Med Genet* 19:113-119, 1984.

58. Buhler EM et al: Chromosome deletion and multiple cartilaginous exostoses, *Eur J Pediatr* 133:163-166, 1980.

59. Buhler EM et al: A final word on tricho-rhino-phalangeal syndromes, *Clin Genet* 31:273-275, 1987.

60. Burgio GR, Belloni C, Beluffi G: Nanisme pseudodiastrophique: etude de deux soeurs nouveau-nes, *Arch Fr Pediatr* 31:681-696, 1974.

61. Byers PH: Molecular heterogeneity in chondrodysplasias, *Am J Hum Genet* 45:1-4, 1989.

62. Caffey J: Chondroectodermal dysplasia (Ellis-van Creveld disease): report of three cases, *Am J Roentgenol* 68:875-886, 1952.

63. Caffey J, Silverman W: Infantile cortical hyperostosis: preliminary report on new syndrome, *Am J Roentgenol* 54:1-16, 1945.

64. Canki-Klain N et al: Pseudodiastrophic dysplasia, evolution with age and management: report of two new cases and review of the literature, *Ann Genet* 33:129-136, 1990.

65. Carbonell Juanico M, Vineta Teixido J: Otro caso de discondroteosis generalizada congenita, tipo Ollier, *Rev Esp Pediatr* 18:91-99, 1962.

66. Carlson DH, Wilkinson RH: Variability of unilateral epiphyseal dysplasia (dysplasia epiphysealis hemimelica), *Radiology* 133:369, 1979.

67. Carnevale A et al: Autosomal dominant craniometaphyseal dysplasia: clinical variability, *Clin Genet* 23:17-22, 1983.

68. Castro DJ et al: Multicentric fibromatosis of familial inheritance, *Arch Pathol Lab Med* 111:867-869, 1987.

69. Cedarbaum SD et al: The chondroosseous dysplasia of adenosine deaminase deficiency with severe combined immunodeficiency, *J Pediatr* 89:737-742, 1976.

70. Chan D, Cole WG: Low basal transcription of genes for tissue-specific collagens by fibroblasts and lymphoblastoid cells: application to the characterization of glycine 997 to serine substitution in alpha 1(II) collagen chains of the patient with spondyloepiphyseal dysplasia, *J Biol Chem* 266:12487-12494, 1991.

71. Chang TK: Skeletal growth in Ancon sheep, *Growth* 13:221, 1949.

72. Charrow J, Poznanski AK: The Jansen type of metaphyseal chondrodyplasia: confirmation of dominant inheritance and review of radiographic manifestations in the newborn and adult, *Am J Med Genet* 18:321-327, 1984.

73. Chemke J, Graff G, Lancet M: Familial thanatophoric dwarfism *Lancet* 1:1358 (only), 1971.

74. Chen H, Liu CT, Yang SS: Achondrogenesis: a review with special consideration of achondrogenesis type II (Langer-Saldino), *Am J Med Genet* 10:379-394, 1981.

75. Chen H et al: Short rib–polydactyly syndrome, Majewski type, *Am J Med Genet* 7:215-222, 1980.

76. Chen H et al: A lethal, Larsen-like multiple joint dislocation syndrome, *Am J Med Genet* 13:149-161, 1982.

77. Chomette B et al: A peculiar form of osteodysplasia: cherubism, *Arch Anat Cytol Pathol* 35:69-75, 1987.

78. Chung EB, Enzinger FM: Infantile myofibromatosis, *Cancer* 48:1807-1818, 1981.

79. Chung KF et al: Acromegaly and hyperprolactinemia in McCune-Albright syndrome: evidence of hypothalamic dysfunction, *Am J Dis Child* 137:134-136, 1983.

80. Clayton-Smith J, Dinnai D: A further patient with the lethal type of Larsen syndrome, *J Med Genet* 25:499-500, 1988.

81. Cobb SR et al: CT of the temporal bone in achondroplasia, *Am J Neurol Radiol* 9:1195-1199, 1988.

82. Coccia PF et al: Successful bone-marrow transplantation for infantile malignant osteopetrosis, *New Engl J Med* 302:701-708, 1980.

83. Cooke CT et al: Campomelic dysplasia with sex reversal: morphological and cytogenetic studies of a case, *Pathology* 17:526-529, 1985.

84. Cooper CP, Hall CM: Lethal short-rib polydactyly syndrome of the Majewski type: a report of three cases, *Radiology* 144:513-517, 1982.

85. Cooper RR, Ponseti IV: Metaphyseal dysostosis: description of an ultrastructural defect in the epiphyseal plate chondrocytes. *J Bone Joint Surg* 55(A):485-495, 1973.

86. Cooper RR, Ponseti IV, Maynard JA: Pseudoachondroplastic dwarfism: a rough-surfaced endoplasmic reticulum storage disorder, *J Bone Joint Surg* 55:475-484, 1973.

87. Cornelius EA et al: Cherubism: hereditary fibrous dysplasia of the jaw: roentgenographic features, *Am J Roentgenol* 106:136, 1969.

88. Coste F, Maroteaux P, Chouraki L: Osteodysplasty (Melnick and Needles' syndrome): report of a case, *Ann Rheum Dis* 27:360-366, 1968.

89. Coulter CL et al: Cerebral abnormalities in thanatophoric dysplasia, *Childs Nerv Syst* 7:21-26, 1991.

90. Crisp AJ, Brenton DP: Engelmann's disease of bone: a systemic disorder? *Ann Rheum Dis* 41:183-188, 1982.

91. Curry CJR et al: Inherited chondrodysplasia punctata due to a deletion of the terminal short arm of an X chromosome, *New Engl J Med* 311:1010-1015, 1984.

92. Dawe C, Wynne-Davies R, Fulford GE: Clinical variation in dyschondrosteosis: a report on 13 individuals in eight families, *J Bone Joint Surg* 64(B):377-381, 1982.

93. de la Chapelle A et al: Une rare dysplasie osseuse letale de transmission recessive autosomique, *Arch Fr Pediatr* 29:759-770, 1972.

94. DeHaas WHD, DeBoer W, Griffionene F: Metaphyseal dysostosis: a late follow-up of the first reported case, *J Bone Joint Surg* 51(B):290-299, 1969.

95. Dennis JP, Rosenberg HS, Alvord EC Jr: Megalencephaly, internal hydrocephalus and other neurological aspects of achondroplasia, *Brain* 84:427-445, 1961.

96. Dent CE, Normand ICS: Metaphyseal dysostosis : type Schmid, *Arch Dis Child* 39:444-454, 1964.

97. Desbuquois G, Grenier B, Michel J: Nanisme chondrodystrophique avec ossification anarchique et polymalformations chez deux soeurs, *Arch Fr Pediatr* 23:573-587, 1966.

98. Dipierri JE, Guzman JD: A second family with autosomal dominant osteosclerosis: type Stanescu, *Am J Med Genet* 18:13-18, 1984.

99. Dodinval P, Le Marec B: Genetic counseling in unexpected familial recurrence of achondroplasia, *Am J Med Genet* 28:949-954, 1987.

100. Donalson JS et al: Osteochondroma of the distal femoral epiphysis, *J Pediatr* 43:212-216, 1953.

101. Donnenfeld AE et al: Melnick-Needles syndrome in males: a lethal multiple congenital anomalies syndrome, *Am J Med Genet* 27:159-173, 1987.

102. Dyggve HV, Melchior JC, Clausen J: Morquio-Ulrich's disease: an inborn error of metabolism? *Arch Dis Child* 37:525-534, 1962.

103. Eastman JR, Bixler D: Generalized cortical hyperostosis (Van Buchem disease): nosologic considerations. *Radiology* 125:297-304, 1977.

104. Eicher EM et al: Hypophosphatemic (vitamin D–resistant) rickets, *Proc Natl Acad Sci USA* 73:4667, 1976.

105. El Khazen et al: Lethal osteopetrosis with multiple fractures in utero, *Am J Med Genet* 23:811-819, 1986.

106. Ellis RWB: Osteopetrosis (marble bones: Albers-Schönberg's disease, osteosclerosis fragilis generalisata, congenital osteosclerosis), *Proc Roy Soc Med* 27:1563-1571, 1934.

107. Emmery L et al: Familial infantile cortical hyperostosis, *Eur J Pediatr* 141:56-58, 1983.

108. Enell H, Pherson M: Studies on osteopetrosis. I. Clinical report of three cases with genetic considerations, *Acta Pediatr* 47:279-287, 1958.

109. Eng CEL, Pauli RM, Strom CM: Nonrandom association of a type II procollagen genotype with achondroplasia, *Proc Natl Acad Sci* 82:5465-5469, 1985. (Retraction, *Proc Natl Acad Sci USA* 83:5354 only, 1986.)

110. Epstein JA, Malis LJ: Compression of spinal cord and cauda equina in achondroplastic dwarfs, *Neurology* 5:875-881, 1955.

111. Eroglu M et al: Congenital hyperphosphatasia (juvenile Paget's disease): eleven-year follow-up of three sisters, *Ann Radiol (Paris)* 20:145-150, 1977.

112. Erzen M et al: Comparative histopathology of the growth cartilage in short-rib polydactyly syndromes type I and type III and in chondroectodermal dysplasia, *Ann Genet* 31:144-150, 1988.

113. Espiritu C, Chen H, Woolley PV Jr: Mesomelic dwarfism as the homozygous expression of dyschondrosteosis, *Am J Dis Child* 129:375-377, 1975.

114. Eteson DJ et al: Fibrochondrogenesis: radiologic and histologic studies, *Am J Med Genet* 19:277-290, 1984.

115. Eteson DJ et al: Pseudodiastrophic dysplasia: a distinct newborn skeletal dysplasia, *J Pediatr* 109:635-641, 1986.

116. Eyre DR et al: Nonexpression of cartilage type II collagen in a case of Langer-Saldino achondrogenesis, *Am J Hum Genet* 39:52-67, 1986.

117. Eyring EJ, Eisenberg E: Congenital hyperphosphatasia: a clinical, pathological and biochemical study of two cases, *J Bone Joint Surg* 50(A):1099-1117, 1968.

118. Fairbank HAT: *An atlas of general affections of the skeleton*, Edinburgh, 1951, E & S Livingstone.

119. Fairbank T: Dysplasia epiphysialis multiplex, *Br J Surg* 34:225-232, 1947.

120. Fasanelli S et al: Dyssegmental dysplasia: report of two cases with a review of the literature, *Skeletal Radiol* 14:173-177, 1985.

121. Faye-Peterson OM, Knisely AS: Neural arch stenosis and spinal cord injury in thanatophoric dysplasia, *Am J Dis Child* 145:87-89, 1991.

122. Felman AH, Kirkpatrick JA Jr: Madelung's deformity: observations in 17 patients, *Radiology* 93:1037-1042, 1969.

123. Fennell SJ et al: Partial deletion 8q without Langer-Giedion syndrome: a recognizable syndrome, *J Med Genet* 26:167-171, 1989.

124. Feshchenko SP et al: The absence of type II collagen and changes in proteoglycan structure of hyaline cartilage in a case of Langer-Saldino achondrogenesis, *Hum Genet* 82:49-54, 1989.

125. Finklestein JE et al: Analysis of the chondroitin sulfate proteoglycan core protein (CSPGCP) gene in achondroplasia and pseudoachondroplasia, *Am J Hum Genet* 48:97-102, 1991.

126. Fischer A et al: Bone-marrow transplantation for immunodeficiencies and osteopetrosis: European survey 1968-1985, *Lancet* 2:1080-1084, 1986.

127. Fitch N, Jequier S, Gorlin R: The oto-palato-digital syndrome, proposed type II, *Am J Med Genet* 15:655-664, 1983.

128. Folz SJ, Trobe JD: The peroxisome and the eye, *Surv Ophthalmol* 35:353-368, 1991.

129. Fontaine G et al: La dysplasie spondylaire pure ou brachyolmie: a propos d'une observation, *Arch Fr Pediatr* 32:695-708, 1975.

130. Ford N, Silverman FN, Kozlowski K: Spondylo-epiphyseal dysplasia (pseudo-achondroplasia type), *Am J Roentgenol* 86:462-472, 1961.

131. Forland M: Cleidocranial dysostosis: a review of the syndrome and report of a sporadic case with hereditary transmission, *Am J Med* 33:792-799, 1962.

132. Fraccaro M: Cuntributo allo studio delle malattie del mesenchima osteopoietico: L'acondrogenesi, *Folia Hered Path* 1:190-208, 1952.

133. Francomano CA, Pyeritz RE: Achondroplasia is not caused by mutation in the gene for type II collagen, *Am J Med Genet* 29:955-961, 1988.

134. Francomano JE, Torjak JE, McKusick VA: Cartilage hair hypoplasia in the Amish: increased susceptibility to malignancy, *Am J Hum Genet* 35:89A only, 1983.

135. Francomano CA et al: The Stickler syndrome: evidence for close linkage to the structural gene for type II collagen, *Genomics* 1:293-296, 1987.

136. Fraser GR et al: Dysplasia spondyloepiphysaria and related generalized skeletal dysplasias among children with severe visual handicaps, *Arch Dis Child* 44:490-498, 1969.

137. Freire de Paes Alves A et al: Sclerosteosis: a marker of Dutch ancestry? *Rev Brasil Genet* 4:825-834, 1982.

138. Friede H et al: Craniofacial and mucopolysaccharide abnormalities in Kniest dysplasia, *J Craniofac Genet Devel Biol* 5:267-276, 1985.

139. Friedman SI et al: A lethal form of diastrophic dwarfism. In Bergsma D, editor: *Skeletal dysplasias*, Amsterdam, 1974, Excerpta Medica, pp 43-49.

140. Frydman M et al: Possible heterogeneity in spondylo-echondrodysplasia: quadriparesis, basal ganglia calcifications, and chondrocyte inclusions, *Am J Med Genet* 36:279-284, 1990.

141. Fryns JP, van den Berghe H: Langer type of mesomelic dwarfism as the possible homozygous expression of dyschondrosteosis, *Hum Genet* 46:21-27, 1979.

142. Fryns JP, van den Berghe H: 8q24.12 interstitial deletion in trichorhinophalangeal syndrome type I, *Hum Genet* 74:188-189, 1986.

143. Fryns JP, van den Berghe H: Facial paralysis at the age of 2 months as a first clinical sign of van Buchem disease (endosteal hyperostosis), *Eur J Pediatr* 147:99-100, 1988.

144. Fryns JP et al: Prenatal diagnosis of campomelic dwarfism, *Clin Genet* 19:199-201, 1981.

145. Gardner DL: Familial canine chondrodystrophia foetalis (achondroplasia), *J Pathol Bacteriol* 77:243, 1959.

146. Gardner RJM: A new estimate of the achondroplasia mutation rate, *Clin Genet* 11:31-38, 1977.

147. Giedion A: Das tricho-rhino-phalageale syndrome, *Helv Padiatr Acta* 21:475-485, 1966.

148. Giedion A et al: Autosomal dominant transmission of the trich-rhino-phalangeal syndrome: report of four unrelated families, review of 60 cases, *Helv Pediatr Acta* 28:249-259, 1973.

149. Giedion A et al: The widened spectrum of multiple cartilaginous exostosis (MCE), *Pediatr Radiol* 3:93, 1975.

150. Gilbert EF et al: Chondrodysplasia punctata-rhizomelic form: pathologic and radiologic studies of three infants, *Eur J Pediatr* 12:89-109, 1976.

151. Gilbert EF et al: Pathologic changes of osteochondrodysplasia in infancy: a review, *Pathol Ann* 22:283-345, 1987.

152. Giovannelli G, Bernasconi S, Banchini G: McCune-Albright syndrome in a male child: a clinical and endocrinologic enigma, *J Pediatr* 92:220-226, 1978.

153. Girdany BR: Englemann's disease (progressive diaphyseal dysplasia): a nonprogressive familial form of muscular dystrophy with characteristic bone changes, *Clin Orthop* 14:102-109, 1959.

154. Glass L et al: Audiologic findings in patients with achondroplasia, *Int J Otorhinolaryngol* 3:129-135, 1981.

155. Godfrey M, Hollister D: Type II achondrogenesis-hypochondrogenesis: identification of abnormal type II collagen, *Am J Hum Genet* 43:904-913, 1988.

156. Godfrey M et al: Type II achondrogenesis-hypochondrogenesis: morphologic and immunohistopathologic studies, *Am J Hum Genet* 43:894-903, 1988.

156a. Golbus MS: Personal communication, 1979.

157. Golbus MS et al: Prenatal diagnosis of achondrogenesis, *J Pediatr* 91:464-466, 1977.

158. Goldblatt J et al: Heterozygous manifestations of Langer mesomelic dysplasia, *Clin Genet* 31:19-24, 1987.

159. Goodman RM et al: Evidence for an autosomal recessive form of cleidocranial dysostosis, *Clin Genet* 8:20-29, 1975.

160. Gorlin RJ, Cohen MM Jr: Frontometaphyseal dysplasia: a new syndrome, *Am J Dis Child* 118:487-494, 1969.

161. Gorlin RJ, Glass L: Autosomal dominant osteosclerosis, *Radiology* 125:547-548, 1977.

162. Gorlin RJ, Langer LO Jr: Dyssegmental dwarfism(?s): lethal anisospondylic camptomicromelic dwarfism, *Birth Defects (Original Article Series)* 14(6B):193-197, 1978.

163. Gorlin RJ, Langer LO Jr: Melnick-Needles syndrome: radiographic alterations in the mandible, *Radiology* 128:351-353, 1978.

164. Gorlin RJ, Meskin LH, St Geme JW: Oculodentodigital dysplasia, *J Pediatr* 63:69-75, 1963.

165. Gorlin RJ, Spranger J, Koszalka MF: Genetic craniotubular bone dyspasia and hyperostoses: a critical analyses. In Bergsma D, editor: *Clinical delineation of birth defects. IV. Skeletal dysplasias*, New York, 1969, National Foundation, March of Dimes, pp 79-95.

166. Gorlin RJ, Winter RB: Frontometaphyseal dysplasia: evidence for X-linked inheritance, *Am J Med Genet* 5:81-84, 1980.

167. Goumy P et al: Syndrome de transmission recessive autosomique, associant un diabete congenital et des desordres de la croissance des epiphyses, *Arch Fr Pediatr* 37:323-328, 1980.

168. Graff G, Chemke J, Lancet M: Familial recurring thanatophoric dwarfism, *Obstet Gynecol* 39:515-520, 1972.

169. Gram PB et al: Metaphyseal chondrodysplasia of Jansen, *J Bone Joint Surg* 41(A):951-959, 1959.

170. Grebe H: *Chondrodysplasie*, Rome, 1955, Gregor Mendel Institute.

171. Greenberg CR et al: A new autosomal recessive lethal chondrodystrophy with congenital hydrops, *Am J Med Genet* 29:623-632, 1988.

172. Gregory PW: Genetic interrelationships of bovine chondrodystrophies In Bergsma D, editor: *Clinical delineation of birth defects. IV. Skeletal dysplasias*, New York, 1969, National Foundation, March of Dimes, pp 207-213.

173. Grischke EM et al: Prenatal sonographic diagnosis of a case of Desbuquois familial osseous dysplasia, *Z Geburtshilfe Perinatal* 193:195-197, 1989.

174. Grote W et al: Prenatal diagnosis of short-rib polydactyly syndrome type Saldino-Noonan at 17 weeks gestation, *Eur J Pediatr* 140:63-66, 1983.

175. Gruber HE, Lachman RS, Rimoin DL: Ultrastructural abnormalities in bone and calcifying cartilage in the short rib polydactyly syndromes, *J Bone Min Res* 4:(suppl 1):242, 1989.

176. Gruber HE, Lachman RS, Rimoin DL: Calcospherite (calcification nodule) size in the short rib polydactyly syndromes, *Scanning Microsc* 4:775-780, 1990.

177. Gruber HE et al: Lenz-Majewski syndrome: evidence for abnormally high bone formation and defective coupling, *J Bone Min Res* 3(suppl 1):164, 1988.

178. Gruber HE et al: Ultrastructural abnormalities in bone and calcifying cartilage in two siblings with a newly described recessive lethal chondrodysplasia, *Ultrastructural Pathol* 14:343-355, 1990.

179. Gruneberg H: *The pathology of development: a study of inherited skeletal disorders in animals*, New York, 1964, John Wiley and Sons.

180. Gustavson KH, Holmgren G, Probst F: Spondylometaphyseal dysplasia in two sibs of normal parents, *Pediatr Radiol* 7:90-96. 1978.

181. Gustavson KH et al: Lethal and nonlethal diastrophic dysplasia: a study of 14 Swedish cases, *Clin Genet* 28:321-334, 1985.

182. Hall BD, Spranger JW: Hypochondroplasia: clinical and radiological aspects in 39 cases, *Radiology* 133:95-100, 1979.

183. Hall BD, Spranger JW: Campomelic dysplasia: further elucidation of a distinct entity, *Am J Dis Child* 134:285-289, 1980.

184. Hall JG: Pseudoachondroplasia, *Birth Defects (Original Article Series)*. 11(6):187-202, 1975.

185. Hall JG, Dorst JP: Four types of pseudo-achondroplastic spondyloepiphyseal dysplasia (SED). In Bergsma D, editor: *Clinical delineation of birth defects. IV Skeletal dysplasias*, New York, 1969, National Foundation, March of Dimes, pp 242-259.

186. Hall JG, Froster-Iskenias UG, Manson JE: *Handbook of normal physical measurements*, Oxford, 1989, Oxford Medical Publications, p 408.

187. Hall JG et al: Two probable cases of homozygosity for the achondroplasia gene, *Birth Defects (Original Article Series)* 5(4):24-34, 1969.

188. Hall JG et al: Failure of early prenatal diagnosis in classic achondroplasia, *Am J Med Genet* 3:371-375, 1979.

189. Hall JG et al: Gonadal mosaicism in pseudoachondroplasia, *Am J Med Genet* 28:143-151, 1987.

190. Hall JG et al: Familial multiple exostosis: no chromosome 8 deletion observed, *Am J Med Genet* 82:327-329, 1989.

191. Hamidi-Toosi S, Maumenee IH: Vitreoretinal degeneration in spondyloepiphyseal dysplasia congenita, *Arch Ophthalmol* 100:1104-1107, 1982.

192. Handmaker SD et al: Dyssegmental dwarfism: a new syndrome of lethal dwarfism, *Birth Defects (Original Article Series)* 13(3D):79-90, 1977.

193. Hansen HG: Sklerosteose. In Opitz H, Schmid F, editors: *Hanbuch de Kinderheilkunde*, vol 6, Berlin, 1967, Springer-Verlag, pp 351-355.

194. Hansen HJ: A pathologic-anatomical study on disc degeneration in dog: with special reference to the so-called enctiondrosis intervertebralis, *Acta Orthop Scand* 11(suppl):4, 1952.

195. Hansen HJ: *Acta Orthop Scand* 43(suppl):5, 1972.

196. Happle R: X-linked dominant chondrodysplasia punctata, *Hum Genet* 53:65-73, 1979.

197. Happle R: The McCune-Albright syndrome: a lethal gene surviving by mosaicism, *Clin Genet* 29:321-324, 1986.

198. Happle R et al: Homologous genes for X-linked chondrodysplasia punctata in man and mouse, *Hum Genet* 63:24, 1983.

199. Harris R, Cullen CH: Autosomal dominant inheritance in Larsen's syndrome, *Clin Genet* 2:87-90, 1971.

200. Harris R, Patton JT: Achondroplasia and thanatophoric dwarfism in the newborn, *Clin Genet* 2:61-72, 1971.

201. Harris R, Patton JT, Barson AJ: Pseudo-achondrogenesis with fractures, *Clin Genet* 3:435-441, 1972.

202. Harris RE et al: Cartilage-hair hypoplasia, defective T-cell function, and Diamond-Blackfan anemia in an Amish child, *Am J Med Genet* 8:291-297, 1981.

203. Harrod MJE, Sherrod PS: Warfarin embryopathy in siblings, *Obstet Gynecol* 57:673-676, 1981.

204. Hastbacka J et al: Diastrophic dysplasia gene maps to the distal long arm of chromosome 5, *Proc Natl Acad Sci USA* 87:8056-8059, 1990.

205. Hawkin H, Golden A, Fox S: Familial osteoectasia with macrocranium. *Am J Roentgenol* 91:609-617, 1964.

206. Hecht JT, Butler IJ: Neurologic morbidity associated with achondroplasia, *J Child Neurol* 5:84-97, 1990.

207. Hecht JT et al: Computerized tomography of the foramen magnum: achondroplastic values compared to normal standards, *Am J Med Genet* 20:355-360, 1985.

208. Hecht JT et al: Obesity in achondroplasia, *Am J Med Genet* 31:597-602, 1988.

209. Hecht JT et al: Growth of the foramen magnum in achondroplasia, *Am J Med Genet* 32:528-535, 1989.

210. Heikoop JC et al: Peroxisomes of normal morphology but deficient in 3-oxoacyl-CoA thiolase in rhizomelic chondrodysplasia punctata fibroblasts, *Biochim Biophys Acta*, 1097:62-70, 1991.

211. Hennekam R: Hereditary multiple exostoses, *J Med Genet* 28:262-266, 1991.

212. Hennekam R: Short rib syndrome—Beemer type in sibs, *Am J Med Genet* 40:230-233, 1991.

213. Hensinger RN et al: Familial dysplasia epiphysealis hemimelica associated with chondromas and osteochondromas: report of a kindred with variable presentations, *J Bone Joint Surg* 56(A):1513-1516, 1974.

214. Herdman RC, Langer LO: The thoracic asphyxiant dystrophy and renal disease, *Am J Dis Child* 116:192-201, 1968.

215. Herdman RC, Langer LO, Good RA: Dyschondrosteosis: the most common cause of Madelung's deformity, *J Pediatr* 68:432-441, 1966.

216. Herman GE, Walton SJ: Close linkage of the murine locus bare patches to the X-linked visual pigment gene: implications for mapping human X-linked dominant chondrodysplasia punctata, *Genomics* 7:307-312, 1990.

217. Herrmann J et al: The Stickler syndrome (hereditary arthrophthalmopathy), *Birth Defects (Original Article Series)* 11(2):76-103, 1975.

218. Herzberg AJ et al: Variant of atelosteogenesis? Report of a 20-week fetus, *Am J Med Genet* 29:883-890, 1988.

219. Heselson NG, Cremin BJ, Beighton P: Pseudoachondroplasia, a report of 13 cases, *Br J Radiol* 50:473-482, 1977.

220. Heymans HSA et al: Rhizomelic chondrodysplasia punctata: another peroxisomal disorder, *New Engl J Med* 2:187-188, 1985.

221. Hille JJ et al: Cherubism: two case reports and a review of the literature, *J Dent Assoc S Afr* 41:461-466, 1986.

222. Hinkel CL, Beiler DD: Osteopetrosis in adults, *Am J Roentgenol* 74:46-64, 1955.

223. Hirata G, Rimoin DL, Poole AR: Biochemical and immunochemical studies of pseudoachondroplasia : abnormalities in posttranslational processing, *Trans Orthoped Res Soc* 15(11):303, 1990.

224. Hirsch S: Generalized osteochondrodystrophy, *J Bone Joint Surg* 19:297-313, 1937.

225. Hirschhorn R et al: Adenosine deaminase deficiency: frequency and comparative pathology in autosomally recessive severe combined immunodeficiency, *Clin Immunol Immunopathol* 14:107-129, 1979.

226. Ho KL: Neuropathologic findings in thanatophoric dysplasia, *Acta Neuropathol* 63:218-228, 1984.

227. Hobaeck A: *Problems of hereditary chondrodysplasia*, Oslo, Norway, 1961, Oslo University.

228. Hoefnagel D et al: Camptomelic dwarfism associated with XY-gonadal dysgenesis and chromosome anomalies, *Clin Genet* 13:489-499, 1978.

229. Holt JF: The evolution of cranio-metaphyseal dysplasia, *Ann Radiol* 9:209-214, 1966.

230. Horan FT, Beighton PH: Osteopathia striata with cranial sclerosis: an autosomal dominant entity, *Clin Genet* 13:201-206, 1978.

231. Horan F, Beighton P: *Orthopaedic problems in inherited skeletal disorders*, Berlin, 1982, Springer-Verlag.

232. Horton WA: Histochemical, immunohistochemical and lectin studies in decalcified iliac crest growth plate in skeletal dysplasias, *Prog Clin Biol Res* 104:401-410, 1982.

233. Horton WA, Harris DJ, Collins DL: Discordance for the Kleeblattschadel anomaly in monozygotic twins with thanatophoric dysplasia, *Am J Med Genet* 15:97-101, 1983.

234. Horton WA, Rimoin DL: Kniest dysplasia: a histochemical study of the growth plate, *Pediatr Res* 13:1266-1270, 1979.

235. Horton WA et al: The phenotypic variability of diastrophic dysplasia, *J Pediatr* 93:609-613, 1978.

236. Horton WA et al: Standard growth curves for achondroplasia, *J Pediatr* 93:435-438, 1978.

237. Horton WA et al: Diastrophic dwarfism: a histochemical and ultrastructural study of the endochondral growth plate, *Pediatr Res* 613:904-909., 1979.

238. Horton WA et al: Further heterogeneity within lethal neonatal short-limbed dwarfism: the platyspondylic types, *J Pediatr* 94:736-742, 1979.

239. Horton WA et al: Brachyolmia, recessive type (Hobaek): a clinical, radiographic and histochemical study, *Am J Med Genet* 16:201-211, 1983.

240. Horton WA et al: Achondrogenesis type II: abnormalities of extracellular matrix, *Pediatr Res* 22:324-329, 1987.

241. Horton WA et al: Abnormal ossification in thanatophoric dysplasia, *Bone* 9:53-61, 1988.

242. Horton WA et al: Tissue and cell studies of the growth plate in the chondrodyplasias, *Am J Med Genet* 34:91-95, 1989.

243. Houston CS, Awen CF, Kent HP: Fatal neonatal dwarfism, *J Can Assoc Radiol* 23:45-61, 1972.

244. Houston CS, Gerrard JW, Ives EJ: Dysosteosclerosis, *Am J Roentgenol* 130:988-991, 1978.

245. Houston CS, Reed MH, Desansch JEL: Separating Larsen's syndrome from the 'arthrogryposes,' *J Can Assoc Radiol* 32:206-214, 1981.

246. Houston CS et al: The campomelic syndrome: review, report of 17 cases, and follow-up on the currently 17-year-old boy first reported by Maroteaux et al. in 1971, *Am J Med Genet* 15:3-28, 1983.

247. Hovmoller ML et al: Camptomelic dwarfism: genetically determined mesenchymal disorder combined with sex reversal, *Hereditas* 86:51-62, 1977.

248. Hower J et al: Familiaere kongenitale generalisierte Fibromatose bei zwei Halbschwestern, *Schweiz Med Wschr* 101:1381-1385, 1971.

249. Hsu NG et al: The radiological manifestations of metaphyseal dysplasia (Pyle disease), *Br J Radiol* 52:431-440, 1979.

250. Hulvey JT, Keats TE: Multiple epiphyseal dysplasia: contribution to the problem of spinal involvement, *Am J Roentgenol* 106:170-177, 1969.

251. Hunter AG, Carpenter BF: Atelosteogenesis I and boomerang dysplasia: a question of nosology, *Clin Genet* 39:471-480, 1991.

252. Hurko O et al: Craniocervical decompression for cervicomedullary compression in pediatric patients with achondroplasia, *J. Neurol* 73:375-382, 1990.

253. Iceton JA, Horne G: Spondylo-epiphyseal dysplasia tarda: the X-linked variety in three brothers, *J Bone Joint Surg* 68(B):616-619, 1986.

254. Ilizarov GA: Clinical application of the tension-stress effect for limb lengthening, *Clin Orthop Rel Res* 250:8-26, 1990.

255. Iverson J: Cleidocranial dysostosis, *Acta Obstet Gynecol Scand* 41:93-99, 1962.

256. Jackson WPU: An irregular, familial chondro-osseous defect, *J Bone Joint Surg* 33(B):420-429, 1951.

257. Jackson WPU: Osteo-dental dysplasia (cleido-cranial dysostosis): The 'Arnold head'. *Acta Med Scand* 139:292-307, 1951.

258. Jackson WPU, Hanelin J, Albright F: Metaphyseal dysplasia, epiphyseal dysplasia, diaphyseal dysplasia, and related conditions: familial metaphyseal dysplasia and craniometaphyseal dysplasia: their relation to leontiasis ossea and osteopetrosis: disorders of 'bone remodeling.' *Arch Intern Med* 94:871-885, 1954.

259. Jacobsen AW: Hereditary osteochondrodystrophia deformans: a family with 20 members affected in five generations, *JAMA* 113:121-124, 1939.

260. Jaffe HL: Hereditary multiple exostoses, *Arch Pathol* 36:335-357, 1943.

261. Jansen M: Ueber atypische Chondrodystrophie Achondroplasia und ueber eine noch nicht beschriebene angeborene Wachstumsstörung des Knochensystems: Metaphysare Dysostosis, *Z Orthop Chir* 61:255, 1934.

262. Jarvis JL et al: Cleidocranial dysostosis: a review of 40 new cases, *Am J Roentgenol* 121:5-16, 1974.

263. Jennings TA et al: Infantile myofibromatosis: evidence for an autosomal dominant disorder, *Am J Surg Pathol* 8:529-538, 1984.

264. Jeune M, Beraud C, Carron R: Dystrophie thoracique asphyxiante de caractere familial, *Arch Fr Pediatr* 12:886-891, 1955.

265. Johnston CC Jr et al: Osteopetrosis: a clinical, genetic, metabolic, and morphologic study of the dominantly inherited benign form, *Medicine* 47:149-167, 1968.

266. Jones WA: Cherubism: a thumbnail sketch of its diagnosis and a conservative method of treatment, *Oral Surg* 20:648-653, 1965.

267. Joseph R et al: Dysplasie craniodiaphysaire progressive: ses relations avec la dysplasie progressive de Camurati-Englemann, *Ann Radiol* 1:477-490, 1958.

268. Juberg RC, Holt JF: Inheritance of multiple epiphyseal dyplasia tarda, *Am J Hum Genet* 20:549-563, 1968.

269. Kahanovitz N, Rimoin DL, Sillence DO: The clinical spectrum of lumbar spine disease in achondroplasia. *Spine* 7:137-140, 1982.

270. Kaibara N et al: Torrance type of lethal neonatal short-limbed dwarfism, *Skeletal Radiol* 10:17-19, 1983.

271. Kaitila I, Rimoin DL: Histologic heterogeneity in the hyperostotic bone dysplasias, *Birth Defects (Original Article Series)* 12(6):71-79, 1976.

272. Kaitila I et al: Craniodiaphyseal dysplasia, *Birth Defects (Original Article Series)* 11(6):359-362, 1975.

273. Kalliala E, Taskinen PJ: Cleidocranial dysostosis: report of six typical cases and one atypical case, *Oral Surg* 15:808-822, 1962.

274. Kalter DC, Atherton DJ, Clayton PT: X-linked dominant Conradi-Hünermann syndrome presenting as congenital erythroderma, *J Am Acad Dermatol* 21:248-256, 1989.

275. Kashler SG, Burns JA, Aylsworth AS: A mild autosomal recessive form of osteopetrosis, *Am J Med Genet* 17:451-464, 1984.

276. Kaufmann E: *Untersuchungen über die sogenannten fötale Rachitis (Chondrodystrophia foetalis)*, Berlin, 1892, Reimer.

277. Kaufmann E: Die chondrodystrophia hyperplastica: ein Beitrag zu den fötalen Skeleterkrankungen, *Beitr Path Anat* 13:32, 1893.

278. Keats TE, Smith TH, Sweet DE: Craniofacial dysostosis with fibrous metaphyseal defects, *Am J Roentgenol* 124:271-275, 1975.

279. Keith, Sir A: The nature of the structural alteration in this disorder known as multiple exostoses, *J Anat* 54:10-113, 1919-1920.

280. Keizer DRR, Schilder JH: Ectodermal dysplasia, achondroplasia and congenital morbus cordis, *Am J Dis Child* 82:341-344, 1951.

281. Kelley RI et al: Osteoglophonic dwarfism in two generations, *J Med Genet* 20:436-440, 1983.

282. Kelling C, Goldsmith LA, Baden HP: Biophysical and biochemical studies of the hair in cartilage-hair hypoplasia, *Clin Genet* 4:500-506, 1973.

283. Kelly TE, Wells HH, Tuck KB: The Weissenbacher-Zweymuller syndrome: possible neonatal expression of the Stickler syndrome, *Am J Med Genet* 11:113-119, 1982.

284. Kennedy LA: Metachondromatosis, *Radiol* 148:117-118, 1983.

285. Kenny AB, Hitzig WH: Bone marrow transplantation for severe combined immunodeficiency disease: reported from 1968-1977, *Eur J Pediatr* 131:155-176, 1979.

286. Key L et al: Treatment of congenital osteopetrosis with high dose calcitriol, *New Engl J Med* 310:409-414, 1984.

287. Khajavi A et al: Heterogeneity in the campomelic syndromes: long and short bone varieties, *Radiology* 120:641-647, 1976.

288. Kim HJ et al : Kniest syndrome with dominant inheritance and mucopolysacchariduria, *Am J Hum Genet* 27:755-764, 1975.

289. Kimata K et al: Absence of proteoglycan core protein in cartilage from the cmd/cmd (cartilage matrix deficiency) mouse, *J Biol Chem* 256:2691-6968, 1981.

290. Kirkpatrick DB. et al: The craniotubular bone modeling disorders: a neurosurgical introduction to rare skeletal dysplasias with cranial nerve compression, *Surg Neurol* 4:221-232, 1977.

291. Knisely AS: Thanatophoric dysplasia in identical twins, *J Med Genet* 26:735-736, 1989.

292. Knowles S, Winter R, Rimoin DL: A new category of short limbed dwarfism, *Am J Med Genet* 25:41-46, 1986.

293. Knowlton RG et al: Genetic linkage analysis of hereditary arthro-ophthalmopathy (Stickler syndrome) and the type II procollagen gene, *Am J Hum Genet* 45:681-688, 1989.

294. Knowlton RG et al: Genetic linkage of polymorphism in the type II procollagen gene (COL2A1) to primary osteoarthritis associated with mild chondrodysplasia, *New Engl J Med* 322:536-530, 1990.

295. Kopits S: Orthopedic complications of dwarfism, *Clin Orthop Rel Res* 114:153-179, 1976.

296. Kousseff BG et al: Spondyloepiphyseal dysplasia tarda and deutan color blindness in a family (abstract), *Seventh International Congress on Human Genetics*, Berlin, 1986, p 258.

297. Kozlowski K, Beighton P: Radiographic features of spondylo-epimetaphyseal dysplasia with joint laxity and progressive kyphoscoliosis, *Fortschr Roentgenstr* 141:337-341, 1984.

298. Kozlowski K, Kennedy J, Lewis IC: Radiologic features of progressive pseudorheumatoid arthritis, *Australas Radiol* 30:244-250, 1986.

299. Kozlowski K, Maroteaux P, Spranger JW: La dysostose spondylometaphysaire. *Presse Méd* 75:2769-2774, 1967.

300. Kozlowski K et al: Mandibular and para-mandibular tumors in children: report of 16 cases, *Pediatr Radiol* 11:183-192, 1981.

301. Kozlowski K et al: Spondylo-metaphyseal dysplasia: report of 7 cases and essay of classification. In Papadatos CJ, Bartsocas CS, editors: *Skeletal dysplasias*, New York, 1982, Alan R Liss, pp, 89-101.

302. Kozlowski K et al: Case report: boomerang dysplasia, *Br J Radiol* 369-371, 1985.

303. Kozlowski K et al: A new type of spondylometaphyseal dysplasia: Algerian type, *Pediatr Radiol* 18:221-226, 1988.

304. Krajewska-Walasek M, Winkielman J, Gorlin RJ: Melnick-Needles syndrome in males, *Am J Med Genet* 27:153-158, 1987.

305. Kraut JR et al: Isoenzyme studies in transient hyperphosphatasemia of infancy: ten new cases and a review of the literature, *Am J Dis Child* 139:736, 1985.

306. Krecak J, Starshak RJ: Cervical kyphosis in diastrophic dwarfism: CT and MR findings, *Pediatr Radiol* 17:321-322, 1987.

307. Krooth RS, Macklin MAP, Hillbish TF: Diaphysial aclasis (multiple exostoses) on Guam, *Am J Hum Genet* 13:340-397, 1961.

308. Kunze J, Klemm T: Mesomelic dysplasia, type Langer: a homozygous state for dyschondrosteosis, *Eur J Pediatr* 134:269-272, 1980.

309. Labat ML: A new approach to the study of the origin of genetic diseases: retroviral etiology of osteopetrosis, *Biomed Pharmacother* 45:23-27, 1991.

310. Labat ML et al: Retroviral expression in mononuclear blood cells isolated from a patient with osteopetrosis (Albers-Schönberg disease), *J Bone Min Res* 5:425-435, 1990.

311. Lachman RS, Rappaport V: Fetal imaging in the skeletal dysplasias, *Clin Perinatol* 17:703-722, 1990.

312. Lachman RS, Rimoin DL, Hollister DW: Arthrography of the hip: a clue to the pathogenesis of the epiphyseal dysplasia, *Radiology* 108:317-322, 1973.

313. Lachman RS, Rimoin DL, Spranger J: Metaphyseal chondrodysplasia, Schmid type: clinical and radiographic delineation with a review of the literature, *Pediatr Radiol* 18:93-102, 1988.

314. Lachman RS et al: Metachondromatosis, *Birth Defects (Original Article Series)* 10(9):171-178, 1974.

315. Lachman RS et al: The Kniest syndrome, *Am J Roentgenol* 123:805-814 1975.

316. Lachman RS et al: The spondylometaphyseal dysplasias: clinical, radiologic and pathologic correlation, *Ann Radiol* 22:125-135, 1979.

317. Lachman RS et al: Diastrophic dysplasia: the death of a variant, *Radiology* 140:79-86, 1981.

318. Lamy M, Maroteaux P: *Les chondrodystrophies genotypiques*, Paris, 1960, L'Expansion Scientifique Francaise.

319. Lamy M, Maroteaux P: Le nanisme diastrophique, *Presse Méd* 68:1977-1980, 1960.

320. Lamy M, Maroteaux P: Acro-osteolyse dominante, *Arch Fr Pediatr* 18:693-702, 1961.

321. Lamy M et al: Trois cas de maladie d'Ollier dans une fratrie, *Bull Mèm Soc Méd Hôp Paris* 70:62-70, 1954.

322. Landauer W: Malformations occurring in the creeper stocks, *J Genet* 30:303, 1935.

323. Landauer W: *Studies on fowl paralysis. III. A condition resembling osteopetrosis (marble bone) in the common fowl,* Storrs Agricultural Experiment Station Bull no 222, Storrs, Conn, 1938, University of Connecticut.

324. Landauer W: *Studies on the creeper fowl. XII. Size of body, organs and long bone of late homozygous creeper embryos,* Storrs Agricultural Experiment Station Bull no 232, Storrs, Conn, 1939, University of Connecticut.

325. Landing BH, Wells TR, Claireaux AD: Morphometric analysis of liver lesions in cystic diseases of childhood, *Hum Pathol* 11(suppl):549-560, 1980.

326. Langer LO Jr: Spondyloepiphyseal dysplasia tarda: hereditary chondrodysplasia with characteristic vertebral configuration in an adult, *Radiology* 82:833-839, 1964.

327. Langer LO Jr: Dyschondrosteosis: a hereditable bone dysplasia with characteristic roentgenographic features, *Am J Roentgenol* 95:178-188, 1965.

328. Langer LO Jr: Mesomelic dwarfism of the hypoplastic ulna, fibula, mandible type, *Radiology* 89:654-660, 1967.

329. Langer LO Jr: Thoracic-pelvic-phalangeal dystrophy, asphyxiating thoracic dystrophy of the newborn, infantile thoracic dystrophy, *Radiology* 91:447-456, 1968.

330. Langer LO Jr, Baumann PA, Gorlin RJ: Achondroplasia, *Am J Roentgenol* 100:12-26, 1967.

331. Langer LO Jr, Baumann PA, Gorlin RJ: Achondroplasia: clinical radiologic features with comments on genetic implications, *Clin Pediatr* 7:474, 1968.

332. Langer LO Jr et al: Thanatophoric dwarfism: a condition confused with achondroplasia in the neonate, with brief comments on achondrogenesis and homozygous achondroplasia, *Radiology* 92:285-294, 1969.

333. Langer LO Jr et al: The tricho-rhino-phalangeal syndrome with exostoses (or Langer-Giedion syndrome): four additional patients without mental retardation and review of the literature, *Am J Med Genet* 19:81-111, 1984.

334. Langer LO Jr et al: Thanatophoric dysplasia and cloverleaf skull, *Am J Med Genet* 3 (suppl):167-179, 1987.

335. Langer LO Jr et al: Spondylometaphyseal dysplasia, corner fracture type: a heritable condition associated with coxa vara, *Radiology* 175:761-766, 1990.

336. Langier R et al: Osteopoikilosis: a radiological and pathological study, *Skeletal Radiol* 11:161-168, 1984.

337. Larsen LJ, Schottstaedt ER, Bost FC: Multiple congenital dislocations associated with characteristic facial abnormality, *J Pediatr* 37:574-581, 1950.

338. Larson NE et al: Hereditary multiple exostoses with compression of the spinal cord, *Proc Mayo Clin* 32:729-734, 1957.

339. Laxova R et al: Family with probable achondrogenesis and lipid inclusions in fibroblasts, *Arch Dis Child* 48:212-216, 1973.

340. Lazzaroni-Fossati F et al: La fibrochondrogenese, *Arch Fr Pediatr* 35:1096-1104, 1978.

341. Lee B et al: Identification of the molecular defect in a family with spondyloepiphyseal dysplasia, *Science* 244:978-980, 1989.

342. Lee FA, Issacs H, Strauss J: The 'campomelic' syndrome: short life-span dwarfism with respiratory distress, hypotonia, peculiar facies, and multiple skeletal and cartilaginous deformities, *Am J Dis Child* 124:485-496, 1972.

343. Leeds NE: Epiphyseal dysplasia multiplex, *Am J Roentgenol* 84:506-510, 1960.

344. Lemli L: Fibrous dysplasia of bone: report of female monozygotic twins with and without the McCune-Albright syndrome, *J Pediatr* 91:947-949, 1977.

345. Lenz WD, Holt JF: Discussion: Murk Jansen type of metaphyseal dysostosis, *Birth Defects (Original Article Series)* 4:71-75, 1969.

346. Lenz WD, Majewski F: A generalized disorder of the connective tissues with progeria, choanal atresia, symphalangism, hypoplasia of dentine and craniodiaphyseal hyperostosis, *Birth Defects (Original Article Series)* 10(12):133-136, 1974.

347. Léri A, Weill J: Une affection congenitale et asymetrique du developpment osseux: la dyschondrosteose, *Bull Soc Méd Hôp Paris* 53:1491-1494, 1929.

348. Liberfarb RM, Goldblatt A: Prevalence of mitral-valve prolapse in the Stickler syndrome, *Am J Med Genet* 24:387-392, 1986.

349. Lichtenstein JR, Sundaram M, Burdge R: Sex-influenced expression of Madelung's deformity in a family with dyschondrosteosis, *J Med Genet* 17:41-43, 1980.

350. Lichtenstein L, Jaffe HL: Fibrous dysplasia of the bone: a condition affecting one, several or many bones, the graver of which may present abnormal pigmentation of skin, premature sexual development, hyperthyroidism or still other extraskeletal abnormalities, *Arch Pathol* 33:777-816, 1942.

351. Lièvre JA, Fischgold H: Leontiasis ossea chez l'enfants (osteopétrose partiele probable), *Presse Méd* 64:763-765, 1956.

352. Loewinger RJ et al: Maffucci's syndrome: a mesenchymal dysplasia and multiple tumour syndrome, *Br J Dermatol* 96:317-322, 1977.

353. Loria-Cortès R, Quesada-Calvo E, Cordero-Chaverri E: Osteopetrosis in children: a report of 26 cases, *J Pediatr* 91:43-47, 1977.

354. Lowry RB et al: Epiphyseal dysplasia, microcephaly nystagmus, and retinitis pigmentosa, *Am J Med Genet* 33:341-345, 1989.

355. Lundar T, Bakke SJ, Nornes H: Hydrocephalus in an achondroplastic child treated by venous decompression at the jugular foramen, *J Neurosurg* 73:138-140, 1990.

356. Lux SE et al: Neutropenia and abnormal cellular immunity in cartilage-hair hypoplasia, *New Engl J Med* 282:234-236, 1970.

357. MacDonald RM et al: Growth and development in thanatophoric dysplasia, *Am J Med Genet* 33:508-512, 1989.

358. MacKenzie WG et al: Avascular necrosis of the hip in multiple epiphyseal dysplasia, *J Pediatr Orthop* 9:666-671, 1989.

359. Mackler B, Bargman GJ, Shepard TH: Etiology of achondroplasia in the rabbit: a defect in oxidative metabolism, *Teratology* 5:261, 1972.

360. MacLachlan AK et al: Familial infantile cortical hyperostosis in a large Canadian family, *Can Med Assoc J* 130:1172-1174, 1984.

361. Maclean RN, Prater WK, Lozzio CB: Skeletal dysplasia with short, angulated femora (kyphomelic dysplasia), *Am J Med Genet* 14:373-380, 1983.

362. Macpherson RI, Wood BP: Spondyloepiphyseal dysplasia congenita: a cause of lethal neonatal dwarfism, *Pediatr Radiol* 9:217-224, 1980.

363. Mainzer F et al: The variable manifestations of multiple enchondromatosis, *Radiology* 99:377-388, 1971.

364. Majewski F et al: Polysyndaktylie, verkuerzte Gliedmassen und Genetitalfehlbildunger: Kennzeichen eines selbstaendigen Syndrome? *Z Kinderheilk* 111:118-138, 1971.

365. Mandell GA et al: Identification of avascular necrosis in the dysplastic proximal femoral epiphyses, *Skeletal Radiol* 18:273-281, 1989.

366. Manger H, Kruse K, Spranger J: Spondyloenchondrodysplasia, *J Med Genet* 26:93-99, 1989.

367. Maraia R, Saal HM, Wangsa D: A chromosome 17q de novo paracentric inversion in a patient with campomelic dysplasia: case report and etiologic hypothesis, *Clin Genet* 39:401-408, 1991.

368. Maroteaux P: La metachondromatose, *Z Kinderheilk* 109:246-261, 1971.

369. Maroteaux P: *Bone diseases of children*, Philadelphia, 1979, Lippincott.

370. Maroteaux P: Brachytelephalangic chondrodysplasia punctata: a possible X-linked recessive form, *Hum Genet* 82:167-170, 1989.

371. Maroteaux P, Lamy M: Les formes pseudo-achondroplastiques des dysplasies spondyloepiphysaires, *Presse Méd* 67:383-386, 1959.

372. Maroteaux P, Lamy M: La pycnodysostose, *Presse Méd* 70:999-1002, 1962.

373. Maroteaux P, Lamy M: Achondroplasia in man and animals, *Clin Orthop* 33:91-103, 1964.

374. Maroteaux P, Lamy M: The malady of Toulouse-Lautrec, *JAMA* 191:715-717, 1965.

375. Maroteaux P, Lamy M, Robert JM: Le nanisme thanatophore, *Presse Méd* 75:2519-2524, 1967.

376. Maroteaux P, Spranger J: The spondylometaphyseal dysplasias: a tentative classification, *Pediatr Radiol* 21:293-297, 1991.

377. Maroteaux P, Spranger JW, Weidemann HR: Der metatropische Zwergwuchs, *Arch Kinderheilk* 173:211-226, 1966.

378. Maroteaux P, Stanescu V, Stanescu R: Hypochondrogenesis, *Eur J Pediatr* 141:14-22, 1983.

379. Maroteaux P et al: Le syndrome campomelique, *Presse Méd* 22:1157-1162, 1971.

380. Maroteaux P et al: L'hyperostose corticale generalisee a transmission dominante, *Arch Fr Pediatr* 28:685-698, 1971.

381. Maroteaux P et al: The mild form of pseudoachondroplasia: Identification of the morphological and biochemical alterations of growth cartilage with those of typical pseudoachondroplasia, *Eur J Pediatr* 133:227-231, 1980.

382. Maroteaux P et al: Atelosteogenesis, *Am J Med Genet* 13:15-25, 1982.

383. Maroteaux P et al: Opsismodysplasia: a new type of chondrodysplasia with predominant involvement of the bones of the hand and the vertebrae, *Am J Med Genet* 19:171-182, l984.

384. Maroteaux P et al: Recessive lethal chondrodysplasia, "round femoral inferior epiphysis type," *Eur J Pediatr.* 147:408-411, 1988.

385. Martin JR et al: Platyspondyly, polyarticular osteoarthritis and absent β_2-globulin in two brothers, *Arthritis Rheum* 13:53-67, 1970.

386. Martinez-Frias ML, Ramos-Arroyo MA, Salvador J: Thanatophoric dysplasia: an autosomal dominant condition, *Am J Med Genet* 31:815-820, 1988.

387. Maumenee IH, Traboulsi EI: The ocular findings in Kniest dysplasia, *Am J Ophthalmol* 100:155-160, 1985.

388. Maynard JA, Cooper RR, Ponseti IV: A unique rough surface endoplasmic reticulum inclusion in pseudoachondroplasia, *Lab Invest* 26:40-44, 1972.

389. McCune DJ, Bradley C: Osteopetrosis (marble bones) in an infant: review of the literature and report of a case, *Am J Dis Child* 48:949-1000, 1934.

390. McCune DJ, Bruch H: Progress in pediatrics: osteodystrophia fibrosa, *Am J Dis Child* 54:806-848, 1937.

391. McKusick VA: *Heritable disorders of connective tissue*, ed 4, St Louis, 1972, Mosby–Year Book.

392. McKusick VA: *Mendelian inheritance in man*, ed 9, Baltimore, 1990, Johns Hopkins University.

393. McKusick VA, Kelly TE, Dorst JP: Observations suggesting allelism of the achondroplasia and hypochondroplasia genes, *J Med Genet* 10:11-16, 1973.

394. McKusick VA, Milch RA: The clinical behavior of genetic disease: selected aspects, *Clin Orthop* 33:22-39, 1964.

395. McKusick VA et al: Dwarfism in the Amish, *Trans Assoc Am Physicians* 77:151-168, 1964.

396. McKusick VA et al: Dwarfism in the Amish. I. The Ellis-van Creveld syndrome, *Bull Hopkins Hosp* 115:306-336, 1964.

397. McKusick VA et al: Medical genetics 1963, *J Chronic Dis* 17:1077-1215, 1964.

398. McKusick VA et al: Dwarfism in the Amish. II. Cartilage-hair hypoplasia, *Bull Hopkins Hosp* 116:285-326, 1965.

399. McLennan TW, Steinbach HL: Shwachman's syndrome: the broad spectrum of bony abnormalities, *Radiology* 112:167-173, 1974.

400. McPeak CN: Osteopetrosis: report of eight cases occurring in three generations of one family, *Am J Roentgenol* 37:816-829, 1936.

401. Meinecke P, Hayek H: Orofaciodigital syndrome type IV (Mohr-Majewski syndrome) with severe expression expanding the known spectrum of anomalies, *J Med Genet* 27:200-202, 1990.

402. Melnick JC, Needles CF: An undiagnosed bone dysplasia: a two-family study of four generations and three generations, *Am J Roentgenol* 97:39-48, 1966.

403. Mena HR, et al: Multiple epiphyseal dysplasia: a family case report, JAMA 236:2629, 1976.

404. Mills KLG, Johnston AW: Pycnodysostosis, *J Med Genet* 25:550-553, 1988.

405. Milroy CM, Michaels L: Temporal bone pathology of adult-type osteopetrosis, *Arch Otolaryngol Head Neck Surg* 116:79-84, 1990.

406. Morch ET: Chondrodystrophic dwarf in Denmark, *Opera ex Domo Biol Hered Hum Univ Hafn*, vol 3, 1941.

407. Morgan JP, Carlson WD, Adams OR: Hereditary multiple exostosis in the horse, *J Am Vet Med Assoc* 140:1320-1322, 1962.

408. Morris JM et al: Melorheostosis: review of the literature and report of an interesting case with 19-year follow-up, *J Bone Joint Surg* 45(A):1191, 1963.

409. Mostello D et al: Prenatal diagnosis of recurrent Larsen syndrome: further definition of a lethal variant, *Prenat Diagn* 11:215-225, 1991.

410. Mueller RF et al: X-linked dominant chondrodysplasia punctata, *Am J Med Genet* 20:137-144, 1985.

411. Murdoch JL et al: Achondroplasia: a genetic and statistical survey, *Ann Hum Genet* 33:227-244, 1970.

412. Murray L, Hollister DW, Rimoin DL: Diastrophic dysplasia: evidence against a defect of type II collagen, *Matrix* 9:459-467, 1989.

413. Murray L, Rimoin DL: Abnormal type II collagen in the spondyloepiphyseal dysplasias, *Pathol Immunopathol Res* 7:99-103, 1988.

414. Murray L et al : Type II collagen defects in the chondroysplasias. I. Spondyloepiphyseal dysplasias, *Am J Hum Genet* 45:5-15, 1989.

415. Murray RO, et al: Melorheostosis and sclerotome: a radiological correlation, *Skeletal Radiol* 4:57, 1979.

416. Murray TG, et al: Spondyloepiphyseal dysplasia congenita: light and electron microscopic studies of the eye, *Arch Ophthalmol* 103:407-411, 1985.

417. Naffah J: The Dyggve-Melchior-Clausen syndrome, *Am J Hum Genet* 28:607-614, 1976.

418. Nager GT et al: Sclerostosis involving the temporal bone: clinical and radiologic aspects, *Am J Otolaryngol* 4:1-17, 1983.

419. Naito M et al: Abnormal differentiation of tissue macrophage populations in 'osteopetrosis' (op) mice defective in the production of macrophage colony-stimulating factor, *Am J Pathol* 139:657-667, 1991.

420. Naumoff P et al: Short-rib–polydactyly syndrome type III, *Radiology* 122:443-447, 1977.

421. Naveh Y et al: Progressive diaphyseal dysplasia: genetics and clinical and radiologic manifestations, *Pediatrics* 74:399-405, 1984.

422. Naveh Y et al: Progressive diaphyseal dysplasia: evaluation of corticosteroid therapy, *Pediatrics* 75:321-323, 1985.

423. Nelson FW et al: Neurological basis of respiratory complications in achondroplasia, *Ann Neurol* 24:89-93, 1988.

424. Nicoletti B et al: *Human achondroplasia: a multidisciplinary approach*, New York, 1986, Plenum.

425. Ogilvie D et al: Evidence against the structural gene encoding type II collagen (COL2A1) as the mutant locus in achondroplasia, *J Med Genet* 23:19-22, 1986.

426. Ohlsson A et al: Carbonic anhydrase II deficiency syndrome: recessive osteopetrosis with renal tubular acidosis and cerebral calcification *Pediatrics* 77:371-381, 1986.

427. Olge RF et al: Multiple exostoses in a patient with t(8;11)(q24.llp15.5), *J Med Genet* 28:881-883, 1991.

428. Opitz JM: Delayed mutation in achondroplasia. In Bergsma D, editor: *Clinical delineation of birth defects. IV. Skeletal dysplasias*, New York, 1969, National Foundation, March of Dimes, pp 20-23.

429. Opitz JM: Ocular anomalies in malformation syndromes, *Trans Am Acad Ophthalmol Otolaryngol* 76:1193-1202, 1972.

430. Opitz JM: Unstable premutation in achondroplasia: penetrance vs. phenotrance, *Am J Med Genet* 19:251-254, 1984.

431. Orioli M, Castilla EE, Barbosa-Neto JG: The birth prevalence rates for the skeletal dysplasias, *J Med Genet* 23:328-332, 1986.

432. Orkin RW, Pratt RM, Martin GR: Undersulfated chondroitin sulfate in the cartilage matrix of brachymorphic mice. *Dev Biol* 50:82, 1976.

433. Ornoy A et al: The role of mesenchymal-like tissue in the pathogenesis of thanatophoric dysplasia, *Am J Med Genet* 21:613-630, 1985.

434. Ornoy A et al: *Atlas of fetal skeletal radiology*, St Louis, l988, Mosby– Year Book.

435. Owen OE et al: Resting metabolic rate and body composition of achondroplastic dwarfs, *Medicine* 69:56-67, 1990.

436. Palotie A et al: Predisposition to familial osteoarthrosis linked to type II collagen gene, *Lancet* 1:924-927, 1989.

437. Parenti GC: La anosteogenesi (una varieta della osteogenesi imperfecta), *Pathologica* 28:447-664, 1936.

438. Partington MW et al: Cloverleaf skull and thanatophoric dwarfism: report of four cases, two in the same sibship, *Arch Dis Child* 46:656-664, 1971.

439. Pasquino AM et al: Precocious puberty in the McCune-Albright syndrome, *Acta Pediatr Scand* 76:841-843, 1987.

440. Patrone NA, Kredich DW: Arthritis in children with multiple epiphyseal dysplasia, *J Rheumatol* 12:145-149, 1985.

441. Patton MA, Laurence KM: Three new cases of oculodentodigital (ODD) syndrome: development of the facial phenotype, *J Med Genet* 22:386-389, 1985.

442. Pauli RM et al: Apnea and sudden unexpected death in infants with achondroplasia, *J Pediatr* 104:342-348, 1984.

443. Pearce L, Brown WH: Hereditary osteopetrosis in the rabbit, *J Exp Med* 88:579-597, 1928.

444. Penchaszadeh VB, Gutierriz ER, Figeueroa EP: Autosomal recessive craniometaphyseal dysplasia, *Am J Med Genet* 5:43-55, 1980.

445. Penrose LS: Parental age and mutation, *Lancet* 2:312-313, 1955.

446. Perez-Vicente JA et al: Autosomal dominant endosteal hyperostosis: report of a Spanish family with neurological involvement, *Clin Genet* 31:161-169, 1987.

447. Peters WJN: Cherubism: a study of twenty cases from one family, *Oral Surg* 47:307-311, 1979.

448. Petit C et al: An interstitial deletion in Xp22.3 in a family with X-linked recessive chondrodysplasia punctata and short stature, *Hum Genet* 85:247-250, 1990.

449. Pettifor JM, Benson R: Congenital malformations associated with the administration of oral anticoagulants during pregnancy, *J Pediatr* 86:459-462, 1975.

450. Pfeiffer RA: Langer-Giedion syndrome and additional congenital malformations with interstitial deletion of the long arm of chromosome 8 46, XY, del 8 (q13-22), *Clin Genet* 18:142-146, 1980.

451. Pfeiffer RA, Diekmann L, Stock HJ: Aplasia of the thumbs and great toes as the outstanding feature of Yunis and Varon syndrome: a new entity, a new observation, *Ann Genet* 31:241-243, 1988.

452. Philip N et al: Achondroplasia in sibs of normal parents, *J Med Genet* 25:857-859, 1988.

453. Pierce GF, Polmar SH: Lymphocyte dysfunction in cartilage-hair hypoplasia: evidence for an intrinsic defect in cellular proliferation, *J Immunol* 129:570-575, 1982.

454. Pierre-Kahn A et al: Hydrocephalus and achondroplasia: a study of 25 observations, *Child's Brain* 7:205-219, 1980.

455. Polmar SH, Pierce GF: Cartilage hair hypoplasia: immunological aspects and their clinical implications, *Clin Immunol Immunopathol* 40:87-93, 1986.

456. Polmar SH et al: Enzyme replacement thereapy for adenosine deaminase deficiency and severe combined immunodeficiency, *New Engl J Med* 295:1337-1343, 1976.

457. Ponseti IV: Skeletal growth in achondroplasia, *J Bone Joint Surg* 52A:701, 1970.

458. Poole AR et al: Kniest dysplasia is characterized by an apparent abnormal processing of the C-propeptide of type II cartilage collagen resulting in imperfect fibril assembly, *J Clin Invest* 81:579-589, 1988.

459. Poulos A et al: Rhizomelic chondrodysplasia punctata: clinical, pathologic and biochemical findings in two patients, *J Pediatr* 113:685-690, 1988.

460. Prendiville JS, Zaparackas ZG, Esterly NB: Normal peroxisomal function and absent skeletal manifestations in Conradi-Hünermann syndrome, *Arch Dermatol* 127:539-542, 1991.

461. Prins HW, Van den Hamer JA: Primary biochemical defect in copper metabolism in mice with a recessive X-linked mutation analogous to Menkes disease in man, *J Inorg Biochem* 10:19, 1979.

462. Pulst SM et al: The achondroplasia gene is not linked to the locus for neurofibromatosis 1 on chromosome 17, *Hum Genet* 85:12-14, 1990.

463. Pyeritz RE, Sack GH Jr, Udvarhelyi GB: Thoracolumbosacral laminectomy in achondroplasia: long-term results in 22 patients, *Am J Med Genet* 28:433-444, 1987.

464. Ratech H et al: Pathologic findings in adenosine deaminase deficient–severe combined immunodeficiency disease. I. Kidney, adrenal and chondroosseous tissue alterations, *Am J Pathol* 120:157-169, 1985.

465. Rawlinson PS et al: Malignant osteopetrosis: hypercalcaemia after bone marrow transplantation, *Arch Dis Child* 66:638-639, 1991.

466. Rezza E, Iannaccone G, Lendvai D: Familial congenital bowing with short thick bones and metaphyseal changes, a distinct entity: report of the clinical and radiological findings in two siblings, *Pediatr Radiol* 14:323-327, 1984.

467. Ribbing S: Studien ueber hereditare, multiple Ephiphysen-storungen, *Acta Radiol* 34, 1937.

468. Ribbing S: Hereditary multiple diaphyseal sclerosis, *Acta Radiol* 31:522-536, 1949.

469. Rieth KG et al: Pituitary and ovarian abnormalities demonstrated by CT and ultrasound in children with features of the McCune-Albright syndrome, *Radiology* 153:389-393, 1984.

470. Rimoin DL: The chondrodystrophies: In Harris H, Hirschhorn K, editors: *Advances in human genetics*, vol 5, New York, 1975, Plenum, pp 1-118.

471. Rimoin DL: Symposium on the skeletal dysplasias, *Clin Orthop Rel Res* , 114:2-179, 1976.

472. Rimoin DL: Variable expressivity in the skeletal dysplasias, *Birth Defects, (Original Article Series)* 15(5B):91-112, 1979.

473. Rimoin DL: Clinical variability in achondroplasia, *Basic Life Sci* 48:123-127, 1988.

474. Rimoin DL, Eteson DJ, Sillence DO: Comparisons and correlations of skeletal defects in mouse and human, *Pathol Immunopathol Res* 7:139-145, 1988.

475. Rimoin DL, Horton WA: Short stature. I and II. *J Pediatr* 92:523-528, 697-704, 1978.

476. Rimoin DL, Lachman RS: The chondrodysplasias. In Emery AE, Rimoin DL, editors: *The principles and practice of medical genetics*, ed 2, Edinburgh, 1990, Churchill Livingstone, pp 895-932.

477. Rimoin DL, Woodruff SL, Holman BL: Craniometaphyseal dysplasia (Pyle's disease): autosomal dominant inheritance in a large kindred, *Birth Defects (Original Article Series)* 5(4):96-104, 1969.

478. Rimoin DL et al: Endochondral ossification in achondroplastic dwarfism, *New Engl J Med* 283:728-735, 1970.

479. Rittler M, Menger H, Spranger J: Chondrodysplasia punctata, tibia-metacarpal (MT) type, *Am J Med Genet* 37:200-208, 1990.

480. Robinow M, Johanson AJ, Smith TH: The Lenz-Majewski hyperostotic dwarfism: a syndrome of multiple congenital anomalies, mental retardation and progressive skeletal sclerosis, *J Pediatr* 91:417-421, 1977.

481. Robinson D et al: Spondyloepiphyseal dysplasia associated with progressive arthropathy: an unusual disorder mimicking juvenile rheumatoid arthritis, *Arch Orthop Trauma Surg* 108:397-399, 1989.

482. Rolland JC et al: Nanisme chondrodystrophique et division palatine chez un nouveau-ne, *Ann Pediatr* 19:139-43, 1972.

483. Rosenbloom AL, Smith DW: The natural history of metaphyseal dysostosis, *J Pediatr* 66:857-868, 1965.

484. Rossberg A: Zur Erblichkeit der Knochenchondromatose, *Fortschr Roentgenstr* 90:138-139, 1959.

485. Royer P et al: Maladie d'Engelmann: resultat du traitement par la prednisone, *Arch Fr Pediatr* 24:693-702, 1967.

486. Rubin P: *Dynamic classification of bone dysplasias*, St Louis, 1964, Mosby–Year Book.

487. Sabry A: Thanatophoric dwarfism in triplets, *Lancet* 2:533 only, 1974.

488. Saldino RM: Lethal short-limbed dwarfism: achondrogenesis and thanatophoric dwarfism, *Am J Roentgenol* 112:185-197, 1971.

489. Saldino RM, Noonan CD: Severe thoracic dystrophy with striking micromelia, abnormal osseous development, including the spine, and multiple visceral abnormalities, *Am J Roentgenol* 114:257-263, 1972.

490. Salzano FM: Osteopetrosis: review of dominant cases and frequency in a Brazilian state, *Acta Genet Med Gemellol* 10:353-358, 1961.

491. Salzano FM, Ebling H: Cherubism in a Brazilian kindred, *Acta Genet Med Gemellol* 15:296-301, 1966.

492. Sande R, Bingel S: *Vet Clin North Am Small Anim Pract* 13:71, 1982.

493. Schaffer B et al: Dominantly inherited craniodiaphyseal dysplasia: a new craniotubular dysplasia, *Clin Genet* 30:381-391, 1986.

494. Schantz K, Anderson PE Jr, Justesen P: Spondyloepiphyseal dysplasia tarda: report of a family with autosomal dominant transmission, *Acta Orthop Scand* 59:716-719, 1988.

495. Schmid F: Beitrag zur Dysostosis enchondralis metaphys-area, *Mschr Kinderheilk* 97:393-397, 1949.

496. Schmidt BJ et al: Metaphyseal dysostosis: review of literature, study of a case with cytogenetic analysis, *J Pediatr* 63:106-112, 1963.

497. Schorr S, Legum C, Ochshorn M: Spondyloenchondrodysplasia: enchondromatosis with severe platyspondyly in two brothers, *Radiology* 118:133-139, 1976.

498. Schreiber F, Rosenthal H: Paraplegia from ruptured lumbar discs in achondroplastic dwarfs, *J Neurosurg* 9:648-651, 1952.

499. Schwartz HS et al: The malignant potential of enchondromatosis, *J Bone Joint Surg* 69(A):269-274, 1987.

500. Schwartz NB et al: Defective PAPS-synthesis in epiphyseal cartilage from brachymorphic mice, *Biochem Biophys Res Commun* 82:173, 1978.

501. Schwarz E, Fish A: Roentgenographic features of a new congenital dysplasia, *Am J Roentgenol* 84:511-517, 1960.

502. Scriver C et al: *The metabolic basis of inherited disease*, ed 6, New York, 1989, McGraw-Hill.

503. Sear WR: The congenital bone dystrophies and their corelation, *J Fac Radiologists* 4:221-234, 5:140 only, 1953.

504. Sedano HP, Gorlin RJ, Anderson VE: Pycnodysostosis: clinical and genetic considerations, *Am J Dis Child* 116:70-77, 1968.

505. Semble EL et al: Successful symptomatic treatment of melorheostosis with nifedipine, *Clin Exp Rheumatol* 4:277-280, 1986.

506. Shapiro F: Ollier's disease, *J Bone Joint Surg* 64(A):95-103, 1982.

507. Shaul WL, Emery H, Hall JG: Chondrodysplasia punctata and maternal warfarin use during pregnancy, *Am J Dis Child* 129:360-362, 1975.

508. Sheffield LJ et al: Chondrodysplasia punctata: 23 cases of a mild and relatively common variety, *J Pediatr* 89:916-923, 1976.

509. Shepard TH, Fry LR, Moffett BC Jr: Microscopic studies of achondroplastic rabbit cartilage, *Teratology* 2:13, 1969.

510. Sher C et al: Mild spondyloepiphyseal dysplasia (Namaqualand type): genetic linkage to the type II collagen gene COL2A1, *Am J Hum Genet* 48:518-524, 1991.

511. Shibuya H et al: The radiological appearances of familial metaphyseal dysplasia, *Clin Radiol* 33:439-444, 1982.

512. Shigematsu H et al: Neuropathological and golgi study on a case of thanatophoric dysplasia, *Brain Dev* 7:628-632, 1985.

513. Shmerling DH et al: The syndrome of exocrine pancreatic insufficiency, neutropenia, metaphyseal dysostosis and dwarfism, *Helv Paediat Acta* 24:547-575, 1969.

514. Shohat M, Lachman R, Rimoin DL: Odontoid hypoplasia with vertebral cervical spine subluxation and ventriculomegaly in metatropic dysplasia, *J Pediatr* 114:239-243, 1989.

515. Shohat M et al: Brachyolmia: radiographic and genetic evidence of heterogeneity, *Am J Med Genet* 33:209-219, 1989.

516. Shohat M et al: Geleophysic dysplasia: a storage disorder affecting the skin, bone, liver, heart and trachea *J Pediatr* 117:227-232, 1990.

517. Shohat M et al: Perinatal lethal hypophosphatasia: clinical, radiographic and morphologic findings, *Pediatr Radiol* 21:421-427, 1991.

518. Shohat M et al: Hearing loss and temporal bone structure in achondroplasia, *Am J Med Genet*, 1992 (in press).

519. Shokeir MHK, Houston CS, Awen CF: Asphyxiating thoracic chondrodystrophy: association with renal disease and evidence for possible heterozygous expression, *J Med Genet* 8:107-112, 1971.

520. Shwachman H et al: The syndrome of pancreatic insufficiency and bone marrow dysfunction, *J Pediatr* 65:645-663, 1964.

521. Siebens AA, Hungerford DS, Kirby NA: Curves of the achondroplastic spine: a new hypothesis, *Johns Hopkins Med J* 142:205-210, 1978.

522. Sieff CA et al: Allogeneic bone-marrow transplantation in infantile malignant osteopetrosis, *Lancet* 1:437-441, 1983.

523. Siggers DC, et al: The Kniest syndrome, *Birth Defects (Original Article Series)* 10(9):193-208, 1974.

524. Silengo MC, Luzzati L, Silverman FN: Clinical and genetic aspects of Conradi-Hünermann disease: a report of three familial cases and review of the literature, *J Pediatr* 97:911-917, 1980.

525. Silengo MC et al: Oro-facial-digital syndrome. II. Transitional type between the Mohr and the Majewski syndromes: report of 2 new cases, *Clin Genet* 31:331-336, 1987.

526. Sillence DO: Non-Majewski short rib–polydactyly syndrome, *Am J Med Genet* 7:223-229, 1980.

527. Sillence DO, Horton WA, Rimoin DL: Morphologic studies in the skeletal dysplasias, *Am J Pathol* 96:813-870, 1979.

528. Sillence DO, Ritchie HE, Selby PB: Skeletal anomalies in mice with cleidocranial dysplasia, *Am J Med Genet* 27:75-85, 1987.

529. Sillence DO et al: Spondylohumerofemoral hypoplasia (giant cell chondrodysplasia): a neonatally lethal short-limb skeletal dysplasia, *Am J Med Genet* 13:7-14, 1982.

530. Sillence DO et al: Atelosteogenesis: evidence for heterogeneity, *Pediatr Radiol* 17:112-118, 1987.

531. Sillence DO et al: Perinatally lethal short rib–polydactyly syndrome, *Pediatr Radiol* 17:474-480, 1987.

532. Silverthorn KG et al: Mark Jansen's metaphyseal chondrodysplasia with long-term follow-up, *Pediatr Radiol* 17:119-123, 1987.

533. Simon D et al: Une osteosclerose axiale de transmission dominant autosomique: nouvelle entite? *Rev Rhum* 46:375-382, 1979.

534. Simril WA, Thurston D: Normal interpediculate space in spines of infants and children, *Radiology* 64:340-347, 1955.

535. Singh I et al: Rhizomelic chondrodysplasia punctata: biochemical studies of peroxisomes isolated from cultured skin fibroblasts, *Arch Biochem Biophys* 286:277-283, 1991.

536. Sly WS et al: Carbonic anhydrase II deficiency identified as the primary defect in the autosomal recessive syndrome of osteopetrosis with renal tubular acidosis and cerebral calcification, *Proc Natl Acad Sci* 80:2752-2756, 1983.

537. Sly WS et al: Carbonic anhydrase II deficiency in 12 families with the autosomal recessive syndrome of osteopetrosis with renal tubular acidosis and cerebral calcification, *New Engl J Med* 313:139-145, 1985.

538. Smits B, Bubenik GA: Congenital osteopetrosis in white-tailed deer (Odocoileus virginianus), *J Wildl Dis* 26:567-571, 1990.

539. Sommer A, Young-Wee T, Frye T: Achondroplasia-hypochondroplasia complex, *Am J Med Genet* 26:949-957, 1987.

540. Sorell M et al: Marrow transplantation for juvenile osteopetrosis, *Am J Med* 70:1280-1287, 1981.

541. Spahr A, Spahr-Hartmann I: Dysostose metaphysaire familiale: etude de 4 cas dans une fratrie, *Paediat Acta* 16:836-849, 1961.

542. Sparkes RS, Graham CB: Camurati-Engelmann disease: genetics and clinical manifestations with a review of the literature, *J Med Genet* 9:73-85, 1972.

543. Spranger JW: Hereditary arthro-ophthalmopathy, *Ann Radiol* 11:359-364, 1968.

544. Spranger JW: Pattern recognition in bone dysplasias, *Prog Clin Biol Res* 200:315-342, 1985.

545. Spranger JW: Radiologic nosology of bone dysplasias, *Am J Med Genet* 34:96-104, 1989.

546. Spranger JW, Bierbaum B, Herrmann J: Heterogeneity of Dyggve-Melchior-Clausen dwarfism, *Hum Genet* 33:279-287, 1976.

547. Spranger JW, Langer LO Jr: Spondyloepiphyseal dysplasia congenita, *Radiology* 94:313-322, 1970.

548. Spranger JW, Langer LO: Spondyloepiphyseal dysplasias, *Birth Defects (Original Article Series)* 10(9):19-61, 1974.

549. Spranger JW, Langer LO, Wiedemann HR: *Bone dysplasias: an atlas on constitutional disorders of skeletal development*, Philadelphia, 1974, WB Saunders.

550. Spranger JW, Maroteaux P: The lethal osteochondrodysplasias, *Adv Hum Genet* 19:1-103, 1990.

551. Spranger JW, Maroteaux P, Der Kaloustian VM: The Dyggve-Melchior-Clausen syndrome, *Radiology* 114:415-422, 1975.

552. Spranger JW, Opitz JM, Bidder U: Heterogeneity of chondrodysplasia punctata, *Humangenetik* 11:190-212, 1971.

553. Spranger JW, Paulsen K, Lehmann W: Die kraniometaphysaere Dysplasie (Pyle), *Z Kinderheilk* 93:64-79, 1965.

554. Spranger JW, Paulsen K, Lehmann W: Die kraniometaphysare Dysplasie (Pyle), *Z Humangenetik* 11:190-212, 1971.

555. Spranger JW, Wiedemann HR: Dysplasia spondyleopiphysaria congenita, *Helv Paediatr Acta* 21:598-611, 1966.

556. Spranger JW et al: Die dysosteosklerose: Eine sonderform der generalisierten osteoklerose, *Fortschr Roentgenstr* 109:504-512, 1968.

557. Spranger JW et al: Short rib–polydactyly (SRP) syndromes, types Majewski and Saldino-Noonan, *Z Kinderheilk* 116:73-94, 1974.

558. Spranger JW et al: Progressive pseudorheumatoid arthritis of childhood (PPAC): a hereditary disorder simulating rheumatoid arthritis, *Eur J Pediatr* 1490:34-40, 1983.

559. Spranger JW et al: Geleophysic dysplasia, *Am J Med Genet* 19:487-499, 1984.

560. Spranger JW et al: International nomenclature of constitutional disorders of bone, *Eur J Pediatr* 151:407-417, 1992.

561. Stanescu R, Stanescu V, Maroteaux P: Abnormal pattern of segment long spacing (SLS) cartilage collagen in diastrophic dysplasia, *Collagen Rel Res* 2:111-116, 1982.

562. Stanescu R, Stanescu V, Maroteaux P: Homozygous achondroplasia: morphologic and biochemical study of cartilage, *Am J Med Genet* 37:412-421, 1990.

563. Stanescu V, Maroteaux P, Stanescu R: The biochemical defect of pseudoachondroplasia, *Eur J Pediatr* 138:221-522, 1982.

564. Stanescu V, Stanescu R, Maroteaux P: Morphological and biochemical studies of epiphyseal cartilage in dyschondroplasias, *Arch Fr Pediatr* (suppl 3), 1977.

565. Stanescu V, Stanescu R, Maroteaux P: Pathogenic mechanisms in osteochondrodysplasias, *J Bone Joint Surg* 66:817-836, 1984.

566. Stanescu V et al: Syndrome hereditaire dominant, reunissant une dysostose cranio-faciale de type particular, une insuffisance de croissance d'aspect chondrodystrophique et un epaississement massif de la corticale des os longs, *Rev Fr Endocr Clin* 4:219-231, 1963.

567. Stanley CS, Thelin JW, Miles JH: Mixed hearing loss in Larsen syndrome, *Clin Genet* 33:395-398, 1988.

568. Steel HH, Kohl J: Multiple congenital dislocations associated with other skeletal anomalies (Larsen's syndrome) in three siblings, *J Bone Joint Surg* 54(A):75-82, 1972.

569. Stein SA et al: Sclerosteosis: neurogenetic and pathophysiologic analysis of an American kinship, *Neurology* 33:267-277, 1983.

570. Stephens FE: An achondroplastic mutation and the nature of its inheritance, *J Hered* 34:229-235, 1943.

571. Stern HJ et al: Atelosteogenesis type III: a distinct skeletal dysplasia with features overlapping atelosteogenesis and oto-palato-digital syndrome, type II, *Am J Med Genet* 36:183-195, 1990.

572. Stickler GB et al: Hereditary arthro-ophthalmopathy, *Mayo Clin Proc* 40:433-455, 1965.

573. Stoll CG et al: Birth prevalence rates of skeletal dysplasias, *Clin Genet* 35:88-92, 1989.

574. Stoll CG, Collin D, Dreyfus J: Osteomesopyknosis: an autosomal dominant osteosclerosis, *Am J Med Genet* 8:349-353, 1981.

575. Stoner CN, Hayes JG, Holt JF: Diastrophic dwarfism, *Am J Roentgenol* 89:914-922, 1963.

576. Stoss H et al: Wolcott-Rallison syndrome: diabetes mellitus and spondyloepiphyseal dysplasia, *Eur J Pediatr* 138:120-129, 1982.

577. Stout AP: Juvenile fibromatosis, *Cancer* 7:953-978, 1954.

578. Streeten E et al: Extended laminectomy for spinal stenosis in achondroplasia. In Nicoletti AB et al, editors: *Human achondroplasia*, New York, 1986, Plenum, pp 261-274.

579. Strom CM: Achondroplasia due to DNA insertion into the type II collagen gene, *Pediatr Res* 18:226A only, 1984.

580. Stromme Koppang H et al: Oral abnormalities in the Saldino-Noonan syndrome, *Virchows Arch* 398:247-262, 1983.

581. Stuve A, Weidemann HR: Congenital bowing of the long bones in two sisters, *Lancet* 1:495 only, 1971.

582. Sugarman GI: The Larsen syndrome: autosomal dominant form, *Birth Defects Original Article Series* 11(5):121-129, 1975.

583. Sun TC et al: Chondrosarcoma in Maffucci's syndrome, *J Bone Joint Surg* 67(A):1214-1219, 1985.

584. Superti-Furga A, Gimelli F: Fronto-metaphyseal dysplasia and the oto-palato-digital syndrome, *Dysmorph Clin Genet* 1:2-5, 1987.

585. Szpiro-Tapia S et al: Spondyloepiphyseal dysplasia tarda: linkage with genetic markers from the distal short arm of the X chromosome, *Hum Genet* 81:61-63, 1988.

586. Tager JM et al: Genetic relationship between the Zellweger syndrome and other peroxisomal disorders characterized by an impairment in the assembly of peroxisomes, *Prog Clin Biol Res* 321:545-558, 1990.

587. Taybi H: Diastrophic dwarfism, *Radiology* 80:1-10, 1963.

588. Taybi H, Lachman R: *Radiology of syndromes and metabolic disorders and skeletal dysplasias*, ed 3, St Louis, 1990, Mosby–Year Book.

589. Taybi H, Mitchell AD, Friedman GD: Metaphyseal dysostosis and the associated syndrome of pancreatic insufficiency and blood disorders, *Radiology* 93:563-571, 1969.

590. Temple IK et al: Kyphomelic dysplasia, *J Med Genet* 26:457-468, 1989.

591. Tiller GE et al: Tandem duplication within a type II collagen gene (COL2A1) exon in an individual with spondyloepiphyseal dysplasia, *Proc Natl Acad Sci USA* 87:3889-3893, 1990.

592. Tips RL, Lynch HT: Malignant congenital osteopetrosis resulting from a consanguineous marriage, *Acta Paediat* 51:585-588, 1962.

593. Toledo SPA et al: Recessively inherited, late onset, spondylar dysplasia and peripheral corneal opacity with anomalies in urinary mucopolysaccharides: a possible error of chondroitin-6-sulfate synthesis, *Am J Med Genet* 2:385-395, 1978.

594. Toledo SPA et al: Dyggve-Melchior-Clausen syndrome: genetic studies and report of affected sibs, *Am J Med Genet* 4:255-261, 1979.

595. Tonoki H: A boy with thanatophoric dysplasia surviving 212 days, *Clin Genet* 32:415-416, 1987.

596. Toutain A et al: Reinhardt-Pfeiffer mesomelic dysplasia or dyschondrosteosis? Is the distinction well-founded? Apropos of a familial case with variable expression, *Ann Pediatr (Paris)* 38:37-45, 1991.

597. Treble NJ et al: Development of the hip in multiple epiphyseal dysplasia: natural history and susceptibility to premature osteoarthritis, *J Bone Joint Surg* 72:1061-1064, 1990.

598. Trevor D: Tarso-epiphysial aclasis: a congenital error of epiphyseal development, *J Bone Joint Surg* 32(B):204-213, 1950.

599. Tucker AS et al: Craniodiaphyseal dysplasia: evolution over a 5-year period, *Skeletal Radiol* 1:47, 1976.

600. Turkel SB, Diehl EJ, Richmond JA: Necropsy findings in neonatal asphyxiating thoracic dystrophy, *J Med Genet* 22:112-118, 1985.

601. Urteaga BO et al: Craniometaphyseal dysplasia (Pyle's disease) in an ancient skeleton from the Mochica culture of Peru, *Am J Roentgenol* 99:712, 1967.

602. Van Buchem FSP: Hyperostosis corticalis generalisata: eight new cases, *Acta Med Scand* 189:257-267, 1971

603. Van Buchem FSP et al: Hyperostosis corticalis generalisata: report of seven cases, *Am J Med* 33:387-397, 1962.

604. Vandenberg P et al: Expression of a partially deleted gene of human type II procollagen (COL2A1) in transgenic mice produces a chondrodysplasia, *Proc Nat Acad Sci USA* 88:7640-7644, 1991.

605. Vanek VJ: Metachondromatose: 3 Beobachtungen mit erblichen Vorkommen, *Beitr Orthop Traumatol* 29:103-107, 1982.

606. Vaz RM, Turner C: Ollier disease (enchondromatosis) associated with ovarian juvenile granulosa cell precocious pseudopuberty, *J Pediatr* 108:945-947, 1986.

607. Verbov J, Graham R: Buschke-Ollendorff syndrome-disseminated dermatofibrosis with osteopoikilosis, *Clin Exp Dermatol* 11:17-26, 1986.

608. Verma IC, Bhargava S, Agarwal S: An autosomal recessive form of lethal chondrodystrophy with severe thoracic narrowing, rhizoacromelic type of micromelia, polydactyly and genital anomalies, *Birth Defects (Original Article Series)* 11(6):167-174, 1975.

609. Villarrubias JM, Ginebreda I, Jimeno E: Lengthening of the lower limbs and correction of lumbar hyperlordosis in achondroplasia, *Clin Orthoped Rel Res* 250:143-149, 1990.

610. Vinstein AL, Franken EA Jr: Hereditary multiple exostoses: report of a case with spinal cord compression, *Am J Roentgenol* 112:405-407, 1971.

611. Virolainen M et al: Cellular and humoral immunity in cartilage-hair hypoplasia, *Pediatr Res* 12:961-966, 1978.

612. Vissing H et al: Glycine to serine substitution in the triple helical domain of pro 1(II) collagen results in a lethal perinatal form of short-limbed dwarfism, *J Biol Chem* 264:18265-18267 1989.

613. Vogl A, Osborne R: Lesions of the spinal cord (transverse myelopathy) in achondroplasia, *Arch Neurol Psychiatr* 61:644-662, 1949.

614. Voorhoeve N: L'image radiologique non encore decrite d'une anomalie du squelette; ses raports avec la dyschondroplasie et l'osteopathia condensans disseminata, *Acta Radiol* 3:407-417, 1924.

615. Voutsinas S, Wynne-Davies R: The infrequency of malignant disease in diaphyseal aclasis and neurofibromatosis, *J Med Genet* 20:345-349, 1983.

616. Wackerle B et al : Radiologic findings in cherubism: Orthopantomography, CT, MRI, *Roentgenpraxis* 40:104-107, 1987.

617. Wadia R: Achondroplasia in two first cousins, *Birth Defects (Original Article Series)* 5(4):227-230, 1969.

618. Walker BA et al: Hypochondroplasia, *Am J Dis Child* 122:95-104, 1971.

619. Walker BA et al: Diastrophic dwarfism, *Medicine* 51:41-59, 1972.

620. Walker DG: Osteopetrosis. In Bergsma D, editor: *Clinical delineation of birth defects. IV. Skeletal dysplasias*, New York, 1969 National Foundation, March of Dimes, pp 308-311.

621. Walker DG: Osteopetrosis cured by temporary parabiosis, *Science* 180:875 only, 1973.

622. Walker DG: Bone resorption restored in osteopetrotic mice by transplants of normal bone marrow and spleen cells, *Science* 190:784-785, 1975.

623. Walpole I, Manners PJ: Clinical considerations in Buschke-Ollendorff syndrome, *Clin Genet* 37:59-63, 1990.

624. Walpole I, Nicoll A, Goldblatt J: Autosomal dominant osteopetrosis type II with "malignant" presentation: further support for heterogeneity? *Clin Genet* 38:257-263, 1990.

625. Wardinsky TD et al: Rhizomelic chondrodysplasia punctata and survival beyond one year: a review of the literature and five case reports, *Clin Genet* 38:84-93, 1990.

626. Weinstein LS et al: Activating mutations of the stimulatory G protein in the McCune-Albright syndrome, *New Engl J Med* 325:1688-1695, 1991.

627. Whalen JP et al: Calcitonin treatment in hereditary bone dysplasia with hyperphosphatasemia: a radiographic and histologic study of bone, *Am J Roentgenol* 129:29-35, 1977.

628. Whitley CB, Gorlin RJ: Achondrogenesis: new nosology with evidence of genetic heterogeneity, *Radiology* 148:693-698, 1983.

629. Whitley CB et al: Fibrochondrogenesis: lethal autosomal recessive chondrodysplasia with distinctive cartilage histopathology, *Am J Med Genet* 19:265-275, 1984.

630. Whitley CB et al: De la Chapelle dysplasia, *Am J Med Genet* 25:29-39, 1986.

631. Whyte MP, Murphy WA: Osteopathia striata associated with familial dermopathy and white forelock: evidence for postnatal development of osteopathia striata, *Am J Med Genet* 5:227-234, 1980.

632. Whyte MP et al: Osteopetrosis, renal tubular acidosis and basal ganglia calcification in three sisters, *Am J Med* 69:64-74, 1980.

633. Weidemann HR: *Die Grossen Konstitutions-Krankheiten des Skeletts*, Stuttgart, 1960, Gustav Fischer Verlag.

634. Wilson DJ, Weleber RG, Beals RK: Retinal dystrophy in Jeune's syndrome, *Arch Opthalmol* 105:651-657, 1987.

635. Winter RM, Thompson EM: Lethal, neonatal, short-limbed platyspondylic dwarfism: a further variant? *Hum Genet* 61:269-272, 1982.

636. Winter RM et al: Osteopathia striata with cranial sclerosis: highly variable expression within a family including cleft palate in two neonatal cases, *Clin Genet* 18:462-474, 1980.

637. Winter RM et al: The Weissenbacher-Zweymuller, Stickler and Marshall syndromes: further evidence for their identity, *Am J Med Genet* 16:189-199, 1983.

638. Wirth CR et al: Diaphyseal dysplasia (Engelmann's syndrome), *Clin Orthop* 171:186-195, 1982.

639. Wolcott CD, Rallison ML: Infancy-onset diabetes mellitus and multiple epiphyseal dysplasia, *J Pediatr* 80:292-297, 1972.

640. Worth HM, Wolin DG: Hyperostosis corticalis generalisata congenita, *J Can Assoc Radiol* 17:67-74, 1966.

641. Wynne-Davies R, Hall C, Ansell BM: Spondylo-epiphyseal dysplasia tarda with progressive arthropathy: a 'new' disorder of autosomal recessive inheritance, *J Bone Joint Surg* 64(B):442-445, 1982.

642. Wynne-Davies R, Hall CM, Apley AG: *Atlas of skeletal dysplasias*, Edinburgh, 1985, Churchill Livingstone.

643. Wynne-Davies R, Hall CM, Young ID: Pseudoachondroplasia: clinical diagnosis at different ages and comparison of autosomal dominant and recessive types: a review of 32 patients (26 kindreds)., *J Med Genet* 23:425-434, 1986.

644. Yang SS, Heidelberger KP, Bernstein J: Intracytoplasmic inclusion bodies in the chondrocytes of type I lethal achondrogenesis, *Hum Pathol* 7:667-673, 1976.

645. Yang SS et al: Two types of heritable lethal achondrogenesis, *J Pediatr* 85:796-801, 1974.

646. Yang SS et al: Lethal short-limbed chondrodysplasia in early infancy, *Perspect Pediatr Pathol* 3:1-40, 1976.

647. Yang SS et al: Upper cervical myelopathy in achondroplasia, *Am J Clin Pathol* 68:68-72, 1977.

648. Yang SS et al: Short-rib polydactyly syndrome, type III with chondrocytic inclusions: report of a case and review of the literature, *Am J Med Genet* 7:205-213, 1980.

649. Yang SS et al: Spondyloepiphyseal dysplasia congenita: a comparative study of chondrocytic inclusions, *Arch Pathol Lab Med* 104:208-211, 1980.

650. Yang SS et al: Two lethal chondrodysplasias with giant chondrocytes, *Am J Med Genet* 15:615-625, Aug 1983.

651. Yang SS et al: Three conditions in neonatal asphyxiating thoracic dysplasia (Jeune) and short rib−polydactyly syndrome spectrum: a clinicopathologic study, *Am J Med Genet* 3(suppl):191-207, 1987.

652. Yoshida H et al: The murine mutation osteopetrosis is in the coding region of the macrophage colony stimulating factor gene, *Nature* 345:442-444, 1990.

653. Young ID, Patel I, Lamont AC: Thanatophoric dysplasia in identical twins, *J Med Genet* 26:276-279, 1989.

654. Yulish BS et al: Partial resolution of bone lesions: a child with severe combined immunodeficiency disease and adenosine deaminase deficiency after enzyme-replacement therapy, *Am J Dis Child* 134:61-63, 1980.

655. Yunis E, Varon H: Cleidocranial dysostosis, severe micrognathism, bilateral absence of thumbs and first metatarsal bone, and distal aphalangia: a new genetic syndrome, *Am J Dis Child* 134:649-653, 1980.

656. Zangwill KM, Boal DKB, Ladda RL: Dandy-Walker malformation in Ellis-van Creveld syndrome, *Am J Med Genet* 31:123-129, 1988.

657. Zonana J et al: A unique chondrodysplasia secondary to a defect in chondrosseous transformation. In Bergsma D, Lowry RB, editors: *Embryology and pathogenesis and prenatal diagnosis, Birth Defects (Original Article Series)* 13(3D):155-163, 1977.

CHAPTER 15

Future Prospects

Victor A. McKusick

John S. O'Brien[2] usefully indicated the following levels of sophistication, or five usual stages, in the understanding of a genetic disorder:

1. *Description of the phenotype* includes not only clinical signs and symptoms but also the natural history (age of onset, rate of progression, and age at death) and the signs elicited by special means, that is, the radiographic and gross histologic and cellular morphology, as well as physiologic abnormalities.

2. *Delineation of the mendelian nature* of the condition involves establishing the mode of inheritance and peculiarities of distribution and transmission in families.

3. *Discovery of the general biochemical nature* of the disorder, by means of identification of substances excreted in the urine or stored in tissues in excess or identification of other chemical alterations, is usually the next step.

4. *Identification of a defect in a specific enzyme or other protein gene product* is the penultimate level of sophistication.

5. *Determination of the precise nature of the gene mutation* is the ultimate level of understanding in the O'Brien staging.

In the first edition of *Heritable Disorders of Connective Tissue* (1956), the five main categories of disorders discussed were Marfan syndrome, Ehlers-Danlos syndrome (EDS), osteogenesis imperfecta (OI), pseudoxanthoma elasticum (PXE), and Hurler syndrome. With the exception of PXE, at least one entity within each of the categories has been elucidated at the level of the gene. For example, in the Marfan syndrome, in EDS type IV,

in several forms of OI, and in the several forms of mucopolysaccharidoses, including the entity now specifically designated as Hurler syndrome, the gene that is the site of the point mutation has been cloned and mutations within the gene characterized. Comparable advances have been made in some of the other conditions that have been added to the collection of heritable disorders of connective tissue in later editions of the book, notably, homocystinuria, the spondyloepiphyseal dysplasia class of skeletal dysplasias, and Stickler syndrome. The notable laggard among the original "Big Five" is PXE. The intractable physical properties of elastic tissue, which appears to be the site of the basic defect in PXE, may be responsible.

The fruitfulness of cell-culture methods in the study of heritable disorders of connective tissue predicted in the first edition of this book[1] was fulfilled in several of the disorders—most particularly, in the case of the mucopolysaccharidoses. But even in the fourth edition (1972) I could not predict the extent to which molecular genetic methods, which were just then being developed, would advance this field.

Definition of the basic defect in the heritable disorders of connective tissue has followed O'Brien's scheme: demonstration of mendelian nature, which justified the conclusion that a unitary basic defect would be found; description of biochemical derangements by analysis of tissues and body fluids; study of the essence of the disease in cultured cells; cloning of the wide-type versions of the gene by *functional cloning* (working back from the protein gene product to the gene, as in the case of the collagens or fibrillin involved in EDS, OI, or Marfan syndrome, or from the specific enzymes deficient in homocystinuria and some of the mucopolysaccharidoses), or by *positional cloning* (first, mapping the gene to a specific chromosomal site and then identifying its nature, either by the candidate gene approach or by an expedition—"walking" or "jumping"—through that region of the genome).

Possibly, a sixth step in the elucidation of genetic disorders should be added to the O'Brien five: the elucidation in full detail of the pathogenetic mechanisms. Having gotten back to the mutant gene—sometimes by short-cutting directly to the gene through positional cloning—it is necessary to return to the phenotype to work out the pathogenetic steps that connect the mutation with a clinical disorder, the steps from gene to phene. Efforts to ameliorate or eliminate the ill effects of the mutant gene can usefully be directed at these steps. Transgenic methods involving the transfer of the mutant gene into cultured cells or into whole organisms, as in the case of transgenic mice, will probably play an important role in working out the effects of mutant genes.

As pointed out by British biostatistician A. Bradford Hill, clinical medicine involves seeking the answer to three questions: What is wrong? (diagnosis); What is going to happen? (prognosis); What can be done about it? (treatment). Rich opportunity for further study of heritable disorders of connective tissue at the clinical level remains. A "two-way street" connects clinical studies and basic investigations. It is easy to argue the importance of basic understanding to precise molecular (DNA) diagnosis, to prognosis, and increasingly in the future, to effective treatment. Much remains to be done on the clinical side that can aid in the search for the basic gene defect. Search for further genetic heterogeneity, correlation of phenotype with the particular nature of the gene mutation, and exploration of therapeutic measures based on the newfound basic information are all useful areas for future clinical research.

REFERENCES

1. McKusick VA: *Heritable disorders of connective tissue*, ed 1, St Louis, 1956, Mosby–Year Book, p 210.
2. O'Brien JS: Ganglioside storage diseases. In Hirschorn K, Harris H, editors: *Advances in human genetics*, vol 3, New York, 1971, Plenum.

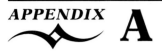
Glossary of Genetic Terms

Allele	Alternative forms of a gene found at the same locus on homologous chromosomes.
Aneuploid	A chromosome number that is not an exact multiple of the haploid number; an individual with an aneuploid chromosome number.
Association	The occurrence of a particular allele in a group of patients more often than accounted for by chance.
Autosome	Any chromosome other than a sex chromosome. Humans have 22 pairs of autosomes.
Carrier	An unaffected individual who is heterozygous at a particular locus for a normal gene and an abnormal gene that, although it may be detectable by laboratory tests, is not expressed phenotypically.
Centimorgan (cM)	The unit of genetic distance between linked loci as measured by the probability of a cross-over occurring between them at meiosis.
Centromere	The dark-staining (heterochromatic) region within a chromosome at the junction of the chromatids.
Chorionic villus sampling (CVS)	A technique used to obtain fetal cells for prenatal diagnosis by means of a biopsy of the placenta preformed at approximately 8 to 10 weeks of gestation.
Chromatid	During mitosis each chromosome replicates into two DNA strands called *chromatids* just before cell division.
Chromosome	Threadlike, deep-staining bodies situated in the nucleus. They are composed of DNA and protein and carry the genetic information.

Cis	On the same chromosome, usually quite close. The opposite of *trans*.
Clone	An animal cell line or bacterial colony derived from a single cell.
Codominant	When both alleles are expressed in the heterozygote.
Codon	The group of three adjacent nucleotides that codes for amino acids and polypeptide chain initiation.
Complementary	Two nucleotide sequences are complementary when they can form a perfect double helix because the bases and their orientation are exactly matched.
Consanguinity	Relationship by descent from a common ancestor; a consangineuous mating is between individuals who have one or more common ancestors.
Cosmid	A cloning vector capable of accommodating large fragments of foreign DNA.
Coupling	When two linked alleles are known to be on the same chromosome; the opposite of *repulsion*.
Cross-over	The exchange of genetic information between members of a chromosome pair during meiosis.
DNA	Deoxyribonucleic acid. The long, double-stranded molecule whose sequence of nucleotide bases determines genetic information.
Deletion	Loss of a portion of a gene or chromosome.
Diploid	Containing two chromosome sets; the normal condition of all human cells except gametes.
Dominant	A trait that is expressed by the heterozygote.
Exon	The regions of a gene containing the coding sequences.
Expressivity	The extent to which a genetic defect is expressed.
Gene	The unit responsible for transmitting an inherited character; the region of DNA that specifies the synthesis of a polypeptide.
Genetic distance	The separation of loci in terms of the probability of a cross-over occurring between them.
Genetic fingerprint	A pattern of restriction fragments detected by a probe that recognizes many highly polymorphic loci and is unique to an individual.

Genetic marker A feature used in following the inheritance pattern of genes in the study of cell lines, pedigrees, or populations.

Genome The complete genetic composition of an individual; the complete set of genes characteristic of a species.

Genotype The alleles present at a locus in an individual.

Haploid Containing one chromosome set. The normal situation for gametes.

Hemizygous The condition of cells with respect to genes when only one set is present, as in genes on the male X-chromosome.

Heterozygote An individual with two different alleles at a particular locus (adjective, heterozygous).

Homozygous An individual with two identical alleles at a particular locus.

Hybridization The artificial conjunction of two complementary DNA (cDNA) strands, one of which usually carries a radioactive marker.

Insertion Addition of DNA to a gene or chromosome.

Intron The regions of a gene that contain noncoding sequences.

Karyotype The chromosome set; the number, size, and shape of the chromosomes of a somatic cell.

Kilobase (kb) A thousand bases. A unit of measure commonly used to specify the size of genes and physical distances along a DNA region.

Linkage The study of linked loci. Linked loci are within a measurable genetic distance of one another on the same chromosome.

Locus A precise position on a chromosome; usually that of a gene.

LOD The term *LOD* is derived from "log of the odds"; it is a numeric expression of the likelihood that two loci are linked at a particular genetic distance.

Lyonization Random inactivation of one X chromosome in the somatic cells of female mammals during early embryonic life.

Mapping The process of determining the location of a gene.

Mendelian A trait obeying Mendel's law of independent genetic segregation.

Meiosis The type of cell division that occurs during gamete formation and results in the halving of the somatic number of chromosomes so that each gamete is haploid.

Mitosis	The type of cell division that occurs in somatic cells.
Monogenic	A trait governed by a single gene.
Mosaic	An individual with two or more cell lines, differing in genotype or karyotype, derived from a single zygote.
Multifactorial	Inheritance determined by many small additive effects of both genes and the environment.
Mutation	A permanent and heritable change in genetic material (includes point mutations, deletions, and changes in number or structure of chromosomes).
Nondisjunction	Failure of two members of a chromosome pair to disjoin (separate) during cell division.
Oligonucleotide	A short piece of DNA (typically 5 to 50 nucleotides)
Open reading frame (ORF)	A stretch of DNA following an initiation codon that does not contain a stop codon. ORFs in a nucleotide sequence indicate the presence of a gene.
Polymerase chain reaction (PCR)	A useful method of amplifying a particular piece of DNA without cloning.
Pedigree	A diagrammatic representation of a family history.
Penetrance	The frequency of expression of a trait or genotype.
Phage	A virus that infects bacteria and is a useful cloning vector for medium-sized pieces of DNA (between 5 and 25 kb).
Phenocopy	An environmentally induced mimic of a genetic disorder.
Phenotype	The appearance (physical, biochemical, and physiologic) of an individual, which results from the interaction of environment and genotype.
Plasmid	Extrachromosomal, small, circular DNA molecule capable of autonomous replication with a bacterium. Commonly used as a cloning vector for small pieces of DNA. (typically 50 to 5000 bases)
Polygenic	Inheritance determined by many genes at different loci, each with small additive effects.
Polymorphism	The occurrence in a population of two or more genetically determined forms in such frequencies that the rarest of them could not be maintained by mutation alone.

Prenatal diagnosis   Determination of the status (genetic and otherwise) of the fetus by means of a variety of techniques (chromosomal, biochemical, DNA, structure, and the like) using a variety of procedures (chorionic villus sampling, amniocentesis, ultrasonic examination, fetal cord blood sampling, and so forth), usually after 9 weeks of gestation and before viability (i.e., 28 weeks of gestation). Prenatal diagnosis is used when there is reason to suspect that the fetus might have a detectable abnormality.

Proband (propositus)   The affected individual who brings the family to medical attention.

Probe   A fragment of DNA radioactively labeled or fluorescently used to identify a complementary sequence.

RNA   Ribonucleic acid. The nucleic acid found mainly in cytoplasm. *Messenger RNA* (mRNA) transfers genetic information from the nucleus to the ribosomes in the cytoplasm and acts as a template for the synthesis of polypeptides; *transfer RNA* (tRNA) transfers activated amino acids from the cytoplasm to mRNA; *ribosomal RNA* (rRNA) is a component of the ribosomes that functions as a nonspecific site of polypeptide synthesis.

Recessive   A trait that is expressed only in individuals who are homozygous for a particular gene, not in those who are heterozygous.

Recombinant DNA   DNA that is artificially transferred from the genome of one organism into the genome of another.

Repulsion   When alleles at two linked loci are on different chromosomes. The opposite of *coupling*.

Restriction endonuclease   A group of enzymes in which each enzyme cleaves DNA at a specific base sequence (recognition site)

Restriction fragment length polymorphism (RFLP)   The occurrence of two or more alleles in a population differing in the lengths of fragments produced by a restriction endonuclease.

Reverse transcriptase   An enzyme which can make complementary DNA (cDNA) from mRNA.

Segregation   Separation of allelic genes at meiosis.

Sex chromosome   The chromosomes that primarily govern sex determination (XX in women and XY in men).

Sibship	A set of brothers and sisters.
Synteny	Loci of the same chromosome that may or may not be linked.
Southern blotting	The eponymous technique used for transferring DNA to a backing sheet before hybridization. Northern and western blots are non-eponymous variations.
Trans	On different chromosomes, usually quite close. The opposite of *cis*.
Translocation	The transfer of genetic material from one chromosome to another, nonhomologous chromosome.
Trisomy	The state of having three of a given chromosome instead of the usual pair, as in trisomy 21 (Down syndrome).
Triploid	A cell with 3 times the haploid number of chromosomes, that is, three copies of all chromosome types.
Vector	A vehicle into which DNA is inserted before it is cloned in bacteria. Includes plasmids, phage, and cosmids.
X-linked	Genes carried on the X chromosome.

Molecular Nosology of Heritable Disorders of Connective Tissue

Peter Beighton

The molecular nosology of the heritable disorders of connective tissue in Appendix B represents a systematic tabulation of abnormalities at the loci for collagen genes I through III. Loci for genes other than collagens have also been listed if there is reason to suppose that they might be involved with these disorders. Information concerning the corresponding protein change and the clinical phenotype is provided, together with key references.

The nosology was developed by an expert committee and subsequently published in the American Journal of Medical Genetics. *It is reproduced by kind permission of the editor, Dr. John Opitz. The main contents of the molecular nosology, with the names of the individual contributors, are as follows:*

COL1A1, D.W. Hollister
COL1A2, P. Tsipouras
COL2A1, D.W. Hollister
COL3A1, F.M. Pope and A. De Paepe
Other gene loci, R.E. Pyeritz

CONVENTIONS USED FOR TABULAR DATA

The data summarized below are listed by individual gene loci, which are designated by the protein product. The locus symbol, size, and chromo-

somal location of the gene are indicated. Known molecular defects are then presented in tabular form, followed by provisional defects and linkage data (which include instances in which a disease has been excluded from linkage with the locus in question). An abbreviated format has been adopted for the tabular data, and the reader should refer to the following information regarding the abbreviations used:

i) Diseases: (refer to Beighton et al., [1988] for clinical subtypes)
OI = osteogenesis imperfecta
EDS = Ehlers-Danlos syndrome
SEDc = spondyloepiphyseal dysplasia congenita
Ach-Hyp = achondrogenesis II (or IB)-hypochondrogenesis
OP = osteoporosis
OA = osteoarthritis
Stickler syndrome = hereditary progressive arthro-ophthalmopathy

ii) MIM #: Accession number for specific disease as listed in Mendelian Inheritance in Man, 9th ed. [McKusick, 1990].

iii) Zygosity:
Homo = homozygous or compound, implying autosomal recessive inheritance
Hetero = heterozygous, implying autosomal dominant inheritance
Hemi = hemizygous implying inheritance on the X chromosome

iv) Mutation:
PMm = point mutation, missense

Modified from Beighton P et al: *Am J Med Genet* 42:431-448, 1992.

PMs = point mutation, splicing

LMd = length mutation, deletion

LMi = length mutation, insertion (secondary effects of LM: s = splicing; f = frameshift)

Nucleotide(s) changes are denoted by the normal base followed by a number indicating the position within the designated exon or intron, and the abnormal nucleotide observed.

v) Protein change: The normal amino acid and position within the designated protein domain is given, followed by the abnormal amino acid observed or inferred from the mutant RNA and/or DNA sequence, aa = amino acid.

vi) Domain: N-propeptide = amino-terminal precursor-specific peptide; N-telopeptide = amino-terminal nonhelical junctional peptide linking N-propeptide to the helical domain; helical = large central triple helical domain; C-telopeptide = carboxyl-terminal nonhelical junctional peptide uniting the helical domain with the C-propeptide;

C-propeptide = carboxyl-terminal precursor-specific peptide.

TYPE I COLLAGEN COL1A1

Gene: alpha 1 chain of type I collagen; alpha 1(I)

Locus symbol: COL1A1

Size: 18 kilobases

Chromosomal location: 17q21-22 [Myers and Emanuel, 1987]

Linkage Data

Disorders linked to COL1A1:

OI, Type I and Type IV [Sykes et al., 1986; Sykes et al., 1990].

Disorders *not* linked to COL1A1:

Marfan syndrome [Ogilvie et al., 1987; Boileau et al., 1990; Schwartz et al., 1990]

Mitral valve prolapse syndrome [Wordsworth et al., 1989]

OI (some forms) [Aitchison et al., 1988]

Table I. COL1A1: Known mutations

Disease	MIM #	Zygosity	Mutation	Protein change	Domain	References	Comments
OI, Type I/EDS	166200	Hetero	PMm; exon 7 G(1) to T	Gly(19) to Cys	Helical	Nicholls et al., 1990	Jt. hypermobility, osteoporosis, no fractures Rediagnosed as OI
OI, Type I	166200	Hetero	PMm; exon 12	Gly(94) to Cys	Helical	Starman et al., 1989	Presumably G(10) to T
OI, Type I	166200	Hetero	PMm; exon 48 G(52) to T	Gly(3) to Cys	C-telopeptide	Cohn et al., 1988 Labhard et al., 1988	
OI, Type I	166200	Hetero	LMd,f; exon 52 del of GAATT after G(108)	Additional 84 missense aa	C-propeptide	Willing et al., 1990	Frameshift
OI, Type II	166210	Homo	PMm,s; intron 14 G(5) to A	Del exon 14 (18 aa)	Helical	Bonadio et al., 1990	Alternative splicing
OI, Type II	166210	Hetero	LMi: insertion approx. 600 bp between exons 13-19	Insertion of 50-70 aa	Helical	Byers et al., 1988	
OI, Type II	166210	Hetero	PMm; exon 20 G(2) to T	Gly(256) to Val	Helical	Patterson et al., 1989	

Table I. COL1A1: Known mutations—cont'd

Disease	MIM #	Zygosity	Mutation	Protein change	Domain	References	Comments
OI, Type II	166210	Hetero	LMd; del exons 23-25	84 aa deleted	Helical	Barsh et al., 1985 Chu et al., 1985	Intron to intron deletion
OI, Type II	166210	Hetero	PMm; exon 25	Gly(391) to Arg	Helical	Bateman et al., 1987	Presumably G(37) to C
OI, Type II	166210	Hetero	PMm; exon 32	Gly(541) to Asp	Helical	Zhang et al., 1990	Presumably, G(29) to A
OI, Type II	166210	Hetero	PMm; exon 32 G(55) to A	Gly(550) to Arg	Helical	Wallis et al., 1990a	Father mosaic
OI, Type II	166210	Hetero	PMm; exon 33	Gly(568) to Asp	Helical	Cohn et al., 1990c	Parent mosaic; presumably G(2) to A
OI, Type II	166210	Hetero	PMm; exon 33	Gly(598) to Ser	Helical	Westerhausen et al., 1990	Presumably, G(91) to A
OI, Type II	166210	Hetero	PMm; exon 35	Gly(631) to Ser	Helical	Westerhausen et al., 1990	Presumably, G(28) to A
OI, Type II	166210	Hetero	PMm; exon 36 G(82) to A	Gly(667) to Arg	Helical	Bateman et al., 1988; Baker et al., 1989	
OI, Type II	166210	Hetero	PMs; exon 36	Gly(673) to Asp	Helical	Cohn et al., 1990c	Parent mosaic; presumably G(101) to A
OI, Type II	166210	Hetero	PMm; exon 37	Gly(691) to Cys	Helical	Prockop, 1990	Presumably G(46) to T
OI, Type II	166210	Hetero	PMm; exon 39	Gly(718) to Cys	Helical	Starman et al., 1989	Presumably, G(19) to T
OI, Type II	166210	Hetero	PMm; exon 39 G(109) to T	Gly(748) to Cys	Helical	Vogel et al., 1987	
OI, Type II	166210	Hetero	PMm; exon 41 G(92) to A	Gly(832) to Asp	Helical	Cohn et al., 1990a	Father mosaic
OI, Type II	166210	Hetero	PMm; exon 43	Gly(847) to Arg	Helical	Wallis et al., 1990b	Presumably G(28) to A or C
OI, Type II	166210	Hetero	LMd; exon 43 del 9 bp	Del aa 874-876	Helical	Wallis et al., 1990b	
OI, Type II	166210	Hetero	PMm; exon 43	Gly(883) to Asp	Helical	Cohn et al., 1990c	Parent mosaic; presumably G(83) to A
OI, Type II	166210	Hetero	PMm; exon 44 G(37) to T	Gly(904) to Cys	Helical	Constantinou et al., 1989	Mother mosaic
OI, Type II	166210	Hetero	PMm; exon 45	Gly(913) to Ser	Helical	Cohn et al., 1990b	Presumably G(10) to A
OI, Type II	166210	Hetero	PMm; exon 45 G(56) to C	Gly(928) to Ala	Helical	Lamande et al., 1989	
OI, Type II	166210	Hetero	PMs; del exon 47	Del exon 47 (36 aa)	Helical	Wallis et al., 1990b	+1 or +2 mutation, intron 47
OI, Type II	166210	Hetero	PMm; exon 47	Gly(964) to Ser	Helical	Wallis et al., 1990b	
OI, Type II	166210	Hetero	PMm; exon 47 G(29) to T	Gly(973) to Val	Helical	Lamande et al., 1989	
OI, Type II	166210	Hetero	PMm; exon 47 G(37) to A	Gly(976) to Arg	Helical	Lamande et al., 1989	
OI, Type II	166210	Hetero	PMm; exon 47 G(73) to T	Gly(988) to Cys	Helical	Cohn et al., 1986	

Continued.

Table I. COL1A1: Known mutations—cont'd

Disease	MIM #	Zygosity	Mutation	Protein change	Domain	References	Comments
OI, Type II	166210	Hetero	PMm; exon 48	Gly(1003) to Ser	Helical	Cohn et al., 1990b	Presumably, G(10) to A
OI, Type II	166210	Hetero	PMm; exon 48 G(20) to T	Gly(1006) to Val	Helical	Lamande et al., 1989	
OI, Type II	166210	Hetero	LMi,f; exon 49 i(T) after T(57)	Truncated, missense C-propeptide	C-propeptide	Bateman et al., 1989	Frameshift
Variable OI I/IV/III		Hetero	PMm; exon 17 G(1) to T	Gly(175) to Cys	Helical	Wirtz et al., 1990	
OI, Type III	259420*	Hetero	PMm; exon 31	Gly(526) to Cys	Helical	Starman et al., 1989	Presumably G(82) to T
OI, Type III	259420*	Hetero	PMm; exon 42 G(19) to A	Gly(844) to Ser	Helical	Pack et al., 1989	
OI, Type III-IV	259420*	Hetero	PMm; exon 26 G(10) to T	Gly(415) to Cys	Helical	Nicholls et al., 1990	
OI, Type III	259420*	Hetero	PMm; exon 48	Gly(1009) to Ser	Helical	Cohn et al., 1990b	Presumably G(28) to A
OI, Type IV/I	166220	Hetero	PMm; exon 17	Gly(178) to Cys	Helical	Cetta et al., 1990	
OI, Type IV	166220	Mosaic	PMm; exon 32 G(55) to A	Gly(550) to Arg	Helical	Wallis et al., 1990a	Gonadal, other mosaicism, offspring with lethal OI
OI, Type IV	166220	Hetero	PMm; exon 41 G(91) to A	Gly(832) to Ser	Helical	Marini et al., 1989	
EDS, Type VIIA	130060	Hetero	PMm,s; exon 6 G(72) to A	24 aa of exon 6 deleted	N-telopeptide	Weil et al., 1989	Alternative splicing

*Although OI-III is classified as a recessive condition in *Mendelian Inheritance in Man* (McKusick, 1990), these patients clearly have a dominant disorder, as do many persons with this phenotype.

Table II. COL1A1: Provisional data

Disease	Evidence	References
OP	Increased bone type III collagen; increased content of alpha 1(I) trimers	Batge et al., 1990
OP	Heterozygous Gly(661) to Ser substitution in an alpha 2(I) chain	Spotila et al., 1990
OI, Type I	Half normal amounts of alpha 1(I) mRNA in fibroblasts	Rowe et al., 1985

TYPE I COLLAGEN COL1A2

Locus name: alpha 2 chain of type I collagen; alpha 2(1)
Locus symbol: COL1A2
Size: 38 kilobases [de Wet et al., 1987]
Chromosomal location: 7q22 [Henderson et al., 1983]

Linkage Data

Disorders linked to COL1A2:
OI, Type IV [Tsipouras et al., 1984; Sykes et al., 1990]

Table III. COL1A2: Known mutations

Disease	MIM #	Zygosity	Mutation	Protein change	Domain	References	Comments
OI, Type I	166200	Hetero	LMd; s; exon 13; IVS 13, del between nt +4 to +22	Residues 209-223 deleted	Helical	Zhuang et al., 1990	
OI, Type II	166210	Hetero	PMm; exon 45 G(47) to A	Gly(907) to Asp	Helical	Baldwin et al., 1989	
OI, Type II	166210	Hetero	PMm; exon 39 G(1) to A	Gly(694) to Arg	Helical	Tsuneyoshi et al., 1990	
OI, Type II	166210	Hetero	PMm; exon 29 G(19) to T	Gly(472) to Cys	Helical	Edwards et al., 1990	The mildly affected parent is mosaic for mutation in the germline and somatic tissues
OI, Type II	166210	Hetero	PMm; exon 44 G(28) to A	Gly(865) to Ser	Helical	Lamande et al., 1989	
OI, Type II	166210	Hetero	PMm; exon 28 G(28) to C	Gly(457) to Arg	Helical	Bateman et al., 1990	
OI, Type II	166210	Homo	PMm; s; exon 28 g to A at 3' consensus of IVS27	Residues 548-566 deleted	Helical	Tromp et al., 1988	The proband is a compound heterozygote. Other allele is silent.
OI, Type III	259400	Hetero	PMm; exon 20 G(10) to A	Gly(259) to Cys	Helical	Wenstrup et al., 1990	
OI, Type III	259420	Homo	LMd; f; exon 52. Del 4bp resulting in out-of-frame reading	Alpha(1) trimer	C-propeptide	Dickson et al., 1984 Pihlajaniemi et al., 1984	Parents are heterozygous for the mutation and are phenotypically normal.
OI, Type IV	166220	Hetero	PMm; exon 34 G(2) to T	Gly(586) to Val	Helical	Bateman et al., 1990	
OI, Type IV	166220	Hetero	PMm; exon 49 G(38) to C	Gly(1012) to Arg	Helical	Wenstrup et al., 1988	
OI, Type IV	166220	Hetero	PMm; exon 37 G(19) to T	Gly(646) to Cys	Helical	Wenstrup et al., 1991	
OI, Type I/EDS (unclassified)		Hetero	LMd; s; exon 11 del 19 bp at the junction of IVS 10 and exon 11	Residues 73-90 deleted	Helical	Kuivaniemi et al., 1988	Significant variability of expression among affected individuals. Phenotype is a mixture of OI and mild EDS.
EDS, Type VIIB	130060	Hetero	PMm; s; exon 6 G(54) to A	Residues 1-18 deleted	N-telopeptide	Weil et al., 1989	
EDS, Type VIIB	130050	Hetero	PMm; s; exon 6 T(2) to C in IVS6	Residues 1-18 deleted	N-telopeptide	Weil et al., 1988, 1990 Vasan et al., 1991	
OI, Type II	166210	Hetero	LMd; s; exon 33 G(5) to A, IVS 33	Residues 667-684 deleted	Helical	Ganguly et al., 1990	

TYPE II COLLAGEN COL2A1

Gene: alpha 1 chain of type II collagen, alpha 1(II)
Locus symbol: COL2A1
Size: 30 kilobases [Sangiorgi et al., 1985]
Chromosomal location: 12q12.1-12.3 [Myers and Emanuel, 1987]

Linkage Data

Disorders linked to COL2A1:
SEDc [Anderson et al., 1990a]
SEDc, Namaqualand type [Sher et al., 1991]
Osteoarthritis [SEDc] [Palotie et al., 1989; Knowlton et al., 1990]
Stickler syndrome (some families) [Francomano et al., 1988a; Knowlton et al., 1989]
Disorders not linked to COL2A1:
Achondroplasia [Wordsworth et al., 1988; Francomano and Pyeritz, 1988b]
Diaphyseal aclasis [Wordsworth et al., 1988]
Hypochondroplasia [Wordsworth et al., 1988]
Marfan syndrome [Ogilvie et al., 1987; Boileau et al., 1990]
Multiple epiphyseal dysplasia [Wordsworth et al., 1988]

Pseudoachondroplasia [Wordsworth et al., 1988]
SED tarda [Wordsworth et al., 1988]
SED type Kimberley [Anderson et al., 1990b]
Stickler syndrome (some families) [Knowlton et al., 1989]
Trichorhinophalangeal syndrome [Wordsworth et al., 1988]

TYPE III COLLAGEN COL3A1

Gene: alpha 1 chain of type III collagen; alpha 1(III)
Locus symbol: COL3A1
Size: 38 kilobases
Chromosomal location: 2q31-32.3 [Huerre-Jeanpierre et al., 1986]

Linkage Data

Disorders linked to COL3A1:
EDS, Type IV variable type III collagen [Tsipouras et al., 1986; Nicholls et al., 1988]
Disorders not linked to COL3A1:
Marfan syndrome [Dalgleish et al., 1987; Ogilvie et al., 1987; Francomano et al., 1988]

Table IV. COL2A1: Known mutations

Disease	MIM #	Zygosity	Mutation	Protein change	Domain	References	Comments
SEDc	183900	Hetero	LMd; deletion of exon 48	36 aa del (exon 48)	Helical	Lee et al., 1989	Intron to intron del
SEDc	183900	Hetero	LMi; 45 bp ins in exon 48	15 aa duplicated	Helical	Tiller et al., 1990	Partial exon duplication
SEDc	183900	Hetero	PMm; exon 31	Arg(519) to Cys	Helical	Ala-Kokko et al., 1990	Initially reported as OA. Now regarded as mild SEDc.
Stickler syndrome	108300	Hetero	PMm; exon 39 C to T	Arg(732) to STOP	Helical	Ahmad et al., 1990 Knowlton et al., 1989	Disease linked to COL2A1
Ach-Hyp	200610	Hetero	PMm; exon 46 G to A	Gly(943) to Ser	Helical	Vissing et al., 1989	

Table V. COL2A1: Provisional data

Disease	MIM #	Evidence	References
Kniest syndrome	156500	Intracellular retention of the C-propeptide of type II collagen	Poole et al., 1988
SEDc	183900	Overmodification of type II collagen and constituent CNBr peptides	Murray et al., 1989

Table VI. COL3A1: Known mutations

Disease	MIM #	Zygosity	Mutation	Protein change	Domain	References	Comments
EDS, Type IV	130050	Hetero	LMd; 2 kb deletion near 5′ end	normal and shortened protein	Helical	McGookey et al., 1989	Paternal mosaicism. Equal amount (10%) of normal/shortened type III collagen
EDS, Type IV	130050	Hetero	LMd; 7.5 kb; exon 9 to intron 24	342 aa deleted aa(46) to aa(387)	Helical	Superti-Furga et al., 1988, 1989 Lee et al., 1991a	Classical EDS IV shortened/normal type III collagen secreted Affected father and son
EDS, Type IV	130050	Hetero	LMd; 9.0 kb intron 33 to exon 48	414 aa deleted aa(586) to aa(999)	Helical	Superti-Furga et al., 1989 Vissing et al., 1991	Mild EDS IV Uncomplicated pregnancy Short and long trimers equally well secreted Heterotrimers retained; collagen cleavage site deleted
EDS, Type IV	130050	Hetero	LMd; 27 bp in exon 37	9 aa deleted	Helical	Nicholls et al., 1988 Narcisi et al., 1989 Richards et al., 1992	Variable type III collagen Linkage with COL3A1
Arterial aneurysms/ EDS, Type IV		Hetero	PMm; intra-exonic	Gly(619) to Arg	Helical	Kontusaari et al., 1990a	Moderate joint laxity, minimal skin changes Familial aneurysms
Arterial aneurysms/ EDS, Type IV		Hetero	PMm; intra-exonic	Gly(790) to Ser	Helical	Tromp et al., 1989a Stolle et al., 1985	Classical, severe EDS IV
EDS, Type IV	130050	Hetero	PMm; intra-exonic	Gly(883) to Asp	Helical	Tromp et al., 1989b	Mild EDS IV Affected father and daughter
EDS, Type IV	130050	Hetero	PMm; intra-exonic	Gly(910) to Val	Helical	De Paepe et al., 1991 Richards et al., 1991	Mild EDS IV bowel perforation Poor secretion of collagen III; decreased thermal stability

Continued.

Table VI. COL3A1: Known mutations—cont'd

Disease	MIM #	Zygosity	Mutation	Protein change	Domain	References	Comments
EDS, Type IV		Hetero	PMs; IVS16+1 splice junction G to A		Helical	Kuivaniemi et al., 1990a	Aneurysm of cervical artery Soft skin
EDS, Type IV		Hetero	PMs; IVS20+1 splice junction G(1) to A		Helical	Kontusaari et al., 1990b Kuivaniemi et al., 1990	Aortic aneurysm Easy bruisability Soft skin 50% normal type III collagen
EDS, Type IV	130050	Hetero	PMs; IVS41+1 splice junction G to A		Helical	Cole et al., 1990	Poor secretion of type III collagen Collagenase cleavage site deleted
EDS, Type IV	130050	Hetero	PMs; IVS42+1 splice junction G to A		Helical	Kuivaniemi et al., 1990	Severe EDS Aortic aneurysm Soft skin
EDS, Type IV	130050	Hetero	PMs; IVS 27+5 G to T		Helical	Thakker-Varia et al., 1990	10% type III collagen secreted
EDS, Type IV	130050	Hetero	PMs; IVS 25+5 G to T		Helical	Superti-Furga et al., 1989 Lee et al., 1991b	Severe, sporadic EDS IV, decreased thermal stability of COLIII, temperature-dependent alternative splicing

Table VII. COL3A1: Provisional data

Disease	MIM #	Evidence	References	Comments
Familial cerebral aneurysms		Type III collagen deficiency in cultured skin fibroblasts in some patients with congenital berry aneurysms	Pope et al., 1981, Pope, 1989 Pope et al., 1990 Leblanc et al., 1989	In some patients with cerebral aneurysms normal type III collagen levels were present Genetic heterogeneity?

Table VIII. Other gene loci: mapped human gene loci for which both a heritable disorder of connective tissue and a component of the extracellular matrix are known

Map position	Symbol	Locus name	Disorder(s) assoc. with locus
1p36.2-p34	ALPL	Alkaline phosphatase [171760] (Chodirker et al., 1987)	Hypophosphatasia, infantile [241500] Hypophosphatasia, adult [146300]
1p34	FUCA1	Alpha-L-fucosidase-1 (Fowler et al., 1986 Willems et al., 1988a)	Fucosidosis [230000] (Willems et al., 1988b)
2q31-qter	ELN	Elastin	Osteopoikilosis [166700] (Berlin et al., 1967)
2q34-q36	FN1	Fibronectin-1 (Jhanwar et al., 1986)	?EDS, type X [225310] (Arneson et al., 1980) Plasma fibronectin deficiency (Shirakami et al., 1986)
3p21-p142	GLB1	Beta-D-galactosidase-1 [230500] (Geihl et al., 1989)	MPS IVB [253010](Morquio B) also G_{m1}-gangliosidosis (van der Horst et al., 1983)
4q21-q23	GNPTA	N-acetyl-alpha-glucos-aminylphosphotransferase (Mueller et al., 1987)	Mucolipidosis II; mucolipidosis III [252500] (Ben-Yoseph et al., 1987)
4q21-qter	AGA	Aspartylglucosaminidase (Aula et al., 1984)	Aspartylglucosaminuria [208400] (Mononen et al., 1991)
5q11-q13	ARSB	Arylsulfatase B	MPS VI [253200]
5q23-q31	FBN2	Fibrillin-like protein (Lee et al., 1991)	Congenital contractural arachnodactyly [121050]
7q21.1-q22	GUSB	Beta-glucuronidase (Allanson et al., 1988)	MPS VII [253220]
11q11-23	CLG	Collagenase (Gerhard et al., 1987)	Epidermolysis bullosa dystrophica, recessive [226600] (Bauer & Eisen, 1978)
12q14	G6S	N-acetylglucosamine-6-sulfatase	MPS IIID [252940]
15q21.1	FBN1	Fibrillin (Maslen et al., 1991)	Marfan syndrome (Hollister et al., 1990; Kainulainen et al., 1990; Dietz et al., 1991a,b; Lee et al., 1991)
19p13.2-q.12	MANB	Alpha-D-mannosidosis B (Kaneda et al., 1987)	Mannosidosis [248500]
21q22.3	CBS	Cystathionine-beta-synthase (Skovby et al., 1982, 1948)	Homocystinuria [236200] pyridoxine—nonresponsive; pyridoxine—responsive (Munke et al., 1988)
22q11	IDUA	Alpha-L-iduronidase (Schuchman et al., 1984)	MPS IH, IH/S. IS [252800] (Hurler, Scheie, & Hurler-Scheie syndromes) (Schuchman & Desnick, 1988)
Xq22	COL4A5	Collagen IV, alpha-5 (Barker et al., 1990; Myers et al., 1990)	Alport syndrome [301050] (Hasstadt and Atkin, 1983)
Xq27.3	FRAXA	Fragile site Xq27.3 (Thibodeau et al., 1988; Sutherland & Baker, 1989)	Martin-Bell syndrome [309550] (Pyeritz et al., 1982) (Hagerman & Synhorst, 1984; Hagerman et al., 1984; Opitz et al., 1984)
Xq28	IDS	Sulfoiduronate sulfatase	MPS II [309200] (Hunter syndrome)

Table IX. Mapped human phenotypes for which the basic defect is unknown

Map position	Symbol	Disorder(s) assoc. with locus
1q21-q24	EBS2	Epidermolysis bullosa simplex, Koebner type [131900]
2p	AKE	Acrokeratoelastoidosis [101850]
4q13-q21	DGI1	Dentinogenesis imperfecta-1 [125490] (Ball et al., 1982)
5q33.1	CMD1	Campomelic dysplasia with sex reversal [211970] also 8q21.4 (balanced translocation)
6p21.3	PDB	Paget disease of bone [167250]
8q23.2-q24.11	LGCR	Langer-Giedion syndrome [150230] (Ludecke et al., 1989)
8q24	EBS1	Epidermolysis bullosa simplex-1 [131950]
9q34	NPS1	Nail-patella syndrome [161200] (Renwick & Schulze, 1965; Westerveld et al., 1976; Puffenberger et al., 1990)
16p13.31-	PKD1	Adult polycystic kidney disease [173900] (Reeders et al., 1985, 1987, 1988; Ryynanen et al., 1987; Watson et al., 1987; Kimberling et al., 1988; Bachner et al., 1989; Mc-Parland et al., 1989)
18	DD	Diastrophic dysplasia [222600] (Holmgren et al., 1984)
20p11.23-p12.1	AHD	Arteriohepatic dysplasia [118450] (Byrne et al., 1986; Shrimpton et al., 1989)
Xpter-p22.32	CPXR	Chondrodysplasia punctata, recessive [302950] (Bick et al., 1989)
Xp22	SEDL	Spondyloepiphyseal dysplasia tarda [313400] (Szpiro-Tapia et al., 1988)
Xp22	AIH	Amelogenesis imperfecta [301200] [301100] (Lagerstrom et al., 1989)
Xp22.2-p22.1	CLS	Coffin-Lowry syndrome [303600] (Hanauer et al., 1988; Gilgenkrantz et al., 1988)
Xq12-q13	MNK	Menkes disease [309400] (Tonnesen et al., 1986)
Xq28	CPXD	Chondrodysplasia punctata, dominant [302960]
Xq28	MRSD	Mental retardation and skeletal dysplasia [309620]
X		Occipital horn syndrome [304150] (formerly Ehlers-Danlos syndrome type IX) (Byers et al., 1980; Peltonen et al., 1983; Storis et al., 1984)

Table X. Candidate loci: mapped components of the extracellular matrix without known phenotypic associations

Map position	Symbol	Matrix component assoc. with locus
1q31	LAMB2	Laminin B2 [150290]
1q43	NID	Nidogen (entactin) [131390] (Mattei M-G, 1989)
2	VNRA	Vibronectin receptor, alpha polypeptide [193210]
4	OPN	Osteopontin [166490]
4p14.8-q21	BMP3	Bone morphogenic protein-3 [112263]
5q31-q33	ON	Osteonectin [182120] (Naylor et al., 1989)
7q11.2	ELN	Elastin [130160] (Fazio et al., 1991)
7q31.1-q31.3	LAMB1	Laminin B1 [150240]
10p11.2	FNRB	Fibronectin receptor, beta subunit [135630]
10q21.3-q23.1	PO4HA	Prolyl-4-hydroxylase, alpha [176710]
10q22.1	PRG	Proteoglycan, secretory granule [177040]
11q12.1-q13.5	FNL2	Fibronectin-like-2 [135610]
12p	ELA1	Elastase-1 [130120]
12p12.1-qter	DCN	Decorin [125255]
12q11-q13	FNRA	Fibronectin receptor, alpha subunit [135620]
12q11-q21	KRTA	Keratin, acid or alpha [139350]
13q14	BMP1	Bone morphogenic protein-1 [112264]
13q34	COL4A1	Alpha 1 (IV) procollagen [120130]
13q34	COL4A2	Alpha 2 (IV) procollagen [120090]
14	BMP2A	Bone morphogenic protein-2a [112261]
15	COL1AR	Collagen I, alpha, receptor [120340]
15	CSPG1	Chondroitin sulfate proteoglycan core protein [155769] (Rettig et al., 1984; Finkelstein et al., 1991)
16q21	CLG4A	Collagenase type IVA [120360] (Fan Y-S et al., 1989)
17q11-q21	KRTB	Keratin, basic or beta [148030]
17q25	P4HB	Prolyl-4-hydroxylase, beta subunit [176790]
18p11.31	LAMA	Laminin A chain [150320] (Mattei M-G et al., 1989)
20	BMP2B1	Bone morphogenic protein-2b1 [112262]
Xp	AMEL	Amelogenin [301200]
Xq13qter	BGN	Biglycan [301870]

Table XI. Unmapped candidate loci for components of the extracellular matrix

Symbol	Locus name	Disorder(s) assoc. with locus
CSPGLP	Chondroitin sulfate proteoglycan link protein	Not linked to achondroplasia and pseudoachondroplasia (Finkelstein et al., 1991)
	Collagen galactosyl transferase	
	Collagen glucosyl transferase	
ELA2	Elastase-2	
	Lysyl hydroxylase	EDS VI [225400]
	Lysyl hydroxylase	
	Lysyl oxidase	
	Procollagen C-proteinase	
	Procollagen N-proteinase	EDS VII [225410]
	Prolyl-3-hydroxylase	
	Signal peptidase (procollagen)	

REFERENCES

Beighton P, de Paepe A, Danks D, Finidori G, Gedde-Dahl T, Goodman R, Hall JG, Hollister DW, Horton W, McKusick, VA, Opitz JM, Pope FM, Pyeritz RE, Rimoin DL, Sillence D, Spranger JW, Thompson E, Tsipouras P, Viljoen D, Winship I, Young I (1988): International nosology of heritable disorders of connective tissue, Berlin, 1986. Am J Med Gen 29:581-594.

McKusick VA (1990): "Mendelian Inheritance in Man," 9th ed. Baltimore: Johns Hopkins University Press.

COL1A1

Aitchison K, Ogilvie D, Honeyman M, Thompson E, Sykes B (1988): Homozygous osteogenesis imperfecta unlinked to collagen I genes. Hum Genet 78:233-236.

Baker AT, Ramshaw JAM, Chan D, Cole WG, Bateman JF (1989): Changes in collagen stability and folding in lethal perinatal osteogenesis imperfecta: The effect of alpha 1 (I)-chain glycine-to-arginine substitutions. Biochem J 261:253-257.

Barsh GS, Roush CL, Bonadio J, Byers PH (1985): Intron-mediated recombination may cause a deletion in an alpha 1 type collagen chain in a lethal form of osteogenesis imperfecta. Proc Natl Acad Sci USA 82:2870-2874.

Bateman JF, Chan D, Walker ID, Rogers JG, Cole WG (1987): Lethal perinatal osteogenesis imperfecta due to the substitution of arginine for glycine at residue 391 of the alpha 1(I) chain of type I collagen. J Biol Chem 262:7021-7027.

Bateman JF, Lamande SR, Dahl H-HM, Chan D, Cole WG (1988): Substitution of arginine for glycine 664 in the collagen alpha 1(I) chain in lethal perinatal osteogenesis imperfecta. J Biol Chem 263:11627-11630.

Bateman JF, Lamande SR, Dahl H-HM, Chan D, Mascara T, Cole WG (1989): A frameshift mutation results in a truncated nonfunctional carboxylterminal pro alpha 1(I) propeptide of type I collagen in osteogenesis imperfecta. J Biol Chem 264:10960-10964.

Batge B, Diebold J, Stein H, Muller PK (1990): First evidence for an altered bone matrix in osteoporosis. In Abstracts of the Third International Conference on the Molecular Biology and Pathology of Matrix, III-14.

Boileau C, Jondeau G, Bonaiti C, Coulson M, Delorme G, Dubourg O, Bourdarias J-P, Junien C (1990): Linkage analysis of five fibrillar collagen loci in a large French Marfan syndrome family. J Med Genet 27:78-81.

Bonadio J, Ramirez F, Barr M (1990): An intron mutation in the human alpha 1(I) collagen gene alters the efficiency of pre-mRNA splicing and is associated with osteogenesis imperfecta type II. J Biol Chem 265:2262-2268.

Byers PH, Starman BJ, Cohn DH, Horwitz AL (1988): A novel mutation causes a perinatal lethal form of osteogenesis imperfecta. J Biol Chem 263:7855-7861.

Cetta G, Tenni R, Rossi A, Antoniazzi F, Vitellaro-Zuccarello L, Valli M (1990): The substitution of cys for gly 178 in alpha 1(I) triple helical domain; mutual influence of the mutation with neighboring amino acids. IV International conference on Osteogenesis Imperfecta, abstract 8.

Cohn DH, Byers PH, Steinmann B, Gelinas RE (1986): Lethal osteogenesis imperfecta resulting from a single nucleotide change in one human pro alpha 1(I) collagen allele. Proc Natl Acad Sci USA 83:6045-6047.

Cohn DH, Starman BJ, Blumberg B, Byers PH (1990a): Recurrence of lethal osteogenesis imperfecta due to parental mosaicism for a dominant mutation in a human type I collagen gene (COL1A1). Am J Hum Genet 46:591-601.

Cohn DH, Wallis G, Zhang X, Byers PH (1990b): Serine for glycine substitutions in the alpha 1(I) chain of Type I collagen: Biological plasticity in the gly-pro-hyp clamp at the carboxy-terminal end of the triple helical domain. Abstracts of the Third International Conference on the Molecular Biology and Pathology of Matrix, III-2.

Cohn DH, Wallis GA, Edwards MJ, Starman BJ, Byers PH (1990c): Germline and somatic mosaicism in osteogenesis imperfecta. IV International Conference on Osteogenesis Imperfecta. Abstract 47.

Constantinou CD, Nielsen KB, Prockop DJ (1989): A lethal variant of osteogenesis imperfecta has a single base mutation that substitutes cysteine for glycine 904 of the alpha 1(I) chain of type I procollagen. J Clin Invest 83:574-584.

Labhard ME, Wirtz MK, Pope FM, Nicholls AC, Hollister DW (1988): A cysteine for glycine substitution at position 1017 in an alpha 1(I) chain of type I collagen in a patient with mild dominantly inherited osteogenesis imperfecta. Mol Biol Med 5:197-207.

Lamande SR, Dahl H-HM, Cole WG, Bateman JF (1989): Characterization of point mutations in the collagen COL1A1 and COL1A2 genes causing lethal perinatal osteogenesis imperfecta. J Biol Chem 264:15809-15812.

Marini JC, Grange DK, Gottesman GS, Lewis MB, Koeplin DA (1989): Osteogenesis imperfecta type IV: Detection of a point mutation in one alpha 1(I) collagen allele (COL1A1) by RNA/RNA hybrid analysis. J Biol Chem 264:11893-11900.

Myers JC, Emanuel BS (1987): Chromosomal localization of human collagen genes. Coll Rel Res 7:149-159.

Nicholls AC, Oliver J, Renouf D, Pope FM (1990): Type I collagen mutations in osteogenesis imperfecta and inherited osteoporosis. In IV International Conference on Osteogenesis Imperfecta, abstract 48.

Ogilvie DJ, Wordsworth BP, Priestley LM, Dalgleish R, Schmidtke J, Zoll B, Sykes BC (1987): Segregation of all four major fibrillar collagen genes in the Marfan syndrome. Am J Hum Genet 41:1071-1082.

Pack M, Constantinou CD, Kalea K, Nielsen KB, Prockop DJ (1989): Substitution of serine for alpha 1-glycine 844 in a severe variant of osteogenesis imperfecta minimally destabilizes the triple helix of type I procollagen. J Biol Chem 264:19694-19699.

Patterson E, Smiley E, Bonadio J (1989): RNA sequence analysis of a perinatal lethal osteogenesis imperfecta mutation. J Biol Chem 264:10083-10087.

Prockop DJ (1990): Mutations in collagen genes, The lessons of rare diseases applied to common diseases. In IV International Conference on Osteogenesis Imperfecta, abstract 50.

Rowe DW, Shapiro JR, Poirier M, Schlesinger S (1985): Diminished type I collagen synthesis and reduced alpha 1(I) collagen messenger RNA in cultured fibroblasts from patients with dominantly inherited (type I) osteogenesis imperfecta. J Clin Invest 76:604-611.

Schwartz RC, Blanton SH, Hyde CA, Sottile TR Jr., Hudgins L, Sarfarazi J, Tsipouras P (1990): Linkage analysis in Marfan syndrome. J Med Genet 27:86-90.

Spotila LD, Constantinou CD, Sereda L, Riggs BL, Prockop DJ (1990): Substitution of serine for gly alpha 2-661 in the gene for type I procollagen (COL1A2) as a cause of postmenopausal osteoporosis. In Abstracts of the Third International Conference on the Molecular Biology and Pathology of Matrix, III-46.

Starman BJ, Eyre D, Charbonneau H, Harrylock M, Weis MA, Weiss L, Graham JM Jr., Byers PH (1989): Osteogenesis imperfecta—The position of substitution for glycine by cysteine in the triple helical domain of the pro alpha 1(I) chains of type I collagen determines the clinical phenotype. Am Soc Clin Invest 84:1206-1214.

Sykes B, Ogilvie D, Wordsworth P, Anderson J, Jones N (1986): Osteogenesis imperfecta is linked to both type I collagen structural genes. Lancet 2:69-72.

Sykes B, Ogilvie D, Wordsworth P, Wallis G, Mathew C, Beighton P, et al. (1990): Consistent linkage of dominantly inherited osteogenesis imperfecta to the type I collagen loci COL1A1 and COL1A2. Am J Hum Genet 46:293-307.

Vogel BE, Minor RR, Freud M, Prockop DJ (1987): A point mutation in a type I procollagen gene converts glycine 748 of the alpha 1 chain to cysteine and destabilizes the triple helix in a lethal variant of osteogenesis imperfecta. J Biol Chem 262:14737-14744.

Wallis GA, Starman BJ, Zinn AB, Byers PH (1990a): Variable expression of osteogenesis imperfecta in a nuclear family is explained by somatic mosaicism for a lethal point mutation in the alpha 1(I) gene (COL1A1) of type I collagen in a parent. Am J Hum Genet 46:1034-1040.

Wallis GA, Starman BJ, Chessler SD, Willing MC, Byers PH (1990b): Mutations in the CB6 and carboxyl-terminal regions of COL1A1 causing lethal OI have different effects on the stability and secretion of the type I collagen molecule. In IV International Conference on Osteogenesis Imperfecta, abstract 55.

Weil D, D'Alessio M, Ramirez F, de Wet W, Cole WG, Chan D, Bateman JF (1989): A base substitution in the exon of a collagen gene causes alternative splicing and generates a structurally abnormal polypeptide in a patient with Ehlers-Danlos syndrome type VII. EMBO J 8:1705-1710.

Westerhausen A, Kishi J, Prockop DJ (1990): Mutations that substitute serine for glycine alpha 1-631 in type I procollagen. The effects of thermal unfolding of the triple helix are position-specific and demonstrate that the protein unfolds through a series of cooperative blocks. In Abstracts of the Third International Conference on the Molecular Biology and Pathology of Matrix, III-53.

Willing M, Cohn DH, Byers PH (1990): Frameshift mutation near the 3' end of the COL1A1 gene of type I collagen predicts an elongated pro alpha 1(I) chain and results in osteogenesis imperfecta type I. J Clin Invest 85:282-290.

Wirtz MK, Rao VH, Glanville RW, Labhard ME, Pretorius PJ, de Vires WN, de Wet WJ, Hollister DW (1990): A cysteine for glycine substitution at position 175 in an alpha 1(I) chain of type I collagen in a clinically heterogeneous form of osteogenesis imperfecta. In Abstracts of the Third International Conference on the Molecular Biology and Pathology of Matrix, III-42.

Wordsworth P, Ogilvie D, Akhras F, Jackson G, Sykes B (1989): Genetic segregation analysis of familial mitral valve prolapse shows no linkage to fibrillar collagen genes. Br Heart J 61:300-306.

Zhuang J, Constantinou CD, Prockop DJ (1990): A single base mutation in type I procollagen that converts glycine alpha 1-541 to aspartate in a lethal variant of osteogenesis imperfecta. Detection of the mutation with carbodiimide reaction. In Abstracts of the Third International Conference on the Molecular Biology and Pathology of Matrix, III-54.

COL1A2

Baldwin CT, Constantinou CD, Dumars KW, Prockop DJ (1989): A single base mutation that converts glycine 907 of the alpha 2(I) chain of type I procollagen to aspartate in a lethal variant of osteogenesis imperfecta. J Biol Chem 264:3002-3006.

Bateman JF, Mascara T, Lamande SR, Wu H, Rudnicki M, Jaenisch R (1990): Collagen defects produced by site-directed mutagenesis of COL1A1. In Abstracts of the IV International Conference on Osteogenesis Imperfecta, Pavia Italy.

de Wet W, Bernard M, Benson-Chanda V, Chur M-L, Dickson L, Weil D, Ramirez F (1987): Organization of the human pro alpha 2(I) collagen gene. J Biol Chem 262:16032-16036.

Dickson LA, Pihlajaniemi T, Deak S, Pope FM, Nicholls A, Prockop DJ, Myers JC (1984): Nuclease S1 mapping of a homozygous mutation in the carboxyl-propeptide-coding region of the pro alpha 2(I) collagen gene in a patient with osteogenesis imperfecta. Proc Natl Acad Sci USA 81:4524-4528.

Edwards MJ, Byers PH, Cohn DH (1990): Mild osteogenesis imperfecta produced by somatic mosaicism for a lethal mutation in a type I collagen gene. Am J Hum Genet 47:A215.

Ganguly A, Baldwin CT, Conway D, Prockop DJ (1990): Use of a carbodiimide reaction to locate single-base mutations. Detection of a single-base mutation in an intron of a type I procollagen gene (COL1A2) that causes abnormal RNA processing in a proband with lethal osteogenesis imperfecta (type II). Am J Hum Genet 47:A217 (abstract).

Henderson AS, Myers JC, Ramirez F (1983): Localization of the human alpha 2(I) collagen gene (COL1A2) to chromosome 7q22. Cytogenet Cell Genet 36:586-587.

Kuivaniemi H, Sabol C, Tromp G, Sippola-Thiele M, Prockop DJ (1988): A 19-base pair deletion in the pro alpha 2(I) gene of type I procollagen that causes in-frame RNA splicing from exon 10 to exon 12 in a proband with atypical osteogenesis imperfecta and in his asymptomatic mother. J Biol Chem 263:11407-11413.

Lamande SR, Dahl H-HM, Cole WG, Bateman JF (1989): Characterization of point mutations in the collagen COL1A1 and COL1A2 genes causing lethal perinatal osteogenesis imperfecta. J Biol Chem 264:15809-15812.

Molyneaux K, Byers PH, Dalgleish R (1990): A new mutation in the alpha 2(I)gene of a patient with non-lethal osteogenesis imperfecta. In Abstracts of the IV International Conference on Osteogenesis Imperfecta, Pavia, Italy.

Pihlajaniemi T, Dickson LA, Pope FM, Korhonen VM, Nicholls A, Prockop DJ, Myers JC (1984): Osteogenesis imperfecta: Cloning of a pro-alpha-2(I) collagen gene with a frameshift mutation. J Biol Chem 259:12941-12944.

Sykes B, Ogilvie D, Wordsworth P, Wallis G, Mathew C, Beighton P, et al., (1990): Consistent linkage of dominantly inherited osteogenesis imperfecta to the type I collagen loci: COL1A1 and COL1A2. Am J Hum Genet 46:293-307.

Tromp G, Prockop DJ (1988): Single base mutation in the pro alpha 2(I) collagen gene that causes efficient splicing of RNA from exon 27 to exon 29 and synthesis of a shortened but in-frame pro alpha 2(I) chain. Proc Natl Acad Sci USA 85:5254-5258.

Tsuneyoshi T, Constantinou CD, Mikkelsen M, Prockop DJ (1990): A substitution of arginine for glycine a2-694 in a gene for type I procollagen (COL1A2) that causes lethal osteogenesis imperfecta. Further definition of a cooperative block for micro-unfolding of the triple helix between about residues 637 and 775. Am J Hum Genet 47:A240.

Vasan NS, Kuivaniemi H, Vogel BE, Minor RR, Wootton JAM, Tromp G, Weksberg R, Prockop DJ (1991): A mutation in the pro-alpha-2(I) gene (COL1A2) for type I procollagen in Ehlers-Danlos syndrome type VII: Evidence suggesting that skipping of exon 6 in RNA splicing may be a common cause of the phenotype. Am J Hum Genet 48:305-317.

Weil D, Bernard M, Combates N, Wirtz MK, Hollister DW, Steinmann B, Ramirez F (1988): Identification of a mutation that causes exon skipping during collagen pre-mRNA splicing in an Ehlers-Danlos Syndrome variant. J Biol Chem 263:8561-8564.

Weil D, D'Alessio M, Ramirez F, Steinmann B, Wirtz MK, Glanville RW, Hollister DW (1989): Temperature-dependent expression of a splicing defect in the fibroblasts of a patient with Ehlers-Danlos Syndrome Type VII. J Biol Chem 264:16804-16809.

Weil D, D'Alessio M, Ramirez F, Eyre DR (1990): Structural and functional characterization of a splicing mutation in the Pro-alpha2(I) collagen gene of an Ehlers-Danlos syndrome type VII patient. J Biol Chem 265:16007-16011.

Wenstrup RJ, Cohn DH, Cohen T, Byers PH (1988): Arginine for glycine substitution in the triple-helical domain of the products of one alpha 2(I) collagen allele (COL1A2) produces the osteogenesis imperfecta type IV phenotype. J Biol Chem 263:7734-7740.

Wenstrup RJ, Shrago-Howe AW, Lever LW, Phillips CL, Byers PH, Cohn DH (1990): The effects of different cysteine for glycine substitutions within alpha 2(1) chains. J Biol Chem 266(4): 2590-2594.

Willing MC, Cohn DH, Starman B, Holbrook KA, Greenberg CR, Byers PH (1988): Heterozygosity for a large deletion in the alpha 2(I) collagen gene has a dramatic effect on type I collagen secretion and produces prenatal lethal osteogenesis imperfecta. J Biol Chem 263:8398-8404.

Zhuang J, Constantinou CD, Prockop DJ (1990): A single base mutation in type I procollagen that converts glycine 1-541 to aspartate in a lethal variant of osteogenesis imperfecta. Detection of the mutation with carbodiimide reaction. In Abstracts of the Third International Conference on the Molecular Biology and Pathology of Matrix, III-54.

COL2A1

Ahmad NN, Ala-Kokko L, Knowlton RG, Weaver EJ, Maguire JI, Prockop DJ (1990): A stop codon in the gene for type II procollagen (COL2A1) causes one variant of arthro-ophthalmopathy (the Stickler syndrome). In Abstracts of the Third International Conference on the Molecular Biology and Pathology of Matrix, III-8.

Ala-Kokko L, Baldwin CT, Moskowitz RW, Prockop DJ (1990): Single base mutation in the type II procollagen gene (COL2A1) as a cause of primary osteoarthritis associated with a mild chondroplasia. In Abstracts of the Third International Conference on the Molecular Biology and Pathology of Matrix, III-9.

Anderson IJ, Goldberg RB, Marion RW, Upholt WB, Tsipouras P (1990a): Spondyloepiphyseal dysplasia congenita: Genetic linkage to type II collagen. Am J Hum Genet 46:896-901.

Anderson IJ, Tsipouras P, Scher C, Ramesar RS, Martell RW, Beighton P (1990b): Spondyloepiphyseal dysplasia, mild autosomal dominant type is not due to primary defects of Type II collagen. Am J Med Genet 37:272-276.

Boileau C, Jondeau G, Bonaiti C, Coulson M, Delorme G, Dubourg O, Bourarias J-P, Junien C (1990): Linkage analysis of five fibrillar collagen loci in a large French Marfan syndrome family. J Med Genet 27:78-81.

Francomano CA, Liberfarb RM, Hirose T, Maumenee IH, Streeten EA, Meyers DA, Pyeritz RE (1988a): The Stickler syndrome is closely linked to COL2A1, the structural gene for type II collagen. Pathol Immunopath Res 7:104-106.

Francomano CA, Pyeritz RE (1988b): Achondroplasia is not caused by mutation in the gene for type II collagen. Am J Med Genet 29:955-961.

Knowlton RG, Weaver EJ, Struyk AF, Knobloch WH, King RA, Norris K, Shamban A, Uitto J, Jiminez SA, Prockop DJ (1989): Genetic linkage analysis of hereditary arthro-ophthalmopathy (Stickler syndrome) and the type II procollagen gene. Am J Hum Genet 45:681-688.

Knowlton RG, Katzenstein PL, Moskowitz RW, Weaver EJ, Malemud CJ, Pathria MN, Jiminez SA, Prockop DJ (1990): Genetic linkage of a polymorphism in the type II collagen gene (COL2A1) to primary osteoarthritis associated with mild chondrodysplasia. N Engl J Med 322:526-530.

Lee B, Vissing H, Ramirez F, Rogers D, Rimoin D (1989): Identification of the molecular defect in a family with spondyleopiphyseal dysplasia. Science 244:978-980.

Murray LW, Bautista J, James PL, Rimoin DL (1989): Type II collagen defects in the chondrodysplasias. I Spondyloepiphyseal dysplasia. Am J Hum Genet 45:5-15.

Myers JC, Emanuel BS (1987): Chromosomal localization of human collagen genes. Coll Rel Res 7:149-159.

Ogilvie DJ, Wordsworth BP, Priestley LM, Dalgleish R, Schmidtke J, Zoll B, Sykes BC (1987): Segregation of all four major fibrillar collagen genes in the Marfan syndrome. Am J Hum Genet 41:1071-1082.

Palotie A, Ott J, Elima K, Cheah K, Vaisanen P, Ryhanen L, Vikkula M, Vuorio E, Peltonen L (1989): Predisposition to familial osteoarthritis linked to type II collagen gene. Lancet 1:924-927.

Poole AR, Pidoux I, Reiner A, Rosenberg L, Hollister D, Murray L, Rimoin D (1988): Kniest dysplasia is characterized by an apparent abnormal processing of the C-propeptide of type II collagen resulting in imperfect fibril assembly. J Clin Invest 81:579-589.

Sangiorgi FO, Benson-Chanda V, de Wet WJ, Sobel ME, Tsipouras P, Ramirez F (1985): Isolation and partial characterization of the entire human pro alpha 1(II) collagen gene. Nucleic Acids Res 13:2207-2225.

Sher C, Ramesar R, Martell R, Learmonth I, Tsipouras P, Beighton P (1991): Namaqualand hip dysplasia: Genetic linkage to the type II collagen gene (COL2A1). Am J Hum Genet 48:518-524.

Tiller GE, Rimoin DL, Murray LW, Cohn DH (1990): Tandem duplication within a type II collagen gene (COL2A1) exon in an individual with spondyloepiphyseal dysplasia. Proc Natl Acad Sci USA 87:3889-3893.

Vissing H, D'Alessio M, Lee B, Ramirez F, Godfrey M, Hollister DW (1989): Glycine to serine substitution in the triple helical domain of pro alpha 1(II) collagen results in a lethal perinatal form of short-limbed dwarfism. J Biol Chem 264:18265-18267.

Wordsworth P, Ogilvie D, Priestley L, Smith R, Wynne-Davies R, Sykes B (1988): Structural and segregation analysis of the type II collagen gene (COL2A1) in some heritable chondrodysplasias. J Med Genet 25:521-527.

COL3A1

Cole WG, Chiodo AA, Lamande SR, Janeczko, Ramirez F, Dahl H-HM, Chan D, Bateman JF (1990): A base substitution at a splice site in the COL3A1 gene causes exon skipping and generates abnormal type III procollagen in a patient with Ehlers-Danlos syndrome type IV. J Biol Chem 265:1700-1707.

Dalgleish R, Hawkins JR, Keston M (1987): Exclusion of the alpha 2(I) and alpha 1(III) collagen genes as the mutant loci in a Marfan syndrome family. J Med Genet 24:148-151.

De Paepe A, Nuytinck L, Nicholls AC, Narcisi P, de Roose J, Matton M (1992): Study of a type III collagen protein defect in a patient with ecchymotic EDS: Importance of the analysis of non-cutaneous connective tissues. In Bartsocas

C, Loukopoulos D (eds): "Genetics of Hematological Disorders." Washington D.C.: Hemisphere Publishing Corporation, pp 267-274.

Francomano CA, Streeten FA, Myers DA, Pyeritz RE (1988): Marfan syndrome: Exclusion of genetic linkage to three major collagen genes. Am J Med Genet 29:451-662.

Huerre-Jeanpierre C, Mattei MC, Weil D, Grzeschik KH, Chu ML, Sangiorgi FO, Sobel ME, Ramirez F, Junien C (1986): Further evidence for the dispersion of the human fibrillar collagen genes. Am J Hum Genet 38:26-27.

Kontusaari S, Tromp G, Kuivaniemi H, Romaine A, Prockop DJ (1990a): A mutation in the gene for type III procollagen in a family with aortic aneurysms. J Clin Investigation 86:1465-1469.

Kontusaari S, Tromp G, Kuivaniemi H, Ladda RL, Prockop DJ (1990b): Inheritance of an RNA splicing mutation (G+1, IVS 20) in the type III procollagen gene (COL3A1) in a family having aortic aneurysms and easy bruisability: Phenotypic overlap between familial arterial aneurysms and Ehlers-Danlos syndrome type IV. Am J Hum Genet 47:112-120.

Kuivaniemi H, Kontusaari S, Tromp G, Zhao M, Sabol C, Prockop DJ (1990): Identical G+1 to A mutations in three different introns of the type III procollagen gene (COL3A1) produce different patterns of RNA splicing in three variants of Ehlers-Danlos syndrome IV (1990). An explanation for exon skipping with some mutations and not others. J Biol Chem 265:1206-1207.

Leblanc R, Lozano AM, van der Rest M, Guttmann RD (1989): Absence of collagen deficiency in familial cerebral aneurysms. J Neurosurg 70:837-840.

Lee B, D'Alessio M, Vissing H, Ramirez F, Steinmann B, Superti-Furga A (1991a): Characterization of a large genomic deletion associated with a polymorphic block of repeated dinucleotides in the type III procollagen gene (COL3A1) of a patient with Ehlers-Danlos syndrome type IV. Am J Hum Genet 48:511-517.

Lee B, Vitale E, Superti-Furga A, Steinmann B, Ramirez F (1991b): G to T transversion at position +5 of a splice donor site causes skipping of the preceding exon in the type III procollagen transcripts of a patient with Ehlers-Danlos syndrome type IV. J Biol Chem 266:5256-5259.

McGookey DJ, Smith ACM, Waldstein G, Byers PH (1989): Mosaicism for a deletion in one of the type III collagen alleles indicates that the deletion occurred after identification of cells for recruitment in different cell lineages early in human development. Am J Hum Genet 45:A206 (abstract).

Narcisi P, Nicholls AC, De Paepe A, Pope FM (1989): An alpha 1(1III) CB5 mutation in Ehlers-Danlos syndrome type IV. J Med Genet 26:211 (abstract).

Nicholls AC, De Paepe A, Narcisi P, Dalgleish R, De Keyser F, Matton M, Pope FM (1988): Linkage of a polymorphic marker for the type III collagen gene (COL3A1) to atypical autosomal dominant Ehlers-Danlos syndrome type IV in a large Belgian pedigree. Hum Genet 78:276-281.

Ogilvie DJ, Wordsworth BP, Priestley LN, Dalgleish R, Schmidtke J, Zoll B, Sykes BC (1987): Segregation of all four major fibrillar collagen genes in the Marfan syndrome. Am J Med Genet 41:1071-1082.

Pope FM, Narcisi P, Neil-Dwyer G, Nicholls AC, Bartlett J, Doshi B (1981): Some patients with cerebral aneurysms are deficient in type III collagen. Lancet 1:973-975.

Pope FM (1989): Type III collagen mutations and cerebral aneurysms, Stroke 20:1432.

Pope FM, Limburg M, Schievink WI (1990): Familial cerebral aneurysms and type III collagen deficiency. J Neurosurg 72:156-157.

Richards AJ, Lloyd JC, Narcisi P, Nicholls AC, Ward PN, De Paepe A, Pope FM (1992): A 27bp deletion from one allele of the type III collagen gene COL 3A1 in a large family with atypical Ehlers-Danlos Syndrome type IV. Hum Genet 88:325-380.

Richards AJ, Lloyd JC, Ward PN, De Paepe A, Narcisi P, Pope FM (1991): Characterisation of a glycine to valine substitution at aminoacid position 910 of the triple helical region of type III collagen in a patient with Ehlers-Danlos Syndrome type IV. J Med Genet 28(7):458-463.

Stolle CA, Pyeritz R, Myers GC, Prockop DJ (1985): Synthesis of an altered type III procollagen in a patient with type IV EDS. J Biol Chem 260:1937-1944.

Superti-Furga A, Gugler, E, Gitzelmann R, Steinmann B (1988): Ehlers-Danlos syndrome type IV: A multi-exon deletion in one of the two COL3A1 alleles affecting structure, stability, and processing of type III procollagen. J Biol Chem 263:6226-6232.

Superti-Furga A, Steinmann B, Ramirez F, Byers PH (1989): Molecular defects of type III collagen in Ehlers-Danlos syndrome type IV. Hum Genet 82:104-108.

Superti-Furga A, Lee B, D'Alessio M, Steinmann B, Ramirez F (1990): Identification of a highly polymorphic (CA)n-(TA)n(GT)n element in intron 24 of the COL3A1 gene, Matrix 10:249-250.

Thakker-Varia S, Anderson D, Kuivaniemi H, Tromp G, Prockop DJ, Stolle CA (1990): An exon deletion in type III procollagen mRNA is associated with intracellular degradation of the abnormal protein in a patient with Ehlers-Danlos syndrome IV. Matrix 10:249-250 (abstract).

Tromp G, Kuivaniemi H, Shikata H, Prockop DJ (1989a): A single base mutation that substitutes serine for glycine 790 of the alpha 1(III) chain of type III procollagen exposes an arginine and causes Ehlers-Danlos syndrome IV. J Biol Chem 264:1349-1352.

Tromp G, Kuivaniemi H, Stolle C, Pope FM, Prockop D (1989b): Single base mutation in the type III procollagen gene that converts the codon for glycine 883 to aspartate in a mild variant of Ehlers-Danlos syndrome IV. J Biol Chem 264:19313-19317.

Tsipouras P, Byers PH, Schwartz RC, Chu ML, Weil D, Pepe D, Cassidy SB, Ramirez F (1986): Ehlers-Danlos syndrome type IV: Cosegregation of the phenotype to a COL3A1 allele of type III procollagen. Hum Genet 74:41-46.

Vissing H, D'Alessio M, Lee B, Ramirez F, Byers PH, Steinmann B, Superti-Furga A (1991): Multi-exon deletion in the procollagen III gene is associated with mild Ehlers-Danlos syndrome type IV. J Biol Chem 266:5244-5248.

Other gene loci and candidate proteins

Allanson JE, Gemmill RM, Hecht RK, Johsen S, Wenger DA (1988): Deletion mapping of the beta-glucuronidase gene. Am J Med Genet 29:517-522.

Arneson MA, Hammerschmidt DE, Furcht LT, King RA (1980): A new form of Ehlers-Danlos syndrome: Fibronectin corrects defective platelet function. JAMA 244:144-147.

Aula P, Astin KH, Francke U, Desnick RJ (1984): Assignment of the structural gene encoding human aspartylglucosaminidase to the long arm of chromosome 4 (4q21-4qter). Am J Hum Genet 36:1215-1224.

Bachner L, Vinet MC, Lacave R, Sraer JD, Chevet D, Julier C, Kaplan JC (1989): Linkage analysis of a French family with autosomal dominant polycystic kidney disease (ADPKD) non allelic to PKD1 locus. HGM10 Abstracts: 148.

Bachner L, Vinet MC, Albouze G, Julier C, Le Merrer M, Kaplan J, Mathiew M, Piussan C, Grunfeld JP, Kaplan JC (1989): Linkage analysis of 15 French families with various clinical forms of autosomal dominant polycystic kidney disease (ADPKD). HGM10 Abstracts: 149.

Ball SP, Cook PJL, Mars M, Buckton KE (1982): Linkage between dentinogenesis imperfecta and Gc. Ann Hum Genet 46:35-40.

Barker DF, Hostikka SL, Zhou J, Chow LT, Oliphant AR, Gerken SC, Gregory MC, Skolnick MH, Atkin CL, Tryggvason K (1990): Identification of mutations in COL4A5 collagen gene in Alport syndrome. Science 248:1224-1227.

Bauer EA, Eisen AZ (1978): Recessive dystrophic epidermolysis bullosa: Evidence for increased collagenase as a genetic characteristic in cell culture. J Exp Med 148:1378-1387.

Ben-Yoseph Y, Potier M, Mitchell DA, Pack BA, Malancon GB, Nadler H (1987): Altered molecular size of N-acetylglucosamine 1-phosphotransferase in T-cell disease and pseudo-Hurler polydystrophy. Biochem J 248:697-701.

Berlin R, Hedensin R, Lilja R, Linder L (1967): Osteopoikilosis—a clinical and genetic study. Acta Med Scand 181:305-314.

Bick DP, Snead ML, Yen PH, McGill JR, Schorderet DG, Hejtmancik JF, Ballabio A, Campbell L, Moore CM, Curry CJ, Lau EC, Shapiro LJ (1989): Mapping chondrodysplasia punctata, ichthyosis, Kallmann syndrome and DNA markers in male patients with Xp chromosome deletions HGM10 Abstracts: 32.

Byers PH, Siegel RC, Holbrook KA, Narayanan AS, Bornstein P, Hall JG (1980): X-linked cutis laxa. N Engl J Med 303:61-65.

Byrne JLB, Harod MJE, Friedman JM, Howard-Peebles PN (1986): del (20p) with manifestations of arteriohepatic dysplasia. Am J Med Genet 24:673-678.

Chodirker BN, Evans JA, Lewis M, Coghlan G, Belcher E, Philipps S, Seargeant LE, Sus C, Greenberg CR (1987): Infantile hypophosphatasia—linkage with the RH locus. Genomics 1:280-282.

Curry CJR, Magenis RE, Brown M, Lanman JT Jr., Tsai J, O'Lague P, Goodfellow P, Mohandas T, Bergner EA, Shapiro LJ (1984): Inherited chondrodysplasia punctata due to a deletion of the terminal short arm of an X chromosome. N Engl J Med 311:1010-1015.

Dietz HC, Pyeritz RD, Hall BE, Cadle RG, Hamosh A, Schwartz J, Meyers DA, Francomano CA (1991): The Marfan syndrome locus: Confirmation of assignment to chromosome 15 and identification of tightly linked markers at 15q15-q21.3. Genomics 9:355-361.

Dietz HC, Cutting GR, Pyeritz RE, Maslen CL, Sakai LY, Corson GM, Puffenberger EG, Hamosh A, Nanthakumar EJ, Curristin SM, Stetten G, Meyers DA, Francomano CA (1991b): Defects in the fibrillin gene cause the Marfan syndrome: Linkage evidence and identification of a missense mutation. Nature 352:337-339.

Fan Y-S, Eddy RL, Hyhtala P, Byers MG, Haley LL, Henry WM, Tryggvason K, Shows TB (1989): Collagenase type IV (CLG4) is mapped to human chromosome 16q21. HGM10 Abstracts: 79.

Fazio MJ, Mattei M-G, Passage E, Chu M-L, Black D, Solomon E, Davidson JM, Uitto J (1991): Human elastin gene: New evidence for localization to the long arm of chromosome 7. Am J Hum Genet 48:696-703.

Finkelstein JE, Doege K, Yamada Y, Pyeritz RE, Graham JM, Moeschler JB, Francomano CA (1990): Analysis of chondroitin sulfate proteoglycan core protein (CSPGCP) and link protein (CSPGLP) gene in achondroplasia and pseudoachondroplasia. Am J Hum Genet 48:97-102.

Fowler ML, Nakai H, Byers MG, Fukushima H, Eddy RL, Henry WM, Haley LL, O'Brien JS, Shows TB (1986): Chromosome 1 localization of the human alpha-L-fucosidase structural gene with a homologous site on chromosome 2. Cytogenet Cell Genet 43:103-108.

Gal A, Wirth B, Kaariainen H, Lucotte G, Landaia P, Gillessen-Kaesbach G, Muller Wiefel DE, Zerres K (1989): Childhood manifestation of autosomal dominant polycystic kidney disease: No evidence for genetic heterogeneity. Clin Genet 35:13-19.

Geihl D, Mudd M, O'Brien J, Yamamoto Y, Naylor SL (1989): Regional mapping of the human beta-galactosidase gene using a cDNA probe. HGM10 Abstracts: 47.

Gerhard DS, Jones C, Bauer FA, Eisen AZ, Goldberg GI (1987): Human collagenase gene is localized to 11q. Cytogenet Cell Genet 46:619 (Abstract).

Gilgenkrantz S, Mujica P, Gruet P, Tridon P, Schweitzer F, Nivelon-Chevalilier A, Nivelon JL, Couillault G, David A, Verloes A, Lambotte C, Piussan C, Mathieu M (1988): Coffin-Lowry syndrome: A multicenter study. Clin Genet 34:30-245.

Hagerman RJ, Synhorst DP (1984): Mitral valve prolapse and aortic dilatation in the fragile X syndrome. Am J Med Genet 17:123-131.

Hagerman RJ, Van Housen K, Smith ACM, McGavran L (1984): Consideration of connective tissue dysfunction in the fragile X syndrome. Am J Med Genet 17:111-121.

Hanauer A, Alembik Y, Gilgenkrantz S, Mujica P, Nivelon-Chevallier A, Pembrey ME, Young ID, Mandel JL (1988): Probable localisation of the Coffin-Lowry locus in Xp22.2-p22.1 by multipoint linkage analysis. Am J Med Genet 30:523-530.

Hasstedt SJ, Atkin CL (1983): X-linked inheritance of Alport syndrome: Family P revisited. Am J Hum Genet 35:1241-1251.

Hollister DW, Godfrey M, Sakai LY, Pyeritz RE (1990): Immunohistologic abnormalities of the microfibrillar-fiber system in the Marfan syndrome. N Engl J Med 323:152-159.

Holmgren G, Jagell S, Lagekvist B, Nordenson I (1984): A pair of siblings with diastrophic dysplasia and E trisomy mosaicism. Hum Hered 34:266-268.

Jhanwar SC, Jensen JT, Kaelbling M, Chaganti RSK, Klinger HP (1986): In situ localization of human fibronectin (FN) genes to chromosome regions 2p14-p16, 2q34-q36, and 11q12.1-q13.5 in germ line cells, but to chromosome 2 sites only somatic cells. Cytogenet Cell Genet 41:47-53.

Kainulainen K, Pulkkiner L, Savolainen A, Kaitila I, Peltonen L (1990): Location on chromosome 15 of the gene defect causing Marfan syndrome. N Engl J Med 323:935-939.

Kaneda Y, Hayes H, Uchida T, Yoshida MC, Okada Y (1987): Regional assignment of five genes on human chromosome 19. Chromosoma 95:8-12.

Kimberling WJ, Fain PR, Kenyon JB, Goldgar D, Sujansky E, Gabow PA (1988): Linkage heterogeneity of autosomal dominant polycystic kidney disease N Engl J Med 319:913-918.

Lagerstrom M, Dahl N, Iselius L, Backman B, Pettersson U (1989): Linkage analysis of X-linked amelogenesis imperfecta. HGM10 Abstract: 155.

Lee B, Godfrey M, Vitale E, Hori H, Mattei M-G, Sarfarazi M, Tsipouras P, Ramirez F, Hollister D (1991): Marfan syndrome and a phenotypically related disorder are linked to two different fibrillin genes. Nature 352:330-334.

Ludecke H-J, Senger G, Clauseen U, Horsthemke B (1989): Molecular approach to the Langer-Giedion syndrome chromosome region. HGM10 Abstract: 174.

Maslen CL, Corson GM, Maddox K, Glanville RW, Sakai LF (1991): Partial sequence determination of a candidate gene for the Marfan syndrome. Nature 352:334-337.

Mattei M-G, Passage E, Weil D, Nagayoshi T, Knowlton RG, Chu M-L, Uitto J (1989): Chromosomal mapping of human basement membrane zone genes: Laminin A chain at locus 18p11.31 and Nidogen at locus 1q43. HGM10 Abstracts: 166.

McParland P, Papiha SS, Gale M, Bhattacharya SS (1989): Linkage studies in adult polycystic kidney disease: The question of genetic heterogeneity in Northern England. HGM10 Abstracts: 234.

Mononen I, Heisterkamp N, Kaartinen V, Williams JC, Yates JR, Griffin PR, Hood LE, Groffen J (1991): Aspartylglycosaminuria in the Finnish population: Identification of two point mutations in the heavy chain of glycoasparaginase. Genetics 88:2914-2945.

Munke M, Kraus JP, Ohura T, Francke U (1988): The gene for cystathionine beta-synthase (CBS) maps to the subtelomeric region on human chromosome 21q and to proximal mouse chromosome 17. Am J Hum Genet 42:550-559.

Mueller OT, Wasmuth JJ, Murray JC, Lozzio CB, Lovrien EW, Shows TB (1987): Chromosomal assignment of N-acetylglucosaminylphosphotransferase, the lysosomal hydrolase targeting enzyme deficient in mucolipidosis II and III. Cytogenet Cell Genet 46:664 (Abstract).

Myers JC, Jones TA, Pohjolainen E-R, Kadri AS, Goddar AD, Sheer D, Solomon E, Pihlajaniemi T (1990): Molecular cloning of alpha-5(IV) collagen and assignment of the gene to the region of the X-chromosome containing the Alport syndrome locus. Am J Hum Genet 46:1024-1033.

Naylor SL, Helen-Davis D, Villarreal XC, Long GL (1989): The human osteonectin gene on chromosome 5 is polymorphic. HGM10 Abstract: 45.

Opitz JM, Westphal JM, Daniel A (1984): Discovery of a connective tissue dysplasia in the Martin-Bell syndrome. Am J Med Genet 17:101-109.

Peltonen L, Kivaniemi H, Palotie A, Horn N, Kaitila I, Kivirikko K (1983): Alterations in copper and collagen metabolism in the Menkes syndrome and a new subtype of the Ehlers-Danlos syndrome. Biochemistry 22:6146-6163.

Puffenberger EG, Kwiatkowski DJ, Perman S, Abbott M, Meyers D, Francomano CA (1990): Linkage analysis of nail-patella syndrome with 9q34 markers. Am J Hum Genet 47:A195 (Abstract).

Pyeritz RE, Stamberg J, Thomas GH, Bell BB, Zahka KG, Bernhardt BA (1982): The marker Xq28 syndrome (fragile X syndrome) in a retarded man with mitral valve prolapse. Johns Hopkins Med J 151:231-237.

Reeders ST, Breuning MH, Davies KE, Nicholls RD, Jarman AP, Higgs DR, Pearson PL, Weatherall DJ (1985): A highly polymorphic DNA marker linked to adult polycystic kidney disease on chromosome 16. Nature 317:542-544.

Reeders ST, Breuning MH, Ryynanen MA, Wright AF, Davies KF, King AW, Watson ML, Weatherall DJ. A study of genetic linkage heterogeneity in adult polycystic kidney disease. Hum Genet 76:348-351.

Reeders ST, Keith T, Green P, Germino GG, Barton NJ, Lehmann OJ, Brown VA, Phipps P, Morgan J, Bear JC, Parfrey P (1988): Regional localization of the autosomal dominant polycystic kidney disease locus. Genomics 3:150-155.

Renwick JH, Schulze J (1965): Male and female recombination fractions for the nail patella: ABO linkage in man. Ann Hum Genet 28:379-392.

Rettig WJ, Dracopoli NC, Goetzger TA, Spengler BA, Biedler JL, Oetgen HF, Old LJ (1984): Somatic cell genetic analysis of human cell surface antigens: Chromosomal assignments and regulation of expression in rodent-human hybrid cells. Proc Natl Acad Sci USA 81:6437-6441.

Ryynanen M, Dolata MM, Lampainen F, Reders ST (1987): Localisation of a mutation producing autosomal dominant polycystic kidney disease without renal failure. J Med Genet 24:462-465.

Sartoris DJ, Luzzatti L, Weaver DD, MacFarlane JD, Hollister DW, Parker BR (1984): Type IX Ehlers-Danlos syndrome. Radiology 152:665-670.

Shirakami A, Shigekiyo T, Hirai Y, Takeichi T, Kawauchi S, Saito S, Miyoshi K (1986): Plasma fibronectin deficiency in eight members of one family. Lancet 1:473-474.

Schuchman EH, Astrin KH, Aula P, Desnick RJ (1984): Regional assignment of the structural gene for human alpha-L-iduronidase. Proc Natl Acad Sci USA 81:1169-1173.

Schuchman EH, Desnick RJ (1988): Mucopolysaccharidosis type I subtypes: Presence of immunologically cross-reactive material and in vitro enhancement of the residual alpha-L-iduronidase activities. J Clin Invest 81:98-105.

Shrimpton AE, Vijayalaxmi, Evans HJ (1989): Dominantly inherited spinocerebellar ataxia (SCA1) linkage studies. HGM10 Abstracts: 197.

Skovby F, Krassikoff N, Francke U (1984): Assignment of the gene for cystathionine beta-synthase to human chromosome 21 in somatic cell hybrids. Hum Genet 65:291-294.

Skovby F, Kraus J, Redlich C, Rosenberg LE (1982): Immunochemical studies on cultured fibroblasts from patients with homocystinuria due to cystathionine beta-synthase deficiency. Am J Hum Genet 34:73-83.

Skovby F, Kraus JP, Rosenberg LE (1984): Homocystinuria: Biogenesis of cystathionine beta-synthase subunits in cultured fibroblasts and in an in vitro translation system programmed with fibroblast messenger RNA. Am J Hum Genet 36:452-459.

Sutherland GR, Baker E (1989): The common fragile site (FRAXD) is at Xq27.2 and can be distinguished from the fragile X (FRAXA) at Xq27.3). HGM10 Abstract: 33.

Szpiro-Tapia S, Sefiani A, Guilloud-Bataille M, Heuertz S, LeMarec B, Frezal J, Maroteaux P, Hors.Cayla MC (1988): Spondyloepiphyseal dysplasia tarda: Linkage with genetic markers from the distal short arm of the X-chromosome. Hum Genet 81:61-63.

Tonnesen T, Gerdes AM, Horn N, Friedrich U, Grisar T, Muller A (1986): Localization of the Menkes gene to the long arm of the X-chromosome. In 7th Int Cong Hum Genet, Berlin, 627 (Abstract).

van der Horst GT, Kleijer TJ, Hoogeveen AT, Huijmans JGM, Blom W, van Diggelen Op (1983): Morquio B syndrome: A primary defect in beta-galactosidase. Am J Med Genet 16:261-275.

Watson ML, Wright AF, Macnical AM, Allan PL, Clayton FJ, Dempster M, Jeremiah SJ, Corney G, Hopkinson DA (1987): Studies of genetic linkage between adult polycystic kidney disease and three markers on chromosome 16. J Med Genet 24:457-461.

Westerveld A, Jongsma APM, Meera Khan P, Van Someren H, Bootsma D (1976): Assignment of the AK(1):NP:ABO linkage group to human chromosome 9. Proc Natl Acad Sci USA 73:895-899.

Willems PJ, Darby JK, DiCioccio RA, Nakashima P, Eng C, Kretz KA, Cavalli-Sforza LL, Shooter EM, O'Brien JS (1988): Identification of a mutation in the structural alpha-L-fucosidase gene in fucosidosis. Am J Hum Genet 43:756-763.

Willems PJ, Garcia CA, De Smedt MCH, Martin-Jiminez R, Darby JK, Duenas DA, Grandao-Villar D, O'Brien JS (1988): Intrafamilial variability in fucosidosis. Clin Genet 34:7-14.

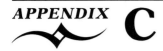

International Nomenclature of Constitutional Disorders of Bone

Osteochondrodysplasias	Mode of inheritance	Chromosomal locus	Gene	Protein	MIM No.
Defects of the tubular (and flat) bones or axial skeleton, or both					
Achondroplasia group					
Thanatophoric dysplasia	AD				187.600
Thanatophoric dysplasia-straight femur and "clover leaf" skull type	AD				187.600
Achondroplasia	AD				100.800
Hypochondroplasia	AD				146.000
Achondrogenesis					
Type IA	AR				200.600
Type IB	AR				200.600
Spondylodysplastic group (perinatally lethal)					
San Diego type	Sp				151.210
Torrance type	Sp				151.210
Luton type	Sp				151.210
Metatropic dysplasia group					
Fibrochondrogenesis	AR				228.520
Schneckenbecken dysplasia	AR				269.250
Metatropic dysplasia	AD				156.530
					250.600
Short-rib dysplasia group (with or without polydactyly)					
SRP Type I, Saldino-Noonan	AR				263.530
SRP Type II, Majewski	AR				263.520
SRP Type III, Verma-Naumoff	AR				263.510
SRP Type IV, Beemer-Langer	AR				269.860
Asphyxiating thoracic dysplasia	AR				208.500
Ellis-van Creveld dysplasia	AR				225.500

Modified from the International Working Group on Constitutional Diseases of Bone: international classification of osteochondrodysplasias, *Eur J Pediatr* 151:407-415, 1992, and *Am J Med Genet* 44:223-229, 1992.

AD, Autosomal dominant; *AR*, autosomal recessive; *MIM*, *Mendelian Inheritance in Man* number; *Sp*, sporadic; *SRP*, short-rib polydactyly; *XLD*, X-linked dominant; *XLR*, X-linked recessive. *Continued.*

Osteochondrodysplasias	Mode of inheritance	Chromosomal locus	Gene	Protein	MIM No.
Atelosteogenesis and diastrophic dysplasia group					
"Boomerang" dysplasia	Sp				—
Atelosteogenesis type I	Sp				108.720
Atelosteogenesis type II (de la Chapelle)	AR				256.050
Omodysplasia I (Maroteaux)	AD				—
Omodysplasia II (Borochowitz)	AR				—
Otopalatodigital syndrome type II	XLR				304.120
Diastrophic dysplasia	AR	5q31-q34			222.600
Pseudodiastrophic dysplasia	AR				264.180
Kniest-Stickler dysplasia group					
Dyssegmental dysplasia, Silverman-Handmaker type	AR				224.410
Dyssegmental dysplasia, Rolland-Desbuquois type	AR				224.400
Kniest dysplasia	AD				156.550
Otospondylomegaepiphyseal dysplasia	AR				215.150
Stickler dysplasia (heterogeneous, some not linked to COL2A1)	AD	12q13.1-q13.3	COL2A1	Type II collagen	108.300
Spondyloepiphyseal dysplasia congenita group					
Langer-Saldino dysplasia (achondrogenesis type II)	AD	12q13.1-q13.3	COL2A1	Type II collagen	200.610 120.140.02
Hypochondrogenesis	AD	12q13.1-q13.3	COL2A1	Type II collagen	120.140.02
Spondyloepiphyseal dysplasia congenita	AD	12q13.1-q13.3	COL2A1	Type II collagen	183.900 120.140.01
Other spondyloepi-(meta)-physeal dysplasias					
X-linked spondyloepiphyseal dysplasia tarda	XLD	Xp22	SEDL		313.400
Other late-onset spondyloepi-metaphyseal dysplasias (i.e., Namaqualand dysplasia, Irapa dysplasia)					
Progressive pseudorheumatoid dysplasia	AR				208.230
Dyggve-Melchior-Clausen dysplasia	AR				223.800
Wolcott-Rallison dysplasia	AR				226.980
Immunoosseous dysplasia	AR				—
Pseudoachondroplasia	AD				177.150
Opsismodysplasia	AR				258.480
Dysostosis multiplex group					
Mucopolysaccharidosis IH	AR	4p16.3	IDA	α-1-Iduronidase	252.800
Mucopolysaccharidosis IS	AR	4p16.3	IDA	α-1-Iduronidase	252.800
Mucopolysaccharidosis II	XLR	Xq27.3-q28	IDS	Iduronate-2-sulfatase	309.900
Mucopolysaccharidosis IIIA	AR			Heparan sulfate sulfatase	
Mucopolysaccharidosis IIIB	AR			N-Ac-α-D-glucosaminidase	
Mucopolysaccharidosis IIIC	AR			Ac-CoA:α-glucosaminidase-N-acetyltransferase	
Mucopolysaccharidosis IIID	AR	12q14	GNS	N-Ac-glucosamine-6-sulfate-sulfatase	252.940
Mucopolysaccharidosis IVA	AR			Galactosamine-6-sulfatase	
Mucopolysaccharidosis IVB	AR	3p21-p14.2	GLBI	β-Galactosidase	230.500
Mucopolysaccharidosis VI	AR	5q13.3	ARSB	Arylsulfatase B	253.200
Mucopolysaccharidosis VII	AR	7q21.11	GUSB	β-Glucuronidase	253.220
Fucosidosis	AR	1p34	FUCA	α-Fucosidase	230.000

Osteochondrodysplasias	Mode of inheritance	Chromosomal locus	Gene	Protein	MIM No.
Dysostosis multiplex group—cont'd					
α-Mannosidosis	AR	19p13.2-q12	MANB	α-Mannosidase	248.500
β-Mannosidosis	AR	4	MNB	β-Mannosidase	248.510
Aspartylglucosaminuria	AR	4q23-q27	AgA	Aspartylglucosaminidase	208.400
gM1 Gangliosidosis, several forms	AR	3p21-p14.2	GLB1	β-Galactosidase	230.500
Sialidosis, several forms	AR	6p21.3	NEU	α-Neuraminidase	256.550
Sialic storage disease	AR				269.920
Galactosialidosis, several forms	AR	20	NgBE	Neur/Gal expression protein	256.540
Mucosulfatidosis	AR			Multiple sulfatases	272.200
Mucolipidosis II	AR			N-Ac-Gluc-phosphotransferase	252.500
Mucolipidosis III	AR			N-Ac-Gluc-phosphotransferase	252.600
Mucolipidosis IV	AR				252.650
Spondylometaphyseal dysplasias					
Spondylometaphyseal dysplasia, Kozlowski type	AD				271.660
Spondylometaphyseal dysplasia, corner fracture type (Sutcliffe)	AD				—
Spondyloenchondrodysplasia	AR				271.550
Epiphyseal dysplasias					
Multiple epiphyseal dysplasia Fairbanks and Ribbing	AD				132.400
Chondrodysplasia punctata (stippled epiphyses) group					
Rhizomelic type	AR			Peroxisome	215.100
Conradi-Hünermann type	XLD	Xq28	CPXD		302.950
X-linked recessive type	XLR	Xpter-p22.32	CPXR		302.940
MT type	Sp				—
Others, including CHILD syndrome, Zellweger syndrome, warfarin embryopathy, chromosomal abnormalities, fetal alcohol syndrome					
Metaphyseal dysplasias					
Jansen type	AD				156.400
Schmid type	AD				156.500
Spahr type	AR				250.400
McKusick type (cartilage-hair hypoplasia)	AR				250.250
Metaphyseal anadysplasia	XLR?				—
Shwachman type	AR				260.400
Adenosine deaminase deficiency	AR	20q13.11	ADA		102.700
Brachyrachia (short-spine dysplasia)					
Brachyolmia, several types					113.500
					271.530
Mesomelic dysplasias					
Dyschondrosteosis	AD				127.300
Langer type	AR				249.700
Nievergelt type	AD				163.400
Robinow type	AD				180.700
Acromelic and acromesomelic dysplasias					
Acromicric dysplasia	Sp				102.370
Geleophysic dysplasia	AR				231.050
Acrodysostosis	AD				101.800
Trichorhinophalangeal dysplasia, type I	AD	8q24.12	TQPS1		190.350

Continued.

Osteochondrodysplasias	Mode of inheritance	Chromosomal locus	Gene	Protein	MIM No.
Acromelic and acromesomelic dysplasias—cont'd					
Trichorhinophalangeal dysplasia, type II	AD	8q24.11-q24.13	TQPS2		150.230
Saldino-Mainzer dysplasia	AR				266.920
Pseudohypoparathyroidism,					103.580
several types	AD				139.320
	AR?				203.330
	XLD?				300.800
Cranioectodermal dysplasia	AR				218.330
Acromesomelic dysplasia	AR				201.250
Grebe dysplasia	AR				200.700
Dysplasias with significant (but not exclusive) membranous bone involvement					
Cleidocranial dysplasia	AD				119.600
Osteodysplasty, Melnick-Needles	XLD				309.350
Bent-bone dysplasia group					
Campomelic dysplasia	AR		CMO1		211.970
Kyphomelic dysplasia	AR				211.350
Stüve-Wiedemann dysplasia	AR				—
Multiple dislocations with dysplasias					
Larsen syndrome	AD				150.250
Desbuquois syndrome	AR				215.200
Spondyloepimetaphyseal dysplasia with joint laxity	AR				271.640
Osteodysplastic primordial dwarfism group					
Type I	AR				210.710
Type II	AR				210.720
Dysplasias with decreased bone density					
Osteogenesis imperfecta, several types	AD	17q21.31-q22.05	COL1A1	Collagen type I	120.150
	AD	7q21.3-q22.1	COL1A2	Collagen type I	120.160
					166.210-60
	AR				259.110
					259.420
Osteoporosis with pseudoglioma	AR				259.770
Idiopathic juvenile osteoporosis	Sp				259.750
Bruck syndrome	AR				259.450
Homocystinuria	AR	21q22.3	CBS	Cystathionine-β-synthase	236.200
Singleton-Merten syndrome	Sp				182.250
Geroderma osteodysplastica	AR				231.070
Menkes syndrome	XLR	Xq12-q13	MNK		309.400
Dysplasias with defective mineralization					
Hypophosphatasia	AD	1p36.1p34	ALPL	alkaline phosphatase	146.300
					171.760
					241.500
					241.510
Hypophosphatemic rickets	XR				370.800
Pseudodeficiency rickets, several types	AR				264.700
					277.420
					277.440
Neonatal hyperparathyroidism	AR				239.200
Dysplasias with increased bone density					
Osteopetrosis					
Precocious type	AR				259.700
Delayed type	AD				166.600
Intermediate type	AR				259.710

Osteochondrodysplasias	Mode of inheritance	Chromosome	Gene	Protein	MIM No.
Dysplasia with increased bone density—cont'd					
Osteopetrosis—cont'd					
With renal tubular acidosis	AR	8q22	CA2	Carbonic anhydrase II	259.730
Dysosteosclerosis	AR				224.300
Pyknodysostosis	AR				265.800
Osteosclerosis, Stanescu type	AD				122.900
Axial osteosclerosis					
Osteomesopyknosis	AD				166.450
with Bamboo hair (Netherton syndrome)	AR				256.500
Trichothiodystrophy	AR				242.170
Osteopoikilosis	AD				166.700
Melorheostosis	Sp				155.950
Osteopathia striata	Sp				—
Osteopathia striata with cranial sclerosis	AD				166.500
Diaphyseal dysplasia, Camurati-Engelmann	AD				131.300
Craniodiaphyseal dysplasia	AD				122.860
	AR				218.300
Lenz-Majewski dysplasia	Sp				151.050
Craniometadiaphyseal dysplasia	Sp				—
Endosteal hyperostoses					
van Buchem disease	AR				239.100
Sclerosteosis	AR				269.500
Worth disease	AD				144.750
With cerebellar hypoplasia	AR				—
Pachydermoperiostosis	AD				167.100
Frontometaphyseal dysplasia	XLR				305.620
Craniometaphyseal dysplasia					
Severe type	AR				218.400
Mild type	AD				123.000
Pyle (disease) dysplasia	AR				265.900
Osteoectasia with hyperphosphatasia	AR				239.000
Oculodentoosseous dysplasia					
Severe type	AR				257.850
Mild type	AD				164.200
Familial infantile cortical hyperostosis, Caffey	AD				114.000

Disorganized development of cartilaginous and fibrous components of the skeleton

Dysplasia epiphysealis hemimelica	Sp				127.800
Multiple cartilaginous exostoses	AD	8q23-q24.1			133.700
Enchondromatosis, Ollier	Sp				166.000
Enchondromatosis with hemangiomata, Maffucci	Sp				166.000
Metachondromatosis	AD				156.250
Osteoglophonic dysplasia	Sp				166.250
Fibrous dysplasia (Jaffe-Lichtenstein)	Sp				174.800
Fibrous dysplasia with pigmentary skin changes and precocious puberty (McCune-Albright)					

Continued.

Osteochondrodysplasias	Mode of inheritance	Chromosome	Gene	Protein	MIM No.
Disorganized development of cartilaginous and fibrous components of the skeleton—cont'd					
Cherubism	AD				118.400
Myofibromatosis (generalized fibromatosis)	AR				228.550
Idiopathic Osteolyses					
Predominantly phalangeal					
Hereditary acroosteolysis, several forms					102.400
Hajdu-Cheney type	AD				102.500
Predominantly carpal and tarsal					
Carpal-tarsal osteolysis with nephropathy	AD				166.300
Francois syndrome (dermo-chondrocorneal dystrophy)	AR				221.800
Multicentric					
Winchester syndrome	AR				277.950
Torg type	AR				259.600
Mandibuloacral dysplasia	AR				248.370
Other					
Familial expansile osteolysis	AD				174.810

Index

A